THE ESSENTIALS

Walsh & Hoyt's
Clinical Neuro-Ophthalmology

Fifth Edition
Neil R. Miller
Nancy J. Newman

THE ESSENTIALS

Walsh & Hoyt's
Clinical Neuro-Ophthalmology

5th Edition

THE ESSENTIALS

Walsh & Hoyt's
Clinical Neuro-Ophthalmology

5th Edition

EDITORS

Neil R. Miller, M.D.

Professor of Ophthalmology, Neurology and Neurosurgery
Frank B. Walsh Professor of Neuro-Ophthalmology
Wilmer Eye Institute
Johns Hopkins Medical Institutions,
Baltimore, Maryland

Nancy J. Newman, M.D.

Cyrus H. Stoner Professor of Ophthalmology
Associate Professor of Ophthalmology and Neurology
Instructor in Neurological Surgery
Emory University School of Medicine, Atlanta, Georgia
Lecturer in Ophthalmology
Harvard Medical School, Boston, Massachusetts

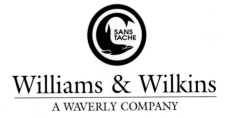

Williams & Wilkins
A WAVERLY COMPANY

BALTIMORE • PHILADELPHIA • LONDON • PARIS • BANGKOK
BUENOS AIRES • HONG KONG • MUNICH • SYDNEY • TOKYO • WROCLAW

Editor: Charles W. Mitchell
Managing Editor: Grace E. Miller
Marketing Manager: Adam Glazer
Project Editor: Robert D. Magee

Copyright © 1999 Williams & Wilkins

351 West Camden Street
Baltimore, Maryland 21201-2436 USA

Rose Tree Corporate Center
1400 North Providence Road
Building II, Suite 5025
Media, Pennsylvania 19063-2043 USA

Printed in the United States of America

First Edition, 1999

Library of Congress Cataloging-in-Publication Data

The essentials : Walsh & Hoyt's clinical neuro-ophthalmology, 5th
   edition / editors, Neil R. Miller, Nancy J. Newman. — 1st ed.
      p. cm.
   Condensed clinical information found in the 1st volume of: Walsh
and Hoyt's clinical neuro-ophthalmology, 5th ed. c1998.
   Includes index.
   ISBN 0-683-30682-0
   1. Neuroophthalmology. I. Miller, Neil R. II. Newman, Nancy J.
III. Walsh and Hoyt's clinical neuro-ophthalmology.
   [DNLM: 1. Eye Diseases. 2. Neurologic Manifestations. WW
140E787 1999]
RE725.E86 1999
617.7—dc21
DNLM/DLC
for Library of Congress   98-21736
                                        CIP

The publishers have made every effort to trace the copyright holders for borrowed material. If they have inadvertently overlooked any, they will be pleased to make the necessary arrangements at the first opportunity.

To purchase additional copies of this book, call our customer service department at **(800) 638-0672** or fax orders to **(800) 447-8438.** For other book services, including chapter reprints and large quantity sales, ask for the Special Sales department.

Canadian customers should call **(800) 665-1148**, or fax **(800) 665-0103.** For all other calls originating outside of the United States, please call **(410) 528-4223** or fax us at **(410) 528-8550.**

Visit Williams & Wilkins on the Internet: **http://www.wwilkins.com** or contact our customer service department at **custserv@wwilkins.com**. Williams & Wilkins customer service representatives are available from 8:30 am to 6:00 pm, EST, Monday through Friday, for telephone access.

99 00 01 02 03
1 2 3 4 5 6 7 8 9 10

To Simmons Lessell, M.D., who taught me how to be a teacher.

NJN

To Bill Hoyt, M.D., who taught me how to be a student.

NRM

Preface

The 5th edition of Walsh and Hoyt's Clinical Neuro-Ophthalmology was a 2-year whirlwind project involving multiple contributors and culminating in 5 volumes, 6000 pages, comprehensively researched and referenced. When the dust had settled, we were pleased to find that we had accomplished our goal—to provide an up-to-date extensive review of medicine from the point of view of the neuro-ophthalmologist. We recognized, however, that not every practitioner requires such an in-depth exposure to neuro-ophthalmology, especially as regards the detailed referencing. We felt there was a need to distill the material found primarily in the first volume of the 5th edition down to the basics of neuro-ophthalmic disease, to "just the essentials."

The Essentials consists of a single text, divided into five sections: the afferent visual system, the pupil, the efferent (ocular motor) system, the eyelid, and nonorganic disorders. As in the 5th edition, to help readers peruse chapters for content, there is a summary of major and minor headings at the beginning of each chapter. In addition, the various portions of the five volumes of the 5th edition pertinent to a particular chapter in *The Essentials* are referenced at the end of each chapter.

In this age of easily accessible computer literature searches, and with the comprehensively referenced full five volumes of the 5th edition available, we have chosen not to include specific bibliographic entries. Readers who desire more in-depth information on the topics discussed in *The Essentials* are encouraged to consult the larger comprehensive textbook.

Acknowledgments

We wish to thank the Williams & Wilkins team for embracing this project and letting us run with it, allowing for production of this "little" book in record time. At the helm was Charley Mitchell, Executive Editor, admirably supported by Grace Miller, Managing Editor, Bob Magee as Production Editor, and Diane Harnish in marketing. We wish to especially acknowledge Valerie Biousse, M.D. for her critical review of the entire manuscript. Most importantly, we wish to thank our authors of the 5th edition, especially those contributing to the first volume.

Contributors to the 5th Edition

Anthony C. Arnold, MD
Associate Professor of Ophthalmology
Chief, Neuro-Ophthalmology Division
Jules Stein Eye Institute
Department of Ophthalmology
UCLA School of Medicine
Los Angeles, California

Lea Averbuch-Heller, MD
Assistant Professor
Department of Neurology
University Hospitals of Cleveland
Case Western Reserve University
Cleveland, Ohio

Robert S. Baker, MD, FRCP, FRCS
Professor and Chairman of Ophthalmology
Professor of Neurosurgery, Neurology, and
Pediatrics
Kentucky Clinic
Lexington, Kentucky

Jason J.S. Barton, MD
Beth Israel Deaconess Medical Center
Harvard Medical School
Boston, Massachusetts

Roy W. Beck, MD, PhD
Director, Jaeb Center for Health Research
Clinical Professor of Ophthalmology and
Adjunct Professor of Epidemiology and
Biostatistics
University of South Florida
Tampa, Florida

Mark S. Borchert, MD
Associate Professor of Clinical Ophthalmology and
Neurology
Children's Hospital Los Angeles
School of Medicine, University of Southern
California
Los Angeles, California

Paul W. Brazis, MD
Associate Professor of Neurology
Mayo Medical School
Consultant in Neurology and Neuro-Ophthalmology
Mayo Clinic, Jacksonville
Jacksonville, Florida

Michael C. Brodsky, MD
Professor of Ophthalmology and Pediatrics
University of Arkansas for Medical Sciences
Chief of Pediatric Ophthalmology
Arkansas Children's Hospital
Little Rock, Arkansas

Wayne T. Cornblath, MD
Kellogg Eye Institute
Assistant Professor of Ophthalmology and
Neurology
University of Michigan
Ann Arbor, Michigan

Shelley Ann Cross, MD
Consultant in Neurology
Mayo Clinic
Assistant Professor of Neurology
Mayo Medical School
Rochester, Minnesota

Jon N. Currie, MBBS, FRACP
Director, Drug and Alcohol Services
Western Sydney Area Health Services
Head, Neuro-Ophthalmology Service
Westmead Hospital
Sydney, New South Wales, Australia

Kathleen B. Digre, MD
Associate Professor of Neurology and
Ophthalmology
Director of Neuro-Ophthalmology Clinic
Moran Eye Center
University of Utah
Salt Lake City, Utah

**Dominic E. Dwyer, BSc, MBBS, FRACP,
FRCPA**
Department of Virology
Center for Infectious Diseases and Microbiology
Laboratory Services
ICPMR, Westmead Hospital
Westmead, New South Wales, Australia

Eric R. Eggenberger, DO
Michigan State University Clinical Center
Assistant Professor
Michigan State University
East Lansing, Michigan

Craig Evinger, PhD
Professor, Department of Neurology and Behavior
Associate Professor, Department of Ophthalmology
University Hospital and Medical Center at Stony
Brook
SUNY Stony Brook
Stony Brook, New York

Warren L. Felton III, MD
Associate Professor
Departments of Neurology and Ophthalmology
Chairman, Division of Neuro-Ophthalmology
Medical College of Virginia
Virginia Commonwealth University
Richmond, Virginia

William A. Fletcher, MD
Foothills Hospital
Associate Professor
Department of Clinical Neurosciences
Division of Ophthalmology
University of Calgary
Calgary, Alberta, Canada

Benjamin M. Frishberg, MD
Clinical Professor of Ophthalmology
Assistant Clinical Professor of Neurology
Howard University School of Medicine
Assistant Clinical Professor of Neurology
Georgetown University Medical Center
Director of Neuro-Ophthalmology
Howard University Hospital
Washington, D.C.
North County Neurology Associates
La Jolla, California

Steven L. Galetta, MD
Professor of Neurology and Ophthalmology
Director, Neuro-Ophthalmology Service
University of Pennsylvania School of Medicine
Philadelphia, Pennsylvania

James A. Garrity, MD
Associate Professor of Ophthalmology
Mayo Medical School
Consultant, Department of Ophthalmology
Mayo Clinic
Rochester, Minnesota

John W. Gittinger, Jr., MD
Professor and Chair, Department of Ophthalmology
Professor of Neurology
University of Massachusetts Medical School
Worcester, Massachusetts

Robert A. Goldberg, MD
Chief, Orbital and Ophthalmic Plastic Surgery
Division
Jules Stein Eye Institute
Associate Professor of Ophthalmology
UCLA School of Medicine
Los Angeles, California

Karl C. Golnik, MD
Assistant Professor of Ophthalmology and
Neurosurgery
University of Cincinnati
The Cincinnati Eye Institute
Cincinnati, Ohio

Steven R. Hamilton, MD
Eye Associates Northwest
Assistant Clinical Professor of Neurology and
Ophthalmology
University of Washington School of Medicine
Seattle, Washington

Thomas R. Hedges III, MD
Professor of Ophthalmology
Associate Professor of Neurology
Tufts University School of Medicine
Director of Neuro-Ophthalmology, New England
Eye Center
Boston, Massachusetts

Paul N. Hoffman, MD, PhD
Associate Professor of Ophthalmology and
Neurology
Johns Hopkins School of Medicine
Baltimore, Maryland

Saunders L. Hupp, MD
Professor, Ophthalmology and Neuro-
Ophthalmology
Department of Ophthalmology
University of South Alabama College of Medicine
Mobile, Alabama

Daniel M. Jacobson, MD
Director, Neuro-Ophthalmology Service
Departments of Neurology and Ophthalmology
Marshfield Clinic
Marshfield, Wisconsin
Clinical Associate Professor
Departments of Ophthalmology and Visual
Sciences, and Neurology
University of Wisconsin Medical School
Madison, Wisconsin

Chris A. Johnson, PhD
Professor, Department of Ophthalmology
Director, Optics and Visual Assessment Lab
(OVAL)
UC Davis Medical Center
Sacramento, California

Randy H. Kardon, MD, PhD
Director of Neuro-Ophthalmology
Associate Professor
University of Iowa Hospitals and Clinics
Veterans Administration Medical Center
Iowa City, Iowa

Barrett J. Katz, MD
Professor of Ophthalmology, Neurology, and
Neurosurgery
University of Rochester School of Medicine
Strong Memorial Hospital
Rochester, New York

David I. Kaufman, DO
Director, Clinical Neurosciences Unit
Michigan State University
Sparrow Hospital
Professor, Neuro-Ophthalmology
East Lansing, Michigan

James R. Keane, MD
Professor of Neurology
University of Southern California
Los Angeles, California

Shalom E. Kelman, MD
Associate Professor of Ophthalmology
University of Maryland School of Medicine
Baltimore, Maryland

John L. Keltner, MD
Chairman, Department of Ophthalmology
Professor of Ophthalmology, Neurology, and
Neurological Surgery
UC Davis Medical Center
Sacramento, California

**Christopher Kennard, PhD, BSc, MBBS, FRCP,
FRCOphth**
Chairman and Head of the Neuroscience and
Psychological Medicine Divisions
Imperial College School of Medicine
Charing Cross Hospital
London, United Kingdom

John S. Kennerdell, MD
Chairman, Department of Ophthalmology
Professor, Allegheny University Health Sciences at
Allegheny General Hospital
Adjunct Professor of Ophthalmology
University of Pittsburgh
Pittsburgh, Pennsylvania

Lanning B. Kline, MD
Professor of Clinical Ophthalmology
Combined Program in Ophthalmology Eye
Foundation Hospital
University of Alabama School of Medicine
Birmingham, Alabama

Gregory S. Kosmorsky, DO
Head, Section of Neuro-Ophthalmology
Division of Ophthalmology
The Cleveland Clinic Foundation
Cleveland, Ohio

Ralph W. Kuncl, MD, PhD
Professor of Neurology
Neuromuscular Division
Johns Hopkins Hospital
Baltimore, Maryland

Andrew G. Lee, MD
Cullen Eye Institute
Assistant Professor of Ophthalmology, Neurology
and Neurosurgery
Baylor College of Medicine
Neuro-Ophthalmology Consultant
Division of Neurosurgery
M.D. Anderson Cancer Center
Houston, Texas

R. John Leigh, MD
Staff Neurologist
Cleveland Veterans Affairs Medical Center
Professor
Department of Neurology, Neurosciences,
Otolaryngology, and Biomedical Engineering
Case Western Reserve University
Cleveland, Ohio

Simmons Lessell, MD
Massachusetts Eye and Ear Infirmary
Professor of Ophthalmology
Harvard Medical School
Boston, Massachusetts

Robert L. Lesser, MD
Associate Clinical Professor of Ophthalmology
Department of Ophthalmology and Visual Science
Yale University School of Medicine
New Haven, Connecticut
Clinical Professor of Neurology and Neurosurgery
University of Connecticut School of Medicine
Farmington, Connecticut

Grant T. Liu, MD
Assistant Professor of Neurology and
Ophthalmology
Division of Neuro-Ophthalmology
Departments of Neurology and Ophthalmology
Hospital of the University of Pennsylvania
Children's Hospital of Philadelphia
Scheie Eye Institute
Philadelphia, Pennsylvania

Joseph C. Maroon, MD
Professor and Chairman, Division of Neurosurgery
Allegheny University of the Health Sciences
Allegheny Campus
Pittsburgh, Pennsylvania

Linda Kirschen McLoon, PhD
Associate Professor, Department of Ophthalmology
University of Minnesota
Minneapolis, Minnesota

Neil R. Miller, MD
Professor of Ophthalmology, Neurology, and
Neurosurgery
Frank B. Walsh Professor of Neuro-Ophthalmology
Johns Hopkins Medical Institutions
Baltimore, Maryland

Mark L. Moster, MD
Professor and Senior Associate Chairman
Department of Neurology
Temple University School of Medicine
Chairman, Department of Neurosensory Sciences
Albert Einstein Medical Center
Philadelphia, Pennsylvania

Golnaz Moazami, MD
Instructor in Clinical Ophthalmology
Edward S. Harkness Eye Institute
Columbia-Presbyterian Medical Center
New York, New York

Nancy J. Newman, MD
Cyrus H. Stoner Professor of Ophthalmology
Associate Professor of Ophthalmology and
Neurology
Instructor in Neurological Surgery
Emory University School of Medicine
Atlanta, Georgia
Lecturer in Ophthalmology
Harvard Medical School
Boston, Massachusetts

Steven A. Newman, MD
Associate Professor of Ophthalmology and
Neurological Surgery
Department of Ophthalmology
University of Virginia Medical Center
Charlottesville, Virginia

Jeffrey G. Odel, MD
Associate Clinical Professor of Ophthalmology
Edward S. Harkness Eye Institute
Columbia-Presbyterian Medical Center
New York, New York

Kimberly Peele Cockerham, MD
Director, Oculoplastics, Orbital Disease, and
Reconstruction
Staff, Neuro-Ophthalmology
Walter Reed Army Medical Hospital
Washington, District of Columbia

Stephen C. Pollock, MD
Associate Professor of Ophthalmology
Duke University Eye Center
Durham, North Carolina

Jonathan D. Porter, PhD
Departments of Anatomy and Neurobiology
Professor of Anatomy, Neurobiology, and
Ophthalmology
University of Kentucky Medical Center
Lexington, Kentucky

Valerie A. Purvin, MD
Chief, Neuro-Ophthalmology Section
Midwest Eye Institute
Associate Clinical Professor of Ophthalmology and
Neurology
Indiana University Medical Center
Indianapolis, Indiana

Michael X. Repka, MD
Wilmer Eye Institute
Johns Hopkins Hospital
Associate Professor
Johns Hopkins University School of Medicine
Baltimore, Maryland

Joseph F. Rizzo, III, MD
Massachusetts Eye and Ear Infirmary
Assistant Professor
Department of Ophthalmology
Harvard Medical School
Boston, Massachusetts

Matthew Rizzo, MD
University of Iowa
Professor of Neurology and Public Policy
Adjunct Professor of Engineering
Director of the Visual Function Laboratory
Division of Behavioral Neurology and Cognitive
Neuroscience
Iowa City, Iowa

Alfredo A. Sadun, MD, PhD
Professor, Departments of Ophthalmology and
Neurological Surgery
Doheny Eye Institute
University of Southern California School of
Medicine
Los Angeles, California

John B. Selhorst, MD
Professor and Chairman
Department of Neurology
Saint Louis University
St. Louis, Missouri

James A. Sharpe, MD, FRCPC
Professor of Neurology and Head, Division of
Neurology
University of Toronto
Head of Neurology, The Toronto Hospital
Toronto, Ontario, Canada

William T. Shults, MD
Chief of Neuro-Ophthalmology
Devers Eye Institute
Department of Ophthalmology
Portland, Oregon

Patrick A. Sibony, MD
Professor, Department of Ophthalmology
University Hospital and Medical Center at Stony
Brook
SUNY Stony Brook
Stony Brook, New York

Barry Skarf, MD, PhD
Director, Neuro-Ophthalmology Unit
Departments of Eye Care Services, Neurology and
Neurosurgery
Henry Ford Health Sciences Center
Detroit, Michigan

Thomas L. Slamovits, MD
Montefiore Medical Center
Professor of Ophthalmology, Neurology, and
Neurosurgery
Albert Einstein College of Medicine
Bronx, New York

Craig H. Smith, MD
Director, Neuro-Ophthalmology Research Unit
Swedish Hospital Medical Center
Clinical Professor of Medicine, Neurology and
Ophthalmology
University of Washington
Seattle, Washington

Kenneth D. Steinsapir, MD
Assistant Clinical Professor
Jules Stein Eye Institute
UCLA School of Medicine
Los Angeles, California

H. Stanley Thompson, MD
University of Iowa Hospitals and Clinics
Professor of Ophthalmology
University of Iowa
Iowa City, Iowa

B. Todd Troost, MD
Professor of Neurology and Anesthesia
Chairman, Department of Neurology
Bowman Gray School of Medicine
Wake Forest University
Winston-Salem, North Carolina

Michael Wall, MD
Professor of Neurology and Ophthalmology
University of Iowa College of Medicine
Veterans Administration Hospital
Iowa City, Iowa

Joel M. Weinstein, MD
Associate Clinical Professor of Ophthalmology,
Neurology, and Neurosurgery
University of Wisconsin School of Medicine
Madison, Wisconsin

Jacqueline M.S. Winterkorn, MD, PhD
Clinical Professor
Departments of Ophthalmology, Neurology and
Neuroscience
Cornell University Medical College
Attending in Ophthalmology and Neurology
The New York Hospital Cornell Medical Center
New York, New York

Jonathan D. Wirtschafter, MD
Professor of Ophthalmology, Neurology, and
Neurosurgery
University of Minnesota Medical School
Minneapolis, Minnesota

Rochelle S. Zak, MD
New York Hospital, Westchester Division
White Plains, New York

David S. Zee, MD
Professor, Departments of Neurology and
Ophthalmology
Johns Hopkins Hospital
Baltimore, Maryland

Contents

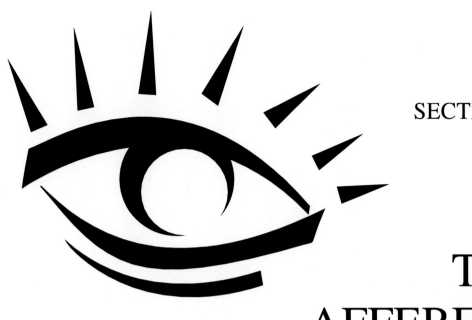

SECTION I

THE
AFFERENT
VISUAL SYSTEM

CHAPTER 1

Approach to the Patient: Examination of the Visual Sensory System

HISTORY	Fundus Examination
CLINICAL OFFICE EXAMINATION	Other Procedures
Refraction and Visual Acuity	PSYCHOPHYSICAL TESTS
Stereoacuity	Visual Acuity
Color Vision and Brightness Comparison	Contrast Sensitivity
Visual Field Examination	Perimetry and Visual Field Testing
Photostress Test	Color Vision
Pulfrich Phenomenon	Dark Adaptation
Pupillary Examination	ELECTROPHYSIOLOGIC TESTS
Cranial Nerves, Exophthalmometry, External	Electroretinogram
Examination, and Anterior Segment	Electro-oculogram
Examination	Visual-Evoked Potential

Despite continuous advances in neurodiagnostic imaging and other new techniques, the examination of the afferent visual sensory system is still the core of the neuro-ophthalmologic examination. This chapter describes the most common subjective and objective testing parameters used in the afferent visual system examination. In addition, it discusses recent developments in perimetry, clinical psychophysics, and electrophysiology.

Evaluation of the afferent system begins with a thorough medical history, followed by an ophthalmologic examination (refraction, slit lamp examination, funduscopy, assessment of pupillary function, etc.), evaluation of selected psychophysical visual functions (acuity, stereoacuity, color vision, visual fields, contrast sensitivity, etc.) and relevant ancillary test procedures. Once the examiner has performed these functions, providing a diagnosis, or at least a differential diagnosis, for the etiology of an afferent visual system deficit should be possible.

HISTORY

An examination of patients experiencing dysfunction of the afferent visual system begins with a careful history about the details of the visual loss. A thorough history is one of the most important parts of the examination, because it determines the initial strategy for differential diagnostic evaluation. It is essential to establish if the visual loss is monocular or binocular; if its location is central, peripheral, altitudinal, or hemianopic; and if the onset of the loss is gradual, sudden, or intermittent. If it is intermittent, does it last for seconds, minutes, or hours? If the visual loss is unilateral, it is important to determine if there is pain on motion of the eye or if there are other associated neurologic symptoms, such as decreased vision with exercise or overheating (Uhthoff symptom), the feeling of an electric shock going down the spine when the neck is flexed (Lhermitte's symptom), or other symptoms for demyelinating disease or other neurologic disorders (e.g., paresthesias, weakness, dizziness, bladder or bowel dysfunction).

It is also important to ask about photopsias—visual phenomena such as flashing black squares, flashes of lights, or showers of sparks—distortions in vision such as metamorphopsia or micropsia, and positive scotomas. A positive scotoma is one that is seen by the patient, like the purple spot that is often seen after a flash bulb goes off, whereas a negative scotoma refers to a nonseeing area of the visual field. Metamorphopsia, micropsia, and positive scotomas often occur in patients with maculopathies, but they can also occur during a migraine attack. Photopsias may be present in patients with retinal disease, optic nerve dysfunction, or cerebral dysfunction from migraine and other disorders.

The history of visual loss in young children deserves special attention because it is usually obtained indirectly through the parents. The parents of a blind infant often do not realize that the child has a visual problem until the infant is 3 to 4 months of age. Typically, it is the mother who notices that the infant fails to follow her face or notice toys, mobiles, and other items in the crib. The parents should be questioned about eye movement abnormalities (particularly nystagmus) and about behavior suggesting photophobia, such as squinting in sunlight or in a brightly lit room.

The patient's past medical history is also critical in establishing a diagnosis of afferent visual pathway disorders. Medications that the patient may be taking, previous operations, injuries, illnesses, and other medical problems may be related to the patient's visual problems. Work, recreational activities, and social activities of the patient can provide additional pertinent information, as can a history of smoking, alcohol intake, nutritional habits, and an exposure to toxins. Finally, the patient's family history is very important, particularly for such conditions as retinitis pigmentosa, Leber's hereditary optic neuropathy, dominant optic atrophy, and other genetic disorders. Patients are often reluctant to disclose such genetic problems because of denial, hoping that by not disclosing it to the examiner, they will not be diagnosed as having the condition.

CLINICAL OFFICE EXAMINATION

Clinical evaluation of the afferent visual system for each eye incorporates the items in Table

Table 1.1.

Components of the Clinical Neuro-Ophthalmologic Examination

I. REFRACTION
  Retinoscopy
  Keratometry
  Manifest Refraction
  Cycloplegic Refraction
II. VISUAL FUNCTION
  Visual Acuity (Distance and Near)
  Stereoacuity
  Color Vision, Color Comparison
  Brightness Comparison
  Photostress Test
  Pulfrich Phenomenon
  Visual Fields
    Confrontation Fields
    Amsler Grid
    Tangent Screen
    Manual Kinetic Perimetry (Goldmann Perimeter)
    Automated Static Perimetry
III. PUPILS
  Size
  Direct and Consensual Response
  Accommodation Response
  Afferent Pupillary Defect
IV. CRANIAL NERVES
  I, III, IV, V, VI, VII, VIII
V. EXOPHTHALMOMETRY
  Right Eye
  Left Eye
VI. EXTERNAL AND ANTERIOR SEGMENT
  External Examination
  Slit Lamp Examination
  Applanation Tonometry
VII. FUNDUS
  Optic Nerve Head and Nerve Fiber Layer
  Macula and Retinal Vessels
  Peripheral Retina

1.1. These procedures can be performed in the office. In this section, we present a brief discussion of each component. A more detailed discussion of several visual function tests (visual acuity, contrast sensitivity, color vision, and perimetry) and ancillary procedures (dark adaptation and clinical electrophysiology) is presented later in this chapter, and other aspects of the clinical examination are covered in subsequent chapters of this book.

The first goal for the neuro-ophthalmologic examination is to determine if the visual loss is caused by a disorder anterior to the retina (ocular media), in the retina, in the optic nerve, in the optic chiasm, in the retrochiasmal pathways, or is nonorganic (i.e., hysteria or malingering). The second goal is to establish a differential and working diagnosis. By assessing various parameters of afferent visual function, the examiner can frequently make a determination as to the anatomic site of the afferent system abnormality and the most probable cause or causes.

REFRACTION AND VISUAL ACUITY

A thorough refraction is an important part of all clinical neuro-ophthalmologic examinations. Identification of a previously undetermined refractive error, corneal pathology, or a subtle lens problem can prevent initiation of an expensive, time-consuming, and exhaustive work-up. It is essential to have the best refraction possible when measuring visual acuity to distinguish if loss of vision is caused by optical factors or damage to neural elements in the visual system. Refractive problems not only can cause loss of visual acuity but also may produce symptoms such as monocular diplopia. A cycloplegic refraction is important, not only to obtain the correct refraction, but also to observe the red reflex through the retinoscope as a means of identifying corneal irregularities and lens opacities that may not be apparent during a slit lamp examination. Visual acuity measurements obtained with the patient viewing through a pinhole can also help identify problems with the optics of the eye. In many instances, it is useful to dilate the patient in conjunction with the use of a pinhole to maximize the likelihood of finding a clear pinhole region around an opacity. Improvement of visual acuity with the use of a pinhole indicates that the cause of the visual loss is optical in nature, whereas worsening of visual acuity with a pinhole may indicate a central posterior subcapsular cataract or a maculopathy. The Potential Acuity Meter (PAM), which uses the pinhole principle, can be helpful. Keratoconus and surface irregularities of the cornea can be diagnosed by improvement in visual acuity with the use of a hard contact lens. A Placido disk, keratometry readings, or corneal topography maps can also help to identify corneal surface irregularities and associated problems.

Subtle central vision loss can often be identified by the use of low-contrast visual acuity charts or contrast sensitivity measurements.

Low-luminance visual acuity can be compared with similar measures made under standard lighting conditions. For example, placing a 2.0 log unit neutral density filter before the eye (i.e., producing a 100-fold reduction in the luminance of the visual acuity chart) causes a normal eye to be reduced from 20/20 to 20/40 visual acuity (a factor of 2 or 0.3 logMAR). Patients with optic neuropathies characterized by a disturbance of conduction, such as optic neuritis or compressive optic neuropathy, have a disproportionately greater reduction in visual acuity (e.g., from 20/30 down to 20/200) when the neutral density filter is placed before the affected eye. Other anomalies such as amblyopia do not demonstrate this disproportionate drop in visual acuity with the neutral density filter.

Measuring visual acuity in children requires skill, patience, and an enthusiastic attitude. By creating a friendly, relaxed environment for the child in which vision testing is presented as a game, the chances of success will be greater. A system of positive rewards, ranging from a verbal "Hooray!" or "That's terrific!" to the use of mechanical animal toys and projected cartoons, is essential (Fig. 1.1).

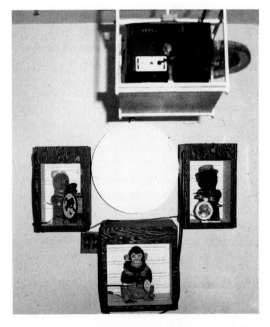

Figure 1.1. Wall-mounted mechanical animals and video projection system for providing fixation targets and "rewards" for pediatric patients during the examination.

During any neuro-ophthalmologic examination, it is essential to measure not only distance visual acuity but also near visual acuity. In some instances (e.g., when performing an in-hospital consultation on a patient who is unable to come to the examination room), near visual acuity is the only measurement that is possible. Near visual acuity measurements can be performed with any of the standard near acuity cards, which are held 13 to 14 inches from the eyes with the patient wearing an appropriate near refractive correction. Because these cards are not standardized, the same near card should be used for serial measurements in the same patient. In patients with normal visual function, there is little or no difference between distance and near visual acuity. A discrepancy between near and distance visual acuity suggests several possible etiologies. Patients with nuclear sclerotic cataracts often have better near acuity than distance acuity, whereas patients with central posterior subcapsular cataracts often have better distance acuity than near acuity. Young patients with head trauma may complain of reading problems from loss of accommodation, resulting in poorer near acuity than distance acuity. Patients with nonorganic loss of vision may not understand the relationship between near and distance acuity and may provide inconsistent responses with the two measurements. One must be careful, however, to ensure that optical factors (e.g., cataract, presbyopia) are not responsible for the differences.

STEREOACUITY

Stereoacuity requires good visual acuity in both eyes and normal cortical development. As such, stereoacuity can be helpful in establishing if a patient has visual loss from longstanding amblyopia or monofixation syndrome, as well as verifying the extent of any monocular visual acuity loss. Using the Titmus Stereo Tester, stereoacuity in normal observers with good binocular function and visual acuity should be 40 seconds of arc or better when both eyes have 20/20 visual acuity. If plus lenses are placed before one eye, stereoacuity is reduced to 60 seconds of arc when that eye is blurred to 20/40 and 100 seconds of arc when the eye is blurred to 20/100. Although this correlation does not hold for all clinical conditions, it provides a useful reference for cross-checking a mild loss of monocular visual acuity, especially when nonorganic visual loss is suspected (see Chapter 23).

COLOR VISION AND BRIGHTNESS COMPARISON

Color vision testing, using pseudoisochromatic plates or the Farnsworth Panel D-15 test, can be helpful in detecting subtle signs of optic neuropathy or macular disease. In general, **Kollner's rule** applies to acquired dyschromatopsias: acquired blue-yellow or pure blue (tritan) dyschromatopsias are produced by diseases affecting the retina, whereas acquired red-green dyschromatopsias (protan and deutan, respectively) are produced by diseases affecting the optic nerve and beyond. It should be kept in mind, however, that there are many exceptions to Kollner's rule. Blue-yellow or tritan deficits occur in many patients with dominant optic atrophy and glaucoma, protan deficits occur in patients with serous retinal detachments, and patients with acute optic neuritis have a mixture of red-green and blue-yellow deficits. It should also be kept in mind that **congenital** red-green deficits occur in approximately 8% of the male population and in 0.4% of females. Congenital blue-yellow deficits are much less common, occurring in 0.005% of the population. Nevertheless, both types of congenital color vision deficits need to be distinguished from **acquired** color vision loss. A comparison of color vision between the two eyes can be helpful in this regard, because both the type and severity of congenital color vision deficits are the same for each eye, a situation that is often not true for acquired color vision loss. In addition, congenital color vision deficits are stable over time and are almost always red-green deficits. Congenital tritan (blue) color vision deficits are extremely rare.

A comparison of the saturation of colors between eyes and across the vertical midline can sometimes identify subtle optic nerve dysfunction or chiasmal lesions. The same is true for brightness comparisons between the two eyes and across the vertical midline. Although such tests can be used to corroborate other evidence of optic neuropathy, an isolated subjective brightness difference between the two eyes of a patient with an otherwise normal examination is, in and of itself, often of no significance.

VISUAL FIELD EXAMINATION

Examination of the visual field is one of the most important parts of the evaluation of the afferent visual system. This section provides a brief overview of clinical visual field testing, with a more extensive discussion provided later in the chapter. A variety of visual field test procedures can be employed, including confrontation fields, the Amsler grid, the tangent (Bjerrum) screen, manual kinetic testing using a Goldmann perimeter, and automated static perimetry. When evaluating a patient with an afferent system deficit, it is important to keep in mind the advantages and disadvantages of the various procedures.

Confrontation visual fields should be part of every afferent system examination. Although testing by confrontation may lack the sophistication of modern techniques, it is the most flexible form of visual field testing and can be performed almost anywhere. In some instances, it may be the only form of visual field testing that is possible. When performed by a skilled individual, confrontation testing can provide information equivalent to that obtained with more extensive forms of visual field testing.

The **Amsler grid** is particularly useful in identifying patients with retinal pathology. The grid is held 30 cm from the patient, at which distance each 5 mm square subtends 1° of visual angle (total extent is 20° diameter, or 10° radius). The patient is shown the Amsler grid and told to look at the center spot and report: 1) if there is absence or distortion of the central fixation spot, 2) if any portions of the grid are missing, and 3) if any of the lines are wavy or bent (metamorphopsia). This type of image distortion is usually indicative of macular disease (Fig. 1.2*A*), whereas inability to see the central fixation point may indicate a central scotoma (Fig. 1.2*B*).

Tangent screen testing permits evaluation of the central 30° radius of the visual field. A 1-meter tangent screen can be placed on the wall of an examining room for easy use. It can provide more detailed, quantitative visual field information than that afforded by confrontation field testing. In the hands of a skilled perimetrist, the tangent screen examination provides information that is equal to that obtained with automated perimetric test procedures.

Sophisticated, quantitative evaluations can be achieved with **kinetic perimetry** using a Goldmann or similar perimeter. One advantage is

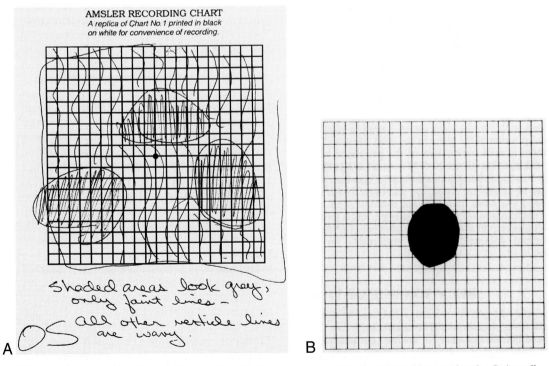

Figure 1.2.   Amsler grid defects. *A.* Metamorphopsia and paracentral scotomas in a patient with a maculopathy. *B.* A small central scotoma in a patient with optic neuritis.

greater flexibility afforded by close interaction between the patient and the perimetrist to obtain the most accurate responses from the patient. In children, the elderly, or patients with dementia, this may be the only form of quantitative visual field test that can be performed. The Goldmann perimeter also makes it possible to evaluate efficiently the peripheral visual field beyond a radius of 30°. This information can be useful in determining the extent of visual field loss and in establishing a differential diagnosis. The major disadvantages of this form of perimetry include the lack of standards and normative values and the high dependence on the skills of the perimetrist.

Automated perimetry is the most popular form of visual field testing. Although both projection and nonprojection (light-emitting diode, fiber optics targets) automated perimeters are available, nonprojection perimeters are most commonly used for screening purposes, and projection perimeters are employed for quantitative threshold determinations. The major advantages of automated perimetry include standardized test procedures, age-related normal population values, and statistical analysis procedures for evaluating the data. Its major disadvantages include long testing times, inflexibility, and learning and fatigue effects. In addition, many physicians assume that patients undergoing automated perimetry cannot provide nonorganic responses without it being evident that they are doing so—but this is not the case!

PHOTOSTRESS TEST

The differentiation between unilateral retinal disease and retrobulbar optic neuropathy may be aided using the **photostress recovery test**. This test is based on the principle that visual pigments bleach when exposed to an intense light source, resulting in a transient state of sensitivity loss and reduced central visual acuity. Recovery of retinal sensitivity is dependent upon regeneration of visual pigments, which is determined by the anatomic and physiologic apposition of the photoreceptors and retinal pigment epithelium. It is independent of neural mechanisms. Diseases that produce visual loss by damaging the photoreceptors or the adjacent retinal pigment epithelium cause a lag in regeneration of pigment, resulting in a delay in visual recovery following light stress; disorders that produce visual loss from damage to ganglion cells or their axons

produce no delay in pigment regeneration, and thus are associated with a normal visual recovery time after light stress.

The photostress test is performed by determining best-corrected visual acuity, shielding one eye, and then asking the patient to look directly at a bright focal light held 2 to 3 cm from the eye for about 10 seconds. The time needed to return to within one line of best-corrected visual acuity level is called the photostress recovery time (PSRT). The PSRT in normal eyes averages 27 seconds with a standard deviation of 11 seconds. Ninety-nine percent of normal eyes have a PSRT of 50 seconds or less. In eyes with macular disease, the PSRT is likely to be significantly prolonged, even when the retina appears to be relatively normal, whereas the PSRT is relatively normal in eyes with optic neuropathies. The photostress test thus is especially useful in the differentiation of subtle macular disease from a subtle optic neuropathy.

PULFRICH PHENOMENON

When a small target oscillating in a frontal plane is viewed binocularly with one eye covered with a filter to reduce light intensity, the target appears to move in an elliptic, rather than a to-and-fro, path—the **Pulfrich phenomenon.** When the filter is placed over the right eye, the rotation appears counterclockwise; if it is placed over the left eye, the rotation appears clockwise. The explanation for this stereo phenomenon is that the covered eye is more weakly stimulated than the uncovered eye, resulting in a delay in the transmission of visual signals to the striate cortex. This disparity in latency between eyes results in a difference in the apparent position of the target in the two eyes, thereby producing a retinal disparity cue underlying the stereoscopic effect. The magnitude of the effect is determined by the velocity of the target, the difference in retinal illumination between the two eyes, the level of retinal illumination, and the distance of the observer from the target.

Because optic nerve damage results in delayed transmission of impulses to the occipital cortex, patients with unilateral or markedly asymmetric optic neuropathy observe the Pulfrich phenomenon under natural viewing conditions without a filter in front of one eye. This can present difficulties for the patient with regard to driving and mobility over uneven terrain and with certain recreational activities, such as tennis, volleyball, and baseball. As with brightness comparisons between eyes, the presence of a Pulfrich phenomenon in a patient with a normal examination and no other visual or neurologic symptoms or signs should be regarded with caution (like an isolated difference in brightness between the two eyes—see above).

PUPILLARY EXAMINATION

Examination of the pupils is an essential part of the evaluation of the afferent system. Pupil size for each eye should be noted, as should the magnitude and latency of the direct and consensual responses to light and near stimulation. The presence of a relative afferent pupil defect (RAPD) is the hallmark of a unilateral afferent sensory abnormality or bilateral asymmetric visual loss. The etiology is usually an optic neuropathy, but other abnormalities such as a central or branch retinal artery occlusion, retinal detachment, or a large macular scar may be responsible (see Chapter 2). In the case of a retrobulbar optic neuropathy with a relatively normal appearing fundus examination, **the RAPD may be the only objective sign of anterior visual pathway dysfunction.** Cataracts, refractive errors, and nonorganic visual loss do not cause an RAPD. A patient with a dense strabismic or anisometropic amblyopia (visual acuity of 20/200 or worse) may demonstrate a mild RAPD, but the clinical history will be of a long-standing visual deficit rather than a progressive or sudden onset of visual loss. The RAPD can be quantified by placing graded neutral density filters over the normal or less-affected eye until the RAPD can no longer be appreciated. The examination of the pupils is discussed in more detail in Chapter 14 of this text.

CRANIAL NERVES, EXOPHTHALMOMETRY, EXTERNAL EXAMINATION, AND ANTERIOR SEGMENT EXAMINATION

Cranial nerves I, III, IV, V, VI, VII, and VIII should be tested as part of the afferent visual system examination, because lesions in the orbit, cavernous sinus, suprasellar cistern, and brainstem may directly or indirectly produce afferent system dysfunction. Exophthalmometry is essential for someone who may have an orbital mass or thyroid orbitopathy causing visual loss. External examination of the eye and anterior segment evaluation may suggest various causes of afferent visual loss, such as a carotid-cavernous sinus fistula or thyroid eye disease. A slit lamp examination will establish whether or not corneal or anterior segment problems are the cause of the visual loss. It may also demonstrate iris abnormalities, such as transillumination defects characteristic of albinism or Lisch nodules seen in neurofibromatosis type 1. Applanation tonometry should also be performed. This test not only will establish the intraocular pressure (IOP) but also will detect a significant asymmetry of IOP between the two eyes, such as occurs in patients with unilateral severe carotid artery stenosis or carotid-cavernous sinus fistula.

FUNDUS EXAMINATION

The clinical examination must include an assessment of the macula, retina, nerve fiber layer, and optic nerve. This can be performed by several methods, including direct ophthalmoscopy using a hand-held ophthalmoscope and indirect ophthalmoscopy with a 20-diopter hand-held lens. Examination of the macula with a 78- or 90-diopter hand-held lens or a corneal contact lens viewed through a slit lamp may also be helpful, particularly in patients with suspected macular disease (see Chapter 2).

Performing a fundus examination on infants and young children can be a challenge. In preparation for the examination, the parents should bring an assortment of treats for young children and plenty of feeding bottles for infants during the evaluation. It is best to leave the room after performing the afferent system and motility evaluations, allowing a nurse or technician to administer dilating drops to preserve your rapport with the child. In the case of infants, it is best to ask the parents to withhold a feeding bottle until you return to the room. Most infants will readily accept a bottle at this point and will be cooperative as a cycloplegic refraction and dilated fundus examination are performed. The soporific effect of the cycloplegic drops may also cause them to fall asleep. After completing the cycloplegic refraction, the physician should perform a dilated fundus examination using both a hand-held direct ophthalmoscope and a 20-diopter lens in conjunction with an indirect ophthalmoscope. Both assessments are best accomplished with a low level of illumination. A lid speculum is not necessary for most pediatric neuro-ophthalmologic examinations, because the macula and optic disc are the primary areas of interest. If a child becomes uncooperative at this point, it may be necessary for the parents to hold the child in a ''lock-down'' position (one parent holding the arms outstretched over the ears with the other parent holding the feet) to complete the examination. This is a stressful and difficult situation for all concerned, and all rapport with the child is gone when this occurs. If it is not possible to perform an adequate dilated examination of the infant or child, it may be necessary to conduct an evaluation with light sedation.

OTHER PROCEDURES

Other tests beyond a conventional office examination may be needed to establish the site of the pathology in the afferent visual system. Fluorescein angiography and indocyanine green angiography (ICG) may be necessary to identify retinal pathology. A full-field electroretinogram (ERG), focal or maculoscope ERG, pattern electroretinogram (PERG), electro-oculogram (EOG), dark adaptation study, visual-evoked potential (VEP), or a combination of these tests may be needed to establish the locus of the afferent system disorder. Finally, neuroimaging with magnetic resonance imaging (MRI) or computed tomographic (CT) scanning may be needed to establish the anatomic site of the afferent system abnormality.

PSYCHOPHYSICAL TESTS

Light, a very small portion of the electromagnetic spectrum (wavelengths between 400 and 700 nm), is emitted by natural and artificial sources and is reflected by objects in the environment, thereby serving as the stimulus for vision. Light entering the eye is first refracted by the tear film, cornea, and lens to form an inverted image on the retina. Photoreceptors convert this light energy into electric signals that are subsequently processed by neural elements in the retina, optic nerve, and higher visual centers of the brain. The relationship between the physical properties of light and perceptual and behavioral responses is known as **visual psychophysics,** which serves as the foundation for the clinical assessment of visual function.

A variety of specialized neural mechanisms and visual centers are responsible for encoding motion, form, color, depth, and other fundamental properties of the visual image, with new information about neural processing of visual information accumulating rapidly. Beginning at the ganglion cell level, there are two major visual processing streams whose pathways run in parallel.

- *P-cells,* the ganglion cells that project to the parvocellular layers of the lateral geniculate nucleus, are most prevalent in central vision, tend to have smaller diameter axons with lower conduction velocities, and are most effectively stimulated by low temporal frequencies and high spatial frequencies. Some P-cells respond most effectively to chromatic information, whereas others have achromatic responses to luminance and contrast. The P-cell pathway appears to be primarily involved in the processing of color, form, acuity, and related functions.
- *M-cells,* the ganglion cells that project to the magnocellular layers of the lateral geniculate nucleus, are distributed rather uniformly throughout the visual field, tend to have larger diameter axons and higher conduction velocities, and are most effectively stimulated by high temporal frequencies and low spatial frequencies. The M-cell pathway appears to be primarily involved in the processing of motion, high frequency flicker, and related functions.

Both of the major pathways described above can be further divided into more specific subgroups with distinct response properties. The M-cell and P-cell dichotomy carries through to higher visual centers, with specific projections to a large number of cortical sites that have highly specialized functions, although there is considerable overlap of these pathways at the cortical level (see Chapter 13).

Because these subpopulations of neural elements have such distinct response characteristics to particular visual attributes, it is possible to design psychophysical tests that isolate (or at least are dominated by) the activity of specific visual mechanisms. These psychophysical tests thus can serve as probes to evaluate different neural populations throughout the visual pathways. Early detection of eye disease, differential diagnosis of various ocular and neurologic disorders, and monitoring the efficacy of therapeutic regimens are just a few of the purposes that psychophysical tests can serve in a clinical setting. This section provides a brief overview of some of the more common psychophysical test procedures that can be used in the clinical evaluation of patients.

VISUAL ACUITY

The most common measurement of visual function in a clinical setting is visual acuity. It is the primary method of assessing the integrity of the optics of the eye and the neural mechanisms subserving the fovea, because good visual acuity is obtained only when both the optics and the neural components of the visual system are functioning properly. Visual acuity is used to monitor central visual function in patients, is an essential part of clinical refraction procedures, and is important to the patient for reading, face recognition, and other tasks involving fine visual detail. Visual acuity is specified in terms of the visual angle subtended by the finest spatial detail that can be identified by the observer. The physical size of an object and its distance from the observer determines its visual angle.

There are three basic types of visual acuity measurements: detection acuity, resolution acuity, and identification acuity.

1. **Detection acuity** is the smallest stimulus object or pattern of elements (the minimum angle of detection) that can be distinguished from a uniform field, and it is primarily limited by stimulus contrast. The optics of the eye are the main factors limiting detection acuity for normal human foveal vision, producing an attenuation of contrast for small stimuli imaged on the retina.

2. **Resolution acuity** is the smallest spatial detail that can be discriminated to permit one stimulus pattern to be distinguished from another (e.g., distinguishing horizontal from vertical stripes), and it is usually measured by grating patterns of alternating light and dark lines of varying widths. Resolution acuity also is limited by contrast. It is primarily constrained by the properties of the photoreceptor mosaic and underlying neural mechanisms in normal human foveal vision and is specified in terms of the minimum angle of resolution (MAR). By examining the relationships between detection acuity and recognition acuity, visual acuity deficits that are caused by optical factors may be distinguished from those that are caused by neural losses.

3. **Identification acuity**, the measure used for clinical purposes, is the smallest spatial detail that can be resolved in order to recognize objects (e.g., letters of the alphabet). It is specified in terms of MAR, log MAR, or values such as Snellen notation or metric equivalents that are based on MAR.

Table 1.2 presents a comparison of the various methods of designating visual acuity. For clini-

Table 1.2
Visual Acuity Notation Systems

DISTANCE (FEET)	SNELLEN	DISTANCE (METERS)	METRIC	MAR (MINUTES)	LogMAR	CYCLES/ DEGREE
10	20/10	3.0	6/3	0.50	−0.3	60.0
12	20/12	3.6	6/3.8	0.60	−0.2	50.0
16	20/16	4.8	6/4.8	0.80	−0.1	38.0
20	20/20	6.0	6/6	1.00	0.0	30.0
25	20/25	7.5	6/7.5	1.25	0.1	24.0
30	20/30	9.0	6/9	1.50	0.2	20.0
40	20/40	12.0	6/12	2.00	0.3	15.0
50	20/50	15.0	6/15	2.50	0.4	12.0
60	20/60	18.0	6/18	3.00	0.5	10.0
80	20/80	24.0	6/24	4.00	0.6	7.5
100	20/100	60.0	6/60	5.00	0.7	6.0
200	20/200	120.0	6/120	10.00	1.0	3.0
400	20/400	240.0	6/240	20.00	1.3	1.5

MAR = Minimum angle of resolution

cal visual acuity charts, the MAR is the angle subtended by the thickness or stroke of a letter, with the overall height and width of the letter typically being 5 times larger than the thickness. Figure 1.3 presents an example of a typical eye chart used for clinical evaluation of visual acuity. This design represents the most common form of reporting visual acuity, the so-called "Snellen notation," consisting of a fraction in which the numerator is the testing distance (20

feet or 6 meters) and the denominator is the distance at which a "normal" observer is able to read the letter. By definition, a visual acuity of 20/20 (6/6) refers to a MAR of 1 minute of arc letter thickness. The standard of 20/20 for "normal" vision was developed more than 100 years ago, and with today's high-contrast eye charts and better light sources, many normal persons under 50 years of age can be corrected to better than 20/20.

Another type of visual acuity chart is known by various names, including the Early Treatment for Diabetic Retinopathy Study (ETDRS) Chart, the Bailey-Lovie chart, and the logMAR chart (Fig. 1.4). This chart has several advantages over the standard Snellen chart. First, the letters used are equally detectable for normal observers. Second, each line has an equal number of letters. Third, the spacing between letters is proportional to the letter size. Fourth, the change in visual acuity from one line to another is in equal logarithmic steps. Fifth, better specification of visual acuity with Snellen notation, MAR, or logMAR values can be achieved. Finally, certain methods of scoring responses can be implemented that produce greater sensitivity and reliability.

A number of stimulus parameters affect visual acuity measurements in normal persons, including background adaptation luminance, stimulus contrast, refractive error, pupil size, stimulus eccentricity, duration of stimulus presentation, the type of optotype used, and interaction effects from adjacent visual contours, or "crowding." Factors such as "crowding," luminance level, contrast, and type of optotype used can sometimes have an even greater influence on visual acuity measurements for specific patient populations with ocular disorders than for normal persons. If test parameters are varied in a consistent manner, they can potentially be used for diagnostic purposes. However, the unintentional variation of background luminance or other test parameters (from one examination room to another or from one visit to another) can produce problematic outcomes when monitoring the visual status of patients.

The measurement of visual acuity in special populations (e.g., young children and physically challenged persons) is not always possible with a standard letter chart. Testing of central visual function of infants begins with an assessment of how well the infant fixes and follows the exam-

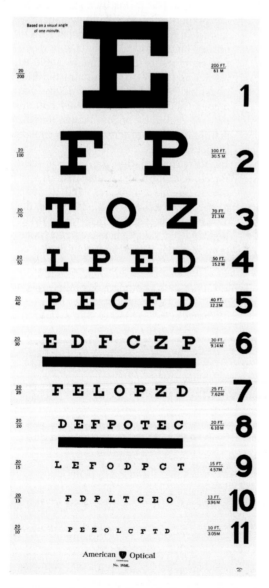

Figure 1.3. An example of a standard eye chart for visual acuity testing.

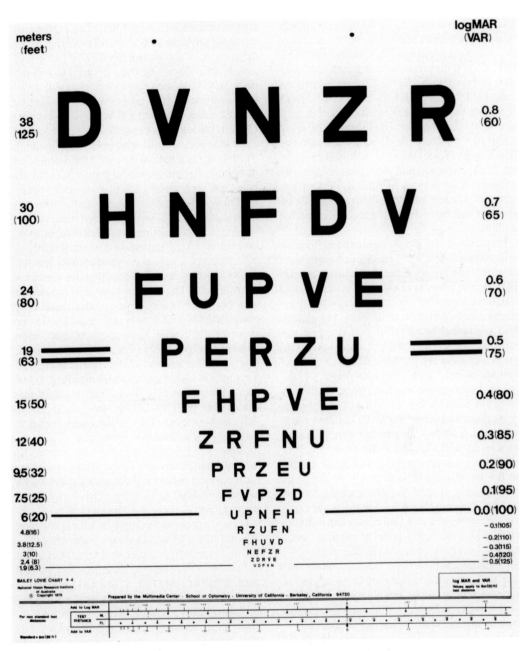

Figure 1.4.   An example of the Bailey-Lovie LogMAR visual acuity chart.

iner's face, a small toy, or other objects of interest. For older children, the "Tumbling E Cube" can be used for visual acuity testing. This cube is a white block with black E letters of different sizes on each of its sides. By rotating the cube, an individual E can be presented in four different orientations to test the patient's ability to distinguish the direction of the E. The cube can be placed at various distances from the patient, and different-sized E targets can be evaluated to make a determination of visual acuity. The Tumbling E Cube thus relies on a child's ability to orient the hand according to the direction of the E. For older children, the "E game" can be performed using a projected "E" acuity chart. The "HOTV" test involves matching each test letter to one of four letters (H, O, T, or V) printed on a card held by the child. A number of visual acuity tests use pictures or symbols. These may be more reliable than the HOTV test. The most popular of the picture visual acuity tests are the Allen Cards. Projector slides with the familiar cake, bird, telephone, and other pictures are also available. Other devices like the B-VAT vision tester can generate many random sequences of characters and figures to avoid memorization by the child.

"Preferential looking" techniques, ocular motor responses such as optokinetic nystagmus, and electrophysiologic measures such as the VEP can also be used to estimate visual acuity. In addition, a number of eye charts and behavior test procedures can be used to assess visual acuity in nonverbal or physically challenged patients. These tests use patterned stimuli and caricatures of faces (e.g., Mr. Happy Face) or common objects with "critical detail" (e.g., Cheerios) that can be used to obtain an indication of the individual's level of visual acuity.

Visual acuity measurements in children present special problems, in part because the child wants to do well and please the examiner. It is therefore important for the examiner to ensure that the nontested eye is properly occluded to avoid peeking (Fig. 1.5). The examiner must work quickly, may need to use more than one procedure to establish visual acuity capabilities, and should continually provide positive feedback to the child to maintain cooperation.

In patients suspected of having nonorganic visual loss, several additional methods of assessing visual acuity may be useful (see Chapter 23). The Tumbling E Cube can be used as a cross-check of the eye chart visual acuity determination (e.g., a patient who can see the 20/200 E on the eye chart at 20 feet should be able to see an E that is 5 times smaller at a distance of 4 feet, because the Es subtend the same visual angle). By moving the cube from one distance to another, the consistency of visual acuity responses can be ascertained. If this is done quickly, it is extremely difficult for a patient with nonorganic visual loss to maintain consistent responses (i.e., select appropriate target sizes for different distances to maintain a con-

stant visual angle), and the patient will often pick the same physical target size, irrespective of the distance at which it is presented.

A helpful device that can be used to test patients with suspected nonorganic monocular visual acuity loss is a cross-Polaroid projection chart (the American Optical Vectograph Project-O-Chart slide). This consists of a projector eye chart that is combined with polarizing material. The left or right half of the eye chart is projected through horizontally polarized material, and the other half is projected through vertically polarized material. The patient views the chart wearing a pair of glasses with polarized material that has different orientations over the two eyes (e.g., horizontal left eye polarization, vertical right eye polarization). Thus, one eye sees only the left half of the eye chart, and the other eye sees only the right half. The chart is viewed by the patient with both the "good" eye and the "bad" eye open. Patients with nonorganic visual loss in one eye will often read all of the eye chart, even though the "good" eye can only see half of the chart. Another portion of the American Optical Vectograph slide has randomly arranged visual acuity letters (ranging from 20/20 to 20/40) that can be seen with the left eye only, the right eye only, or both eyes. This is especially useful in patients with nonorganic monocular visual acuity loss.

In normal observers, visual acuity is highest for the foveal region and decreases rapidly with increasing visual field eccentricity. In many instances, central visual field loss and reduced visual acuity appear to be closely related. However, visual acuity is also reduced when there is generalized depression of the central visual field, and no scotoma is present. There are also several conditions for which the visual field may be at or near normal sensitivity, but visual acuity may be dramatically reduced. These conditions include refractive errors, corneal surface irregularities, cataract, retinal edema, serous detachment of the retina, and amblyopia.

CONTRAST SENSITIVITY

Visual acuity defines the smallest spatial detail that can be resolved for high-contrast stimuli, but it does not specify the responses of the visual system to objects of different sizes and contrasts. Measurement of the spatial contrast sensitivity function is necessary to obtain this information (Fig. 1.6). The contrast sensitivity

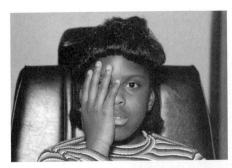
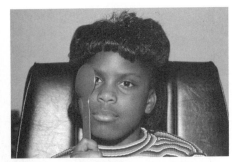
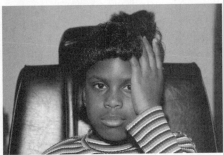
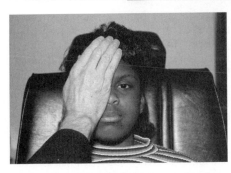
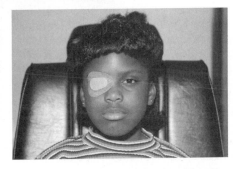

Figure 1.5. Peeking techniques that may be used by children whose visual acuity is being tested and techniques to avoid this problem. *Top left:* The examiner is attempting to test vision in the left eye. The child is supposed to be covering the right eye with her fingers, but the fingers are spread, allowing her to view with the right eye. *Top right:* The examiner is attempting to test vision in the left eye. The child is supposed to be covering the right eye with an occluder but is holding the occluder to one side, allowing her to view with the right eye. *Middle:* The examiner is attempting to test vision in the right eye. The child is supposed to be covering the left eye with the palm of her hand but is holding the hand to one side, allowing her to view with the right eye. *Bottom left:* The examiner uses his or her own hand to occlude one of the child's eyes. In this way, the examiner can be certain that the child is viewing with only one eye. *Bottom right:* Using a patch to occlude one eye is the optimum technique for testing monocular visual function.

function is most commonly determined by measuring contrast thresholds for sinusoidal gratings, an alternating pattern of light and dark bars the luminance of which varies sinusoidally in a direction perpendicular to orientation of the grating. The size of the grating is specified according to spatial frequency, which is the number of cycles (pairs of light and dark bars) of the grating pattern per degree of visual angle.

Typically, between 3 and 10 spatial frequencies from 0.5 to 30 cycles per degree are measured for the contrast sensitivity function. Contrast is defined by the luminance of the peaks (Lmax) and troughs (Lmin) of the sinusoidal grating, according to this equation:

$$\text{Contrast} = \frac{\text{Lmax} - \text{Lmin}}{\text{Lmax} + \text{Lmin}}$$

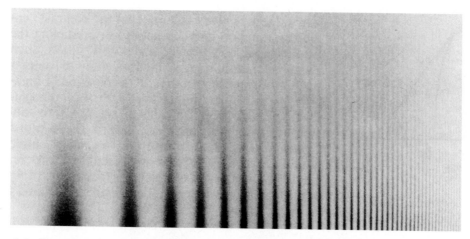

Figure 1.6. Illustration of contrast characteristics of human visual system for sinusoidal gratings. Contrast varies logarithmically along the abscissa and frequency varies logarithmically along the ordinate. Normal contrast sensitivity is greater for middle frequencies and less for high and low frequencies, as indicated by the inverted U shape of the pattern above. (Reprinted with permission from Hess RF. Application of contrast-sensitivity techniques to the study of functional amblyopia. In: Clinical Applications of Visual Psychophysics. Cambridge: Cambridge University Press, 1981.)

Contrast can vary from a minimum of 0 for a uniform field (Lmax = Lmin) to a maximum of 1 (Lmin = 0). A contrast threshold is the minimum amount of contrast needed to detect the presence of the grating, and contrast sensitivity is the reciprocal of the contrast threshold (Sensitivity = 1/Threshold).

There are several advantages of using sinusoidal gratings to evaluate the contrast sensitivity function. First, blur does not change the shape or appearance of sinusoidal gratings, other than to reduce contrast. Second, the contrast sensitivity function provides a means of characterizing the overall response properties of the visual system to a wide variety of visual images. The spatial contrast sensitivity function for vision makes it possible to determine an individual's ability to process spatial information from complex visual scenes. Fourier analysis demonstrates that all complex waveforms are actually a series of sine waves of various frequencies, amplitudes, and phase (position) relationships. Thus, any complex visual scene can be broken down into a specific combination of sinusoidal distributions of light of different spatial frequencies, amplitudes, and phases in the vertical and horizontal dimensions. If the contrast response characteristics of the human visual system to various spatial frequencies are known, then it should be possible to determine how complex visual scenes are processed by the visual system. It should be emphasized, however, that the contrast sensitivity function describes the behavior of the visual system at **threshold** contrast levels, which is not completely representative of the visual system's characteristics for processing suprathreshold contrast information.

Neurophysiologic findings suggest that neural mechanisms perform spatial frequency analysis and filtering in the early stages of processing of visual information. A number of factors influence the measurement of the normal contrast sensitivity function, including background adaptation luminance, stimulus size, visual field eccentricity, pupil size, temporal characteristics, stimulus orientation, and various optical factors such as defocus, dioptric blur, diffusive blur, and astigmatism.

The contrast sensitivity function can be used to evaluate optical properties of the human eye, including refractive error and defocus, cataract, refractive surgery, intraocular lenses, and the normal aging properties of the optics of the eye. Contrast sensitivity deficits sometimes occur in patients with normal visual acuity and optical conditions that produce subtle changes in the quality of their vision. Contrast sensitivity function losses occur in patients with retinal conditions such as diabetic retinopathy, age-related macular degeneration, and a variety of other disorders. Foveal contrast sensitivity deficits also occur in patients with glaucoma. From a neuro-ophthalmologic standpoint, measurement of the contrast sensitivity function can reveal subtle deficits in patients with optic neuritis and other optic neuropathies, with amblyopia, and with various neurologic or systemic conditions, such as Alzheimer's disease, Parkinson's disease, and cystic fibrosis.

In general, the contrast sensitivity function is clinically useful for detecting early or subtle visual loss (especially when visual acuity is normal), making comparisons between the two eyes, or monitoring the progression or improvement of visual function. One of the shortcomings of the contrast sensitivity function, however, is that sensitivity losses have little specificity for differential diagnostic purposes. In other words, similar patterns of loss are present in a wide variety of conditions, in the same manner that many types of disorders can produce similar amounts of visual acuity loss. The main patterns of contrast sensitivity loss are (Fig. 1.7)

A. Generalized contrast sensitivity loss at all spatial frequencies.

B. Greater high spatial frequency contrast sensitivity loss.
C. Greater low spatial frequency contrast sensitivity loss.
D. A "notch" produced by contrast sensitivity loss for a particular group of spatial frequencies.

Generalized and high-frequency contrast sensitivity deficits are by far the most common patterns of loss across a wide variety of pathologic ocular conditions.

The contrast sensitivity function, which can be measured in infants and young children using either electrophysiologic or behavior techniques, can provide valuable clinical information about the functional visual status in such individuals. The contrast sensitivity function also may be helpful in predicting the performance for various daily tasks, such as the identification of distant objects, reading highway signs and books, recognizing faces, and getting around despite reduced vision. Thus, the contrast sensitivity function is not only useful for revealing subtle visual deficits associated with ocular

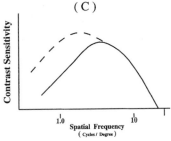

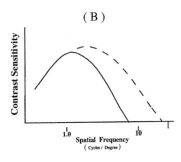

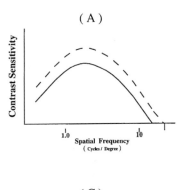

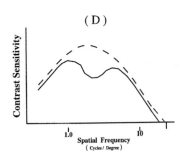

Figure 1.7. Examples of the various types of contrast sensitivity loss. *A.* Generalized depression. *B.* High spatial frequency loss. *C.* Low spatial frequency loss. *D.* Middle spatial frequency loss.

disorders but is also helpful in identifying problems that a patient is likely to encounter during daily activities.

Contrast sensitivity may be measured with a wall chart in a manner similar to the way in which visual acuity is typically measured. One such chart is the Vistech chart (Fig. 1.8). This chart has a series of five rows (A–E), each with a different spatial frequency. Each row consists of a group of nine circular targets containing a sinusoidal grating that is either vertical, tilted to the left, or tilted to the right. From the left side of the chart to the right, there is a successive reduction in the contrast of the grating. Patients are positioned 10 feet from the chart and are asked to read each row from left to right by indicating the orientation of the grating.

A second method of testing contrast sensitivity uses the typical letter charts for testing visual acuity, but there is a low contrast between the letters and the background (Fig. 1.9). Although normal observers show a small reduction in visual acuity for low-contrast targets (about two lines), patients with early or subtle abnormalities sometimes demonstrate quite profound reductions in visual acuity for low-contrast targets compared with high-contrast letters. Thus, this approach to contrast sensitivity testing can reveal mild disturbances of visual sensory function not detectable by standard visual acuity testing. The advantage of a low-contrast acuity chart is that it uses a test procedure that is highly familiar to most patients and clinicians.

A third method of testing contrast sensitivity using a chart is the Pelli-Robson chart, consisting of letters of a fixed size that vary in contrast (Fig. 1.10). Each line consists of six letters, with the three leftmost and three rightmost letters having the same amount of contrast. The patient reads the chart in a manner similar to a standard visual acuity chart, and the minimum contrast at

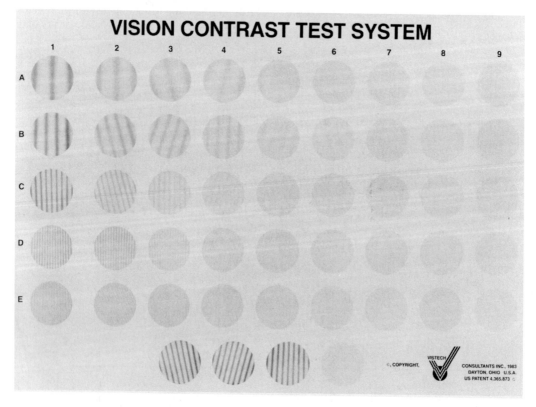

Figure 1.8. The Vistech contrast sensitivity chart.

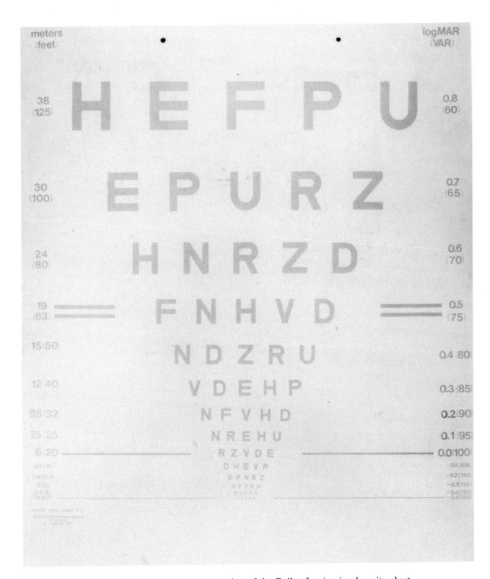

Figure 1.9.   A low-contrast version of the Bailey-Lovie visual acuity chart.

which the letters can be detected is recorded. This method of testing contrast sensitivity is highly reproducible and is capable of detecting disturbances in visual function that are not evident with standard visual acuity testing.

PERIMETRY AND VISUAL FIELD TESTING

General Principles

Perimetry and visual field testing have been clinical diagnostic test procedures for more than 100 years. Although the instrumentation and testing strategies have changed dramatically over this time, the basic principle underlying conventional perimetry has remained the same. Detection sensitivity is determined for a number of locations throughout the visual field using a small target presented against a uniform background. The loss of sensitivity at various visual field locations serves as a noninvasive probe for identifying pathology or dysfunction of the visual pathways.

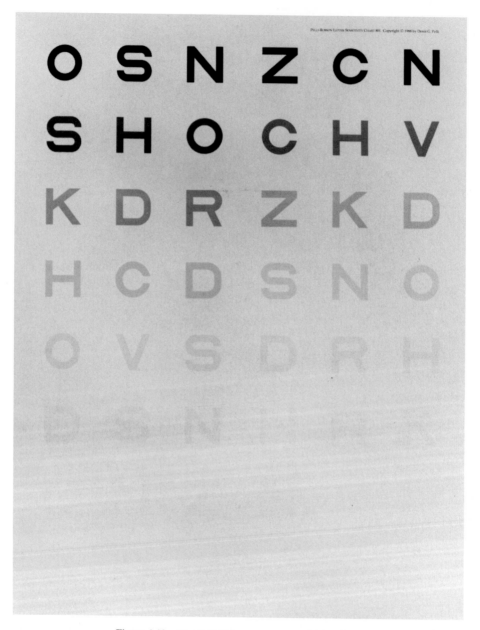

Figure 1.10. The Pelli-Robson contrast sensitivity chart.

The ability of perimetry and visual field testing to provide useful clinical information is responsible for its long-term use as a diagnostic procedure. Because perimetry and visual field testing can provide information about both the probable anatomic locus and disease process or processes for afferent system abnormalities, they remain a vital part of the neuro-ophthalmologic examination. Perimetry and visual field testing fulfill several important diagnostic functions:

1. **Early detection of abnormalities.** Because many ocular and neurologic disorders are initially expressed in the form of sensitivity loss in the periphery of the visual field, perimetry is an important fac-

tor in identifying early signs of afferent system dysfunction. Perimetry is typically the only clinical procedure that evaluates the status of the afferent visual pathways for locations outside the macular region.

2. **Differential diagnosis.** The spatial pattern of visual field deficits and comparison of patterns of visual field loss between the two eyes provide valuable differential diagnostic information. Not only can this information be helpful in defining the location of damage along the visual pathways from the retina to primary visual cortex, it can also assist in identifying the specific type of disease that has caused the damage.

3. **Monitoring progression and remission.** The ability to monitor a patient's visual field over time is important for verifying a working diagnosis, establishing if a condition is stable or progressive, and evaluating the effectiveness of therapy.

4. **Revealing hidden visual loss.** Perhaps the most important role served by perimetry is the ability to find afferent visual pathway loss that may not be apparent to the patient. Changes in foveal visual function are typically symptomatic, whereas peripheral vision loss is often asymptomatic, especially if it is gradual and monocular. Paradoxically, even though a patient may be unaware of peripheral visual field loss, the field loss can significantly affect the performance of daily activities, such as driving, orientation, and mobility.

    Perimetry and visual field testing are therefore important in identifying visual abnormalities that might not otherwise be detected by either a careful history or other parts of a standard eye examination.

Some form of visual field testing should be performed on all patients, particularly those at greater risk of having visual field loss, including:

- Patients over the age of 60.
- Individuals with high myopia, elevated IOP, diabetes, vascular disease, systemic disease, family history of glaucoma or other eye disease, or other risk factors for development of ocular or neurologic disorders.
- Individuals with visual symptoms or complaints but minimal findings on their eye examination.
- Individuals with significant problems involving orientation and mobility, balance, driving, night vision, and related everyday activities.

It is not feasible or necessary to perform a long quantitative visual field examination on all patients; however, a confrontation visual field or brief tangent screen evaluation should be performed as part of a standard neuro-ophthalmologic examination.

When more sensitive measurements of the visual field are needed, automated static perimetry, manual kinetic perimetry, or both can be performed. The choice of test procedures depends on a variety of factors, including the patient's medical history, the suspected disease or diseases, risk factors the patient may have for various diseases, the importance of the perimetric information, the amount of detailed visual field information desired, the setting in which the testing is to be performed, and the patient's ability to comply with the demands of different test procedures.

Although manual kinetic perimetry is used by many physicians, automated perimetry is considered the gold standard for visual field testing. There is no question that automated perimetry has had a dramatic impact on improving the quality of care for patients with ocular disorders. Automatic calibration of instruments, standardized test procedures, high sensitivity and specificity, reliability checks ("catch trials"), and quantitative statistical analysis procedures are some of the many advantages of this method of perimetry; however, there are also disadvantages of automated perimetry, including prolonged test time, increased cognitive demands, fatigue, and lack of flexibility for evaluating difficult patient populations. We believe that there is no single method of visual field testing that is best for all circumstances and all patients. Automated perimetry is but one of many tools that the clinician can use to evaluate peripheral visual function, and the various forms of visual field testing should be regarded as **complementary** techniques, the utility and appropriateness of which are determined by the clinical circumstances and the question that is being addressed. There is no single method of data representation, analysis procedure, visual field index, or other method of evaluating visual field data that provides all of the essential clinical information. It is important to consider all of the information available, including reliability characteristics and the subjective clinical interpretation of the visual field. In addition, it should be kept in mind that although the test may be automated, the patient is not. It is unreasonable to begin an automated visual field test, leave a patient alone in a dark room, and expect the patient to remain alert, energetic, attentive, and interested and to maintain proper alignment and fixation throughout the test procedure. Some patients require periodic rest breaks, encouragement, and personal contact to perform visual field examinations in a reliable manner. It is also important to ensure that proper test conditions, refractive characteristics, and other factors are properly established before initiating the examination. Visual field testing can be a powerful clinical diagnostic tool when these factors are kept in mind.

Psychophysical Basis for Perimetry and Visual Field Testing

The primary psychophysical concept underlying perimetry and visual field testing is the increment or differential light threshold. The increment threshold (Weberian contrast) is the minimum amount of light that must be added to a stimulus (ΔL) to make it just detectable from the background (L). At very low background luminances, the amount of light needed to detect a stimulus is constant. At higher background luminances, the increment threshold increases in direct proportion to the background luminance; for example, a doubling of the background luminance requires a doubling of the stimulus luminance for detection. This relationship, which holds over a large range of background luminance levels, is known as **Weber's Law**.

The standard background luminance used by most perimetric devices is 31.5 apostilbs (asb) or 10 candela per square meter (cd/m^2). This is in the range of background luminance levels for which Weber's Law is valid. There are several advantages to the use of this background luminance level:

1. It is close to the ambient lighting conditions in offices and waiting rooms, thus requiring a minimal amount of adaptation time.

2. The background luminance is one that is comfortable for most patients.

3. Patients have the least amount of response variability at this background luminance.

4. Factors affecting the amount of light reaching the retina (pupil size changes, ocular media transmission loss, etc.) have an equal effect on the background and stimulus luminance.

Thus, over the range of background luminances for which Weber's Law holds, these changes in retinal illumination will not affect the increment threshold measure.

Increment threshold determinations are usually made at a number of visual field locations during quantitative perimetry. For a normal visual field, the increment threshold varies as a function of visual field location. Visual field results are usually represented in terms of sensitivity, the reciprocal of threshold (Sensitivity = 1/ Threshold). At the 31.5 asb background luminance, the fovea has the highest sensitivity and is able to detect both the dimmest and the smallest targets. Sensitivity drops rapidly between the fovea and 3°, decreases gradually out to 30°, and then drops off more rapidly again, especially beyond 50° (Fig. 1.11). The characteristic three-dimensional representation of the visual field sensitivity profile is often called the "hill of vision" or an "island of vision in a sea of blindness." In addition to eccentricity-dependent changes in the slope of the visual field profile, the temporal visual field (to the right of the foveal peak) extends farther than the nasal visual field, and the inferior visual field extends farther than the superior visual field. The location of the blind spot, approximately 15° temporal to the foveal peak, is indicated in most representations by a darkened oval area.

Visual field sensitivity can be affected by many different stimulus attributes, including background luminance, stimulus size, stimulus duration, and chromaticity, as well as other factors unrelated to the stimulus. Of these parameters, stimulus size is the most important for clinical perimetry. Next to stimulus luminance, it is the most common method of adjusting the detectability of perimetric stimuli. Not only does a change in stimulus size affect the overall sensitivity to light, it also changes the slope of the sensitivity profile. Small targets produce steeper sensitivity profiles, and larger

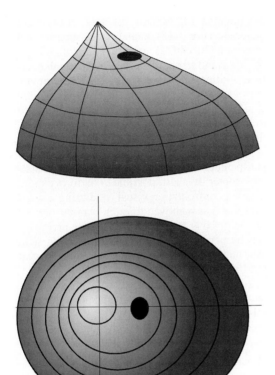

Figure 1.11. Three-dimensional representation of the normal visual field represented as a hill of vision. Sensitivity is plotted as a function of visual field eccentricity.

targets result in a flatter sensitivity profile, especially for the central 30° to 40° eccentricity. Response variability is also reduced as stimulus size is increased.

Certain patient characteristics that are not associated with ocular or neurologic pathology can also influence the increment or differential light threshold. Blur and refractive error, media opacities such as cataract, ptosis, pupil size, and related factors can affect visual field sensitivity characteristics. In addition, procedural circumstances related to trial lens rim obstructions, fixation instability, response errors, and other artifacts of testing can produce the appearance of visual field loss or can obscure visual field deficits that are actually present.

In addition to the influences mentioned above, cognition, attention, practice, learning, and other higher order functions in patients undergoing

visual field testing can influence visual field sensitivity. Fatigue effects can reduce visual field sensitivity, particularly after the test procedure has taken more than 5 to 7 minutes of testing. Patients with visual field loss typically demonstrate greater fatigue effects than those with normal visual fields, and this may be especially true for some conditions, such as optic neuritis.

Techniques for Perimetry and Visual Field Testing

Perimetry and visual field test procedures may be categorized in several different ways:

- The amount of information obtained by the test—screening vs. quantitative
- The type of stimulus used to perform the test—kinetic, static, or suprathreshold static
- The manner in which the test is administered—manually versus computer-driven.

For each of these methods of categorizing various forms of visual field testing, there are both advantages and disadvantages. Automated perimetry, for example, provides greater standardization, calibration, and statistical analysis of results than manual visual field testing, but it is less efficient, less flexible, and too demanding for some patients. Kinetic perimetry, when performed appropriately, is a more efficient method of performing an evaluation of the full visual field than is static perimetry, but the technique varies from one test to another. Quantitative procedures provide a better ability to detect subtle anomalies and monitor changes over time, but they are more time-consuming than screening procedures and may cause fatigue in some patients.

Confrontation Visual Fields

There are nearly as many ways to perform confrontation visual fields as there are persons who perform them. Nevertheless, confrontation visual fields are usually performed with the patient seated in the examination chair and the examiner seated facing the patient at a distance of 2 to 3 feet. One of the patient's eyes is occluded using the palm of the patient's hand, an occluder paddle, or a patch, and the patient is asked to fixate with the uncovered eye on the examiner's nose or opposite eye. The examiner then presents a stimulus or stimuli to various portions of the peripheral visual field and asks the patient to respond in a particular manner. A variety of stimuli can be employed for confrontation visual fields (Fig. 1.12), including hands and fingers, tongue depressors with colored dots, medicine bottle caps, small toys, hat pins stuck on the end of an eraser, pen tips, pen lights, and a host of other items. The basic intent is to use a small, localized target whose presence or absence in the visual field can be readily determined by the patient. The use of a target that can be easily presented or extinguished (e.g., turning a pen light on and off or flipping a tongue depressor with a colored dot on one side) can indicate whether or not the patient can reliably determine when the target appears and disappears. Responses from the patient include signaling the presence or absence of the target, counting the number of fingers presented, saccadic eye movements to a peripheral target, or comparisons of color saturation or brightness of two stimuli presented simultaneously or in an alternating fashion to different parts of the visual field.

A confrontation visual field should include an examination of each of the four visual field quadrants (Fig. 1.13), including the superior and inferior hemifields along the horizontal midline, the nasal and temporal hemifields along the vertical midline, and the central and peripheral visual field. With single stimulus presentation, the examiner typically moves a target from outside the visual field boundary toward fixation until the patient signals detection of the target. This is repeated for all other directions around the perimeter of the visual field to generate a peripheral isopter. It is also possible to perform a more detailed confrontation visual field using a small stimulus that is moved through various parts of the field. Thus, both static and kinetic perimetry can be performed during a confrontation field test, and it is possible to obtain detailed visual field information from this type of testing.

Confrontation visual field techniques for infants and children can be quite challenging (Fig. 1.14). Because of their adaptive abilities, children may demonstrate very good mobility skills and fool the examiner as to the extent of visual field loss. For infants and young children, a vis-

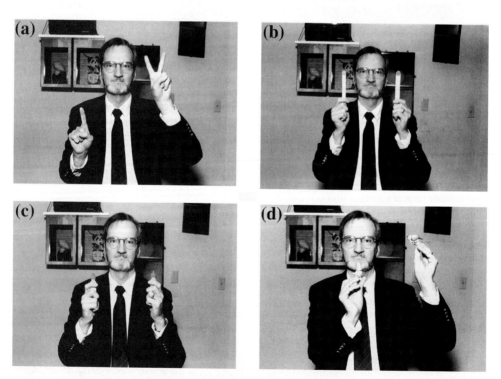

Figure 1.12. Common objects used for confrontation visual field testing. *A.* Hands and fingers. *B.* Tongue depressors with colored dots. *C.* Medicine bottle caps. *D.* Small toys.

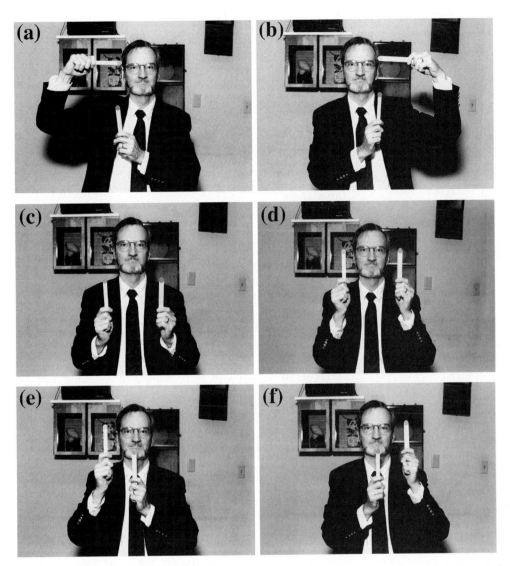

Figure 1.13. Confrontation testing of the visual field. *A–B:* The superior and inferior hemifields along the horizontal midline. *C–D:* The nasal and temporal hemifields along the vertical midline. *E–F:* The central and peripheral visual field.

ually mediated startle response can be used to detect hemianopic defects and other substantial defects in the peripheral field. A child who sees a startle stimulus will look in that direction. For older children, finger mimicking or a "Simon says" game can be used to evaluate the peripheral visual field. The child mimics the examiner by holding up the same number of fingers he or she observes. "Finger puppet perimetry" can be performed, with one puppet used to direct cen-

tral fixation and the other puppet used as a peripheral stimulus for saccadic eye movements. A story with dialogue between the puppets is used to redirect attention from one puppet to the other.

In many instances, simultaneous comparison of color saturation or brightness of stimuli between hemifields is useful in distinguishing subtle anomalies. Similar comparisons between the two eyes are also helpful. When the stimuli are

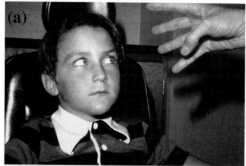

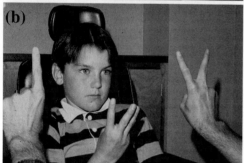

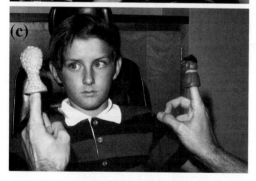

Figure 1.14. Examples of confrontation visual field testing in children. *A.* Startle response. *B.* Finger counting. *C.* Finger puppets.

presented in a double simultaneous fashion to the right and left of fixation, it is possible to detect homonymous defects. Subtle deficits across the vertical midline can be detected by asking the patient to indicate which of the two test objects is clearer or brighter. In addition, double simultaneous presentation can be used to detect the phenomenon of visual extinction—the lack of awareness of an object in a seeing area of the visual field when other seeing areas of the visual field are stimulated simultaneously with that field.

The obvious advantages of confrontation vis-

ual field testing include its simplicity, flexibility, speed of administration, and ability to be performed in any setting, including at the bedside. The disadvantages of confrontation visual field testing include the lack of standardization, the qualitative nature of the results, and the limited ability to detect subtle deficits and monitor progression or remission of visual loss. We believe that because it is quick and easy to perform, **confrontation visual fields should be performed on all patients,** regardless of their visual complaints.

Amsler Grid

Amsler grids are a series of plates consisting of lined and patterned grids that test the central visual field within 10° of fixation when the plates are held at 1/3 meter from the eyes. Each square of the grid subtends 1° of visual angle, making the ability to define the location of small defects rather easy. The patient is asked to fixate a central spot on the grid, using one eye at a time, and is asked if he or she can see the spot. If not, the patient's finger can be placed on the center to help fixation. The patient is then asked to point out any regions in which the lines are missing, blurred, distorted, bent, or irregular.

The Amsler grids can be used to identify and plot the small scotomas and other visual field defects that often occur with macular scars, mild macular degeneration, central serous chorioretinopathy, and related disorders. It is perhaps less well recognized that small central or paracentral scotomas that occur with optic nerve disease can also be identified with these plates (see Fig. 1.2). Indeed, the Amsler grid test may identify small central scotomas and other subtle central visual disturbances that are difficult to detect with more sophisticated automated and manual perimeters. In addition, the Amsler grid is very quick and easy to use. Its main disadvantages are related to the qualitative and subjective nature of the information derived from the test.

Tangent (Bjerrum) Screen

The central visual field can be studied in detail using a tangent or Bjerrum screen. The screen is made of black felt or other black matte material and can be mounted on the wall or hung from the ceiling of an examination room. The screen has several concentric circles and radial lines imprinted on it to provide a reference for the examiner. A dark wand with circular targets of various sizes and colors mounted on the end is used to examine the central visual field, usually within 30° of fixation. In its most common application, testing is performed at a distance of 1 meter, and a light source is employed to provide a relatively uniform illumination of 7 foot-candles on the screen. Targets are specified in terms of their diameter, their color, and the testing distance in millimeters. For example, a 1-mm diameter white target used with the patient located 1 meter from the tangent screen would be designated as 1/1000W, and a 5-mm red target used with the patient located 2 meters from the screen would be designated as 5/2000R.

A kinetic technique is usually used to test the visual field during a tangent screen examination. The patient fixates on a central target, and a stimulus is slowly moved from the periphery toward the center of the screen along a particular meridian until the patient reports detection of the stimulus. By repeating this procedure along different meridians, a contour of equal sensitivity—an **isopter**—can be plotted. The use of several different target sizes generates several different isopters, thus creating a map of the sensitivity of the visual field. Scotomas, areas of low sensitivity or nonseeing areas surrounded by normal visual field regions, are also plotted. A well-performed kinetic tangent screen examination can detect subtle defects and provide quantitative information for the central visual field that is comparable to that obtained by more sophisticated automated procedures.

Suprathreshold static visual field screening can also be accomplished with the tangent screen. Using targets that are white on one side and black on the other, the wand can be rotated to present and then extinguish the stimulus at key locations throughout the visual field. The target size employed is typically one that can be readily detected by persons with normal visual fields. In this manner, it is possible to quickly determine whether or not visual field abnormalities are present.

The main advantages of the tangent screen are its flexibility (i.e., variable distance from the patient, different colored objects, single vs. multiple stimuli used simultaneously), speed, and ease of use. In addition, by varying the distance of the patient from the screen and using appropriate-sized stimuli, the examiner can differentiate organic from nonorganic constriction of the visual field (Fig. 1.15). The main disadvantages are the strong dependence of results on the skill and technique of the perimetrist, the lack of standardization, difficulty in monitoring the patient's fixation while performing the visual field examination, and the need to establish office-specific age-related population norms.

Goldmann Manual Projection Perimeter

The Goldmann perimeter is a white hemispheric bowl of uniform luminance (31.5 asb) onto which a small bright stimulus is projected. It is generally used to perform kinetic perimetry, although static and suprathreshold static perimetry can also be tested with this perimeter. Unlike the Amsler grid and tangent screen, the Goldmann perimeter can be used to evaluate the entire visual field, not just a portion of the central field. With one eye occluded, the patient fixates a small target in the center of the bowl, and the perimetrist monitors eye position by means of a telescope. A particular stimulus size and luminance is projected onto the bowl, the target is moved from the far periphery toward fixation at a constant rate of speed, typically 4° to 5° sec, and the patient is instructed to press a response button when he or she first detects the stimulus. The location of target detection is noted on a chart, and the process is repeated for different meridians around the visual field. Isopters and scotomas are plotted in a manner similar to that described for the tangent screen examination, except that both the target size and luminance can be adjusted to vary stimulus detectability. This process produces a two-dimensional representation of the hill of vision that is basically a topographical contour map of the eye's sensitivity to light (Fig. 1.16). Kinetic testing (at least 1 or 2 isopters) on the Goldmann perimeter can be performed in cooperative children as young as 5 or 6 years of age.

Static Perimetry

Static perimetry uses a stationary target, the luminance of which is adjusted to vary its visibility. Although it can be performed manually using either the Goldmann or Tubinger perimeters, it is most often performed with an automated perimeter, such as the Humphrey Field Analyzer or the Octopus perimeter. Measurements of the increment threshold are obtained at a variety of visual field locations that are usually arranged in a grid pattern or along meridians.

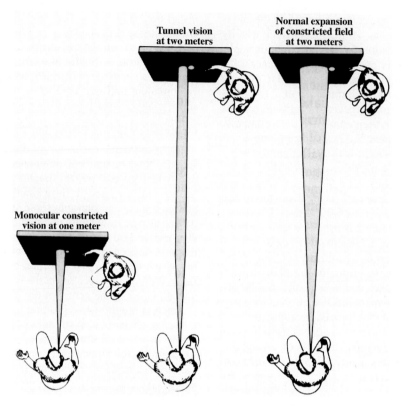

Figure 1.15. A demonstration of physiologically invalid tunnel vision ("tubular vision") associated with nonorganic visual field loss, and the normal cone-shaped expansion of the normal visual field as testing distance is increased. (Reprinted with permission from Beck RW, Smith CH. The neuro-ophthalmologic examination. Neurol Clin 1983;1: 807–830.)

Typically, a bracketing or staircase procedure is used to measure threshold sensitivity. With a staircase procedure, the target luminance is increased if the patient does not detect the target and decreased following detection of the target. Each time the response changes or reverses (from seen to not-seen and vice versa), the amount of the target luminance change becomes smaller. The threshold determination ceases after a criterion number of response reversals, with the average of reversals or the last seen target typically accepted as the detection threshold.

The presentation of visual field sensitivity for grid patterns is typically a gray-scale representation (see Fig. 1.16), rather than the three-dimensional "hill of vision" that is produced during kinetic perimetry. Areas of high sensitivity near the peak of the hill of vision are denoted by lighter shading and areas of low sensitivity by dark shading. Determinations along meridians are usually represented by a sensitivity profile plot (see Fig. 1.16).

The major advantages of automated static perimetry are standardization of test conditions and strategies, quantitative visual field assessment, a normative database and statistical analysis procedures, and automatic calibration. Its major disadvantages include a lengthy amount of time required for testing, limited flexibility, and the need for additional testing space.

Both static and kinetic perimetry are quantitative procedures that require a considerable amount of testing time. **Suprathreshold static perimetry** is a procedure that is faster than quantitative techniques and is typically used for screening purposes. There are a number of variations in test procedures, strategies, and theoretical bases for suprathreshold static perimetry. The basic technique, however, is that targets that

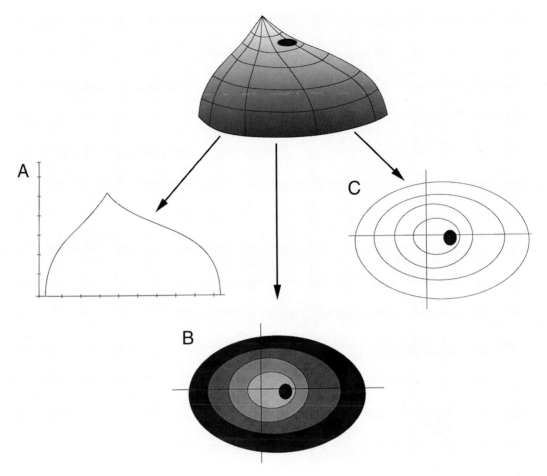

Figure 1.16.   A comparison of the various graphic methods of representing visual field data. *A.* Profile plot. *B.* Gray-scale plot. *C.* Isopter/scotoma plot.

can be easily detected by persons with normal peripheral vision are presented at selected locations throughout the visual field. These locations are usually selected to evaluate areas that are frequently affected by various ocular or neurologic disorders that damage the visual pathways (e.g., glaucoma, chiasmal tumors). Locations at which the target is seen are denoted by one symbol, and locations where the target is not seen are denoted by another. In some instances, two target intensities are presented to each location. If neither target is seen, the deficit is recorded as absolute. If both targets are seen, the location is denoted as normal. If the more intense target is seen, but the lower intensity target is not, the deficit is denoted as relative loss. There are a number of different methods of representing vis-

ual field data from suprathreshold static perimetry, although all of them generally adhere to the aforementioned principles (Fig. 1.17).

Interpretation of Visual Field Information

A large amount of visual field information is derived from perimetric testing, especially from automated perimetry. Test conditions and stimulus parameters used, indicators of patient reliability and cooperation, physiologic factors (pupil size, refractive state, visual acuity, etc.), summary statistics, visual field indices, and other data are presented in conjunction with sensitivity values for various locations in the patient's visual field. Visual field sensitivity can also be represented in many different forms (numerical values, deviations from normal, gray-scale

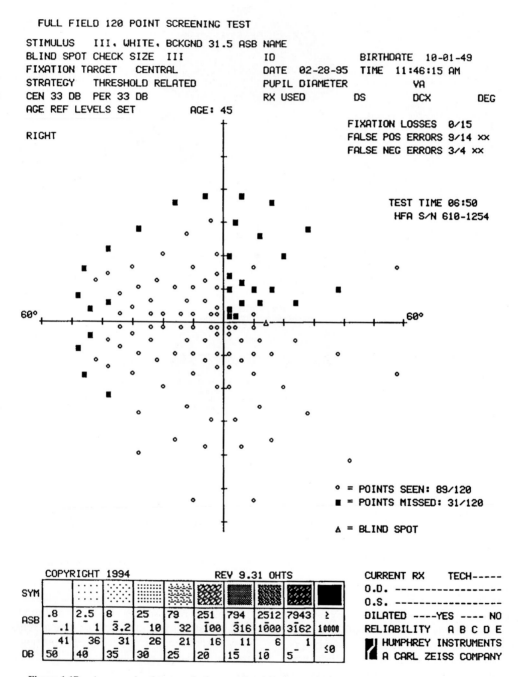

Figure 1.17. An example of test results for suprathreshold static perimetry. (Courtesy of CA Johnson, PhD.)

representations, probability plots, etc.). The following discussion presents a brief overview of the various types of information provided on the final printed outputs.

Graphic Representation of Visual Field Data

In most instances, the numeric representation of visual field information, whether by means of summary values such as visual field indices or by sensitivity values for individual visual field locations, is difficult to interpret. A graphic representation of visual field data makes the data easier to evaluate, particularly for detecting specific patterns of visual field loss or for assessing progression or other visual field changes over time. There are three primary methods of graphically representing visual field data: isopter/scotoma plots, profile plots, and gray-scale plots (see Fig. 1.16).

Ancillary Information

Several important pieces of information that should be checked on each visual field examination are the position of the eyelids, the refractive correction used for testing, the size of the pupil, and the patient's visual acuity. Ptosis can produce a superior visual field defect that may be minimal or significant (Fig. 1.18A). High refractive corrections (greater than 6 diopters spherical equivalent) can sometimes produce trial lens rim artifacts (Fig. 1.18B). When a patient's spherical equivalent correction for perimetric testing exceeds 6 diopters, it is advisable to use a soft contact lens correction that is appropriate for the testing distance to avoid lens rim artifacts. Proper near refractive corrections that are appropriate for the near testing distance of the perimeter bowl and the patient's age must be used to minimize the likelihood of refraction scotomas and sensitivity reductions from blur (Fig. 1.18C). Small pupils (less than 2 mm diameter) can produce spurious test results, especially in older persons who may have early lenticular changes. If pupil size is less than 2 mm, the patient should be dilated to 3 mm or greater to minimize the influence of a small pupil as a confounding variable for visual field interpretation (Fig. 1.18D). Finally, the patient's visual acuity can also provide useful information when assessing generalized visual field sensitivity loss and the potential sources responsible for the loss.

Reliability Indices

The quality of information obtained from perimetry and visual field testing depends on a patient's cooperation, willingness, and ability to respond in a reliable fashion and maintain a consistent response criterion. Thus, it is important to have some type of assessment of patient reliability and consistency in order to properly evaluate the significance of visual field information. With manual perimetry, it is possible to monitor the patient's fixation behavior directly by means of a telescopic viewer that can be used to observe the patient's eye during testing. The use of "catch trials" can be used to determine the patient's response reliability. False-positive errors (responses when no stimulus is presented) and false-negative errors (failure to respond to a stimulus presented in a region previously determined to be able to detect equal or less detectable targets) can be monitored throughout the test procedure.

Automated test procedures not only have the capability of monitoring false-positive errors, false-negative errors, and fixation behavior in the same manner as described above but also can obtain an assessment of response fluctuation by retesting a sample of visual field locations. Also, indirect indicators of fixation accuracy (e.g., whether or not a patient responds to a target presented to the physiologic blind spot) can be monitored. An additional advantage of automated test procedures is that these **reliability indices** (false-positives, false-negatives, fixation losses, short-term fluctuation) can be immediately compared with those of age-adjusted normal control subjects, thereby providing an indication as to whether or not the patient's reliability parameters are within normal population characteristics.

Some of the reliability indices for automated perimetry are not always accurate indicators of a patient's true performance. For example, false-negative rates are correlated with visual field deficits; i.e., there is an increase in false-negative responses with increased field loss. Thus, high false-negative rates may be more indicative of disease severity than of unreliable patient responses. Excessive fixation losses can be caused by factors such as mislocalization of the blind spot during the initial phases of testing, misalignment of the patient midway through testing, or inattention on the part of the technician ad-

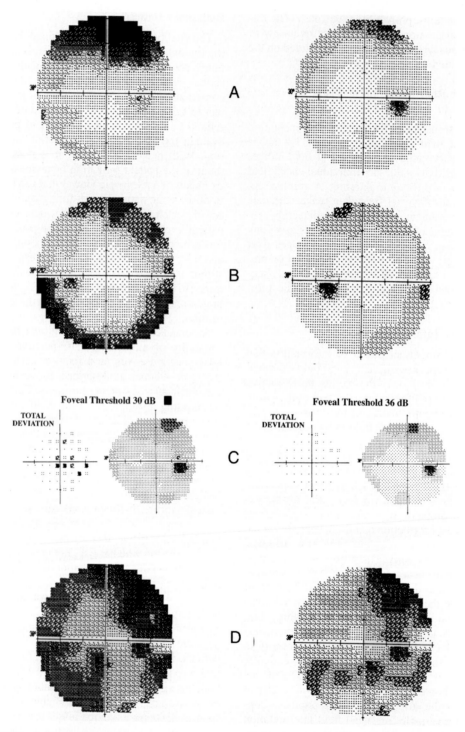

Figure 1.18. Influences on visual field test results. *A.* An example of visual field results for ptosis before (*left*) and after (*right*) taping up the upper lid and brow. *B.* Example of trial lens rim artifact (*left*) and its disappearance (*right*) after re-aligning the patient. *C.* Refractive error introduced by improper lens correction (*left*) and results after proper lens was employed (*right*). *D.* Visual field results obtained in the same eye with a 1-mm (*left*) and a 3-mm (*right*) pupil diameter.

ministering the visual field examination. Also, one should be careful not to consider reliability indices as a replacement for technician interaction and monitoring of patients. Some patients are uncomfortable when left alone in a darkened room during automated perimetry testing. In addition, misalignment of the patient, drowsiness, and related factors can occur during testing and go undetected if the patient is not adequately monitored, thereby producing spurious test results. It is important to remember that, as noted above, it is the test procedure that is automated, not the patient.

Although reliability indices are helpful in determining if the visual field is accurate, they are not sufficient to eliminate the possibility that a visual field defect is nonorganic in nature. It has been shown by numerous investigators that both patients and otherwise normal subjects can "fool" the automated perimeter, producing a variety of abnormal fields despite maintaining reliability indices that are within normal limits.

Visual Field Indices

A distinct advantage afforded by automated perimeters is the ability to provide summary statistics, usually called **visual field indices.** The mean deviation (MD) on the Humphrey Field Analyzer and the mean defect (MD) on the Octopus perimeters refer to the average deviation of sensitivity at each test location from age-adjusted normal population values. They provide an indication of the degree of generalized or widespread loss in the visual field. The pattern standard deviation (PSD) on the Humphrey Field Analyzer and the loss variance (LV) on the Octopus perimeter present a summary measure of the average deviation of individual visual field sensitivity values from the normal slope after correcting for any overall sensitivity differences (i.e., MD). They represent the degree of irregularity of visual field sensitivity about the normal slope and therefore indicate the amount of localized visual field loss, because scotomas produce significant departures from the normal slope of the visual field. Corrected pattern standard deviation (CPSD) and corrected loss variance (CLV) take into account the patient's short-term fluctuation (STF) during testing. STF is derived by testing a sample of 10 locations twice to determine the average deviation of repeated measures. This correction minimizes the influence of patient variability on the local deviation measures.

Probability Plots

One of the advantages of automated static perimetry is that a patient's test results are compared with age-adjusted normal population values. Thus, it is possible to determine the amount of deviation from normal population sensitivity values on a point-by-point basis for all visual field locations tested. A useful means of expressing this information is by means of **probability plots.** The Humphrey Field Analyzer has two methods of presenting this type of information. One is called the "total deviation plot" and the other is called the "pattern deviation plot." For the total deviation plot, each visual field location has one of a group of different symbols indicating if the sensitivity is within normal limits or is below the 5%, 2%, 1%, or 0.5% of normal limits, respectively. In other words, visual field locations or indices that have a probability corresponding to $P < 1\%$ mean that this value is observed less than 1% of the time in a normal population of the same age. This provides an immediate graphic representation of the locations that are abnormal and the degree to which they vary from normal levels.

The pattern deviation plot is similar to the total deviation plot, except that the determinations are performed after the average or overall sensitivity loss has been subtracted, thereby revealing specific locations with **localized** deviations from normal sensitivity values. The value of these representations is twofold. First, they provide an immediate indication of the locations with sensitivity loss. Second, the comparison of the total and pattern deviation plots provides a clear indication of the degree to which the loss is diffuse or localized. If the loss is predominantly widespread, the abnormal locations will appear on the total deviation plot, but all or most of these locations will be within normal limits on the pattern deviation plot (Fig. 1.19A). If the deficit is predominantly localized, the total and pattern deviation plots will look almost identical (Fig. 1.19B). The degree of similarity between the total and pattern deviation plots thus gives an indication of the proportion of loss that is widespread and that which is localized. In a few instances, the total deviation plot may appear to be normal, but the pattern deviation plot reveals a number of abnormal locations (Figs. 1.19C). This occurs when the patient's measured sensitivity is significantly better than normal, and it is most often caused by a patient who presses the response button too often and inappropriately.

Figure 1.19. Patient results as they are depicted on the total deviation and pattern deviation probability plots for the Humphrey Field Analyzer. *A.* Diffuse loss. *B.* Localized loss. *C.* "Trigger happy" patient.

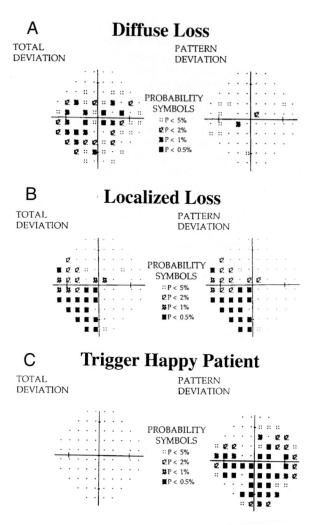

Progression of Visual Field Loss

The determination of whether a patient's visual field improves, worsens, or remains stable over time is probably the most difficult aspect of interpretation of visual fields. Although there are several quantitative analysis procedures available for evaluating visual field progression, none of them enjoys complete acceptance by the clinical ophthalmic community. Nevertheless, the use of quantitative statistical analysis procedures may be helpful in monitoring a patient's visual field status.

There are several important factors to consider when evaluating a patient's visual field status over time. First, it is necessary to review the test conditions that were present for each visual field examination. If different test strategies, target sizes, or other test conditions are different from one examination to another, it is extremely difficult to compare the results, because the type of test procedure and the target size can significantly alter the appearance of the visual field (Figs. 1.20 and 1.21). Second, it is important to determine if there are any differences in patient characteristics from one visual field to another. If there are meaningful differences in pupil size, refractive corrections, visual acuity, time of day, or other factors (e.g., upper lid taped on one occasion and not on another occasion), this can have a dramatic effect on the visual field results obtained on different visits, and an incorrect determination of visual field change may be as-

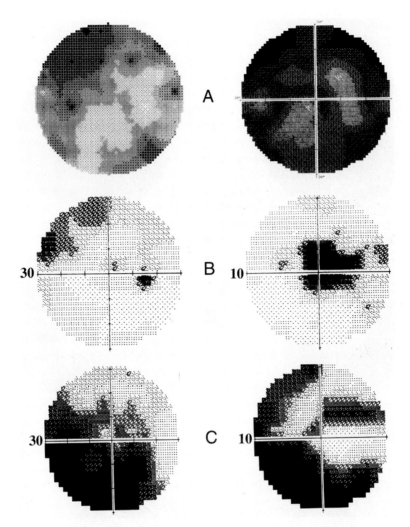

Figure 1.20.   Examples of different fields obtained when patients with a field defect are tested with different strategies on an automated perimeter or with different perimeters. *A.* A patient with an optic neuropathy who was tested on two different automated perimeters. Note marked difference in results. *B.* A macular scotoma using a central 30° test (*left*) and central 10° test (*right*). Note appearance of scotoma when 10° test is performed. *C.* Advanced glaucoma using a central 30° test (*left*) and a central 10° test (*right*).

sessed (see Fig. 1.18). Third, unless the visual field changes are dramatic, it is important to base judgments of visual field progression or stability on the basis of the entire series of visual fields that are available. It is not possible to distinguish subtle visual field changes from long-term variation on the basis of two visual fields (e.g., comparing the current visual field to the previous visual field). In particular, patients with moderate to advanced visual field loss can sometimes exhibit considerable variations from one visual field to another. Also, factors such as fatigue and

experience can produce significant differences in visual field characteristics. If it is suspected that a change in visual field has occurred, it is best to repeat the examination on a separate visit to confirm the suspected change.

Five-Step Approach to Visual Field Interpretation

One of the common errors that occurs in visual field interpretation is the lack of attention to details and specific patterns of visual field loss before obtaining a global evaluation of the visual

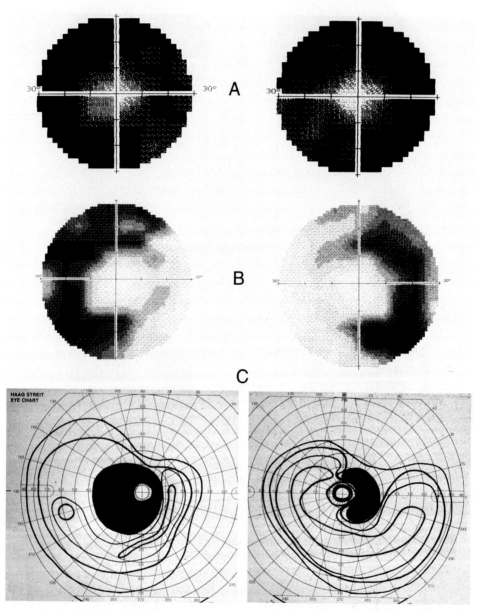

Figure 1.21. Appearance of visual fields obtained by different techniques in a patient with retinitis pigmentosa. *A.* Visual field defects with static perimetry using a Humphrey 30-2 test with a size III target for the left and right eyes shows diffuse reduction in sensitivity in each eye with a small area of central sparing. *B.* Results using a Size V target for the central 30°. Note expansion of the clear central area. *C.* Results obtained by full field kinetic perimetry using a Goldmann perimeter. Note that with static perimetry the true extent of the field defects cannot be appreciated. With kinetic perimetry, the scotomatous nature of the defects can be appreciated.

field. To avoid this tendency, we suggest a simple five-step approach to visual field interpretation:

Step 1. Determine if the visual field is normal or abnormal for each eye separately. Automated perimetry results provide excellent assistance with this task, because they show both point-by-point and overall comparisons of the patient's test results with age-matched normal population values. If both eyes are normal, both in terms of statistical comparison and clinical assessment, further evaluation is not necessary. However, subtle visual field loss can sometimes be present despite visual field indices that are within normal limits. Perhaps the most common of these occurrences are the subtle vertical steps in the superior visual field that may reflect an early bitemporal chiasmal lesion.

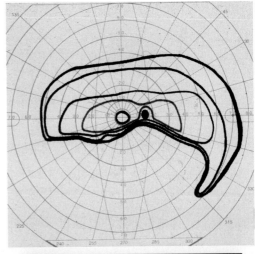

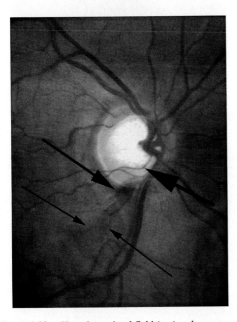

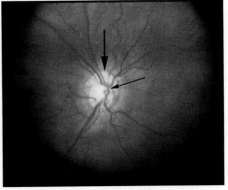

Figure 1.22. Humphrey visual field (*top*) and corresponding fundus photo (*bottom*) from a patient with low tension glaucoma in the right eye. Note moderate cupping (*large arrow*), small peripapillary nerve fiber layer hemorrhage (*medium arrow*), and wedge-shaped nerve fiber layer defect (*small arrows*) that corresponds to the superior arcuate field defect detected by perimetry.

Figure 1.23. Unilateral visual field defect in a patient with segmental hypoplasia of the right optic nerve. Visual acuity was 20/20 in the eye. *Top:* Kinetic perimetry using a Goldmann perimeter shows marked inferior altitudinal defect that does not obey the horizontal midline. Note preservation of the central field to small isopters. *Bottom:* Fundus photograph shows absence of the upper part of the disc substance. The thin arrow indicates the location of the optic disc, and the thick arrow indicates the scleral crescent.

Step 2. If one or both visual fields are abnormal, examine the ancillary information to determine if proper test conditions were employed, the appropriate near correction was used (based on the patient's age, distance refraction, and whether or not the patient was cycloplegled), and the pupil size was sufficiently large. Also, check for patterns of visual field loss that are indicative of a trial lens rim artifact, a ptotic upper eyelid, or other conditions not related to damage to the visual sensory pathway that may account for the visual field loss. Fatigue, drowsiness, and related conditions can also produce apparent visual field loss.

It is crucial that the person who performs the perimetric testing, especially automated perimetric testing, be attentive to these factors, both before and during the examination. A surprising number of visual field deficits can be directly attributed to nonpathologic influences.

Step 3. Determine if the visual field is abnormal in both eyes or in only one eye. If the visual field is abnormal in only one eye, the defect is almost always caused by a disorder anterior to the optic chiasm (Figs 1.22 and 1.23). If the visual field of both eyes is abnormal, either the deficit is at or posterior to the optic chiasm (Figs 1.24 and 1.25) **or**

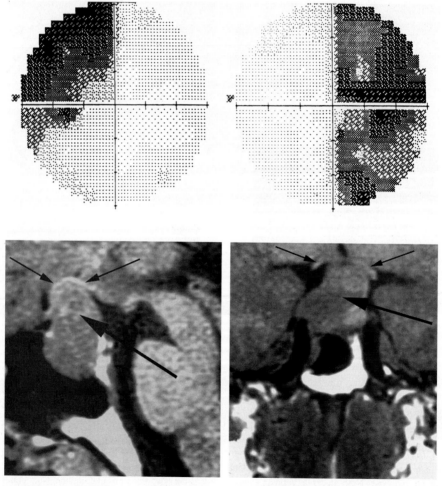

Figure 1.24. Bilateral visual field defect in a patient with a tumor in the region of the optic chiasm. *Top:* Static perimetry reveals a bilateral temporal hemianopia, worse in the right eye (right side of illustration). *Bottom:* Sagittal (*left*) and coronal (*right*) T1-weighted magnetic resonance images show a large mass in the sella turcica with suprasellar extension (*large arrows*). The mass compresses and elevates the optic chiasm (*small arrows*).

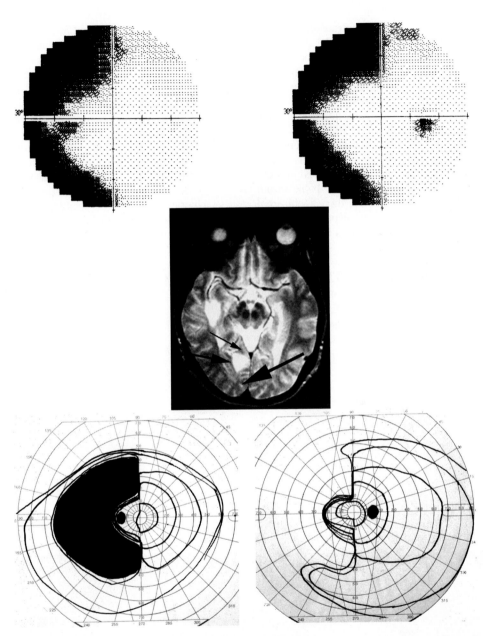

Figure 1.25.   Bilateral visual field defects in a patient with an occipital lobe infarct. *Top:* Static perimetry using a Humphrey visual field analyzer shows a left homonymous field defect with macular sparing. *Middle:* T2-weighted axial magnetic resonance image shows a hyperintense region consistent with an infarct (*medium arrow*) in the right occipital lobe. Note normal appearance of the posterior aspect of the right occipital lobe (*large arrow*), corresponding to the macular sparing. In addition, the deep portion of the calcarine fissure (*thin arrow*), which has only monocular representation and is responsible for the temporal crescent, also appears normal. *Bottom:* Kinetic perimetry confirms a left homonymous hemianopia with macular sparing and sparing of the temporal crescent of the visual field of the left eye.

the patient has bilateral intraocular or optic nerve disease (Figs. 1.26 and 1.27).

Step 4. Determine the general location of the visual field loss for each eye independently. Specifically, determine if the visual field loss is in the superior or inferior hemifield, the nasal or temporal hemifield, or the central portion of the field. This is especially important for the nasal and temporal hemifield assessment. If the loss is extensive, determine where the **greatest** amount of visual field loss is present. If the visual field loss is bitemporal, then a chiasmal locus should be strongly suspected (see Fig. 1.24). If the visual field loss is nasal in one

eye and temporal in the other eye (i.e., homonymous), a retrochiasmal location should be suspected (see Fig. 1.25). Binasal defects or a nasal deficit in only one eye should generate a suspicion of glaucoma, various nonglaucomatous optic neuropathies, or certain types of retinal disorders (see Figs. 1.26 and 1.27). A central deficit in one or both eyes may indicate a macular disorder or an optic neuropathy (Figs. 1.28 and 1.29). With this simple step, a **global** view of visual field properties is generated, and a hierarchy of potential locations of damage along the visual pathway and probable disease entities is hypothesized.

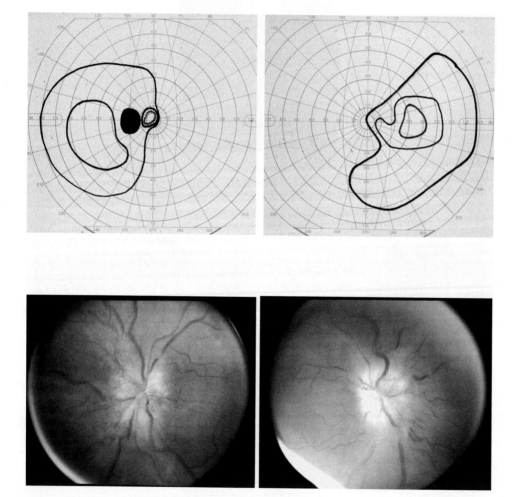

Figure 1.26. Bilateral visual field defects in a patient with pseudotumor cerebri. *Top:* Kinetic perimetry demonstrates complete loss of the nasal visual field of both eyes, with involvement of the temporal fields as well. *Bottom:* Fundus photographs show bilateral chronic papilledema with early atrophy.

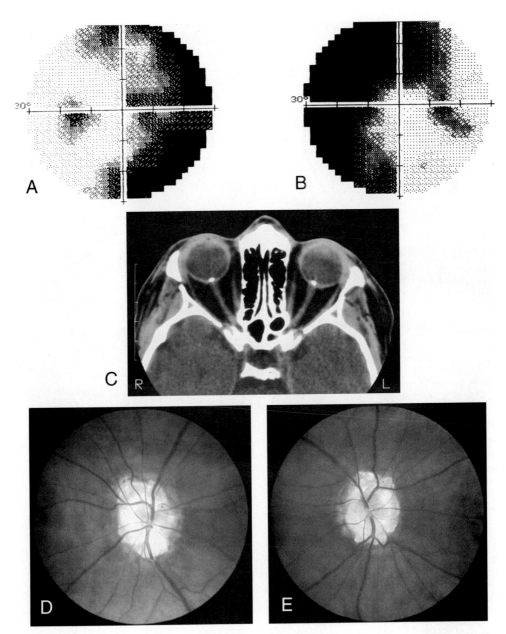

Figure 1.27. Bilateral visual field defects in a patient with bilateral optic disc drusen. *A–B:* Static perimetry reveals significant nasal field loss in both eyes. *C:* Axial computed tomographic scan set at bone window density shows calcified drusen. *D–E:* Fundus photographs show extensive optic disc drusen. Note absence of visible nerve fiber layer and constriction of retinal arteries.

Step 5. Look at the specific shapes, patterns, and features of the visual field loss (Figs. 1.22 through 1.30; Table 1.3). Does the defect respect either the horizontal or vertical meridians? What is the shape of the deficit (arcuate, oval, circular, pie-shaped, irregular, etc.)? Does the deficit "point" to the blind spot or to the fixation? If there is homonymous visual field loss in both eyes, is it congruous (i.e., symmetric in the two

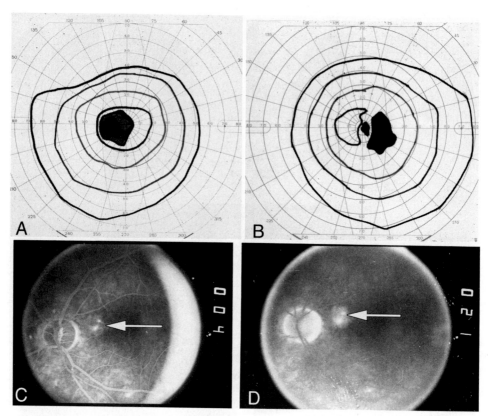

Figure 1.28. Bilateral visual field defects in a patient with bilateral central serous chorioretinopathy. *A–B:* Kinetic perimetry reveals bilateral central defects with normal peripheral fields. *C–D:* Early (*C*) and late (*D*) phases of fluorescein angiography show leakage of dye consistent with central serous chorioretinopathy in the posterior pole of the left eye (*arrows*).

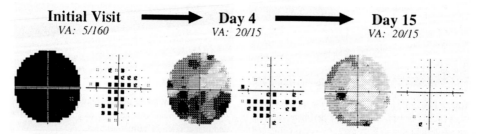

Figure 1.29. Improvement in a visual field defect as detected by static perimetry in a patient with optic neuritis over a 15-day period. (Reprinted with permission from Keltner JL, Johnson CA, Spurr JO, et al. Visual field profile of optic neuritis: one year followup in the Optic Neuritis Treatment Trial. Arch Ophthalmol 1994;112:946–953.)

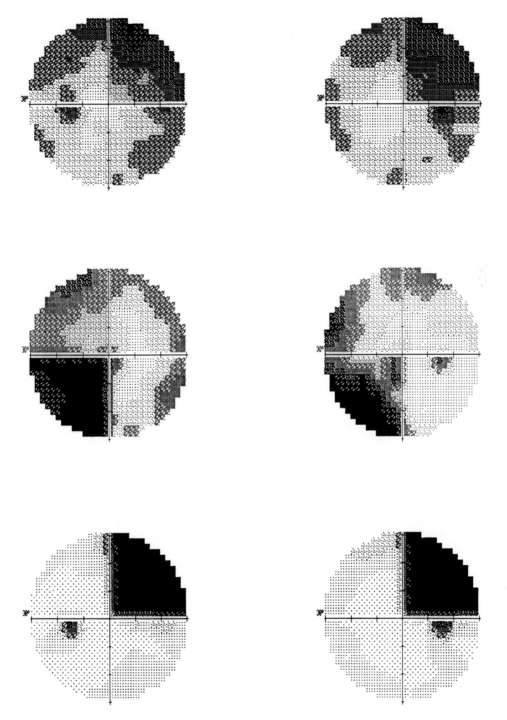

Figure 1.30. Visual field defects caused by postgeniculate lesions in the temporal (*top*), parietal (*middle*), and occipital (*bottom*) lobes as defined by static perimetry. *Top:* Right incomplete incongruous homonymous hemianopia, denser above, from left temporal lobe lesion. *Middle:* Left incom-plete incongruous homonymous hemianopia, denser below, from lesion of the right parietal lobe. *Bottom:* Right con-gruous superior quadrantanopia from lesion of the inferior aspect of the left occipital lobe.

Table 1.3.
Differential Diagnosis of Visual Field Deficits

I. GENERAL DEPRESSION
    A. Cataract (diffuse depression from cataracts may improve with dilation)
    B. Corneal Disease (shows no improvement with dilation)
    C. Other Media Opacities
    D. Some Optic Neuropathies
II. ENLARGED BLIND SPOT
    A. Optic Nerve Disease
        1. Papilledema and Big Blind Spot syndrome
        2. Drusen of the optic nerve head
        3. Congenital optic nerve lesion (coloboma, staphyloma)
        4. Optic neuritis
    B. Retinal Disease
        1. Multiple evanescent white dot syndrome (MEWDS)
        2. Acute zonal occult outer retinopathy (AZOOR)
    C. High Myopia
III. ARCUATE, ALTITUDINAL, NASAL STEP, NASAL DEPRESSION
    A. Optic Nerve Disease
        1. Glaucoma
        2. Papilledema
        3. Drusen of the optic nerve head
        4. Other optic neuropathies (AION, optic neuritis, etc)
    B. Branch Artery Occlusion
IV. CROSSES THE VERTICAL AND HORIZONTAL MERIDIANS
    A. Retinal Disease
        1. Ring scotomas, peripheral depression, "scalloped" field loss
    B. Optic Neuropathy
        1. Generalized depression, sparing of central vision
    C. Fatigue, Poor Testing Ability
        1. Fatigue in conjunction with visual pathology
    D. Malingering
        1. Peripheral depression, square visual fields, spiraling or crossed isopters, inconsistent patterns of loss
V. CENTRAL OR CENTROCECAL DEFECTS
    A. Maculopathy (visual acuity often more affected than visual field)
    B. Optic Neuropathies of All Types
VI. BITEMPORAL DEFECTS
    A. Superior Bitemporal Defects (Pituitary Adenoma)
    B. Inferior Bitemporal Defects (Craniopharyrngioma, Hypothalamic Tumor)
VII. HOMONYMOUS HEMIANOPIA
    A. Complete Homonymous Hemianopia
        1. Retrochiasmal defect with no further localizing value
    B. Tongue- or Keyhole-Shaped Homonymous Defect, or Remaining Visual Field
        1. Lateral geniculate lesion
    C. Incongruous Homonymous Hemianopia (Anterior Optic Tract, Radiations)
        1. Optic tract
        2. Temporal lobe ("pie in the sky" defect)
        3. Parietal lobe ("pie on the floor" defect)
    D. Highly Congruous Homonymous Hemianopia
        1. Occipital lobe lesion
            a. "Cookie cutter" punched-out lesion
            b. Macular sparing
            c. Temporal crescent
            d. Static-kinetic dissociation

eyes) or incongruous (i.e., more extensive visual field loss in one eye than in the other)? Do the edges of the defect have a steep or a gradual sloping profile? These and other specific features of the visual field should provide confirmatory information for the location of the damage determined by step 4 or allow one to differentiate among several possible alternative locations. However, it should not be used as the initial basis for generating a hypothesis about location of damage. Attention to specific features of the visual field before getting a global view of the visual field from step 4 may lead to misinterpretation of visual field information.

The approach to visual field interpretation outlined above is not intended to cover all possible scenarios but rather is meant as a guide to identify most typical kinds of visual field deficits and to avoid many of the common pitfalls in the misinterpretation of visual field information. If there is doubt about the validity of visual field results, the test should be repeated when the patient is well rested. Pathologic visual field changes usually are replicable, whereas nonpathologic visual field changes typically are not. If there is concern about fatigue affecting visual field results, a shorter test procedure (24-2 instead of 30-2, Fastpak instead of Full Threshold, etc.) should be employed.

When evaluating visual field results, it is important for the examiner to realize that it is only one of the many pieces of information needed to establish a diagnosis. The generalizations derived from the five-step approach are helpful, but there is considerable overlap in patterns of visual field loss associated with different disease entities. The rest of the afferent system evaluation needs to be considered in conjunction with the visual field results in order to establish a final differential diagnosis.

Additional Perimetry Tests

In order to improve sensitivity of visual field testing, several test procedures have been modified for use in perimetry. Although the tests vary widely in terms of the visual functions they measure, they have a common objective: by creating a unique stimulus display, these tests attempt to isolate (or strongly bias) threshold responses to be mediated by a specific subpopulation of neu-

ral mechanisms, instead of the wide range of neural mechanisms stimulated by conventional perimetry.

These test procedures have several theoretical advantages. First, because the tests are designed to target specific visual mechanisms, their response properties bear a strong linkage to the underlying physiology and anatomy of the visual pathways. Second, if certain diseases cause selectively greater amounts of damage to some visual mechanisms than others, these procedures may detect early losses or changes in visual function that may not otherwise be detected with conventional perimetry. Finally, because these test procedures are designed to isolate specific subpopulations of neural mechanisms, they eliminate much of the redundancy and overlap that is normally present in the visual pathways. By reducing this redundancy, it becomes easier to detect early, subtle losses or changes in visual function, even if these losses are not selective.

Perimetry tests that appear to have great potential for clinical utility in neuro-ophthalmologic diagnosis include Short Wavelength Automated Perimetry (SWAP), High-Pass Resolution Perimetry (HRP), Flicker Perimetry, Motion and Displacement Perimetry, and Frequency Doubling Perimetry.

COLOR VISION
Normal Color Vision Mechanisms

There are two different theories concerning the mechanisms underlying normal color vision. The trichromatic theory of color vision is that there are three different receptors that are maximally sensitive to wavelengths in different regions of the visual spectrum, with sensitivity peaks at short (blue), middle (green), and long (red) wavelengths, respectively. Although maximally sensitive to a specific part of the spectrum, each of these receptor types are proposed to have some degree of sensitivity to wavelengths throughout most of the visual spectrum. An efficient means of uniquely signaling thousands of different colors should therefore be achieved by examining the ratio of excitation of the three receptors.

An alternate view of color vision, the opponent-process theory, is that there are two chromatic mechanisms (red-green and blue-yellow) and one achromatic mechanism (black-white) that pair sensations in an opposing or antagonistic manner. The opponent-process theory is proposed as a means of accounting for six distinct color sensations (blue, green, yellow, red, black, and white).

Abundant psychophysical and physiologic evidence supports both theories. Initially, visual stimuli are processed by three types of cone photoreceptors, one with peak sensitivity in the short-wavelength region (approximately 440 nm), one with peak sensitivity in the middle-wavelength region (approximately 530 to 540 nm), and one with peak sensitivity in the long-wavelength region (approximately 560 to 580 nm), in accordance with the trichromatic theory. The output from the three cone photoreceptors is then transmitted to neurons in the inner retina that process information according to two opponent chromatic mechanisms (yellow-blue and red-green) and one achromatic mechanism, in accordance with the opponent-process theory. Although there is additional spatial and temporal processing of this information at different levels of the visual pathways, this opponent coding of chromatic information is carried through to the higher visual centers. The processing of color information is conducted by parvocellular mechanisms (see Chapter 13).

Clinical Tests of Color Vision

A wide variety of color vision tests are available to the clinician. Because most of them were designed to evaluate congenital red-green color vision deficiencies, many do not permit adequate testing of blue-yellow deficits or optimum characterization of acquired color vision losses.

As with any test of visual function, it is important that the testing conditions be standardized and performed in the proper manner. Each of the clinically available color vision tests comes with a set of detailed instructions for administering the test and interpreting the results. These instructions should be followed judiciously, because erroneous results can sometimes be obtained if the tests are not properly administered. A particularly important factor for all clinical color vision test procedures is the use of proper lighting, both in terms of having an adequate amount of light for the test and having a light source with the proper spectral distribution.

Pseudoisochromatic Plates

Pseudoisochromatic plates are the most common color vision tests employed in clinical practice. A number of pseudoisochromatic plate tests

are available, although the Ishihara, Hardy-Rand-Rittler, and Dvorine plates are probably the most commonly used versions. Each of these tests consists of a series of plates that contain colored dots of varying size and brightness. The tests are designed so that persons with normal color vision see numbers, shapes, or letters as a consequence of grouping certain colored dots together to form a figure against the background of other dots. Depending on how the particular test is designed, persons with color deficiencies are either unable to see the figure because the figure dots are confused with the background dots, or they see a figure different from that seen by persons with normal color vision because figure dots and background dots are grouped together in an abnormal pattern. The variation in size and brightness of the dots is used to ensure that recognition of figures is made on the basis of color discrimination and not other cues. Other variations of pseudoisochromatic plates include winding paths of colored dots that the patient can trace. These are useful in young children, illiterates, and some neurologically ill patients who are unable to identify letters, numbers, or shapes.

The main advantage of color vision tests using pseudoisochromatic plates is that they are quick and easy to perform and are therefore an excellent screening procedure for distinguishing normal color vision from any type of color vision abnormality. The disadvantages of pseudoisochromatic plate tests are that they have rather limited ability to classify acquired color vision deficits and to determine their severity, and that they have little or no ability (depending on the particular test) to test for either congenital or acquired blue-yellow color vision deficits.

Farnsworth Panel D-15 Test

The Farnsworth Panel D-15 test is a color arrangement test consisting of 15 color caps that form a color circle covering the visual spectrum. A reference cap is permanently fixed in the arrangement tray; the other 15 caps are placed in a scrambled order in front of the patient. The patient's task is to select the cap that is closest in hue to the reference cap and place it next to the reference cap in the tray. The patient is then asked to continue to place the caps in the tray, one at a time, so that they are arranged in an orderly transition of hue. Once all the caps are in the tray, the patient has an opportunity to make final changes in the order of caps. The caps are designed so that persons with normal color vision or very mild color vision deficits (e.g., mild anomalous trichromacy) will arrange the caps in a perfect color circle. Patients with moderate to severe protan, deutan, or tritan color vision deficits will confuse colors across the color circle, so that the arrangement contains misplaced caps. On the back of each cap is a number to assist in scoring the test. By turning the tray over, the number sequence can be determined. On the D-15 scoring chart, the caps along the color circle are connected in a dot-to-dot fashion in the order represented in the tray, and

the specific arrangement indicates the type of color deficiency. The Panel D-15 test does not indicate the degree of color deficiency, other than to separate color normals and mild anomalous trichromats from those with moderate to severe color vision deficiencies.

Farnsworth-Munsell 100 Hues Test

The Farnsworth-Munsell 100 Hues test permits both classification of the type of color vision deficiency and its severity. Despite its name, it consists of **85** colored caps that are arranged in roughly equal small steps around the color circle. The caps are divided into four

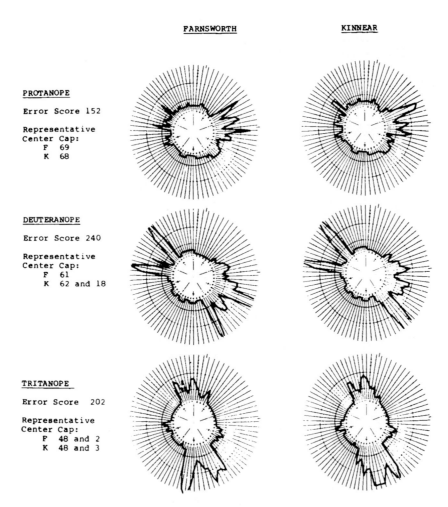

Figure 1.31. Examples of tritan (blue), protan (red), and deutan (green) color vision deficiencies as determined by the Farnsworth-Munsell 100 Hues Test. *Left:* The figures depict the results scored according to the method originally described by Farnsworth. *Right:* The figures depict a modified scoring system. (Reprinted with permission from Kinnear PR. Proposals for scoring and assessing the 100-hue test. Vision Res 1970;10:423–433.)

boxes, and arrangements of caps are performed one box at a time. In each box, there are two reference caps, one at each end, that are permanently attached to the box. The other caps are taken out of the box, scrambled, and placed before the patient. The patient is then asked to arrange the caps so that there is an orderly transition in hue from one reference cap to another. As with the panel D-15 test, the Farnsworth-Munsell 100 Hues test is designed so that certain caps across the color circle will be confused by persons with both congenital and acquired color deficiencies. The caps are numbered on the back, and scoring is determined by the arrangement of the caps in the box. Depending on the type of color deficiency, specific caps across the color circle will be confused, resulting in greater arrangement errors in those locations. In this manner, the type of color vision deficit can be classified (Fig. 1.31).

In addition to classification of the color deficiency, its severity can be quantified by determining an overall error score for arrangement errors. Thus, it is possible to quantify the degree of color vision deficiency and monitor progression and remission of acquired color losses. Normative values for different age groups are also available for the Farnsworth-Munsell 100 Hues test. There is evidence that certain types of optic neuropathies, including optic neuritis, can be diagnosed reliably using only 21 of the 85 chips (chips 22–42) in the set.

General Principles of Color Testing

From a clinical diagnostic standpoint, it is important to distinguish if a color vision deficiency is congenital or acquired (Table 1.4). Congenital color vision deficits are usually easy to classify using standard clinical color vision tests because color discrimination is usually impaired for a specific region of the visual spectrum, and the deficits are long-standing, stable, symmetric in the two eyes, and unassociated with other visual symptoms or complaints. In patients with acquired color vision loss, however, color discrimination may be impaired throughout the visual spectrum or along a specific axis, and the deficits may be mild or severe, of sudden onset, asymmetric, and often associated with other visual symptoms or complaints. In acquired color vision deficiencies, tritan (blue) and blue-yellow deficiencies are most commonly associated with diseases affecting the photoreceptors and the outer plexiform layer, whereas red-green deficiencies are most commonly associated with diseases affecting the optic nerve and posterior visual pathways. Some notable exceptions include glaucoma, dominant hereditary optic atrophy, and chronic papilledema, which demonstrate blue-yellow deficits, and Stargardt's and Best's disease, which produce red-green deficits (Table 1.5). Optic neuritis produces a mixture of red-green and blue-yellow deficits, although one axis is usually more affected than the other.

Table 1.4
Differences Between Congenital and Acquired Color Defects

CONGENITAL	ACQUIRED
Usually color vision loss in specific spectral regions.	Often no specific spectral region of color discrimination loss.
Less marked dependence of color vision on target size and illuminance.	Marked dependence of color vision on target size and illuminance.
Characteristic results obtained on various clinical color vision tests.	Conflicting or variable results may be obtained on various clinical color vision tests.
Many object colors are named correctly, or predictable errors are made.	Some object colors are named incorrectly.
Both eyes are usually affected to the same degree.	The two eyes are often affected to different degrees.
Usually there is no other visual complaint or problems.	Often there are additional visual complaints, reduced visual acuity or visual field loss.
The deficit does not change appreciably over time.	The defect may show clear progression or remission of color discrimination loss.
Are almost always red/green deficits and are mostly found in males.	Are often blue or blue-yellow deficits.

Adapted from Pokorny J, Smith VC, Verriest G, et al. Congenital and Acquired Color Vision Defects. New York, Grune and Stratton, 1979.

Table 1.5
**Acquired Color Vision Deficits Associated with Eye
Disease**

CONDITION	COLOR VISION DEFECT
Glaucoma	B-Y
Retinal Detachment	B-Y
Pigmentary Degeneration of Retina (including RP)	B-Y
Age-Related Macular Degeneration	B-Y
Myopic Retinal Degeneration	B-Y
Chorioretinitis	B-Y
Retinal Vascular Occlusion	B-Y
Diabetic Retinopathy	B-Y
Hypertensive Retinopathy	B-Y
Papilledema	B-Y
Methyl Alcohol Poisoning	B-Y
Dominant Hereditary Optic Atrophy	B-Y
Central Serous Retinopathy	B-Y
Tobacco-Alcohol (ETOH) or Toxic Amblyopia	R-G
Leber's Optic Atrophy	R-G
Lesions of the optic nerve and posterior pathways	R-G
Papillitis	R-G
Stargardt's Disease	R-G
Best's Disease	R-G
Juvenile Macular Degeneration	R-G or B-Y
Optic Neuritis	R-G or B-Y

Adapted from Adams AJ, Verdon WA, Spivey BE. Color vision.
In: Tasman W, Jaeger EA, eds. Duane's Foundations of Clinical
Ophthalmology. Lippincott: Philadelphia, 1996;1:1–43.

Investigations of acquired color vision losses
in retinal and optic nerve disease, using specialized laboratory techniques, suggest that although
many optic nerve and retinal diseases affect
more than just a single opponent pathway, the
magnitude of loss in such disorders is often
greater in one of the opponent channels than in
any of the others. Cerebral dyschromatopsias are
uncommon, but result in severe color vision loss,
sometimes producing a total achromatopsia (vision in black and white only).

It should be emphasized that **color comparison tests**, although only qualitative in nature,
can provide valuable information concerning
subtle visual anomalies. Using pages from the
pseudoisochromatic plates, colored bottle caps,
or other brightly colored objects, comparisons
of color appearance can be very effective in detecting subtle differences between the two eyes.

The brightness or saturation of the colored objects may be less in one eye, making the object's
color appear dim or washed out. Similarly, comparisons within the same eye across the vertical
and horizontal midline or between central vision
and the mid-periphery can detect subtle differences in color appearance that are indicative of
an early visual disturbance.

DARK ADAPTATION

Dark adaptation refers to the change in visual
sensitivity that occurs over time for an observer
in a dark environment. Everyone is familiar with
the problem of entering a dark room, auditorium,
or theater from outside on a bright sunny day.
At first, visual sensitivity in the dark is poor,
and it is difficult to see objects or other people.
After 10 to 20 minutes, however, visual sensitivity recovers, and both objects and people can be
seen more clearly.

Clinically, dark adaptation is usually measured with a perimeter or similar instrument. The
Goldmann-Weekers dark adaptometer is a commercially available device that is also used for
clinical measurement of dark adaptation. As
with perimetry, one eye at a time is tested, with
the fellow eye occluded with an eye patch. The
patient's pupils are usually dilated with mydriatics to minimize the variation in dark adaptation
produced by differences in pupil size. The dark
adaptation test is initiated by pre-adapting the
patient to a fixed background luminance level
(usually a bright photopic light level) for a specific period of time, usually several minutes. The
background luminance is then extinguished, and
the threshold luminance necessary to detect a
flashing target is determined repeatedly over the
next 30 minutes.

The normal dark adaptation curve is produced
by plotting detection threshold (the inverse of
sensitivity) as a function of time. Normal subjects show a rapid decrease in threshold (increase in sensitivity) over the first 2 to 3 minutes
of dark adaptation, followed by a period of time
during which the detection threshold is stable.
This portion of the dark adaptation curve reflects
the recovery in sensitivity of the photopic (cone)
system. In normal eyes, complete recovery of
photopic sensitivity is achieved within about 5
to 7 minutes. Following this period of stable
threshold, there is another decrease in threshold
that occurs after about 7 to 9 minutes of dark
adaptation until full recovery of sensitivity is

achieved after about 25 to 30 minutes. This portion of the curve reflects the recovery of the scotopic (rod) system once its sensitivity surpasses that of the photopic system. The transition from the photopic portion of the curve to the scotopic portion of the curve is called the "rod-cone break." In the fovea, where no rods are present, only the photopic portion of the dark adaptation curve is obtained. In normal eyes, any nonfoveal location should reveal both the photopic and scotopic portions of the dark adaptation curve.

A number of variables affect the rate of dark adaptation and the shape of the dark adaptation curve, including the intensity and duration of the pre-adapting light, pupil size, ocular media absorption, the size of the target, the spectral composition of the stimulus, the duration of the target, and the visual field location tested. Because of the variation introduced by these different parameters, it is important to establish normal standards for different age groups for the particular dark adaptation test procedures being used.

Clinically, the dark adaptation curve is useful for evaluating the function of photopic and scotopic mechanisms in localized regions. Important features include the presence or absence of the rod and cone portions of the dark adaptation curve, the final threshold levels for the rod and cone portions of the curve, the time at which the rod-cone break occurs, and the rate of sensitivity recovery for the rod and cone portions of the curve.

In many instances, dark adaptation provides a visual function measure that simply confirms the results obtained using standard electroretinography. Some patients, however, demonstrate normal ERG findings even though they have localized abnormalities restricted to a small region of the retina. Because dark adaptation stimuli can be placed at any location in the visual field, dark adaptation measures can be obtained for small localized areas to identify rod and cone dysfunction that may not be apparent for standard ERG measures. Dark adaptation can also be useful in confirming patient complaints of night vision problems.

ELECTROPHYSIOLOGIC TESTS

Frequently, the physician is confronted with a patient who has unexplained loss of vision associated with a normal-appearing ocular fundus. Because electrophysiologic testing often provides diagnostic clues as to the etiology of the

Table 1.6

Isolation of Components of the Afferent Visual Pathways Using Electrophysiology

ANATOMICAL STRUCTURE	TECHNIQUE
Retinal pigment epithelium	Electro-oculogram (EOG)
	Electro-retinogram (Flash ERG) c-wave
Photoreceptors	
Rods	Rod-flash ERG (scotopic) a-wave
Cones	Cone-flash ERG (photopic) a-wave
	30 Hz Flicker ERG
Middle retinal layers	Scotopic Threshold Response (STR)
	Flash ERG b-wave
	Oscillatory Potentials
	Pattern ERG (P50)
Ganglion cell layer	Pattern ERG (N95)
Macula or other local region	Focal ERG
	30 Hz Flicker ERG
Optic tract, radiations and cortex	VEP

Reprinted with permission from Weisinger HS, Vingrys AJ, Sinclair AJ, et al. Electrodiagnostic methods in vision. I. Clinical application and measurement. Clin Exp Optom 1996;79:50–61.

unexplained visual loss, it should be part of the neuro-ophthalmologic examination in selected patients. Electrophysiology provides a relatively objective method for evaluating the function of the visual system from the retina to the visual cortex. Several electrodiagnostic methods can be used to evaluate the status of individual components of the afferent visual pathways (Table 1.6).

ELECTRORETINOGRAM

Components of the Electroretinogram

The alteration in the electric potential that occurs when light falls on the retina determines the **electroretinogram** (ERG). There are three main components of the ERG: 1) an early cornea-negative "a-wave," 2) a cornea-positive "b-wave," and 3) a slower, usually cornea-positive "c-wave." The photoreceptors are responsible for the generation of the leading edge of the a-wave. The cellular origin of the b-wave is a combination of cells in the Müller and bipolar cell layers. The retinal pigment epithelium must be present to generate the c-wave, but the photoreceptors also contribute to this part of the ERG.

The rod and cone components of the ERG may be separated on the basis of their respective spectral sensitivities by altering the retinal state of adaptation or by using different flicker rates for the stimulus. Although the rods are more sensitive than the cones across most of the visible spectrum, this difference decreases with increasing wavelength so that it is possible to isolate a cone response if the stimulus wavelength is greater than 680 nm. The rod contribution to the ERG can be separated by recording from a dark-adapted subject and stimulating with a short-wavelength or long-wavelength light that has been scotopically matched for their luminances.

ERGs are often described as having photopic (light-adapted) and scotopic (dark-adapted) responses. ERG waveforms obtained from relatively intense white stimuli usually represent contributions from both the rod and cone systems (mixed response), whereas scotopic ERGs to relatively dim blue light can be generated by the rods alone. Photopic ERGs obtained on an adapting background represent responses from the cone system. The wavelength, intensity, and temporal properties of the stimulus, as well as the state of retinal adaptation are all important

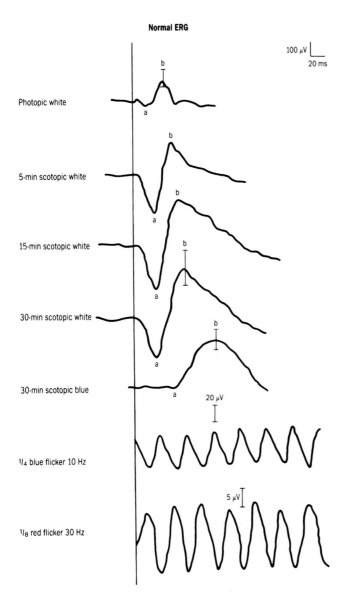

Normal ERG

100 μV
20 ms

Photopic white

5-min scotopic white

15-min scotopic white

30-min scotopic white

30-min scotopic blue

20 μV

¹/₄ blue flicker 10 Hz

5 μV

¹/₈ red flicker 30 Hz

Figure 1.32. Normal electroretinographic response under photopic and scotopic conditions. Cone responses are generally isolated using photopic adaptation conditions and 30 Hz flicker. Rod responses are isolated after 30 minutes of dark adaptation with a low luminance short-wavelength stimulus either as a single flash or with 10 Hz flicker. A dark-adapted scotopic white flash measures a combined rod-cone response. (Reprinted with permission from Fishman GA, Sokol S. Electrophysiologic Testing in Disorders of the Retina, Optic Nerve, and Visual Pathway. San Francisco: American Academy of Ophthalmology, 1990.)

in separating rod and cone system contributions. International standards for ERG testing should be followed.

By stimulating the eye in the presence of a background light sufficient to eliminate the rod response, it is possible to obtain a reasonably isolated cone response (Fig. 1.32). The cone and rod ERG responses have temporal aspects that are dependent on stimulus intensity and state of retinal adaptation. Dim, short-wavelength light elicits slow, small responses from the rod system, and more intense light stimuli result in faster and larger responses. Flickering stimuli presented at 25 to 30 flashes per second (25 to 30 Hz) isolate cone responses. The ERG elicited with a white stimulus of high luminance after 30 minutes of dark adaptation has both rod and cone components. The major contributor to both the increased amplitude and implicit time is the rod component. However, an isolated rod response can be evoked by a low-intensity short-wavelength (blue) stimulus.

In normal persons, low-amplitude, rapid oscillations are superimposed on the ascending limb of the b-wave. These are called the **oscillatory potentials** (OPs). Bandpass filtering over 70 to 300 Hz will extract these oscillations from the underlying a- and b-waves, and they can then be quantified by giving their summed and rectified amplitudes. OPs are thought to reflect activity in the inner retinal layers. They are of clinical importance because they are often absent in patients with diabetic retinopathy and other diseases that are associated with ischemia of the inner retina.

The ERG is described by the temporal characteristics and amplitudes of the recorded waveform (Fig. 1.33). The temporal aspects of the waveform can be described by the latency and implicit times. Latency refers to the time between stimulus onset and response onset, whereas implicit time refers to the time needed for the response to reach maximum amplitude. Waveform amplitudes are measured from the baseline (which is usual for the a-wave) or as a peak-to-peak comparison (which is usual for the b-wave). The b/a wave ratio can be used as an index of inner to outer retinal function.

Testing Conditions and Interpretation

One of the major advances in ERG technology was the development of a low-impedance, user-friendly electrode. The Burian-Allen electrode

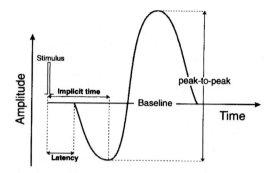

Figure 1.33. Amplitude, latency, and implicit time measurements for the standard single-flash electroretinogram. (Reprinted with permission from Weisinger HS, Vingrys AJ, Sinclair AJ, et al. Electrodiagnostic methods in vision. I. Clinical application and measurement. Clin Exp Optom 1996;79:50–61.)

contains a silver annulus implanted into a plastic (hard) contact lens that is placed on a topically anesthetized cornea. The contact lens is insulated and kept separate from a lid speculum that is used to keep the eyelids open during testing. The speculum is impregnated with silver granules. It thus serves as an inactive electrode, permitting a difference potential to be measured. This is called a bipolar electrode.

The ERG procedure is performed as follows: a drop of topical anesthetic is placed on the patient's cornea, and the contact lens is placed on the anesthetized cornea after 30 minutes of dark adaptation. The patient places the head on a chin rest located at the opening of a Ganzfeld dome, similar to the bowl of a projection perimeter. By using a Faraday cage (a grounded copper enclosure that surrounds the patient and the Ganzfeld dome), it is possible to reduce extraneous levels of electric noise. All recording equipment should be placed outside this enclosure. Rod or cone function is evaluated using a brief (10-microsecond) flash presented at 1-minute intervals. It is recommended that at least 2 to 4 signals be averaged to insure repeatability of the output. Sequential testing of the rods and the cones is then performed according to specific guidelines (see Fig. 1.32).

The ERG can be affected by a number of additional factors. The implicit time of the waveform does not mature until 4 to 6 months of age, and the amplitude may be reduced until 1 year of age. The ERG may be greater in women than in

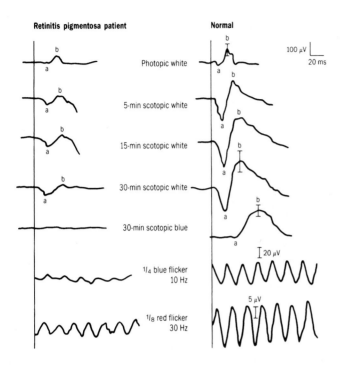

Figure 1.34. An example of electroretinogram (ERG) recordings from a patient with autosomal-dominant retinitis pigmentosa (*left*) compared with normal ERG responses (*right*). (Reprinted with permission from Fishman GA, Sokol S. Electrophysiologic Testing in Disorders of the Retina, Optic Nerve, and Visual Pathway. San Francisco: American Academy of Ophthalmology, 1990.)

men and may be reduced in myopes with more than 6 diopters of refractive error. There may be as much as a 13% reduction in ERG amplitude in the morning, which corresponds to the time of the maximum photoreceptor disk shedding. Systemic drugs and anesthetics may also alter the ERG.

An ERG can provide important information about a number of retinal disorders that may simulate neuro-ophthalmologic problems. These include congenital stationary night blindness, congenital achromatopsia, retinitis pigmentosa (rod-cone dystrophy), retinitis pigmentosa sine pigmenta, cone-rod dystrophy, cone dystrophy, cancer-associated retinopathy (CAR), melanoma-associated retinopathy (MAR), and toxic retinopathies (Figs. 1.34 and 1.35).

The ERG is often helpful in establishing a diagnosis in children with nystagmus or unexplained visual loss. ERGs can be performed on infants without sedation if the infant is sleepy and is given a bottle. In addition, conjunctival electrodes made of thin microfibers (Dawson-Trick-Litzkow electrodes) can be used in children of almost any age. Depending on the procedures employed, however, different laboratories may obtain widely differing results for infants and young children. Thus, it is important that

each laboratory establish normal ERG standards for infants and young children in order to properly interpret the results. When analyzing ERG results for an infant, caution must be exercised. The ERG b-wave amplitude only becomes equivalent to that of adults at 5 to 6 months of age, and some authors believe that b-wave amplitudes do not reach adult levels until 1 year of age.

Focal Electroretinogram

The human ERG recorded at the cornea in response to a full-field stimulus is a mass response generated by cells across the entire retina. Loss of half the retinal photoreceptors across the retina is associated with about a 50% reduction in ERG amplitude. Because the total cone population in the human retina is approximately 7 million, and the number of cones in the macula is at most 440,000, the macula contains only about 7% of the total retinal cone population. The full-field ERG system is thus unable to detect abnormalities confined to the foveola, fovea, or macula, because these structures contribute only about 7% to the total signal. Moreover, recording a foveal or macular ERG using conventional full-field equipment is prevented by the scattered light produced by a focal light

Figure 1.35. Electroretinogram (ERG) recordings from a patient with congenital achromatopsia (*left*) compared with normal ERG responses (*right*). (Reprinted with permission from Fishman GA, Sokol S. Electrophysiologic Testing in Disorders of the Retina, Optic Nerve, and Visual Pathway. San Francisco: American Academy of Ophthalmology, 1990.)

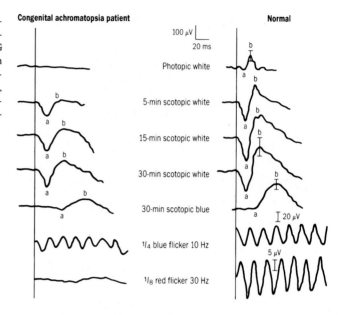

stimulus that evokes a response from many receptors outside of the tested area. The foveal or macular ERG, therefore, cannot be identified in isolation under these conditions. Light is also scattered by the choroid and by small heterogeneities of the ocular media. Indeed, light focused on the optic disc can elicit an ERG response that is equivalent to that derived from stimulation of an adjacent region of functional retina. In addition, the macula contains as many rods as cones, and the macular rod response may obscure the contribution from the macular cones. It thus is apparent that any test that attempts to isolate macular cone responses must consider the reduced response compared with full-field stimulation, stray light artifacts, and perifoveal rod responses.

Focal ERGs that measure macular function can be exceptionally helpful in a neuro-ophthalmologic practice. In our experience, patients with visual loss are frequently referred to the neuro-ophthalmologist by a retinal specialist or general ophthalmologist who can find no abnormalities of the macula or fovea on funduscopic examination or fluorescein angiography. The visual field frequently shows only a mild to modest reduction in foveal threshold or depression in the central field. Because of this, the referring ophthalmologist may suspect that the visual loss is caused by an optic neuropathy or that the patient has nonorganic visual loss. In these

cases, a focal ERG using a hand-held device (sometimes called a "maculoscope") that generates a repetitive, small, focused beam of light can be used to distinguish subtle macular dysfunction from optic neuropathies and nonorganic visual loss.

Pattern Electroretinogram

The **pattern electroretinogram** (PERG) is produced by a phase-reversing patterned stimulus that maintains a constant overall mean luminance. The stimulus may be an alternating pattern of light and dark regions, such as a checkerboard or bar grating generated on a television monitor. When the pattern reverses (light regions become dark and vice versa) once or twice per second, an isolated response is obtained; when faster reversal rates are used (>9 Hz), a steady-state signal is generated.

The isolated PERG has three major components that are reliably used to define it. The first is a negative lobe found at about 30 msec (called N1 or N30). This is followed by a positive lobe at about 50 msec (called P1 or P50) and a second negative lobe at about 95 msec (called N2 or N95). In normal eyes, the P1 occurs between 48 and 55 msec, and the N2 occurs between 87 and 100 msec. Normal persons have exquisite symmetry in the waveforms between the two eyes, and amplitude ratios are typically 0.8 to 0.9 in each eye. It is believed that the N2 reflects ganglion cell activity, whereas the P1 reflects outer retinal function. The PERG is abnormal in a variety of retinal and optic nerve disorders.

Multifocal (Topographical) Electroretinogram

A technique is available for simultaneously recording ERG signals from a large number of retinal locations (up to 256). This **topographical ERG** is able to detect localized abnormalities in a variety of retinal diseases, including age-related macular degeneration, macular holes, retinitis pigmentosa, branch retinal artery occlusion, and other retinal conditions. It thus would seem to be a potential alternative to focal electroretinography. The efficacy of this procedure in clinical practice has yet to be determined.

ELECTRO-OCULOGRAM

The human eye acts as a dipole, with the cornea positive with respect to the retina. If two electrodes are placed near the inner and outer canthi, respectively, movement of the eye will produce a change in the potential measured between the two electrodes, with the electrode closest to the cornea being more positive. A recording of this potential change produced by movement of the eye is called the **electro-oculogram** (EOG). The EOG consists of two different potentials, one that is sensitive to light and the other that is insensitive to light.

For typical recording, the EOG is measured under conditions of dark adaptation after previous exposure to a pre-adapting illumination. The patient is asked to make saccades every second between two stimuli (usually light-emitting diodes) that are spaced about 30° apart and alternately illuminated. These saccadic eye movements produce the change in potential that comprises the EOG signal, with the average of several saccades being taken as the potential at that time. The light-insensitive potential (also called the standing potential) decreases slightly over a period of 8 to 9 minutes, at which time the lowest potential recorded in the dark-adapted state can be measured (the dark trough). Following reexposure to light, the potential gradually increases and reaches its peak in another 10 to 15 minutes (the light peak). The amplitude of the light peak is approximately twice that of the dark trough (light rise of the EOG) in normal persons. Because the standing potential can vary considerably, in part related to the placement of the electrodes, the EOG is most appropriately represented as a ratio of the light peak to the dark trough. This ratio is called the **Arden ratio** and is typically greater than 1.8 in normal persons. The International Society for Clinical Electrophysiology of Vision (ISCEV) has established standards for EOG testing.

The results of clinical studies indicate that the retinal pigment epithelium is probably responsible for generating the EOG. The light-sensitive, large, slow, cornea-positive component must depend upon the activity of the photoreceptors and on cells in the inner nuclear layers of the retina, because it is induced by light and eliminated by central retinal artery occlusion. Based on studies of the action spectrum of the EOG in both dark-adapted and light-adapted states, as well as the observation that human subjects without rod function may have a large, light-rise response, this response is thought to represent both rod and cone activity. The light-insensitive potential of the EOG provides a way to measure the function of the pigment epithelium without having to stimulate the photoreceptors. The EOG probably should not be used in patients with poor fixation because their poor ability to make accurate saccades can affect the results of the test.

The EOG has limited usefulness in the diagnosis of visual dysfunction. When the EOG is abnormal, the ERG is also usually abnormal. There are four exceptions, however, in which patients may have a normal or nearly normal ERG with an abnormal EOG light-rise to dark-trough ratio. The conditions are 1) butterfly-shaped pigment dystrophy of the fovea, 2) Stargardt's disease (fundus flavimaculatus), 3) advanced drusen, and 4) vitelliform dystrophy or Best's disease. From a neuro-ophthalmologic standpoint, the EOG is more important for the recording and analysis of ocular motility than in diagnosing causes of visual loss.

VISUAL-EVOKED POTENTIAL

If the spontaneous occipital electroencephalogram (EEG) is recorded while brief flashes of light are presented to an eye, changes result in the occipital potential. These changes are called the **visual-evoked potential** (VEP), visual-evoked response (VER), or the visual-evoked cortical potential (VECP). The VEP is thus a gross electric potential of the visual cortex in response to visual stimulation. The VEP is lim-

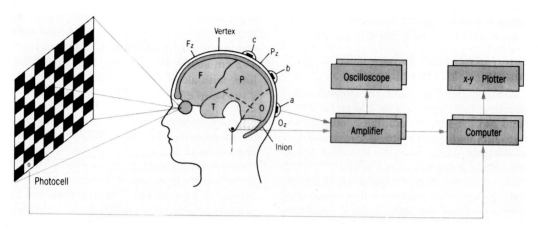

Figure 1.36. Method for generating and recording the visual-evoked potential. (Reprinted with permission from Fishman GA, Sokol S. Electrophysiologic Testing in Disorders of the Retina, Optic Nerve, and Visual Pathway. San Francisco: American Academy of Ophthalmology, 1990.)

ited mainly to the occipital region of the brain, with an amplitude between 1 and 20 microvolts.

The VEP depends on the integrity of the entire visual pathway, although it remains to be determined if its components can truly be separated into anatomic correlates. The precise origin and pathways through which the VEP is mediated are still in question. Nevertheless, the clinical importance of the VEP rests on its usefulness as a relatively objective determinant of the integrity of the visual pathways.

Methodology

The VEP is measured by placing scalp electrodes over the occipital region (O_z) of both hemispheres, with reference electrodes attached to the ear (Fig. 1.36). The patient then views the display, typically a xenon-arc photostimulator for flash VEPs and a television screen display with patterned stimuli for pattern VEPs. Recordings of the VEP may be made from either hemisphere with one or both eyes fixating. Typically, 100 to 150 stimulus presentations are generated, and time-locked signal averaging procedures are used to extract the VEP waveform from the spontaneous EEG activity. The amplitude and latency of the waveform are then measured. A flash stimulus is generally used only when no response is produced using a pattern stimulus. Thus, infants and patients with extremely poor acuity, dense media opacities, or poor fixation are most commonly tested with flash VEP.

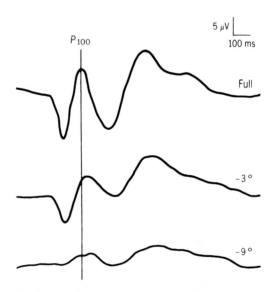

Figure 1.37. Visual-evoked potential waveforms. *Top:* From stimulation of the central 30° visual field. *Middle:* With the central 3° occluded. *Bottom:* With the central 9° occluded. Note that the majority of the waveform is subserved by the central 9° of the visual field. This is consistent with observations that the central 10° of the visual field are represented by at least 50 to 60% of the posterior striate cortex. (Reprinted with permission from Fishman GA, Sokol S. Electrophysiologic Testing in Disorders of the Retina, Optic Nerve, and Visual Pathway. San Francisco: American Academy of Ophthalmology, 1990.)

In most patients, however, a pattern stimulus is preferred for obtaining the VEP, because of the greater clinical utility and more reliable waveform generated with this stimulus. A repetitive pattern of light and dark areas (checkerboards, bar gratings) are phase-reversed every 1 or 2 seconds, similar to the previous description of PERG stimulation (Fig. 1.37 *top*). The pattern VEP is primarily generated from the central 5° of the visual field. Indeed, when the central 3° is occluded (Fig. 1.37 *middle*), there is a dramatic reduction in the amplitude of the pattern VEP, and the waveform almost completely disappears when the central 9° is occluded (Fig. 1.37 *bottom*). These findings are consistent with the anatomic correlates that the central 10° of the visual field is represented by at least 50 to 60% of the posterior striate cortex and that the central 30°

is represented by about 80% of the cortex (see Chapter 12).

The amplitude of the pattern VEP is affected by a number of different factors. The size of the stimulus pattern can affect the amplitude of the VEP signal, as can the rate of alternation of the pattern. At low rates of alternation (1 to 2 reversals per second), the waveform typically contains two negative (N1, N2) and two positive (P1, P2) potentials. This is called the "transient" pattern VEP and is the most commonly used procedure for routine clinical purposes. As the rate of alternation is increased (>6 reversals per second), the response is not able to fully recover between presentations, and only the initial portions of the waveform are observed, similar to the waveforms obtained for ERG with rapidly flickering stimuli. This is called the

Table 1.7
Visual-Evoked Potential Abnormalities

DISORDER	AMPLITUDE	LATENCY	MORPHOLOGY
Optic Nerve and Visual Pathway			
Optic neuritis	A/N	+ + +	N
Ischemic optic neuropathy	− −	+	A
Toxic amblyopia	−	N	A
Dominant optic atrophy	−	N/+	?
Leber's optic atrophy	− −	+	A
Optic nerve hypoplasia	− −	+	A
Glaucoma	N/−	N/−	N
Optic disc drusen	−	+	A
Papilledema	N/−	N/+	N/A
Tumors (anterior pathway)	−	+	A
Neurologic Disorders			
Multiple sclerosis	N/−	+ + +	N/A
Vitamin B_{12} deficiency	N	+	N
Congenital nystagmus	−	+	A
Parkinson's disease	N/−	N/+ +	N
Migraine	N	+	N/A
Down syndrome	−	N	?
Cortical blindness	N/−	N	N
Occipital lobe lesion	−	+	A
Huntington's chorea	−	N	A
Friedreich's ataxia	−	+ +	A
Hereditary spastic ataxia	N	N/+	N
Nonspecific rec. ataxia	N	N	N
Charcot-Marie-Tooth	?	+	N
Phenylketonuria	N	+	N

Reprinted with permission from Fishman GA, Sokol S. Electrophysiologic Testing in Disorders of the Retina, Optic Nerve, and Visual Pathway. San Francisco: American Academy of Ophthalmology, 1990.
N = Normal; A = Abnormal; ? = Information not available; +(−) = Mild increase (decrease); + + (− −) = Moderate increase (decrease); + + + (− − −) = Severe increase (decrease).

"steady-state" VEP. The latencies of the first major positive and negative components of the VEP become increasingly delayed with increasing age in adults. Latency of the response is indirectly related to stimulus intensity, but amplitude tends to reach maximum at only moderate stimulus intensities and varies with electrode placement, scalp thickness, and so on. Infants and young children have quite variable waveforms and prolonged latencies. The VEP also varies with stimulus size and frequency, attention, mental activity, pupil size, fatigue, state of dark adaptation, color of the stimulus, background illumination, and even the emotional content of the stimulus. All of these factors emphasize the importance of using standardized and optimized test conditions (including the best refractive correction) for clinical VEP testing, as well as establishing age-related normative standards for the procedures employed for each laboratory.

Analysis of the VEP waveform is rather complex. For transient pattern VEPs, the amplitude and latency of the N1, P1, and N2 components are typically measured (see Fig. 1.37). For steady-state VEPs, the amplitude and phase of the waveform are measured. The latencies of the pattern VEP are quite consistent both within and among observers, although the amplitudes vary considerably from one person to another. Therefore, the most useful clinical features of the VEP are the latency of its major components and a comparison of the symmetry of the amplitudes between eyes and between hemispheres in the same person.

The Visual-Evoked Potential in Clinical Ophthalmology and Neuro-Ophthalmology

The VEP represents sensory activity in the visual pathways, beginning at the retina and ending at the occipital cortex. A summary of the changes observed in VEP recordings from different visual disorders is provided in Table 1.7. The VEP can be useful in differentiating among retinal, optic nerve, and cortical diseases. It may also be helpful in determining if an infant or young child has intact vision and if a patient has nonorganic visual loss. In general, the VEP should be evaluated for latency, amplitude, waveform, and morphology. The latency and amplitude can be quantified, but waveform morphology is more of a subjective interpretation.

Although the clinical utility and differential diagnostic capabilities of the VEP are limited, there are numerous settings in which the VEP can be quite helpful. In conjunction with retinal electrophysiologic responses, in particular the ERG, the status of visual function from retina to cortex can be evaluated.

FOR FURTHER INFORMATION:
See Walsh & Hoyt's Clinical Neuro-Ophthalmology, 5th edition, Volume 1, Chapter 7, pages 153–235.

CHAPTER 2

Anatomy and Physiology of the Retina and Optic Nerve: Distinguishing Retinal from Optic Nerve Disease

Knowing the anatomy and physiology of the retina and optic nerve is crucial in understanding the similarities and differences in findings in patients with retinal versus optic nerve disease. In this chapter, we discuss these issues.

ANATOMY AND PHYSIOLOGY OF THE RETINA

The retina is a unique part of the nervous system because it can be visualized, allowing the clinician to observe directly the effects of a wide range of diseases such as an infarction in evolution, deposition of metabolic storage products, or slowing of axoplasmic flow. The retina is also a favorite tissue for study by neuroscientists because it is thin and can be easily dissected from the eye, because its cells are segregated into layers, and because there is at least a fundamental appreciation of its anatomic and physiologic organization.

The cellular structure of the retina is enor-mously complex. In humans, it contains over 100 million neurons, among which are about 30 different cell types that use at least 10 different neurotransmitters. Most architectural schemas under-represent the intricacy of the retina because the degree to which information is shared among various cells depends on a variety of factors, including the region of the retina being illuminated, the characteristics of the light stimulus, and the state of adaptation of the retina to light. Given this complexity, one might imagine that a large number of symptoms would result from dysfunction of these many cell types. On the contrary, most clinically recognized diseases of the retina are caused by dysfunction of either photoreceptors or retinal ganglion cells.

The human retina covers an area approximately 2500 mm^2 and extends from the ora serrata to the optic disc (Fig. 2.1). The retina contains six classes of neurons (photoreceptors, horizontal cells, bipolar cells, amacrine cells, interplexiform cells, and ganglion cells) and two

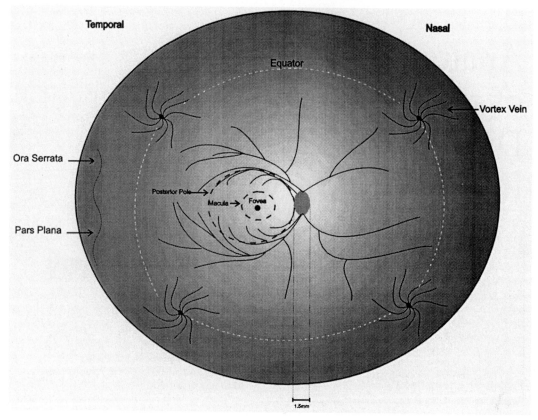

Figure 2.1.   Gross anatomy of the retina. Schematic diagram of overall structure of the retina as viewed by funduscopic examination. The width of the optic nerve is indicated at the bottom of the figure.

Table 2.1
Cellular Organization of the Retina

CELL LAYER	NEURONAL AND GLIAL NUCLEI
Outer nuclear layer	Photoreceptors
Inner nuclear layer	Horizontal cells
	Bipolar cells
	Interplexiform cells
	Amacrine cells
	Müller cells
Ganglion cell layer	Ganglion cells
	Displaced amacrine cells
	Astrocytes

types of glial cells (astrocytes and Müller cells) that are arranged into three parallel layers, except in the perifoveal zone, where the retina thins to a single layer (Table 2.1; Figs. 2.2 and 2.3). The human retina is roughly 120 μm thick over most of its area, with a maximum thickness of 230 μm in the macula and a minimum thickness of 100 μm in the foveal pit.

CELL TYPES AND LAYERS OF THE RETINA

The **retinal pigment epithelium** (RPE) is a monolayer of cells derived from the outer wall of the optic vesicle that is intimately associated with the outer segments of the photoreceptors (Fig. 2.4). The RPE is responsible for several essential functions, most significantly,

1. It is integrally involved in the phototransduction cascade through regeneration of chromophore.
2. It participates in renewal of the proteins and membrane components that are necessary for the health of the photoreceptors.

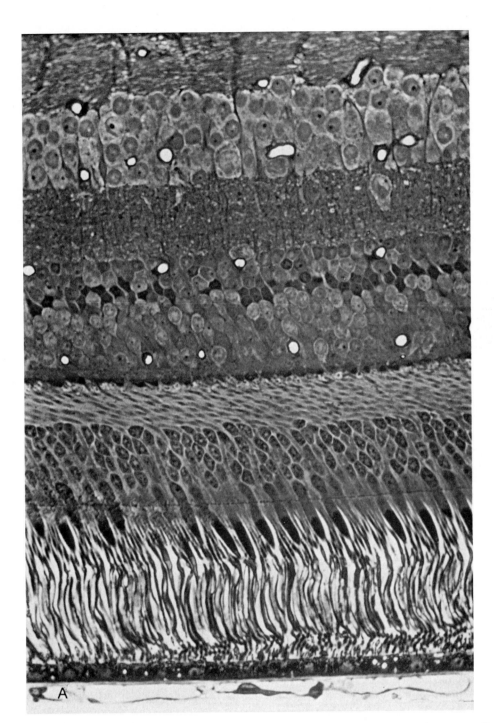

Figure 2.2. The cellular components of the primate retina. *A:* Photomicrograph. *B:* Schematic drawing showing cellular relationships and synapses. *OPL,* outer plexiform layer; *ONL,* outer nuclear layer; *ELM,* external limiting membrane; *IS,* inner segment; *OS,* outer segment; *As,* astrocyte; *G,* ganglion cell; *Am,* amacrine cell; *I,* interplexiform cell; *H,* horizontal cell; *B,* bipolar cell; *C,* cone; *R,* rod; *M,* Müller cell.

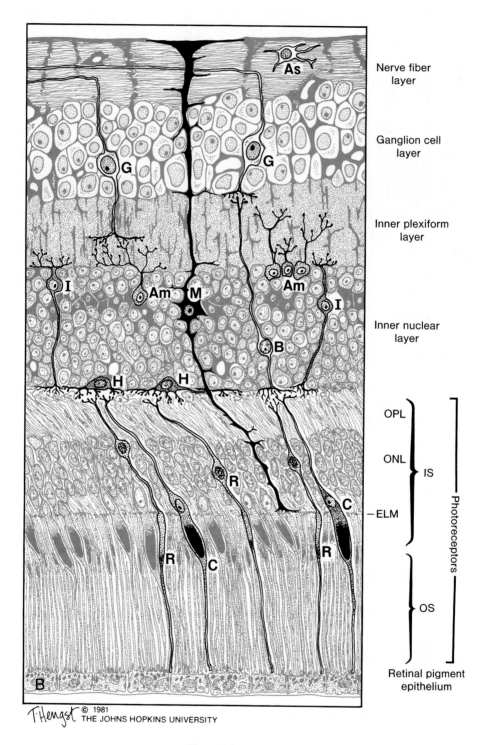

Figure 2.2. *(continued)*

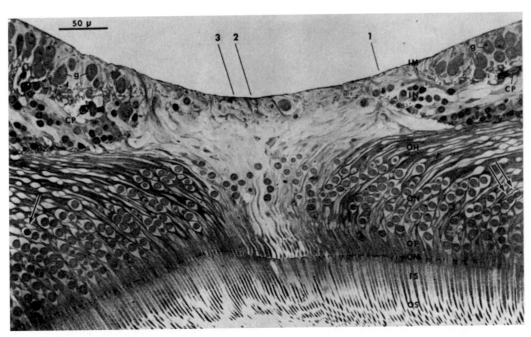

Figure 2.3. Section through center of fovea. Nuclei of rod receptor cells are indicated by arrows. Remaining receptor cells are foveal cone cells. *OS,* outer nuclear layer; *OF,* outer cone fiber; *OH,* outer fiber layer of Henle; *IN,* inner nuclear layer; *g,* ganglion cell; *CP,* capillary; *IM,* internal limiting membrane; *IS,* inner segment; *OM,* outer limiting membrane; *ON,* outer nuclear layer. (Reduced from ×400.) (Reprinted with permission from Yamada E. Some structural features of the fovea centralis in the human retina. Arch Ophthalmol 1969;82:151–159.)

3. It serves as a barrier to transport between the choriocapillaris and the sensory retina.

The visual cycle begins when the outer segment of a photoreceptor absorbs a photon, causing isomerization of 11-*cis*-retinol, the dark-adapted form of rhodopsin, to all-*trans*-retinol. This reaction initiates the phototransduction cascade that ultimately influences propagation of nerve impulses through the retina (Fig. 2.5). The 11-*cis*-retinol must be continuously regenerated to maintain the ability of the photoreceptors to respond to light, and this regeneration is performed by the RPE. Patients in whom regeneration of photopigment is abnormally slow have a prolonged recovery of central vision following exposure of the retina to bright light. This phenomenon, which is present in patients with various macular dystrophies, age-related macular degeneration, and central serous chorioretinopathy, can be detected clinically by performing a photostress test (see Chapter 1).

The second primary function of the RPE—membrane renewal—is just as important as RPE's role in phototransduction. Outer segments of rods and cones are shed on a daily basis. The outer segment of a human rod is entirely replaced over a period of 10 days and, although the timing of cone shedding is more variable, the involvement of the RPE in this process of shedding and renewal is integral. Disruption of the interaction between the RPE and the photoreceptors can lead to retinal degeneration, as occurs in hydroxychloroquine toxicity.

The **photoreceptor cells** of the retina are the sensory transducers for the visual system. They convert electromagnetic energy (i.e., light) into a neural signal. The photoreceptors contain visual pigments that, by absorbing photons of light, initiate the phototransduction process. These pigments have evolved to absorb within the range of electromagnetic wavelengths that pass through the cornea and lens, generally between 400 and 700 nm. The two types of photoreceptors are the rods and the cones.

Photoreceptors have inner and outer segments, both of which are located outside the

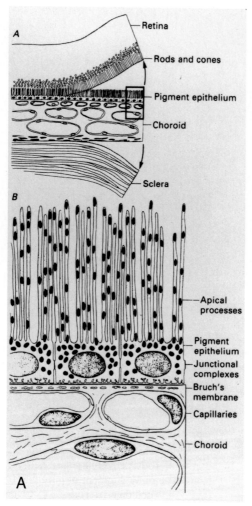

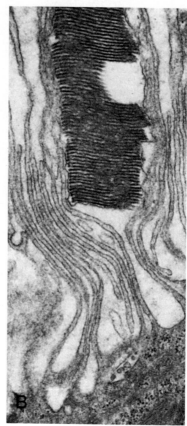

Figure 2.4. The bullfrog retina and retinal pigment epithelium (RPE). *A. Top left:* The relation between the RPE and neural retina. *Bottom left:* Detailed drawing of the RPE and choroid. The basic features of the mammalian RPE, including a convoluted basal membrane (adjacent to Bruch's membrane), junctions between cells, and apical processes, are similar to those illustrated here. (Reprinted with permission from Hughes BA, Steinberg RH. Voltage-dependent currents in isolated cells of the frog retinal pigment epithelium. J Physiol 1990;428:273–297.) *B.* Electron micrograph showing longitudinal section of retinal pigment epithelial cell projections enveloping photoreceptor outer segments. (Reprinted with permission from Anderson DH, Fisher SK. The relationship of primate fovea cones to the pigment epithelium. J Ultrastruct Res 1979;67:23–32.)

boundary of the outer limiting membrane (Fig. 2.6). The inner segment contains the **ellipsoid,** a structure that is richly endowed with mitochondria. The ellipsoid is responsible for the high level of oxidative metabolism that occurs in photoreceptors. The **myoid** is the region between the ellipsoid and the nucleus of the photoreceptor. This region contains numerous cellular organelles. The outer segment is connected to the inner segment by a cilium, which contains nine pairs of microtubules arranged in a pattern that is characteristic of nonmotile cilia.

Rods contain rhodopsin, a molecule that is composed of the apoprotein, opsin, and 11-*cis*-retinol. Rhodopsin is present in very high concentrations within the membranes of the outer

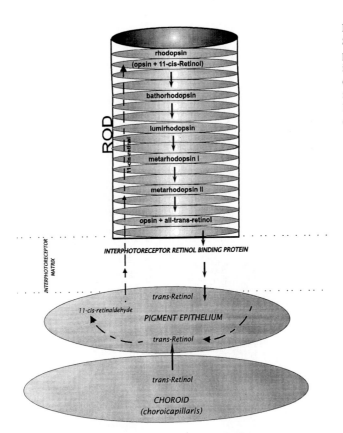

Figure 2.5. Phototransduction cascade. Schematic drawing of junction of rod, retinal pigment epithelium, and choroid to show the interrelationship among those structures required to regenerate photopigment. *trans*-Retinol is carried by the blood to the choriocapillaris where it can then enter the retinal pigment epithelium and contribute to the cycle.

segment discs, which are oriented vertically to maximize capture of incident photons. Activation of the phototransduction cascade causes an intracellular decline in cyclic guanidine monophosphate (GMP) concentration within the rod outer segment, followed by closure of the cyclic GMP-gated cation channel and cessation of inflow of extracellular cations that normally generates the dark current. The rod becomes hyperpolarized upon exposure to light, which decreases the amount of neurotransmitter released at the synaptic terminal.

Vitamin A is used in the process of phototransduction and regeneration of photopigment. Vitamin A must be replenished from the circulation, and failure to do so can result in retinopathy. Because rods are predominately affected in retinopathy caused by deficiency of vitamin A, **nyctalopia** (night blindness) is usually the initial manifestation of this disorder. Hypovitaminosis A is a highly significant problem in developing countries but also occurs in persons who live in developed countries but who have malabsorption syndromes or liver disease, or who adhere to restrictive diets.

Cones also contain 11-*cis*-retinol but have different apoproteins than rods. The variation of the opsin moieties produces three different spectral response curves corresponding to the blue, green, and red cones, which are more appropriately called short (S-), medium (M-), and long (L-) wavelength cones to emphasize that their responsiveness is not limited to a single color but rather is spread across a portion of the visible spectrum. Congenital color blindness almost always results from defects in either the red or green photopigment gene, both of which are located on the X chromosome.

Humans have a cone:rod ratio of approximately 1:20, with each retina containing 140 million rods and 7 million cones. About 50% of the cones are located within the central 30° of the visual field, an area that roughly corresponds to the size of the macula. Rods are absent in the

Figure 2.6. Ultrastructure of photoreceptors. Schematic drawing of photoreceptor cells showing the relationship of the inner and outer segments. The ellipsoid is located at the apex of the inner segment. (Reprinted with permission from Hogan MJ, Alvarado JA, Weddell JC. Histology of the Human Eye: An Atlas and Textbook. Philadelphia: WB Saunders, 1971.)

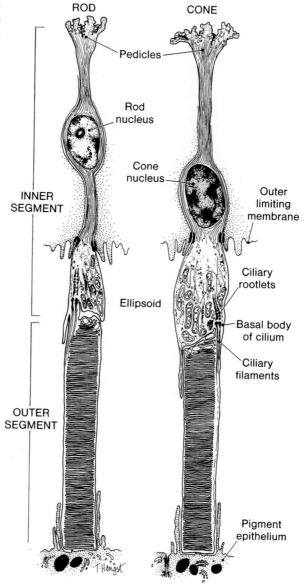

fovea and are in highest density in an elliptical ring, the center of which is the optic nerve head. There is an age-related decline in the number of rods in the human retina, with an annual loss of about 0.2 to 0.4%.

The density of foveal cones poses a problem in regard to their forward connections because their synaptic terminals (called cone pedicles) and the ganglion cells to which they connect have larger diameters than the cone inner segments themselves. Thus, each foveal ganglion cell soma is displaced away from the site of the cone that initiates its visual response. This realignment is accomplished by the nerve fiber layer of Henle, an elongation of cones and rods between their nuclei and synaptic terminals.

The **"midget"** system refers to the anatomic pattern of cone outflow within the most central retina, although there is no specific boundary beyond which the midget pathway cannot be found. The midget system provides the most direct communication of spatial detail from outer to inner retina. In this system, output from one cone passes to one ON-center **and** one OFF-center bipolar cell with each bipolar cell connecting in turn to a single ON- **or** OFF-center ganglion cell. Thus, the divergence of signal from a foveal cone to a ganglion cell is 1:2. In the peripheral retina, by comparison, there is marked convergence of information from outer to inner retina, with perhaps up to 1500 rods influencing the function of one ganglion cell.

The **outer plexiform layer** (OPL) is the zone of synaptic connection between cells whose nuclei are in the outer and inner nuclear layers. Cone pedicles and rod spherules, the synaptic specializations of cones and rods, respectively, have several invaginations into which processes of horizontal and bipolar cells extend, creating "triads" of one bipolar cell and two horizontal cells (Fig. 2.7).

The retina contains two types of **horizontal cells**. The HII cell, the smaller of the two types, makes dendritic contact with cones and axon contact with rods, whereas both ends of the HII cell synapse only with cones. Horizontal cells seem to provide the anatomic substrate for the center-surround response characteristics observed in the physiologic recordings made from ganglion cells and some other inner retinal neurons. Specifically, the response of a ganglion cell to light that falls within the center of its receptive field is opposite to that which occurs to light that falls in the surround (i.e., the portion of the receptive field beyond the center) (Fig. 2.8). The antagonistic center-surround organization em-

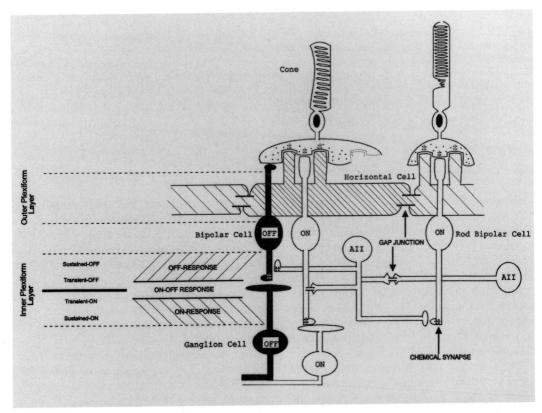

Figure 2.7. Schematic diagram of rod and cone through pathways to the retinal ganglion cells. Both cone pedicles and rod spherules have flat and invaginating surfaces upon which bipolar and horizontal cells make contact within the outer plexiform layer. AII amacrine cells and bipolar cells contact one another within the inner plexiform layer, which is subdivided into zones that contain synapses of either ON-center or OFF-center cells. Sites of chemical (i.e., ribbon) synapses and gap junctions between cells are labeled or indicated by symbols (=, gap junction; :|:, chemical synapse). *AII,* AII amacrine cell.

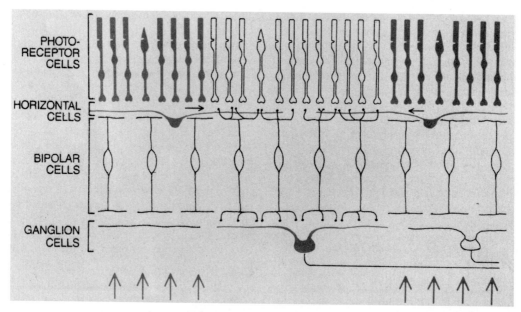

Figure 2.8.   Interactions among retinal cells and their psychophysical result. Lateral interactions can account for such selective features as the antagonistic surround of a receptive field. Suppose the horizontal cells have an effect (*horizontal arrows*) on the bipolar cells opposite to the direct effect of the photoreceptor cells. In this setting, the final signals transmitted to a ganglion cell will have a center and an antagonistic surround (*vertical arrows*). The actual horizontal cell connections that mediate this effect are incompletely known. (Reprinted with permission from Masland RH. The functional architecture of the retina. Sci Am 1986;255:102–111.)

phasizes contrast within the visual scene, which enhances spatial resolution.

Bipolar cells receive input from photoreceptors and provide output to both amacrine cells and ganglion cells. Some bipolar cells receive input from rods, others from cones. Rod bipolar cells are the target of an apparent paraneoplastic immune attack in some patients with cutaneous malignant melanoma, so-called **melanoma-associated retinopathy**. The physiologic consequence of destruction of these cells is loss of the scotopic b-wave of the electroretinogram (ERG).

The major excitatory neurotransmitter in the retina is glutamate, and this substance has a profound effect at the level of the bipolar cells. There are two physiologic types of bipolar cells: hyperpolarizing (OFF-center cells) and depolarizing (ON-center cells). These bipolar cells respond differently to changes in the ambient glutamate concentration within the outer plexiform layer. Release of glutamate by photoreceptors initiates two opposing but parallel signals to the inner retina (Fig 2.9).

Amacrine cells are so-named because they lack axons. Their cell bodies are located primarily in the inner nuclear layer of the retina. Some amacrine cells are interneurons between bipolar and ganglion cells. Others connect to fellow amacrine cells, forming a lateral pathway within the inner plexiform layer similar to that formed by horizontal cells in the outer plexiform layer (see Fig. 2.2). There are numerous subtypes of amacrine cells.

The clinical importance of amacrine cells may be emphasized by the phenomenon of temporary blindness that occasionally occurs following endoscopic surgery of the prostate gland. This condition apparently occurs from the toxic effects of the irrigating solution—which is usually isotonic glycine—on the visual sensory pathway, because affected patients invariably have an increased concentration of glycine in their sera, and glycine readily passes through the blood-brain barrier. There are several hypotheses regarding the site of toxic damage in this condition. The finding of an abnormal ERG that is characterized by a large amplitude a-wave and reduced amplitude and loss of oscillatory potentials of the b-wave in affected patients, coupled with the fact that glycine is an inhibitory neurotransmitter normally present in the inner retina, suggests that the amacrine cells of the inner retina are the most likely targets of the toxicity.

The cell bodies of the **interplexiform cells** reside in the inner plexiform layer. These cells are postsynaptic to amacrine and bipolar cells in the inner plexiform layer and presynaptic to horizontal and bipolar cells in the outer plexiform layer. This cell thus appears to be unique in that it apparently conveys information from the inner to the outer plexiform layer, against the standard direction of neural transmission within the retina.

The retina contains several types of glial cells that have various functions. The most important are Müller cells and astrocytes. Müller cell somas are located in the inner nuclear layer, but processes from these cells extend throughout the entire retina (see Fig. 2.2). The apical processes of **Müller cells** form the outer limiting membrane by making junctional complexes with one another and with photoreceptors. On the vitread side, apposed Müller cell end-feet form the inner limiting membrane. Lateral extensions from Müller cells contact neurons within cellular layers, synapses within plexiform layers, axons within the nerve fiber layer, and blood vessels.

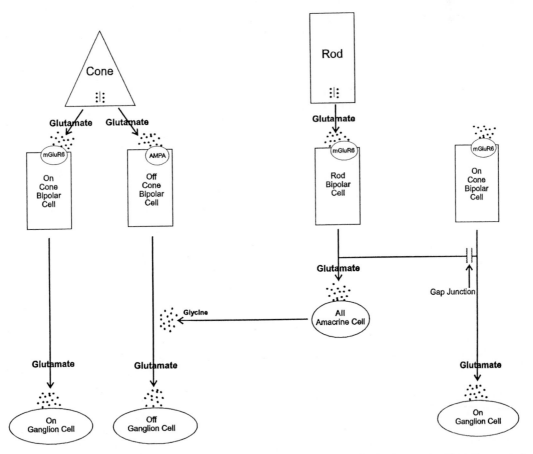

Figure 2.9. Schematic illustration of neurotransmitters used by cells of the rod and cone pathways. The neurotransmitters are released within the outer and inner plexiform layers. The mGluR6 and AMPA receptors of the bipolar cells are also depicted. The former uses a G protein to control the intracellular concentration of cGMP that, in turn, regulates the Na^+-Ca^{2+}-cGMP-gated ion channel.

Despite all their connections, Müller cells are not in the direct pathway of neural signal transfer. However, they exert substantial influence over signal transmission by 1) maintaining the local extracellular environment needed for proper neuronal function, particularly with respect to the extracellular concentration of potassium; 2) adjusting concentrations of extracellular neurotransmitters; and 3) possibly buffering pH levels.

Astrocytes are found only on the vitread side of the retina, within the nerve fiber and ganglion cell layers. Two morphologic types of astrocytes develop from stem cells in the optic nerve. Each cell type preferentially contacts either nerve fiber bundles or blood vessels. Oligodendrocytes are not present in the primate retina, which is consistent with the absence of myelin in these retinas. However, the observation of myelinated nerve fibers in the retinas of about 0.5% of normal persons suggests that such a migration can occur during, and even after, development (see Chapter 3).

The **inner plexiform layer** (IPL), which is much thicker than the outer plexiform layer, is the zone of synaptic connection of bipolar and amacrine cells to ganglion cells. The IPL can be divided into sublaminae a and b. Sublamina a is the more proximal layer. It is nearer the inner nuclear layer and is the zone in which bipolar, amacrine, and ganglion cells of the OFF-center pathway synapse. Sublamina b is the more distal layer. It is nearer the ganglion cell layer and is the site of synaptic connections for the ON-center cell pathway (see Fig. 2.7).

The **retinal ganglion cell layer** is, in fact, composed not only of retinal ganglion cells but also of "displaced" amacrine cells, astrocytes, endothelial cells, and pericytes. The human retina contains about 1.2 million retinal ganglion cells, although there is a very wide inter-individual variability. It has been calculated that 69% of the ganglion cells in the human retina subserve the central 30° of the visual field and are located adjacent to the fovea. The distribution of retinal ganglion cells with respect to the Goldmann visual field map is shown in Figure 2.10.

Dendrites of ganglion cells branch in well-defined strata within the IPL, and the specific region of stratification varies with the particular cell type. ON-center and OFF-center ganglion cells have dendrites that terminate in sublamina b or a of the IPL, respectively (see Fig. 2.7).

Retinal ganglion cell axons terminate in either the magnocellular or parvocellular layers of the lateral geniculate nucleus (LGN), and this also depends on the cell type. In the primate retina, there may be as many as 10 or more subpopulations of ganglion cells.

Retinal ganglion cells can be subdivided into two main types based on cell size. About 80% of the cells are small cells that are called "beta" or "P" cells, for **parvocellular** cells. These cells, as their name implies, synapse in the parvocellular layers of the LGN. From 5 to 10% of primate retinal ganglion cells are large cells that are called "alpha" or "M" cells, for **magnocellular** cells. The axons of these cells synapse in the magnocellular layers of the LGN. Together, the P and M ganglion cells comprise 85 to 90% of all primate retinal ganglion cells. The remainder of the ganglion cells are present in small numbers, are less well studied, and may have functions other than for visual perception, such as the pupillary light reflex and the retinohypothalamic pathway, the latter believed to be an integral part of the pathway that regulates circadian functions.

From a clinical standpoint, the P- and M-cells have great significance. The P-cells are color-opponent (i.e., the center of the receptive field is maximally responsive to either red or green light, whereas the inverse is true for the surround), have small receptive fields, and have low sensitivity to contrast in the visual scene. Color-opponency is generated by connections at both the OPL and IPL. The receptive field center of P ganglion cells near the fovea approximately equals the diameter of a single cone. These cells have linear response characteristics, meaning that their firing rate is proportional to the degree to which the center of the receptive field is stimulated or inhibited. Cells with this response property are also called "X" cells. Given these characteristics, the P-cells are probably the major neural input to the optic nerve for visual functions such as central (i.e., Snellen) acuity, color vision, and fine stereopsis.

The M-cells are spectrally "broad-band." Because of the combined input to these ganglion cells from all three cone types, their peak responsiveness at a given intensity of light is not determined by the wavelength. M-cells have much larger receptive fields and are more responsive to luminance contrast than P-cells. The majority of M-cells have nonlinear responses to light.

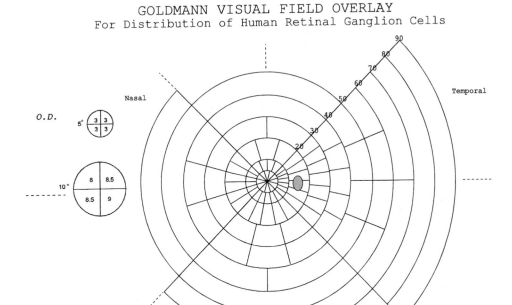

Figure 2.10. Visual field overlay for the distribution of the human retinal ganglion cells for perimetry using a Goldmann perimeter. Each sector of the map equals 1% of the total number of cells. An inset (*left*) has been provided to assist in counting of boxes when a field defect involves the central region. The blind spot is included for orientation only and should not influence the counting of boxes when field defects involve the peripapillary region. The hatched lines extending from the meridia in the nasal quadrants are a reminder that a relatively small number of ganglion cells (<1%) are present beyond the superior, inferior, and nasal borders of the map. (Map constructed by Drs. Joseph F. Rizzo and Anthony C. Castelbuono, using original data from Curcio CA, Allen KA. Topography of ganglion cells in human retina. J Comp Neurol 1990;300:5–25.)

These cells typically show spikes of activity in response to changes in the visual scene, rather than showing activity that is proportional to the intensity of light and that matches the duration of light stimulation, as is the case with P-cells. M-cells with this physiologic profile are also called "Y" cells, to distinguish their responses from the X-like response profile of P-cells. Lesions of the magnocellular pathway in monkeys impair high-temporal-frequency flicker and motion perception.

Parvocellular and magnocellular ganglion cells account for about 90% of anatomically distinct primate retinal ganglion cells. The remainder of ganglion cells include the blue-sensitive ON-center parasol cells and two other types of ganglion cells that can be distinguished by their anatomy. Gamma (γ) cells typically have a small cell body and wide, diffusely branching dendrites, although some γ-cells have a larger soma.

These mixed anatomic traits suggest that the γ-cell class may include more than one physiologic type of cell. Ganglion cells with delta (δ) morphology have a small soma and a diffuse but loosely branching dendritic field.

Most retinal ganglion cells have several physiologic properties in common. First, their receptive fields have a concentric and antagonistic center-surround organization. This property probably derives at least in part from the effect of the lateral inhibition of horizontal, and possibly amacrine, cells. Second, most ganglion cells respond either in an on or off manner to change in the luminance contrast or spectral distribution of light within their receptive field centers (Fig. 2.11). This property is reflected in the location of dendritic ramification within the IPL. ON-center bipolar and ganglion cells ramify in sublamina b of the IPL, whereas OFF-center bipolar and ganglion cells ramify in sublamina a

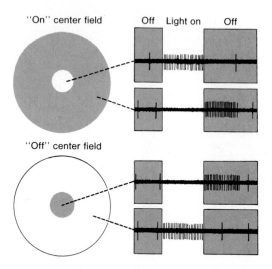

Figure 2.11. Concentric fields are characteristic of retinal ganglion cells. *Top:* Oscilloscope recording shows strong firing by ON-center type of cell when spot of light strikes center of field. If spot hits the OFF surround area, firing is suppressed until the light goes off. *Bottom:* Responses of an OFF-center ganglion cell. Note that it fires only when a spot of light hits the surround area or when a light spot that is hitting its center goes off. (Redrawn from Hubel D. Sci Am 1963;209:58.)

(see Fig. 2.7). Third, the responses to light of most ganglion cells are either sustained or transient, depending on the pattern of interconnections with amacrine cells within the IPL (Fig. 2.12). Fourth, ganglion cells with sustained responses also show linearity of spatial summation; that is, the magnitude of their response is proportional to the degree of illumination within the center of the receptive field. In contrast, transiently responding ganglion cells briefly increase or decrease their firing rates in response to a change in illumination. Lastly, retinal ganglion cells maintain a continuous spontaneous discharge. This activity requires considerable energy but presumably has the advantage of allowing the cell to reflect more precisely the degree of illumination by either increasing or decreasing its firing rate.

It should be emphasized that the two largest classes of retinal ganglion cells (the P- and M-cells) do not alter their mean firing rate in response to a change in the overall level of light striking the retina. Rather, they respond to differences in **contrast** between the center and surround of its receptive field. Hence, it is likely

that neither cell type drives the pupillomotor responses to light.

Retinal ganglion cells can be classified physiologically as well as anatomically. As a general rule, cells classified anatomically as P-cells have an X-cell physiologic profile, whereas M-cells have a Y-cell response. However, just as there are some ganglion cells that are anatomically distinct from P- or M-cells (i.e., γ and δ cells), there is a third physiologic class of ganglion cells called "W" cells. W-cells share many properties with X and Y ganglion cell types, although not all of them have a concentric center-surround organization of their receptive field. On the other hand, some W-cells have unique physiologic properties, such as directional selectivity.

The axon of a retinal ganglion cell is relatively long, and the body of the ganglion cell is the sole site for production of the components needed to maintain the health of the axon. The axon is a dynamic structure that requires nearly constant repair of its membranes, a process that is partly achieved by transport of proteins, enzymes, and other subcellular components (including mitochondria) to, and detritus from, sites up to the synapse.

Axon transport is bidirectional and simultaneous, with velocities that can be broadly divided into fast (i.e., hundreds of mm/day) and slow (<10 mm/day). Slow anterograde transport, which largely carries components that remain within the cell such as cytoskeletal proteins, constitutes the bulk (about 85%) of all movement within the axon. At least five different classes of proteins are transported at different velocities within retinal ganglion cells, and these relationships vary during development. Fast anterograde transport is used to carry neurotransmitter-containing vesicles. Retrograde transport, which is less well understood, proceeds at roughly half the maximum velocity of anterograde transport. It returns to the cell body substances that have been taken into the cell at its terminal synapse. Axon transport, whether anterograde or retrograde, is highly energy dependent, and the adenosine triphosphate (ATP) needed to sustain it is supplied by mitochondria that are distributed along the entire length of the axon.

The final common defect in pathologic swelling of the optic disc from almost any etiology is disruption of anterograde axonal transport of the retinal ganglion cells at the lamina cribrosa

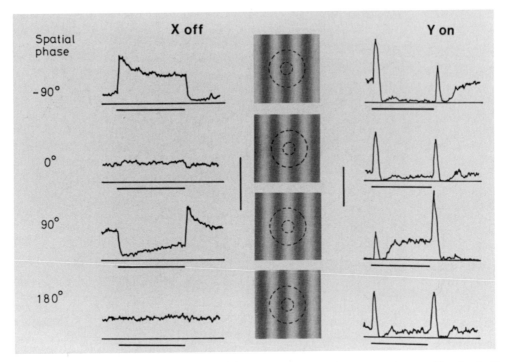

Figure 2.12. Firing-rate records from a cat retinal OFF-center X-cell (*left*) and an ON-center Y-cell (*right*) responding to the appearance and disappearance of a sine-wave grating in different positions. The pictures in the middle show the positions of the stimulus pattern in relation to the receptive field during the period in which the pattern was present (1.1 sec of every 2.2 sec as marked by the bar under each record). When the pattern disappeared, the stimulus screen remained at the same mean luminance. Note that the Y-cell generates a transient excitatory response at both the appearance and disappearance of the stimulus pattern, regardless of its position. The vertical scale bar corresponds to a firing rate of 100 impulses/sec. (Reprinted with permission from Enroth-Cugell C, Robson JG. Functional characteristics and diversity of cat retinal ganglion cells. Invest Ophthalmol Visual Sci 1984;25:250–267.)

(see Chapter 4). The degree to which fast versus slow transport is disrupted probably varies according to the etiology.

Axons of retinal ganglion cells synapse in the LGN, mesencephalon, pretectum, or one of several nuclei in the hypothalamus. The specific site of termination of the axon is related to the anatomy of the ganglion cell body. Generally, P- and M-cell axons synapse in the parvocellular and magnocellular layers, respectively. The γ and δ ganglion cells are probably composed of more than one cell type, and their axons likely terminate in more than one central site. ON-center and OFF-center ganglion cells appear to remain functionally separated at the level of the LGN, although both channels converge at the visual cortex.

The **nerve fiber layer** (NFL) of the retina is composed of axons of ganglion cells, astrocytes, components of Müller cells, and a very small number of efferent fibers to the retina, the functions of which are unknown. The NFL is thinnest in the peripheral retina and thickest adjacent to the superior and inferior margins of the optic disc, where it measures about 200 μm in humans. The temporal and nasal NFL adjacent to the optic disc is about 1/10 as thick.

The gross organization of the NFL is characterized by three main features. The first is the papillomacular bundle, which contains nerve fibers originating from ganglion cells in the foveal area. Papillomacular fibers from ganglion cells on the nasal side of the fovea project directly to the optic disc, whereas those from ganglion cells on the temporal side of the fovea arch around the nasal fibers en route to the optic nerve (Fig. 2.13). The relatively early formation of the central retina relative to the peripheral retina gives

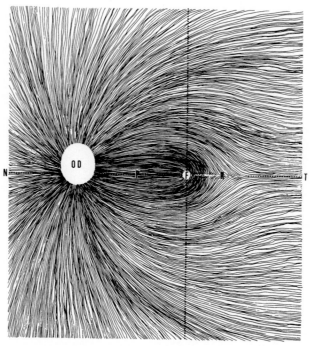

Figure 2.13. Drawing of the retinal nerve axons as they extend from the ganglion cells to the disc. The axons arising from ganglion cells in the nasal macula project directly toward the optic disc (OD) and comprise part of the papillomacular bundle (P). Axons from ganglion cells of the temporal macula have a slight arching pattern around the nasal macular axons. They form the remainder of the papillomacular bundle. Axons from nonmacular ganglion cells that are nasal to the fovea (F) have a straight or gently curved course to the optic disc, whereas axons from ganglion cells temporal to the fovea must arch around the papillomacular bundle and enter the disc at its superior and inferior poles. Note that the superior and inferior portions of the temporal retina are delineated by an anatomic landmark, the temporal raphe (R). The dotted lines delineate the nasal (N), temporal (T), superior, and inferior portions of the retina. Note that the temporal and nasal parts of the retina are defined by a vertical line through the fovea, not the optic disc. (Redrawn from Hogan MJ, Alvarado JA, Weddell JE. Histology of the Human Eye. An Atlas and Textbook. Philadelphia: WB Saunders, 1971.)

rise to the second feature: the arching of axons from midperipheral and peripheral ganglion cells temporal to the fovea around the previously formed papillomacular bundle. A watershed line called the temporal raphe is present on the temporal side of the fovea, and this horizontal demarcation separates axons in the superior temporal retina from those in the inferior temporal retina. The raphe creates not only an anatomic separation but also a physiologic separation between the superior and inferior regions of the temporal retina. The third anatomic feature of the NFL is the radial distribution of nerve fibers that enter the nasal aspect of the optic disc.

The temporal-nasal demarcation of the retina (and, thus, the visual field) is a vertical line that passes through the **fovea,** not the optic disc. In general, fibers from ganglion cells located nasal to the fovea cross to the opposite side within the optic chiasm, whereas fibers from ganglion cells located temporal to the fovea remain uncrossed, passing through the chiasm into the ipsilateral optic tract. This vertical meridian, although reasonably precise from a clinical standpoint, is inexact at a cellular level. There is a small area of nasotemporal overlap on either side of the vertical meridian in which some axons from ganglion cells temporal to the fovea cross within the chiasm, and some axons from ganglion cells nasal to the fovea remain uncrossed. However, the mere presence of an overlap may have no significant visual consequences. A ganglion cell that is located on one side of the fovea does not necessarily receive input from a photoreceptor that is located on the same side. The much larger width of the cone pedicle compared with the foveal cone soma creates a packing problem that is only partly resolved by lateral displacement of cone pedicles and via the nerve fiber layer of Henle (see above). This lateral shift could theoretically connect photoreceptors on one side of the vertical meridian to seemingly displaced ganglion cells on the opposite side. Such an anatomic relationship would have no adverse visual consequences, because it is the position of the photoreceptor and not the ganglion cell body that provides spatial cues to the brain.

There is, in addition to the specific arrangement of fibers in the NFL described above, an orderly arrangement of the fibers in the third dimension—that is, with respect to their vertical orientation as viewed in cross-section. The nerve fibers are generally stratified such that axons from ganglion cells in the peripheral retina occupy a position adjacent to the ganglion cell layer, whereas axons from ganglion cells located more centrally lie more superficially in the NFL, adjacent to the vitreoretinal interface. To achieve this arrangement, fibers from increasingly central ganglion cells must cross fibers from more peripheral ganglion cells. This arrangement is maintained until the fibers are near the optic disc, at which point there is significant intermingling of more central axons with those that originated peripherally. Nevertheless, near the disc margin, most of the axons with a long course (i.e., from peripheral ganglion cells) are located deep within the NFL, whereas axons with a short course (i.e., from central ganglion cells) are located superficially. This arrangement results in the longest axons being positioned in the periphery of the anterior optic disc, and axons from more central ganglion cells being located more centrally in the anterior optic disc.

Table 2.2 provides a list of known neurotrans-mitters for the major classes of retinal cells, and Figure 2.9 shows some of the neurotransmitters used by the intraretinal cone and rod through pathways.

RETINAL BLOOD VESSELS

The human retina receives its essential nutrients—oxygen and glucose—from both the retinal and the choroidal circulations. The border between these circulations is near the outer plexiform layer. The choroidal circulation supplies the photoreceptors; the retinal arteries supply the inner retina, although the latter do not enter a small area composed of the fovea and a varying degree of perifoveal retina. This avascular area is called the **foveal avascular zone**. There is considerable inter-individual variation in the size of the foveal avascular zone. In addition, the degree to which the inner retina is vascularized appears to correlate with the degree of oxidative metabolic demand, rather than with the thickness of the retina.

The retinal vasculature is organized into specific laminae. Generally, four planes of capillaries can be recognized. The two more vitread layers bracket the inner nuclear layer, whereas the two other layers are located more superficially. Superficial retinal capillaries in humans can probably nourish ganglion cell bodies up to 45 μm away.

Retinal blood vessels are barrier vessels, analogous to the blood-brain barrier elsewhere within the central nervous system. These vessels are impermeable to particles larger than 2 nm. Astrocytes and pericytes almost certainly play a role in maintaining this nonspecific low permeability for capillaries within the nerve fiber layer, whereas Müller cells probably play a similar role within deeper retina. The blood-retinal

Table 2.2
Retinal Neurons and Some of Their Associated Neurotransmitters

CELL TYPE	NEUROTRANSMITTER		
Photoreceptors	Glutamate		
Horizontal cells	GABA		
Bipolar cells:			
ON-center (depolarizing)	Glutamate		
OFF-center (hyperpolarizing)	Glutamate		
Interplexiform cells	Dopamine	GABA	
Amacrine cells	Acetylcholine	GABA	Dopamine
	Glycine	Peptides	

barrier is maintained not only by physical factors, such as the cells surrounding the retinal capillaries described above, but also by chemical factors. Specifically, autoregulation of retinal (and choroidal) blood vessels may be at least partially controlled chemically by hormonal products of the local vascular endothelium. These substances include vasodilators, such as nitric oxide and prostaglandins, and vasoconstrictors, particularly endothelin and the products of the renin-angiotensin system that are produced and released via angiotensin-converting enzyme, which is located on the endothelial cell membrane. Additionally, adenosine and α_1-adrenergic receptors in retinal blood vessels have been shown to mediate vasodilation and vasoconstriction, respectively.

ROD AND CONE THROUGH PATHWAYS: FUNCTIONAL CONSIDERATIONS

The complex anatomic and physiologic features of the retina combine to produce a well-defined reaction when the retina is stimulated with light. Light causes the photoreceptors to hyperpolarize, decreasing the release of glutamate from both rod and cone synaptic terminals. Horizontal cells then become hyperpolarized, suppressing the light response of the photoreceptors. Rod and cone outputs then diverge. Rod signals are transmitted to the rod bipolar cells via a sign-inverting signal. Thus, bipolar cells depolarize in response to light. The signal is then carried via the axons of the rod bipolar cells to sublamina b of the IPL, where there is a sign-conserving synapse on amacrine cells. (Rod bipolar cells do not make direct contact with ganglion cells.) The amacrine cells make gap junctions with cone-depolarizing bipolar cells, the axon terminals of which also ramify in sublamina b of the IPL, where the terminal of the amacrine cells contact ON-center ganglion cells via a conventional synapse. The amacrine cells also make conventional synapses on cone-hyperpolarizing bipolar cells through sign-reversing glycinergic synapses, and these bipolar cells terminate in sublamina a of the IPL and then make contact with OFF-center ganglion cells.

Cone output in the central retina uses the midget system of interconnections in which one foveal cone contacts two bipolar cells, each of which then contacts a single ganglion cell. A sign-conserving synapse is made on a cone-hyperpolarizing (OFF-center) bipolar cell, and a sign-conserving synapse is made with a cone-depolarizing (ON-center) bipolar cell. The two bipolar cells then terminate in the proximal (sublamina a) and distal (sublamina b) laminae of the IPL, respectively, wherein they make contact with an OFF-center (sublamina a) or an ON-center (sublamina b) ganglion cell. From this location, visual information is passed to the brain via the optic nerve. Visual information (i.e., spatial detail, color, contrast) is presented in parallel fashion to the brain, with major physiologic cell types in the retina (i.e., X-, Y-, and W-cells) generally maintaining anatomic segregation at the LGN and visual cortex.

ANATOMY AND PHYSIOLOGY OF THE OPTIC NERVE

The **optic nerve** is not really a nerve, as are the peripheral nerves. It is a part of the central nervous system. As such, it is a tract, and its axons are myelinated by oligodendrocytes, not Schwann cells. The optic nerve carries about 1.2 million axons whose cell bodies are the retinal ganglion cells and which synapse in one or more of at least eight primary visual nuclei.

Common nomenclature considers only the anterior portion of this retinofugal fiber projection to be the optic nerve. The optic chiasm is the site of a partial decussation of these fibers, and the optic tract is the posterior continuation of the same fiber tract to its termination in the LGN.

The optic nerve is about 50 mm long (Fig. 2.14), although there is some individual variation in length, especially with regard to its posterior half. It may be described as having four parts:

1. the intraocular portion (the optic nerve head)

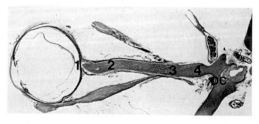

Figure 2.14. Histologic section showing the four topographic sections of the normal optic nerve. *1:* intraocular. *2:* intraorbital. *3:* intracanalicular. *4:* intracranial. *OC:* optic chiasm. (Reprinted with permission from Hogan MJ, Zimmerman LE. Ophthalmic Pathology. An Atlas and Textbook. Philadelphia: WB Saunders, 1962.)

2. the intraorbital portion
3. the intraosseous portion within the optic canal
4. the intracranial portion

The intraocular optic nerve can be further divided into three anatomically distinct zones: the retinal or prelaminar portion (anterior), the choroidal or laminar portion (middle), and the scleral or retrolaminar portion (posterior). These zones have very different microanatomic arrangements, with elements of neuroectoderm and mesoderm intermingled.

OPTIC NERVE HEAD (INTRAOCULAR OPTIC NERVE)

As noted above, axons of the retinal ganglion cells form bundles that constitute the nerve fiber layer, which converges like spokes of a wheel at the optic nerve head (see above). The optic nerve head is about 1 mm long (anterior–posterior); its diameter is 1.5 mm horizontally by 1.8 mm vertically at the level of the retina and a little wider in the retrolaminar space. It is a major zone of transition, because nerve fibers pass from an area of high tissue pressure within the eye to a zone of low pressure that correlates with the intracranial pressure. At the same time, the nerve fibers leave an area in which their blood supply is from the central retinal artery alone to zones supplied by other branches of the ophthalmic artery. In addition, the axons become myelinated immediately at the posterior end of the optic nerve head.

The optic nerve head is composed of four types of cells: ganglion cell axons, astrocytes, capillary-associated cells, and fibroblasts. It also includes an oval grouping of 200 to 300 holes that perforate the choroid and sclera, forming a specialized structure called the **lamina cribrosa,** through which all retinal axons pass to exit the eye.

The anterior surface of the optic nerve head is the clinically visible **optic disc.** The appearance of the disc depends on two important features: the size of the scleral canal and the angle of exit of the canal from the eye. The size of the canal varies somewhat among individuals; however, the volume of tissue passing through the hole appears to be more constant. The scleral canal may be thought of as a hole in the sclera. The larger the scleral canal, the more leftover space is present in the center of the disc, leading

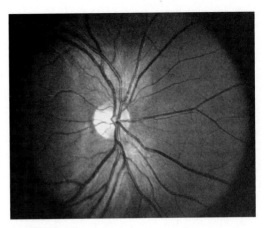

Figure 2.15. Appearance of the "disc at risk." Note that the optic disc is smaller than normal and has no central cup.

to a larger physiologic cup size. The converse is also apt to be true. A small or absent physiologic cup often reflects a small scleral canal and a crowded optic nerve head (Fig. 2.15).

When the optic nerve head exits the sclera at less than a 90° angle, the RPE frequently ends before the edge of the canal proper, exposing a crescent-shaped halo of choroid and sclera (Fig. 2.16). In addition, with an oblique angle of exit at one side of the disc, nerve fibers must make a greater than 90° turn, giving a rolled edge to this rim of the disc that may simulate true swell-

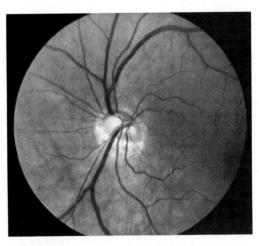

Figure 2.16. Appearance of a tilted optic disc. Note inferior conus.

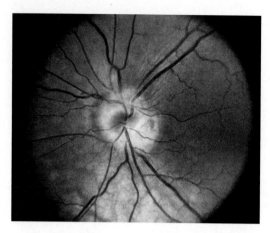

Figure 2.17. Appearance of a tilted optic disc. The elevated superior portion of the disc simulates optic disc swelling. Note inferior conus.

ing (Fig. 2.17). At the opposite side of such a disc, fibers are exiting at less than a 90° angle, and the disc rim appears shallowly sloped.

The retinal NFL turns 90° posteriorly as it enters the optic nerve head. The axons then run in bundles surrounded by glial columns as they pass through the perforations of the lamina cribrosa. The fenestrated connective tissue and glia form a tight seal that helps keep the relatively high intraocular pressure from "leaking" into the retrolaminar tissues.

Within the optic nerve head, there are two types of blood vessels: capillary-sized vessels that directly supply the cells and the central retinal vessels (the central retinal artery and one or more central retinal veins) that pass through the nerve head. The ophthalmic artery originates from the ophthalmic segment of the internal carotid artery just as that vessel emerges from the distal dural ring of the cavernous sinus. It then turns anteriorly and passes through the optic canal along with the optic nerve but separated from it by a covering of dura. Once within the orbit, the ophthalmic artery gives rise to several branches, one of which is the central retinal artery, which pierces the optic nerve sheath 10 to 12 mm behind the globe and runs anteriorly in the central aspect of the optic nerve to emerge in the center of the optic disc. This artery does not contribute directly to the circulation of the optic nerve head. Instead, the blood supply to the optic nerve head derives from the circle of Zinn-Haller which forms a ring about it. The

circle of Zinn-Haller receives three major sources of blood. Much of its blood derives from the choroidal feeder vessels. A second source consists of about four short posterior arteries that feed into the circle directly. The third source of blood to this perineural arteriolar anastomosis is a small contribution from the pial arterial network. Feeding this capillary plexus are subdivisions of the ophthalmic artery via 3rd- and 4th-order branches of posterior ciliary arteries, which enter the lateral aspect of the nerve head and vessels of the pial plexus and retrobulbar optic nerve posteriorly (Fig. 2.18).

The venous drainage of the optic nerve head is primarily via the central retinal venous system. Under certain conditions, however, such as chronic compression of the intraorbital optic nerve or after central retinal vein occlusion, preexisting connections between superficial disc veins and choroidal veins—opticociliary veins—may enlarge and shunt venous blood from the retina to the choroid and then, via the vortex veins, to the superior and inferior ophthalmic veins.

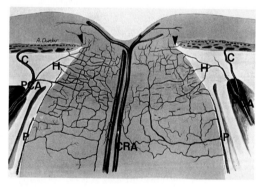

Figure 2.18. Composite illustration to scale of the vascular supply of the optic disc and retrolaminar optic nerve. Venous vessels and superficial central retinal artery are not drawn in full. In the retrolaminar portion of the nerve, branches of the central retinal artery (CRA) and the pial arteries (P) anastomose to supply the nerve tissue. The laminar and immediately prelaminar portions of the nerve are supplied primarily by branches (H) of the posterior ciliary arteries (PCA). Although some arterial branches extend from the choroid to the optic nerve head (*arrowheads*), these are small and inconsequential. C, choroidal branches of the posterior ciliary arteries. (Reprinted with permission from Lieberman MF, Maumenee AE, Green WR. Histologic studies of the vasculature of the anterior optic nerve. Am J Ophthalmol 1976;82:405–423.)

ORBITAL OPTIC NERVE

The orbital portion of the optic nerve is 25 mm in length and thus exceeds the anterior–posterior distance from the back of the eye to the optic foramen by about 8 mm (Fig. 2.19). The redundancy of the sinuous optic nerve permits it to move freely during eye movements. There is also an allowance of up to 9 mm of proptosis before the optic nerve acts as a tether and distorts the globe or is stretched to the point of dysfunction.

The optic nerve increases in diameter from 3 mm just posterior to the globe to about 4.5 mm at the orbital apex. Throughout its orbital course, the nerve is surrounded by dura, arachnoid, and pia mater (Figs. 2.19 and 2.20). The dura is the outermost sheath, a dense collagenous tunic that is continuous anteriorly with the sclera. At the apex of the orbit, the dura fuses with the periosteum and with the annulus of Zinn. The arachnoid lies under the dura and is more cellular, less vascular, and less collagenous. Delicate arachnoidal trabeculae connect this membrane with the dura and underlying pia (Fig. 2.21). The pia is the most vascular of the sheaths covering the optic nerve. It invests the capillaries as they enter the substance of the nerve. The subarach-

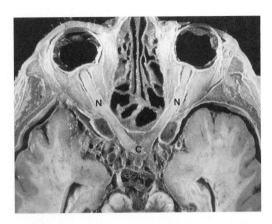

Figure 2.20. Axial section of normal optic nerves (N), showing relationships to other orbital and intracranial structures. Note that the intraorbital and intracanalicular portions of the nerve are covered by a dural sheath that is continuous with the periorbita lining the inner surface of the orbital walls and the dura lining the base of the skull. *C,* optic chiasm. (Reprinted with permission from Unsöld R, DeGroot J, Newton TH. Images of the optic nerve: anatomic-CT correlation. Am J Roentgenol 1980;135:767–773.)

noid space is continuous with the intracranial subarachnoid space and thus contains CSF.

The cellular organization of the myelinated orbital portion of the optic nerve is similar to that of the intraocular optic nerve head, although the retrobulbar nerve is twice as wide because of the addition of myelin. Bundles of nerve fibers are surrounded by connective tissue septa containing small arterioles, venules, and capillaries, forming a meshwork much like that in the lamina cribrosa. Astrocytes are here joined by oligodendrocytes, the specialized glial cells that provide membranes for myelination. All of the visual axons are myelinated from their exit from the eye to their synapse in the LGN. The axons from the largest retinal ganglion cells are surrounded by the thickest myelin sheaths, thus providing them with faster nerve conduction velocities.

With the exception of the central retinal artery, there are few vessels larger than capillaries within the orbital portion of the optic nerve. The arterial input derives chiefly from the surrounding pial plexus.

As the optic nerve leaves the eye, it is surrounded by about four posterior ciliary arteries that are branches of the ophthalmic artery. Within the midportion of the orbit, the ophthal-

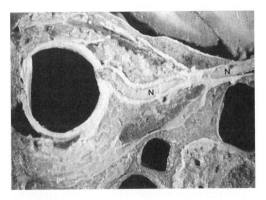

Figure 2.19. Sagittal section through a normal orbit showing the optic nerve (N). Note that the length of the nerve within the orbit appears to exceed the distance from the posterior aspect of the globe to the apex of the orbit. Also note that the intraorbital and intracanalicular portions of the nerve are covered by leptomeninges, the dural sheath of which is continuous with the periorbita lining the inner surface of the orbital walls and the dura lining the base of the skull. (Reprinted with permission from Unsöld R, DeGroot J, Newton TH. Images of the optic nerve: anatomic-CT correlation. Am J Roentgenol 1980;135:767–773.)

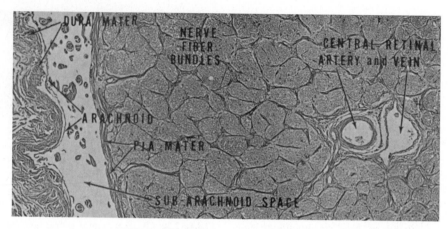

Figure 2.21. Cross-section of human optic nerve, showing relationships of the vaginal sheaths. The nerve fibers are divided into bundles by connective tissue septa that are continuous with both the connective tissue of the pia mater and the adventitia of the central retinal vessels.

mic artery initially runs inferolateral to the optic nerve until it crosses under (or occasionally over) it to proceed medially. At the optic foramen, the ophthalmic artery lies below and lateral to the nerve. The inferior division of the oculomotor nerve, the nasociliary artery, the abducens nerve, and the ciliary ganglion are all located lateral to the optic nerve in the posterior orbit (Figs. 2.22 and 2.23). At the apex of the orbit, the optic nerve is surrounded by the four rectus muscles that originate from the fibrous circle of Zinn.

INTRACANALICULAR (INTRAOSSEOUS) OPTIC NERVE

The optic nerve enters the optic canal through its anterior opening in the apex of the orbital roof about 5 cm posterior and 1.5 cm inferior to the supraorbital margin. This anterior opening is called the **optic foramen**.

The optic canal itself is formed by the union of the two roots of the lesser wings of the sphenoid bone (Fig. 2.24). The proximal (orbital) opening of the optic canal is usually elliptical in shape, with the vertical diameter being consistently greater than the horizontal. The distal (intracranial) opening is always elliptical, but its widest diameter is in the horizontal plane.

The thickness of the bony optic canal wall varies from medial (thinnest in mid-canal) to lateral (thickest in mid-canal) but also from anterior to posterior. The thin medial wall separates the optic nerve from the sphenoid and posterior

ethmoid sinuses. The canal is about 10 mm in length, with the lateral wall being shorter (9 mm) than the medial wall (about 14 mm). Inferolaterally, the optic canal is separated from the superior orbital fissure by a bony ridge that joins the lesser wing of the sphenoid to the body of the sphenoid bone—the **optic strut**.

The relationship between the paranasal sinuses and the optic canal is extremely important, particularly because in about 4% of patients, the nerves have areas covered only by the nerve sheaths and sinus mucosa but without any bone separating the intracanalicular portion of the optic nerve from the adjacent paranasal sinus. The paranasal sinuses may occasionally become ballooned out without erosion of bone. This condition, called "pneumosinus dilatans," may result in the optic canals appearing as tunnels surrounded by sphenoid and posterior ethmoid air cells. Pneumosinus dilatans in this region is usually associated with an adjacent optic nerve sheath meningioma.

The intraorbital optic nerve moves freely as the eye moves; however, the intracanalicular optic nerve is tightly fixed within the optic canal. The dura is adherent to the bone of the canal on one side and the optic nerve on the other (Fig. 2.25). Thus, small lesions arising within the optic canal or at either of its openings may compress and significantly damage the optic nerve while they are still quite small and difficult to visualize, even with thin-section CT scanning and MRI.

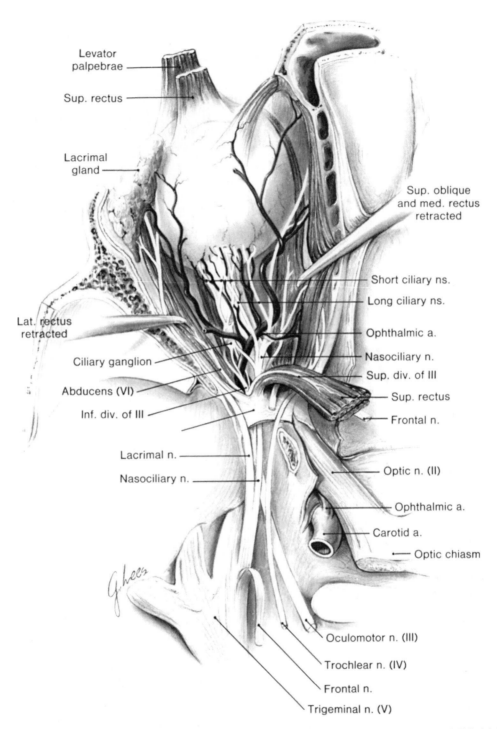

Figure 2.22. View of the intraorbital optic nerve from above showing relationships of the nerve to the ocular motor nerves and the posterior ciliary vessels. (Redrawn from Wolff E. Anatomy of the Eye and Orbit. 6th ed. Philadelphia: WB Saunders, 1968.)

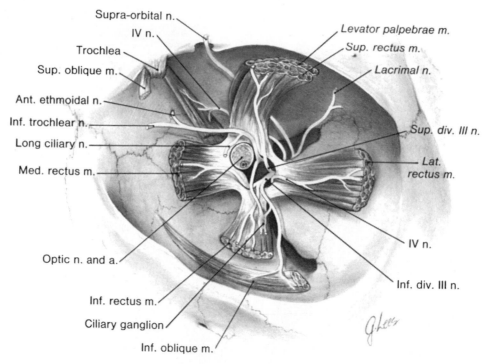

Supra-orbital n.
IV n.
Trochlea
Sup. oblique m.
Ant. ethmoidal n.
Inf. trochlear n.
Long ciliary n.
Med. rectus m.
Optic n. and a.
Inf. rectus m.
Ciliary ganglion
Inf. oblique m.
Levator palpebrae m.
Sup. rectus m.
Lacrimal n.
Sup. div. III n.
Lat. rectus m.
IV n.
Inf. div. III n.

Figure 2.23. View of the posterior orbit showing the relationship of the optic nerve to the ocular motor nerves and extraocular muscles. (Redrawn from Wolff E. Anatomy of the Eye and Orbit. 6th ed. Philadelphia: WB Saunders, 1968.)

INTRACRANIAL OPTIC NERVE

The intracranial portion of each optic nerve exits past a firm fold of dura that covers it superiorly and to some extent on both sides. The distance between the optic nerves as they exit from the optic canal averages 13 mm. The two nerves then extend posteriorly, superiorly, and medially to join at the optic chiasm.

The length of the intracranial segment of the normal optic nerve varies considerably. It is usually about 10 mm long, but it may be as short as 3 mm or as long as 16 mm. This portion of the nerve is about 4.5 to 5.0 mm in average diameter, but it is flattened and thus is wider in the horizontal plane than in the vertical plane (Fig. 2.26). When the intracranial optic nerve is shorter than about 12 mm, the optic chiasm is positioned anteriorly, or "prefixed," and sits directly over the sella turcica. When the intracranial optic nerve is long (over 18 mm), the chiasm is positioned posteriorly to the dorsum sellae, or "post-fixed" (Fig.

2.27). The variation in the length of the optic nerve is extremely important with respect to the visual deficits caused by tumors in the suprasellar region (see Chapter 12).

The gyrus recti of the frontal lobes of the brain are above the optic nerves. On the ventral surface of each frontal lobe, the olfactory tract is separated from the optic nerve by the anterior cerebral and anterior communicating arteries. On the lateral side of the optic nerve, the internal carotid artery sometimes forms an immediate relationship as it emerges from the cavernous sinus. Because the intracranial optic nerve is in the region where the internal carotid artery bifurcates into the anterior cerebral and middle cerebral arteries, these vessels are often immediately adjacent to the optic nerve, as is the proximal portion of the posterior communicating artery.

The internal carotid artery supplies the optic nerve via the ophthalmic artery, which enters the optic canal inferior and lateral to the optic

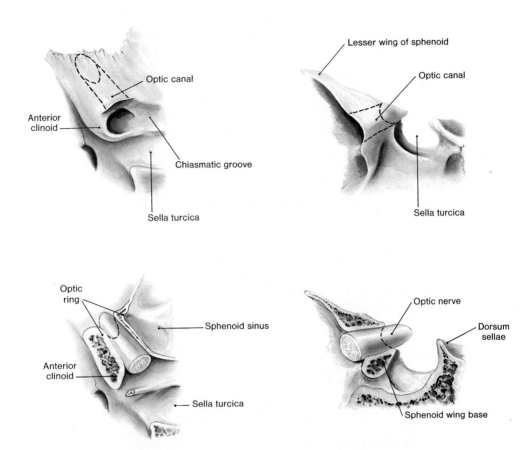

Figure 2.24.   Horizontal and lateral sketches of optic canal anatomy. The canal is shaped like a parallelogram inclined forward into the orbit. The canal arises from the base of the lesser sphenoid wing. (Redrawn from Maniscalco JE, Habal MB. Microanatomy of the optic canal. J Neurosurg 1978; 48:402–406.)

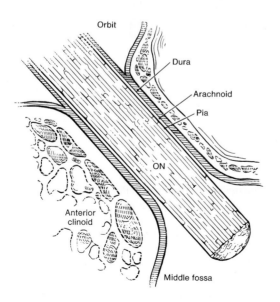

Figure 2.25.   Schematic drawing of the optic nerve sheaths showing their relationship to the optic nerve (ON) and to the surrounding sphenoid bone. The dura is tightly adherent to the bone within the optic canal. Within the orbit it divides into two layers, one of which remains as the outer sheath of the optic nerve, and the other becomes the orbital periosteum (periorbita). Intracranially, the dura leaves the optic nerve to become the periosteum of the sphenoid bone.

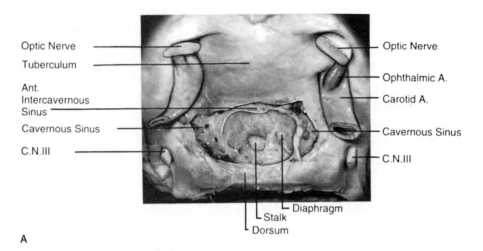

Optic Nerve

Tuberculum

Ant. Intercavernous Sinus

Cavernous Sinus

C.N.III

Optic Nerve

Ophthalmic A.

Carotid A.

Cavernous Sinus

C.N.III

Diaphragm
Stalk
Dorsum

A

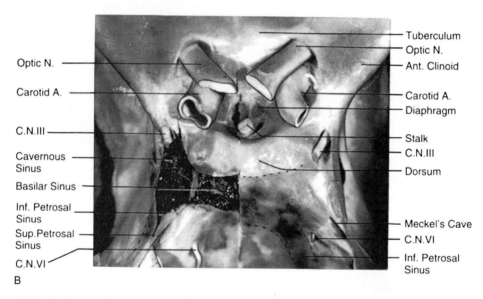

Optic N.

Carotid A.

C.N.III

Cavernous Sinus

Basilar Sinus

Inf. Petrosal Sinus

Sup. Petrosal Sinus

C.N.VI

Tuberculum
Optic N.
Ant. Clinoid

Carotid A.
Diaphragm

Stalk
C.N.III

Dorsum

Meckel's Cave

C.N.VI

Inf. Petrosal Sinus

B

Figure 2.26. The intracranial portions of the optic nerves viewed from above and posteriorly. *A.* Only the proximal portions of the optic nerves are seen as they emerge from the optic canals. Note their flattened appearance. *B.* The optic nerves are seen almost in their entirety. Again note that they have an oval or elliptical shape, with the widest diameter in the horizontal plane. (Reprinted with permission from Renn WH, Rhoton AL Jr. Microsurgical anatomy of the sellar region. J Neurosurg 1975;43:288–298.)

nerve (see Fig. 2.26). It is separated from the nerve, however, by a dural sheath that covers it throughout the length of the canal. The anatomic relationship of the optic nerve and the internal carotid artery and its branches account for the visual deficits that occur in some cases of dolichoectasia or aneurysms of the internal carotid, ophthalmic, and anterior cerebral arteries. Infer-

omedially, the sphenoid sinus has an important relationship to the optic nerve.

OPTIC NERVE PHYSIOLOGY

As noted above, there are at least two classes of retinal ganglion cells in humans. About 80 to 90% of these cells are of small to moderate size, are concentrated in the macula, have small-cali-

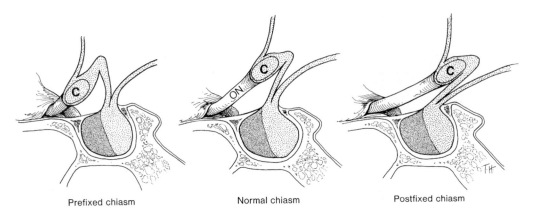

Prefixed chiasm   Normal chiasm   Postfixed chiasm

Figure 2.27.   Schematic drawing of three sagittal sections of the optic chiasm and sellar region. *Left:* The position of a pre-fixed chiasm above the tuberculum sellae. *Center:* The position of a normal chiasm above the diaphragma sellae. *Right:* The position of a post-fixed chiasm above the dorsum sellae. (Redrawn from Rhoton AL Jr, Harris FS, Renn WH. Microsurgical anatomy of the sellar region and cavernous sinus. In: Glaser JS, ed. Neuro-Ophthalmology Symposium of the University of Miami and the Bascom Palmer Eye Institute. St. Louis: CV Mosby, 1977:75–105.)

ber axons, and project to the parvocellular layers of the dorsal LGN (the P-cell system). P-cells have color-opponent physiology and are thought to subserve high-contrast, high-spatial frequency resolution. In contrast, large cells with large, fast-conducting axons comprise about 10 to 20% of the retinal ganglion cell population. These M-cells project to the magnocellular layers of the LGN and are primarily involved with noncolor information of high-temporal and low-spatial frequency. Conduction velocities in optic nerve fibers are much faster than those in the unmyelinated but similar caliber fibers in the retina, ranging from 1.3 to 20 meters per second.

TOPOGRAPHIC ANATOMY OF THE OPTIC NERVE

Fibers from peripheral ganglion cells occupy a more peripheral position in the optic disc, whereas fibers from ganglion cells located closer to the optic disc occupy a more central position. The arrangement of fibers in the optic disc and distal optic nerve corresponds generally to the topographic distribution of fibers in the retina. Fibers from the superior portion of the retina are located in the superior part of the optic nerve head; fibers from the inferior retina are located inferiorly in this region; and nasal and temporal fibers are on their respective sides. The papillomacular bundle is a sector-shaped structure that occupies about one-third of the temporal optic disc, adjacent to the central vessels. This bundle of fibers gradually moves centrally in the more

distal (posterior) portions of the orbital optic nerve. The gradual movement of the macular fibers to the center of the orbital optic nerve allows the uncrossed upper and lower retinal fibers to come together (Fig. 2.28). Dorsal (superior) and ventral (inferior) macular fibers retain their relative positions throughout the nerve, whereas crossed macular fibers lie nasal to the uncrossed fibers. Indeed, all the retinal fibers retain their relative positions throughout the visual pathways; that is, upper fibers remain upper and lower remain lower, except in the optic tract and at the LGN, where there is a rotation of 90° degrees that becomes straightened out in the optic radiations (see Chapter 12).

Within the intracranial portion of the optic nerve, the axons lose their retinotopic order to some extent because some axons decussate within the optic chiasm and some do not. The macular fibers do not have a precise localization in the posterior nerve and the gradual inclination inward of the macular fibers in the most posterior portions of the nerve allows for regrouping of the peripheral visual fibers.

Most of the visual axons, whether crossed or uncrossed, pass directly through the chiasm into the ipsilateral (uncrossed) or contralateral (crossed) optic tract. However, as they enter the chiasm, some ventral crossed fibers, primarily from the inferonasal retina of the contralateral eye and serving the superotemporal portion of the contralateral visual field, are believed to loop anteriorly 1 to 2 mm into the terminal portion

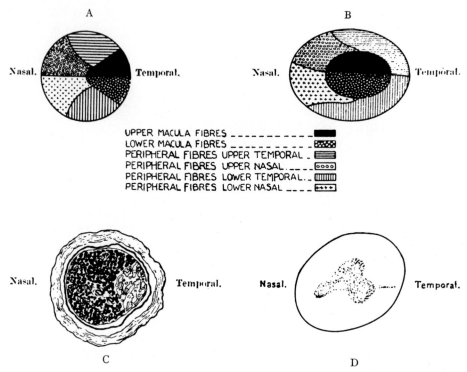

UPPER MACULA FIBRES _____ ▮

LOWER MACULA FIBRES _____ ▨

PERIPHERAL FIBRES UPPER TEMPORAL _ ▤

PERIPHERAL FIBRES UPPER NASAL ____ ⊙⊙⊙⊙

PERIPHERAL FIBRES LOWER TEMPORAL__ ⫿⫿⫿⫿

PERIPHERAL FIBRES LOWER NASAL ____ ⊹⊹⊹

Figure 2.28. Fiber arrangement in the optic nerve. *A.* In the distal portion of the optic nerve. *B.* In the proximal portion of the optic nerve. *C.* A transverse section of the optic nerve in its distal portion in a case of atrophy of the papillomacular bundle. *D.* Secondary degeneration in the proximal portion of the optic nerve after a macular lesion. (Reprinted with permission from Duke-Elder S. Textbook of Ophthalmology. Vol 1. St. Louis: CV Mosby, 1932.)

of the opposite optic nerve before turning posteriorly to continue through the chiasm and into the optic tract. This loop is called **Wilbrand's knee.** There is some evidence that Wilbrand's knee is not a true anatomic structure but is, in fact, an artifact that develops in both humans and nonhuman primates with longstanding unilateral optic atrophy. However, Wilbrand's knee clearly exists from a clinical standpoint. Patients with a monocular optic neuropathy caused by a lesion that has damaged the distal optic nerve at its junction with the optic chiasm not infrequently have an asymptomatic superior temporal defect in the visual field of the contralateral eye. Whether or not this contralateral visual field defect is caused by damage to Wilbrand's knee, the clinical syndrome is of extreme clinical importance in the localization of lesions in this region (see Chapter 12).

TOPOGRAPHIC DIAGNOSIS OF RETINAL LESIONS

Retinal diseases may be divided into two main groups: 1) those affecting the detecting apparatus—the receptor cells and their synapses; and 2) those affecting the conducting apparatus—the ganglion cell and nerve fiber layers. In many cases, the diagnosis is obvious from the appearance of the affected region of the retina. In other cases, however, it is possible to diagnose retinal dysfunction only from other aspects of the clinical examination. Indeed, patients with "unexplained visual loss" may, in fact, have a disorder of the retina that may not be obvious during a clinical examination.

VISUAL ACUITY IN RETINAL DISEASE

Central vision may or may not be affected by disease that damages the retina. Disorders that cause dysfunction only of extramacular retina typically are unassociated with a reduction in central acuity, whereas macular disorders and disorders that damage the entire retina invariably reduce central vision. Most disorders that affect the macula are easily detected by a careful funduscopic examination, particularly when the macula is examined with a slit lamp biomicroscope using a corneal contact lens, a 78- or 90-diopter hand-held lens, or a Hruby lens. Nevertheless, some disorders, such as central serous chorioretinopathy, cystoid macular edema, and epiretinal membrane formation (surface wrinkling retinopathy, cellophane maculopathy) can easily be overlooked (Fig. 2.29). In other diseases that affect the macula, such as macular cone dystrophy, there are often no changes that can be observed in the macula, even though the patient has decreased central vision and a visual field defect. In such cases, the diagnosis of retinal disease may be suspected if there is associated metamorphopsia (an irregularity or distor-

tion in the appearance of viewed objects), photophobia, nyctalopia (night blindness), or hemeralopia (the inability to see as distinctly in a bright light as in a dim one). These symptoms occur much more often in patients with ocular disease than in patients with neurologic disease. Photophobia should be obvious during the examination. Evidence of metamorphopsia may be detected in patients with and without the complaint of distortion of objects by using an Amsler grid (Fig. 2.30). The results of a photostress test usually are abnormal in such patients, as are the results of fluorescein angiography, focal electroretinography, or both (see Chapter 1).

COLOR VISION IN RETINAL DISEASE

Color vision is often but not always abnormal in patients with retinal disease. For instance, patients with central serous chorioretinopathy and epiretinal membrane formation rarely have any significant dyschromatopsia, whereas patients with macular cone or cone-rod dystrophies usu-

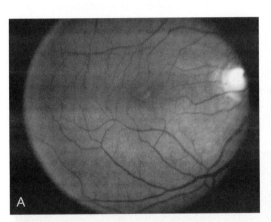

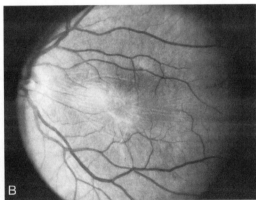

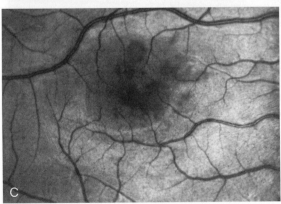

Figure 2.29. Subtle macular lesions causing visual loss. *A.* Pigment changes in the right macula of a patient with ''unexplained'' central visual loss. *B.* Epiretinal membrane in the left macula of a patient complaining of blurred vision in the eye. *C.* Changes in the right macula of a patient who complained of decreased central vision in the eye after blunt ocular trauma. It was initially suspected that he had a traumatic optic neuropathy or was malingering.

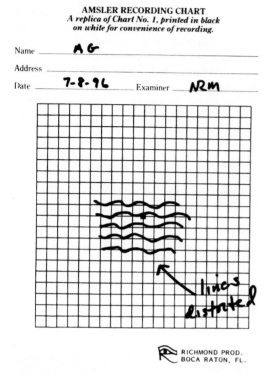

AMSLER RECORDING CHART
*A replica of Chart No. 1, printed in black
on white for convenience of recording.*

Name _____ **A G** _____

Address _____

Date _____ **7-8-96** _____ Examiner _____ **NRM** _____

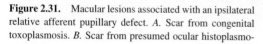

RICHMOND PROD.
BOCA RATON, FL.

Figure 2.30. Distortion of lines on Amsler grid in a patient with unilateral visual loss. The patient had central serous chorioretinopathy.

ally do, and such patients may even develop difficulties with color vision as the initial sign of the disease. In such cases, the correct diagnosis is not made until other studies, such as photostress testing, fluorescein angiography, or electroretinography are performed. Retinal disorders are more likely to produce either generalized loss of color vision or a blue-yellow dyschromatopsia, but there are sufficient exceptions that make the pattern of color vision loss an unreliable diagnostic criterion.

RELATIVE AFFERENT PUPILLARY DEFECT IN RETINAL DISEASE

A relative afferent pupillary defect can be detected clinically as well as with neutral density filters in most patients with unilateral or asymmetric retinal disease. In most cases, the retinal disease is severe, affects most of the retina or the entire macula, and is obvious during a funduscopic examination (Fig. 2.31). If a relative afferent pupillary defect is observed in a patient with decreased visual acuity associated with some macular drusen, central serous chorioretinopathy, cystoid macular edema, an epiretinal membrane, or a normal-appearing fundus, a lesion affecting the optic nerve should be suspected (Fig. 2.32).

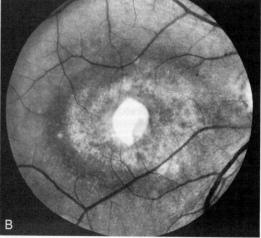

Figure 2.31. Macular lesions associated with an ipsilateral relative afferent pupillary defect. *A.* Scar from congenital toxoplasmosis. *B.* Scar from presumed ocular histoplasmo-

sis. Note that both lesions are quite obvious and would not be overlooked during an ophthalmoscopic examination, even if the pupils were not dilated.

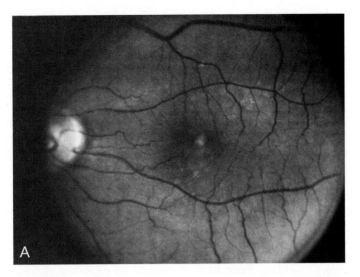

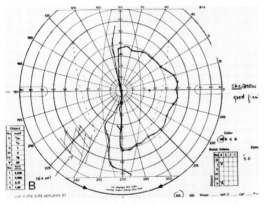

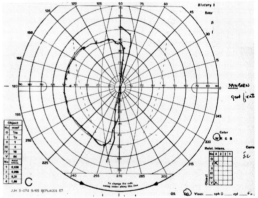

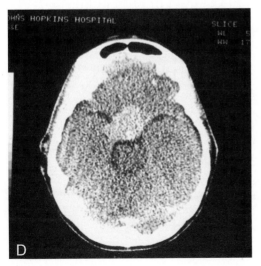

Figure 2.32.   Macular changes in the left fundus of a patient who had visual acuity of 20/50 in the eye associated with an ipsilateral relative afferent pupillary defect. The right ocular fundus appeared normal. The patient was referred for treatment of central serous chorioretinopathy. *A.* There are mild pigmentary disturbances in the left macula; however, it was thought that these abnormalities were not sufficiently severe to account for the relative afferent pupillary defect. *B.* The visual field of the left eye reveals a temporal hemianopia that is almost complete. *C.* The visual field of the right eye also shows a complete temporal hemianopia. *D.* Computed tomographic scan, axial view, after intravenous injection of contrast material, reveals a large suprasellar mass. The lesion was a pituitary adenoma. Following surgery to remove the tumor, the patient's vision improved to 20/30 in the left eye; the relative afferent pupillary defect disappeared; and the visual fields improved.

VISUAL FIELD DEFECTS
IN RETINAL DISEASE

When the photoreceptors are affected, the defect in the visual field corresponds to the retinal defect in position, shape, extent, and intensity. When the ganglion cell or nerve fiber layer is damaged, however, the field defect does not conform to the size and shape of the lesion but rather to the receptive field represented by the ganglion cells whose fibers are damaged. Thus, a small lesion situated close to the optic disc that damages only photoreceptors usually causes a small scotoma, whereas a lesion of the same size that damages the ganglion cells in, and the nerve fibers that pass through, the same area may result in an extensive defect in the visual field (Fig. 2.33). Conversely, a small lesion in the periphery that damages only a few fibers transmitting

impulses from widely separated ganglion cells may produce a small field defect that may be difficult or even impossible to detect.

Diseases that cause photoreceptor damage usually produce a greater loss of the visual field when the field is tested with blue stimuli than when it is tested with red stimuli. This observation is critical because the situation is reversed in disorders that damage the conducting apparatus of the retina. In lesions of the ganglion cells, retinal nerve fiber layer, and optic nerve, there usually is a more pronounced loss of the visual field for red than for blue.

If a lesion superotemporal or inferotemporal to the optic disc damages peripheral visual fibers, the field defect is arcuate in shape because the fibers from peripheral ganglion cells arch around the papillomacular bundle. The field de-

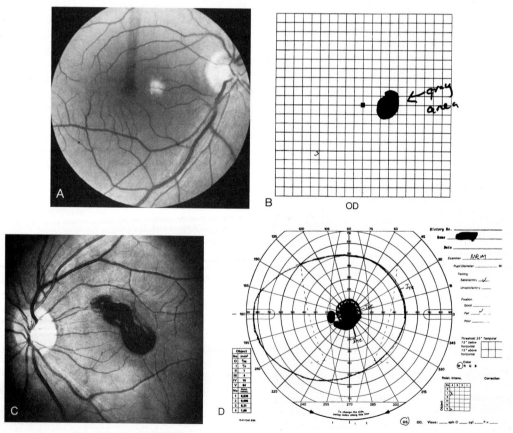

Figure 2.33. Variation in visual fields caused by posterior pole lesions. *A–B:* Small chorioretinal scar adjacent to right fovea. Because this lesion is located in the deep retina at the level of the photoreceptors and retinal pigment epithelium,

it produces only a small central scotoma. *C–D:* Hemorrhage in the left macula in another patient. This lesion has produced a large central scotoma associated with an inferior arcuate defect because of its superficial location in the retina.

fect is, of course, situated nasal to the blind spot. If the lesion is nasal to the optic disc, it damages a nasal bundle. The resultant field defect is temporal and fan-shaped, because fibers from ganglion cells located nasal to the optic disc take a direct path to the disc.

An arcuate defect in the visual field may indicate a defect in the nerve fiber layer. When such a retinal lesion is present, it usually can be identified by ophthalmoscopic examination. Because of the anatomy of the temporal raphe that separates fibers from ganglion cells located above the horizontal midline from those from ganglion cells below the horizontal midline, there is often a sharp dividing line between the area of the scotoma and the functioning upper or lower field. This is particularly evident in large arcuate scotomas, so much so that visual fields performed using a tangent screen or by automated static perimetry may suggest complete loss of the superior or inferior hemifield unless the entire field is tested.

Again, when a retinal lesion affects the receptor cells, the visual field defect corresponds fairly accurately to the extent of the lesion. If the lesion is in the superior temporal retina, the field defect is in the inferior nasal quadrant, and so on. The density of the scotoma depends on the completeness of retinal destruction, and it is this factor that makes quantitative perimetry valuable (see Chapter 1).

Retinal photoreceptors project to ganglion cells, and the axons of the ganglion cells comprise the nerve fiber layer that, in turn, makes up the optic nerve. Clearly, then, any visual field defect that can be produced by an inner retinal lesion can also be produced by a lesion of the optic nerve. Ophthalmoscopic evidence pointing to the retina as the site of the lesion is conclusive, but lack of an ophthalmoscopically visible retinal abnormality does not necessarily indicate that the retina is not the site of the lesion.

Most visual field defects in the central fields that are caused by retinal lesions are associated with ophthalmoscopically visible changes. In patients with macular lesions, the field defects are those already described as resulting from lesions of the receptor cells; that is, the field defect occupies an area consistent with the size of the lesion (Fig. 2.34). However, some macular lesions that produce a central scotoma cannot be easily detected by ophthalmoscopy. In most of these cases, small lesions of the retina or RPE may be diagnosed using red-free ophthalmoscopy, slit lamp biomicroscopy with a contact lens or a 90- or 78-diopter hand-held lens, fluorescein angiography, or a combination of these techniques (Fig. 2.35). In other cases, the diagnosis cannot be made without a focal ERG.

Of course, not all monocular field defects are caused by retinal or optic nerve lesions. Patients with significant opacities of the media (e.g., cataract) may develop such defects. In addition, patients with nonorganic disease can produce spurious central, paracentral, and even quadrantanopic and hemianopic field defects, regardless of whether they are tested with kinetic or static perimetric techniques (see Chapter 23). It should also be emphasized that a spurious central or paracentral scotoma may be charted if the central field of an eye with a high refractive error or under a cycloplegic is plotted without correction for the refractive error (see Chapter 1).

Many patients with various macular dystrophies, macular degeneration, or other disorders affecting the macula (e.g., central serous chorioretinopathy) not only have central defects in the visual fields but also complain of metamorphopsia or micropsia. These symptoms are caused by distortion or displacement of the retinal photoreceptors. **Metamorphopsia**—an irregularity or distortion in the appearance of viewed objects—is usually caused by a distortion of the normal alignment of the photoreceptors. When there is increased separation among cones (and among rods to a lesser extent because of the central position of the lesion), there is an apparent decrease in the size of objects (micropsia). The foveal cones are already so close to each other that it is unlikely that an apparent increase in the size of objects (macropsia) can occur from further crowding together of these cells. We have never heard a patient with a retinal lesion complain of macropsia. Changes in the apparent size of viewed objects usually result from primary retinal damage, but such symptoms may also be described by patients with acquired cerebral disorders that affect perception (see Chapter 13).

Damage to the papillomacular area of the retina results in a central scotoma joined with the physiologic blind spot: a cecocentral scotoma (Fig. 2.36). A cecocentral scotoma may result from damage to the papillomacular bundle alone or may occur in conjunction with peripheral contraction of the visual field.

An arcuate visual field defect usually results from damage to peripheral retinal nerve fibers or ganglion cells in the superior or inferior arcuate nerve fiber bundles, but such a defect may also be produced when specific macular fibers

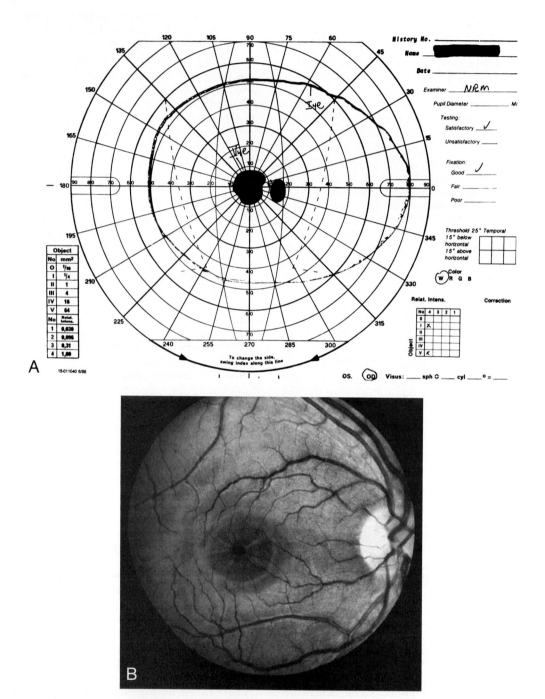

Figure 2.34. Small central scotoma caused by a macular lesion. *A.* Kinetic perimetry reveals a small (7°) central scotoma in the visual field of the right eye of a patient with visual acuity of 20/100 in the eye. *B.* Hole in the right macula of the same patient.

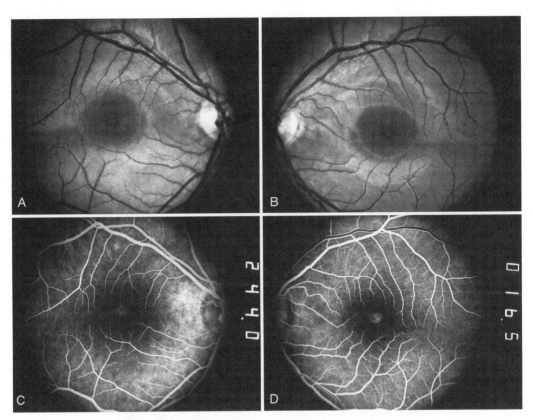

Figure 2.35.   Macular lesions in a 13-year-old girl with unexplained loss of vision in both eyes. Visual acuity was 20/80 OU. *A-B.* The maculae appear fairly normal. *C-D.* However, fluorescein angiography reveals impressive pig-ment epithelial changes in the macula, consistent with the decreased vision. The patient was diagnosed as having a macular dystrophy of unknown cause.

are damaged. In such cases, there is a central field defect that is not circular but instead is limited on one side by the horizontal meridian (Fig. 2.37). This visual field defect may occur in patients with occlusion of the blood supply of the superior or inferior portion of the macula or occasionally in patients with glaucoma. In both settings, the scotoma is associated with normal visual acuity, because it does not completely destroy the macula. Almost any lesion—whether ischemic, inflammatory, infiltrative, or compressive—can cause an arcuate field defect that, as noted above, may be located in either the inner retina or the optic nerve.

A roughly circular pericentral scotoma may be observed in patients with macular or papillomacular disease. Such a scotoma, when unilateral, always indicates damage to the macula. When bilateral pericentral scotomas are present, there is usually bilateral macular disease; how-ever, bilateral "pericentral" scotomas can develop from lesions that damage the posterior aspects of both occipital poles (see Chapter 14). When such lesions occur bilaterally at the occipital tips, bilateral "central" scotomas occur. Actually, however, these visual field defects are bilateral homonymous scotomas, and kinetic or static perimetry will generally disclose a vertical step between the two hemianopic scotomas, indicating their true nature.

Annular or ring scotomas occur in a variety of conditions, most notably in patients with various pigmentary retinopathies. Ring scotomas may also occur in patients with open-angle glaucoma, but in such cases the ring is actually caused by the coalescence of upper and lower arcuate scotomas originating from the physiologic blind spot and extending across the vertical midline into the nasal visual field. Rarer causes of annular or ring scotomas include retinitis, choroiditis,

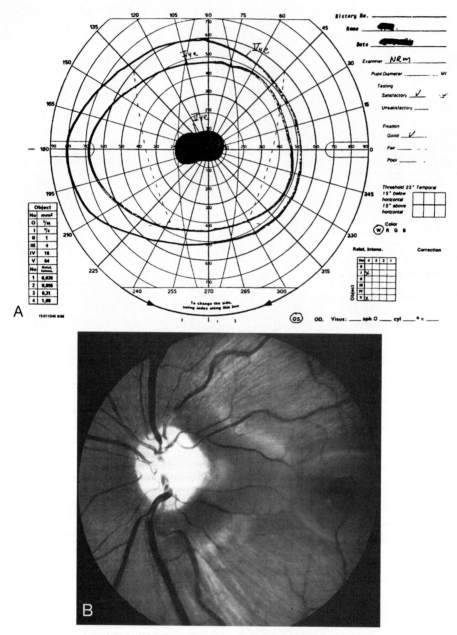

Figure 2.36. Cecocentral scotoma caused by a lesion in the papillomacular bundle. *A.* The patient has a small cecocentral scotoma in the visual field of the left eye. *B.* There is a serous detachment of the retina in the papillomacular bundle of the left eye, associated with a temporal optic pit.

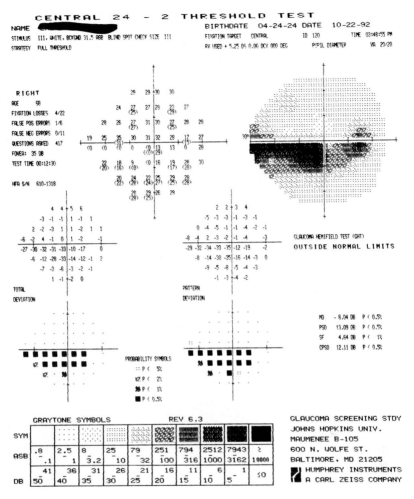

Figure 2.37. ''Central'' scotoma in the right eye of a patient with open-angle glaucoma. Although the visual field defect is central in location, it is actually an arcuate/altitudinal scotoma that is located adjacent but just inferior to the horizontal midline. The visual acuity in this eye is 20/20.

blinding by diffuse light, retinal migraine, malnutrition, and myopia. Similar defects may be seen in various optic neuropathies, particularly those caused by ischemia, compression, and inflammation. A ring scotoma may persist after incomplete resolution of a preexisting central scotoma in patients with retinal or optic nerve disease. Occasionally, ring or annular scotomas are found in patients with nonorganic visual loss (see Chapter 23). In such patients, the scotomas are typically very narrow.

A ring scotoma can be detected in most types of pigmentary retinopathy (e.g., retinitis pigmentosa) if the visual field is carefully examined. In some cases, however, the peripheral field is so contracted and central vision so reduced that the ring scotoma may not be detected even when careful perimetry is performed.

In general, a unilateral temporal or nasal hemianopia that respects the vertical midline is either nonorganic or caused by dysfunction of the optic nerve (see Chapter 4). Nevertheless, in rare instances, a monocular hemianopia is caused by sector retinitis pigmentosa (Fig. 2.38).

APPEARANCE OF THE OPTIC DISC IN RETINAL DISEASE

The optic nerve is composed primarily of axons whose cell bodies are the ganglion cells of the retina. Thus, any retinal disorder that di-

Figure 2.38. Monocular temporal hemianopia with foveal sparing and respect of the vertical midline in the right eye of a patient with a retinal degeneration in that eye. Visual field testing was performed using the Humphrey Central 30-2 Threshold Test. (Reprinted with permission from Johnson LN, Rabinowitz YS, Hepler RS. Hemianopia respecting the vertical meridian and with foveal sparing from retinal degeneration. Neurology 1989;39:872–873.)

CENTRAL 30 - 2 THRESHOLD TEST

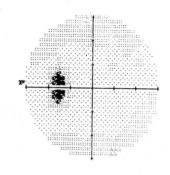
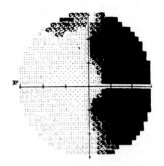

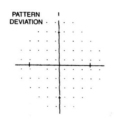
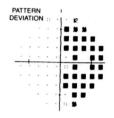

	LEFT		RIGHT	
QUESTIONS ASKED	443	QUESTIONS ASKED	426
FIXATION LOSSES	0/23	FIXATION LOSSES	0/23
FALSE POS ERRORS	0/9	FALSE POS ERRORS	0/12
FALSE NEG ERRORS	1/12	FALSE NEG ERRORS	0/13
TEST TIME 00:12:30		TEST TIME 00:12:42	
FOVEA: 39 DB		FOVEA: 37 DB	

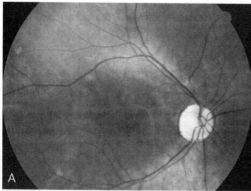
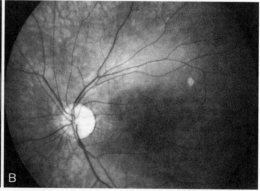

Figure 2.39. Optic atrophy in retinal dystrophy. *A–B:* The right and left optic discs, respectively, of a 20-year-old woman with visual acuity of 20/50 OU, abnormal color vision, and nonspecific visual field defects. Both optic discs show diffuse pallor, and the retinal arteries are somewhat narrowed. The patient was found to have a retinal cone dystrophy. (Reprinted with permission from Newman NJ, Slavin M, Newman SA. Optic disc pallor: a false localizing sign. Surv Ophthalmol 1993;37:273–282.)

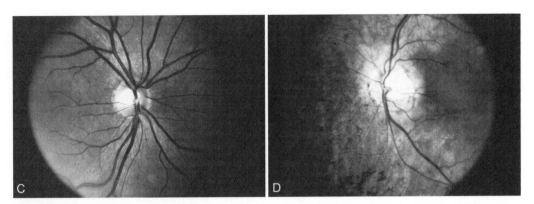

Figure 2.39 *(continued).   C–D:* Optic atrophy in unilateral retinitis pigmentosa. *C.* The right optic disc is normal. Note healthy color of the disc and normal-appearing peripapillary retinal nerve fiber layer. *D.* The left optic disc is pale. Note marked pigmentary change in the posterior pole, as well as marked narrowing of the retinal arteries. (Courtesy of Dr. Daniel Finkelstein.)

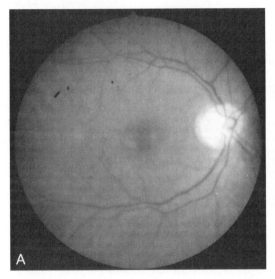
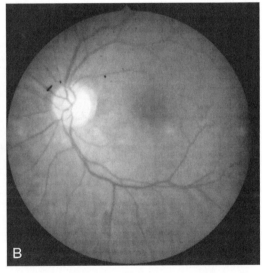

Figure 2.40.   Optic atrophy in vitamin A deficiency. The patient was a woman who developed bilateral visual loss and cecocentral scotomas several years after a jejunoileal bypass for morbid obesity. An electroretinogram revealed evidence of a retinopathy affecting the photoreceptors, and laboratory studies revealed a reduced concentration of vitamin A in the patient's serum. The patient's visual function improved after vitamin A therapy. Both the right (*A*) and left (*B*) optic discs are pale. (Courtesy of Dr. Eric Eggenberger.)

rectly or indirectly damages the ganglion cells or their axons in the retinal nerve fiber layer will eventually produce optic atrophy. Indeed, damage to the ganglion cell body or the NFL is tantamount to damage to the optic nerve; that is, there will be visual loss, a relative afferent pupillary defect if the damage is unilateral or asymmetric, and ultimately optic atrophy. Be-cause the central retinal arterial and venous circulations subserve the inner layers of the retina (including the ganglion cell and nerve fiber layers), retinal vascular occlusive events will result in inner retinal damage, visual loss, and eventual optic atrophy. Acute vascular events involving the retina—including central and branch retinal artery occlusions, ophthalmic artery occlusions,

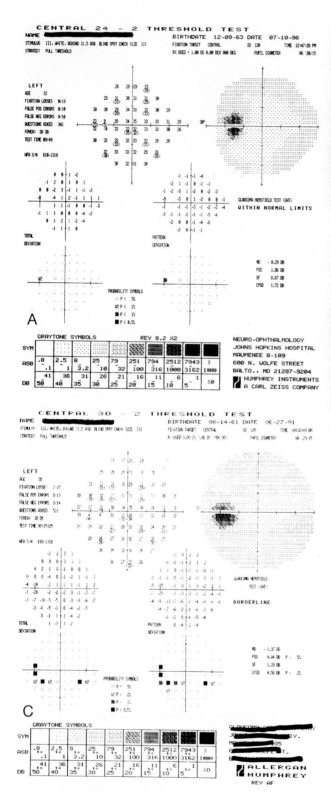

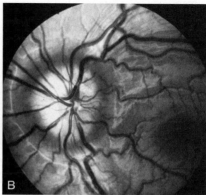

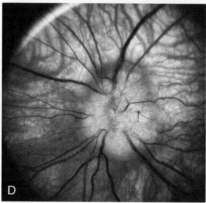

Figure 2.41. Enlargement of the blind spot from congenital and acquired abnormalities of the optic disc. *A.* Enlargement of the blind spot in the visual field of the left eye of a 33-year-old woman with no visual complaints, but who was noted to have an elevated left optic disc. *B.* Appearance of the patient's left optic disc, showing anomalous elevation of the left optic disc. Ultrasonography revealed deep (buried) drusen in the prelaminar portion of the optic nerve. *C.* Enlargement of the blind spot in a 30-year-old obese woman with headaches. *D.* Appearance of left optic disc, showing chronic swelling. An evaluation revealed increased intracranial pressure.

and central retinal vein occlusions—have a dramatic and distinct funduscopic appearance, permitting immediate correct diagnosis. However, over time, the retinal findings resolve, and the optic disc becomes pale. In such cases, subsequent narrowing and sheathing of the retinal arteries or the presence of a visible embolus within the retinal circulation may provide clues as to the etiology of the original event.

Loss of the NFL and optic atrophy are not uncommon in patients with various photoreceptor dystrophies and degenerations, particularly those affecting the cones (Fig. 2.39). Bilateral secondary optic atrophy can be seen in patients with cone dystrophies, rod/cone dystrophies, paraneoplastic retinopathies, and the retinopathy of vitamin A deficiency (Fig. 2.40). Clues that suggest retinal cone dysfunction include profound dyschromatopsia, photophobia and hemeralopia, retinal arterial attenuation, and, eventually, changes in the appearance of the maculae, often resembling a bull's-eye (bull's-eye maculopathy).

BLIND SPOT IN TOPICAL DIAGNOSIS

The blind spot is a negative scotoma that is the projection of the optic disc in the visual field. The optic disc is located nasal to the fovea, and its center is slightly above it. Thus, the blind spot is temporal to the point of fixation, and its center is slightly below it.

The blind spot has both an absolute and a relative portion. The relative portion is a band, about 1° in width, that surrounds the absolute scotoma. In this band, white objects of 1 to 2 mm can be seen when a subject is tested at 2 meters. This zone of relative scotoma is caused by the gradual rather than abrupt termination of the retina at the edge of the optic disc, and in it metamorphopsia can often be demonstrated.

The blind spot becomes enlarged from peripapillary retinal dysfunction. This dysfunction can occur because the peripapillary retina is diseased, as occurs in patients with the so-called "big blind spot syndrome" and related disorders like acute zonal occult outer retinopathy (AZOOR) and the multiple evanescent white dot syndrome (MEWDS), or because expansion of optic disc tissue encroaches on the peripapillary retina, as occurs in optic disc swelling and in pseudopapilledema (Fig. 2.41).

FOR MORE INFORMATION:
See Walsh & Hoyt's Clinical Neuro-Ophthalmology, 5th edition, Volume 1, Chapter 2, pages 25–56; Chapter 3, pages 57–83; and Chapter 8, pages 237–259.

Anomalies of the Optic Disc

The optic nerve and retina are the only portions of the central nervous system (CNS) that can be viewed directly during the clinical examination. The appearance of the optic disc on ophthalmoscopic examination is thus of major importance in the diagnosis of an optic neuropathy and in the differentiation of congenital from acquired abnormalities of the optic nerve.

In acquired disorders, the optic disc initially has only two ways to respond to the many pathologic processes that can damage the optic nerve. It can remain normal in appearance, or it can swell. If the process produces irreversible damage to the optic nerve, the optic disc will eventually become pale, regardless of the underlying process that caused the damage in the first place (see Chapter 4). Although most congenital abnormalities of the optic disc are easily distinguished from acquired optic disc swelling or pallor, some congenital anomalies produce an appearance that mimics acquired disease.

Ophthalmologists and neurologists are frequently asked to evaluate patients with anomalous optic discs. A comprehensive evaluation requires an understanding of the ophthalmoscopic features, associated neuro-ophthalmologic findings, pathogenesis, and appropriate ancillary studies for each anomaly. Increased recognition of the ocular and systemic associations related to each anomaly has advanced our understanding of its pathogenesis. For instance, different forms of excavated optic disc anomalies that were previously lumped together as colobomatous defects are now subclassified. This has enhanced our ability to predict the likelihood of associated CNS anomalies based solely on the appearance of the optic disc. Additionally, the widespread clinical application of computed tomographic (CT) scans and magnetic resonance imaging (MRI) has enabled us to more accurately identify associated CNS anomalies and predict the likelihood of subsequent neurodevelopmental and endocrinologic problems.

Certain general principles are particularly useful in the evaluation and management of patients with anomalous optic discs:

- Children with bilateral optic disc anomalies generally present in infancy with poor vision and nystagmus; those with unilateral optic disc anomalies generally present during their preschool years with sensory esotropia.
- CNS malformations are common in patients with malformed optic discs. Small

discs are associated with a variety of malformations of the cerebral hemispheres, pituitary infundibulum, and midline intracranial structures (septum pellucidum, corpus callosum). Large optic discs of the morning glory configuration are associated with the transsphenoidal form of basal encephalocele, whereas large optic discs with a colobomatous configuration may be associated with systemic anomalies in a variety of coloboma syndromes. MRI is advisable in young children with abnormally small optic discs (unilateral or bilateral) and in young children with large optic discs who have neurodevelopmental deficits, endocrinologic signs, or systemic anomalies (particularly midfacial anomalies suggestive of transsphenoidal encephalocele). The finding of a discrete V- or tongue-shaped zone of infrapapillary retinochoroidal depigmentation adjacent to a malformed optic disc should prompt a search for a transsphenoidal encephalocele.

- Any structural ocular abnormality that reduces visual acuity in infancy may lead to superimposed amblyopia. A trial of occlusion therapy is warranted in young children with unilateral optic disc anomalies and decreased vision. However, prolonged occlusion in children with unilaterally malformed discs who show no early treatment response may be psychologically and developmentally detrimental.

PSEUDOPAPILLEDEMA

The appearance of an optic disc that is anomalously elevated is often similar to that of a truly swollen optic disc. Because anomalously elevated discs are usually associated with normal visual sensory function (particularly visual acuity), the main differential diagnosis is between papilledema and the **pseudopapilledema** caused by anomalous disc elevation. In many instances, a patient is noted to have elevated optic discs or blurred disc margins during the course of a routine examination. The diagnostic uncertainty and alarm created by this finding overshadows the fact that the patient has no other signs or symptoms of increased intracranial pressure. In other cases, the patient is well except for a history of nonspecific headaches or other symptoms thought to be consistent with increased intracranial pressure. Thus, many pa-

tients with pseudopapilledema are subjected to neuroimaging, lumbar puncture, and extensive laboratory studies before the correct diagnosis is made. In fact, the majority of cases of pseudopapilledema can be diagnosed correctly by a careful ophthalmoscopic examination. The remainder can usually be diagnosed correctly using one or more of several noninvasive diagnostic techniques.

Pseudopapilledema is generally separated into cases caused by drusen of the optic disc and cases without optic disc drusen. In the majority of patients, pseudopapilledema occurs as an isolated phenomenon. In some patients, however, pseudopapilledema is associated with a specific retinal disorder, such as pigmented paravenous retinochoroidal atrophy; in other patients it is part of a multisystem disorder, such as Down syndrome, Alagille syndrome (arteriohepatic dysplasia), Kenny syndrome (hypocalcemic dwarfism), or linear sebaceus nevus syndrome. An association of pseudopapilledema and orbital hypotelorism has also been described.

PSEUDOPAPILLEDEMA ASSOCIATED WITH OPTIC DISC DRUSEN

Drusen of the optic disc were first described clinically by Liebreich in 1868. The word "drusen" is of Germanic origin and originally meant tumor, swelling, or tumescence. The word was used in the mining industry about 500 years ago to indicate a crystal-filled space in a rock. Other terms for drusen are **hyaline bodies** and **colloid bodies.** Some drusen are easily visible with the ophthalmoscope; others are located anterior to the lamina cribrosa but are "buried" deep beneath the surface of the optic disc.

Epidemiology

In Scandinavia, the prevalence of drusen in a clinical series was 3.4 per 1000, and the prevalence increased by a factor of 10 in family members of patients with drusen, consistent with an autosomal-dominant mode of transmission. The prevalence of drusen in autopsy series is, as might be expected, somewhat higher than the prevalence in clinical studies, varying from 0.41 to 2.0% among several studies. Men and women are equally affected, and bilateral drusen occur in 67 to 85% of cases. The age at which visible drusen or pseudopapilledema caused by buried drusen is diagnosed varies widely, depending on the population studied. In one series of 98 patients with optic disc elevation and ophthalmoscopic evidence of drusen, for example, the ages of affected persons ranged from 7 to 73 years of age, with a mean age of 22 years.

Pseudopapilledema associated with disc drusen was once thought to occur more frequently in hyperopic eyes than in myopic or emmetropic eyes; however, this does not seem to be the case. The low prevalence of disc drusen in black patients may be attributable to racial variation in the size of the optic disc.

Natural History

The evolution of disc drusen is a dynamic process that is present at birth and continues throughout life. Although it is rare to see visible drusen or significant optic disc elevation in an infant, the involved optic disc begins to appear "full" during childhood and gradually acquires a tan, yellow, or straw color. The buried drusen gradually impart a scalloped appearance to the margin of the disc and produce subtle excrescences on the disc surface that tend to be located nasally. They later enlarge, calcify, and become increasingly visible, eventually deflecting the retinal vessels overlying the disc. Such changes are usually present by the second decade of life. Over time, the optic disc tissue overlying the drusen becomes increasingly thin, optic disc elevation diminishes, the disc gradually becomes pale, and the drusen become obvious to even the most inexperienced observer. Despite this progression, most patients remain asymptomatic and retain normal visual acuity throughout life.

Ophthalmoscopic Appearance of Visible Drusen

In some patients, a few drusen are localized to a particular portion of the optic disc, usually the nasal region. In other patients, they are scattered throughout the disc. In still others, drusen coalesce to form conglomerates that cover the entire disc.

Superficial drusen reflect whitish-yellow light, are globular, and vary in size from minute dots to granules 2 or 3 times the diameter of a retinal vessel. When illuminated directly by a beam of light from a direct or scanning laser ophthalmoscope or a slit lamp, drusen appear as round, slightly irregular excrescences (Fig. 3.1). Such drusen glow brightly at their edges, and uniformly, but less intensely, at their center. In indirect light, the side of a druse that is away from the light appears as a dark crescent in contrast to its glowing central region. Deeply situated drusen lack sharp margins, but they may still be illuminated by indirect light.

Ophthalmoscopic Appearance of Buried Disc Drusen

Optic discs that are elevated because of deep or buried drusen have several distinct features (Fig. 3.2):

1. The disc is not hyperemic, and there are no dilated capillaries on its surface.
2. Despite marked elevation of the disc, the surface vessels—both arteries and veins—are not obscured and are clearly visible as they pass across the disc.
3. The disc is smaller than normal.
4. The physiologic cup is usually absent.
5. The most elevated portion of the disc is usually the central area from which the vessels emerge.
6. Anomalous vascular patterns are often present on the disc surface, including an increased number of otherwise normal vessels, abnormal arterial and venous branchings, increased tortuosity, vascular loops, vascular shunts, and cilioretinal arteries.
7. Elevation is confined to the optic disc and does not extend to the peripapillary nerve fiber layer.
8. The peripapillary retinal nerve fiber layer retains its normal linear pattern of light reflexes or shows abnormalities indicative of nerve fiber atrophy.
9. The disc usually has an irregular border associated with pigment epithelial defects, giving the border a "moth-eaten" appearance.

These features allow most cases of pseudopapilledema caused by buried optic disc drusen to be distinguished from papilledema and other forms of true optic disc swelling (e.g., anterior optic neuritis, anterior ischemic optic neuropathy). For example, in papilledema, the disc swelling extends into the peripapillary retina and obscures the peripapillary retinal vasculature, whereas in pseudopapilledema, there is a discrete, sometimes grayish or straw-colored elevation of the disc without obscuration of vessels or opacification of peripapillary retina (Table 3.1 and Fig. 3.3). The graying or muddying of the peripapillary nerve fiber layer that occurs with

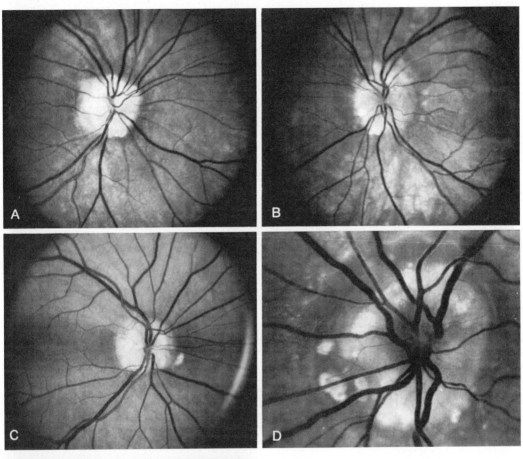

Figure 3.1. Appearance of superficial optic disc drusen. *A–E.* All of the discs show typical glistening, yellow globular excrescences that replace all or part of the disc tissue. The vessels overlying the discs are normal. Note that none of the discs have a central cup. Also note that some of the drusen are actually located outside the disc margins.

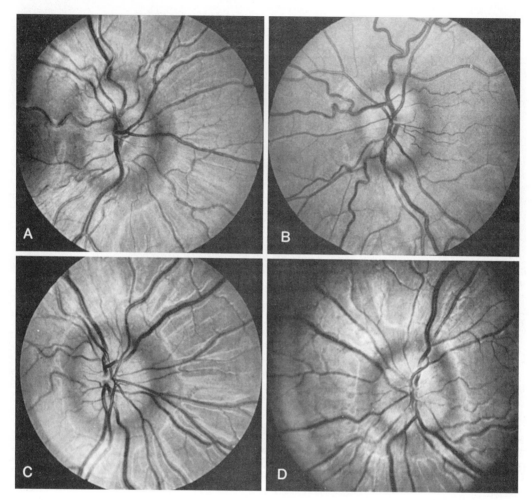

Figure 3.2. *A–D.* Disc elevation presumably caused by nonvisible intrapapillary drusen. In all cases, there is marked disc elevation without disc hyperemia, disturbance of the peripapillary retinal nerve fiber layer, or obscuration of the large vessels that cross the surface of the disc. Note that several of the discs show abnormal branchings of vessels on their surfaces, with absence of the central cup.

swelling of the optic disc from papilledema or other causes also distinguishes true disc swelling from pseudopapilledema associated with buried drusen in which light reflexes of the peripapillary nerve fiber layer appear sharp, and the elevated disc is often haloed by a crescentic peripapillary ring of light that reflects from the concave internal limiting membrane surrounding the elevation (see Fig. 3.2). This crescentic light reflex is absent in papilledema because of diffraction of light from distended peripapillary axons. One or more flame-shaped (splinter), subretinal, or subpigment epithelial hemorrhages are occasionally seen in the peripapillary region in eyes with optic disc drusen, but exudates, cotton-wool spots, hyperemia of the disc, and congestion of retinal veins are conspicuously absent.

Diagnostic Studies

The diagnosis of pseudopapilledema caused by optic disc drusen can be made in most cases by clinical examination alone, either because the drusen can easily be seen ophthalmoscopically or because of the characteristic features described above. In cases in which there remains doubt as to the true nature of the condition, the diagnosis of pseudopapilledema caused by dru-

Table 3.1

Ophthalmoscopic Features Useful in Differentiating Optic Disc Swelling from Pseudopapilledema Associated with Buried Drusen

OPTIC DISC SWELLING	PSEUDOPAPILLEDEMA WITH BURIED DRUSEN
Disc vasculature obscured at disc margins	Disc vasculature remains visible at disc margins
Elevation extends into peripapillary retina	Elevation confined to optic disc
Graying and muddying of peripapillary nerve fiber layer	Sharp peripapillary nerve fiber
Venous congestion	No venous congestion
± exudates	No exudates
Loss of optic cup only in moderate to severe disc swelling	Small cupless disc
Normal configuration of disc vasculature despite venous congestion	Increased major retinal vessels with early branching
No circumpapillary light reflex	Crescentic circumpapillary light reflex
Absence of spontaneous venous pulsations	Spontaneous venous pulsations may be present or absent

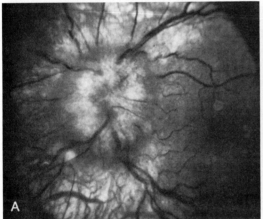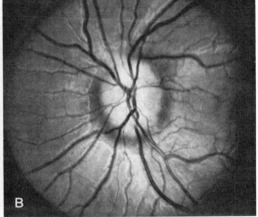

Figure 3.3. Comparison of papilledema and pseudopapilledema. *A.* Papilledema. The disc is elevated and hyperemic. There is distortion of the normal linear light reflexes from the peripapillary nerve fiber layer and obscuration of large vessels as they cross the disc surface. *B.* Pseudopapilledema. The disc is elevated but shows no hyperemia, disruption of the nerve fiber layer reflexes, or obscuration of vessels.

sen is frequently aided by several easily performed diagnostic studies.

In our experience, the most useful and sensitive diagnostic technique for the diagnosis of optic disc drusen is **ultrasonography.** Not only is this procedure extremely sensitive in demonstrating buried disc drusen (Fig. 3.4), it does not expose the patient to radiation. CT scanning, using magnified views of the globe with bone window settings, can also be used to detect calcification within one or both optic discs (Fig. 3.5). Although this technique exposes the patient to some radiation, the amount of exposure is minor, and the technique has the advantage over ultrasonography of providing simultaneous images of the brain. Because both CT scanning and ultrasonography readily detect buried (as well as visible) optic disc drusen, it is not surprising that authors differ as to which imaging modality is preferable. In addition, scanning laser ophthalmoscopy and optical coherence tomography can also be used to identify buried disc drusen. The overall sensitivity of the above noninvasive diagnostic studies in detecting buried optic disc drusen approaches 100%. Thus, there is no longer any reason to subject a patient in whom one or both optic discs are elevated to a lumbar puncture or other invasive test until and unless it is clear that the optic discs are truly swollen.

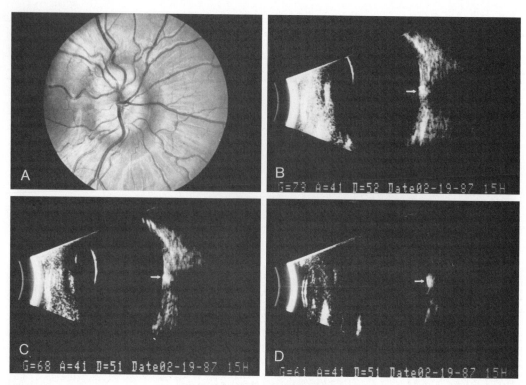

Figure 3.4. Ultrasonography in a patient with deep (buried) optic disc drusen. *A.* Appearance of the right optic disc. Note smooth surface of the optic disc, despite its marked elevation. The vessels overlying the surface of the disc are not obscured. There is an anomalous vascular branching pattern of large vessels on the disc surface. This appearance suggests anomalous elevation of the disc rather than acquired optic disc swelling. *B.* B-scan ultrasonography, low gain, shows elevation of the right optic disc. Note that the area that is elevated has an increased brightness compared with surrounding signal (*arrow*). *C.* B-scan ultrasonography, medium gain, continues to show the region of disc elevation (*arrow*), despite reduced reflection from other ocular tissue. *D.* B-scan ultrasonography, high gain, shows that the area of disc elevation is clearly seen as a focal area of brightness that persists when reflections from the remainder of the posterior segment of the eye are no longer visible (*arrow*). This is consistent with the appearance of calcified drusen. (Courtesy of Cathy DiBernardo, RN, RMDS.)

Special photographic techniques may also be useful in detecting superficial or buried optic disc drusen. For example, monochromatic (red-free) photography can be used to highlight the glistening drusen against the intact or atrophic nerve fiber layer. Alternatively, photographs taken with the filters normally used for fluorescein photography in place but without injection of fluorescein dye show that superficial disc drusen often demonstrate the phenomenon of autofluorescence (Fig. 3.6). Fluorescein angiography can also facilitate the differentiation between true papilledema and pseudopapilledema caused by buried drusen. After intravenous fluorescein injection, drusen exhibit a nodular hyperfluorescence that corresponds to the location of the visible drusen. The late phases may be characterized by some minimal blurring of the drusen that may either fade or maintain fluorescence (i.e., stain). Unlike in papilledema, however, there is no visible leakage along the major vessels. Venous anomalies (venous stasis, venous convolutions, and retinociliary venous communications) and staining of the peripapillary vein walls are occasionally seen in eyes with optic disc drusen.

Electrophysiologic studies give variable results in patients with pseudopapilledema caused

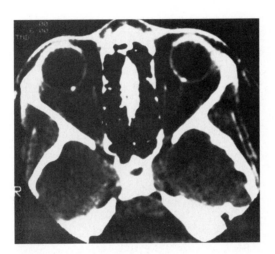

Figure 3.5. Unenhanced CT scan, axial view, in a patient with elevation of the optic disc caused by buried drusen. Note bright signal in the region of both optic discs.

by buried optic disc drusen. Such studies thus add little to the diagnostic evaluation of optic disc elevation.

Ocular Complications Associated with Pseudopapilledema Caused by Optic Disc Drusen

Most patients with optic disc drusen are asymptomatic and remain so throughout life. Nevertheless, patients with optic disc drusen occasionally experience acute loss of central vision, peripheral vision, or both via a variety of different mechanisms.

Visual field defects are present or eventually develop in 71 to 75% of eyes with disc drusen. These defects fall into three general categories:

1. Arcuate, quadrantic, or sector defects
2. Enlargement of the blind spot
3. Concentric visual field constriction

In many cases, the defects are asymptomatic but slowly progressive, reflecting the insidious attrition of optic nerve fibers over decades (Fig. 3.7). However, some patients are aware of a static or slowly progressive visual field disturbance, and others experience episodes of sudden, stepwise visual field loss. Although concentric constriction of the visual field is usually a chronic phenomenon, some patients experience sudden severe visual field constriction with and without

preservation of central vision. In patients with bilateral symmetric field defects, the pupils exhibit a normal reaction to light stimulation; however, a relative afferent pupillary defect is almost always present in patients with unilateral or asymmetric visual field loss.

The pathogenesis of visual field loss in patients with optic disc drusen probably involves one or more of the following mechanisms:

1. Impaired axon transport in an eye with a small scleral canal, leading to gradual atrophy of optic nerve fibers.
2. Direct compression of prelaminar nerve fibers by drusen.
3. Ischemia within the optic nerve head.

The location of visible disc drusen generally does not correlate with the location of the field defects they produce, and some authors have found no correlation between the severity of nerve fiber layer loss by ophthalmoscopy and the severity of visual field abnormality in eyes with disc drusen. Nevertheless, the results of these studies do not eliminate the possibility that the visual field defects produced by optic disc drusen are caused by direct compression of axons.

Loss of visual acuity is a well-documented but extremely rare complication of optic disc drusen. Thus, neither acute nor progressive loss of central vision should be assumed to be related to the effects of optic disc drusen until other causes—including inflammation, ischemia, and compression from orbital or intracranial lesions—are eliminated by appropriate diagnostic studies. In the rare cases in which drusen do produce loss of visual acuity, the loss usually results from a series of episodic, stepwise events that progressively diminish the peripheral visual field.

Prepapillary or peripapillary hemorrhages can develop in eyes with optic disc drusen. These hemorrhages are of three types:

1. Small superficial hemorrhages on the optic disc.
2. Large hemorrhages on the disc, often extending into the vitreous.
3. Deep peripapillary hemorrhages extending from the optic disc under the peripapillary retina (Fig. 3.8).

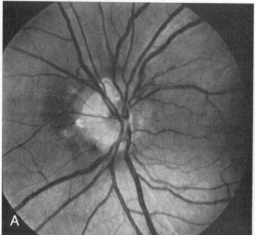

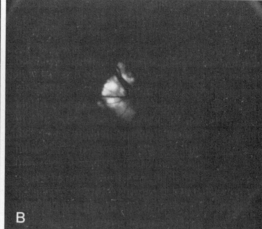

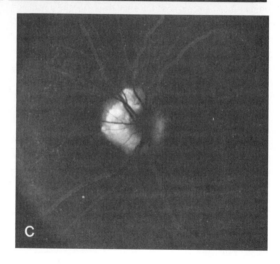

Figure 3.6. Fluorescent characteristics of drusen. *A.* Fundus photograph of optic disc drusen. *B.* Autofluorescence of drusen observed through a fluorescein filter but without injection of fluorescein dye. *C.* Late staining of drusen after fluorescein angiogram.

In our experience, subretinal and subpigment epithelial hemorrhages, although uncommon, are much more frequent in patients with optic disc drusen than are superficial (flame-shaped), subhyaloid, or vitreous hemorrhages. Splinter hemorrhages associated with optic disc drusen tend to be single and prepapillary in location, in contrast to the multiple nerve fiber layer hemorrhages that characterize papilledema (and anterior ischemic optic neuropathy). Deep peripapillary hemorrhages may be located beneath the sensory retina or the retinal pigment epithelium (RPE) and are typically circumferentially oriented around the optic disc.

Subretinal hemorrhages may occur in patients with severe papilledema, but their occur-

rence in mild papilledema is rare. Thus, their appearance in a patient thought to have "early papilledema" should suggest the possibility of disc drusen.

Some patients with optic disc drusen develop a syndrome called **optic disc drusen retinopathy.** The syndrome has five main clinical features:

1. Optic disc drusen
2. Extensive retinal hemorrhages
3. Intraretinal extravasation of serum with or without the presence of blood
4. Elevated mounds lifting the retina and causing striae radiating from the mounds toward the macula and beyond

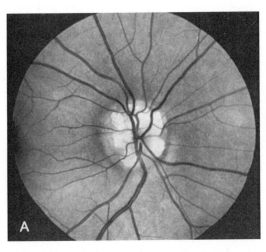

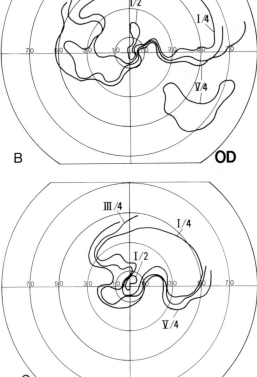

Figure 3.7. Progressive visual field defect in a patient with optic disc drusen. *A.* The optic disc shows numerous drusen and there is generalized loss of the nerve fiber layer. *B.* Visual field defect on initial examination. There is extensive inferior loss. *C.* Four years after initial examination, there has been further loss of the visual field with generalized constriction. Despite severe field loss, the patient's visual acuity remains 20/20.

5. A pigmentary disturbance of the macula or a wider area of papillomacular bundle after the resolution of the acute stages.

Most patients recover normal or near normal vision, even in severe cases.

The pathogenesis of the intraocular hemorrhages that occur in patients with optic disc drusen is unclear. Some may be caused by compression of thin-walled veins by the drusen; others may result from erosion of the vessel wall by the sharp edge of the druse. Some authors postulate that enlarging disc drusen result in circulatory compromise and local hypoxia, thus stimulating the growth of new vessels between the retinal pigment epithelium and Bruch's membrane.

Some patients with optic disc drusen develop a **serous maculopathy** without hemorrhage.

The process can tent the temporal peripapillary retina into striate folds.

Ischemic optic neuropathy may occur as a single episode or as successive episodes of discrete visual loss over years. The optic neuropathy may develop spontaneously, perhaps from crowding of the optic nerve head by drusen, or it may be precipitated by systemic hypotension, such as during peritoneal dialysis.

Retinal vascular occlusions can occur in patients with optic disc drusen. Central retinal artery occlusion, branch retinal artery occlusion, and central retinal vein occlusion have all been reported. Drusen-associated retinal vascular occlusions tend to occur in young adults but may rarely be seen in children. Retinal vascular occlusions that occur in eyes with disc drusen could result from

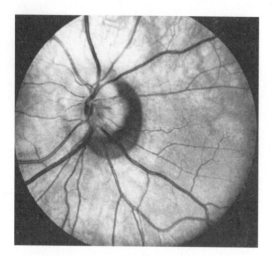

Figure 3.8. Peripapillary subretinal hemorrhage in a patient with intrapapillary drusen. Note the difference between this type of hemorrhage and the superficial nerve fiber layer hemorrhages seen with optic disc swelling.

- Retinal vascular crowding secondary to the small scleral canal size in eyes with drusen.
- Anomalous optic disc vessels that make the disc more susceptible to the effects of disrupted hemodynamics.
- Mechanical displacement of the prelaminar vasculature by the calcified drusen.

Transient visual loss occurred in 8.6% of the patients with disc drusen in one large study. This phenomenon may occur because anomalous elevation of the optic discs, like papilledema, is associated with increased interstitial pressure and decreased perfusion pressure in the intraocular portion of the optic nerve. Thus, minor fluctuations in arterial, venous, or cerebrospinal fluid pressure result in brief but critical decrements in perfusion, leading to transient obscurations of vision. Vitreopapillary traction may be an alternative mechanism in some patients. Rarely, transient visual loss is a harbinger of retinal vascular occlusion in patients with disc drusen.

Peripapillary subretinal neovascularization is a rare but well-documented complication in eyes with disc drusen. Indeed, temporary or permanent visual loss can occur in patients with optic disc drusen who develop subpigment epi-

thelial hemorrhages from subretinal neovascularization. In severe cases, this complication may simulate a juxtapapillary mass lesion or a neuroretinitis. Studies suggest that hemorrhages occurring in the absence of choroidal vascularization tend to produce no symptoms and resolve without sequelae, whereas hemorrhages arising from choroidal neovascularization commonly produce visual symptoms.

Peripapillary central serous choroidopathy rarely can be seen in eyes with optic disc drusen. Fluorescein angiography in affected eyes shows not only the typical findings of the optic disc drusen (see above) but also a bright hyperfluorescent spot corresponding to the area of leakage from the RPE. In some cases, the detachment resolves spontaneously; in others, it may not resolve until the RPE defect is treated with focal laser photocoagulation.

Histology of Optic Disc Drusen

Drusen of the optic disc consist of homogenous, globular concretions, often collected in larger, multilobulated agglomerations (Fig. 3.9). Individual druse usually exhibit a concentrically laminated structure. They are not encapsulated and contain no cells or cellular debris.

Drusen take up calcium salts and must be decalcified before being sectioned for histopathologic study. They appear to be composed predominantly of a mucoprotein matrix with significant quantities of acid mucopolysaccharides and small quantities of ribonucleic acid and occasionally iron. In addition, they stain positively for amino acids and calcium but negatively for amyloid. Drusen are insoluble in most common solvents, including absolute ethanol, ether, chloroform, xylene, acetic acid, hydrochloric acid, nitric acid, sulfuric acid, potassium hydroxide, and sodium hydroxide.

Pathogenesis of Optic Disc Drusen

The primary developmental expression of the genetic trait for drusen is probably a smaller than normal scleral canal. After formation of the optic stalk is complete, mesenchymal elements from the sclera invade the glial framework of the primitive lamina, reinforcing it with collagen. An abnormal encroachment upon the developing optic stalk by sclera, Bruch's membrane, or both would narrow the exit space of optic axons from the eye. The small optic disc size and absent

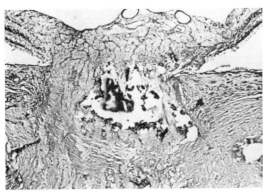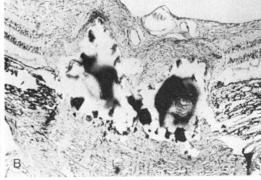

Figure 3.9. Histology of optic disc drusen. *A–B.* Intrapapillary drusen are seen as irregular dark masses within the substance of the prelaminar portion of the optic nerve head. Note elevation of disc tissue overlying the drusen.

central cup in affected eyes are consistent with the mechanism of axonal crowding. The clinical and histopathologic observation that drusen are often first detected at the margins of the optic disc suggests that the rigid edge of the scleral canal may be an aggravating factor in producing a relative mechanical interruption of axonal transport. The lower prevalence of optic disc drusen in African-Americans, who have a larger disc area with less potential for axonal crowding, is also consistent with the concept that axon crowding is a fundamental anatomic substrate for disc drusen.

It is thought that drusen are the products of long-term pathologic alterations in the retinal nerve fibers resulting from disturbances in axon transport. According to this theory, abnormal axon metabolism leads to intracellular mitochondrial calcification. Some axons then rupture, mitochondria are extruded into the extracellular space, and calcium continues to be deposited in the extracellular mitochondria. Small calcified microbodies are then produced, and calcium continues to deposit on the surface of these nidi to form drusen.

Systemic Associations with Optic Disc Drusen

Drusen of the optic disc occur with increased frequency in patients with **retinitis pigmentosa.** Although the drusen associated with retinitis pigmentosa may arise within the optic disc, they are more often located adjacent to the disc margin in the superficial retina. In such cases, the disc is not small and anomalously elevated but of normal size, flat, and waxy yellow. The drusen gradually increase in size, leading some authors to conclude that they are hamartomas rather than drusen; however, histopathologic examinations indicate that the globular excrescences of the optic nerve in retinitis pigmentosa are drusen and not astrocytic hamartomas. Patients with multisystem disorders that include retinitis pigmentosa may also develop optic disc drusen. Photographically documented optic disc and peripapillary drusen were said to be present in 16% of patients with Usher syndrome in one large study. Disc drusen may also occur in patients with Alström syndrome and in patients with pigmented paravenous retinochoroidal atrophy.

Children with retinitis pigmentosa and buried drusen may present with optic disc elevation and be thought to have neurologic disease. In addition, the combination of vitreous cells and optic disc elevation may mimic uveitis in a child with retinitis pigmentosa. In this setting, the finding of attenuated retinal arterioles provides an important (and easily overlooked) clue to the diagnosis, which can be established by electroretinography.

Initial observations suggested that the association of disc drusen with **angioid streaks** was unique to patients with pseudoxanthoma elasticum. In fact, optic disc drusen and angioid streaks occur together with increased frequency irrespective of any other evidence of systemic disease. Bruch's membrane becomes mineralized in eyes with angioid streaks, and mineralization of elastin and adherence of abnormal glycosaminoglycans to elastic fibers (as occurs in the dermis of patients with pseudoxanthoma elasticum) may also affect the lamina cribrosa. Crowding of the laminar portion of the optic nerve and secondary alteration in axonal transport then results. Using ultrasonography, optic disc drusen can be detected in about 20% of patients with pseudoxanthoma elasticum and in 25% of patients with angioid streaks but no evidence of pseudoxanthoma elasticum.

Optic disc drusen may occur as part of the **Riley-Smith syndrome** of macrocephaly, multiple hemangiomata, and pseudopapilledema. If the drusen are not appreciated as such, the combination of the macrocephaly and pseudopapilledema may be mistaken for hydrocephalus, leading to an inappropriate evaluation.

Migraine headaches are said to occur with increased frequency in patients with drusen of the optic disc. However, the concurrence of migraine and optic disc drusen probably reflects the frequent and often expedited referral of patients with headache and elevated discs for evaluation.

Intracranial Masses and Optic Disc Drusen

Patients with optic disc drusen and progressive visual loss can harbor pituitary tumors, meningiomas, craniopharyngiomas, ophthalmic artery aneurysms, cerebral abscesses, and other intracranial masses. No significant relationship between drusen and any of these lesions has ever been established, nor is there any evidence that patients with optic disc drusen have an increased risk of developing such lesions later in life.

Pseudodrusen Associated with Chronic Optic Disc Swelling

The differentiation of papilledema from pseudopapilledema caused by optic disc drusen is confounded by the fact that globular intrapapillary masses that are indistinguishable from hyaline bodies can develop in patients with chronic papilledema. Unlike disc drusen, however, these lesions disappear following regression of papilledema.

ANOMALOUS DISC ELEVATION WITHOUT VISIBLE OR BURIED DRUSEN

Not all anomalously elevated optic discs contain drusen. The morning glory syndrome is characterized by elevation of the optic disc, the nasal aspect of a tilted optic disc is usually elevated, and dysplastic discs may show some degree of elevation (see below). In addition, hypoplastic discs may be elevated out of proportion to the size of the disc. Such discs are often described as "crowded."

Optic discs that are anomalously elevated but that do not contain buried drusen are best diagnosed using ultrasonography in the A- and B-modes. This technique reveals that there are no drusen in the substance of the disc and that the retrobulbar optic nerve is not enlarged.

We believe that anomalously elevated discs unassociated with buried drusen are more common than most physicians realize. The finding of an elevated disc that is neither swollen nor containing buried drusen should not be considered a rare phenomenon.

When the explanation for an elevated optic disc remains in question despite a careful clinical examination and appropriate noninvasive diagnostic studies, we apply the following management guidelines:

1. If nonocular symptoms and signs do not, on their own merit, indicate the need for neurologic or neurosurgical evaluation, we examine the patient at regular weekly or monthly intervals using photographic documentation of disc appearance.
2. Stereoscopic color, red-free, and fluorescein fundus photographs are obtained on each visit.
3. If the appearance of the optic disc in question is stable over time, we inform the patient of the nature of this anomaly, and we provide the patient with a set of stereoscopic color photographs to avoid diagnostic confusion in the future.

OPTIC DISC SWELLING AND PSEUDOPAPILLEDEMA

Patients with pseudopapilledema are not immune to the neurologic and ophthalmologic disorders of the general population. We and others have observed concomitant papilledema, anterior optic neuritis, and anterior ischemic optic neuropathy in patients with anomalously elevated discs. In all cases, however, the history is typical of either increased intracranial pressure or an optic neuropathy, and obvious disc swelling is present.

OPTIC NERVE HYPOPLASIA

Optic nerve hypoplasia is one of the most common optic disc anomalies encountered in ophthalmologic practice.

CLINICAL FEATURES

Ophthalmoscopically, the hypoplastic disc appears as an abnormally small optic nerve head (Fig. 3.10*A*). It may appear gray or pale in color and is often surrounded by a yellowish mottled peripapillary halo, bordered by a ring of increased or decreased pigmentation (dubbed the ''double-ring'' sign), which facilitates recognition of the anomaly (Fig. 3.10*B*). The course of the major retinal vessels is often tortuous.

Optic nerve hypoplasia is characterized histopathologically by a subnormal number of optic nerve axons with normal mesodermal elements and glial supporting tissue. The ''double-ring'' sign correlates to a normal junction between the sclera and lamina cribrosa, which corresponds to the outer ring, and the termination of an abnormal extension of retina and pigment epithelium over the lamina cribrosa, which corresponds to the inner ring.

Visual acuity in optic nerve hypoplasia ranges from 20/20 to no light perception, and affected eyes show localized visual field defects, often combined with generalized constriction. Because visual acuity is determined primarily by the integrity of the papillomacular nerve fiber bundle, it does not necessarily correlate with the overall size of the disc. The strong association

of astigmatism with optic nerve hypoplasia warrants careful attention to correction of refractive errors.

Calculation of the disc-to-macula/disc diameter ratio reveals that in 95% of normals, the ratio is greater than 2.94, in contrast to an average of 2.62 for patients with optic nerve hypoplasia. Calculation of this ratio has the important advantage of eliminating the magnification effect of high refractive errors (myopic refractive errors can make a hypoplastic disc appear normal in size, whereas hyperopic refractive errors can make a normal disc appear abnormally small). However, the notion that one can unequivocally distinguish between the normal and the hypoplastic disc is inherently flawed, because large optic discs can be axonally deficient, and small optic discs do not preclude normal visual function. Theoretically, an extremely small disc is associated with a diminution in axons, but this reasoning has limited applications with regard to mild or borderline cases. Other variables must also be considered, including the size of the central cup, the percentage of the nerve occupied by axons (as opposed to glial tissue and blood vessels), and the cross-sectional area and density of axons. Furthermore, segmental forms of optic nerve hypoplasia (see below) may affect only one sector of the disc and thus not produce a diffuse diminution in the size of the disc. As such, it would seem prudent to reserve the diagnosis of optic nerve hypoplasia for patients with small optic discs who have reduced vision or

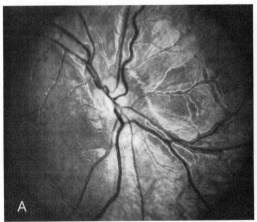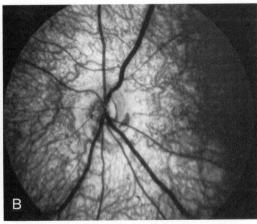

Figure 3.10. Optic nerve hypoplasia. *A.* The disc is small and pale but the retinal vessels are of normal size. *B.* The disc is small and surrounded by a rim of variably pigmented tissue.

visual field loss with corresponding nerve fiber bundle defects.

Electroretinography is normal in the majority of patients with optic nerve hypoplasia. However, a subgroup have decreased amplitudes, suggesting coexistent retinal dysgenesis. Visual-evoked potentials (VEPs) vary from normal to extinguished and may correlate with visual acuity.

ASSOCIATED ENDOCRINOLOGIC DEFICIENCIES

Optic nerve hypoplasia is frequently associated with other CNS anomalies. Septo-optic dysplasia (de Morsier syndrome) refers to the constellation of small anterior visual pathways, absence of the septum pellucidum, and thinning or agenesis of the corpus callosum. The clinical association of septo-optic dysplasia and deficiencies of anterior pituitary hormones as well as diabetes insipidus is well documented. Growth hormone deficiency is the most common endocrinologic deficiency associated with optic nerve hypoplasia, but hypothyroidism, hypocortisolism, diabetes insipidus, and hyperprolactinemia may also occur. Children with an intact septum pellucidum and optic nerve hypoplasia may still have endocrinologic deficiency. Parents should be asked about previous episodes of hypoglycemia in the neonatal period or during periods of illness (which suggest hypocortisolism) and about neonatal jaundice (which suggests hypothyroidism). Growth hormone deficiency may not be clinically apparent within the first 3 to 4 years of life because high prolactin levels can stimulate normal growth over this period. Puberty may be precocious or delayed in children with hypopituitarism. Anterior pituitary hormone deficiencies may evolve over time in some patients; thus, longitudinal reevaluation and periodic monitoring of anterior pituitary hormone function are indicated in children with posterior pituitary ectopia. Estimates of the prevalence of pituitary hormone deficiency in children with septo-optic dysplasia are as high as 62%, but these clinical reports are strongly skewed toward cases with endocrinologic manifestations, and the true prevalence is probably closer to 15%.

Children with septo-optic dysplasia and corticotropin deficiency are at risk for sudden death during febrile illness. This clinical deterioration appears to be caused by an impaired ability to increase corticotropin secretion to maintain blood pressure and blood sugar in response to the physical stress of infection. These children may have coexistent diabetes insipidus that contributes to dehydration during illness and hastens the development of shock. Some also have hypothalamic thermoregulatory disturbances signaled by episodes of hypothermia during well periods and high fevers during illnesses, which may predispose to life-threatening hyperthermia. Children with septo-optic dysplasia who are at risk for sudden death have usually had multiple hospital admissions for viral illnesses. These viral infections can precipitate hypoglycemia, dehydration, hypotension, or fever of unknown origin.

Because corticotropin deficiency is the preeminent threat to life in children with septo-optic dysplasia, a complete anterior pituitary hormone evaluation, including provocative serum cortisol testing and assessment for diabetes insipidus, should be performed in children who have clinical symptoms (history of hypoglycemia, dehydration, or hypothermia) or neuroimaging signs (absent pituitary infundibulum with or without posterior pituitary ectopia) of pituitary hormone deficiency. Subclinical hypopituitarism can manifest as acute adrenal insufficiency following surgery under general anesthesia, and it may thus be prudent to treat children who have optic nerve hypoplasia empirically with perioperative intravenous corticosteroids.

ASSOCIATED CENTRAL NERVOUS SYSTEM MALFORMATIONS

MRI is the optimum noninvasive neuroimaging modality for delineating associated CNS malformations in patients with optic nerve hypoplasia. In optic nerve hypoplasia, coronal and sagittal T1-weighted MR images consistently demonstrate thinning and attenuation of hypoplastic prechiasmatic intracranial optic nerves (Fig. 3.11A). Coronal T1-weighted MRI in bilateral optic nerve hypoplasia shows diffuse thinning of the optic chiasm in patients with bilateral optic nerve hypoplasia (Fig. 3.11B); focal thinning or absence of the side of the chiasm corresponds to the hypoplastic nerve in patients with unilateral optic nerve hypoplasia. When MRI shows a decrease in intracranial optic nerve size accompanied by other features of septo-optic dysplasia, a presumptive diagnosis of optic nerve hypoplasia can be made.

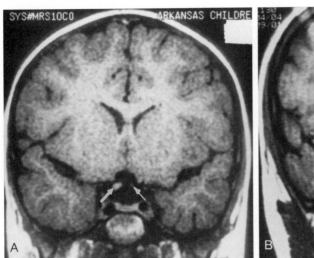 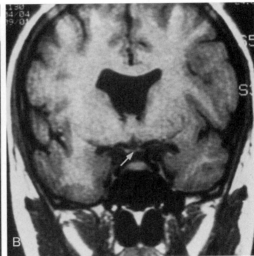

Figure 3.11. Magnetic resonance imaging in optic nerve hypoplasia. *A.* Left optic nerve hypoplasia. *Large arrrow:* normal right optic nerve. *Small arrow:* hypoplastic intracranial prechiasmatic optic nerve. *B.* Bilateral optic nerve hypo-

plasia. *Arrow:* hypoplastic chiasm. (Reprinted with permission from Brodsky MC, Glasier CM, Pollock SC, et al. Optic nerve hypoplasia: identification by magnetic resonance imaging. Arch Ophthalmol 1990;108:562–567.)

The notion of septo-optic dysplasia as a distinct nosologic entity has been challenged because MRI frequently demonstrates structural abnormalities involving the cerebral hemispheres and the pituitary infundibulum. Cerebral hemispheric abnormalities, which are evident on MRI in about 45% of patients with optic nerve hypoplasia, may consist of hemispheric migration anomalies such as schizencephaly, cortical heterotopia, polymicrogyria, as well as evidence of intrauterine or perinatal hemispheric injury such as periventricular leukomalacia, encephalomalacia, or porencephaly. Midline fusion of the cerebral hemispheres (holoprosencephaly) and cerebellar hemispheres is also occasionally seen. Optic nerve hypoplasia may also accompany other intracranial anomalies, including anencephaly, hydranencephaly, and transsphenoidal or frontonasal encephalocele.

Evidence of perinatal injury to the pituitary infundibulum (seen on MRI as posterior pituitary ectopia) is found in approximately 15% of patients with optic nerve hypoplasia. Normally, the posterior pituitary gland appears bright on T1-weighted images (Fig. 3.12A). In posterior pituitary ectopia, MRI demonstrates absence of the normal posterior pituitary bright spot, absence or attenuation of the pituitary infundibulum, and an ectopic posterior pituitary bright

spot where the upper infundibulum is normally located (Fig. 3.12B). It is unclear if posterior pituitary ectopia results from defective neuronal migration during embryogenesis or from a perinatal injury to the hypophyseal-portal system that causes necrosis of the infundibulum.

In a child with optic nerve hypoplasia, posterior pituitary ectopia is almost pathognomonic of anterior pituitary hormone deficiency with normal posterior pituitary function, whereas absence of a normal or ectopic posterior pituitary bright spot predicts coexistent antidiuretic hormone deficiency (i.e., diabetes insipidus). Cerebral hemispheric abnormalities are highly predictive of neurodevelopmental deficits. Absence of the septum pellucidum alone does not portend neurodevelopmental deficits or pituitary hormone deficiency. Thinning or agenesis of the corpus callosum is predictive of neurodevelopmental problems only by virtue of its frequent association with cerebral hemispheric abnormalities. The finding of unilateral optic nerve hypoplasia does not preclude coexistent intracranial malformations. MRI thus provides critical prognostic information regarding the likelihood of neurodevelopmental deficits and pituitary hormone deficiency in the infant or young child with **unilateral** or **bilateral** optic nerve hypoplasia.

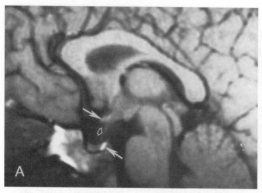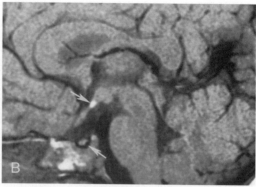

Figure 3.12. Posterior pituitary ectopia. *A.* MRI demonstrating the normal hyperintense signal of the posterior pituitary gland (*lower arrow*), normal pituitary infundibulum (*hollow arrow*), and optic chiasm (*upper arrow*). *B.* MRI demonstrating posterior pituitary ectopia that appears as an abnormal focal area of increased signal intensity at the tuber cinereum (*upper arrow*). Note absence of the pituitary infundibulum and absence of the normal posterior pituitary bright spot (*lower arrow*). (Reprinted with permission from Brodsky MC, Glasier CM. Optic nerve hypoplasia: clinical significance of associated central nervous system abnormalities on magnetic resonance imaging. Arch Ophthalmol 1993;111: 66–74.)

SYSTEMIC AND TERATOGENIC ASSOCIATIONS

Numerous environmental factors that are detrimental to the fetus are sporadically associated with optic nerve hypoplasia. These include

- maternal insulin-dependent diabetes mellitus
- fetal alcohol syndrome
- maternal ingestion of quinine, anticonvulsants, alcohol, or illicit drugs
- fetal or neonatal infection with cytomegalovirus or hepatitis B virus

Optic nerve hypoplasia occurs with increased frequency in firstborn children of young mothers. The majority of cases are sporadic, although a handful of familial cases have been reported in siblings. The growing list of systemic and ocular disorders associated with optic nerve hypoplasia includes aniridia, Dandy-Walker syndrome, Delleman syndrome, Duane syndrome, Klippel-Trenaunay-Weber syndrome, Goldenhar syndrome, linear nevus sebaceous syndrome, Meckel syndrome, hemifacial atrophy, blepharophimosis, osteogenesis imperfecta, chondrodysplasia punctata, Aicardi syndrome, Apert syndrome, Potter syndrome, chromosome 13q– syndrome, trisomy 18, neonatal isoimmune thrombocytopenia, and bilateral microphthalmos.

SEGMENTAL OPTIC NERVE HYPOPLASIA

Some forms of optic nerve hypoplasia are segmental. A pathognomonic superior segmental optic hypoplasia with an inferior visual field defect occurs occasionally in children of insulin-dependent diabetic mothers (Fig. 3.13).

Congenital lesions of the retina, optic nerve, optic chiasm, optic tract, or retrogeniculate pathways are always associated with segmental hypoplasia of the corresponding portions of each optic nerve. The term **homonymous hemioptic hypoplasia** describes the asymmetric form of segmental optic nerve hypoplasia seen in patients with unilateral congenital hemispheric lesions affecting the postchiasmal afferent visual pathways. In this setting, the nasal and temporal aspects of the optic disc contralateral to the hemispheric lesion show segmental hypoplasia and loss of the corresponding nerve fiber layers. This anomaly may be accompanied by a central band of horizontal pallor across the disc. The ipsilateral optic disc may range from normal in size to frankly hypoplastic. Homonymous hemioptic hypoplasia in retrogeniculate lesions results from transsynaptic degeneration.

PATHOGENESIS

The term "optic nerve hypoplasia" implies that the nerve is deficient in axons because of a primary failure of these axons to develop. How-

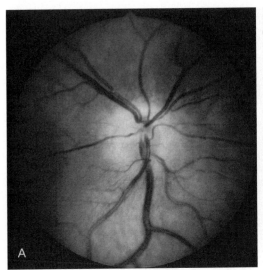
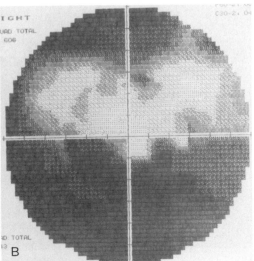

Figure 3.13. Superior segmental optic hypoplasia in a child whose mother had adult-onset diabetes mellitus. *A.* Right optic disc demonstrating an abnormal superior entrance of the central retinal artery, relative pallor of the superior disc, and a superior peripapillary halo. The superior nerve fiber layer is absent, while the inferior nerve fiber layer is clearly seen. *B.* Humphrey visual field in superior segmental hypoplasia showing a nonaltitudinal inferior visual field defect with milder superior depression. (Reprinted with permission from Brodsky MC, Schroeder GT, Ford R. Superior segmental hypoplasia in identical twins. J Clin Neuroophthalmol 1993;13:152–154.)

ever, the known timing of coexistent CNS injuries suggests that some cases of optic nerve "hypoplasia" result from intrauterine destruction of a normally developed structure (i.e., an encephaloclastic event), whereas others represent a primary failure of axons to develop.

In human fetuses, there is a peak of 3.7 million axons at 16 to 17 weeks of gestation, with a subsequent decline to 1.1 million axons by the 31st gestational week. This massive degeneration of supernumerary axons results from a form of programmed cell death called **apoptosis** that occurs as part of the normal development of the visual pathways and that may serve to establish the correct topography of the visual pathways. Toxins or associated CNS malformations may augment or interfere with the usual processes by which superfluous axons are eliminated from the developing visual pathways. Early gestational injuries to midline CNS structures (septum pellucidum, pituitary infundibulum) may directly injure adjacent optic axons or indirectly disrupt their migration. Prenatal hemispheric injuries or malformations that injure the optic radiations can lead to transsynaptic retrograde degeneration and segmental hypoplasia of both optic

nerves. The frequent association of optic nerve hypoplasia with cerebral migration anomalies (e.g., schizencephaly) could also reflect a generalized disruption in normal neuronal guidance mechanisms involved in the migration of both hemispheric neurons and optic axons in utero.

EXCAVATED OPTIC DISC ANOMALIES

Optic disc coloboma, morning glory disc anomaly, and peripapillary staphyloma are examples of excavated anomalies of the optic disc. In the latter two conditions, an excavation of the posterior globe surrounds and incorporates the optic disc. Unfortunately, these terms are often transposed in the literature, causing tremendous confusion regarding their diagnostic criteria, associated systemic findings, and pathogenesis. However, optic disc colobomas, morning glory optic discs, and peripapillary staphylomas are distinct anomalies, each with its own specific embryologic origin—they are not simply clinical variants along a broad phenotypic spectrum.

MORNING GLORY DISC ANOMALY

The **morning glory disc anomaly** is a congenital, funnel-shaped excavation of the pos-

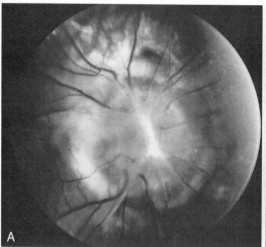

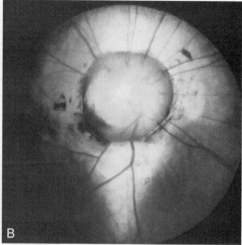

Figure 3.14. Morning glory disc anomaly. *A.* The optic disc shows the classic features of the morning glory syndrome: an enlarged, funnel-shaped, excavated and distorted optic disc that is surrounded by an elevated annulus of chorioretinal pigmentary disturbance. *B.* In another case of morning glory syndrome, a large optic disc is surrounded by an annular zone of pigmentary disturbance and a V-shaped zone of infrapapillary depigmentation. The retinal vessels appear increased in number, appear to emerge from the disc periphery, and have an abnormally straight radial configuration. A tuft of white glial tissue overlies the center of both optic discs.

terior fundus that incorporates the optic disc, resembling the morning glory flower. Ophthalmoscopically, the disc is markedly enlarged, orange or pink in color, and may appear to be recessed or elevated centrally within the confines of a funnel-shaped peripapillary excavation (Fig. 3.14). A wide annulus of chorioretinal pigmentary disturbance surrounds the disc within the excavation. A white tuft of glial tissue overlies the central portion of the disc. The blood vessels appear increased in number and often arise from the periphery of the disc. They often curve abruptly as they emanate from the disc, then run an abnormally straight course over the peripapillary retina. It is often difficult to distinguish arterioles from venules. Close inspection may reveal peripapillary or arteriovenous communications that can be confirmed by fluorescein angiography. The macula may be incorporated into the excavation. Neuroimaging shows a funnel-shaped enlargement of the distal optic nerve at its junction with the globe (Fig. 3.15). Additional findings in patients with the morning glory disc anomaly include diffuse thickening with increased or decreased radiodensity of the orbital optic nerve, cavum vergae, moyamoya vessels, and, most notably, basal encephalocele.

The morning glory disc anomaly usually oc-

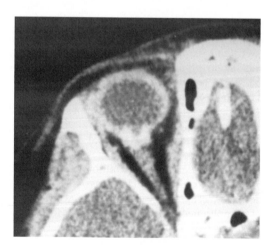

Figure 3.15. CT scan of morning glory disc anomaly. Note calcified funnel-shaped enlargement of the distal optic nerve at its junction with the globe (Reprinted with permission from Brodsky MC. Congenital optic disk anomalies. Surv Ophthalmol 1994;39:89–112.)

curs as a unilateral condition, but bilateral cases have been reported. Visual acuity usually ranges from 20/200 to finger counting, but cases with 20/20 vision occur as do cases with no light perception. As in all congenital optic disc anoma-

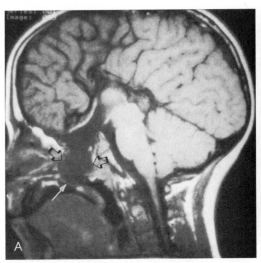
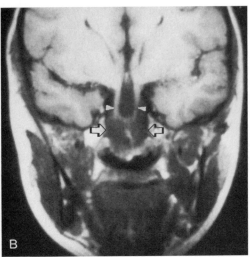

Figure 3.16. MRI in transsphenoidal encephalocele. *A.* Sagittal MRI shows an encephalocele (delimited by hollow arrows) extending down through the sphenoid bone into the nasopharynx with impression on the hard palate (solid arrow). *B.* Coronal MRI shows the 3rd ventricle and hypo-thalamus (solid arrows) extending inferiorly into the encephalocele (delimited inferiorly by hollow arrow) (Reprinted with permission from Brodsky MC. Congenital optic disk anomolies. Surv Ophthalmol 1994;39:89–112.)

lies, functional amblyopia may contribute to visual loss in unilateral cases, and a trial of occlusion therapy is warranted in infants and small children. Unlike optic disc colobomas which have no race or gender predilection (see below), morning glory discs are conspicuously more common in females and rare in African-Americans. With rare exceptions, the morning glory disc anomaly is not part of a multisystem genetic disorder.

The association of morning glory disc anomaly with the transsphenoidal form of basal encephalocele is well established. The finding of V- or tongue-shaped infrapapillary depigmentation adjacent to a morning glory disc anomaly (see Fig. 3.14*B*) is especially suggestive of transsphenoidal encephalocele. Transsphenoidal encephalocele is a rare midline congenital malformation in which a meningeal pouch, often containing the chiasm and adjacent hypothalamus, protrudes inferiorly through a large, round defect in the sphenoid bone (Fig. 3.16). Patients with this occult basal meningocele have a wide head, flat nose, mild hypertelorism, a midline notch in the upper lip, and sometimes a midline cleft in the soft palate (Fig. 3.17). The meningocele protrudes into the nasopharynx, where it may obstruct the airway.

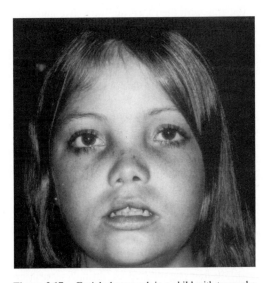

Figure 3.17. Facial photograph in a child with transsphenoidal encephalocele. Note hypertelorism, depressed nasal bridge, and subtle midline upper lip defect (Reprinted with permission from Brodsky MC, Hoyt WF, Hoyt SC, et al. Atypical retinochoroidal coloboma in patients with dysplastic optic discs and transsphenoidal encephalocele. Arch Ophthalmol 1995;113:624–628.)

Symptoms of transsphenoidal encephalocele in infancy include rhinorrhea, nasal obstruction, mouth breathing, or snoring. These symptoms may be overlooked or ignored unless the associated morning glory disc anomaly or the characteristic facial configuration are recognized. A transsphenoidal encephalocele may appear clinically as a pulsatile posterior nasal mass or as a "nasal polyp" high in the nose, and surgical biopsy or excision of the lesion can have severe and even lethal consequences. Associated brain malformations include agenesis of the corpus callosum and posterior dilation of the lateral ventricles. Absence of the chiasm is seen in approximately one-third of patients at surgery or autopsy. Most of the affected children have no overt intellectual or neurologic deficits, but hypopituitarism is common, with growth hormone and antidiuretic hormone deficiencies most common.

Surgery for transsphenoidal encephalocele is considered by many authorities to be contraindicated, because herniated brain tissue may include vital structures such as the hypothalamic-pituitary system, optic nerves and chiasm, and anterior cerebral arteries, and because of the high postoperative mortality, particularly in infants.

Patients with the morning glory disc anomaly are at increased risk for acquired visual loss from several causes. Serous retinal detachments occur in 26 to 38% of eyes with morning glory optic discs. These detachments typically originate in the peripapillary area and extend through the posterior pole, occasionally progressing to total detachments. Although retinal tears are rarely evident, small retinal tears adjacent to or overlying the optic nerve have been described in some patients with morning glory disc–associated retinal detachments. In other cases with acquired visual loss, there is nonattachment and radial folding of the retina within the excavated zone. The sources of subretinal fluid may be multiple.

Several authors have documented contractile movements in a morning glory optic disc, possibly caused by fluctuations in subretinal fluid volume altering the degree of retinal separation within the confines of the excavation. Subretinal neovascularization may occasionally develop within the circumferential zone of pigmentary disturbance adjacent to a morning glory disc.

The embryologic defect leading to the morning glory disc anomaly is widely disputed. Some authors hypothesize that the morning glory disc anomaly results from defective closure of the embryonic fissure and is but one phenotypic form of a colobomatous (i.e., embryonic fissure-related) defect. Others interpret the clinical findings of a central glial tuft, vascular anomalies, and a scleral defect—together with the histologic findings of adipose tissue and smooth muscle within the peripapillary sclera in presumed cases of the morning glory disc—as signifying a primary mesenchymal abnormality. These researchers believe that the presence of associated midfacial anomalies in some patients further supports the concept of a primary mesenchymal defect, because most of the cranial structures are derived from mesenchyme.

Others argue that the fundamental symmetry of the fundus excavation with respect to the disc implicates an anomalous funnel-shaped enlargement of the distal optic stalk at its junction with the primitive optic vesicle as the primary embryologic defect. In this scenario, invagination of the optic vesicle proceeds normally, leading to formation of an embryonic fissure, which extends from the newly formed optic cup into the expanded distal optic stalk. Complete closure of the embryonic fissure follows, but because of the increased dimensions of the distal optic stalk, the process of normal closure fails to obliterate the space within the dysgenetic distal stalk. This results in a persistent excavated defect at the site of entry of the optic nerve into the eye. According to this hypothesis, the glial and vascular abnormalities that characterize the morning glory disc anomaly can be explained as secondary effects of a primary neuroectodermal dysgenesis on the formation of mesodermal elements that arise later in embryogenesis.

OPTIC DISC COLOBOMA

The term *coloboma,* of Greek derivation, means curtailed or mutilated. It is used only with reference to the eye. **Colobomas of the optic disc** result from incomplete or abnormal coaptation of the proximal end of the embryonic fissure.

An optic disc coloboma is characterized by a sharply delimited, glistening white, bowl-shaped excavation that occupies an enlarged optic disc (Fig. 3.18). The excavation is decentered inferiorly, reflecting the position of the embryonic fissure relative to the primitive epithelial papilla. The inferior neuroretinal rim is thin or

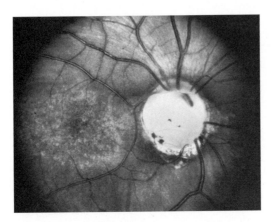

Figure 3.18. Coloboma of the optic disc in an eye with an old serous macular detachment. The disc is enlarged. A deep white excavation occupies most of the disc but spares its superior aspect. Note absence of the inferior retinal nerve fiber layer and a pigment epithelial disturbance in the macula. The patient had a large superior, altitudinal visual field defect.

absent, whereas the superior neuroretinal rim is relatively spared. Rarely, the entire disc appears excavated; however, the colobomatous nature of the defect can still be appreciated ophthalmoscopically because the excavation is deeper inferiorly. The defect may extend farther inferiorly to include the adjacent choroid and retina, in which case microphthalmia is frequently present. Iris and ciliary colobomas often coexist. Axial CT scanning shows a crater-like excavation of the posterior globe at its junction with the optic nerve.

Visual acuity, which depends primarily on the integrity of the papillomacular bundle, may be mildly to severely decreased in patients with a coloboma of the optic disc, but the level of visual function is difficult to predict from the appearance of the disc. Unlike the morning glory disc anomaly, which is usually unilateral, optic disc colobomas occur unilaterally or bilaterally with approximately equal frequency. As with uveal colobomas, isolated optic disc colobomas may be sporadic or inherited. Ocular colobomas may also be accompanied by other systemic anomalies in numerous conditions, including the CHARGE association (coloboma, congenital heart disease, and choanal atresia with multiple anomalies), Walker-Warburg syndrome, Goltz focal dermal hypoplasia, Aicardi syndrome, Goldenhar syndrome, and linear sebaceous

nevus syndrome. Optic disc coloboma was linked to a mutation of the PAX2 gene in a family with renal anomalies and vesicoureteral reflux.

An optic disc coloboma may be associated with other ocular malformations, including large orbital cysts that communicate with atypical dark excavations of the disc that may be colobomatous in nature, retinal venous malformations, and macular hole.

Histopathologic examination of an optic disc coloboma typically demonstrates intrascleral smooth muscle strands oriented concentrically around the proximal optic nerve. Presumably, this pathologic finding accounts for the contractility of the optic disc seen in rare cases of optic disc coloboma. Heterotopic adipose tissue is also present within and adjacent to some optic disc colobomas. Eyes with an isolated optic disc coloboma can develop a serous macular detachment (see Fig. 3.18) (in contrast to the rhegmatogenous retinal detachments that complicate retinochoroidal colobomas).

Unfortunately, many uncategorizable dysplastic optic discs (see below) are indiscriminately labeled as optic disc colobomas. This practice complicates the nosology of coloboma-associated genetic disorders.

Although the phenotypic profiles of optic disc coloboma and the morning glory disc anomaly occasionally overlap, the ophthalmoscopic features of the optic disc coloboma are most consistent with a primary structural dysgenesis of the proximal embryonic fissure, as opposed to an anomalous dilation confined to the distal optic stalk in the morning glory disc anomaly (Table 3.2). The profound differences in associated ocular and systemic findings between the two anomalies (Table 3.3) lend further credence to this hypothesis. The concept of ''an optic disc coloboma with a morning glory configuration'' should be abandoned.

PERIPAPILLARY STAPHYLOMA

A **peripapillary staphyloma** is an extremely rare, usually unilateral, anomaly, in which a deep fundus excavation surrounds the optic disc (Fig. 3.19). In this condition, the disc is seen at the bottom of the excavated defect and may appear normal or show temporal pallor. The walls and margin of the defect may show atrophic changes in the RPE and choroid. Unlike the morning glory disc anomaly, there is no central

Table 3.2
Ophthalmoscopic Findings That Distinguish the Morning Glory Disc Anomaly from Optic Disc Coloboma

MORNING GLORY DISC	OPTIC DISC COLOBOMA
Optic disc lies within the excavation	Excavation lies within the optic disc
Symmetric defect (disc lies *centrally* within the excavation)	Asymmetric defect (excavation lies *inferiorly* within the disc)
Central glial tuft	No central glial tuft
Severe peripapillary pigmentary disturbance	Minimal peripapillary pigmentary disturbance
Anomalous retinal vasculature	Normal retinal vasculature

Table 3.3
Associated Ocular and Systemic Findings That Distinguish the Morning Glory Disc from Isolated Optic Disc Coloboma

MORNING GLORY DISC	OPTIC DISC COLOBOMA
More common in females; rare in African-Americans	No sex or race predilection
Rarely familial	Often familial
Rarely bilateral	Often bilateral
No iris, ciliary, or retinal colobomas	Iris, ciliary, and retinal colobomas common
Rarely associated with multisystem genetic disorders	Often associated with multisystem genetic disorders
Basal encephalocele common	Basal encephalocele rare

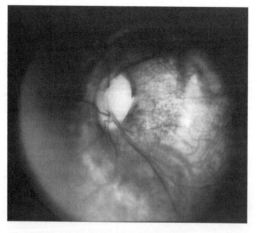

Figure 3.19. Peripapillary staphyloma. The left optic disc is positioned along the nasal margin of a deep, bowl-shaped peripapillary staphyloma. The temporal aspect of the disc is pale and tilted posteriorly relative to the nasal portion.

glial tuft overlying the disc, and the retinal vascular pattern remains normal, apart from reflecting the essential contour of the lesion. The staphylomatous excavation in peripapillary staphyloma is also notably deeper than that seen in the morning glory disc anomaly. Several cases of contractile peripapillary staphyloma have been documented.

Visual acuity is usually markedly reduced in eyes with a peripapillary staphyloma, but cases with nearly normal acuity occur. Affected eyes are usually emmetropic or slightly myopic, and eyes with decreased vision frequently have cecocentral scotomas. Although the peripapillary staphyloma is clinically and embryologically distinct from the morning glory optic disc, these conditions are frequently transposed in the literature. Table 3.4 contrasts the ophthalmoscopic features that distinguish these two anomalies.

Unlike the other excavated disc anomalies, a peripapillary staphyloma is rarely associated with systemic or intracranial disease. Exceptions to this generalization include the description of

Table 3.4
Ophthalmoscopic Findings That Distinguish Peripapillary Staphyloma from the Morning Glory Disc Anomaly

PERIPAPILLARY STAPHYLOMA	MORNING GLORY DISC
Deep, cup-shaped excavation	Less depth, funnel-shaped excavation
Relatively normal, well-defined optic disc	Grossly anomalous, poorly defined optic disc
Absence of glial and vascular anomalies	Central glial bouquet, anomalous vascular pattern

peripapillary staphyloma in one child with linear nevus sebaceous syndrome and in another child with 18q– (de Grouchy) syndrome.

The fairly normal appearance of the optic disc and retinal vessels in eyes with a peripapillary staphyloma suggests that the development of these structures is complete before the staphylomatous process begins. The clinical features of peripapillary staphyloma are most consistent with diminished peripapillary structural support, perhaps resulting from incomplete differentiation of sclera from posterior neural crest cells in the 5th month of gestation. Staphyloma formation presumably occurs when establishment of normal intraocular pressure leads to herniation of unsupported ocular tissues through the defect. Thus, the peripapillary staphyloma and the morning glory disc anomaly appear to be pathogenetically distinct both in the timing of the insult (5 months' gestation vs. 4 weeks' gestation), and in the embryologic site of structural dysgenesis (posterior sclera vs. distal optic stalk).

MEGALOPAPILLA

Megalopapilla is a generic term that connotes an abnormally large optic disc that lacks the inferior excavation of an optic disc coloboma or the numerous anomalous features of the morning glory disc anomaly. In its current usage, megalopapilla comprises two phenotypic variants.

The first is a common variant in which an abnormally large optic disc (greater than 2.1 mm in diameter) retains an otherwise normal configuration. This form of megalopapilla is usually bilateral and is often associated with a large cup-to-disc ratio, which almost invariably raises the diagnostic consideration of low-tension glaucoma (Fig. 3.20A). However, the optic cup is usually round or horizontally oval with no vertical notching or encroachment, so the quotient of horizontal to vertical cup-to-disc ratio remains normal, in contrast to the decreased quotient that characterizes glaucomatous optic atrophy. Because the axons are spread over a larger surface area, the neuroretinal rim may also appear pale, mimicking optic atrophy.

Less commonly, the normal optic cup is replaced by a grossly anomalous noninferior excavation that obliterates the adjacent neuroretinal rim (Fig. 3.20B). The inclusion of this rare variant under the rubric of megalopapilla serves the nosologically useful function of distinguishing it from a colobomatous defect with the latter's attendant systemic implications. Cilioretinal arteries are common in eyes with megalopapilla. A high prevalence of megalopapilla was observed in natives of the Marshall Islands.

Visual acuity is usually normal with megalopapilla, but it may be mildly decreased. The visual field is also usually normal, except for an enlarged blind spot, allowing the examiner to distinguish this condition from low-tension glaucoma or compressive optic atrophy. Colobomatous discs are distinguished from megalopapilla by their predominant excavation of the inferior optic disc. Aside from glaucoma and optic disc coloboma, the differential diagnosis of megalopapilla includes orbital optic glioma, which in children can cause progressive enlargement of a previously normal-sized optic disc.

Pathogenetically, most cases of megalopapilla may simply be a statistical variant of normal. However, it is likely that megalopapilla occasionally results from altered migration of optic axons early in embryogenesis, as evidenced by two reports of megalopapilla in patients with anterior encephaloceles. Nevertheless, the rarity of an association between megalopapilla and CNS abnormalities suggests that neuroimaging is unwarranted in a patient with megalopapilla, unless midline facial anomalies (e.g., hypertelor-

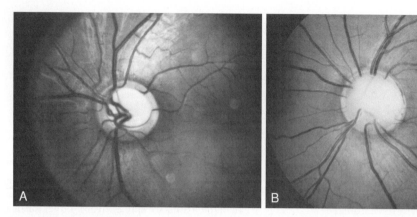

Figure 3.20. Megalopapilla. *A.* A common variant of megalopapilla in which an abnormally large optic disc contains a large central cup. Unlike glaucomatous optic atrophy, the cup is horizontally oval with an intact neuroretinal rim, and there is no nasalization of vessels at their point of origin.

B. An uncommon variant of megalopapilla in which an anomalous superior excavation obliterates much of the temporal neuroretinal rim. (Reprinted with permission from Brodsky MC. Congenital optic disk anomolies. Surv Ophthalmol 1994;39:89–112.)

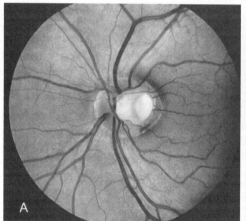

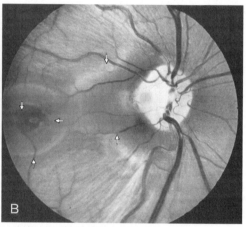

Figure 3.21. Optic pit. *A.* Oval white excavation occupies the temporal portion of the disc. *B.* Grayish temporal optic disc with adjacent retinoschisis cavity (*large arrows*), serous macular detachment (*small arrows*) and outer layer hole (*hollow arrow*).

ism, cleft palate, cleft lip, depressed nasal bridge) coexist.

OPTIC PIT

An **optic pit** is a round or oval, gray, white, or yellow depression in the optic disc (Fig. 3.21*A*). The estimated frequency of optic pits is approximately 1 in 11,000.

Optic pits commonly affect the temporal portion of the optic disc but may be situated in any sector. Such temporally located pits are often accompanied by adjacent peripapillary pigment epithelial changes. One or two cilioretinal arteries emerge from the bottom or the margin of the pit in more than 50% of cases. Although optic pits are typically unilateral, bilateral pits are present in 15% of cases. In unilateral cases, the affected disc is slightly larger than the normal disc. Visual acuity is typically normal unless there is fluid within or beneath the macula (see below). Although visual field defects are variable and often correlate poorly with the location of the pit, the most common defect appears to be a paracentral arcuate scotoma connected to an enlarged blind spot. Optic pits do not portend additional CNS malformations, although rare exceptions exist. Acquired depressions in the optic disc that are indistinguishable from optic pits are said to occur in low-tension glaucoma.

Serous macular elevations develop in 25 to 75% of eyes with optic pits. Optic pit–associated maculopathy generally becomes symptomatic in the third and fourth decades of life. Vitreous traction on the margins of the pit and traction changes in the roof of the pit may be the inciting events that ultimately lead to late-onset macular detachment (Fig. 3.21*B*). The following progression of events has been proposed:

1. A schisis-like inner layer retinal separation initially forms in direct communication with the optic pit, producing a mild, relative, cecocentral scotoma.
2. An outer layer macular hole develops beneath the boundaries of the inner layer separation and produces a dense central scotoma.
3. An outer layer retinal detachment develops around the macular hole, presumably from influx of fluid from the inner layer separation. This outer layer detachment ophthalmoscopically resembles an RPE detachment but fails to hyperfluoresce on fluorescein angiography.
4. The outer layer detachment may eventually enlarge and obliterate the inner layer separation. At this stage, it is no longer ophthalmoscopically or histopathologically distinguishable from a primary serous macular detachment.

The risk of optic pit–associated macular detachment is greatest in eyes with large optic pits and in eyes with temporally located pits. Spontaneous reattachment occurs in about 25% of cases. Bed rest and bilateral patching lead to retinal reattachment in some patients, presumably by decreasing vitreous traction. Laser photocoagulation to block the flow of fluid from the pit to the macula is usually unsuccessful, perhaps because of the inability of laser photocoagulation to seal a retinoschisis cavity. Vitrectomy with internal gas tamponade and laser photocoagulation can produce long-term improvement in acuity.

Histologically, optic pits consist of herniations of dysplastic retina into a collagen-lined pocket extending posteriorly, often into the subarachnoid space, through a defect in the lamina cribrosa. The source of intraretinal fluid in eyes with optic pits is controversial. Possible sources include the vitreous cavity via the pit, the subarachnoid space, the blood vessels at the base of the pit, and the orbital space surrounding the dura.

Although the pathogenesis of optic pits is unclear, many authorities view optic pits as the mildest variant in the spectrum of optic disc colobomas. This widely accepted hypothesis is probably untenable for the following reasons:

- Optic pits are usually unilateral, sporadic, and unassociated with systemic anomalies, whereas colobomas are bilateral as often as unilateral, commonly autosomal dominant, and may be associated with a variety of multisystem disorders.
- Optic pits rarely coexist with iris or retinochoroidal colobomas.
- Optic pits usually occur in locations unrelated to the embryonic fissure.

Although colobomas may contain focal crater-like deformations that resemble optic pits, and the distinction between an inferiorly located pit and a small optic disc coloboma is difficult at times, there appears to be sufficient evidence to conclude that most optic pits are fundamentally distinct from colobomas in their pathogenesis. The presence of one or more cilioretinal arteries emerging from the majority of optic pits must somehow also be pathogenetically relevant.

CONGENITAL TILTED DISC SYNDROME

The **tilted disc syndrome** is a nonhereditary, usually bilateral condition in which the superotemporal optic disc is elevated and the inferonasal disc is posteriorly displaced, resulting in an oval-appearing optic disc, with its long axis obliquely oriented (Fig. 3.22). This configuration is accompanied by situs inversus of the retinal vessels, congenital inferonasal conus, thinning of the inferonasal RPE and choroid, and a bitemporal hemianopia that does not respect the vertical midline. Histopathologically, the optic nerve enters at an extremely oblique angle, the

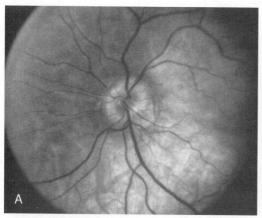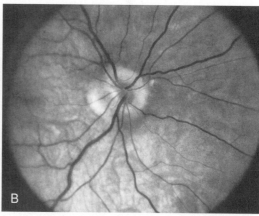

Figure 3.22. Congenital tilted disc syndrome. Both optic discs are oval with relative elevation of the superior-temporal portion compared to the inferior-nasal portion. This eleva-tion is often mistaken for true disc swelling. Note situs inver-sus of the vessels and inferior retinochoroidal hypopigmenta-tion.

superior or superotemporal portion of the disc is elevated, and there is posterior ectasia of the inferior or inferonasal fundus and optic disc. Affected patients often have myopic astigmatism, with the plus axis oriented parallel to the ectasia. The ocular imagery resulting from a tilted retina creates a type of curvature of field that may subjectively simulate astigmatic blur. The inferior crescent is created by a disparity between the size of the retinal and scleral openings. The congenital tilted disc syndrome is bilateral in about 80% of cases. The cause of the tilted disc syndrome is unknown, but the inferonasal or inferior location of the excavation suggests a pathogenetic relationship to retinochoroidal coloboma.

Familiarity with the tilted disc syndrome is crucial for the ophthalmologist, because affected patients may present with a bitemporal hemianopia, suggesting a chiasmal syndrome. The bitemporal hemianopia in patients with tilted discs, however, is typically incomplete, is confined primarily to the superior quadrants, and does not respect the vertical midline as do field defects caused by lesions that damage the optic chiasm (see Chapter 12). It is, in fact, a refractive scotoma, secondary to regional myopia localized to the inferonasal retina. Furthermore, the superotemporal depression is selectively detected with midsized isopters, whereas the large and small isopters give fairly normal results because the ectasia that occurs in such cases is confined

to the midperipheral fundus (Fig. 3.23). In some cases, perimetry with a spectacle lens in place to correct myopic astigmatism may reduce or eliminate the superotemporal defect, confirming its refractive nature. In other cases, retinal sensitivity is decreased in the area of the ectasia, and the defect thus persists to some degree despite appropriate refractive correction. Other quadrants also show mildly decreased sensitivities on threshold perimetry, suggesting that the tilted disc syndrome may actually include some degree of diffuse retinal or optic nerve hypoplasia.

In some cases, elevation of the superior portion of the tilted optic disc mimics true optic disc swelling. However, in patients with tilted discs, the peripapillary retinal nerve fiber layer shows no evidence of disruption, there are no hemorrhages or exudates, and the retinal vessels appear from beneath the normal portion of the disc. In most cases, the superior vessels course superiorly and nasally over the top of the disc. Some then turn temporally, and others continue nasally to supply the superior retina. The inferior vessels generally run inferiorly and may turn slightly nasally before some turn temporally to supply the temporal inferior retina.

Some patients with tilted optic discs develop a serous detachment of the macula caused by subretinal leakage of fluid.

It should be emphasized that a true bitemporal hemianopia may occur in patients with the tilted disc syndrome who also harbor a congenital su-

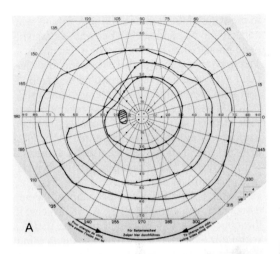

A   B

Figure 3.23. Kinetic perimetry demonstrates a supero-temporal visual field defect in both (A) left and (B) right eyes. Note that the defect is confined to the midperipheral isopter and does not respect the vertical meridian.

prasellar tumor. As with optic nerve hypoplasia, these two seemingly disparate lesions may reflect the disruptive effect of a suprasellar lesion on the migration of optic axons during embryogenesis. This sinister association mandates neuroimaging in any patient with a tilted disc syndrome whose bitemporal hemianopia respects the vertical meridian, fails to preferentially involve the midperipheral isopter on kinetic perimetry, or progressively worsens. The tilted disc syndrome also occurs in some patients with craniofacial anomalies, including Crouzon disease and Apert disease.

Tilted discs without retinal ectasia occur in patients with transsphenoidal encephalocele, congenital tumors of the anterior visual pathways, X-linked congenital stationary night blindness, Ehlers-Danlos syndrome (type III), and familial dextrocardia. In addition, there is one report of a patient who had bilaterally tilted discs, facial hemiatrophy, and congenital horizontal gaze paralysis.

OPTIC DISC DYSPLASIA

The term **optic disc dysplasia** should not be viewed as a diagnosis. Rather, it is a descriptive term that connotes a markedly deformed optic disc that fails to conform to any recognizable diagnostic category (Fig. 3.24). The distinction between a nonspecifically "anomalous" disc and a "dysplastic" disc is somewhat arbitrary and based primarily upon the severity of the lesion.

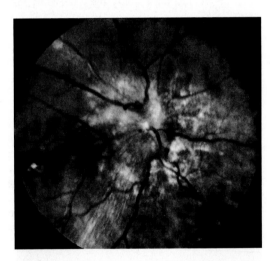

Figure 3.24. Optic disc dysplasia. The optic disc is grossly malformed, and the retinal vessels emerge from the region of the disc in an anomalous pattern.

Dysplastic optic discs in patients with transsphenoidal encephalocele tend to be associated with a discrete infrapapillary zone of V- or tongue-shaped retinochoroidal depigmentation (see Fig. 3.14). These juxtapapillary defects differ from typical retinochoroidal colobomas, which widen inferiorly and are not associated with basal encephalocele. Unlike the typical retinochoroidal coloboma, this distinct juxtapapillary defect is associated with minimal scleral excavation and no visible disruption in the integrity of the overlying retina.

CONGENITAL OPTIC DISC PIGMENTATION

Congenital optic disc pigmentation is a condition in which melanin deposition anterior to or within the lamina cribrosa imparts a slate-gray appearance to the entire optic disc (Fig. 3.25). True congenital optic disc pigmentation is extremely rare, but it has been described in a child with an interstitial deletion of chromosome 17, in children with Aicardi syndrome, and in patients who also have optic nerve hypoplasia (see Fig. 3.25). Congenital optic disc pigmentation is compatible with good visual acuity but may be associated with coexistent optic disc anomalies that decrease vision. The effects of abnormal pigment deposition on optic nerve embryogenesis may explain the frequent coexistence of congenital optic disc pigmentation with other anomalies, particularly optic nerve hypoplasia.

The majority of patients with gray optic discs do not have congenital optic disc pigmentation. For reasons that are poorly understood, the optic discs of infants with delayed visual maturation and albinism often have a diffuse gray tint when viewed ophthalmoscopically. In these conditions, the gray tint usually disappears within the first year of life without visible pigment migration. Indeed, gray optic discs have been observed

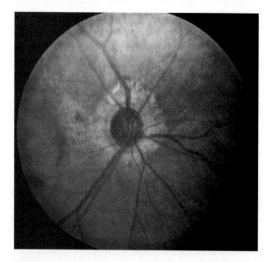

Figure 3.25. Congenital optic disc pigmentation. The entire disc is gray and hypoplastic with a surrounding zone of depigmentation, suggesting migration of peripapillary pigment onto the disc.

in premature infants and in albinotic infants who appeared to be blind at birth but who later developed good vision as the gray color disappeared. The gray appearance of these neonatal discs has been attributed to delayed optic nerve myelination with preservation of the "embryonic tint." It should be noted, however, that gray optic discs may also be seen in normal neonates with no evidence of either delayed myelination or albinism, in whom such discs are usually a nonspecific finding of little diagnostic value. Myelinated peripapillary nerve fibers may impart a gray cast to the optic disc, as may pseudopapilledema associated with buried drusen. A grayish cast to the optic discs was described in three patients with Pelizaeus-Merzbacher disease, in an infant with maple syrup urine disease, and in a child with partial trisomy 10q syndrome.

Optically gray optic discs and congenital optic disc pigmentation can usually be distinguished ophthalmoscopically, because melanin deposition in true congenital optic disc pigmentation is often discrete, irregular, and granular in appearance. True optic disc pigmentation may also be acquired, as in cases of melanocytoma or malignant melanoma of the optic nerve head, following removal of the retrobulbar optic nerve for optic nerve glioma, and following presumed infectious optic neuritis.

AICARDI SYNDROME

Aicardi syndrome is a congenital, uniformly fatal, cerebroretinal disorder of unknown etiology that occurs almost exclusively in females. Its salient clinical features are infantile spasms, agenesis of the corpus callosum, a modified form of the electroencephalographic pattern termed hypsarrhythmia, and a pathognomonic optic disc appearance consisting of multiple depigmented "chorioretinal lacunae" clustered around the disc (Fig. 3.26). Histologically, the chorioretinal lacunae consist of well-circumscribed, full-thickness defects limited to the RPE and choroid. The overlying retina remains intact but is often histologically abnormal.

Congenital optic disc anomalies, including optic disc coloboma, optic nerve hypoplasia, and congenital optic disc pigmentation, may be present in patients with Aicardi syndrome. Other ocular abnormalities in this disorder include microphthalmos, retrobulbar cyst, pseudoglioma, retinal detachment, macular scar, cataract, pupillary membrane, iris synechiae, iris coloboma,

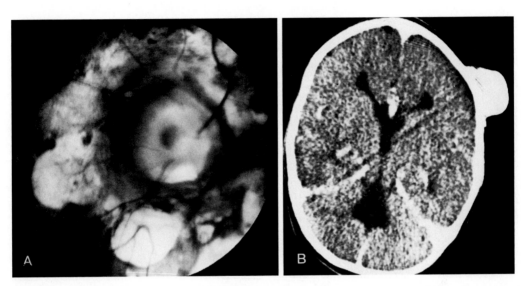

Figure 3.26. Aicardi syndrome. *A.* An enlarged, malformed optic disc is surrounded by numerous, well-circumscribed, chorioretinal lacunae. *B.* CT scan shows agenesis of the corpus callosum.

and persistent hyperplastic primary vitreous. The most common systemic findings associated with Aicardi syndrome are vertebral malformations (fused vertebrae, scoliosis, spina bifida) and costal malformations (absent ribs, fused or bifurcated ribs). Other systemic manifestations include muscular hypotonia, microcephaly, dysmorphic facies, cleft lip and palate, auditory disturbances, and auricular anomalies. There also seems to be an association between choroid plexus papilloma and Aicardi syndrome. Severe mental retardation is present in almost all cases. Aicardi syndrome is associated with decreased life expectancy, but some patients survive into their teenage years. The size of the largest chorioretinal lacuna correlates with neurologic outcome.

CNS anomalies in Aicardi syndrome include agenesis of the corpus callosum, cortical migration anomalies (pachygyria, polymicrogyria, cortical heterotopias), and multiple structural CNS malformations (cerebral hemispheric asymmetry, Dandy-Walker variant, colpocephaly, midline arachnoid cysts) (Fig. 3.27). This complex cerebral malformation suggests a problem in nerve cell proliferation and migration. An overlap between Aicardi syndrome and septo-optic dysplasia has been recognized in several patients.

Aicardi syndrome is thought to result from an X-linked mutational event that is lethal in males. Parents should therefore be asked about a previous history of miscarriages. Parental gonadal mosaicism for the mutation may be an additional mechanism of inheritance. With rare exceptions, cytogenetic testing with special attention to the X chromosome gives normal results in Aicardi syndrome. It is speculated that an insult to the CNS must occur between the 4th and 8th week of gestation.

DOUBLING OF THE OPTIC DISC

Doubling of the optic discs is a rare anomaly in which two optic discs are seen ophthalmoscopically and presumed to be associated with a duplication or separation of the distal optic nerve into two fasciculi. Most cases have a "main" disc and a "satellite" disc, each with its own vascular system (Fig. 3.28). Most examples are present in only one eye and are associated with decreased acuity in the affected eye.

Documented separation of the optic nerve into two or more strands is rare in humans but common in some lower vertebrates. More commonly, an apparent doubling of the optic disc results from focal juxtapapillary retinochoroidal colobomas, which may display abnormal vascular anastomoses with the optic disc. Neuroimaging should allow in vivo confirmation of true optic nerve diastasis.

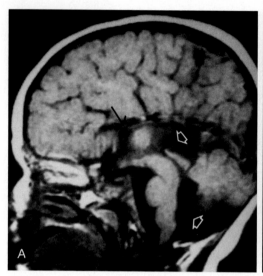

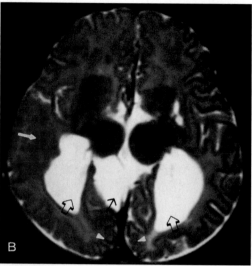

Figure 3.27. Aicardi syndrome. *A.* Sagittal MRI demonstrating agenesis of the corpus callosum (*black arrow, normal* position of the corpus callosum), an arachnoid cyst in the region of the quadrigeminal cistern (*hollow arrow*), and hypoplasia of the cerebellar vermis with cystic dilation of the 4th ventricle (Dandy-Walker variant). *B.* Axial T1-weighted MRI demonstrates gray matter heterotopias in the right temporal lobe (*white arrow*), small areas of probable polymicrogyria medial to occipital poles (*white arrowheads*), an arachnoid cyst in the region of the quadrigeminal cistern (*black arrow*), and dilation of the posterior horns of the lateral ventricles (colpocephaly) (*hollow arrows*). (Reprinted with permission from Carney SH, Brodsky MC, Good WV, et al. Aicardi syndrome: more than meets the eye. Surv Ophthalmol 1993;37:419–424.)

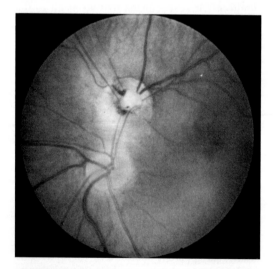

Figure 3.28. Doubling of the optic disc. Note "main" disc and "satellite" disc. (Reprinted with permission from Donoso LA, Magargal LE, Eiferman RA, Meyer D. Ocular anomalies simulating double optic discs. Can J Ophthalmol 1981;16:84–87.)

OPTIC NERVE APLASIA

Optic nerve aplasia is a rare nonhereditary malformation, that is seen most often in a unilaterally malformed eye of an otherwise healthy person. In its current usage, the term implies absence of the optic nerve (including the optic disc), retinal ganglion and nerve fiber layers, and optic nerve vessels. Histopathologic examination usually demonstrates a vestigial dural sheath entering the sclera in its normal position, as well as retinal dysplasia with rosette formation (Fig. 3.29).

Ophthalmoscopically, optic nerve aplasia may take on any of the following appearances:

1. Absence of a normally defined optic nerve head or papilla in the ocular fundus, without central blood vessels and with an absence of macular differentiation.
2. A whitish area corresponding to the optic disc, without central vessels or macular differentiation.
3. A deep avascular cavity in the site corre-

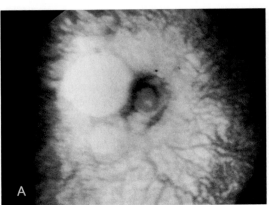

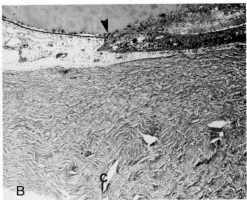

Figure 3.29.   Optic nerve aplasia. *A.* Note absence of optic disc and retinal vessels. (Reprinted with permission from Little LE, Whitmore PV, Wells TW Jr. Aplasia of the optic nerve. J Pediatr Ophthalmol 1976;13:84–88.) *B.* Histologic appearance of optic nerve aplasia. The edge of the choroid and retinal pigment epithelium is marked by an arrowhead.

Fibroglial tissue (*asterisk*) occupies the colobomatous area. A ciliary vessel (*C*) traverses the sclera, but optic nerve tissue is absent. (Reprinted with permission from Hotchkiss ML, Green WR. Optic nerve aplasia and hypoplasia. J Pediatr Ophthalmol Strabismus 1979;16:225–240.)

sponding to the optic disc, surrounded by a whitish annulus.

Visual fields are normal in the unaffected eye. Fluorescein angiography shows absent retinal blood vessels in the affected eye and normal retinal circulation in the opposite eye. The electroretinographic waveform may be flat; if present, the a- and b-waves are diminished. Neuroimaging may show the globe and bony orbit to be smaller than normal, associated with absence of the optic nerve on the affected side. The cause of optic nerve aplasia is unknown.

Although one might logically assume optic nerve aplasia to be the most severe form of optic nerve hypoplasia, optic nerve aplasia seems to fall within a malformation complex that is fundamentally distinct from that seen with optic nerve hypoplasia. This is evidenced by the proclivity of optic nerve aplasia to occur unilaterally and its frequent association with malformations that are otherwise confined to the affected eye (microphthalmia, malformations in the anterior chamber angle, hypoplasia or segmental aplasia of the iris, cataracts, persistent hyperplastic primary vitreous, anterior colobomas, macular staphyloma, retinal dysplasia, or pigmentary disturbance). However, when optic nerve aplasia occurs bilaterally, it is usually associated with severe and widespread congenital CNS malformations.

In patients with unilateral optic nerve aplasia, the intracranial course of the "intact" optic nerve may vary. In one patient with unilateral optic nerve aplasia and microphthalmos, MRI demonstrated true unilateral optic nerve aplasia, hemichiasmal hypoplasia on the affected side, but bilateral optic tracts. VEPs were increased over the occipital lobe contralateral to the intact optic nerve, suggesting chiasmal misdirection of axons from the temporal retina of the normal eye, as seen in albinos. It was speculated that this abnormal decussation may represent an atavistic form of neuronal reorganization.

MYELINATED RETINAL NERVE FIBERS

Myelination of the anterior visual system begins centrally at the lateral geniculate body at 5 months of gestation. It proceeds distally and reaches the optic chiasm by 6 to 7 months of gestation, the retrobulbar optic nerve by 8 months, and the lamina cribrosa at term, although in some cases, myelination continues for a short time after birth. Normally, myelin does not extend intraocularly; however, **intraocular myelination of retinal nerve fibers** occurs in 0.3 to 0.6% of the population by ophthalmoscopy and in 1% by postmortem examinations. In most eyes, myelination is continuous with the optic disc, and the majority of patients have normal visual acuity. The pathogenesis of myelinated nerve fibers remains largely speculative, but it has been proposed that a defect in the lamina cribrosa may allow oligodendrocytes to gain access to the retina and produce myelin there.

Ophthalmoscopically, myelinated nerve fibers usually appear as white striated patches at the upper and lower poles of the optic disc (Fig. 3.30). In these locations, they may impart a gray appearance to the optic disc, and they may also simulate papilledema, both by elevating the adjacent portions of the disc and by obscuring the disc margin and underlying retinal vessels. Distally, they have an irregular fan-shaped appearance that facilitates their recognition. Small slits

or patches of normal-appearing fundus color are occasionally visible within areas of myelination. Myelinated nerve fibers are bilateral in 17 to 20% of cases, and clinically they are discontinuous with the optic nerve head in 19%. The papillomacular bundle is classically spared. Isolated patches of myelinated nerve fibers are occasionally found in the peripheral retina (Fig. 3.31). Retinal vascular abnormalities, including mild telangiectasis and even frank neovascularization, can occur within areas of myelinated nerve fibers.

Myelinated retinal nerve fibers usually do not reduce visual acuity; however, relative scotomas

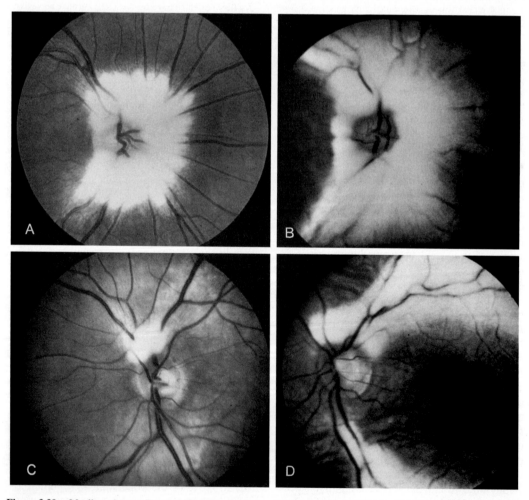

Figure 3.30. Myelinated nerve fibers. *A.* The optic disc is surrounded by myelinated, feathery nerve fibers. *B.* Nerve fiber myelination not only surrounds the disc but also extends temporally along the arcuate nerve fibers surrounding the macula and nasally as well. *C.* A small patch of myelinated nerve fibers is present adjacent to the superior disc margin. *D.* Myelinated nerve fibers extend superiorly and inferiorly from the optic disc along the arcuate nerve fiber bundles.

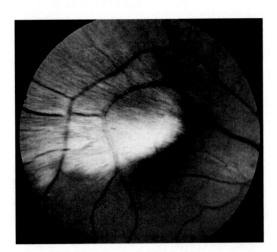

Figure 3.31.   Peripheral myelinated nerve fibers.

may be charted if a sufficient number of myelinated fibers are present. The scotomas are invariably smaller than the size of the myelinated patch would suggest. Because myelinated fibers are usually adjacent to the optic disc, the blind spot is often enlarged in such patients. When the nerve fibers surround the macula, there may be a ring scotoma, and isolated patches in the retinal periphery may produce isolated peripheral scotomas. If the macula is affected, there may be a central scotoma, but this is exceedingly rare.

Extensive unilateral (or rarely bilateral) myelination of nerve fibers can be associated with high myopia and severe amblyopia. Unlike other forms of unilateral high myopia that characteristically respond well to occlusion therapy, the amblyopia that occurs in children with myelinated nerve fibers is notoriously refractory to this treatment. In such patients, myelination surrounds most or all of the circumference of the disc. Additionally, the macular region (although unmyelinated) usually appears abnormal, showing a dulled reflex or pigment dispersion.

Myelinated nerve fibers occur in association with the Gorlin syndrome (multiple basal cell nevi). This autosomal-dominant disorder can often be recognized by the finding of numerous tiny pits in the hands and feet, which produce a "sandpaper" irregularity. Multiple cutaneous tumors develop in the second or third decades, but they may occasionally develop in the first few years of life. When present in childhood, these lesions remain quiescent until puberty, when they increase in number and demonstrate a more rapid and invasive growth pattern. Additional features include jaw cysts, rib anomalies, mild mental retardation, and facial abnormalities (including hypertelorism, prominent supraorbital ridges, frontoparietal bossing, a broad nasal root, and mild mandibular prognathism). Ectopic calcification, especially of the falx cerebri, is an almost constant finding. Medulloblastomas develop in some patients.

Myelinated nerve fibers may be familial, in which case the trait is usually inherited in an autosomal-dominant fashion. Isolated cases of myelinated nerve fibers may also occur in association with abnormal length of the optic nerve (oxycephaly), defects in the lamina cribrosa (tilted disc), anterior segment dysgenesis, and neurofibromatosis type 2. An autosomal-dominant vitreoretinopathy associated with myelination of the nerve fiber layer is characterized by congenitally poor vision, bilateral extensive myelination of the retinal nerve fiber layer, severe degeneration of the vitreous, high myopia, a retinal dystrophy with night blindness, reduction of the electroretinographic responses, and limb deformities.

Rarely, areas of myelinated nerve fibers are acquired after infancy and even in adulthood. Conversely, myelinated nerve fibers may disappear as a result of tabetic optic atrophy, pituitary tumor, glaucoma, central retinal artery occlusion, branch retinal artery occlusion, and various optic neuropathies.

FOR MORE INFORMATION:
See Walsh & Hoyt's *Clinical Neuro-Ophthalmology,* 5th edition, Volume 1, Chapter 8, pages 266–274 and Chapter 18, pages 775–823.

CHAPTER 4

Topical Diagnosis of Acquired Optic Nerve Disorders

APPEARANCE OF THE DISC
  Optic Disc Swelling
  Infiltration of the Optic Disc
  Optic Atrophy
SYNDROMES OF UNILATERAL OPTIC NERVE
  DYSFUNCTION
  Optociliary Shunts and the Syndrome of Chronic
    Optic Nerve Compression
  Prechiasmal Optic Nerve Compression Syndrome
  Distal Optic Nerve Syndrome

Foster Kennedy Syndrome
BILATERAL LESIONS OF THE OPTIC NERVES
  Bilateral Superior or Inferior Hemianopia
  Bilateral "Checkerboard" Altitudinal Hemianopia
    and the Vertical Hemifield Slide Phenomenon
  Nasal Hemianopia
CHRONIC OPEN-ANGLE GLAUCOMA

Damage to an optic nerve classically causes an abnormality in visual sensory function, a relative afferent pupillary defect, and, if the damage is irreversible, a change in the appearance of the optic disc. Acquired optic neuropathies can produce any type of visual field defect, including a central scotoma, cecocentral scotoma, arcuate field defect, altitudinal defect, or even a temporal or nasal hemianopic defect. Unless the optic neuropathy is bilateral or the lesion is located near the optic chiasm, the field defect produced by an optic nerve lesion is always monocular.

The visual field defects that occur with various optic neuropathies are not in themselves localizing. Rather, it is the history of visual loss (rapid vs. slow onset, progressive vs. stable), the presence or absence of other neurologic or ocular signs (relative afferent pupillary defect, acquired color deficit, ocular motor paresis, proptosis, optociliary shunt veins, optic disc swelling, optic pallor), and, occasionally, the results of electrophysiologic testing that most often allow the examiner to diagnose an optic neuropathy, to localize the pathology along the course of the nerve, and to determine its etiology.

APPEARANCE OF THE DISC

The optic disc has only two ways to respond to the many acquired pathologic processes that may affect the optic nerve. It can swell, or it can remain normal in appearance. If the pathologic process causes irreversible damage to the optic nerve, the disc will eventually become pale.

OPTIC DISC SWELLING

Swelling of the optic disc occurs when there is obstruction of axon transport at the lamina cribrosa (Fig. 4.1). This may result from compression, ischemia, inflammation, metabolic dysfunction, or toxic damage (Table 4.1). In some cases, infiltration of the proximal portion of the disc by inflammatory or malignant processes causes an appearance that is indistinguishable from true swelling. Anomalies of the optic disc that produce an appearance that mimics true swelling are discussed in Chapter 3 of this text.

Appearance

Useful funduscopic signs of early swelling of the optic disc include blurring of the nerve fiber layer around the disc, especially superiorly and

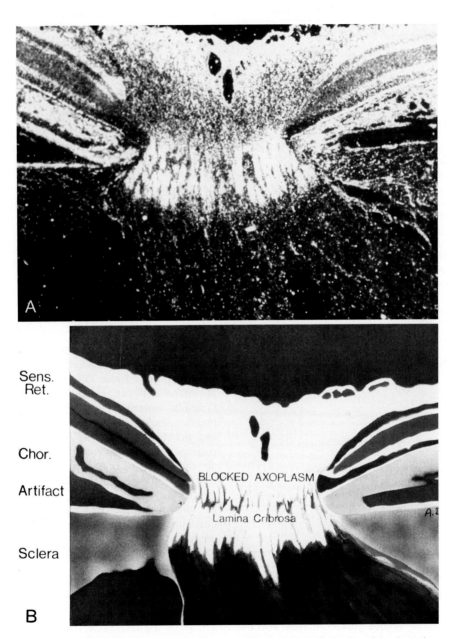

Figure 4.1. The final common denominator of optic disc swelling: obstruction of axon transport. *A.* Phase-contrast photomicrograph of a swollen optic disc in an animal with experimental papilledema shows accumulation of axon products (seen as white material) in the region of the lamina cribrosa. *B.* Artist's drawing of the photomicrograph. *Sens. Ret.:* sensory retina. *Chor.:* choroid. (Reprinted with permission from Miller NR, Fine SL. The Ocular Fundus in Neuro-ophthalmologic Diagnosis: Sights and Sounds in Ophthalmology. Vol 3. St. Louis: CV Mosby, 1977.)

Table 4.1
The Differential Diagnosis of the "Swollen Disc"

Disc Elevation Without True Swelling
• Optic disc anomalies
  Drusen
  Tilted disc
  Crowded disc
• Optic disc infiltration

True Disc Swelling
• Elevated intracranial pressure
• Inflammatory
  Infectious
  Demyelinating
  Sarcoidosis
• Vascular
  Anterior ischemic optic neuropathy
    Arteritic
    Nonarteritic
  Central retinal vein occlusion
• Compressive
  Neoplastic
    Meningioma
    Hemangioma
  Non-neoplastic
    Thyroid ophthalmopathy
• Infiltrative
  Neoplastic
    Leukemia
    Lymphoma
    Glioma
  Non-neoplastic
    Sarcoidosis
• Toxic/Metabolic/Nutritional deficiency
• Hereditary
  Leber's hereditary optic neuropathy
• Traumatic
• Hypotony

inferiorly, and a tendency for the increasingly swollen and opaque nerve fibers to obscure segments of blood vessels, especially arteries, as they approach or cross the disc edge (Fig. 4.2) (see Chapter 5). Disc hyperemia and absence of spontaneous venous pulsations may also be noted. When disc swelling is fully developed, additional funduscopic changes can appear, including intraretinal hemorrhages and infarcts (cotton-wool spots) within the nerve fiber layer, hard exudates (sometimes in a star figure around or on the nasal half of the macula), and subhyaloid hemorrhage, occasionally breaking out into the vitreous cavity (Figs. 4.2 and 4.3).

When disc swelling persists for several

months or longer, the hemorrhages and exudates tend to resolve, and the initial hyperemia is replaced by a milky gray appearance that reflects supervening gliosis, often accompanied by the development of "drusen-like" hard exudates in the superficial substance of the disc itself (Fig. 4.4). Neovascular membranes with subretinal hemorrhages and serous fluid can progressively develop. Optic atrophy with narrowed, often sheathed, retinal vessels may supervene in patients with chronic disc swelling. Optociliary shunt vessels may also appear on the optic disc, presumably secondary to chronic obstruction of normal retinal venous drainage through the central retinal vein by chronic disc swelling.

Optic disc swelling may not develop if significant optic atrophy is already present: dead axons can't swell. This is particularly important to remember when the ophthalmoscopic appearance of an atrophic optic disc is being used to determine recurrence or exacerbation of a condition such as pseudotumor cerebri (see Chapter 5).

Specific Etiologies

Patients with increased intracranial pressure may develop optic disc swelling. This condition is called **papilledema**. The symptoms and signs in patients with papilledema generally are those typically associated with raised intracranial pressure, including headache, nausea, vomiting, and pulsatile tinnitus. Visual symptoms in such patients include transient obscurations of vision and diplopia. Loss of central vision, dyschromatopsia, a relative afferent pupillary defect, and visual field defects other than enlargement of the blind spot caused by the swollen disc are uncommon in patients with acute papilledema unless the lesion causing the increased intracranial pressure also directly damages the visual sensory system in some way, or there are hemorrhages or exudates in the macula.

The optic disc swelling in papilledema is usually bilateral and symmetric (see Fig. 4.3), but it may be asymmetric or even unilateral (Fig. 4.5). It may be very mild or extremely severe (see Fig. 4.2). Papilledema is discussed in Chapter 5 of this text.

Inflammation of the proximal portion of the optic nerve produces swelling of the optic disc. This condition, called **anterior optic neuritis** or **papillitis**, is characterized by sudden visual loss, usually in one eye; it is almost always associated with pain around or behind the eye. The pain is

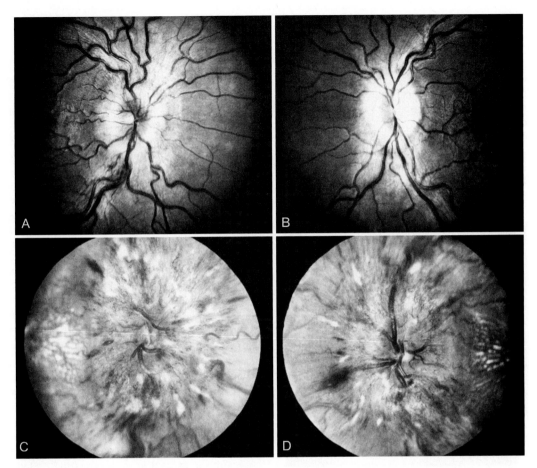

Figure 4.2. Variability in severity of papilledema. *A–B.* Mild papilledema in a 14-year-old boy with hydrocephalus caused by congenital aqueductal stenosis. The right disc (*A*) is somewhat more hyperemic and swollen than the left (*B*). *C–D.* Severe papilledema in a 32-year-old woman with pseudotumor cerebri. Note numerous hemorrhages and cotton-wool spots surrounding the markedly swollen right (*C*) and left (*D*) optic discs. Also note hard exudates (lipid) in both maculae.

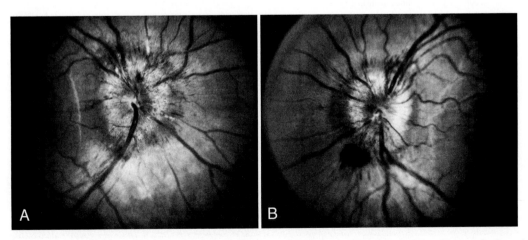

Figure 4.3. Bilateral symmetric papilledema in a young man with a posterior fossa mass. *A.* Right optic disc is moderately swollen and hyperemic. Several flame-shaped intraretinal hemorrhages and soft exudates surround the swollen disc. *B.* The left optic disc is also swollen and hyperemic. Several small flame-shaped hemorrhages and a larger round hemorrhage surround the disc.

often exacerbated by eye movement. The appearance of the optic disc ranges from very mild to severe swelling (Fig. 4.6). Vitreous cells may be present, particularly overlying the swollen disc, but peripapillary hemorrhages are rarely seen (Fig. 4.7).

In most cases of anterior optic neuritis, vision continues to decline for several hours to several

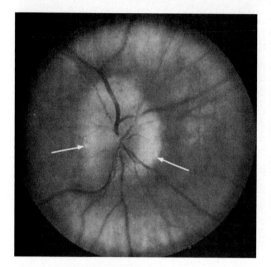

Figure 4.4. Drusen-like bodies (*arrows*) in chronic atrophic papilledema. (Reprinted with permission from Hoyt WF, Beeston D. The Ocular Fundus in Neurologic Disease. St. Louis: CV Mosby, 1966.)

days. It then stabilizes and, after several days to several weeks, begins to improve.

Anterior optic neuritis typically occurs in young adults and is most often caused by demyelination, although it may also develop in patients with a variety of systemic disorders, such as cat-scratch disease, syphilis, Lyme disease, and sarcoidosis. Vitreous cells tend to be absent in demyelinating optic neuritis, whereas they are more likely to be present and significant in patients with underlying systemic inflammatory or infectious disease. Patients who develop optic neuritis that is unassociated with a systemic inflammatory or infectious disorder have an increased risk of developing clinical evidence of multiple sclerosis (MS) compared with the normal population.

A special form of anterior optic neuritis called **neuroretinitis** is characterized ophthalmoscopically by optic disc swelling associated with a macular star figure composed of lipid (Fig. 4.8). This form of optic neuritis is almost never caused by demyelination and occurs most often in the setting of cat-scratch disease or in association with other systemic infectious diseases such as Lyme disease, syphilis, toxoplasmosis, and tuberculosis, as well as with sarcoidosis. Optic neuritis is discussed in Chapter 6 of this text.

Ischemia that affects the laminar or prelaminar portions of the optic nerve produces swelling of the optic disc. This condition, called **anterior**

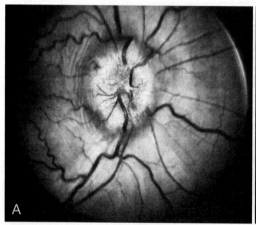
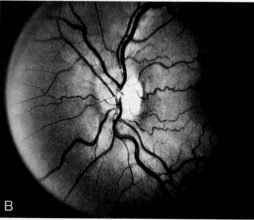
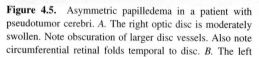

Figure 4.5. Asymmetric papilledema in a patient with pseudotumor cerebri. *A.* The right optic disc is moderately swollen. Note obscuration of larger disc vessels. Also note circumferential retinal folds temporal to disc. *B.* The left optic disc is minimally swollen. It was thought to be normal when the patient was examined; however, the photograph shows mild hyperemia of the disc and blurred disc margins from 6 to 12 o'clock.

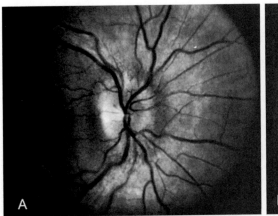
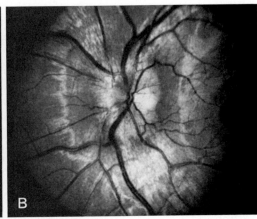
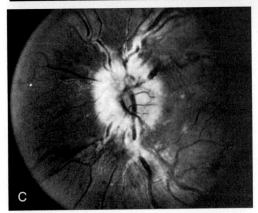

Figure 4.6.   Variability in appearance of the optic disc in patients with anterior optic neuritis. *A.* Mild swelling of right optic disc in a 13-year-old girl with acute loss of vision in the right eye, a central visual field defect, and an ipsilateral relative afferent pupillary defect. *B.* Moderate swelling of the left optic disc in a 20-year-old woman with a similar history. *C.* Severe swelling with exudates and sheathing in a 25-year-old man with syphilis.

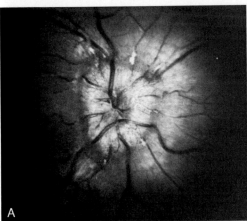
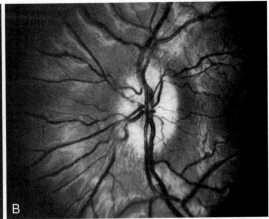

Figure 4.7.   The appearance of a ''choked disc'' caused by papilledema compared with a ''choked disc'' in a patient with anterior optic neuritis. *A.* Right optic disc in a young woman with papilledema. There is moderate swelling of the disc, which is surrounded by several intraretinal hemorrhages and soft exudates. *B.* Left optic disc in a patient with anterior optic neuritis. The disc is moderately swollen, and there are mild circumferential retinal folds temporal to the disc. Note that both optic discs appear similar in appearance. It is impossible to determine the cause of optic disc swelling in most cases unless one obtains a complete medical and ocular history and performs a complete ocular examination (e.g., tests of visual acuity, color vision, visual field).

Figure 4.8. Neuroretinitis. The patient was a young woman who developed acute visual loss in the right eye while visiting Connecticut. The right optic disc is swollen, and there is a star figure composed of lipid (hard exudate) in the macula. An evaluation revealed serologic evidence of Lyme disease. Neuroretinitis is not associated with the subsequent development of multiple sclerosis, but is most often caused by an underlying systemic infection, such as cat-scratch disease, Lyme disease, syphilis, or sarcoidosis.

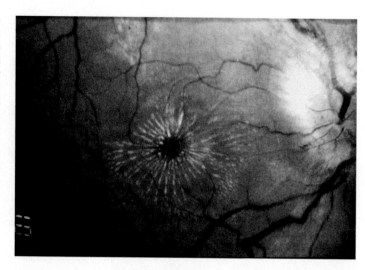

ischemic optic neuropathy (AION), is characterized by sudden, monocular, and usually painless visual loss associated with a relative afferent pupillary defect and a visual field defect that is most often altitudinal or arcuate in nature. The loss of vision usually occurs over several hours to several days. It then stabilizes and remains stable in many cases; however, about 40% of patients with the nonarteritic form of the condition improve spontaneously over weeks to months.

AION occurs most often in patients over 50 years of age who have underlying systemic vasculopathies, particularly diabetes mellitus, systemic hypertension, and giant cell arteritis. Younger patients with hypertension, diabetes mellitus, systemic vasculitis, or migraine are also at increased risk to develop AION.

The optic disc swelling that occurs in AION may be hyperemic or pallid and is usually accompanied by one or more flame-shaped hemorrhages near the margins of the disc (Fig. 4.9). When the swelling is pallid, visual loss is usually very severe and incapable of improving.

Patients with nonarteritic AION invariably have a congenitally small optic disc with an absent or small central cup (Fig. 4.10), and this congenital abnormality is thought to be the major predisposing factor for the development of the disorder. Patients with arteritic AION, on the other hand, may have any sized optic disc. Thus, if a patient with AION has a normal optic disc in the opposite eye, one can be fairly certain that the AION is arteritic in origin; however, if

the contralateral optic disc is small, with little or no cup, the AION may be arteritic or nonarteritic. AION is discussed in Chapter 7 of this text.

Compression of the proximal portion of the optic nerve may produce optic disc swelling. The compression may be caused by a tumor, such as a cavernous hemangioma, meningioma, or schwannoma. In other cases, enlargement of structures normally in the orbit, such as the extraocular muscles in dysthyroid ophthalmopathy, causes optic nerve compression. Patients in whom such compression occurs initially may have no visual complaints and may have few, if any, signs of optic nerve dysfunction other than an enlarged blind spot on visual field testing. Alternatively, they may complain of insidious and slowly progressive visual loss. In such cases, there is invariably some degree of dyschromatopsia, a relative afferent pupillary defect, and a defect in the visual field of the affected eye. The optic disc is generally only mildly to moderately swollen and hyperemic (Fig. 4.11). Peripapillary hemorrhages are usually absent, but chorioretinal striae are present in some cases, particularly when the compressive lesion is adjacent to the globe. The diagnosis of anterior compressive optic neuropathy is made by ultrasonography or neuroimaging of the orbit. Compressive optic neuropathy is discussed in Chapter 8 of this text.

Toxic and metabolic disorders may cause swelling of the optic disc. In such cases, the swelling is usually bilateral and mild (Fig. 4.12). Central vision is often reduced, with visual loss progressing slowly over several weeks to

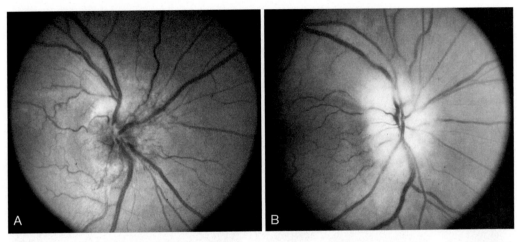

Figure 4.9.   Optic disc swelling in anterior ischemic optic neuropathy. *A*. Hyperemic swelling. *B*. Pallid swelling. Eyes with pallid disc swelling usually have worse visual function than eyes with hyperemic disc swelling.

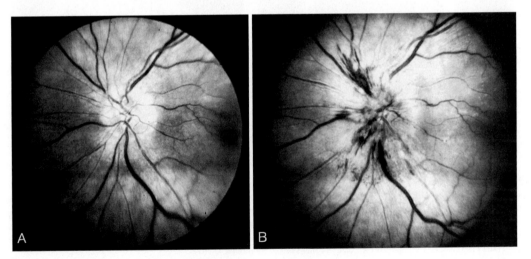

Figure 4.10.   The "disc at risk" in nonarteritic anterior ischemic optic neuropathy (NAION). *A*. Small left optic disc with no cup in a patient who had experienced an attack of NAION in the right eye several months earlier. *B*. NAION characterized by hyperemic disc swelling and peripapillary hemorrhages in the same eye several months later.

months. Color vision is almost always markedly abnormal, regardless of the level of central vision. Bilateral central or cecocentral scotomas are the rule, in some cases being associated with mild to severe constriction of the peripheral visual field. In many but not all cases, eliminating the source of the toxicity or reversing the metabolic abnormality is associated with partial or complete recovery of visual function. Toxic and metabolic optic neuropathies are discussed in Chapter 10 of this text.

Intraocular **hypotony** may induce optic disc swelling. Lowering the intraocular pressure in experimental animals causes ipsilateral disc swelling. Following a penetrating wound of the eye or following an intraocular operation in which the wound is not tightly closed, there may be development of disc swelling (Fig. 4.13). Blunt trauma to the eye may result in damage to the ciliary body and reduction of aqueous humor formation with subsequent development of hypotony and disc swelling despite an intact globe.

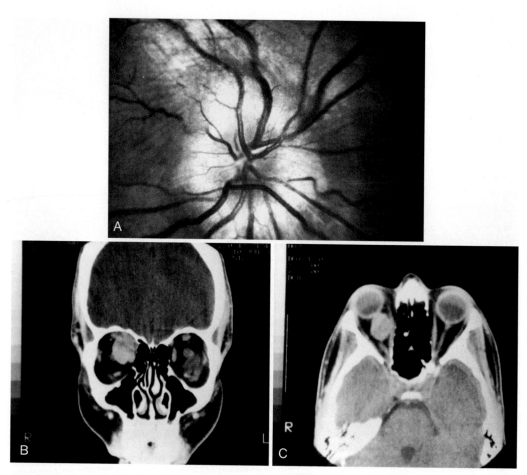

Figure 4.11. Optic disc swelling from compression of the anterior portion of the orbital optic nerve. *A.* Right optic disc of a 25-year-old man who noted mildly decreased vision in the right eye. Visual acuity was 20/25 and there was an ipsilateral relative afferent pupillary defect. The optic disc is moderately swollen. *B.* Noncontrast CT scan, coronal view, shows that the mass compresses the nasal and superior portions of the optic nerve, displacing it downward. *C.* Noncontrast CT scan, axial view, shows a well-circumscribed orbital mass compressing the optic nerve. Note distortion and irregularity of the nerve. The patient's vision returned to normal, and the optic disc swelling resolved after the mass was removed.

In such cases, the hypotony resolves spontaneously as does the disc swelling. Although visual acuity is impaired in such cases, the visual disturbance appears to be related primarily to increased corneal thickness from the hypotony rather than to a true optic neuropathy. As with other forms of true disc swelling, the pathophysiology of disc swelling in patients with ocular hypotony appears to be blockage of axon transport at the lamina cribrosa.

INFILTRATION OF THE OPTIC DISC

Infiltration of the proximal portion of the optic nerve by tumor or inflammatory cells can produce an appearance similar to true swelling of the optic disc (Fig. 4.14). The disc changes may be asymptomatic or associated with variable visual loss, dyschromatopsia, and a visual field defect. The infiltration may be unilateral or bilateral, and a relative afferent pupillary defect may be present if the infiltration is either unilateral or bilateral but asymmetric. Infiltration of the optic nerve occurs most frequently in patients with malignant tumors, such as leukemia, lymphoma, and various carcinomas that spread to the central nervous system, but it may also occur in patients with systemic inflammatory

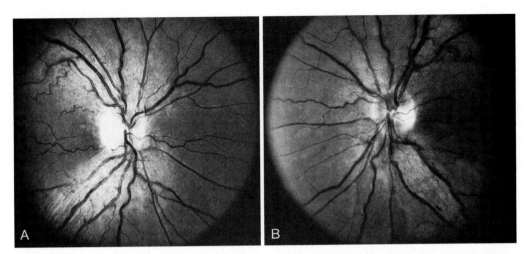

Figure 4.12.   Optic disc swelling in nutritional optic neuropathy. The patient was a 34-year-old alcoholic man who had a poor diet and who developed progressive loss of vision in both eyes. Visual acuity was 20/200 OU, and there were bilateral cecocentral scotomas. The concentration of folic acid in the patient's red blood cells was low. *A.* The right optic disc is pale temporally and hyperemic nasally. There is atrophy of the papillomacular bundle. *B.* The left optic disc is hyperemic and mildly swollen. An assay of the patient's blood for mitochondrial mutations of Leber's optic neuropathy was negative. The patient's vision improved and the disc swelling resolved after he reduced his alcohol intake, improved his diet, and was treated with vitamin supplements that included folic acid.

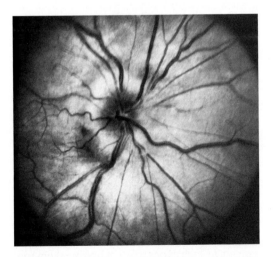

Figure 4.13.   Optic disc swelling in hypotony. The patient was a 43-year-old woman who developed hypotony in the right eye after a glaucoma filtering operation. Note moderate swelling and hyperemia of the right optic disc. The appearance of this disc is similar to that which may occur in papilledema, anterior optic neuritis, and other conditions that produce optic disc swelling.

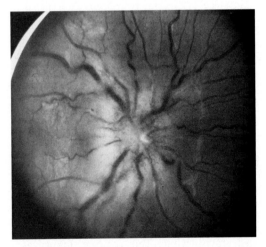

Figure 4.14.   Optic disc elevation from infiltration of the orbital portion of the optic nerve. The patient was an 11-year-old boy with acute lymphocytic leukemia that was thought to be in remission when he developed mild blurred vision in the right eye. Note moderate elevation of the right optic disc, associated with dilation of small disc vessels. Malignant cells were detected in the patient's cerebrospinal fluid. The disc elevation resolved and visual acuity improved after radiation therapy.

disorders, including sarcoidosis, tuberculosis, and syphilis. Infiltrative optic neuropathies are discussed in Chapter 8 of this text.

OPTIC ATROPHY

Optic atrophy is not a disease. It is a morphologic sequela of disease—any disease—that causes irreversible damage to ganglion cells and axons of the optic nerve. The term "optic atrophy" is, therefore, a pathologic generalization applied to optic nerve shrinkage from any process that produces degeneration of axons in the anterior visual system (the retinogeniculate pathway), including ischemia, inflammation, compression, infiltration, and demyelination. Although the pathologist can make the diagnosis of optic atrophy by direct observation of histopathologic changes in the optic nerve, the clinical diagnosis of atrophy is usually based on (1) ophthalmoscopic abnormalities of color and structure of the optic disc with associated changes in the retinal vessels and nerve fiber layer, and (2) defective visual function that can be localized to the optic nerve.

Nonpathologic Pallor of the Optic Disc

An absolute prerequisite to recognition of the abnormal disc is familiarity with normal disc color. The temporal side of the normal disc usually has less color than the nasal side. The degree of this temporal pallor is primarily related to the size of the physiologic cup, to the thin translucent character of the temporal nerve fiber layer, and possibly to the relative sparseness of capillaries on that side of the disc.

The normal physiologic cup may vary in size. When it extends almost to the temporal edge of the disc, the temporal side of the disc is pale. In addition, the temporal margins of some large physiologic cups are steep-walled. When the margins slope gradually downward from the margin of the disc, the crescent of sclera adjacent to the temporal, and occasionally to the inferior, margin of the disc is visible and appears a mottled grayish white. This crescent, known as a temporal (or sometimes inferior) conus, is exposed by retraction of the dark retinal pigment epithelium from the disc margin. It enhances the white appearance of the disc.

Marked recession or excavation of a physiologic cup makes the center of a disc pale. The retinal vessels at the base of the cup are partially obscured as they pass through a thin rim of neural tissue that borders the excavation. It may be difficult to distinguish this type of cup from a glaucomatous cup. The pallor of the floor of a physiologic cup is directly related to the glistening whiteness of the lamina cribrosa or cribriform plate, a connective and elastic tissue structure with small sieve-like openings through which transparent nerve fiber bundles pass (see Chapter 2). Because the openings are irregular, direct light entering them is reflected in many directions, and the holes appear as grayish yellow ovals or dots. When this dotting is seen, it signifies that no abnormal opaque connective tissue is present over the surface of the cribriform plate.

A white-appearing disc is common in an eye with axial myopia. Because the optic nerve enters the globe obliquely, the contents of the disc, including the nerve fibers and the retinal vessels, are displaced nasally. The physiologic cup is shallow, and its extension to the temporal margin produces relative temporal pallor that is often exaggerated by a temporal conus.

In infants, ophthalmoscopic examinations are made with difficulty. Efforts to keep the lids separated produce inadvertent pressure on the eye and may account for apparent pallor of the optic discs seen in such cases. In addition, many infants have generally pale fundi; the optic discs in such cases also appear pale.

An illusory impression of whiteness may be caused merely by fresh batteries or a new bulb in the examiner's ophthalmoscope (thus providing a brighter light source). Conversely, true pallor of an optic disc may be overlooked when the light source is weak. The color of the disc also varies with the color temperature of the light source and the age of the lens. Finally, removal of the natural lens with cataract extraction causes an illusion of pallor in the aphakic or pseudophakic eye.

Pathology and Pathophysiology of Optic Atrophy

Because the axons in the optic nerve arise from the ganglion cells located in the retina, damage to such axons may occur from numerous sources at several locations:

- From disease within the eye that damages the ganglion cells, the retinal nerve fiber layer, or the optic disc.
- From disease within or surrounding the in-

traorbital, intracanalicular, or intracranial portions of the optic nerve
- From disorders that damage the optic chiasm, optic tracts, or lateral geniculate bodies.
- From disorders of the retrogeniculate pathways that produce transsynaptic (transneuronal) degeneration.

A disease may be focal, multifocal, or diffuse. It may destroy axons directly or by its effects on their investing glia or capillary blood supply. Focal disruption anywhere along an axon causes degeneration of the entire axon and its cell body, the retinal ganglion cell. When large numbers of axons undergo such degeneration, gross shrinkage or atrophy of the optic nerve becomes evident.

When an axon is irreversibly damaged, it undergoes two types of degeneration: anterograde and retrograde. Anterograde degeneration occurs in the distal portion of the axon that has been separated from its cell body, whereas retrograde degeneration occurs in the proximal segment of the nerve that remains in contact with the cell body.

When a visual axon is severed, its distal (ascending) segment, being separated from its nutrient ganglion cell body, quickly disintegrates and disappears, and its investing myelin sheath undergoes a slower breakdown into simpler lipids that are eventually catabolized. This process is called **anterograde** or **wallerian** degeneration. Nerve fibers in the optic nerve undergo wallerian degeneration at a rate proportional to their thickness. Large axons show varicosities as early as 30 hours from the time of severance from the cell body. Within 4 to 8 days, they break up into shorter oval or spherical fragments that progressively disintegrate and disappear. In medium-sized myelinated fibers, the axon is still in the varicose or beaded stage at the end of a week and breaks up from the 14th to 15th day onward. In fine fibers, the process is even slower, with many axons showing little change during the first 10 days.

An essential feature of wallerian degeneration is the swelling and degeneration of the terminal buttons (bouton terminaux) of axons within the lateral geniculate bodies. This consists of globular thickening or swelling of the terminals of visual axons that can be identified within layers of the lateral geniculate body as early as 24 hours

after a lesion of the axon. Wallerian degeneration and the optic pallor it produces can only be observed clinically when retinal axons are damaged within the eye.

Although anterograde degeneration begins and becomes nearly complete within 7 days after injury, the portion of the axon still connected to the cell body, and the cell body itself, remain normal in appearance for 3 to 4 weeks. During this time, orthograde axonal transport continues in a normal manner. After about 3 to 4 weeks, however, the entire remaining structure (the cell body and axon from the point of injury) degenerates rapidly, so that by about 6 to 8 weeks after severe optic nerve injury, no affected ganglion cells remain viable.

A most fascinating feature of this **retrograde degeneration** of the optic nerve (and other nerves as well) is that the time course of this degeneration is apparently independent of the distance of the injury from the ganglion cell body. Damage to the retrobulbar portion of the optic nerve, the optic chiasm, and the optic tract all cause pathologic and visible degeneration of the ganglion cell bodies at about the same time.

Regeneration of axons in the optic nerve in human and nonhuman primates is quite limited and abortive. However, some degree of remyelination does occur after injury. This remyelination results from the activity of uninjured, injured but surviving, and newly generated oligodendroglia.

Transsynaptic (transneuronal) **degeneration** is a secondary degenerative reaction of neurons that occurs in a number of areas of the brain. For example, transneuronal degeneration is a well-established phenomenon in the cells of the lateral geniculate body following destruction of parts of the retina. However, the most profound transsynaptic changes occur following lesions in the immature brain. This type of transsynaptic degeneration occurs most often in patients with occipital lobe damage in utero or during early infancy. Although it has been suggested that transsynaptic degeneration may occur in mature adult human and nonhuman primate visual systems if enough time has elapsed, clinically apparent transsynaptic degeneration probably does not occur after injury in adult humans.

Loss of function within the central nervous system is consistently associated with a reduction of blood supply to the affected tissue, regardless of the primary pathogenetic process.

When the optic nerve degenerates, its blood supply is reduced, and small vessels that were once visible in the normal nerve can no longer be seen with an ophthalmoscope. In addition to reduction of blood supply, formation of glial tissue is said to occur with optic atrophy. These two factors—reduction of blood supply and formation of glial tissue—are presumed by most authors to account for the pallor that is associated with optic nerve atrophy.

Other factors that may account for the normal pink appearance of the optic disc are its thickness and the cytoarchitecture of nerve fiber bundles passing between glial columns containing capillaries. Light entering the disc is normally conducted along the transparent nerve fiber bundles, much like fiberoptic pathways. The light diffuses among adjacent columns of glial cells and capillaries and acquires the pink color of the capillaries. Thus, light rays that exit through the tissue via the nerve fiber bundles are pink and give the disc its characteristic color. The axon bundles of an atrophic optic disc have been destroyed, and the remaining astrocytes are arranged at right angles to the entering light. Thus, little light passes into the disc substance to traverse the capillaries that, although still present, are surrounded by layers of astrocytes. Because the light is reflected from opaque glial cells and does not pass through capillaries, it remains white, and the optic disc thus appears pale. In some areas, loss of tissue also allows light to pass directly to the opaque scleral lamina, and this adds to the pale color of the disc.

Ophthalmoscopic Features of Optic Atrophy

The evaluation of optic disc color is a routine but often perplexing problem. It is precisely the lack of color in an optic disc that is most difficult to assess, record, compare, and describe. The normal color of the optic disc depends on its composition, the relationship of the components to each other, and the light that strikes them and is either reflected or refracted from the disc surface.

Pallor of the optic disc is often graded as mild, moderate, or severe; however, such distinctions are subjective and unreliable. More objective evaluation of the pale optic disc can be obtained by detailed observation of its configuration and neural tissue; its veins, arteries, and capillaries; and the peripapillary retinal nerve fiber layer that

surrounds it. Pallor of the optic disc may be diffuse or confined to one sector (Fig. 4.15).

In the early stages of atrophy, the optic disc loses its reddish hue, and the substance of the disc slowly disappears, leaving a pale, shallow, concave meniscus: the exposed lamina cribrosa (Fig. 4.16). In the end stages of the atrophic process, retinal vessels of normal caliber still emerge centrally through the otherwise avascular-appearing disc. In many cases, the changes that develop during the progression to atrophy do not result in a significant change in the central cup of the optic disc. In some cases, however, pathologic optic disc cupping develops in patients with normal intraocular pressures and optic atrophy from various causes, including ischemia, compression, inflammation, and trauma (Figs. 4.17 and 4.18). There is significant controversy as to whether or not the cupping in such cases is identical to that seen with glaucoma.

We would stress that despite the occasional confusion between glaucomatous and nonglaucomatous optic neuropathy that occurs in patients with pathologic cupping and pallor of the optic disc, a careful clinical examination almost always results in the correct diagnosis. Glaucomatous visual field defects occur only after extensive cupping is present, and acuity loss usually occurs even later. In such cases, there is usually absence of at least a portion of the neuroretinal rim, and any remaining rim tissue has a normal color (see Figs. 4.17A–B and 4.18B). In nonglaucomatous optic neuropathies, significant loss of visual acuity, color vision, and field may occur in combination with only mild cupping. In addition, the optic discs in such cases rarely have any areas in which the neuroretinal rim is completely absent, and the remaining rim is often pale (see Figs. 4.17E and 4.18A). The appearance of the neuroretinal rim is thus a crucial factor in determining if cupping is caused by glaucomatous or nonglaucomatous optic nerve damage. Pallor of the neuroretinal rim is 94% specific for nonglaucomatous atrophy and cupping, whereas focal or diffuse obliteration of the neuroretinal rim with preservation of color of any remaining rim tissue is 87% specific for glaucoma.

Focal destruction of nerve fiber bundles is one of the common pathologic denominators of disease that affects the inner retinal layers, optic disc, retrobulbar optic nerve, or a combination of these structures. The normal appearance of

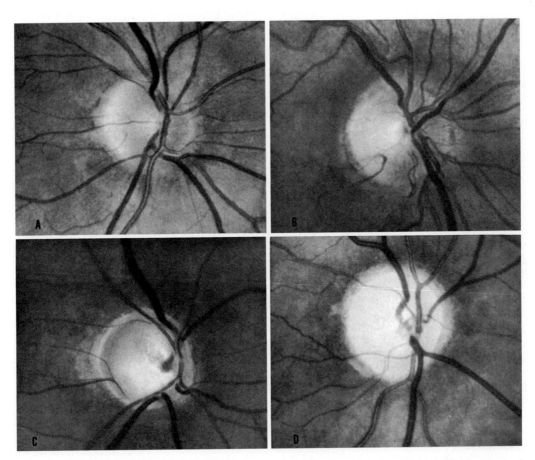

Figure 4.15.   Pallor of the optic disc. *A.* Mild temporal pallor in a patient with multiple sclerosis but who denied acute optic neuritis. *B.* Temporal pallor in a patient with toxic amblyopia. *C.* Pallor with glaucomatous cupping. Note preservation of small nasal neuroretinal rim. *D.* Diffuse pal-lor in a patient with retrograde (descending) optic atrophy from the effects of an intracranial mass. (Reprinted with permission from Hoyt WF, Beeston D. The Ocular Fundus in Neurologic Disease. St. Louis: CV Mosby, 1966.)

the peripapillary retinal nerve fiber layer consists of fine curvilinear striations that overlie the retinal vessels, causing them to be seen slightly out of focus. Early focal loss of axons is represented by the development of dark slits or wedges in the peripapillary retinal nerve fiber layer. These slits or bands appear darker or redder than the adjacent normal tissue in which the normal linear or curvilinear nerve fiber layer striations can easily be seen (Fig. 4.19*A–B*). The slit defects are most easily identified in the superior and inferior arcuate regions where the nerve fiber layer is particularly thick. With increasing distance from the disc, the defects gradually lose contrast and cannot be identified. When only a few nerve fiber bundle defects are present, they

can be identified only by the appearance of a dark, linear, arching region among the lighter, linear nerve fiber reflexes; however, when multiple nerve fiber bundle defects are present, they impart a "raked" appearance to the nerve fiber layer.

As nerve fiber bundle defects increase, they may coalesce, producing a large wedge pattern (Fig. 4.19*C–E*). A similar pattern occurs when a large region of nerve fiber layer is simultaneously damaged (e.g., after ischemic optic neuropathy). Within the wedge, the entire retina takes on a flat granular appearance with no striations being appreciated (Fig. 4.19*E–F*). In addition, vessels in this area, having lost their surrounding nerve fiber covering, appear darker

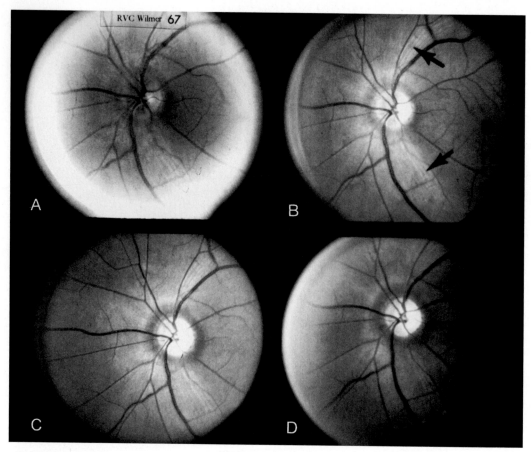

Figure 4.16. Development of pallor of the optic disc in a patient with retrograde (descending) optic atrophy. *A.* The optic disc is normal in the early stage of the process. *B.* With time, the optic disc loses its reddish hue, and the substance of the disc slowly disappears, leaving a pale, shallow concave meniscus, the exposed lamina cribrosa. As these changes occur, the peripapillary retinal nerve fiber layer begins to show defects that appear as dark linear striations (*arrows*). *C.* With more time, the disc becomes more diffusely pale, and the peripapillary nerve fiber layer becomes less visible. *D.* In the end stage of the atrophic process, retinal vessels of normal caliber still emerge centrally through the otherwise avascular-appearing disc, and the peripapillary retinal nerve fiber layer is no longer visible. (Reprinted with permission from Miller NR, Fine SL. The Ocular Fundus in Neuro-Ophthalmologic Diagnosis: Sights and Sounds in Ophthalmology. Vol 3. St. Louis: CV Mosby, 1977.)

than normal and stand out sharply in relief. A prominent light reflex usually emanates from alongside the vessels, presumably as a result of draping of the inner limiting membrane directly over the vessels (Fig. 4.19*G*).

Diffuse thinning of the nerve fiber layer around the optic disc is difficult to recognize in the early stages. In more advanced stages, signs of atrophy include decreased opacity of the arcuate fiber bundles, enhanced linear highlights on large and small retinal blood vessels, reduced caliber of blood vessels, and pallor of the optic

disc with decreased visibility of disc capillaries (see Fig. 4.19*F*). In many instances, diffuse thinning of the nerve fiber layer accompanies focal atrophy (slit defects) and ultimately causes disappearance of the defects as the entire nerve fiber layer atrophies (see Fig. 4.19*E*).

These abnormalities may be difficult to observe unless the illumination of the ophthalmoscope is sufficiently bright. Visualization of the nerve fiber layer is much improved when long (red) wavelengths are selectively filtered from the white light emitted from the ophthalmo-

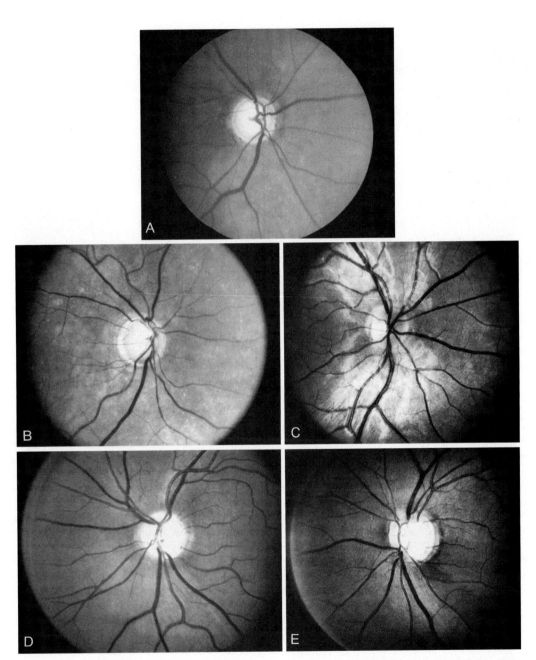

Figure 4.17. Appearance of optic disc in patients with glaucomatous field loss, compared with varied appearances of optic discs with nonglaucomatous field loss. *A.* Right optic disc in an eye with glaucomatous field loss. Note moderate cupping with preservation of normal color of remaining neuroretinal rim. *B.* In another patient with glaucoma, the right optic disc is markedly cupped, but remaining neuroretinal rim (from about 12 to 7 o'clock) retains its normal color. *C.* In a patient with 20/20 visual acuity and visual field loss similar to that seen in glaucoma, the right optic disc is normal in appearance. The patient had experienced an attack of retrobulbar neuritis several days earlier. *D.* Appearance of left optic disc in a patient with good visual acuity but significant visual field loss in the left eye after an attack of optic neuritis. Note diffuse pallor of the disc without obvious cupping. *E.* Appearance of the left optic disc after an attack of anterior ischemic optic neuropathy in the setting of temporal arteritis. The disc is diffusely pale and cupped. Note that the remaining neuroretinal rim, particularly temporally, is as pale as the cupped portion of the disc.

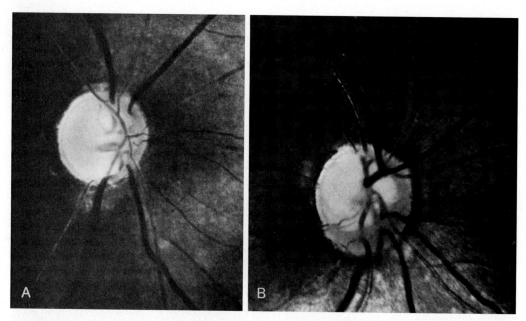

Figure 4.18. Optic disc cupping in glaucomatous and non-glaucomatous optic atrophy. *A.* Nonglaucomatous cupping. Note pallor and thinning of the neuroretinal rim. *B.* Glauco-matous cupping. Note normal appearance of the remaining neuroretinal rim.

scope, slit lamp biomicroscope, and fundus camera. Clinical detection of nerve fiber layer atrophy is possible in nonhuman primates after loss of 50% of the neural tissue in a given area. The detectability of nerve fiber layer atrophy is directly affected both by the pattern of nerve fiber loss and by the zone of the retina in which the loss has occurred.

In most cases of optic atrophy, the retinal arteries are narrowed or attenuated. In some instances, the narrowing is minor in nature; in others, such as severe nonarteritic AION, the vessels appear thread-like or are completely obliterated (Fig. 4.20). Not all cases of optic atrophy are associated with retinal vascular changes, however. Indeed, in eyes with optic atrophy from damage to the retrolaminar optic nerve, the retinal vessels are often unaffected. Thus, eyes in which significant retinal vascular narrowing is associated with optic atrophy presumably have suffered an additional insult directly affecting the retinal vasculature.

Differential Diagnosis of Optic Atrophy

When optic atrophy is complete, it is often impossible to determine its etiology solely from the appearance of the optic disc. However, the atrophy caused by central retinal artery occlusion and ischemic optic neuropathy can often be differentiated from other entities because of the associated retinal arteriolar attenuation and sheathing.

Acquired temporal pallor is the most common expression of segmental optic atrophy (see Fig. 4.19*A–B*). The white area, which generally extends from the temporal edge of the disc to the central vessels, may appear totally devoid of capillaries. Margins of this white area tend to blend gradually with the reddish-yellow of the surrounding disc tissue. Sharply demarcated wedge-shaped temporal pallor is a consequence of discrete papillomacular bundle lesions that occur in the retina between the macula and the disc or within the core of the optic nerve. Superior, inferior, or nasal sector-shaped pallor seldom appears as sharply circumscribed as temporal pallor. Acquired temporal pallor is usually caused by optic neuropathies that selectively affect central vision and field, sparing the peripheral field. Such optic neuropathies include toxic and nutritional optic neuropathies, autosomal-dominant and Leber's hereditary optic neuropa-

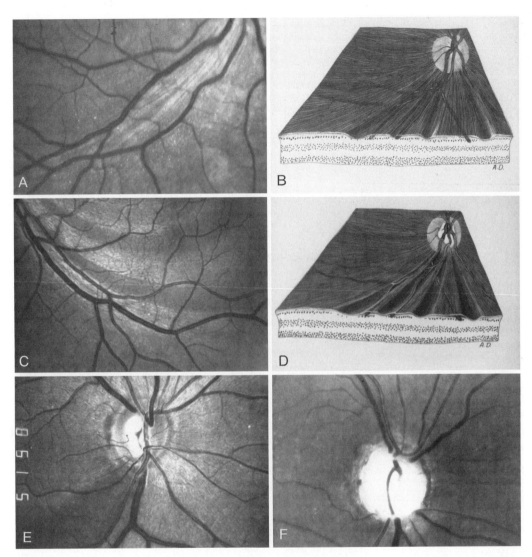

Figure 4.19.   Appearance of atrophy of the peripapillary retinal nerve fiber layer. *A.* Monochromatic red-free photograph shows mild nerve fiber bundle defects in the inferior arcuate fiber bundle. They are seen as thin dark streaks interrupting the normal linear light reflexes. *B.* Artist's drawing of the thin defects in the peripapillary retinal nerve fiber layer that occur in patients with mild optic neuropathies. *C.* Monochromatic red-free photograph shows two large defects in the peripapillary retinal nerve fiber layer in the inferior arcuate region of the left eye in a patient with radiation-induced optic neuropathy. Note that compared with *A,* the defects in this photograph are darker, wider, and more distinct from the surrounding nerve fiber layer. *D.* Artist's drawing of moderate defects in the peripapillary retinal nerve fiber layer. Note that the darker appearance results from both widening and deepening of the defects. *E.* Monochromatic red-free photograph shows a single broad defect in the peripapillary retinal nerve fiber layer in the inferior arcuate region of the right eye in a patient with early glaucoma and inferior extension of the optic cup. The defect is dark and quite distinct from the otherwise normal peripapillary nerve fiber layer. Note the granular appearance of the fundus within the defect. This appearance is caused by loss of the axons. Also note that the vessels crossing the defect are seen more clearly than are other vessels because of loss of the overlying nerve fibers. *F.* Complete loss of the peripapillary retinal nerve fiber layer in a patient with severe glaucoma. No linear striations can be seen, the peripapillary region has a distinct granular appearance, and the retinal vessels are seen clearly because of absence of overlying nerve fibers.

Figure 4.19. *(continued)*. *G.* Artist's drawing of complete loss of the nerve fiber layer in a large sector. Note draping of the inner limiting membrane over the retinal vessels.

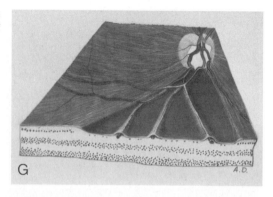

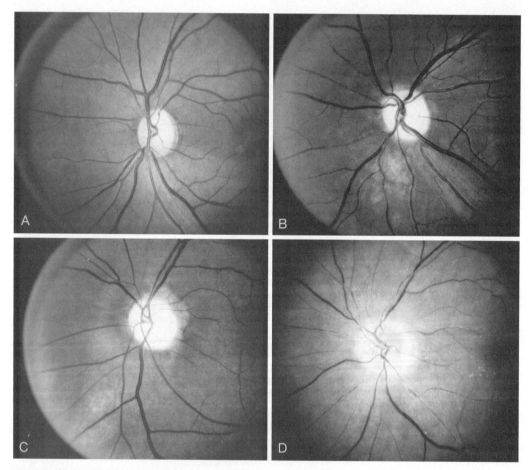

Figure 4.20. Appearance of retinal arteries in optic atrophy. *A.* Minimal narrowing of retinal arteries in left eye of a patient with optic atrophy from compression of the intracranial optic nerve by a suprasellar meningioma. *B.* Minimal narrowing of retinal arteries in the left eye of a patient after an episode of severe retrobulbar optic neuritis. *C.* Moderate narrowing of retinal arteries in the left eye of a patient who experienced an attack of nonarteritic anterior ischemic optic neuropathy. *D.* Marked narrowing of retinal arteries in the left eye of another patient who experienced an attack of nonarteritic anterior ischemic optic neuropathy.

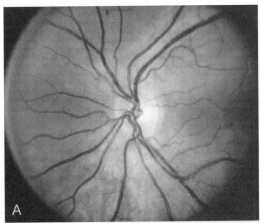

Figure 4.21. Temporal pallor of the optic disc in various optic neuropathies. *A.* After acute retrobulbar optic neuritis. *B.* In a patient with dominant hereditary optic atrophy. *C.* In a patient with Leber's optic neuropathy. *D.* In a patient with toxic optic neuropathy from ethambutol. *E.* In a patient with Cuban epidemic optic neuropathy. Note selective loss of the nerve fiber layer in the papillomacular bundle in several of these photographs.

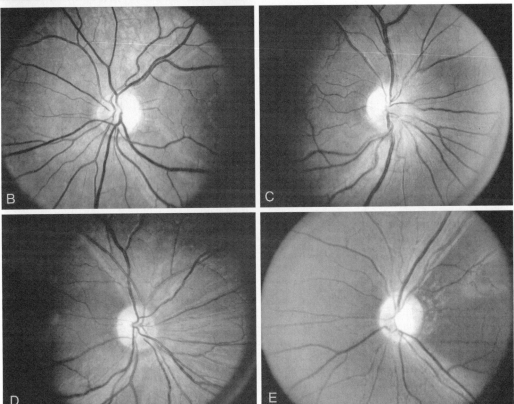

thies, and optic neuritis (Fig. 4.21). When superior or inferior disc pallor is present, an ischemic etiology is more likely.

The specific organization of the retinal nerve fiber layer results in specific patterns of nerve fiber layer and optic atrophy in patients with visual loss from optic chiasmal and retrochias-

mal-pregeniculate lesions. In patients with chiasmal lesions, for example, temporal field defects are mirrored by loss of fibers from ganglion cells nasal to the fovea. The atrophy is most impressive directly nasal and temporal to the disc, because the superior and inferior arcuate nerve fiber bundles are composed of fibers from gan-

Figure 4.22. "Band" or "bow-tie" atrophy of the right optic disc in a patient with a temporal hemianopia caused by a pituitary adenoma. Note horizontal band of atrophy across the right disc, with preservation of the superior and inferior portions of the disc.

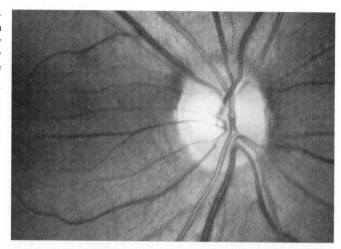

glion cells both temporal and nasal to the fovea. Thus, the arcuate bundles are relatively spared compared with other areas. The optic pallor is primarily nasal and temporal with sparing superiorly and inferiorly. This "band" or "bow-tie" atrophy is characteristic of temporal field loss (Fig. 4.22). Patients with optic chiasmal syndromes and bitemporal hemianopic field defects ultimately develop "band" optic disc pallor and characteristic nerve fiber layer atrophy in both eyes.

In patients with congenital or neonatally acquired homonymous hemianopia, or in patients with pregeniculate homonymous hemianopias, the eye contralateral to the lesion has temporal field loss and shows the pattern of nerve fiber and optic nerve atrophy described above—band atrophy of the optic disc. The eye ipsilateral to the lesion has a complete nasal field loss with loss of ganglion cells temporal to the fovea. Because the nerve fibers from these ganglion cells primarily comprise the superior and inferior arcuate bundles, these regions show extensive loss of nerve fibers, and the disc atrophy is more diffuse. The characteristic features of the fundi of such individuals are thus a bow-tie or band atrophy in the contralateral eye and reduced visibility of the superior and inferior arcuate nerve fiber bundles in the ipsilateral eye compared with the contralateral eye.

Although the presence or absence of pathologic pallor of the optic disc cannot be directly equated with visual function, it should be obvious that no judgment of pallor is meaningful until and unless the pallor is correlated with

optic nerve function. The data should be obtained from careful testing of visual acuity, contrast sensitivity, and color vision, as well as quantitative perimetry, examination of the pupils, and electrophysiologic studies when appropriate (see Chapter 1). An optic disc may appear to be pale, yet meticulous clinical and electrophysiologic testing of visual function may fail to disclose any abnormality. In such cases, it is most likely that the pallor is physiologic rather than pathologic. Conversely, an optic disc occasionally appears normal despite severe and even long-standing visual acuity or field loss caused by optic nerve dysfunction. In most of these cases, careful evaluation of the optic disc as well as the peripapillary retinal nerve fiber layer will provide evidence of retinal nerve fiber atrophy, either too focal or too mild and diffuse to produce obvious optic pallor.

SYNDROMES OF UNILATERAL OPTIC NERVE DYSFUNCTION

Although the appearance of the optic disc alone is usually insufficient to permit an accurate diagnosis of the cause of an optic neuropathy, the combination of a complete history and meticulous examination can provide the correct localization and explanation for many cases of acquired optic nerve dysfunction.

OPTOCILIARY SHUNTS AND THE SYNDROME OF CHRONIC OPTIC NERVE COMPRESSION

Chronic optic nerve compression may cause a specific syndrome characterized by progressive loss of vision, optic disc swelling that is followed or accompanied by optic atrophy, and the appearance of dilated venous channels called **optociliary shunt veins**. These shunt veins are congenital connections between the retinal and choroidal venous circulations. When there is chronic compression of the optic nerve, particularly when the lesion is within the orbit, these veins enlarge and shunt blood from the retinal to the choroidal venous circulation, thus allowing the retinal venous blood to bypass the obstructed central retinal vein and exit the orbit via the choroidal circulation, vortex veins, and ophthalmic veins (Fig. 4.23). Spheno-orbital meningiomas most commonly cause this syndrome, although it may also be caused by chronic papilledema, optic gliomas, arachnoid cysts of the optic nerve, or craniopharyngioma. Acquired optociliary shunt veins also develop in patients after central retinal vein occlusion and in patients with orbital vascular malformations.

PRECHIASMAL OPTIC NERVE COMPRESSION SYNDROME

Prechiasmal optic nerve compression syndrome is characterized by slowly progressive monocular dimming of vision with near-normal acuity (initially), poor color vision, a relative afferent pupillary defect, and a normal-appearing optic disc. In such patients, there are usually subtle central or arcuate visual field defects that can be detected by static perimetry or careful tangent screen examination and that are themselves slowly progressive. Neuroimaging in such patients almost always detects a compressive lesion.

DISTAL OPTIC NERVE SYNDROME (DISTAL OPTIC NEUROPATHY; ANTERIOR OPTIC CHIASMAL SYNDROME)

Where the optic nerve joins the chiasm, at the anterior angle of the chiasm, its particular fiber anatomy provides another opportunity for anatomic diagnosis. The crossed and uncrossed fibers are separated at this level but are quite compact, and a small lesion affecting either the crossed or the uncrossed fibers may produce a unilateral hemianopic defect. Such a defect is called a ''junctional scotoma.'' In such cases, it is not uncommon to find an asymptomatic scotoma in the upper temporal field of the **opposite** eye (Fig. 4.24). This scotoma results from damage to ventrally located fibers originating from

ganglion cells located inferior and nasal to the fovea that, upon reaching the distal end of the optic nerve, are thought to loop anteriorly about 1 to 2 mm into the contralateral optic nerve. This loop, called **Wilbrand's knee**, is vulnerable to damage from lesions that affect the distal aspect of an optic nerve. There is some evidence that Wilbrand's knee is not a normal anatomic structure but rather is an artifact that develops when there is atrophy of the ipsilateral optic nerve. Although this may be true, Wilbrand's knee clearly exists from a clinical standpoint: a patient with evidence of an optic neuropathy in one eye and a superior temporal defect in the visual field of the opposite eye has a lesion of the distal optic nerve at its junction with the optic chiasm.

A point of confusion regards the terminology of the superior temporal field defect that is so critical to topical diagnosis of lesions of the distal optic nerve. The term ''junctional scotoma'' was originally used to refer to the temporal hemianopic scotoma produced by damage to nasal fibers of the intracranial optic nerve at its junction with the optic chiasm. Thus, the term was used when a strictly unilateral visual field defect was present, and the assumption was made that the lesion was near the optic chiasm. However, it is common practice to use the term ''junctional scotoma'' to refer not to the field defect in the eye with other evidence of an optic neuropathy but rather to the superior temporal field defect seen in the **opposite** eye. In this setting, the location of the lesion is definite rather than assumed.

Most monocular temporal field defects, whether quadrantanopic or hemianopic, are caused by damage to the distal optic nerve near the optic chiasm. However, such defects can be produced voluntarily by normal individuals and by malingerers with no organic disease. The physician who detects a monocular defect in the temporal visual field that respects the vertical midline should assume that a lesion of the distal optic nerve is present and evaluate the patient appropriately, beginning with neuroimaging; however, he or she should not be surprised when, on rare occasions, no such lesion is detected (see Chapter 23).

FOSTER KENNEDY SYNDROME

Intracranial lesions that exert direct pressure on one optic nerve usually produce optic atrophy. As these lesions enlarge, they may eventually produce increased intracranial pressure. When the compressed optic nerve is signifi-

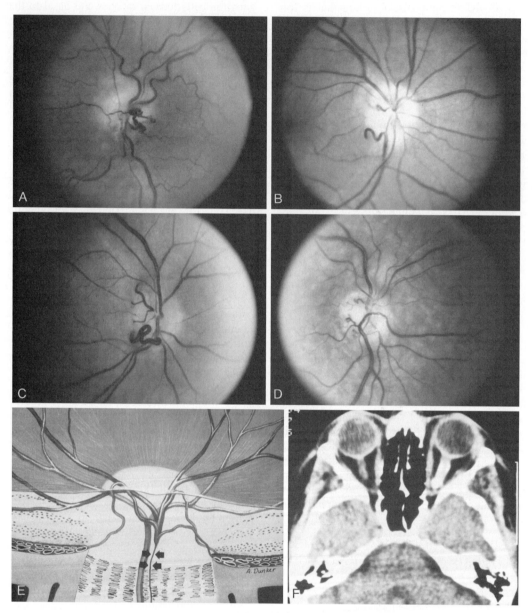

Figure 4.23. Acquired optociliary (retinochoroidal) shunt veins. *A–D.* Four fundus photographs showing optociliary shunt veins in patients with optic atrophy from chronic compression of the optic nerves. Note varying size of the vessels, which are shunting venous blood from the retinal to the choroidal circulation so that it can exit the eye via the vortex veins to the superior and inferior ophthalmic veins rather than via the central retinal vein. *E.* Artist's drawing of acquired retinochoroidal shunt veins that are, in fact, **con-** **genital** structures that simply enlarge in the setting of chronic compression of the optic nerve. *F.* CT scan, axial view, shows the appearance of a left optic nerve sheath meningioma in the patient whose fundus appearance is shown in *A.* Note that the nerve is thickened and brighter than the opposite optic nerve. (Schematic drawing reprinted with permission from Miller NR, Fine SL. The Ocular Fundus in Neuro-Ophthalmologic Diagnosis: Sights and Sounds in Ophthalmology. Vol 3. St. Louis: CV Mosby, 1977.)

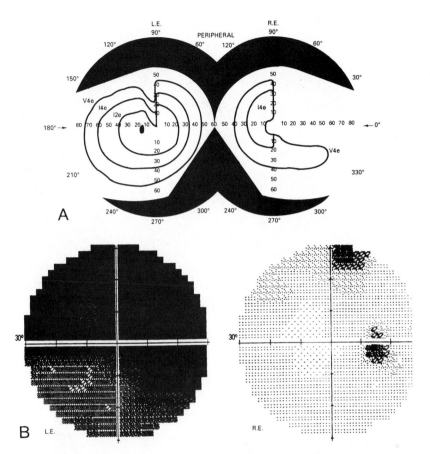

Figure 4.24.   Two examples of the syndrome of the distal optic nerve (anterior chiasmal syndrome). *A.* Kinetic perimetry in a patient with decreased vision in the right eye from a pituitary adenoma shows a dense temporal defect with a central scotoma in that eye. In addition, however, there is a superior temporal defect in the visual field of the contralat-

eral eye. *B.* Static perimetry in another patient with loss of vision in the left eye from a pituitary adenoma shows almost complete loss of the central field in that eye as well as a small superior temporal defect in the visual field of the right eye.

cantly atrophic by the time intracranial pressure becomes increased, the increased intracranial pressure produces papilledema only in the contralateral eye. Homolateral optic atrophy and contralateral papilledema, when associated with anosmia, are the hallmarks of the so-called **Foster Kennedy syndrome** (Fig 4.25). This syndrome occurs most often with frontal lobe tumors and olfactory groove meningiomas.

In some cases, this syndrome of optic atrophy in one eye and papilledema in the other eye is falsely localizing; that is, the optic atrophy is not on the side ipsilateral to the tumor but on the contralateral side. More importantly, how-

ever, we would emphasize that a true Foster Kennedy syndrome is extremely rare. It is much more common to see optic atrophy on one side with optic disc swelling on the opposite side in cases of bilateral nonsimultaneous optic neuritis or ischemic optic neuropathy. In such cases, the symptoms and signs are profoundly different and should cause no difficulty in diagnosis. It should also be emphasized that a "Foster Kennedy syndrome" consisting of optic atrophy on one side and optic disc swelling on the other may result from asymmetric optic nerve compression from an intracranial mass in the absence of increased intracranial pressure.

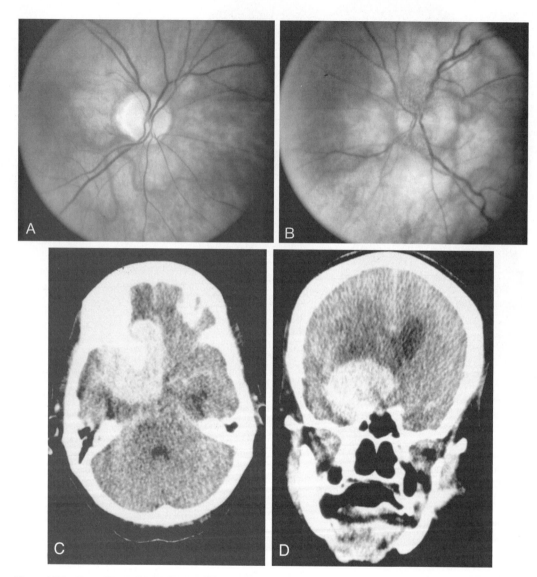

Figure 4.25. Foster Kennedy syndrome of unilateral optic atrophy, contralateral papilledema, and anosmia. The patient was a 34-year-old woman with severe headaches and progressive loss of vision in the right eye. A neurologic examination revealed anosmia and some degree of confusion. Visual acuity was 20/400 OD and 20/25 OS. There was a right relative afferent pupillary defect. *A.* The right optic disc is diffusely pale. *B.* The left optic disc shows chronic swelling. *C.* CT scan, axial view, after intravenous injection of contrast material, reveals a large enhancing mass along the right sphenoid wing, consistent with a meningioma. *D.* CT scan, coronal view, after intravenous injection of contrast material, shows the upward extension of the mass as well as enlargement of the lateral ventricles.

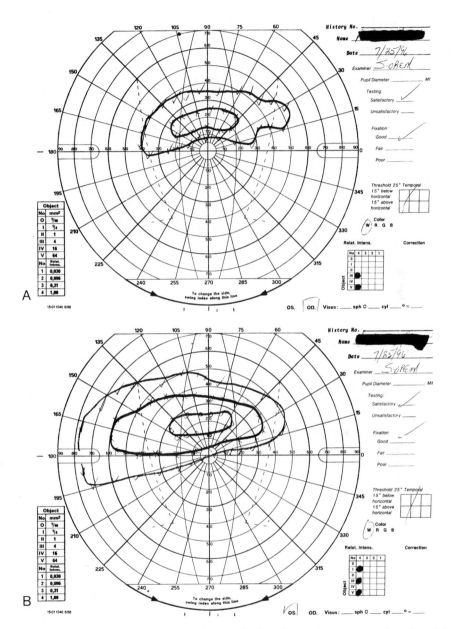

Figure 4.26. Bilateral altitudinal visual field defects in a patient with simultaneous bilateral anterior ischemic optic neuropathy. The patient was a 67-year-old man who awoke from cardiac surgery with loss of vision in both eyes. Visual acuity was 5/200 OD and 20/300 OS. *A.* Kinetic perimetry in the right eye shows complete loss of the inferior field and constriction of the remaining superior field. *B.* Kinetic perimetry in the visual field of the left eye shows almost complete loss of the inferior field with preservation of the superior field.

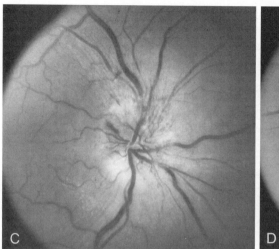

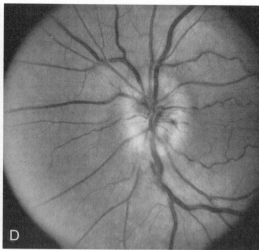

Figure 4.26. *(continued). Right (C)* and left *(D)* optic discs are swollen and hyperemic, and there are flame-shaped hemorrhages at the margins of both discs. It was subsequently discovered that the patient's hematocrit had dropped over 40% during the surgery and that his blood pressure had also dropped substantially during part of the procedure.

BILATERAL LESIONS OF THE OPTIC NERVES

The visual fields of both eyes may be altered not only by a single lesion posterior to the optic chiasm but also by a lesion affecting the chiasm itself. Thus, the question often arises in a patient with bilateral visual field defects if a single lesion accounts for the field defects or if there are bilateral optic nerve lesions. In a majority of cases, the problem is not a difficult one to solve. Bilateral central, cecocentral, and arcuate defects all suggest dysfunction of both optic nerves. Probably, ring scotomas do the same when there is no visible retinal abnormality to account for them. Bitemporal visual field defects are usually produced by a single lesion affecting the optic chiasm, whereas homonymous visual field defects are invariably produced by a single lesion affecting the visual sensory pathway posterior to the optic chiasm. Bilateral altitudinal field defects usually are caused by bilateral retinal or optic nerve lesions, but they may also be caused by postgeniculate lesions (see Chapter 12).

BILATERAL SUPERIOR OR INFERIOR (ALTITUDINAL) HEMIANOPIA

A unilateral visual field defect in all or most of the upper or lower portion of the field is always caused by a lesion of the retina or optic nerve. Similarly, bilateral visual field defects of this type usually represent bilateral lesions damaging the retinas or optic nerves. In many of these cases, one eye is affected before the other. In such cases, the pathology is ischemia, and most patients have an underlying systemic vasculopathy, such as giant cell arteritis, diabetes mellitus, or systemic hypertension that has caused nonsimultaneous bilateral ischemic optic neuropathy. In other cases, acute hemorrhage with resultant anemia; acute intraoperative, postoperative, or spontaneous hypotension; or a combination of these phenomena may cause a simultaneous bilateral ischemic optic neuropathy (Fig. 4.26).

Rarely, a large prechiasmal lesion compresses both optic nerves, producing bilateral altitudinal field defects. In most of these cases, the etiology is a pituitary adenoma that compresses the inferior aspects of both optic nerves, producing bilateral superior altitudinal defects. In other cases, however, compression of the optic nerves from below elevates them against the dural shelves extending out from the intracranial end of the optic canals. Pressure from the dura against the superior aspects of the nerves subsequently produces bilateral inferior altitudinal defects.

BILATERAL "CHECKERBOARD" ALTITUDINAL HEMIANOPIA AND THE VERTICAL HEMIFIELD SLIDE PHENOMENON

Patients with bilateral altitudinal field defects do not necessarily lose the superior or inferior field in both eyes. Some patients with bilateral optic neuropathies—particularly those who develop bilateral simultaneous or nonsimultaneous anterior ischemic optic neuropathy—develop a superior altitudinal defect in one eye and an inferior altitudinal defect in the other. In addition to the expected difficulties with visual function that result from loss of visual acuity, color vision, and visual field, such patients may experience binocular diplopia or difficulty reading caused by decompensation of a preexisting vertical or horizontal phoria. The problems encountered by

these patients result from loss of the normal partial overlap of the superior or inferior fields of the two eyes. This overlap normally permits fusion of images and helps stabilize ocular alignment in patients with vertical or horizontal phorias. Because their remaining visual fields represent only the superior projection from one eye and the inferior projection from the other, patients with a superior hemianopia in one eye and an inferior hemianopia in the other do not have a physiologic linkage between the two remaining altitudinal hemifields. In such patients,

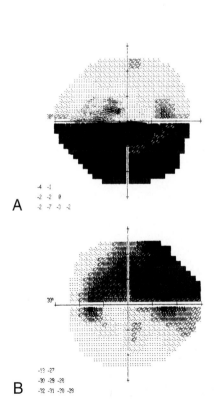

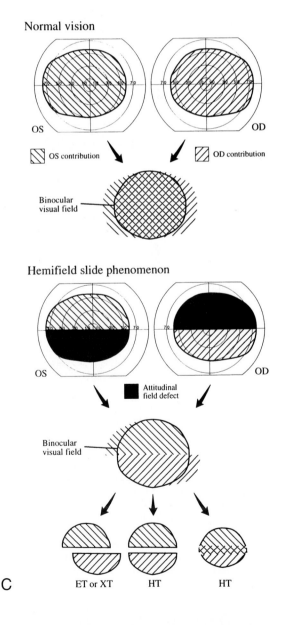

Figure 4.27.   Hemifield slide phenomenon from bilateral optic neuropathy. Inferior altitudinal defect in the visual field of the right eye (*A*) and superior altitudinal defect in the visual field of the left eye (*B*) from bilateral ischemic optic neuropathy. *C.* Artist's drawing shows that such defects can produce a vertical or horizontal hemifield slide phenomenon from loss of overlapping portions of the visual fields. Affected patients may complain of vertical, horizontal, or diagonal diplopia.

a preexisting asymptomatic phoria becomes a tropia because of vertical or horizontal separation or overlap of the two remaining hemifields. Patients thus complain of diplopia and may have difficulty reading because of doubling or inability to see printed letters or words. This condition, called the **hemifield slide phenomenon**, was initially described in patients with bitemporal hemianopic field defects, and it is in such patients that it most often occurs (see Chapter 12). However, the hemifield slide phenomenon can also occur in patients with heteronymous **altitudinal** or broad **arcuate** field defects (Fig. 4.27).

NASAL HEMIANOPIA

Most organic nasal visual field defects are actually arcuate in nature. In some cases, however, a true unilateral hemianopia or bilateral nasal hemianopias develops, with the defects having no connection to the blind spot and respecting the vertical meridian. Such field defects are never caused by direct damage to the lateral aspects of the optic chiasm. Rather, they result from damage to the temporal aspects of one or both optic nerves.

A unilateral nasal hemianopia may occur in association with suprasellar aneurysms, pituitary

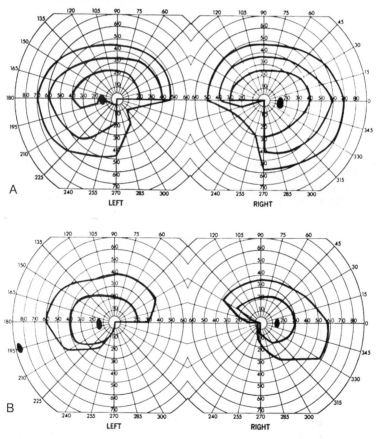

Figure 4.28. Bilateral nasal quadrantic field defects in two patients with intracranial lesions. In both cases, the defects respect the vertical midline. *A.* Kinetic perimetry reveals bilateral inferior nasal quadrantic defects in a 61-year-old man with bilateral dolichoectatic internal carotid arteries. *B.* Kinetic perimetry reveals bilateral inferior nasal quadrantic defects in a 43-year-old woman with a right-sided olfactory groove meningioma. At surgery, it was found that the menin-gioma was pushing the right optic nerve downward and laterally against the right internal carotid artery. The mass also caused displacement of the left internal carotid artery against the lateral aspect of the left optic nerve. (Reprinted with permission from Manor RS, Ouaknine GE, Matz S, et al. Nasal visual field loss with intracranial lesions of the optic nerve pathways. Am J Ophthalmol 1980;90:1–10.)

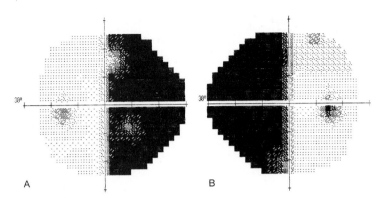

Figure 4.29.   Bilateral complete nasal hemianopia in a 34-year-old woman with a suprasellar aneurysm that displaced both optic nerves laterally against the supraclinoid portion of the internal carotid arteries. The field defect resolved after clipping of the aneurysm. *A.* Visual field of the left eye. *B.* Visual field of the right eye.

adenoma, and ischemia. A binasal hemianopia, however, is an exceedingly infrequent visual field defect. Although a "binasal hemianopia" is sometimes said to occur in patients with intracranial tumors that grow between the intracranial optic nerves, pushing them laterally against the anterior cerebral or internal carotid arteries, the field defects in such cases are usually arcuate, not hemianopic, and do not respect the vertical midline. True binasal quadrantic or hemianopic defects occur in rare patients with a variety of intracranial lesions, including pituitary tumors, meningiomas, suprasellar aneurysm, dolichoectatic internal carotid arteries, optochiasmatic arachnoiditis, and primary empty sella syndrome (Figs. 4.28 and 4.29).

Bilateral nasal field defects also occur in patients with both primary hydrocephalus and with hydrocephalus caused by intracranial tumors. In such cases, enlargement of the 3rd ventricle causes lateral displacement of the optic nerves against the supraclinoid portion of the internal carotid arteries.

Most of the nasal defects resulting from intracranial optic nerve damage affect the inferior, rather than the superior, visual field. The underlying pathogenesis of these defects may be vascular or compressive, and this may explain the inconsistent improvement following decompression.

Bilateral irregular nasal field defects are commonly associated with drusen of the optic discs. Such defects do not obey the vertical midline and, in fact, are generally arcuate in nature.

CHRONIC OPEN-ANGLE GLAUCOMA (GLAUCOMATOUS OPTIC NEUROPATHY)

Chronic open-angle glaucoma requires comment here not so much for its intrinsic importance, but because the clinical manifestations it produces, particularly the visual field defects, are identical with the field defects produced by other types of optic neuropathy.

Most patients with chronic open-angle glaucoma develop loss of visual field long before they experience loss of central vision, although exceptions occur. Color vision deficits are typically of the blue-yellow type but, again, exceptions regularly occur, and red-green deficits are not uncommon. A relative afferent pupillary defect is almost always present in cases of unilateral or asymmetric glaucoma.

The visual field defects in chronic open-angle glaucoma occur from damage to nerve fiber bundles at the level of the sclera within the optic nerve head. This damage seems to occur focally in its initial stages and is thus expressed in the visual field as isolated scotomas appearing between 5° and 30° from fixation in the arcuate or Bjerrum area (Fig. 4.30). About two-thirds of these isolated paracentral or arcuate scotomas are accompanied by a depression in sensitivity in the upper or lower half of the field. This loss of sensitivity appears initially as a step in a plotted isopter, usually at the nasal, horizontal meridian (the nasal step of Rönne) (Fig. 4.31*A*). One-third of early paracentral scotomas that

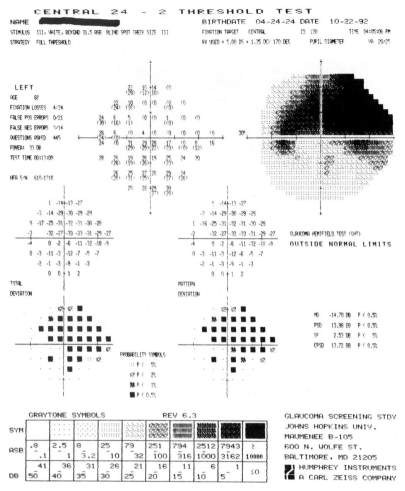

Figure 4.30. Arcuate visual field defect in a 68-year-old woman with open-angle glaucoma. Static perimetry, using a Humphrey perimeter to perform a 24–2 Threshold Test, reveals a superior arcuate defect located within the central 30° from fixation.

occur in patients with chronic open-angle glaucoma have no associated nasal step. Even less frequently, a nasal step is present without a paracentral scotoma (see Fig. 4.31*B*).

As damage proceeds, the paracentral scotoma becomes deeper, wider, or both, and new scotomas may develop in the same arcuate region. As these defects coalesce, they take on an arching shape between the nasal horizontal meridian and the blind spot. Isolated enlargement or elongation of the blind spot is a relatively nonspecific finding and is not diagnostic of glaucomatous damage, although it may indicate a general depression in visual sensitivity. Defects in the field temporal to the blind spot occur in early glaucomatous damage but are much less frequent. As arcuate scotomas enlarge and affect both the upper and lower regions, they may meet at the horizontal meridian and produce a ring-shaped scotoma. Further damage results in the breaking out of the scotoma to the peripheral field, so-called "baring" to the periphery. Thus, patients with advanced glaucoma may retain only the central 5° and a temporal island of vision.

Although the visual field defects that occur in chronic open-angle glaucoma are identical with defects that result from various types of nonglau-

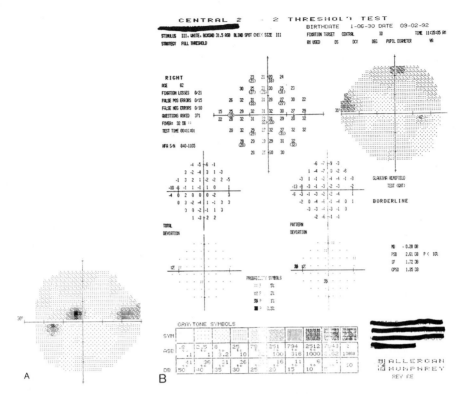

Figure 4.31. Nasal steps in the visual fields of patients with early open-angle glaucoma, detected with static perimetry. *A.* Nasal step of reduced sensitivity just superior to the horizontal meridian, combined with a paracentral scotoma just temporal to fixation in the visual field of the left eye of a patient with early open-angle glaucoma. *B.* Isolated nasal step in the visual field of the right eye in another patient with early glaucoma.

comatous optic neuropathy, the differentiation between glaucoma and nonglaucomatous optic neuropathy should be easily made by a careful ophthalmoscopic examination using a 90- or 78-diopter hand-held lens or a contact lens. Patients with glaucoma develop visual field defects only after there is extensive damage to the optic disc. As noted above, the ophthalmoscopic appearance of such a disc is typical. In nearly every such case, there is substantial cupping of the disc, with the remaining neuroretinal rim appearing relatively normal, without evidence of pallor and with diffuse thinning of the retinal nerve fiber layer (see Fig. 4.17*A–B*). This is in contrast to other types of optic nerve disease producing similar visual field defects, in which the optic

disc may appear normal (see Fig. 4.17*C*), diffusely or sectorially pale without enlargement in the size of the cup (see Fig. 4.17*D*), or pale with substantial cupping but also with pallor of the remaining neuroretinal rim (see Fig. 4.17*E*). Thus, when the optic disc and retinal nerve fiber layer are carefully examined in an eye with a visual field defect consistent with chronic open-angle glaucoma, it is rarely difficult to differentiate glaucoma from other diseases capable of producing such a defect.

FOR MORE INFORMATION:

See Walsh & Hoyt's *Clinical Neuro-Ophthalmology*, 5th edition, Volume 1, Chapter 8, pages 253–306; Volume II, Chapter 38, pages 1798–1804.

Papilledema

The term *papilledema* is often mistakenly applied to any type of swelling of the optic disc regardless of the etiology. Although it is true that swelling of the optic papilla can theoretically be denoted as ''papilledema,'' the term has a particular, ingrained meaning to most clinicians. It should be used *only* for optic disc swelling that results from increased intracranial pressure (ICP). Other forms of disc swelling caused by local or systemic processes should be designated with respect to the presumed etiology—for example, ''anterior ischemic optic neuropathy'' or ''anterior optic neuritis''—or in general terms, such as ''optic disc swelling.''

Normal cerebrospinal fluid (CSF) pressure in persons in the lateral recumbent position varies between 100 and 250 mm of water and is not related to weight or height (Fig. 5.1), although pressure readings may appear higher than they actually are when a patient coughs, strains, or holds his or her breath during the procedure. In addition, ICP in normal persons and in patients with increased ICP can vary within wide limits from one moment to the next.

In addition to problems relating to artifactitiously elevated ICP and temporal variations in ICP, one must be aware of other issues in the assessment of ICP. For example, the CSF pres-

sure is often lower than the ICP in patients with infratentorial tumors that block communication between the ventricular system and the spinal subarachnoid space. These patients may have true papilledema despite normal or low intrathecal pressures. In such cases, only ventricular pressure readings give accurate information regarding the ICP, but even ventricular pressure may be low in patients with intracranial tumors.

The dangers involved in diagnostic lumbar puncture in patients with increased ICP are well known. Removal of fluid from the spinal canal may allow a compressed brain to shift downward and to impact at the tentorial incisura or the foramen magnum, often with fatal results. It is estimated that the overall complication rate of lumbar puncture in patients with intracranial masses and increased ICP is about 1.2%. The risk of a fatal herniation of intracranial contents after lumbar puncture is certainly not nearly as great in patients with pseudotumor cerebri (PTC) (see below) as it is in patients with an intracranial mass, but it is still a possibility.

The availability of computed tomographic (CT) scanning and magnetic resonance imaging (MRI) has greatly improved both the diagnosis and the management of patients with suspected increased ICP with and without papilledema and

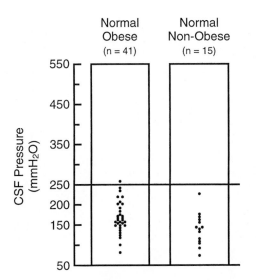

Normal Obese (n = 41)   Normal Non-Obese (n = 15)

CSF Pressure (mmH₂O)

Figure 5.1. Range of normal cerebrospinal fluid pressure in nonobese and obese adults. Note that normal intracranial pressure does not exceed 250 mm of water. (Reprinted with permission from Corbett JJ, Mehta MP. Cerebrospinal fluid pressure in normal obese subjects and patients with pseudotumor cerebri. Neurology 1983;33:1386–1388.)

has reduced the complication rate after lumbar puncture in such patients. Both neuroimaging procedures are rapid and effective methods of noninvasively assessing the intracranial contents and the state of the ventricular system, allowing the physician to decide whether to perform a lumbar puncture. If the physician decides to do so, he or she will at least be prepared for the possibility of a complication. In addition, in cases where the physician cannot decide if the elevation of the optic disc is true papilledema or pseudopapilledema, CT scanning or MRI can be obtained immediately to determine if an intracranial mass is present or the ventricles are enlarged, following which a decision can be made regarding the need for further diagnostic testing.

OPHTHALMOSCOPIC APPEARANCE

Papilledema may be classified into four types: (1) early, (2) fully developed, (3) chronic, and (4) atrophic.

EARLY PAPILLEDEMA

The early phase of papilledema consists of the incipient disc changes that occur before the de-

velopment of obvious disc swelling. Several features distinguish early papilledema, including hyperemia of the optic disc, blurring of the peripapillary retinal nerve fiber layer, swelling of the optic disc, blurring of the disc margins, peripapillary flame-shaped hemorrhages, and absent spontaneous venous pulsations (Fig. 5.2). Dilation of retinal veins is a comparatively late phenomenon and not a sign of early papilledema.

Hyperemia develops from dilation of capillaries on the surface of the disc and is always an early sign of papilledema. However, hyperemia of the disc as well as capillary dilation and development of microaneurysms on the disc surface may appear *after* disc swelling and blurring of the peripapillary retinal nerve fiber layer. In addition, the color of normal discs varies, and this in itself may result in difficulty with interpretation. Obviously, if there is evidence that the optic discs have changed in color, then hyperemia is of definite importance.

With the increasing use of brighter direct ophthalmoscopes and hand-held 90- or 78-diopter lenses at the slit lamp biomicroscope, and with an increasing awareness of the improvement in nerve fiber layer detail when a red-free filter is used during ophthalmoscopy or slit lamp biomicroscopy, subtle **changes in the peripapillary retinal nerve fiber layer** can be observed in early papilledema. In eyes with early papilledema, the peripapillary retina loses its superficial linear and curvilinear light reflexes and appears deep red and without luster.

In patients with papilledema, **swelling of the optic disc** typically appears first at the lower pole, then at the upper pole. The nasal and temporal portions of the disc swell later. Early swelling of the optic disc is best detected clinically by careful direct ophthalmoscopy or slit lamp biomicroscopy. Although **indistinct optic disc margins** clearly occur in early papilledema, numerous congenital anomalies of the optic disc are also characterized by indistinct disc margins. We therefore do not find blurring of the disc margins a particularly useful sign of early papilledema unless it is associated with other changes, or there is definite evidence that the appearance of the disc margins has changed.

A small **nerve fiber layer hemorrhage** in the peripapillary region may be an extremely important sign of early papilledema. Such a hemorrhage appears as a thin, radial streak on the disc

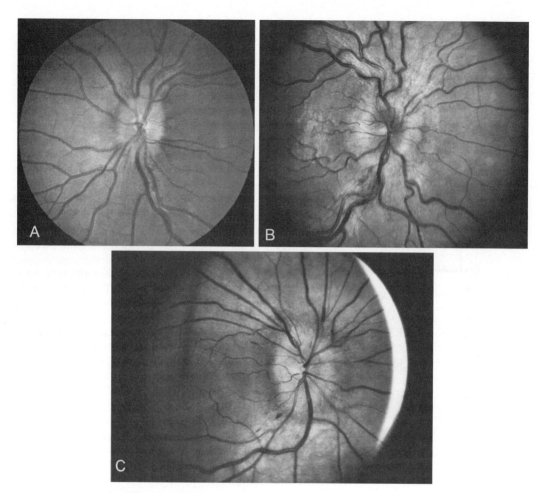

Figure 5.2. Early papilledema. *A.* The disc shows slight hyperemia and blurring of the peripapillary nerve fiber layer at the superior and inferior poles of the disc. *B.* This disc is hyperemic and mildly swollen. Note the inferior peripapil-lary nerve fiber hemorrhages. *C.* The disc is moderately swollen, and there are small ''splinter'' hemorrhages adjacent to the disc margins at 7 and 10 o'clock.

or near its margins and is presumably caused by rupture of a distended capillary within or surrounding the disc (Fig. 5.3). Although peripapillary nerve fiber layer hemorrhages can be seen using routine direct ophthalmoscopy, they are often more apparent with the magnification provided by slit lamp biomicroscopy using a hand-held or contact lens.

The **absence of spontaneous retinal venous pulsations** is thought by some investigators to be an early sign of papilledema. According to several authors, pulsations cease when ICP exceeds about 200 mm of water. Thus, if spontaneous venous pulsations are present, ICP must

be below this figure. However, as noted above, marked fluctuations in ICP can occur in patients with increased ICP, and in such patients the ICP may occasionally drop into the normal range. A patient could therefore have increased ICP but be examined at a time when ICP was transiently reduced at the trough of a pressure wave, at which time spontaneous venous pulsations might be observed. In addition, spontaneous venous pulsations occur in only about 80% of normal subjects. Thus, 20% of patients without increased ICP lack spontaneous venous pulsations. For this reason, the absence of spontaneous venous pulsations does not necessarily argue for a

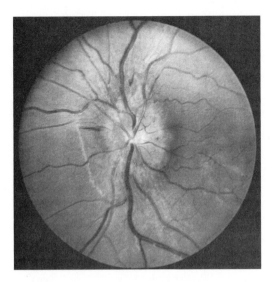

Figure 5.3. Early papilledema. Two splinter hemorrhages can be seen in the nerve fiber layer adjacent to the disc margin at 9 o'clock and 12 o'clock. Gray edema surrounds the disc, and the optic cup is partially obliterated by hyperemic disc tissue. Both veins and venules are engorged. (Reprinted with permission from Hoyt WF, Beeston D. The Ocular Fundus in Neurologic Disease. St Louis: CV Mosby, 1966.)

cases, circumferential retinal folds (Paton's lines) often develop, linear or curvilinear choroidal folds may be observed, and both hard exudates and hemorrhages may occur in the peripapillary region and in the macula, producing decreased central vision (Fig. 5.6). Because nerve fibers in the macula have a radial fan-shaped appearance, hemorrhages and exudates in this region can assume a fan or star shape; because vascular compromise on and around the optic disc is responsible for these macular changes, the star figure in such cases is usually asymmetric, being more prominent on the nasal side of the fovea toward the disc.

When the increase in ICP is rapid, subhyaloid hemorrhages may be present in addition to the more common intraretinal hemorrhages (Fig. 5.7). These hemorrhages break into the vitreous in some cases. Severe posterior pole hemorrhages or prominent subhyaloid and vitreous bleeding occur in about 4% of patients with papilledema. In these patients, the subhyaloid and vitreous hemorrhages are thought to result from forward dissection of severe peripapillary hemorrhage, whereas scattered posterior pole hemorrhages are believed to represent central retinal

diagnosis of papilledema, and the observation of spontaneous venous pulsations indicates only that ICP is below 200 mm of water *at that time,* not that the patient does not have papilledema.

FULLY DEVELOPED PAPILLEDEMA

As papilledema develops, disc swelling becomes more obvious. The veins of the retina become engorged and dusky, and numerous splinter hemorrhages may appear at or adjacent to the disc margin (Fig. 5.4). With continued progression of papilledema, the surface of the disc becomes grossly elevated above the surface of the retina. At this stage, microaneurysm formation and capillary dilation on the disc surface are quite obvious (Fig. 5.5).

Blurring of the disc margin also becomes obvious, and the surface vessels become obscured by the now opaque nerve fiber layer as they pass across and off the disc. There are often numerous flame-shaped hemorrhages, the number of which may relate to the rapidity with which ICP became increased, and there may also be cotton-wool spots (focal retinal infarcts) and tortuous vessels on or surrounding the disc. In severe

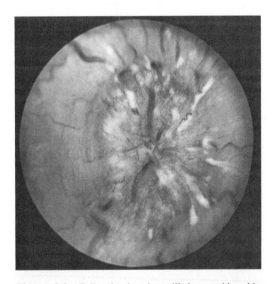

Figure 5.4. Fully developed papilledema with white "fleck" exudates (small infarcts) among the nerve fibers, retinal wrinkling, and intraretinal exudates in the macular area (on the left). Note the corkscrew-like venules on the surface of the swollen tissue. (Reprinted with permission from Hoyt WF, Beeston D. The Ocular Fundus in Neurologic Disease. St Louis: CV Mosby, 1966.)

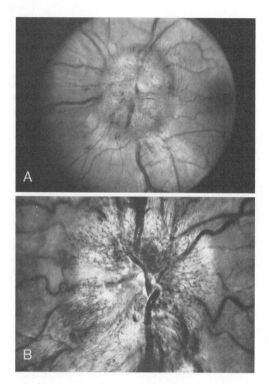

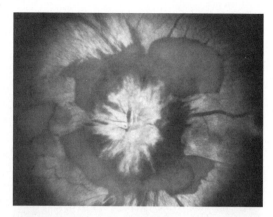

Figure 5.7. Subhyaloid hemorrhage with papilledema. The patient had a severe, subarachnoid hemorrhage from an intracranial aneurysm.

Figure 5.5. Fully developed papilledema with marked dilation of disc vessels and formation of microaneurysms. *A.* Fundus photograph. *B.* Red-free photograph.

vein compromise from the swollen optic nerve head. Rarely, patients with papilledema develop macular and peripapillary subretinal neovascularization, especially when the papilledema is chronic (Fig. 5.8).

CHRONIC PAPILLEDEMA

When papilledema persists, hemorrhages and exudates slowly resolve, and the disc develops a rounded appearance (Fig. 5.9). The central cup, which initially is retained even in severe acute papilledema, ultimately becomes obliterated. The initial disc hyperemia changes to a milky gray color, with hard exudates becoming apparent in the superficial disc substance. These exudates resemble optic disc drusen and can result in a misdiagnosis of pseudopapilledema. When these exudates are present, it is likely that papilledema has been present for at least several months.

Most patients with chronic papilledema have evidence of nerve fiber layer atrophy. The appearance of the atrophy ranges from slit-like defects to diffuse loss (see Chapter 4). Nerve fiber layer atrophy can be appreciated most easily by viewing through the red-free filter in a direct ophthalmoscope or slit lamp biomicroscope.

Cases are occasionally seen in which papilledema persists over many years without significant visual symptoms. This occurs primarily in patients with PTC, but it also occurs in patients with intracranial tumors.

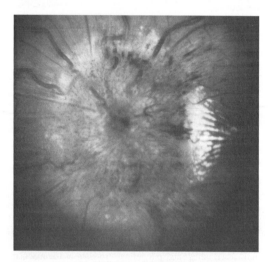

Figure 5.6. Macular star figure in fully developed papilledema. The incomplete star in this position is characteristic, but occasionally a complete star figure is seen.

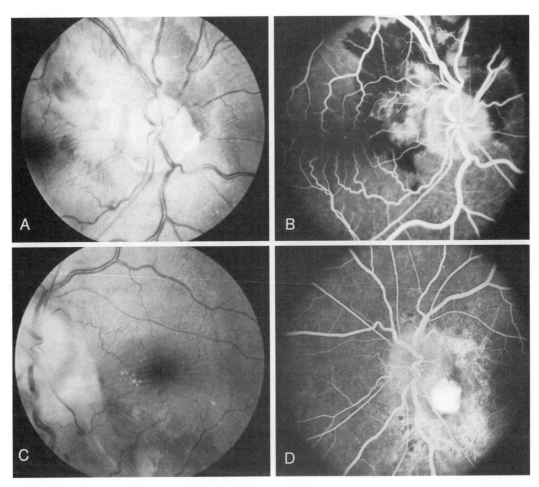

Figure 5.8. Subretinal neovascularization in chronic papilledema. *A.* Right eye shows a marked subretinal neovascular membrane superior-temporal to the optic disc, with subretinal hemorrhage, serous subretinal fluid, and retinal striae. *B.* Late stage fluorescein angiogram of right eye shows marked staining of subretinal neovascular membrane and hyperfluorescence of the disc. *C.* Left eye with elevated disc and an inferior-temporal subretinal neovascular membrane with surrounding hemorrhage, hard exudate, and retinal striae. *D.* Fluorescein angiogram of the left eye shows the residual subretinal neovascular membrane with a surrounding area of mottled disruption of the retinal pigment epithelium. (Reprinted with permission from Morse PH, Leveille AS, Antel JP, et al. Bilateral juxtapapillary subretinal neovascularization associated with pseudotumor cerebri. Am J Ophthalmol 1981;91:312–317.)

POSTPAPILLEDEMA ATROPHY

Over time, untreated papilledema subsides, the disc becomes pale, and the retinal vessels become narrow and sheathed (Fig. 5.10). In such cases, the nerve fiber layer can no longer be visualized by either direct ophthalmoscopy or slit lamp biomicroscopy. Some patients have persistent pigmentary changes or choroidal folds in the maculae (Fig. 5.11), and if the papilledema has been particularly severe, these changes may resemble those caused by a hamartoma of the pigment epithelium.

The time required for papilledema to evolve into optic atrophy depends on many factors, including the severity and constancy of the increased ICP. Atrophic changes can appear within several weeks and even days following the initial observation of acute papilledema, particularly if the rise in ICP is rapid, severe, and sustained. In such cases, the appearance of the

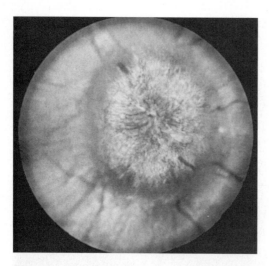

Figure 5.9.   Chronic papilledema. Note round compact appearance of the optic disc and lack of hemorrhages.

disc may rapidly progress to fully developed papilledema and then to postpapilledema optic atrophy without ever having gone through a stage of chronic papilledema. In other cases, the appearance of the optic disc gradually progresses over several months through the stages of early papilledema, fully developed papilledema, and chronic papilledema before becoming atrophic. In still other cases, many months or even years elapse before atrophy develops. In such cases, the appearance of the fundus is typically that of chronic papilledema that gradually melts away into atrophy. Finally, there are patients who appear to have stable chronic papilledema for many months to years until, for unclear reasons, they rapidly develop optic atrophy.

In some cases, as papilledema evolves from the fully developed stage to the chronic stage and then to the atrophic stage, optociliary shunt veins develop and then disappear. These vessels, which are preexisting veins that connect the retinal and choroidal venous circulations, enlarge because the increased ICP either directly compresses the central retinal vein or indirectly compresses it by compressing the optic nerve (Fig. 5.12). In either case, the vessels shunt venous blood from the retinal to the choroidal venous circulations, thus allowing the blood to exit the eye and orbit via the vortex veins to the superior and inferior ophthalmic veins, bypassing the obstructed central retinal vein. At this stage, patients usually have significant visual field defects, diminished color vision, and variably reduced visual acuity (see below). When the ICP is reduced or shunted from the anterior optic nerve, the optociliary veins may disappear.

Optic atrophy that results from chronic papilledema has a specific pattern of axon loss—a selective loss of peripheral axons with sparing of central axons. This pattern of axon dropout is consistent with the preservation of good central visual acuity despite severe papilledema and optic atrophy that is the rule in most patients with chronic papilledema.

UNILATERAL OR ASYMMETRIC PAPILLEDEMA

In most patients, papilledema is bilateral and relatively symmetric in the two eyes. In some instances, however, it is strictly unilateral or at least much more pronounced in one eye than in the other (Fig. 5.13). In some of these patients, optic atrophy has occurred in one eye before the development of increased ICP (the Foster Kennedy syndrome). If there are not enough nerve fibers to swell, papilledema cannot occur. In many cases of optic atrophy, however, sufficient nerve fibers remain such that even though the optic disc is pale, papilledema may still develop. A particularly interesting pattern of papilledema can occur in patients with optic atrophy from previous damage to the optic chiasm or optic tract. In such patients, an eye with a temporal hemianopia and atrophy of nasal fibers has band atrophy with preservation of the majority of the upper and lower (temporal) arcuate fibers. When papilledema develops, the swelling is thus limited to the superior and inferior poles of the disc. In an eye with a nasal hemianopia, atrophy of temporal fibers has occurred and most of the swelling is confined to the nasal portion of the disc.

In the Foster Kennedy syndrome, patients with frontal lobe or olfactory groove tumors develop optic atrophy in one eye with papilledema in the other (as well as anosmia) (see Chapter 4). On the side of the optic atrophy, the spaces about the optic nerve may be closed off by compression. Because a rise in CSF pressure in the optic nerve sheath is a prerequisite condition for development of papilledema, a combination of absence of elevated intravaginal sheath pressure and atrophy of nerve fibers from optic nerve compression prevent the development of papilledema on that side. In addition to optic atrophy

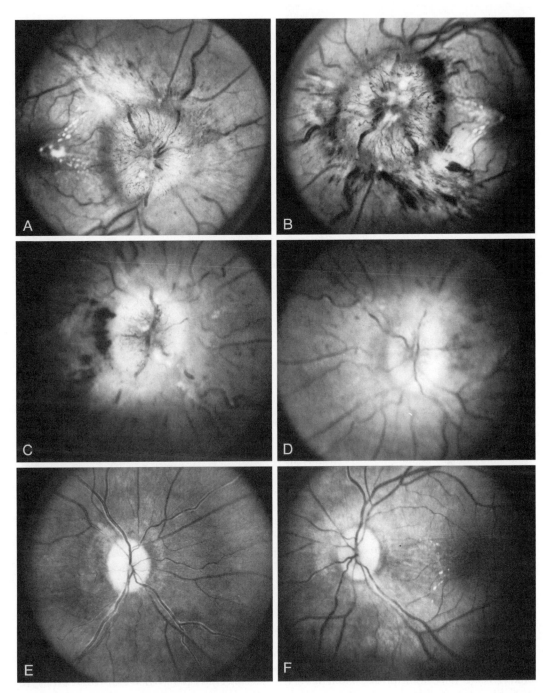

Figure 5.10. Progression from fully developed papilledema to postpapilledema optic atrophy. *A–B.* Right and left fundi showing fully developed papilledema. Note extensive peripapillary hemorrhages and exudates, including star figure of lipid in both maculae. *C–D.* Two weeks later, both optic discs are less swollen but pale. The hemorrhages and exudates are resolving. *E–F.* Four months later, both optic discs are diffusely pale, the retinal vessels are sheathed, and the nerve fiber layer is absent.

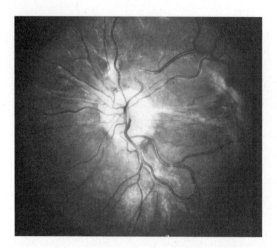

Figure 5.11. Pigmentary changes in the left macula of a patient who previously had severe papilledema. Note pallor of left optic disc, narrowed sheathed retinal vessels, and extensive pigmentary changes in left macula.

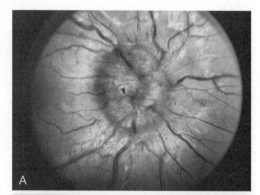
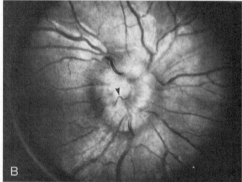
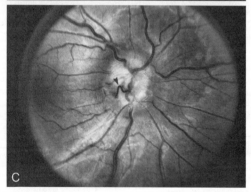

Figure 5.12. Development of optociliary shunt vein in a patient with chronic papilledema from pseudotumor cerebri. *A.* Fully developed papilledema. Note the small vessel located on the surface of the disc at 8 o'clock (*arrowhead*). *B.* As disc swelling resolves, the previously noted vessel becomes more apparent (*arrowhead*). *C.* Disc swelling has almost completely resolved. Vessel at 8 o'clock appears larger than previously and clearly represents a retinal-choroidal shunt (*arrowhead*).

as a condition preventing development of papilledema, we have also examined several patients with unilateral optic disc dysplasia who developed papilledema only on the side of the previously normal disc.

When unilateral papilledema occurs in a patient with an apparently normal optic disc on the opposite side, it probably results from some congenital anomaly of the optic nerve sheath that prevents transmission of pressure to the optic nerve head on the side on which papilledema is absent. Other authors believe that the anatomic arrangement of the venous sinuses is somehow responsible for unequal or unilateral papilledema in patients with previously normal optic discs. If congenital anomalies of the optic nerve sheaths or venous sinuses are responsible for unilateral papilledema, they may also explain the absence of papilledema in at least some patients with significantly elevated ICP.

In most patients with apparent unilateral papilledema, careful observation of the "normal" optic disc often discloses minimal hyperemia, blurred nerve fiber layer, or disc swelling that is easily overlooked in the face of significant papilledema on the opposite side. Nevertheless, purely unilateral papilledema as determined by both careful ophthalmoscopic examination and fluorescein angiography can occur, probably in about 2% of cases.

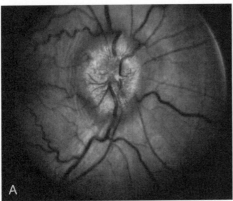
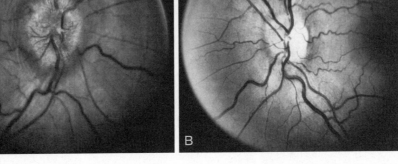

Figure 5.13. Unilateral papilledema in a 34-year-old woman with pseudotumor cerebri. *A.* The right optic disc shows fully developed papilledema. *B.* The left optic disc is normal.

Papilledema that is unilateral, or at least more pronounced on one side than on the other, may be of significance in many cases of intracranial mass lesions, particularly abscesses. The papilledema is usually ipsilateral to the lesion, but this is not always the case.

The following generalizations seem appropriate regarding unilateral or asymmetric papilledema:

1. Unilateral optic disc swelling is unlikely to be true papilledema. More frequently, it is caused by local pathology (e.g., inflammation, ischemia, or compression of the optic nerve within the orbit).
2. When an optic disc is significantly atrophic or anomalous, it may not develop papilledema, or papilledema will develop only in the regions of functioning axons.
3. Most patients with apparent unilateral papilledema actually have bilateral asymmetric papilledema.

DIAGNOSIS

The most important method of diagnosing papilledema is by a careful ophthalmoscopic examination. If, after performing a careful clinical examination that includes red-free ophthalmoscopy, the examiner cannot determine if the patient does or does not have true optic disc swelling, there are several options.

Many authors recommend the use of fluorescein angiography to diagnose early papilledema. The test is easily performed in an outpatient setting. Five milliliters of 10% fluorescein sodium

are rapidly injected into a superficial arm vein. The passage of dye through retinal vessels is then observed and photographed at rapid intervals, with a cobalt blue filter interposed in front of the light source to visualize the fluorescence of the dye. If photographic facilities are lacking, the examiner can observe the ocular fundus using an indirect ophthalmoscope or a slit lamp and a hand-held or contact lens. The earliest frames of the fluorescein angiogram in patients with early papilledema show dilation of disc capillaries, dye leakage, and microaneurysm formation; later frames show leakage of dye beyond the disc margins (Fig. 5.14).

Echography (ultrasonography) can be performed in cases of questionable papilledema. This test reliably determines whether the diameter of the optic nerve is increased, and if so, whether the increase is caused by CSF surrounding the nerve. It can also easily detect buried optic disc drusen (see Chapter 3). Alternatively, CT scanning can be used to determine if there are buried drusen causing an appearance mimicking papilledema, and both CT scanning and MRI can be used to detect evidence of an intracranial mass or hydrocephalus.

Finally, the ICP can be measured directly by lumbar puncture. This procedure should be performed only after neuroimaging has determined if an intracranial mass is present.

The **differential diagnosis of papilledema** includes anomalous elevation of one or both optic discs and true optic disc swelling from a cause other than increased ICP (see Chapter 4 and Table 4.1). In most cases, the patients have

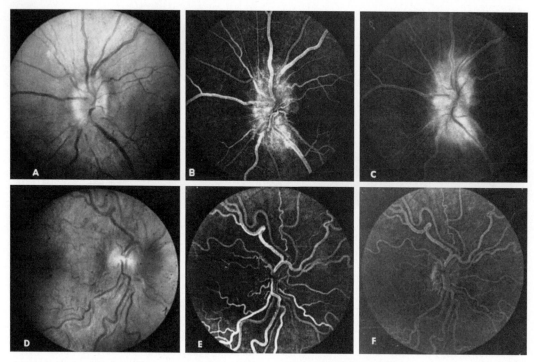

Figure 5.14. Fluorescein angiogram of mild papilledema (*A–C*) and pseudopapilledema (*D–F*). *A.* Reproduction of color photograph of the left fundus showing blurred disc margins. No hemorrhages are visible. *B.* In arteriovenous phase, fluorescein angiogram shows early leakage of dye into peripapillary region. *C.* Ten minutes after fluorescein injection, angiogram shows residual hyperfluorescence of disc and surrounding region. *D.* Optic disc shows tortuous vessels and mild elevation. *E.* Fluorescein angiogram in early arteriovenous phase shows no disc fluorescence or leakage into the peripapillary region. *F.* Eight minutes after fluorescein injection shows no evidence of disc leakage or hyperfluorescence. (Courtesy of Dr. Michael Sanders.)

no neurologic or systemic symptoms or signs referable to increased ICP, and this lack of manifestations should help the physician focus on other possibilities. When the patient has other complaints such as headaches, however, the differentiation of papilledema from other causes of optic disc elevation becomes more complex.

Anomalous elevation of the optic discs is probably caused most often by buried optic disc drusen; however, hypoplastic discs may be anomalously elevated, and tilted optic discs often show elevation of their superior and nasal portions. In addition, some optic discs are anomalously elevated but do not contain drusen, nor are they small or tilted. In all cases, a careful ophthalmoscopic examination combined with ultrasonography, CT scanning, or both should differentiate anomalously elevated optic discs from true optic disc swelling.

True optic disc swelling that mimics papille-

dema may be caused by local ocular disease, such as intraocular inflammation. Eyes in which optic disc swelling occurs in the setting of inflammation invariably show other evidence of inflammation, particularly aqueous or vitreous cells and, in some cases, sheathing of retinal vessels. Retinal vascular disturbances can also produce optic disc swelling. In such cases, there may be no way to determine the cause of the disc swelling without performing appropriate neuroimaging studies and a lumbar puncture. Patients with optic perineuritis (perioptic neuritis) have optic disc swelling that is also indistinguishable from papilledema unless there is associated intraocular inflammation. Nonarteritic anterior ischemic optic neuropathy can mimic papilledema, particularly when it is asymptomatic. Rare patients with anterior optic neuritis have normal central visual acuity; however, such patients invariably complain that they have decreased vision, and other tests of visual function in such patients (e.g., contrast sensitivity, color vision, visual fields) usually reveal an abnormality inconsistent with papilledema. Finally, optic discs infiltrated by inflammatory or neoplastic cells may appear similar to papilledema. The diagnosis in such cases can usually be made by neuroimaging, with or without a lumbar puncture.

COURSE

The rapidity with which papilledema can develop depends to a large extent on the etiology of the increased ICP. Papilledema may develop within 2 to 8 hours when there is sudden intracranial or epidural hemorrhage. In addition, minimal papilledema may exist and suddenly become fully developed over several hours in certain settings, such as encephalitis associated with a cerebral abscess. Occasionally, there is the apparently paradoxical development, or increase in the severity, of papilledema several days to a week after normalization of increased ICP.

Fully developed papilledema may disappear completely within hours, days, or weeks, depending on the way in which ICP is lowered (Fig. 5.15). For instance, papilledema can resolve 6 to 8 weeks after a successful craniotomy to remove a brain tumor. We have observed resolution of papilledema within 2 to 3 weeks after lumboperitoneal shunting in patients with PTC and within several days after optic nerve sheath fenestration.

In most cases, retinal venous as well as disc capillary dilations begin to regress as soon as ICP is lowered to a normal level. During the next few days to weeks, presumably because of the change in hemodynamics at the disc, new hemorrhages may appear; but these are of no significance and disappear within a short time. Gradually, disc hyperemia and elevation resolve. The last abnormalities to disappear are blurring of the disc margins and abnormalities of the peripapillary retinal nerve fiber layer. In some cases, optic atrophy appears as papilledema resolves. There may be extensive sheathing of vessels and gliosis indicating the nature of the etiology in such cases; however, in many cases, the atrophy is indistinguishable from that caused by inflammation, vascular disease, or trauma.

It is difficult to predict the visual prognosis in a patient with papilledema. Generally speaking, the more rapid the development of papilledema, the greater the danger to sight. Similarly, the more severe the papilledema, the worse the visual prognosis. Ominous signs include narrowing of the retinal arteries, often with sheathing, and loss of the peripapillary retinal nerve fiber layer. When these changes are seen, irreversible damage to optic nerve tissue has already occurred. Disc pallor that becomes evident while papilledema is still present is also an indication that the visual prognosis is poor, even if ICP is lowered immediately, because the pallor is caused by loss of axons. Most patients with these changes have clinical evidence of visual dysfunction, including decreased color vision, visual field defects, and abnormal contrast sensitivity. Loss of visual acuity is the last visual parameter to be affected, much as is the case in patients with chronic open-angle glaucoma. Once a patient with papilledema begins to experience, or is found to have, deficits in these parameters, the visual prognosis is extremely tenuous. On the other hand, severe venous engorgement, retinal hemorrhages, and hard and soft exudates have no prognostic significance.

Papilledema may be observed at any age. Not only is there no upper age limit, but there is abundant evidence that papilledema occurs frequently in infants and children. This phenomenon is remarkable because we explain the absence of papilledema in most cases of congenital hydrocephalus on the basis of expansibility of the skull. If this were true, one would expect a lower prevalence of papilledema in infants and children with intracranial tumors. Nevertheless, studies have found papilledema or postpapilledema optic atrophy in 56 to 90% of children with brain tumors.

PATHOGENESIS

Although the pathogenesis of papilledema remains unclear, there are some general points of agreement. First, papilledema occurs only when there is patency of the meningeal spaces surrounding the optic nerve and intracranial structures. Blockage of these spaces by adhesions or tumor prevents papilledema from occurring on the side of the obstruction. Second, papilledema does not occur in an eye in which antecedent optic atrophy has destroyed most or all of the nerve fibers. Finally and most importantly, axon transport is clearly abnormal in patients with

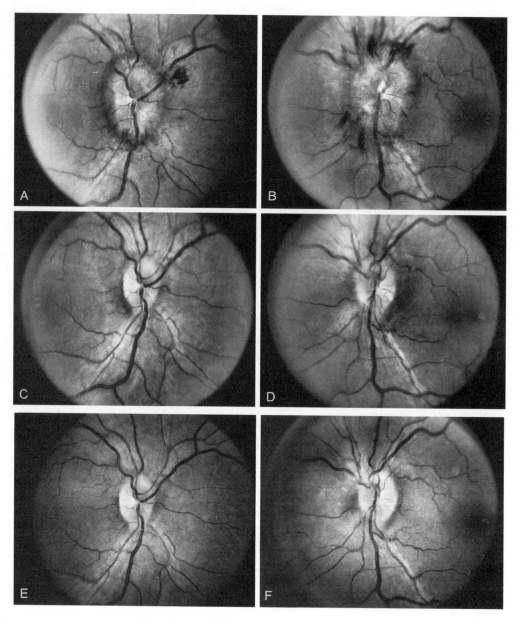

Figure 5.15. Resolution of papilledema in a patient with pseudotumor cerebri. *A–B.* Right and left optic discs prior to treatment. *C–D.* One month after beginning treatment with dehydrating agents, much of the disc swelling has re- solved in both eyes, and no hemorrhages are evident. *E–F.* Three months after beginning treatment, both discs show complete resolution of swelling and now appear normal.

papilledema as well as in patients with disc swelling from other causes (ischemia, inflammation, hypotony, etc.). Accumulation of axoplasm results in the swelling of axons.

Numerous questions still exist regarding the pathogenesis of papilledema:

1. Is there a relationship between the severity of axon transport obstruction and the clinical degree of optic disc swelling? Although it is clear that even in early experimental papilledema, disc swelling is due to blockage of axon transport, resulting

in secondary axon distention, no studies relating severity of the block to severity of disc swelling have yet been performed.

2. Is obstruction of axon transport compatible with normal conduction of nerve impulses? Transport and conduction are two separate, although related, processes. Abundant evidence suggests that conduction can continue along an axon in which there is partial blockage of axon transport. Nevertheless, it is not clear how long an axon can survive and continue to conduct action potentials when there is sustained, though partial, blockage of axon transport. In addition, although detailed psychophysical testing in patients with papilledema often reveals a variety of deficits in vision not detected on routine visual acuity, color vision, or visual field testing, the marked difference in visual function among patients with optic disc swelling from different causes (e.g., papilledema vs. anterior optic neuritis) suggests that either the degree of axon transport blockage is different in different types of optic disc swelling or that obstruction of axon transport is not, in and of itself, sufficient to cause loss of visual function.

3. What is the cause of axon transport obstruction in papilledema? This is the critical question that has yet to be answered. Although the direct cause of optic disc swelling is blockage of axon transport, the cause of the blockage is still unknown. Some investigators believe that the cause is mechanical, from transmission of raised ICP to retinal ganglion cell axons in the optic nerve. In this scheme, visual loss occurs in the setting of chronic papilledema from prelaminar ischemia secondary to the mechanically induced optic disc swelling. Other investigators believe that ischemia caused by disturbances of autoregulation in the prelaminar, laminar, and retrolaminar regions of the optic nerve head contributes to axon transport obstruction.

SYMPTOMS AND SIGNS

Both nonvisual and visual symptoms occur in patients with papilledema. As a general rule, the nonvisual symptoms are more severe and bothersome to the patient, although visual symptoms can be both distressing and indicative of impending permanent visual dysfunction.

NONVISUAL MANIFESTATIONS

Headache is one of the earliest symptoms of increased ICP, although there may be a considerable increase in ICP without headache. Neither the severity of the headache nor its location has any value in determining whether an intracranial mass is present, and if so, its location. An exception to this rule is the meningioma that infiltrates the dura over the convexity of the cerebral hemispheres and produces a palpable swelling and local pain at the site of the lesion. In some patients, headache associated with increased ICP is increased by coughing, straining, and so on. This is an inconstant phenomenon, but its presence may suggest a ball-valve action of the lesion within the ventricular system. It is believed that headache associated with increased ICP is caused by stretching of the meninges, whereas sharply localized pains in such cases may be explained on the basis of damage to sensory nerves at the base of the skull or localized dysfunction of meningeal nerves.

Nausea and vomiting are frequently associated with significantly increased ICP, although so-called projectile vomiting is rare. Vomiting, bradycardia, difficulty in swallowing, and eventual respiratory failure may all be explained by herniation of the medulla into the foramen magnum.

Loss of consciousness, generalized motor rigidity, and pupillary dilation are terminal effects of increased ICP. Loss of consciousness presumably occurs from compression of the cerebral cortex and the reduction of its blood supply. Herniation of the hippocampal gyrus through the tentorium from increased ICP results in crowding of the temporal lobe into the incisura of each side. Tentorial herniation thus places pressure on the crura cerebri, resulting in generalized motor rigidity. Finally, direct pressure on the oculomotor nerves or dorsal midbrain produces bilaterally dilated pupils that do not respond to light stimulation.

Patients with increased ICP may, on occasion, develop spontaneous **CSF rhinorrhea.** In some cases, there is a history of previous trauma; in others, there is a congenital anomaly at the base of the skull. When spontaneous, CSF fistulas are usually located in the region of the cribriform plate.

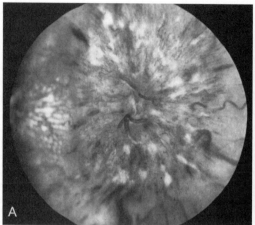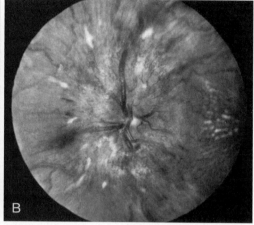

Figure 5.16. Papilledema associated with bilateral visual loss related to macular hard exudate. The patient was a 35-year-old woman with headaches and decreased vision in both eyes. Visual acuity was 20/50 OU. Visual fields showed marked enlargement of the blind spots. *A.* The right optic disc is markedly swollen. There are numerous hemorrhages and soft exudates on and surrounding the disc, and there is a star figure composed of hard exudate (lipid) in the right macula. *B.* The left optic disc and macula appear similar to the right.

VISUAL MANIFESTATIONS

Patients with early, and even fully developed, papilledema are usually visually asymptomatic, with neither visual acuity nor color vision being affected. In some of these patients, the only abnormality found on careful testing is mild to moderate enlargement of the physiologic blind spot. Other patients may be aware of the physiologic blind spot, and such patients may complain of a negative scotoma in the field of vision of one or both eyes. Still other patients have variable loss of visual acuity, color vision, visual field, or a combination of these visual parameters. Some of these patients have retinal or vitreous hemorrhages or exudates that reduce central acuity (Fig. 5.16). In others, an intracranial mass produces a visual sensory deficit in one or both eyes by one or more mechanisms, including direct compression of a portion of the visual sensory pathway (e.g., compression of the occipital lobe by a meningioma, producing a homonymous field defect), indirect compression of part of the pathway via a secondary effect on surrounding brain (e.g., gyrus rectus compression of the optic nerves producing a bilateral optic neuropathy in a patient with a frontal lobe tumor), and infiltration of a part of the pathway (e.g., infiltration of the optic chiasm by a germinoma, producing a bitemporal hemianopia).

Transient Visual Obscurations

Patients with papilledema may experience brief, transient obscurations of vision. During these episodes, vision may vary from mildly blurred to complete blindness. Some patients describe a rapid gray-out of vision, whereas others experience positive visual phenomena—such as photopsias, phosphenes, and even scintillating scotomas—that obscure their vision. In all cases, recovery of vision is invariably rapid and complete. The obscurations may affect only one eye, alternate eyes, or both eyes simultaneously. They usually last only a few seconds, although attacks lasting several hours sometimes occur. Some patients experience up to 20 to 30 such episodes a day, with the obscurations often precipitated by changes in posture, particularly from sitting to standing or from lying down to sitting or standing; rare patients experience gaze-evoked amaurosis, a phenomenon much more commonly observed in patients with orbital lesions that compress and deform the optic nerve.

Transient visual obscurations have little prognostic value. Indeed, in many patients with transient obscurations, papilledema resolves completely without producing any detectable visual deficit. Conversely, patients with papilledema may develop permanent visual damage without ever having experienced any transient visual obscurations. The cause of these obscurations is most likely related to transient compression or ischemia of the optic nerve.

Visual Field Defects

Concentric enlargement of the blind spot is the most common—and frequently the only—visual field defect in patients with papilledema. Compression, detachment, and lateral displacement of the peripapillary retina appear to be the major reasons that the blind spot increases in size in patients with papilledema; however, the blind spot may be enlarged even when there is no obvious retinal displacement or detachment. In this setting, the enlarged blind spot represents a refractive scotoma caused by acquired peripapillary hyperopia, which in turn results from elevation of the retina by peripapillary subretinal fluid.

Early visual field defects in eyes with papilledema are not uncommon on automated static perimetry and are often present when standard kinetic perimetry gives normal results. These early defects are generally arcuate scotomas or nasal steps, whereas constriction of the visual fields is invariably a late sign of papilledema, occurring during the chronic stage as it progresses to optic atrophy. The field defects are usually worse nasally than temporally (Figs. 5.17 and 5.18). Thus, an eye may have only a temporal island of vision before becoming completely blind.

Loss of visual field in the setting of papilledema is usually slow and progressive. Sudden loss of visual field in this setting suggests a local cause, such as ischemia. Superimposed ischemic optic neuropathy presumably occurs from occlusion of prelaminar disc arterioles caused by increased tissue pressure in the optic disc. These vessels may be more sensitive to increased intraocular pressure than are other vessels in the ocular fundus.

Loss of Central Vision

Patients with papilledema caused by intracranial mass lesions or meningitis (septic, aseptic, carcinomatous, lymphomatous) can lose central vision acutely or progressively from the effects of the underlying process on the optic nerves.

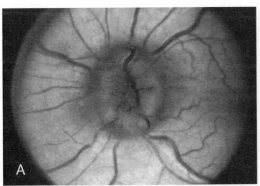

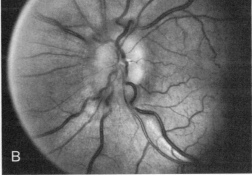

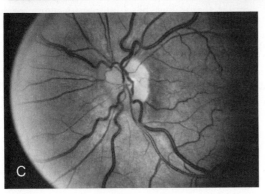

Figure 5.17.   Progression of visual field defect in a patient with chronic papilledema. *A–C.* Progression of chronic papilledema to optic atrophy.

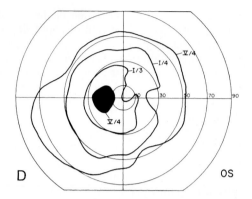

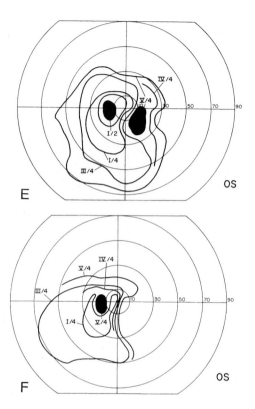

Figure 5.17. *(continued). D–F.* Progression of the visual field defects. Note progressive loss of nasal field and associated constriction with preservation of visual acuity.

In other cases, permanent loss of central vision results from the nonspecific effects of increased ICP on the optic nerve and begins with visual field constriction that is slowly progressive. In such cases, loss of central acuity is usually a late phenomenon, although it may occur over several weeks in cases with markedly increased ICP.

Acute loss of vision occurs in some patients with papilledema. In most of these cases, local causes are responsible. Some patients lose central vision because they develop hemorrhages or exudates in the maculae. Others develop ischemic optic neuropathy or retinal vascular occlusions that may be related to the underlying process (e.g., a coagulopathy) or to the rapid rate at which the ICP has risen. In addition, rare patients, many of them children, seem to have a fulminant course characterized by a rapid progression from normal vision to profound and permanent visual loss.

As in other types of optic neuropathies, papilledema may be associated with abnormalities of visual sensation that can be detected when specific tests are performed. For example, patients with visual acuity of 20/20, a full visual field, and normal color perception may nevertheless have abnormal contrast sensitivity. Such patients also may have delayed latency of the P100 wave when visual-evoked potentials are measured.

Diplopia

Increased ICP may result in compression or stretching of the abducens nerve at the base of the skull. The damage may be unilateral or bilateral. Trochlear nerve palsies may also occur in patients with increased ICP, presumably from compression of either the dorsal midbrain or the nerves themselves by a ballooned suprapineal recess. Such palsies are often misdiagnosed as skew deviation if quantitative testing of eye movements or a Bielschowsky head tilt test is not performed, although true skew deviation can also occur in patients with increased ICP. Only very rarely does an oculomotor nerve paralysis result from raised ICP.

ETIOLOGY

The craniospinal cavity is an almost rigid bony enclosure completely filled by tissue, CSF, and circulating blood. Within this enclosure,

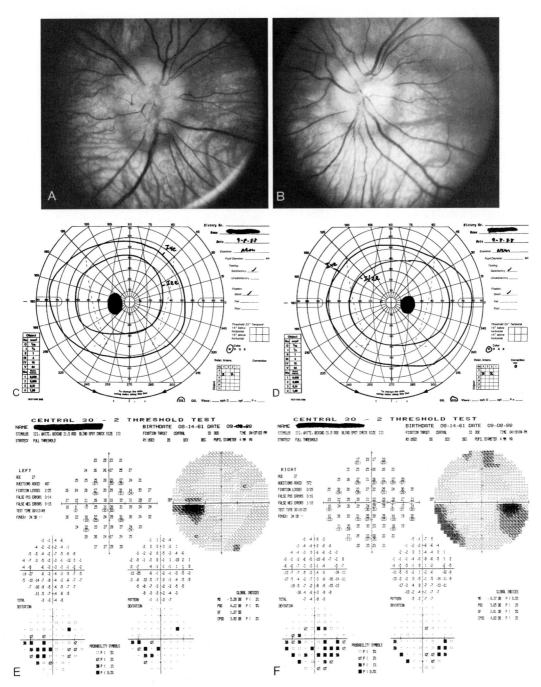

Figure 5.18. Difference in sensitivity of kinetic versus static perimetry in chronic papilledema. *A–B.* Right and left optic discs show chronic papilledema. *C–D.* Kinetic perimetry shows no abnormalities except for mildly enlarged blind spots. *E–F.* Static perimetry in the same patient shows nasal steps, inferior arcuate defects, and reduction in sensitivity in both eyes.

CSF is constantly produced at the rate of about 0.37% per minute, primarily inside the ventricular system. Almost all of the production is by the choroid plexus within the lateral ventricles, although the choroid plexuses of the 3rd and 4th ventricles and the ependymal cells lining the ventricular system also contribute a small amount.

CSF flows from the lateral ventricles through the interventricular foramina into the 3rd ventricle and mixes with the CSF produced in that ventricle. The CSF then flows through the cerebral aqueduct (of Sylvius) into the 4th ventricle and out into the subarachnoid space through the foramina of Luschka and Magendie. In the subarachnoid space, CSF flows rostrally from the posterior fossa through the lower ventral basal cisterns and tentorial notch to reach the interpeduncular and chiasmatic cisterns. The CSF then flows dorsally through the communicating cisterns to reach the dorsal cisterns and laterally and superiorly from the chiasmatic cistern into the cisterns of the sylvian fissure. From the cisterns and sylvian fissures, CSF moves outward and superiorly over the cerebral convexities, where it is absorbed. The chief route of absorption of CSF is through the arachnoid granulations that protrude into the venous sinuses and diploic veins. These vessels drain to the internal jugular vein and other extracranial veins.

Under appropriate circumstances, as little as 80 cc of rapidly added volume (CSF, blood, edema, tissue, etc.) will raise ICP to a level incompatible with life. Increased ICP occurs from several mechanisms (Table 5.1):

- An increase in the total amount of intracranial tissue by a space-occupying lesion.
- An increase in intracranial tissue volume by focal or diffuse cerebral edema.
- A decrease in total volume within the cranial vault by thickening of the skull.
- Blockage of the flow of CSF within the ventricular system (obstructive or noncommunicating hydrocephalus) or within the arachnoid granulations (nonobstructive or communicating hydrocephalus).
- Reduced absorption of CSF from obstruction or compromise of venous outflow both intracranially and extracranially.
- Increased production of CSF by an intracranial tumor at a rate that precludes ade-

Table 5.1
Causes of Increased Intracranial Pressure

Space-Occupying Lesions
- Neoplasms
- Abscesses
- Inflammatory masses
- Hemorrhages
- Infarctions
- Arteriovenous malformations

Focal or Diffuse Cerebral Edema

Reduction in the Size of the Cranial Vault
- Craniosynostosis
- Thickening of the skull

Blockage of CSF Flow
- Noncommunicating hydrocephalus

Reduction in CSF Resorption
- Communicating hydrocephalus
- Meningeal processes
- Elevated venous pressure

Increased CSF Production

Idiopathic Intracranial Hypertension (Pseudotumor Cerebri)

quate absorption for maintenance of normal ICP.

INTRACRANIAL MASSES

Intracranial masses produce increased ICP through most of the mechanisms mentioned above. They may act solely as space-occupying lesions; they may produce focal or diffuse cerebral edema; they may block the flow of CSF by occluding the normal CSF drainage pathways by direct compression or infiltration of the arachnoid villi or the cerebral venous sinuses and by producing increased protein or blood products that secondarily block the arachnoid villi; and they may produce CSF.

Papilledema develops in about 60% of patients with cerebral tumors. Tumors that are located below the tentorium (infratentorial) are more likely to produce papilledema than those situated above it (supratentorial). Supratentorial tumors usually produce papilledema by deflection of the falx and pressure upon the great vein of Galen, whereas tumors below the tentorium usually produce papilledema by obstruction of the aqueduct. Some infratentorial masses do not obstruct the aqueduct but still produce papilledema, possibly by compression of the vein of Galen or the posterior superior sagittal sinus.

Brain tumors in certain locations may produce papilledema without lateralizing or localizing signs. Such tumors are usually supratentorial and are located within the nondominant hemisphere or within one of the lateral ventricles. Not all intracranial tumors cause a pressure rise sufficient to produce papilledema. Neither the type of intracranial tumor nor its rate of growth correlate well with the development of papilledema.

Papilledema may occur with any type of intracranial mass, including primary and secondary (metastatic) brain tumors, hamartomas, teratomas, hematomas, giant aneurysms, arteriovenous malformations, cysticercus cysts, and granulomas (e.g., in syphilis, tuberculosis, or sarcoidosis). In rare cases, the entire brain is infiltrated by a glioma—cerebral gliomatosis. In such cases, the diffusely infiltrated brain may appear normal on neuroimaging, and the CSF may have a normal concentration of protein and glucose and may contain no cells even when large amounts are obtained for cytopathologic examination. Such patients may initially be thought to have PTC until further growth of tumor cells occurs, and the true diagnosis becomes evident.

DISORDERS OF CSF FLOW

Aqueductal stenosis often presents in childhood. It may be congenital, in which case it may or may not be associated with a Chiari malformation, or it may be acquired from intracranial infections such as toxoplasmosis or mumps ependymitis. Presentation in infancy is with macrocephaly. Adult presentations include headache, dorsal midbrain syndrome, meningitis, hemorrhage, endocrine disturbances from compression of the pituitary gland, seizures, gait disturbances, and CSF rhinorrhea.

Subarachnoid hemorrhage usually produces papilledema either by blocking CSF flow within the ventricular system or by blocking CSF absorption at the arachnoid granulations. Papilledema occurs in 10 to 24% of patients with ruptured intracranial aneurysms. The papilledema does not vary significantly by sex, age, or site of aneurysm. Papilledema can develop within several hours after the hemorrhage, or it may develop only after several weeks of increased ICP.

Hydrocephalus is a known complication of the inherited disorders of mucopolysaccharide metabolism called the **mucopolysaccharidoses,** and papilledema occurs in some of these cases. Increased ICP in these patients probably results from an obstruction to the distal circulation of CSF over the cerebral convexities, in the arachnoid villi, or both, by the deposition of mucopolysaccharide in the meninges, leading to delayed CSF absorption.

MENINGITIS AND ENCEPHALITIS

The mechanism producing increased ICP in patients with meningitis or encephalitis is commonly diffuse cerebral edema, although aqueductal stenosis or obstruction of CSF resorption through the arachnoid granulations may also be responsible. Papilledema occurs in about 2.5% of patients with **meningitis.** It is more likely to occur in patients with tuberculous meningitis (25% of cases) than any other type of bacterial meningitis, although it is also common in patients with cryptococcal meningitis. The papilledema associated with meningitis is usually mild and transient, although patients with cryptococcal meningitis may have fulminant papilledema.

The CNS is involved in about 5% of cases of **sarcoidosis.** In such cases, granulomas may develop in the meninges, causing nodular masses or, more commonly, an adhesive meningitis. Less frequently, granulomas develop within brain parenchyma. Papilledema that occurs in this setting may result either from obstruction of CSF flow or from a mass effect. These mechanisms also apply to syphilis and tuberculosis.

Papilledema may occur with any form of **encephalitis.** Approximately 19% of patients with viral encephalitis have papilledema, and papilledema occurs not uncommonly in both herpes simplex encephalitis and herpes zoster encephalitis. ICP is frequently elevated in measles encephalitis, and papilledema may also occur in such patients; however, rubella encephalitis is rarely associated with papilledema, and the encephalitides produced by mumps and varicella also seem to be unassociated with papilledema in the majority of cases. Papilledema occurs in some cases of California encephalitis, lymphocytic choriomeningitis, infectious mononucleosis, and Coxsackie meningoencephalitis. Patients with poliomyelitis may develop increased ICP during both the acute and convalescent phases of the disease, and papilledema may develop in such cases. In most of these cases, CSF protein is elevated, and there is a moderate lymphocytic or mixed pleocytosis. Patients with subacute sclerosing panencephalitis (Dawson's encephalitis) usually show signs of slowly progressive dementia and myoclonus, often preceded by or associated with macular pigmentary changes. Rare patients develop papilledema.

It must be emphasized that in almost all CNS infections and inflammations, swelling of the optic disc may occur without elevated ICP, presumably from inflammation of the optic nerve; i.e., optic perineuritis. In such cases, differentiating between papilledema and optic perineuritis is impossible, because in both cases there is normal visual function. Only when a lumbar puncture is performed in a patient with a CNS infection and disc swelling, and the CSF is found to be under normal pressure with an increased protein and a pleocytosis, can the true inflammatory etiology of the disc swelling be ascertained.

Increased ICP, often associated with papilledema, occurs in patients with diffuse spread of a variety of tumors throughout the CNS. These tumors include carcinomas, lymphomas, leukemias, and leptomeningeal gliomatosis. The increased pressure is usually caused by tumor cells that either obstruct CSF outflow across the arachnoid villi or CSF flow in the basal cisterns.

SYNDROMES OF ELEVATED VENOUS PRESSURE

Obstruction of cerebral venous drainage may result in increased ICP and papilledema (Table 5.2). The obstruction is most often caused by compression or thrombosis, with the vessels most often affected being the superior sagittal and transverse (lateral) sinuses.

Tumors that obstruct the superior sagittal sinus are usually extra-axial lesions, such as meningiomas. The transverse sinus can be occluded by acoustic neuromas, meningiomas, and metastatic tumors.

Septic thrombosis of the transverse sinus tends to occur in the setting of acute or chronic otitis media, in which there is extension of the infection to the mastoid air cells and then to the adjacent lateral sinus. In such cases, papilledema usually occurs early and tends to be bilateral and symmetric. A similar appearance occurs in patients with septic thrombosis of the superior sagittal sinus, a much less common condition. Septic thrombosis of the cavernous sinus may also be associated with papilledema, although the papilledema develops late in the course of the process.

Table 5.2

Etiologies of Obstruction/Impairment of Cerebral Venous Drainage

Primary Hematologic
- Antiphospholipid antibody syndrome
- Thrombophilia (antithrombin III deficiency, protein S deficiency, resistance to activated protein C, etc.)
- Thrombocythemia
- Polycythemia
- Disseminated intravascular coagulation

Systemic Conditions Associated with Coagulopathy
- Behçet's disease
- Systemic lupus erythematosus
- Neurosarcoidosis
- Cancer
- Pregnancy/postpartum
- Renal disease (nephrotic syndrome)
- Infections

Local Infections
- Mastoiditis
- Cellulitis

Traumatic

Tumors

Dural Arteriovenous Fistula

Occlusion of Internal Jugular Vein
- Iatrogenic
    Indwelling catheter
    Surgery
- Traumatic
- Tumors (extravascular)

Aseptic thrombosis usually occurs in the nonpaired sinuses of both adults and children, with the superior sagittal sinus most frequently affected. In such cases, there may be pronounced engorgement of the vessels of the scalp, retina, and conjunctiva in addition to papilledema. Many of these patients have a coagulopathy from a primary hematologic disorder (e.g., protein C or S deficiency, antiphospholipid antibody syndrome, essential thrombocythemia) or associated with a systemic process (e.g., renal disease, pregnancy, cancer); others have a systemic inflammatory or infectious disease (e.g., systemic lupus erythematosus, Behçet's syndrome, paroxysmal nocturnal hemoglobinuria, trichinosis, sarcoidosis).

Ligation of one jugular vein (if it is the principal vein draining the intracranial area) or both jugular veins may produce papilledema. In most instances, occlusion of the jugular veins occurs during radical neck dissection for regional tumors; in other cases, the veins become thrombosed from the effects of indwelling catheters. The papilledema in such cases usually does not appear for a week or two. It is almost always bilateral and severe; however, it typically resolves in 2 to 3 months as collateral venous drainage from the head develops to meet the demands of cerebral blood flow.

Cerebral venous thrombosis can present with an isolated syndrome of raised ICP indistinguishable from idiopathic intracranial hypertension (see below), or other neurologic manifestations may make the diagnosis more apparent. Examples of the latter include severe headache, seizures, somnolence, disturbances of consciousness, and focal neurologic signs such as hemiparesis.

TRAUMA

Papilledema occurs in 20 to 30% of persons who have suffered severe cranial injuries, both with and without an associated skull fracture. In most of these cases, the increased ICP is caused by a severe subarachnoid hemorrhage or a significant intracerebral, subdural, or epidural hematoma. In other cases, the increased ICP is caused by cerebral venous thrombosis or by diffuse or localized cerebral edema.

Papilledema that develops in patients after head trauma is usually mild and may develop immediately, several days after the injury, or up to 2 weeks later. A sudden, severe, but transient increase in ICP is usually responsible for the immediate development of papilledema, whereas sustained but mild to moderately elevated ICP accounts for papilledema that appears during the first week after injury. Papilledema in the second week or later results from impaired CSF absorption and consequent communicating hydrocephalus or delayed focal or diffuse cerebral swelling.

CRANIOSYNOSTOSES

The intracranial vault may become smaller in certain types of craniosynostoses. Among patients with premature synostosis of the cranial sutures, 12 to 15% eventually develop papilledema. However, simple cranial synostosis (oxycephaly, scaphocephaly, trigonocephaly, or plagiocephaly) is almost never associated with papilledema, whereas about 40% of patients with craniofacial dysostosis (Crouzon's syndrome) or acrocephalosyndactyly (Apert's syndrome) develop papilledema.

If papilledema is going to develop in a patient with a craniosynostosis, it usually does so before the age of 10 years. It is often chronic by the time it is detected, possibly because such patients may not undergo a careful examination of the ocular fundi unless they complain of visual disturbances. However, papilledema may develop at any age.

EXTRACRANIAL LESIONS

The association of increased ICP and papilledema with **tumors in the spinal canal** is an unusual but well-documented phenomenon. Most of these tumors are intradural; however, extradural spinal tumors can also cause increased ICP associated with papilledema. In some cases, the tumors are located in the high cervical region, and the explanation for the increased ICP in such cases is thought to be upward swelling of the tumor with compression of the cerebellum and obstruction of CSF flow through the foramen magnum. This mechanism seems unlikely to be the explanation in the majority of cases, however, because over 50% of spinal cord lesions associated with papilledema are ependymomas or neurofibromas that are usually located in the thoracic and lumbar regions. These tumors can produce extremely high concentrations of protein in the CSF, and it is therefore likely that increased ICP and papilledema in such cases is caused by the decreased CSF absorption that results from blockage of the arachnoid granulations by protein. In other cases, recurrent subarachnoid hemorrhage, which occurs commonly from bleeding from the surface of ependymomas, may also cause reduced CSF absorption from blockage of the arachnoid villi by blood or blood products.

Papilledema is an uncommon complication of the **Landry-Guillain-Barré syndrome** (GBS). Its pathogenesis remains uncertain, although it is postulated that protein in the arachnoid villi and granulations alters cerebral venous dynamics or causes partial venous thrombosis, leading to increased ICP. Increased ICP, often associated with papilledema, occurs more often in patients with **chronic inflammatory demyelinating polyneuropathy (CIDP)** than in patients with acute GBS. It seems to be caused in most cases by the markedly increased protein concentration that is one of the laboratory hallmarks of the disease; however, patients with CIDP can develop papilledema even with only a mildly increased concentration of protein in the CSF.

The **POEMS syndrome** is an unusual multisystem disorder that is characterized by polyneuropathy (*P*), organomegaly (*O*), endocrinopathy (*E*), monoclonal gammopathy (*M*), and skin changes (*S*). Patients with POEMS syndrome not infrequently develop ICP associated with papilledema. In addition, optic disc swelling may occasionally occur in patients without evidence of increased ICP. The POEMS syndrome may be a variant of multiple myeloma, and the associated monoclonal immunoglobulin may mediate the multiple systemic manifestations. Patients with multiple myeloma can also develop increased ICP and papilledema, but the mechanism is unknown.

PSEUDOTUMOR CEREBRI AND IDIOPATHIC INTRACRANIAL HYPERTENSION

Definition

Pseudotumor cerebri (PTC), also called benign intracranial hypertension, is the term used for a syndrome that is defined by four criteria: (1) increased ICP, (2) normal or small ventricles by neuroimaging, (3) no evidence of an intracranial mass lesion, and (4) normal CSF composition. Most, but not all patients have papilledema. About 10% of cases of PTC are caused by an identifiable process (see below). In the remaining 90% of cases, no cause is found, although most of these patients are obese young women, suggesting an endocrinologic disturbance. In such cases, the terms "idiopathic pseudotumor cerebri" or "idiopathic intracranial hypertension" (IIH) are appropriate.

Epidemiology

The overall incidence of PTC is unknown and the incidence of IIH varies throughout the world. It approaches zero in countries in which the incidence of obesity, a significant factor in the condition, is low, and it is common in countries or regions within countries with an increased incidence of obesity. In Iowa, the incidence is 0.9 per 100,000 in the general population; 3.5 per 100,000 in women aged 20 to 44 years; 13 per 100,000 in women who are 10% over ideal weight; and 19 per 100,000 in women who are 20% over ideal weight. There is a similar incidence in Louisiana. The incidence of IIH in Rochester, Minnesota, is 1 per 100,000 in the general population; 1.6 in the female population; and 7.9 per 100,000 in obese women (defined as body mass index greater than 26). The annual incidence of IIH in Benghazi, Libya, is 2.2 per 100,000 in the general population; 4.3 per 100,000 in women; and 21.4 per 100,000 in women aged 15 to 44 years who are 20% over ideal weight.

The age range in patients with PTC in general and IIH in particular is broad. Children and even infants are not infrequently affected, and such patients may have a higher incidence of permanent visual loss. The peak incidence of the disease, however, seems to occur in the third decade of life, with a female preponderance that ranges from 2 to 1 in some studies to 8 to 1 in others.

The occurrence of IIH in family members is uncommon but well recognized. No common metabolic or endocrinologic abnormalities have been found in such patients.

Clinical Manifestations

The most common presenting symptom in patients with PTC is headache, occurring in more than 90% of cases. The headache is usually generalized, worse in the morning, and aggravated when cerebral venous pressure is increased by some type of Valsalva maneuver (coughing, sneezing, etc.). Other common nonvisual manifestations of PTC include nausea, vomiting, dizziness, and pulsatile tinnitus. Focal neurologic deficits in patients with PTC are extremely uncommon, and their occurrence should make one consider alternative diagnoses. Patients with chronic PTC may occasionally develop persistent disturbances in cognition and depression.

Visual manifestations of PTC are usually preceded by headache and occur in 35 to 70% of patients. These symptoms are identical with those described by patients with increased ICP from other causes, including:

- Transient visual obscurations
- Loss of vision from macular hemorrhages, exudates, pigment epithelial changes, retina striae, choroidal folds, subretinal neovascularization, or optic atrophy.
- Horizontal diplopia from unilateral or bilateral abducens nerve paresis.
- Rarely, vertical or oblique diplopia from trochlear nerve paresis, oculomotor nerve paresis, or skew deviation.

The papilledema that occurs in over 90% of patients with PTC is identical with that which occurs in patients with other causes of increased ICP. There is no correlation between severity of optic disc swelling and age, race, or body weight in patients with PTC, although men may have worse swelling than women. Postpapilledema optic atrophy occurs in untreated or inadequately treated patients after a variable period of time, usually over several months, but occasionally within weeks of the onset of symptoms. Some patients have persistent chronic papilledema without development of atrophy. Postpapilledema optic atrophy in patients with PTC usually develops symmetrically; but just as papilledema may be asymmetric, so postpapilledema optic atrophy can be asymmetric, and some patients develop a pseudo-Foster Kennedy syndrome characterized by postpapilledema optic atrophy on one side and papilledema on the other.

Etiology

IIH, which, as noted above, accounts for 90% of cases of PTC, occurs primarily in young obese women, and occasionally men, with no evidence of any underlying disease. In about 10% of patients, particularly in men and nonobese women, PTC develops in a number of different settings, including obstruction or impairment of cerebral venous drainage (see above), endocrine and metabolic dysfunction, exposure to exogenous drugs and other substances, withdrawal of certain drugs, and systemic illnesses. Tables 5.2 through 5.5 list some of these purported associations. Except for those cases in which venous occlusive disease can be demonstrated, the exact mechanisms of increased ICP in these settings remain undetermined and a definite causal association unproven.

As noted above, uncompensated **obstruction of cerebral venous drainage** may cause PTC. Such patients may be thought to have IIH unless the cerebral veins and venous sinuses are imaged using standard MRI, MR angiography, or CT angiography (see Table 5.2). Patients with **endocrine and metabolic dysfunction** can also develop PTC (Table 5.3). Obesity is the most common finding in patients with IIH, and recent weight gain has been associated with worsening of vision in such patients. In many of these patients, there is also a history of menstrual irregularity. However, attempts to uncover specific underlying endocrinologic disturbances in patients

with this form of PTC have been unsuccessful. PTC not infrequently occurs during **pregnancy.**

Patients who are exposed to, or ingest, a variety of **exogenous substances** can develop PTC (Table 5.4). For some of these substances, a causative relationship is supported by only a single case report and is tenuous at best. For example, some authors report that PTC can develop in patients taking **oral contraceptives** or estrogen replacement after hysterectomy; however, a precise causal relationship between drug intake and increased ICP has not yet been established.

For other drugs, the association between exposure or ingestion and the development of increased ICP is well documented in numerous reports and investigations. For example, chronic functional suppression of the adrenal cortex with systemic **corticosteroid** therapy can cause PTC, especially in children. Within days or weeks after a change in the dosage or type of steroid, and sometimes associated with an intercurrent infection, the patients complain of headache, often accompanied by nausea and vomiting, less

Table 5.3

Endocrine and Metabolic Disturbances Associated with Pseudotumor Cerebri

Addison's disease	Menarche
Hypoparathyroidism	Menopause
• Primary	Obesity (idiopathic)
• Secondary	Pregnancy
Hyperthyroidism	Turner's syndrome
Hypothyroidism	

Table 5.4

Exogenous Substances Whose Exposure or Ingestion Is Associated with Pseudotumor Cerebri

Amiodarone	Growth hormone
Antibiotics	Indomethecin
• Nalidixic acid	Ketoprofen
• Penicillin	Lead
• Tetracyclines	Leuprolide acetate (Lupron)
Carbidopa/Levodopa	Levonorgestrel implants
(Sinemet)	(Norplant)
Chlordecone (Kepone)	Lithium carbonate
Corticosteroids	Oral contraceptives
• Systemic	Oxytocin (intranasal)
• Topical	Perhexiline maleate
Cyclosporine	Phenytoin
Danazol	Vitamin A

commonly by diplopia, and occasionally drowsiness or stupor.

Several **antibiotics** are associated with the development of PTC (see Table 5.4). The most well known of these drugs are the tetracyclines. These antibiotics can produce the syndrome in infants, children, and both younger and older adults. The mechanism of the reaction is obscure. There is no correlation between the onset of the syndrome and either the dosage of the drug or the length of therapy. Cessation of tetracycline administration causes prompt regression of symptoms.

Daily ingestion of 100,000 or more units of **vitamin A** may, within a few months, produce PTC. Patients may ingest the vitamin itself, or excessive amounts of calf, bear, chicken, or shark liver. Some of these patients exhibit other manifestations of hypervitaminosis A, including fissuring of the angles of the lips, loss of hair, migratory bone pain, hypomenorrhea, hepatosplenomegaly, and dryness, roughness, and desquamation of the skin. Reduction of the excessive vitamin intake is associated with resolution of all symptoms and signs, although resolution of disc swelling may take 4 to 6 months.

Severe cerebral edema with increased ICP occurs with **lead encephalopathy**. Although the incidence of lead intoxication is fairly low, it remains a serious health hazard in children. In over 80% of cases, there is a history of pica.

PTC can also occur after **withdrawal** or **deficiency** of certain substances, especially withdrawal of steroids following chronic use. A deficiency of vitamin A can also cause raised ICP. A deficiency of vitamin D produces nutritional rickets and can be associated with PTC in infants and young children.

We have already commented on increased ICP with papilledema in patients with meningitis and encephalitis. In many of these cases, the ventricular system is blocked in some location and is thus dilated, and the CSF contains white blood cells or an elevated protein content. Such cases are not, by definition, examples of PTC. In other cases, such as meningeal carcinomatosis and lymphomatosis, Whipple's disease, neuroborreliosis, and neurosarcoidosis, the ventricular system appears normal, although the CSF contains white blood cells, malignant cells, an increased protein content, or a combination of these. These cases also are not examples of PTC because the CSF content is abnormal. Nevertheless, some

Table 5.5
Systemic Illnesses Associated with Pseudotumor Cerebri

Anemia
Chronic respiratory insufficiency
• Pickwickian syndrome
• Obstructive sleep apnea
Familial Mediterranean fever
Hypertension
Multiple sclerosis
Polyangiitis overlap syndrome
Psittacosis
Renal Disease
Reye's syndrome
Sarcoidosis
Systemic lupus erythematosus
Thrombocytopenic purpura

systemic diseases produce increased ICP, papilledema, normal-sized ventricles, and normal CSF content—a clinical picture consistent with PTC (Table 5.5).

Papilledema is a rare finding in patients with microcytic or iron deficiency **anemia.** The mechanism of increased ICP in these patients is not known, but the syndrome responds to correction of the underlying disorder.

Chronic respiratory insufficiency may be associated with increased ICP and papilledema. Affected patients have chronic hypercapnia, with retention of carbon dioxide (CO_2), reduced blood oxygen (O_2) levels, polycythemia, increased venous pressure, and increased ICP. Respiratory acidosis causes an accumulation of CO_2 in brain tissue, which, in turn, causes dilation of cerebral capillaries and increases intracranial blood volume. In most cases of increased ICP related to pulmonary insufficiency, the pulmonary dysfunction is caused by primary pulmonary disease. In other patients, respiratory insufficiency is caused by a systemic myopathy, such as muscular dystrophy. In still others, hypoventilation from extreme obesity causes a typical cardiopulmonary syndrome—the Pickwickian syndrome. The obesity causes diminished vital capacity, polycythemia, and cyanosis. Severe drowsiness is common, and many patients have obstructive sleep apnea. The neurologic manifestations of respiratory failure include somnolence, asterixis, other movement disorders, and in severe cases, coma. Supportive respiratory therapy and prompt treatment of the acute physiologic, metabolic, and electrolyte abnormalities can significantly prolong survival and improve the quality of survival time.

Optic disc swelling occurs in some patients with severe **hypertension.** Some of these patients have neurologic symptoms of an encephalopathy; others do not. Among the patients with evidence of an encephalopathy, almost all have increased ICP caused by cerebral edema. In addition, some patients without symptoms of encephalopathy nevertheless have evidence of cerebral edema by neuroimaging and increased ICP on lumbar puncture. In patients with optic disc swelling associated with normal ICP, the swelling may be caused by breakdown of the blood-retinal barrier, or it may represent hypertensive retinopathy or an anterior ischemic optic neuropathy.

The incidence of PTC associated with **renal insufficiency** is probably low, and the cause is probably multifactorial. Some patients are obese, an important association with IIH. Fluid overload and increased cerebral blood flow may play a role in the development of raised ICP in others. Hypervitaminosis A, a condition associated with elevated ICP, occurs in some patients with renal failure. Vitamin A, in the form of retinol, is carried in the serum by retinol-binding protein. This protein is normally excreted by the kidney; however, in the setting of renal failure, the protein is not excreted, and the concentration of the protein in the serum rises, as do the concentrations of both bound and unbound vitamin A. Although bound retinol is nontoxic, unbound retinyl esters cause hypervitaminosis A.

Papilledema that occurs in **sarcoidosis** is usually associated with evidence of an aseptic meningitis. Occasionally, however, sarcoidosis is associated with true PTC; that is, there is no evidence of a mass lesion, the ventricles are normal in size, the ICP is elevated, and the CSF contains no cells and has a normal concentration of glucose and protein. Some of these cases may be caused by dural venous sinus thrombosis. In other cases, the etiology is unclear. Papilledema associated with sarcoidosis often responds to treatment with systemic corticosteroids.

PTC can occur in patients with **systemic lupus erythematosus.** In some of these cases, the pathogenesis is occlusion of one of the dural venous sinuses, usually the superior sagittal sinus. In other cases, the pathogenesis is unclear. Because the condition usually resolves when the

patients are treated with systemic corticosteroids, it is possible that inflammation and tissue necrosis in the region of the arachnoid villi interferes with CSF absorption, thereby raising ICP.

Course

In the 10% of patients with PTC in which an underlying cause can be found and treated, the PTC generally resolves. IIH may, in some cases, be a self-limited condition, but in most cases, the ICP remains elevated for many years, even if systemic and visual symptoms resolve. In one study, 57 patients with a diagnosis of IIH were followed for 5 to 41 years. Severe visual impairment occurred in one or both eyes in 14 patients (26%). In seven patients, the visual loss occurred *months to years* after initial symptoms appeared. In over 80% of the patients in this study, CSF pressure remained elevated, regardless of the treatment the patients had received.

The effects of even self-limited IIH on the visual system may be catastrophic. Studies have shown that up to 50% of patients with IIH have visual field or visual acuity deficits, with severe, legally blinding deficits in up to 26%. Some authors believe that children with IIH are even more likely than adults to develop permanent visual loss despite early therapy, emphasizing the importance of close ophthalmic surveillance.

Patients with chronic PTC may develop a secondary empty sella syndrome, characterized by extension of the subarachnoid space into the sella turcica. It seems likely that in these patients, the empty sella is produced by chronically elevated ICP in a setting of an incompetent diaphragma sella, a not uncommon finding.

Pathophysiology

The etiology of increased ICP in some patients with the clinical features of PTC is clear (e.g., in patients with obstruction of the cerebral venous sinuses or in patients with hypervitaminosis A). In most patients, however, the pathogenesis of increased ICP is unknown or controversial. Evidence exists to suggest both diminished absorption of CSF and cerebral edema. Indeed, patients with IIH may have both a defect in CSF resorption and an increased cerebral volume associated with a noncompliant ventricular system that resists dilation. A number of patients with IIH may have partial venous outflow obstruction that produces increased intracranial venous pressure that, in turn, leads to reduction of CSF absorption. What causes this obstruction, however, remains unclear.

Diagnosis

The diagnosis of PTC, as noted above, is based on three crucial findings.

1. The patient must have normal or small ventricles and no intracranial mass lesion or other intracranial abnormalities.
2. The ICP must be increased.
3. The CSF must have no cells and a normal protein and glucose concentration.

It is inappropriate to diagnose PTC in a patient with a "slightly elevated" concentration of protein or a pleocytosis in the CSF.

To satisfy the criteria required to diagnose PTC, a patient *must* undergo some type of neuroimaging study followed by a lumbar puncture. CT scanning is probably adequate to detect any intracranial mass lesion that could produce increased ICP and to determine the size of the ventricles, but it is not as sensitive as MRI in detecting cerebral venous thrombosis or in detecting an enlarged elongated subarachnoid space around the optic nerve. We thus prefer to obtain MRI initially, whenever possible.

Lumbar puncture should be performed in the lateral decubitus position. The opening pressure should be measured with a manometer, and adequate CSF should be obtained for assessment of cellular content, concentrations of protein and glucose, and any other tests deemed appropriate by the treating physician. We find that the easiest method of performing a lumbar puncture in obese patients is with fluoroscopic guidance.

Most patients with PTC have ICPs greater than 250 mm of H_2O (25 cm of H_2O); however, rare patients with an otherwise typical clinical picture of PTC have normal pressures on multiple occasions and improve when the pressure is lowered by medicine or surgery. This phenomenon appears to be the neurologic counterpart of so-called low-tension glaucoma.

Making a diagnosis of PTC without both neuroimaging studies and lumbar puncture is inappropriate and dangerous, even if the clinical setting appears straightforward. We have examined several obese patients in whom a tentative diagnosis of idiopathic PTC (i.e., IIH) was made after they developed headaches and papilledema and were found to have normal results on neuroimaging studies but in whom the increased ICP was found to have been caused by septic or aseptic meningitis, by cerebral gliomatosis, or by leptomeningeal carcinomatosis, lymphomatosis, or gliomatosis. We also have even seen obese patients with brain tumors in whom an initial diagnosis of IIH was made on the basis of headaches and papilledema alone, *without the patient having had either neuroimaging or lumbar puncture.*

Once a diagnosis of PTC is made by CT scanning or MRI followed by lumbar puncture, the physician should attempt to determine if a cause can be found. This is particularly important in nonobese women and in men, regardless of age or body habitus, because such patients are much less likely to have IIH. A particularly careful history is necessary in such patients, with special attention given to any underlying systemic inflammatory or infectious disease, or ingestion or exposure to an inciting agent. We also believe that nonobese men and women with presumed IIH should undergo an assessment of the cerebral venous system. Such an assessment can be performed with standard MRI, MR angiography, CT angiography, or conventional angiography.

Most patients with PTC have papilledema but, as noted above, some do not. In obese young women with headaches, pulsatile tinnitus, and normal CT scans or MRI, it is imperative that a lumbar puncture be performed before making a diagnosis of "pseudotumor cerebri sine papilledema."

MONITORING

Patients with papilledema most often develop progressive loss of visual function in a manner similar to that which occurs in chronic open-angle glaucoma. Loss of central vision is usually a late phenomenon, whereas visual field defects (usually arcuate scotomas and nasal steps) are an early finding and defects in color vision can occur at any stage. Patients with papilledema, regardless of the cause of the increased ICP, should be followed at regular intervals to detect the earliest evidence of an optic neuropathy, because most visual defects associated with papilledema are reversible if ICP is lowered before there is severe visual loss, chronic papilledema, or optic atrophy.

Such patients should undergo testing of best-corrected visual acuity at distance and near, color vision testing using pseudoisochromatic plates or a similar method, visual field testing using kinetic perimetry for the peripheral field and automated static perimetry for the central field, and ophthalmoscopic examination of the optic discs.

Although all patients with papilledema should be tested to determine if there is a relative afferent pupillary defect, papilledema tends to be a bilateral symmetric condition (see above). Thus, when a relative afferent pupillary defect is present in a patient with papilledema, it generally indicates damage to the retina or optic nerve of the eye with the defect. However, the absence of a relative afferent pupillary defect cannot be taken as evidence that there is no optic nerve damage from increased ICP.

In addition to standard clinical testing, stereo color photographs of the optic discs should be obtained on a regular basis on any patient with papilledema to provide the examiner with objective evidence of the appearance of the optic discs. Other tests of visual sensory function—such as contrast sensitivity testing, motion perimetry, or visual-evoked potentials—are not routinely performed, but these tests may be useful in individual patients in whom issues of management develop.

The intervals between clinical assessments of patients with papilledema must be individualized. We examine some patients every 1 to 2 weeks until we have a sense of the progression or stability of their condition. Other patients are examined every 1 to 3 months, and patients with stable papilledema may only be examined every 4 to 12 months.

Patients with papilledema should be monitored not only with respect to their clinical manifestations but also with respect to their increased ICP. In some patients, simple assessment of the optic discs is sufficient; in others, ultrasonography can be used to assess the diameter of the retrobulbar optic nerves as a measure of ICP. Although ICP can be measured directly by performing a lumbar puncture, this is potentially dangerous in patients with an intracranial mass. Performing a lumbar puncture on patients with IIH may be difficult when the patient is obese, but it usually is straightforward when the procedure is performed under fluoroscopy.

TREATMENT

If increased ICP is directly related to a mass lesion, or if a lesion is blocking either the ven-

tricular system or venous outflow, removal of the lesion is the obvious treatment of choice. If the lesion cannot be removed, or treated in some other fashion (e.g., radiosurgery) or if the CSF absorption is reduced at the level of the arachnoid villi, treatment is directed toward shunting of CSF into the atrial or peritoneal cavities. If there is cerebral edema, then osmotic agents, diuretics, or corticosteroids may reduce swelling, particularly in the acute period.

The treatment of PTC depends on whether or not an underlying cause can be identified and treated. If so, treatment of the causative process should result in normalization of ICP and resolution of papilledema. On the other hand, if no etiology can be identified—that is, if the patient has IIH—then treatment is directed at lowering ICP.

There are generally only two reasons to treat patients with IIH: severe intractable headache and evidence of optic neuropathy. Methods of treatment include weight loss, medical therapy, serial lumbar punctures, and surgery. No single procedure is completely effective in this regard.

The optimum treatment for obese patients is **weight loss.** When possible, the weight loss should be achieved through a combination of diet and exercise prescribed by a registered dietitian or nutritionist. When weight loss is achieved in this fashion, the patient's symptoms and signs almost always resolve. When this method fails, as it often does, or the patient is morbidly obese, then gastric bypass surgery can be performed. Although it has significant potential complications, including anastomotic leaks, small bowel obstruction, and gastrointestinal bleeding, such surgery is generally followed by reduction in weight, normalization of ICP, and resolution of papilledema.

Patients with PTC in the setting of morbid obesity (i.e., the Pickwickian syndrome) and who have sleep apnea may respond not only to weight loss but also to low-flow oxygen and positive airway ventilation using either continuous positive airway pressure (CPAP) or bilevel positive airway pressure (bi-PAP).

Although weight loss is, in our opinion, the optimum way to treat IIH, it is often difficult to achieve. Indeed, we find that even though patients understand the need to lose weight and the consequences of not doing so, they simply cannot lose weight or, if they do, they subsequently gain it back. Thus, other methods of treatment need to be considered.

A number of **drugs** can be used to lower ICP. By far the most effective is acetazolamide (Diamox). This drug decreases production of CSF by inhibition of carbonic anhydrase, resulting in decreased sodium ion transport across the choroidal epithelium. Acetazolamide should be started at a dose of 1 gram per day, given in divided doses of either 250 mg 4 times a day or 500 mg sequels 2 times a day. Theoretically, the dose can be increased up to a maximum of 4 grams per day, but most patients cannot tolerate dosages over about 2 grams per day because of the side effects, which include paresthesias of the extremities, lethargy, decreased libido, and a metallic or dry taste in the mouth. These side effects can be reduced but not eliminated by using sequels.

Patients who cannot tolerate or do not respond to acetazolamide may be treated with an alternative carbonic anhydrase inhibitor, such as methazolamide (Neptazane), but we have not been impressed with the efficacy of this drug in such patients. Similarly, most dehydrating drugs, such as furosemide, are not particularly efficacious in lowering ICP in patients with IIH, although it may be appropriate to try them before pursuing surgical alternatives. Although systemic corticosteroids are clearly beneficial in the treatment of raised intracranial pressure associated with various systemic inflammatory disorders such as sarcoidosis and systemic lupus erythematosus, they are not generally recommended for use in patients with IIH and may actually compound the problem by inducing weight gain or preventing weight loss.

Multiple **lumbar punctures** are advocated as a nonmedical, nonsurgical method of relieving the increased ICP of IIH. The theory behind this treatment is that the needle used for the lumbar puncture creates an opening in the dura through which CSF leaks. With several lumbar punctures, one creates a ''sieve'' that allows sufficient egress of CSF that ICP is normalized. The procedure can be painful, and most patients (and their doctors) find multiple lumbar punctures intolerable as a chronic treatment plan. Nevertheless, by performing the lumbar punctures under fluoroscopy, the discomfort can be minimized, and we have encountered several patients who have preferred this form of management rather than medical or surgical therapy.

Surgical decompression procedures are generally used for patients with PTC only when patients initially present with severe optic neuropathy or when other forms of treatment have failed, and the patients are incapacitated by headache or have begun to develop evidence of progressive optic neuropathy. Subtemporal decompression was advocated in the past, but most neurosurgeons favor some form of shunting procedure. Ventriculoperitoneal shunting is quite effective in lowering ICP in patients with PTC, but this procedure can be difficult unless some type of stereotactic method is used, because the ventricles in such patients are normal in size rather than being enlarged. Thus, the preferred technique is the lumboperitoneal shunt, in which a silicone tube is placed percutaneously between the lumbar subarachnoid space and the peritoneal cavity. Complications of the shunt procedure are minimal and usually benign but include spontaneous obstruction of the shunt, usually at the peritoneal end, excessive low pressure, infection, radiculopathy, and migration of the tube, resulting in abdominal pain. Some patients also develop a Chiari malformation that may or may not be symptomatic. At least one shunt revision is necessary in over 50% of patients. Nevertheless, most patients treated with a lumboperitoneal shunt experience rapid return of ICP to normal and resolution of papilledema, often with improvement in visual function.

In the procedure known as optic nerve sheath fenestration (ONSF), a window or multiple slits are made in the dural sheath of the optic nerve immediately behind the globe. A successful ONSF results in resolution of papilledema on that side—and occasionally on the other—with improvement in visual function in many cases. Most surgeons prefer a medial approach, but some advocate a lateral approach. Regardless of the technique used, the procedure immediately reduces pressure on the nerve by creating a filtration apparatus that controls the intravaginal pressure surrounding the orbital segment of the optic nerve; however, it does not consistently reduce ICP and therefore does not treat the underlying condition. It is probably for this reason that over 80% of patients with IIH develop recurrent papilledema within 6 years of the procedure.

The risks of ONSF, although low, are nevertheless significant. They include hemorrhage, diplopia, infection, and loss of vision from vascular occlusion. Because of these potential complications, the low permanent success rate of the procedure, and the difficulty in performing repeat ONSF on patients in whom the initial procedure has failed, we favor lumboperitoneal shunt as the surgical treatment of choice in most patients with IIH who fail or cannot tolerate medical therapy. Nevertheless, long-term benefit from ONSF does occur, and the procedure may be appropriate for patients with IIH who refuse, cannot undergo, or do not respond to lumboperitoneal shunting. It may also be the treatment of choice for patients with severe papilledema caused by a malignant brain tumor in whom a long-term solution is not required, and for patients with IIH and severe visual loss on presentation in whom immediate decompression of the optic nerve is mandatory. These latter patients may benefit from a combined lumboperitoneal shunt and optic nerve sheath fenestration.

Women who develop IIH during pregnancy can be treated in much the same way as nonpregnant women except that caloric restriction and the use of diuretics are contraindicated. Lumboperitoneal shunting can be performed with little or no maternal or fetal risk, and this treatment should not be withheld simply because the patient is pregnant.

FOR MORE INFORMATION:
See Walsh & Hoyt's *Clinical Neuro-Ophthalmology,* 5th edition, Volume 1, Chapter 10.

Optic Neuritis

Optic neuritis is a term used to refer to inflammation of the optic nerve. When it is associated with a swollen optic disc, it is called *papillitis* or *anterior optic neuritis.* When the optic disc appears normal, the terms *retrobulbar optic neuritis* or *retrobulbar neuritis* are used. In the absence of signs of multiple sclerosis (MS) or other systemic disease, the optic neuritis is referred to as isolated, monosymptomatic, or idiopathic. The pathogenesis of isolated optic neuritis is presumed to be demyelination of the optic nerve, similar to that seen in MS. It is likely that most cases of isolated acute optic neuritis are a forme fruste of MS.

Optic neuritis does not always present as acute loss of vision. It may develop as insidious progressive or nonprogressive visual dysfunction, and it may even be asymptomatic. Patients with asymptomatic optic neuritis have laboratory evidence of optic nerve dysfunction and may also have subtle clinical evidence of optic nerve damage if appropriate studies are performed.

Optic neuritis can be caused by disorders other than MS and related demyelinating diseases. In addition, two variants of optic neuritis occasionally occur. *Neuroretinitis* is a term used to describe inflammatory involvement of both the intraocular optic nerve and the peripapillary retina. *Optic perineuritis,* also called "perioptic neuritis," describes inflammatory involvement of the optic nerve sheaths, without inflammation of the nerve itself.

IDIOPATHIC DEMYELINATING OPTIC NEURITIS

Optic neuritis usually is a primary demyelinating process. It almost always occurs as an isolated phenomenon or in patients with MS. Patients in whom optic neuritis occurs as an isolated phenomenon have a higher risk of the subsequent development of MS than the normal population. There are three forms of primary demyelinating optic neuritis: acute, chronic, and subclinical.

ACUTE IDIOPATHIC DEMYELINATING OPTIC NEURITIS

Acute demyelinating optic neuritis is by far the most common type of optic neuritis that occurs throughout the world and is the most frequent cause of optic nerve dysfunction in the young adult population. Much of our knowledge regarding this form of optic neuritis was obtained from an ongoing study begun in 1988 called the Optic Neuritis Treatment Trial (ONTT). The ONTT was a multicenter controlled clinical trial funded by the National Eye Institute of the National Institutes of Health in the United States. The investigators in this trial enrolled 455 patients with acute unilateral optic neuritis. Although the primary objective of the trial was the assessment of the efficacy of corticosteroids in the treatment of optic neuritis, the trial also provided invaluable information about the clinical profile of optic neuritis, its natural history, and its relationship to MS.

When evaluating the data from the ONTT, it should be noted that the entry criteria in the trial included a clinical syndrome consistent with unilateral optic neuritis (including a relative afferent pupillary defect and a visual field defect in the affected eye), visual symptoms of 8 days or less, no previous episodes of optic neuritis in the affected eye, no previous corticosteroid treatment for optic neuritis or MS, and no evidence of a systemic disease other than MS as a cause for the optic neuritis.

Demographics

The annual incidence of acute optic neuritis is estimated in population-based studies to be between 1 and 5 per 100,000. In Olmstead County, Minnesota, where the Mayo Clinic is located, the incidence rate is estimated to be 5.1 per 100,000 person-years and the prevalence rate 115 per 100,000.

The majority of patients with acute optic neuritis are between the ages of 20 and 50 years, with a mean age of 30 to 35 years. Nevertheless, optic neuritis can occur at any age. We have encountered it in children in the first and second decades of life and in adults in their sixth and seventh decades. Females are affected more commonly than males by a ratio of approximately 3:1.

Symptoms

The two major symptoms in patients with acute optic neuritis are loss of central vision and pain in and around the affected eye. Loss of central visual acuity is reported by over 90% of patients. Vision loss is typically abrupt, occurring over several hours to several days. Progression over a longer period of time can occur but should make the clinician suspicious of an alternative disorder. The degree of visual loss varies widely from minimal reduction to complete blindness with no perception of light. The majority of patients describe diffuse blurred vision, although some recognize that the blurring is predominantly central. Occasionally, patients complain of a loss of a portion of peripheral field,

such as the inferior or superior region, often to one side. The visual loss is monocular in most cases, but in a small percentage, particularly in children, both eyes are simultaneously affected.

Pain in or around the eye is present in more than 90% of patients with acute optic neuritis. It is usually mild, but it may be extremely severe and may even be more debilitating to the patient than the loss of vision. It may precede or occur concurrently with visual loss, usually is exacerbated by eye movement, and generally lasts no more than a few days. The presence of pain is a helpful differentiating feature from anterior ischemic optic neuropathy, particularly when it is severe and when it occurs or worsens during movement of the eyes, features uncommon in the 10 to 12% of ischemic optic neuropathy patients with pain (see Chapter 7).

Up to 30% of patients with optic neuritis experience positive visual phenomena, called *photopsias,* both at the onset of their visual symptoms and during the course of the disorder. These phenomena are spontaneous flashing black squares, flashes of light, or showers of sparks, sometimes precipitated by eye movement or certain sounds.

Signs

Examination of a patient with acute optic neuritis reveals evidence of optic nerve dysfunction. Visual acuity is reduced in most cases, but varies from a mild reduction to no light perception. Contrast sensitivity and color vision are impaired in almost all cases. The reduction in contrast sensitivity often parallels the reduction in visual acuity, although in some cases, it is much worse. The reduction in color vision is often much worse than would be expected from the level of visual acuity. Standard color vision testing with the Ishihara or Hardy-Rand-Rittler pseudoisochromatic plates commonly reveals abnormalities in the affected eye, whereas the more sensitive Farnsworth-Munsell 100-Hues test can reveal more subtle defects. Even when the patient can detect all the pseudoisochromatic figures correctly, careful comparison of the appearance of a single plate by each eye may reveal a striking difference in color and brightness between the two eyes.

Visual field loss can vary from mild to severe, may be diffuse or focal, and can involve the central or peripheral field. Indeed, almost any type

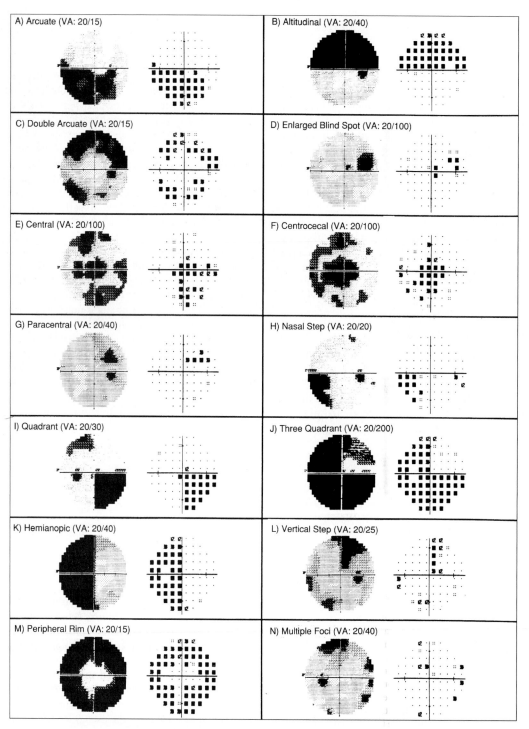

Figure 6.1. Visual field defects in acute optic neuritis. Fourteen types of localized monocular visual field defects that may occur in acute optic neuritis, as defined by static perimetry as performed with a Humphrey automated perimeter using a 30–2 program incorporating the full-threshold test strategy, a 31.5-apostilb background, and size III targets for the test and blind spot checks. The foveal threshold and fluctuation tests were turned on. Note that central, cecocentral, arcuate, altitudinal, quadrantic, and even hemianopic defects may develop. *VA:* visual acuity. (Reprinted with permission from Keltner JL, Johnson CA, Spurr JO, et al. Baseline visual field profile of optic neuritis: the experience of the Optic Neuritis Treatment Trial. Arch Ophthalmol 1993; 111:231–234.)

of field defect can occur in an eye with optic neuritis. Among 415 patients in the ONTT with baseline visual acuity of hand motions or better, automated perimetry of the central 30° of visual field revealed diffuse visual field loss in 48% of patients and focal loss in 52%. Focal nerve fiber bundle type defects (altitudinal, arcuate, and nasal step) were present in 20% of patients; pure central or centrocecal defects in 8%; and hemianopic defects in 5% (Fig. 6.1).

A relative afferent pupillary defect is demonstrable with the swinging flashlight test in all unilateral cases of optic neuritis. When such a defect is not present, either there is a coexisting optic neuropathy in the fellow eye (e.g., from previous or concurrent asymptomatic optic neuritis) or the visual loss in the affected eye is not caused by optic neuritis or any other form of optic neuropathy. The use of neutral density filters may help uncover a subtle relative afferent pupillary defect.

Patients with optic neuritis also can be shown to have a reduced sensation of brightness in the affected eye, either by simply asking them to compare the brightness of a light shined in one eye and then the other, or by more complex tests using polarized lenses or flickering lights of varying frequencies.

About one-third of patients with acute optic neuritis have some degree of disc swelling (Fig. 6.2). The optic disc may be slightly or markedly blurred. At times, the disc swelling is so severe that it mimics the choked disc seen in patients

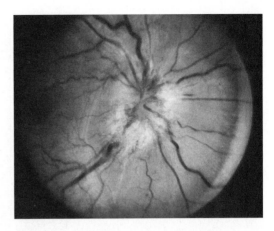

Figure 6.3.   Severe anterior optic neuritis mimicking papilledema. Note hyperemia and elevation of the disc and several peripapillary retinal hemorrhages.

with papilledema (Fig. 6.3). The degree of disc swelling does not correlate with the severity of either visual acuity or visual field loss. Disc or peripapillary hemorrhages and segmental disc swelling are less common in eyes with acute optic neuritis than in eyes with anterior ischemic optic neuropathy.

Slit lamp biomicroscopy in eyes with demyelinating optic neuritis is almost always normal. In some patients with anterior optic neuritis, vitreous cells may be observed, particularly in the vitreous overlying the optic disc. Sheathing of retinal veins may also occur, especially in patients with MS. Indeed, patients with acute optic neuritis and uveitis or retinal phlebitis have an increased risk of developing MS than patients with isolated optic neuritis. When the cellular reaction is extensive, etiologies other than demyelination should be considered, including sarcoidosis, syphilis, cat-scratch disease, and Lyme disease (see below).

The majority of patients with idiopathic acute optic neuritis have a normal optic disc in the affected eye (''the doctor sees nothing when the patient sees nothing''), unless they have had a previous attack of acute or asymptomatic optic neuritis or have ongoing chronic optic neuritis. Over approximately 4 to 6 weeks, the optic disc becomes pale, even as the visual acuity and other parameters of vision improve (Fig. 6.4). The pallor may be diffuse or located to a particular portion of the disc, most often the temporal region.

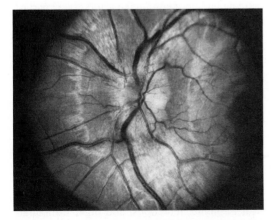

Figure 6.2.   Anterior optic neuritis. There is significant swelling and hyperemia of the disc with dilated surface capillaries.

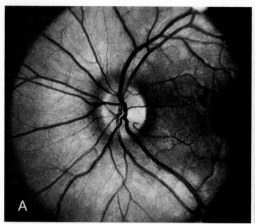
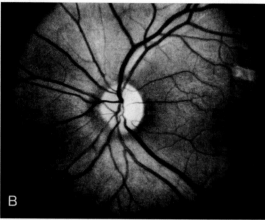

Figure 6.4. Optic atrophy after acute, retrobulbar optic neuritis. *A.* In acute phase, visual acuity in the left eye is 20/300 with a central scotoma, but the optic disc is normal.

B. Three months later, visual acuity has returned to 20/30, but the optic disc is pale, particularly temporally, and there is mild nerve fiber layer atrophy.

Visual Function in the Fellow Eye

In adults, bilateral, clinically simultaneous acute optic neuritis is uncommon, although the relative frequency increases when evaluating populations of patients with established MS. One of the surprising findings in the ONTT was the relatively high percentage of presumably asymptomatic fellow eye deficits at baseline: 14% with visual acuity abnormalities, 22% with color vision abnormalities, and 48% with visual field defects. The majority of the fellow eye deficits resolved over several months, suggesting that such abnormalities may be caused by subclinical but concurrent acute demyelination in the fellow optic nerve. In contrast to adults, acute optic neuritis is often symptomatically bilateral and simultaneous in children. In such cases, the optic neuritis is presumed to be related to infection (see below).

Diagnostic and Prognostic Studies

Studies in patients with presumed acute optic neuritis are usually performed for one of three reasons:

1. To determine if the cause of the optic neuropathy is something other than inflammation, particularly a compressive lesion.
2. To determine if a cause other than demyelination is responsible for inflammation of the optic nerve.

3. To determine the visual and neurologic prognosis of optic neuritis.

With the widespread availability of magnetic resonance imaging (MRI), computed tomographic (CT) scanning has little or no role in the evaluation of patients with presumed optic neuritis. Furthermore, as regards the detection of lesions that compress the optic nerve, although MRI is a sensitive technique, its usefulness in the patient with clinically typical acute optic neuritis is minimal. Indeed, only 2 of 455 patients enrolled in the ONTT had compressive lesions as the cause of their visual loss. If these patients had not been imaged initially as part of the study, it is likely that their lack of visual improvement would have resulted in neuroimaging within several weeks. In the patient with a typical history and findings suggestive of optic neuritis, MRI to rule out a compressive lesion is unwarranted from the standpoint of both clinical yield and cost-effectiveness.

MRI can also detect demyelinating lesions of the optic nerve, manifesting as foci of T2-bright signal, areas of enhancement, and even optic nerve enlargement (Fig. 6.5). Unfortunately, the appearance of these lesions is nonspecific, and a similar appearance can be observed in patients with ischemic, infectious, and other inflammatory optic neuropathies.

Other tests are similarly nonspecific in differentiating acute demyelinating optic neuritis from

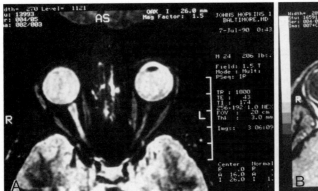

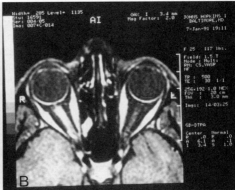

Figure 6.5. Magnetic resonance imaging (MRI) of the optic nerve in acute demyelinating optic neuritis. *A.* Unenhanced proton density-weighted axial MRI in a 24-year-old man with right optic neuritis shows diffuse hyperintensity of the right optic nerve. *B.* T1-weighted axial MRI after intravenous injection of paramagnetic contrast material in a 25-year-old woman with right optic neuritis shows marked thickening and enhancement of the orbital portion of the right optic nerve.

the less common systemic and local infectious and inflammatory optic neuropathies. The vast majority of patients with optic neuritis caused by such disorders can be identified simply by performing a thorough history. In patients without a history of (or consistent with) syphilis, sarcoidosis, cat-scratch disease, Lyme disease, or systemic lupus erythematosus, the likelihood of such a condition being responsible for optic neuritis is low. In the ONTT, antinuclear antibody assay, fluorescent treponemal antibody adsorbent test for syphilis, chest radiograph, and cerebrospinal fluid (CSF) analysis did not yield any unsuspected information. We agree that none of these tests are warranted in a patient with presumed acute optic neuritis unless the history or examination suggest that the patient has an underlying systemic or local infection or inflammation or the patient's course does not follow that of typical optic neuritis (see below).

The most important application of MRI in patients with optic neuritis is the identification of signal abnormalities in the white matter of the brain, usually in the periventricular region, consistent with demyelination (Fig. 6.6). Two or more brain lesions on MRI of patients with isolated optic neuritis are reported in 27 to 64% of patients, depending on the referral population and the timing of the MRI. The presence of multiple lesions on MRI in the periventricular or other white matter in the brain of a patient with presumed acute optic neuritis suggests not only

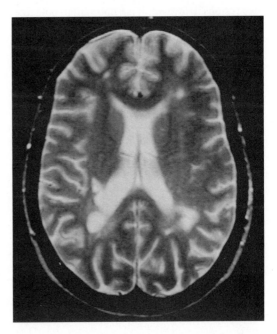

Figure 6.6. Magnetic resonance imaging (MRI) of the brain of a patient with isolated optic neuritis and no previous history of neurologic dysfunction. T2-weighted axial MRI shows multiple ovoid periventricular white-matter lesions in both hemispheres. These lesions are identical with those seen in patients with acute multiple sclerosis.

that the diagnosis of optic neuritis is correct but that the cause of the optic neuritis is demyelination.

The role of various studies in establishing the patient's **neurologic prognosis** is a separate issue. A substantial percentage of patients with isolated optic neuritis develop MS within months to years after the onset of optic neuritis (see below). It would be helpful if there were certain studies that could be performed in a patient with isolated optic neuritis that would allow accurate prediction of the odds of subsequent development of MS.

It is clear that the results of MRI in the patient with isolated acute optic neuritis correlate with the eventual development of MS. Multiple lesions in the periventricular and other white matter on MRI are the most significant risk factor associated with an increased likelihood of developing MS (Fig. 6.7). Among patients with isolated optic neuritis in the ONTT, the cumulative percentage developing MS within 5 years of the onset of the optic neuritis was 16% in patients with normal MRI, 37% in patients with one or two lesions, and 51% in patients with more than two lesions. However, it is important to note that

an abnormal MRI is not completely predictive of, nor is a normal scan completely protective from, the subsequent development of MS. Further follow-up is ongoing to determine if patients who have normal brain MRI at the time of optic neuritis remain at low risk for developing MS.

Immunologic abnormalities in the CSF are common in patients with optic neuritis, occurring in up to 79% of cases. As in patients with MS, CSF pleocytosis, elevated protein concentration, elevated levels of myelin basic protein, increased IgG ratio and IgG synthesis, oligoclonal bands, κ light chains, and increased concentrations of cytokines may be detected. Although the predictive value of these CSF findings for the development of MS is somewhat controversial, there appear to be certain CSF and even serologic risk factors that increase the likelihood that a patient with isolated optic neuritis will eventually develop MS. These include CSF oligoclonal banding and elevated levels of myelin basic protein, CSF and serum elevations of cytokines, and positivity for certain HLA types (see below). However, the robust predictive value of the baseline MRI diminishes the relative usefulness of these other studies in the individual patient

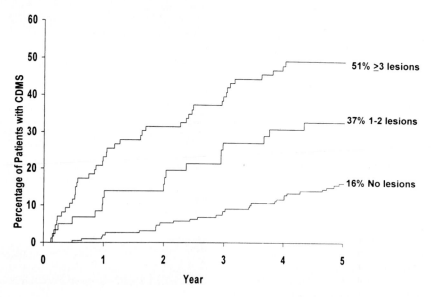

Figure 6.7. Graph showing the 5-year cumulative incidence of development of clinically definite multiple sclerosis (CDMS) correlated with MRI of the brain in patients with acute isolated optic neuritis enrolled in the Optic Neuritis Treatment Trial and Longitudinal Optic Neuritis Study. Note that the risk of developing CDMS increases with increasingly abnormal MRI at the time of the episode of optic neuritis. (Reprinted with permission from Optic Neuritis Study Group. The 5-year risk of MS after optic neuritis: experience of the Optic Neuritis Treatment Trial. Neurology 1997;49: 1404–1413.)

with acute optic neuritis who wishes to have some idea of prognosis for the development of MS.

Visual Prognosis

The natural history of acute demyelinating optic neuritis is to worsen over several days to 2 weeks, and then to improve. The improvement initially is fairly rapid. It then levels off, but further improvement can continue to occur 1 year after the onset of visual symptoms. Among patients in the ONTT who received placebo, visual acuity began to improve within 3 weeks of onset in 79% and within 5 weeks in 93%. For most patients in this study, recovery of visual acuity was nearly complete by 5 weeks after onset (Fig. 6.8). The mean visual acuity 1 year after an attack of otherwise uncomplicated optic neuritis is 20/15, and less than 10% of patients

have permanent visual acuity less than 20/40. Other parameters of visual function, including contrast sensitivity, color perception, and visual field, improve in conjunction with improvement in visual acuity.

The visual improvement that occurs in patients with acute optic neuritis tends to do so regardless of the degree of visual loss, although there is some correlation between the severity of visual loss and the degree of eventual recovery. In the ONTT, of the 167 eyes in which the baseline visual acuity was 20/200 or worse, only 10 (6%) had this level of vision 6 months later. Of 28 patients whose initial visual acuity in the affected eye was light perception or no light perception, 18 (64%) recovered to 20/40 or better. Factors such as age, gender, optic disc appearance, and pattern of the initial visual field defect do not appear to have any appreciable effect on the visual outcome.

Even though the overall prognosis for visual acuity after an attack of acute optic neuritis is extremely good, some patients have persistent severe visual loss after a single episode. Furthermore, even patients with improvement in visual function to "normal" may complain of movement-induced photopsias or transient loss of vision with overheating or exercise (Uhthoff symptom) and may have persistent visual deficits when tested using more sensitive clinical, electrophysiologic, or psychophysical tests. Indeed, following an attack of acute optic neuritis, disturbances of visual acuity (10 to 30%), contrast sensitivity (56 to 100%), color vision (33 to 100%), visual field (32 to 100%), stereopsis (89%), light brightness sense (89 to 100%), pupillary reaction to light (54 to 92%), optic disc appearance (60 to 80%), and the visual-evoked potential (VEP) (63 to 100%) may all persist.

Subjectively, patients with recovered optic neuritis frequently complain that their vision in the affected eye is "not right" or "remains fuzzy," or that colors are "washed out." One cause of these symptoms is probably related to subtle abnormalities in the visual field in which patients experience abnormally rapid disappearance of focal visual stimuli and abnormally rapid fatigue in sensitivity. These patients typically complain that when they look at something, it appears as if they have "holes" in their vision, some of which fill in while other new ones appear: a so-called "Swiss cheese" visual field. This phenomenon is not limited to optic neuritis,

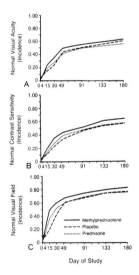

Figure 6.8.   Graphs of speed of visual recovery in patients with acute optic neuritis treated with intravenous high-dose methylprednisolone (1 g/day × 3 days) followed by a 2-week course of oral prednisone (1 mg/kg/day) (*solid line*), compared with patients treated with oral prednisone alone (*dotted line*) and untreated patients given placebo (*dashed line*) in the Optic Neuritis Treatment Trial. Note that improvement in (*A*) visual acuity, (*B*) contrast sensitivity, and (*C*) visual field occur more rapidly in patients treated with the intravenous regimen than in patients given either low-dose oral prednisone or untreated patients. (Reprinted with permission from Beck RW, Cleary PA, Anderson MM Jr, et al. A randomized, controlled trial of corticosteroids in the treatment of acute optic neuritis. N Engl J Med 1992;326:581–588.)

however; it can occur in other optic neuropathies.

Following an episode of optic neuritis, some patients experience transient visual blurring during exercise, during a hot bath or shower, or during emotional stress. This phenomenon, called **Uhthoff symptom,** is most common in patients with other evidence of MS, but it is also experienced by otherwise healthy patients after optic neuritis, by patients with chronic or subclinical optic neuritis, by patients with Leber's hereditary optic neuropathy, and by patients with optic neuropathies from other causes. It occurs in approximately 10% of patients after an attack of demyelinating optic neuritis and, when present, may be a marker for abnormal brain MRI and for the subsequent development of MS. Some patients with Uhthoff symptom note that their visual symptoms improve in colder temperatures or when drinking cold beverages. Two major hypotheses regarding Uhthoff symptom are that (1) elevation of body temperature interferes directly with axon conduction, and (2) exercise or a rise in body temperature changes the metabolic environment of the axon which, in turn, interferes with conduction.

Recurrent attacks of optic neuritis occur in 11 to 24% of patients and may occur in either eye. Recurrences were reported within 5 years in 28% of the patients in the ONTT. Patients who experience one or two recurrent attacks of optic neuritis nevertheless usually experience substantial improvement in vision, often to normal; however, after multiple attacks of optic neuritis, visual function may improve little or not at all.

Neurologic Prognosis

Optic neuritis occurs in about 50% of patients with MS and is the presenting manifestation in about 20%. Available evidence suggests that the pathogenesis of isolated optic neuritis is no different that that of MS in general. In fact, a strong case can be made for optic neuritis being a forme fruste of MS, based on similarities between the two in incidence, CSF findings, histocompatibility data, results of MRI, and family history as well as other features. Both isolated optic neuritis and MS are more common in northern latitudes, among certain racial populations, and in females compared with males. From 27 to 64% of patients with isolated optic neuritis have changes in the brain on MRI that are indistinguishable from the lesions seen in MS. Immuno-

logic changes in the CSF similar to those in MS, such as elevation of CSF IgG and oligoclonal banding, may also occur in up to 79% of patients with optic neuritis. Up to 75% of patients with isolated optic neuritis have abnormalities on somatosensory-evoked potentials, brainstem-evoked potentials, or CSF protein electrophoresis. There is an increased prevalence of MS among family members of patients with optic neuritis, and certain HLA types are more prevalent in both diseases.

Both retrospective and prospective studies have been performed to determine the prognosis for the development of MS in patients who experience an attack of acute optic neuritis. Although retrospective studies provide figures ranging from 11.5 to 85%, most prospective studies support the higher figures. The risk of developing MS is about 30% in patients followed 5 to 7 years after an attack of optic neuritis, and eventually increases to about 75% in women and 34% in men with 15 to 20 years of follow-up. Among 95 incident cases of optic neuritis in Olmstead County, Minnesota, the estimated risk of MS was 39% by 10 years, 49% by 20 years, 54% by 30 years, and 60% by 40 years. The average time interval from an initial attack of optic neuritis until other symptoms and signs of MS develop varies considerably; most studies found that the majority of persons who develop MS after optic neuritis do so within 7 years of the onset of visual symptoms. It therefore seems appropriate to consider most cases of optic neuritis a limited form of MS and to counsel patients appropriately. We believe that most patients should be told about the relationship between optic neuritis and MS and that this conversation should include a frank discussion of MS and its prognosis. It is our experience that most patients appreciate this approach and are able to handle this information much better than most physicians anticipate.

There appear to be certain risk factors that increase the likelihood that a patient with isolated optic neuritis will eventually develop MS. Without question, the most highly predictive baseline factor is multiple lesions in the periventricular white matter on MRI, a phenomenon noted in 27 to 64% of patients with isolated optic neuritis. Among patients with isolated optic neuritis in the ONTT, the cumulative percentage developing MS within 5 years was 16% in patients with normal MRI and 51% in patients with more than two lesions. Other risk factors for the development of MS among ONTT patients were caucasian race, a family history of MS, history of previous ill-defined neurologic complaints, and a previous episode of optic neuritis. However, none of these factors affected the risk of developing MS as much as the results of MRI. Among patients with normal MRI, negative risk factors included male gender, absence of pain, mild visual acuity loss, and optic disc swelling. Although the ONTT did not support any correlation between age of onset and the development of MS, other studies suggest that the younger the age of onset of optic neuritis, the greater the subsequent risk for MS. Winter onset of optic neuritis may also be a risk factor.

Although evidence of immunologic dysfunction (especially oligoclonal banding) in the CSF is common in patients with either optic neuritis or MS, whether or not their presence in patients with clinically isolated optic neuritis increases the risk for the subsequent development of MS remains controversial. Studies indicate that 25 to 50% of patients with isolated acute optic neuritis and abnormal CSF remain free of neurologic manifestations of MS for many years (if not for life), whereas 10 to 50% of patients with optic neuritis and normal CSF nevertheless develop other manifestations of MS during the same period of time. In view of these findings, it seems likely that CSF abnormalities alone are not a primary risk factor in determining whether or not a patient with acute optic neuritis eventually develops clinical evidence of disseminated demyelination. There may be some added value of the detection of CSF abnormalities in conjunction with MRI of the brain, but data from the ONTT suggest that the presence of CSF abnormalities has little predictive value for the development of MS over and above the powerful predictive value of MRI.

There is considerable evidence that genetic factors play a role in the development of MS. This is based on the familial incidence of the disease, twin studies, and HLA typing patterns. The major predisposing genes in MS are the HLA class II molecules, in particular the haplotype HLA-DR2, which is especially common among MS patients of northern and western European ancestry. This haplotype represents a susceptibility locus in specific populations, but a direct contribution to the pathogenesis of the disease is likely small and presence of the haplotype is not necessary for disease expression in all patients. Indeed, patient groups with MS in different ethnic populations are immunogenetically distinct and thus have HLA polymorphisms that are common within each population but that are different from other populations. HLA type does not seem to strongly influence the subsequent risk for MS in patients with isolated optic neuritis. Although the combination of HLA typing and MRI may slightly increase predictive ability, MRI is a much stronger and reliable indicator of risk.

Some studies suggest that patients in whom optic neuritis is the initial manifestation of MS tend to have a more benign course than patients in whom MS presents with nonvisual symptoms and signs. Other studies, however, report no difference in the eventual outcome of the disease.

Treatment

Studies of the treatment of acute optic neuritis have typically used adrenocorticotrophic hormone (ACTH) or various preparations of corticosteroids delivered orally (prednisone), intravenously (methylprednisolone), or via retrobulbar injection (triamcinolone). Although visual recovery may be more rapid with treatment, in no study is there any evidence that the ultimate visual outcome is modified by any treatment.

In the ONTT, patients with acute optic neuritis were randomized to one of three treatment groups: (1) oral prednisone (1 mg/kg/day) for 14 days; (2) intravenous methylprednisolone sodium succinate (250 mg 4 times a day for 3 days) followed by oral prednisone (1 mg/kg/day) for 11 days; (3) oral placebo for 14 days. Each regimen was followed by a short oral taper (20 mg on day 15, 10 mg on days 16 and 18). Most patients in all three treatment groups had a good recovery of vision with only 10% of patients in each group having a visual acuity of 20/50 or worse in the affected eye at 6 months of follow-up. Among the three groups 1 year after onset of visual symptoms, there was no significant difference in mean visual acuity, contrast sensitivity, color vision, or visual field. However, patients treated with the regimen of intravenous methylprednisolone followed by oral prednisone recovered vision faster than patients in the other two groups. The benefit of this treatment regimen was greatest in the first 15 days of follow-up and decreased subsequently. Patients treated

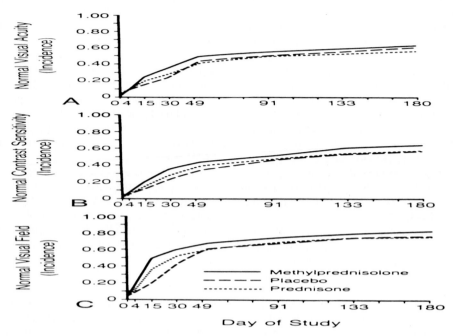

Figure 6.9. Graph showing the 5-year probability of recurrent attacks of optic neuritis in the previously affected eye and new attacks of optic neuritis in the fellow eye of patients enrolled in the Optic Neuritis Treatment Trial and Longitudinal Optic Neuritis Study by treatment groups. Note that patients who were treated with oral prednisone alone, in a dose of 1 mg/kg/day for 14 days, had a much higher incidence of such attacks than patients who were given oral placebo or patients who were treated with intravenous methylprednisolone in a dose of 250 mg every 6 hours for 3 days followed by an 11-day course of oral prednisone in a dose of 1 mg/kg/day. (Reprinted with permission from The Optic Neuritis Study Group. Visual function 5 years after optic neuritis: experience of the Optic Neuritis Treatment Trial. Arch Ophthalmol 1997;115:1545–1552.)

with oral prednisone alone did not recover vision any faster and had no better visual outcome. Importantly, patients treated with oral prednisone alone had an increased rate of recurrent attacks of optic neuritis in the previously affected eye and an increased rate of new attacks of optic neuritis in the fellow eye compared with patients in the other two groups (Fig. 6.9).

The ONTT also evaluated the rate of development of MS in the three treatment groups and found that the patients treated with the intravenous followed by oral corticosteroid regimen had a reduced rate of development of clinically definite MS during the first 2 years. The benefit of treatment was seen only in patients who had significantly abnormal brain MRI at the time of onset of the optic neuritis, and the clinical benefit of the intravenous treatment lessened over time such that by 3 years of follow-up, there was no significant difference in the rate of development of MS among treatment groups.

In summary, there is no treatment for acute demyelinating optic neuritis that has been shown to improve the ultimate visual prognosis compared with the natural history of the disorder. A short course of intravenous methylprednisolone (250 mg 4 times a day for 3 days) followed by a 2-week course of oral prednisone (11 days of 1 mg/kg/day followed by a 3-day taper) may result in an increase in the speed of recovery of vision by 2 to 3 weeks compared with no treatment when the steroids are begun within 1 to 2 weeks of the onset of visual loss, but the ultimate visual function at 1 year is the same as it would have been if no treatment were given. Because treatment with oral corticosteroids at a dose of 1 mg/kg/day does not improve visual outcome or speed recovery and is associated with a higher incidence of recurrent and new attacks of optic neuritis, it is **inappropriate** to treat any patient with acute demyelinating optic neuritis with oral corticosteroids alone at this dosage.

Management Recommendations

In a patient with typical features of optic neuritis, a clinical diagnosis can be made with a high degree of certainty without the need for ancillary testing. Brain MRI is a powerful predictor of the short-term probability of MS (for at least the first 5 years). Until there is clear evidence that the knowledge from MRI is needed for proper patient management, it is most reasonable for the decision to obtain brain MRI to be made on an individual patient basis.

Based on the results of the ONTT, it is reasonable to consider treatment with intravenous methylprednisolone, 250 mg every 6 hours for 3 days or 1 gram per day in a single dose for 3 days, followed by a 2-week course of oral prednisone, 1 mg/kg/day, with a rapid taper for patients with acute optic neuritis, particularly if brain MRI demonstrates multiple signal abnormalities in the periventricular white matter consistent with MS, or if a patient has a need to recover vision faster than the natural history of the condition. Because the potential beneficial effects on the visual and neurologic courses are short term and not lasting, prescribing no treatment is also a reasonable approach. However, oral prednisone alone in standard dosages (e.g., 1 mg/kg/day or less) should be avoided. The visual recovery is excellent without treatment, and the long-term vision does not appear to be any better when corticosteroids are prescribed.

CHRONIC DEMYELINATING OPTIC NEURITIS

It was once stated that, for all intents and purposes, chronic optic neuritis does not occur. The reason for this dogmatic statement was that too many patients with mass lesions compressing the intracranial portion of the optic nerve were being diagnosed as having chronic optic neuritis, leading to delayed treatment of the underlying lesion with resultant permanent visual loss. Thus, the statement that chronic optic neuritis was never a tenable diagnosis was made in an effort to raise the consciousness of the majority of physicians to look for another, potentially treatable cause of unilateral progressive optic neuropathy.

In reality, chronic optic neuritis not only oc-

curs but is not uncommon. In any group of patients with MS, one can find numerous patients who have no history of acute visual loss (painful or otherwise) but who nevertheless complain that the vision in one or both eyes is not normal and who have evidence of unilateral or bilateral optic nerve dysfunction. Such patients may complain of a static disturbance of vision, a slowly progressive loss of vision in one or both eyes, or, occasionally, a stepwise loss of vision unassociated with periods of recovery. Some patients with MS complain of blurred or distorted vision even though visual acuity is 20/20 or better in both eyes. Such patients often can be found to have evidence of chronic optic neuritis by clinical testing (e.g., color vision, visual fields, ophthalmoscopy), electrophysiologic testing (VEPs), psychophysical testing (e.g., contrast sensitivity), or a combination of these methods.

Most patients with chronic unilateral or bilateral demyelinating optic neuropathies develop visual symptoms after other signs and symptoms of MS have developed, and it is for this reason that the percentage of patients with MS and evidence of chronic progressive optic neuritis increases the longer patients are followed. Nevertheless, slowly progressive visual loss or complaints of blurred or distorted vision in one or both eyes are the first symptoms underlying neurologic disease in some patients. We are unaware of any efficacious treatment for chronic progressive demyelinating optic neuritis. As new therapies for other forms of chronic progressive MS become available, it is possible that the symptoms and signs of chronic optic neuritis also may respond to treatment.

ASYMPTOMATIC (SUBCLINICAL) OPTIC NEURITIS

A substantial percentage of patients with MS have clinical or laboratory evidence of optic nerve dysfunction even though they have no visual complaints and believe their vision to be normal. This is not surprising given that the anterior visual pathways show damage in up to 100% of patients with MS in autopsy studies. Pathologic evidence of demyelination is not uncommon in the optic nerves of patients who never had visual complaints during life. Evidence for optic neuritis in a patient who is visually asymptomatic may be clinical, electrophysiologic, psychophysical, or a combination of these.

A careful clinical examination may reveal that

despite having visual acuity of 20/20 or better, the patient has a subtle disturbance of color perception when tested with color plates, the Farnsworth-Munsell 100-Hues test, or some other method. There may be subtle visual field defects in one or both eyes detected using automated (static) perimetry. A relative afferent pupillary defect may be present, or the patient may have subtle optic nerve fiber layer atrophy. The ONTT found that 48% of patients with apparently unilateral optic neuritis and no history of previous optic neuritis in the contralateral eye nevertheless had an abnormal visual field unexplained by intraocular pathology in their asymptomatic, fellow eye. A substantial percentage of these eyes also had disturbances of visual acuity, color vision, and contrast sensitivity. In some cases, MRI showed enhancement of the asymptomatic optic nerve.

Visually asymptomatic patients suspected or known to have MS may be demonstrated to have disturbances of the visual sensory pathways by electrophysiologic testing. VEPs seem to be a particularly sensitive indicator of optic nerve and other visual sensory pathway disturbances in such patients. Psychophysical tests of visual function, such as contrast sensitivity using a Peli-Robson chart, Arden gratings, oscilloscope screen projections, or similar techniques, may reveal abnormalities in patients with MS who are visually asymptomatic. Some psychophysical tests, such as measurements of sustained visual resolution and assessment of chromatic, luminance, spatial, and temporal sensitivity, give similar results but are too complex and time-consuming to be of use in screening patients in clinical practice. Other tests—such as assessing the presence or absence of the Pulfrich phenomenon (by having the patient gaze at a pendulum swinging at right angles to the line of sight and determining if the pendulum appears to the patient to be swinging in a elliptical path) and the "flight of colors" test (in which a bright light is aimed directly in one eye at a distance of 2.5 cm for 10 seconds while the other eye is covered and the patient then closes both eyes and reports the sequences of colors and duration of the afterimage)—give little more information that one can obtain by an otherwise complete clinical and electrophysiologic examination.

OPTIC NEURITIS IN OTHER PRIMARY DEMYELINATING DISEASES

NEUROMYELITIS OPTICA (DEVIC'S DISEASE)

The association of acute or subacute loss of vision in one or both eyes caused by acute optic neuropathy preceded or followed within days to weeks by a transverse or ascending myelopathy is known as **neuromyelitis optica** or **Devic's disease**.

Epidemiology

Neuromyelitis optica occurs primarily in children and young adults, but all ages may be affected, and the condition has been described in patients over the age of 60 years. Both sexes are equally affected. It does not seem to be inherited, but there are reports in monozygotic twins. Although most patients who develop this condition are otherwise healthy, a neuromyelitis picture may develop in patients with systemic lupus erythematosus (SLE), pulmonary tuberculosis, sarcoidosis, and after chickenpox.

Pathology

The brain, optic nerves, and spinal cord are affected by scattered lesions of demyelination that principally affect the white matter but that also may affect the gray matter. In some cases, the cerebrum may be only slightly affected or completely spared, but the optic nerves and the spinal cord are invariably damaged. Liquefaction and formation of cavities are common. There is widespread destruction of myelin sheaths, and axis cylinders may also be destroyed. There may be small areas of perivascular lymphocytosis in both brain and spinal cord. Formation of glial tissue occurs in mild or moderately severe cases.

Although some investigators believe that neuromyelitis optica is simply a rare and aggressive variant of MS, there are several important differences in the pathologic findings in the two conditions:

1. The cerebellum is almost never affected in patients with neuromyelitis optica, whereas it is frequently affected in MS.
2. Excavation of affected tissue with formation of cavities is rare in MS, but it is

common in neuromyelitis optica, where there is often liquefaction of tissue.

3. Gliosis is characteristic of MS but is almost never present or is minimal in neuromyelitis optica.

4. The arcuate fibers located in the cerebral subcortex are relatively unaffected in patients with neuromyelitis optica, but they are severely damaged in most patients with MS.

5. Evidence of a necrotizing rather than a demyelinating process is noted in the spinal cords of some patients with neuromyelitis optica.

It remains unclear why the lesions of neuromyelitis optica selectively affect the optic nerves, the optic chiasm, and the spinal cord.

Clinical Manifestations

The primary features of neuromyelitis optica are visual loss caused by damage to the anterior visual sensory pathways and paraplegia caused by damage to the spinal cord. Other visual and neurologic manifestations are much less common.

Many patients with neuromyelitis optica develop a mild febrile illness several days or weeks before the onset of visual or neurologic manifestations. Typical symptoms of this prodrome include sore throat, headache, and fever. In rare cases, there is a clear history of an antecedent viral illness, such as mumps, varicella, or infectious mononucleosis, or of a recent viral vaccination.

Visual loss is almost always bilateral, although unilateral cases occur. One eye is often affected first, but the second eye usually is affected within hours, days, or rarely weeks after onset. The loss of vision is typically rapid and usually severe. It is not uncommon for complete blindness to develop. In such cases, the pupils become dilated and nonreactive to light. When some vision remains, the size of the pupils and their reactivity to light stimulation are related to the severity of visual acuity and visual field loss.

The rapid, bilateral loss of vision that occurs in patients with neuromyelitis optica is in sharp contrast to the loss of vision in optic neuritis, which tends to be unilateral and not as severe, and to the loss of vision in Leber's hereditary optic neuropathy, which tends to be more slowly

progressive. Pain in or around the eyes precedes the loss of vision in a minority of cases, again distinguishing the condition from optic neuritis in which pain is an almost universal feature.

Because the foci of demyelination that affect the optic nerves are irregular and occur in a variety of different locations, the visual field defects that develop in patients with neuromyelitis optica are similarly variable. In many instances, vision is so poor when the patient is first examined that it is impossible to plot the field defect. Nevertheless, central scotomas seem to be the most common defect observed, with some patients developing concentric contraction of one or both fields.

The ophthalmoscopic appearance of the optic discs varies considerably. A majority of patients have mild swelling of both optic discs. Some patients, however, have substantial disc swelling that may be associated with dilation of retinal veins and extensive peripapillary exudates, and others have normal-appearing optic discs. With time, most patients develop pallor of the discs regardless of their initial appearance (Fig. 6.10). In some of these cases, there is slight narrowing of retinal vessels.

Some recovery of vision usually occurs in patients with neuromyelitis optica. Visual acuity usually begins to improve within 1 to 2 weeks after visual symptoms begin, with maximum improvement occurring within several weeks to months. The peripheral fields usually begin to recover before there is noticeable improvement in the central field defects. Nevertheless, some patients have severe and permanent visual loss in both eyes.

There is some controversy about the relationship of visual loss to the onset of paraplegia. Most studies indicate that the loss of vision precedes the onset of paraplegia in the majority of cases, whereas others find that paraplegia usually precedes the loss of vision. Regardless of which manifestation develops first, the interval between manifestations may be days, weeks, or months. In some cases, the blindness and paraplegia occur simultaneously.

The onset of the paraplegia, like that of visual loss, usually is sudden and severe, and it may be associated with a mild fever. Some patients develop an ascending paralysis that simulates Guillain-Barré syndrome; however, the presence of associated sensory symptoms and signs and

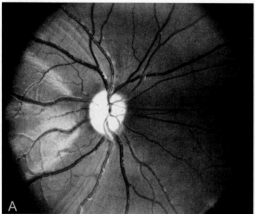
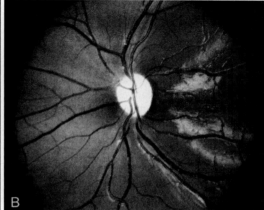

Figure 6.10. Ophthalmoscopic appearance in neuromyelitis optica (Devic's disease). The patient was a 13-year-old girl who developed transverse myelitis, followed several months later by bilateral visual loss. Visual acuity decreased to 20/400 OD and hand motions at 2 feet OS over 72 hours. The pupils were sluggishly reactive to light, and both optic discs appeared normal. The patient was treated with intravenous corticosteroids and gradually recovered both neurologic and visual function. Visual acuity eventually stabilized at 20/40 OD and 20/70 OS associated with small cecocentral scotomas. *A–B.* Ophthalmoscopic appearance of the right and left ocular fundi, respectively, shows symmetric pallor of the optic discs associated with atrophy of the retinal nerve fiber layer, especially in the papillomacular bundles.

the lack of peripheral nerve involvement should be sufficient to eliminate Guillain-Barré syndrome from consideration. The paraplegia of neuromyelitis optica varies from paraplegia in flexion to paraplegia in extension to paraplegia with loss of all deep-tendon reflexes. There may be severe root pains, and urinary retention may be present or develop shortly after the onset of motor weakness. Ascending paralysis may paralyze respiration and cause death at an early stage of the disease. Rarely, there is peripheral nerve involvement. Most patients recover motor function to some extent but have residual paraparesis, some have persistent and complete paralysis, and rare patients have complete recovery.

The mortality rate in patients with neuromyelitis optica was reported in the past to be as high as 50%, but improvements in supportive care have greatly reduced this rate, and we would estimate that death occurs in less than 10% of cases now. The disease tends to occur as a single episode without recurrences, unlike MS. Nevertheless, occasional recurrences of both visual loss and paraplegia, both separate and simultaneous, can occur.

Diagnosis

During the active stage of neuromyelitis optica, the CSF usually shows evidence of an inflammatory process. There often is a mild lymphocytic pleocytosis, rarely a dramatic one. The concentration of protein in the CSF may be increased, but intrathecal synthesis of IgG is usually not increased and oligoclonal bands are rarely detected. The CSF glucose concentration invariably is normal. Rare cases have been recorded in which there was raised intracranial pressure. Neuroimaging rarely shows intracranial lesions, aside from the anterior visual pathways. However, MRI may show abnormal T2-weighted signals and enhancement with gadolinium in the optic nerves, chiasm, and spinal cord (Fig. 6.11).

It may be impossible to differentiate between neuromyelitis optica and MS on clinical grounds alone, and some investigators believe that they are simply variants of the same disease. Nevertheless, not only are there important pathologic differences and differences in CSF findings between the two diseases (see above), but also there are important clinical differences. First, neuromyelitis optica is not uncommon in the first decade of life, whereas MS rarely occurs in patients under 10 years of age. Second, the occurrence of bilateral optic neuritis associated with myelitis is rarely recorded in cases of pathologically proven MS. Third, bilateral

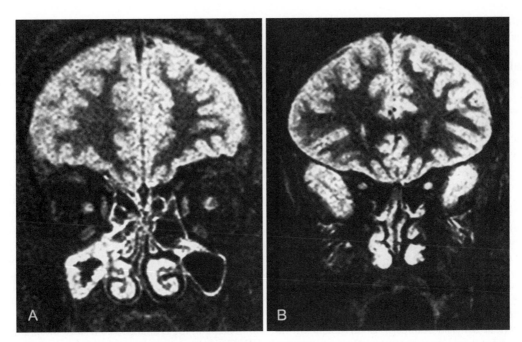

Figure 6.11.   Neuroimaging in neuromyelitis optica (Devic's disease). The patient was a 39-year-old man who developed loss of vision in the left eye 4 days after developing paraparesis. *A.* Proton density–weighted coronal MRI performed several hours after the onset of visual symptoms shows enlargement of the left optic nerve. *B.* Proton density-weighted coronal MRI at a slightly different setting shows marked hyperintensity of the left optic nerve. (Reprinted with permission from Barkhof F, Scheltens P, Valk J, et al. Serial quantitative MR assessment of optic neuritis in a case of neuromyelitis optica, using gadolinium-''enhanced'' STIR imaging. Neuroradiology 1991;33:70–71.)

blindness is extremely unusual in MS but is the rule in neuromyelitis optica.

Treatment

There is no specific treatment for neuromyelitis optica. Supportive care is crucial to ensure survival in patients with severe myelitis. The use of intravenous corticosteroids may lessen the severity of the attack and increase the speed of recovery of both visual and motor function. Administration of intravenous gamma globulin also may be considered.

MYELINOCLASTIC DIFFUSE SCLEROSIS (ENCEPHALITIS PERIAXIALIS DIFFUSA, SCHILDER'S DISEASE)

Although original descriptions of **Schilder's disease** may have inadvertently included examples of adrenoleukodystrophy and subacute sclerosing panencephalitis, there remains a characteristic group of patients with a noninherited demyelinating disease related to MS that is most commonly referred to now as **myelinoclastic diffuse sclerosis**. The characteristic lesion in these patients is a large, sharply outlined, asymmetric focus of demyelination with severe, selective myelinoclasia that often affects an entire lobe or cerebral hemisphere. There is typically extension across the corpus callosum and damage to the opposite hemisphere. Both hemispheres are symmetrically affected in some cases. Careful examination of the optic nerves, brainstem, cerebellum, and spinal cord often discloses typical discrete lesions consistent with MS, and histopathologic examination of both large and small foci reveals the characteristic features reminiscent of MS, including fibrillary gliosis with formation of giant multinucleated or swollen astrocytes and perivascular cuffing with inflammatory infiltrates containing plasma cells. The axons themselves may show little damage. Indeed, both the clinical and histopathologic features of myelinoclastic diffuse sclerosis disease suggest that it is closely related to MS and probably is a variant of it.

Myelinoclastic diffuse sclerosis occurs most

often in children and young adults, but it occasionally occurs in older persons. It is characterized by a progressive course that may be steady and unremitting or punctuated by a series of rapid worsening. A change in personality may be the first evidence of the disease. Irritability, peevishness, unprovoked laughter or crying, and general apathy may be present. Cerebral blindness may be an early feature of the disease, particularly in adults. Central deafness may also occur. Other manifestations include dementia, homonymous visual field defect, varying degrees of hemiparesis and quadriparesis often culminating in plegia, and pseudobulbar palsy. The brainstem and cerebellum are affected in some cases, resulting in nystagmus, intention tremor, scanning speech, and spastic paraplegia.

Visual loss occurs in approximately 60% of cases, most often a result of damage to the postchiasmal visual pathways, producing homonymous hemianopic or quadrantic visual field defects or cerebral blindness. Involvement of the visual association areas may also cause visual difficulties. Occasional patients develop demyelination in the optic chiasm, producing bitemporal field defects. Optic neuritis occurs less frequently than in patients with MS, although the true incidence is not known. Rarely, papilledema occurs.

The CSF may show changes similar to those seen in typical MS. The intracranial pressure is usually normal, but in some patients the pressure is elevated. The protein concentration of the CSF is usually slightly increased, and there may be a mild lymphocytic pleocytosis. The IgG content is often increased, as is the CSF IgG index. Oligoclonal bands may be present, and myelin basic protein may be extremely elevated. Neuroimaging studies show large, multifocal areas of extensive demyelination. In some cases, these lesions are similar in appearance to tumors or abscesses.

The diagnosis of myelinoclastic diffuse sclerosis may be suspected when a child or young adult develops evidence of a subacute or chronic progressive neurologic disease with neuroimaging and laboratory evidence of focal hemispheric demyelinating disease but without adrenal dysfunction or abnormal long-chain fatty-acids.

Most patients with myelinoclastic diffuse sclerosis follow a progressive unremitting course that ends in death within a few months or years. A few cases have been reported in which there was temporary or permanent spontaneous improvement, and rare patients survive for a decade or longer. Some patients improve after being treated with intravenous or oral corticosteroids, ACTH, or immunosuppressants. Patients who improve clinically generally show disappearance or shrinkage of the lesions seen on neuroimaging studies.

ENCEPHALITIS PERIAXIALIS CONCENTRICA (CONCENTRIC SCLEROSIS OF BALÓ)

Encephalitis periaxialis concentrica clinically resembles myelinoclastic diffuse sclerosis but differs from it pathologically. Patients rapidly develop a variety of neurologic symptoms and signs separated in time and space, including visual loss and diplopia. The visual loss is usually caused by damage to postgeniculate visual pathways and is characterized by homonymous field defects or cerebral blindness, although optic nerve involvement can occur.

The pathologic changes consist of alternating bands of demyelination and preserved myelin in a series of concentric rings in the cerebral white matter. The predominant feature of the bands of myelin is remyelination. The lesion likely originates as a small focus of acute demyelination around a perivascular inflammatory cuff, and the concentric bands are actually alternating areas of demyelination and remyelination. Some patients not only have pathologic changes consistent with encephalitis periaxialis concentrica but also have lesions typical of acute MS, suggesting that the former disease may actually be a variant of the latter.

Neuroimaging studies initially may be normal in patients with encephalitis periaxialis concentrica; however, eventually both CT scanning and MRI show multiple lesions consistent with demyelination. Similarly, analysis of the CSF at an early stage of the disease may reveal normal findings, but later analysis may show mild to moderate pleocytosis, increased protein, an increased IgG index, and multiple oligoclonal bands. The diagnosis can only be made conclusively by pathologic examination, either by biopsy or on postmortem studies.

Without treatment, encephalitis periaxialis concentrica usually progresses inexorably and is invariably fatal within a few weeks to a year. Treatment with systemic corticosteroids, however, may result in both immediate and long-term improvement in neurologic symptoms and signs. Early diagnosis thus is extremely important, supporting the use of stereotactic biopsy in some cases.

CAUSES OF OPTIC NEURITIS OTHER THAN PRIMARY DEMYELINATION

In a small percentage of cases, a primary demyelinating process in the optic nerve or the central nervous system is not the cause of unilateral or bilateral anterior or retrobulbar optic neuritis. Instead, the condition develops in the setting of, or as the presenting manifestation of, an underlying or recent systemic infection, vaccination, or systemic inflammatory disease.

INFECTIOUS AND PARAINFECTIOUS OPTIC NEURITIS

Inflammation of the optic nerve can result from direct infection of the nerve by a variety of infectious agents such as viruses and bacteria. In addition, systemic or central nervous system infection can trigger an immune response that results in inflammation of the optic nerve. Distinguishing between these two pathogeneses is not always possible.

Parainfectious optic neuritis typically follows the onset of a viral, or less often a bacterial, infection by 1 to 3 weeks. It is more common in children than in adults and is thought to occur most often on an immunologic basis, producing demyelination of the optic nerve. The optic neuritis may be unilateral, but it is often bilateral (Fig. 6.12). The optic discs may appear normal or swollen. Swelling of the peripapillary retina may be observed in patients with anterior optic neuritis. If a star figure composed of lipid and exudate develops in the macula of the affected eye, the condition is called *neuroretinitis* (see below). If there is evidence of optic nerve dysfunction and the intracranial pressure is normal, the inflammation is assumed to be affecting the periphery of the nerve and is called *perioptic neuritis* or *optic perineuritis* (see below).

Parainfectious optic neuritis, whether viral or bacterial, may occur in patients with no evidence of neurologic dysfunction or in association with a meningitis, meningoencephalitis, or encephalomyelitis—so-called acute disseminated encephalomyelitis. When neurologic manifestations are present, patients have typical abnormalities in the CSF, such as a lymphocytic pleocytosis and an elevated protein concentration. Patients with encephalitis usually have disturbances on electroencephalography, and they may also have lesions on brain imaging, whereas patients with encephalomyelitis may show lesions in both the brain and spinal cord. Both enlargement and enhancement of the optic nerves may be demonstrated on MRI.

Visual recovery following parainfectious optic neuritis is usually excellent without treatment. Whether corticosteroids hasten recovery in patients with postviral optic neuritis is unknown, but this treatment is reasonable to consider, particularly in cases in which visual loss is bilateral and severe.

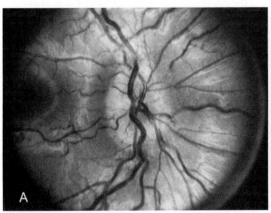 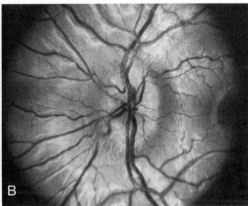

Figure 6.12.   Bilateral anterior optic neuritis. The patient is a 19-year-old girl who suffered bilateral visual loss 2 weeks following a flu-like illness. *A–B*. Both optic discs show moderate swelling without hemorrhages. Visual acuity is 20/400 in the right eye and 20/300 in the left eye, and there are bilateral central scotomas. Visual acuity returned to normal within 6 weeks, and disc swelling completely resolved.

Optic neuritis may occur in association with infections by a large number of both deoxyribonucleic (DNA) and ribonucleic (RNA) viruses including adenovirus, coxsackievirus, cytomegalovirus, hepatitis A virus, human herpes virus 4 (Epstein-Barr virus), human immunodeficiency virus (HIV) type 1, and the measles, mumps, rubeola, rubella, and varicella-zoster (in both chickenpox and herpes zoster) viruses. Bacterial infections can also produce optic neuritis and include syphilis, Lyme disease, cat-scratch disease, anthrax, β-hemolytic streptococcal infection, brucellosis, meningococcal infection, tuberculosis, typhoid fever, and Whipple's disease.

Optic neuritis in **syphilis** is not rare, but it is particularly common in patients also infected with HIV. The optic neuritis of syphilis can be unilateral or bilateral and anterior or retrobulbar. When the condition is anterior, there is usually some cellular reaction in the vitreous, which serves to distinguish it (and other systemic inflammatory diseases that cause anterior optic neuritis) from demyelinating optic neuritis in which the vitreous is usually clear. The diagnosis of syphilis is established using a variety of serologic and CSF assays. Treatment with intravenous penicillin produces visual recovery in many cases; however, the disease may be difficult to cure, particularly in patients who are HIV-positive or who have the acquired immune deficiency syndrome (AIDS). Syphilis can also cause both neuroretinitis and optic perineuritis (see below).

Optic neuritis can occur in patients with Lyme borreliosis (**Lyme disease**). This disorder is a spirochetal infection that is transmitted through the bite of a tick infected with the etiologic agent, *Borrelia burgdorferi*. It can produce a multitude of ocular and neurologic findings, including both anterior and retrobulbar optic neuritis. The diagnosis of Lyme disease is made by serologic detection of infection or by finding the organism or its nucleic acid in the serum, CSF, or both. Treatment with antibiotics is usually effective, particularly in the early stages of the disease. As is the case with other systemic infectious processes that can cause optic neuritis, Lyme disease can also cause neuroretinitis (see below).

Many infectious agents that do not normally cause optic neuritis can do so in patients who are immunocompromised from drugs or disease.

Such optic neuritis is particularly common in patients who are infected with **HIV** and in patients with AIDS. Optic neuritis, both anterior and retrobulbar, is an occasional finding in HIV-infected patients with cryptococcal meningitis, cytomegalovirus infection, herpesvirus infections, syphilis, tuberculous meningitis, and a variety of fungal infections. Rare patients with toxoplasmosis also develop optic neuritis. In some cases, such infections cause neuroretinitis, whereas in others, optic perineuritis occurs. Some patients with AIDS develop optic neuritis that is probably caused by infection with HIV itself, although it is not clear if the pathogenesis is direct infection or an immune-mediated parainfectious process.

In the pre-antibiotic era, spread of infection from the paranasal sinuses to the optic nerve was not unusual. However, this is now a rare occurrence, and most cases of **sinusitis** in patients with optic neuritis are fortuitous. Nevertheless, some patients with acute severe sinusitis develop a secondary optic neuritis from spread of infection. When the infection originates from the ethmoid or maxillary sinuses, there are usually obvious signs of orbital inflammation; however, spread of infection from the sphenoid sinus to the posterior optic nerve in the apex of the orbit or within the optic canal can be silent except for the loss of vision. Aspergillosis and other fungal infections are considerations in this clinical setting. Neuroimaging techniques, particularly CT scanning and MRI, generally can be used to diagnose paranasal sinus disease. Even when sinus disease is present in the setting of optic neuritis, one must be wary of attributing the optic neuritis to this cause. Obviously, patients with retrobulbar neuritis and suppurative sinusitis with signs of orbital inflammation should be actively treated not only to eradicate the infection but also for the possible beneficial effects of treatment on the optic neuritis. In our opinion, however, operative intervention is not warranted in patients with radiologic evidence of sinus disease that normally would not require surgical therapy.

POST-VACCINATION OPTIC NEURITIS

Optic neuritis can occur after vaccinations against both bacterial and virus infections. Most cases are bilateral, and both anterior and retrobulbar forms of optic neuritis may occur. Optic neuritis may develop after vaccinations with *Bacille Calmette-Guérin* (BCG), hepatitis B virus, rabies virus, tetanus toxoid, and variola virus; combined smallpox, tetanus, and diphtheria vaccine; and combined measles, mumps, and rubella vaccine. Influenza vaccine is commonly associated with the development of optic neuritis. Most cases of post-vaccination optic neuritis appear to be of the anterior variety and typically occur within 1 to 3 weeks of the vaccination. Visual recovery is common but may occur over several months.

INFLAMMATORY OPTIC NEURITIS

Granulomatous inflammation of the optic nerve may occur in **sarcoidosis,** producing a typical anterior or retrobulbar optic neuritis. In some cases, the optic neuritis occurs during the course of the disease, whereas in others it is the presenting manifestation. Clinical findings may be indistinguishable from those of demyelinating optic neuritis. However, the optic disc may have a characteristic lumpy, white appearance that suggests a granulomatous etiology, and there may be an inflammatory reaction in the vitreous or even the anterior chamber.

Unlike primary demyelinating optic neuritis that does not respond dramatically to systemic corticosteroids, the optic neuritis associated with sarcoidosis is usually extremely sensitive to steroids. In most cases, recovery of vision is rapid after treatment is instituted, although vision may decline again once steroids are tapered or stopped. Indeed, it must be emphasized that rapid recovery of vision with corticosteroid treatment and subsequent worsening when the steroids are tapered is atypical for demyelinating optic neuritis and suggests an infiltrative or non-demyelinating inflammatory process, such as sarcoidosis.

Patients with possible sarcoid optic neuritis should undergo an evaluation that includes a careful history and physical examination, a chest radiograph, serum chemistries, an assay for angiotensin converting enzyme (ACE) in the serum and possibly the CSF, and, in some cases, a gallium scan and tissue sampling via bronchoscopic lavage or biopsy of skin, conjunctiva, lacrimal gland, mediastinal tissue, lung, liver, or other organs looking for noncaseating granulomas.

Patients with systemic lupus erythematosus, polyarteritis nodosa, and other **vasculitides** can experience an attack of what seems clinically to be typical acute optic neuritis. This phenomenon occurs in about 1% of patients with SLE. In rare cases, the optic neuropathy is the presenting sign of the disease. The pathogenesis is not a true infection or inflammation of the nerve tissue itself, but is likely related to ischemia which may produce demyelination alone, axonal necrosis, or a combination of the two. The clinical profile of optic neuropathy in SLE and other vasculitides can be an acute anterior or retrobulbar optic neuropathy associated with pain or a slowly progressive loss of vision that mimics a compressive lesion.

The diagnosis of SLE or other vasculitides as a cause of optic neuropathy is established by identification of systemic symptoms and signs of the disease as well as by serologic testing. Treatment with corticosteroids is indicated, but steroid dependency is a not uncommon problem (vision worsens when steroids are tapered), that often requires the chronic use of other immunosuppressive agents.

MISCELLANEOUS CAUSES OF OPTIC NEURITIS

Optic neuritis can rarely occur in a large variety of conditions other than bacterial or viral infections, including acute posterior multifocal placoid pigment epitheliopathy, bee or wasp sting, birdshot retinochoroidopathy, Creutzfeldt-Jakob disease, cysticercosis, familial Mediterranean fever, Guillain-Barré syndrome, inflammatory bowel disease, intraocular nematode infection, presumed histoplasmosis, Reiter's syndrome, toxocariasis, toxoplasmosis, and *Mycoplasma pneumoniae* infection. As is true for optic neuritis associated with bacterial or viral infections, some of these cases are isolated, whereas others are associated with other evidence of central nervous system dysfunction.

Intraocular inflammation alone may cause optic disc swelling; however, in such cases, visual acuity is usually not significantly affected from damage to the optic nerve (Fig. 6.13). In such patients, visual acuity is limited only by the degree of vitreous inflammation or by secondary changes that occur in the macula (e.g., cystoid edema). Perhaps the most common form of disc swelling that occurs as part of an ocular inflammatory syndrome is the Irvine-Gass syndrome, which occurs after cataract extraction and is associated with moderately decreased visual acuity and cystoid macular edema.

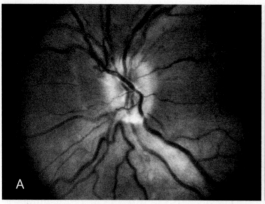
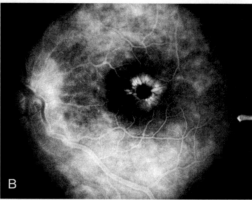

Figure 6.13. Optic disc swelling in a patient with pars planitis (chronic cyclitis). The patient was initially believed to have papilledema. *A.* The left optic disc is hyperemic and slightly swollen. The hazy appearance is due to the presence of vitreous cells. *B.* Fluorescein angiogram of the left macula shows cystoid macular edema, characteristic of this disorder. The opposite eye had a similar ophthalmoscopic appearance.

OPTIC NEURITIS IN CHILDREN

Optic neuritis in children has several unique characteristics that distinguish it from optic neuritis in adults:

1. It is more often anterior, with disc swelling in more than 70% of cases.
2. It is more often a bilateral simultaneous condition (in up to 60% of cases).
3. It often seems to occur within 1 to 2 weeks after a known or presumed viral infection or vaccination.
4. It is less often associated with the development of MS (15 to 44% of cases).
5. It is often **steroid-sensitive and steroid-dependent.**

As in adult optic neuritis, the visual prognosis in children with optic neuritis appears to be quite good, but not all children achieve a good visual result. It is our policy to evaluate all patients with optic neuritis under 15 years of age with MRI and a lumbar puncture. Unless there is a contraindication to doing so, we then treat these children with intravenous methylprednisolone 1–2 mg/kg/day for 3 to 5 days, followed by a slow taper of oral prednisone, often over several months.

NEURORETINITIS

Neuroretinitis is characterized by acute unilateral visual loss in the setting of optic disc swelling and hard exudate arranged in a star figure around the fovea (Fig. 6.14). Some cases of neuroretinitis are associated with particular infectious diseases, whereas others occur as apparently isolated phenomena, designated "Leber's idiopathic stellate neuroretinitis."

Neuroretinitis affects persons of all ages, although it occurs most often in the third and fourth decades of life, with no gender predilection. The condition is usually painless, but some patients complain of an eye ache that may worsen with eye movements. Visual acuity at the time of initial examination can range from 20/20 to light perception. The degree of color deficit is usually worse than the degree of visual loss would suggest. The most common field defect is a cecocentral scotoma, but central scotomas, arcuate defects, and even altitudinal defects may be present, and the peripheral field may be nonspecifically constricted. A relative afferent pupillary defect is present in most patients, unless the condition is bilateral. The degree of optic disc swelling ranges from mild to severe, depending in part on the timing of the first examination. In severe cases, splinter hemorrhages may be present. Segmental disc swelling has been reported but is uncommon. A macular star figure composed of lipid (hard exudates) may not be present when the patient is examined soon after visual symptoms begin, but it becomes apparent within days to weeks and tends to become more prominent even as the optic disc swelling

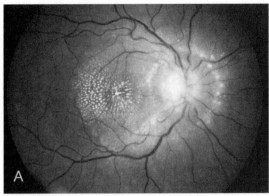 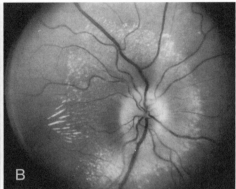

Figure 6.14. Neuroretinitis. *A.* The right optic disc is swollen, there is peripapillary edema, and there is a star figure composed of hard exudate in the macula. This is a form of optic neuritis that is *not* associated with multiple sclerosis.

B. In another case, the star figure is incomplete and located nasal but not temporal to the fovea. Note the extensive exudate surrounding the swollen optic disc. (Courtesy of Dr. J.M. Christiansen.)

resolves (see Fig. 6.14). Small, discrete, usually white, chorioretinal lesions may occur in both the symptomatic and asymptomatic eyes. Posterior inflammatory signs consisting of vitreous cells and venous sheathing, as well as occasional anterior chamber cell and flare may occur. Fluorescein angiography in patients with acute neuroretinitis demonstrates diffuse disc swelling and leakage of dye from vessels on the surface of the discs. The retinal vessels may show slight staining in the peripapillary region; however, the macular vasculature is entirely normal.

Neuroretinitis is usually a self-limited disorder with a good visual prognosis. Typically over 6 to 8 weeks, the optic disc swelling resolves, and the appearance of the disc becomes normal or mildly pale. The macular exudate progresses over about 7 to 10 days, then remains stable for several weeks before gradual resolution occurs over 6 to 12 months. Most patients ultimately recover good visual acuity, although some complain of persistent metamorphopsia or nonspecific blurred vision from mild disruption of the macular architecture. Most patients do not experience a subsequent attack in the same eye, and only a small percentage of patients develop a similar attack in the fellow eye.

Neuroretinitis is thought to be an infectious or parainfectious (i.e., immune-mediated) process that may be precipitated by a number of different agents. In our experience, cat-scratch disease, a systemic infection caused by the pleomorphic gram-negative bacillus *Bartonella henselae*, is

the most common infectious process associated with neuroretinitis. Patients with cat-scratch fever usually have a history of contact with a cat, especially a kitten. They complain of malaise, fever, muscle aches, and headache. Examination typically reveals local lymphadenopathy. Some patients also have symptoms of arthritis, hepatitis, meningitis, or encephalitis; others are systemically and neurologically asymptomatic.

Other common infections that cause neuroretinitis are the spirochetoses, especially syphilis, Lyme disease, and leptospirosis. Neuroretinitis frequently occurs in patients with secondary and tertiary (late) syphilis. There is usually a history of previous sexual contact, a chancre, or prior treatment for syphilis or other sexually transmitted diseases. Neuroretinitis may develop in patients with secondary syphilis as part of the syndrome of syphilitic meningitis. In such cases, it is usually bilateral and associated with evidence of meningeal irritation and multiple cranial neuropathies. It may also occur as an isolated phenomenon in patients with secondary syphilis, in which case it is often associated with uveitis and may be either unilateral or bilateral. Neuroretinitis occasionally occurs in patients with late syphilis, usually in patients with meningovascular neurosyphilis.

When neuroretinitis occurs in Lyme disease, it may be unilateral or bilateral, but when bilateral it is usually simultaneous and symmetric. Almost all cases occur in patients with second-stage (early-disseminated) Lyme disease. The patients usually live or work in an endemic area and may give a history of a tick bite within the last 6 months. They often have cutaneous, cardiac, or neurologic manifestations. The most common cutaneous manifestation is a solitary red or violaceous abnormality that may be small or several centimeters in diameter, appearing at the site of the tick bite or remote from it (e.g., on the ear lobe in children or on the nipple in adults). Cardiac manifestations occur in about 5 to 8% of patients with early-disseminated Lyme disease and include atrioventricular block, myocarditis, cardiomyopathy, and pericarditis. Neurologic manifestations occur in 10 to 15% of cases and include meningitis, myelitis, encephalitis, cranial neuropathies, meningoradiculitis, and peripheral neuropathies. Ocular manifestations in addition to neuroretinitis include unilateral or bilateral granulomatous iridocyclitis, choroiditis, pars planitis, vitreitis, panophthalmitis; and intraocular vascular disturbances, such as retinal perivasculitis, branch retinal artery occlusion, recurrent vitreous hemorrhage, sheathing of retinal vessels, and intraretinal hemorrhages. Like the neuroretinitis associated with syphilis, the neuroretinitis that occurs in Lyme disease may recover spontaneously but also resolves rapidly once the patient is treated with appropriate antibiotics.

Neuroretinitis is commonly associated with an antecedent viral syndrome, suggesting a possible viral etiology for up to 50% of cases; however, viruses are rarely cultured from the CSF of such patients, and serologic evidence of a concomitant viral infection is usually lacking. Proposed causative viral agents include herpes simplex, hepatitis B, mumps, and the herpes viruses associated with the acute retinal necrosis (ARN) syndrome. Other presumed etiologies for neuroretinitis include toxoplasmosis, toxocariasis, and histoplasmosis.

Certain noninfectious and noninflammatory conditions should not be called neuroretinitis even though they are characterized by optic disc swelling that may on occasion be associated with the development of a macular star figure. These mimicking conditions include papilledema, anterior ischemic optic neuropathy, and infiltration of the optic disc by tumor. Systemic hypertension may also produce both optic disc swelling and a macular star figure, but fluorescein angiography in such cases shows leakage from macular vessels. A similar phenomenon may occur in the condition called diffuse unilateral subacute neuroretinitis (DUSN), thought to be caused by one or more types of helminths.

One condition that is *not* associated with neuroretinitis is MS. Although the rate of development of MS after an attack of typical optic neuritis is substantial (see above), there is no increased tendency for patients who experience an attack of neuroretinitis to develop MS. Thus, the designation of an attack of acute optic neuropathy as an episode of neuroretinitis rather than anterior optic neuritis substantially alters the neurologic prognosis in the patient being evaluated.

Investigation into the etiology of neuroretinitis should begin with a careful history including questioning regarding sexually transmitted diseases, cat scratches, skin rashes, tick bites, lymphadenopathy, fever, and flu-like illnesses. Complete physical and ocular examinations are essential. If there is no history suggesting an underlying infectious or inflammatory disease, and the patient has no clinical evidence of such a process, it probably is reasonable to forgo any serologic testing, analysis of CSF, neuroimaging, or other evaluation. On the other hand, in the appropriate setting, screening with serologic testing for treatable diseases such as cat-scratch disease, syphilis, and Lyme disease may certainly be desirable in the individual patient with neuroretinitis.

Treatment of neuroretinitis depends on whether there is an underlying infectious or inflammatory condition that requires therapy. Cat-scratch disease is usually treated with ciprofloxacin, trimethoprim-sulfa, or tetracycline. Such treatment is almost always associated with improvement of the associated neuroretinitis, although whether or not the neuroretinitis would resolve spontaneously without treatment is unknown. Patients with neuroretinitis and secondary or late syphilis should be treated with intravenous penicillin, and patients with Lyme disease should also be treated with an appropriate antibiotic, such as ceftriaxone, amoxacillin, or tetracycline. Patients with presumed viral or idiopathic neuroretinitis may or may not require treatment. Some authors advocate the use of systemic corticosteroids or ACTH to treat isolated neuroretinitis, but there is no definite evidence that such treatment alters either the speed of re-

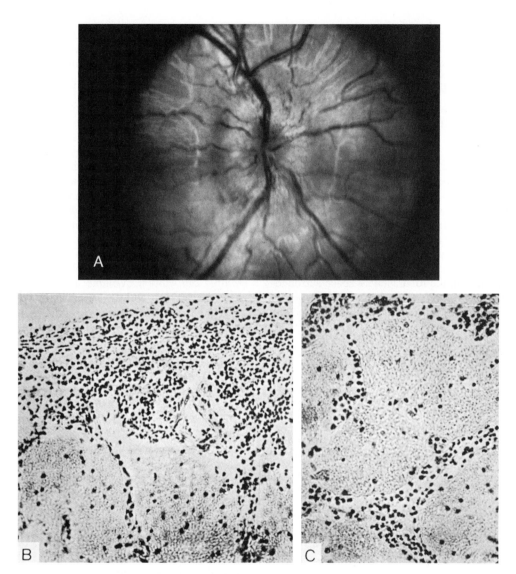

Figure 6.15.   Optic perineuritis. *A.* The optic disc is hyper-emic and swollen (as was the left disc). The patient was a 15-year-old boy complaining of a headache and stiff neck. He had a moderate fever. Visual acuity was 20/15 in both eyes, color vision was normal, and visual fields were full. The patient was believed to have papilledema. A lumbar puncture, however, revealed normal intracranial pressure, an increased concentration of protein in the cerebrospinal fluid (CSF), and a significant CSF lymphocytosis. *B.* Histologic appearance of optic perineuritis in a case of fatal meningitis. Polymorphonuclear leukocytes (PMNs) are infiltrating the leptomeninges surrounding the optic nerve and are present in the subarachnoid space. *C.* Magnified view of affected area of peripheral optic nerve. PMNs extend from the pia in the septal system deep into the nerve. There is no invasion of the nerve tissue, however. (Specimen courtesy of Dr. S.T. Orion.)

covery or the ultimate outcome. The prognosis for most cases of idiopathic neuroretinitis is excellent.

OPTIC PERINEURITIS

Optic perineuritis, also called perioptic neuritis, is a condition in which only the periphery of the optic nerve is inflamed. Optic perineuritis can occur in two forms: exudative and purulent. The exudative form, representing a localized, nonsuppurative pachymeningitis, occurs infrequently, most often in association with syphilis, sarcoidosis, and viral encephalitides. The purulent form, actually a leptomeningitis, arises as an extension from the cerebral meninges. Pathologically, the pia and arachnoid are infiltrated by polymorphonuclear leukocytes that are also found free in the subarachnoid space surrounding the optic nerve (Fig. 6.15). From the leptomeninges, the infiltration may spread into the substance of the optic nerves without at first affecting the nerve fibers themselves.

In many cases of optic perineuritis, there are neither ocular symptoms nor signs other than disc swelling that is usually bilateral. Apparently, the absence of visual dysfunction occurs because the infiltration is loose and disorganized. When vitreous cells are present, the differentiation from papilledema is easy; when there are no intraocular signs of inflammation, it may be necessary to perform neuroimaging and lumbar puncture for diagnosis. Enlargement of the optic nerve sheath on neuroimaging may simulate optic nerve sheath meningioma.

FOR MORE INFORMATION:

See Walsh & Hoyt's *Clinical Neuro-Ophthalmology,* 5th edition, Volume 1, Chapter 12, pages 599–647; Volume 5, Chapter 71, pages 5581–5590 and 5632–5639.

Ischemic Optic Neuropathies

The term **ischemic optic neuropathy** (ION) is used as a general and inclusive term to refer to all presumed ischemic causes of optic neuropathy. The term "anterior ischemic optic neuropathy" (AION) indicates visible optic disc pathology; i.e., swelling of the disc and peripapillary hemorrhages whereas "posterior (or retrobulbar) ischemic optic neuropathy" (PION) indicates that no disc swelling or other abnormality is evident (at least initially). AION is much more common than PION, accounting for about 90% of cases of ION.

Many different systemic diseases are associated with AION, most notably giant cell (temporal) arteritis; however, the majority of patients are healthy or may only have associated hypertension or diabetes mellitus. Because it is crucial to differentiate the arteritic form of AION from the nonarteritic type, most authors refer to the more common variety as "nonarteritic anterior ischemic optic neuropathy" (NAION). The clinical characteristics, natural history, and management of patients with arteritic and nonarteritic AION are substantially different. Most of the conditions associated with both arteritic and nonarteritic AION also are associated with PION.

ANTERIOR ISCHEMIC OPTIC NEUROPATHY

NONARTERITIC ANTERIOR ISCHEMIC OPTIC NEUROPATHY

Demographics

The majority of studies of NAION are retrospective chart reviews using nonstandardized collections of data on relatively few patients with variable and generally poor follow-up. A notable exception is the Ischemic Optic Neuropathy Decompression Trial (IONDT), a multicenter prospective study of newly diagnosed patients with NAION begun in 1992. The baseline history and examination, which took place within 14 days of onset of symptoms, used standardized methods and diagnostic criteria to collect data on factors that were possibly related to the etiology of NAION. Hence, the immediacy and reliability of the historic data gathered by the IONDT are unique, compared with those of any previous reports.

NAION is a common disorder. The annual incidence of NAION is 2.3 to 10.2 per 100,000 persons over 50 years of age and 0.54 per 100,000 for all ages. About 55% of patients are male. NAION may affect patients as young as 11 years old and as old as 90 years. The average age of onset in most studies ranges from 57 to 65 years, with peak age ranging typically from 55 to 70 years.

Patients with some conditions such as diabetes mellitus, migraine, and hypertension may develop AION relatively early in life, and some studies suggest that patients who are current or previous smokers have an earlier onset of AION than nonsmokers.

Of patients with NAION, 95% are Caucasians. Although there are few data on the incidence of NAION in any group, it is our general impression that NAION is rare among African-Americans. It is possible that differences in optic nerve anatomy, including smaller cup-to-disc ratios (see below) in Caucasians, predispose them to NAION.

Risk Factors and Associated Conditions

In the IONDT, 60% of patients had conditions associated with small-vessel occlusive cerebrovascular disease, including hypertension, diabetes mellitus, and cigarette use. The percentage of NAION patients with hypertension and diabetes mellitus ranges from 34 to 50% and 10 to 25%, respectively. A history of cigarette use seems to be significant for an earlier onset of NAION and may be an additional risk factor. Other possible risk factors include elevated fibrinogen, cholesterol, and triglyceride levels.

A small cup-to-disc ratio and small optic discs are noted much more frequently in patients with NAION than in control populations. This morphologic finding is perhaps the most important risk factor in the development of NAION (see below).

There appear to be three major categories of diseases associated with NAION:

1. Diseases, such as hypertension and diabetes mellitus, that produce vascular changes in optic nerve head blood vessels. These disorders most likely play a causal role in the pathogenesis of NAION.
2. Diseases that show a significant association with, but do not directly relate to, the development of NAION. Instead, such disorders are a manifestation of diseases common to both. For example, although small-vessel cerebrovascular occlusive disease occurs with increased incidence in patients with NAION, the two disorders are not causally related. They do, however, share common risk factors for atherosclerosis, such as hypertension and diabetes mellitus.
3. Disorders that occur in isolated or small groups of patients with NAION but that have no obvious pathogenetic connections.

From 35 to 50% of patients with NAION have systemic **hypertension,** a figure that is higher than the expected frequency in the general population. Indeed, NAION may be the optic nerve equivalent of the lacunar infarcts that occur in the brains of patients with hypertension from progressive hyalinosis of vessel walls induced by long-standing hypertension. Another theory is that chronic hypertension adversely affects au-toregulation of blood flow to the optic nerve head. In longstanding hypertension, the vascular tone of arterioles feeding the optic nerve head may be increased. Because of this increased tone, arteriolar sphincters that regulate blood flow through the posterior ciliary arteries may be unable to relax rapidly enough to maintain perfusion pressure when there is a drop in systemic blood pressure. Hyalinosis of vessel walls in chronic hypertension may also contribute to a loss of autoregulation. Chronic hypertensive patients are thus at increased risk to develop optic nerve head ischemia when systemic blood pressure falls.

Diabetes mellitus occurs in 10 to 25% of patients with NAION. As is the case with hypertension, some studies report higher than expected prevalence rates of diabetes mellitus in patients with NAION when compared with control populations. Indeed, in some studies, diabetes mellitus is the only systemic vasculopathy that is associated with the development of NAION.

The relationship between NAION and **cerebrovascular disease** is unclear. Even when there is an increased association, confounding factors such as concurrent hypertension or diabetes make conclusions problematic. Some investigators have identified an association between subcortical and periventricular white matter lesions observed with magnetic resonance imaging (MRI) as a marker for small vessel cerebrovascular disease and NAION. Patients with hypertension, diabetes mellitus, cardiovascular disease, and cerebrovascular disease have an increased prevalence of such lesions, which are believed to represent focal perivascular ischemic demyelination and gliosis. Other studies, however, have found no such association in patients with NAION compared with control patients. An increased incidence of **cardiac disease** has been found among NAION patients in only a few studies.

NAION may occur in patients with a variety of **coagulopathies,** including those caused by increased serum concentrations of circulating antiphospholipid antibodies and those caused by decreased concentrations of protein C, protein S, or antithrombin III. The precise relationship of these factors to the development of NAION is unclear.

The relationship between NAION and **carotid artery disease** also is unclear. Ipsilateral carotid artery disease is implicated as the causative factor in some cases of AION. In some of these cases, the optic nerve infarction results from reduced blood flow to the nerve because of a combination of carotid stenosis or occlusion, poor collateral blood supply, and local changes in the pial circulation of the optic nerve. In a few cases, the optic neuropathy results from emboli to multiple posterior ciliary arteries.

AION caused by carotid artery disease can be associated with other neurologic manifestations, including ipsilateral head pain, transient ischemic attacks, and cerebral infarction. The phenomenon of simultaneous ipsilateral AION (or PION) and internal carotid artery occlusion has been called the **optico-pyramidal syndrome,** or perhaps more appropriately, the **optico-cerebral syndrome.**

In some instances, AION caused by carotid artery disease is associated with evidence of diffuse ocular ischemia but no neurologic symptoms. The finding of iris neovascularization or stasis retinopathy in conjunction with NAION or PION, in the absence of diabetic retinopathy or central retinal vein obstruction, strongly suggests concomitant (and causative) carotid occlusive disease. Slowly progressive NAION may occur in patients with carotid occlusive disease.

On the other hand, studies investigating the degree of carotid stenosis in groups of patients with NAION compared with age-matched controls found no difference between groups and concluded that ipsilateral carotid artery disease is uncommon in patients with NAION and that if there truly is an increased risk of stroke in patients with NAION, it is most likely caused by occlusion of *small* vessels and not by stenosis or occlusion of the extracranial portion of the internal carotid artery.

In summary, although NAION may be caused by disease of the extracranial portion of the internal carotid artery, and although this mechanism should be considered in any patient with other symptoms or signs of carotid artery disease (particularly transient ischemic attacks), we believe that when carotid artery stenosis or occlusion is found in a patient with NAION, the carotid disease in most cases is not causative but is instead evidence of widespread atherosclerosis affecting both large and small vessels.

We alluded above to AION thought to be directly caused by **embolism** from the ipsilateral carotid artery. Embolic NAION also occurs in other settings, such as coronary bypass surgery,

cardiac catheterization, and metastatic cancer. Evidence of concurrent retinal embolism is typically present.

The syndrome of visual loss in the setting of acute, severe **blood loss** typically represents either AION or PION, although in some cases, the visual loss is secondary to retinal or occipital lobe infarction, and in some, multiple areas of the pre- and postgeniculate visual sensory system are damaged. Visual loss following acute blood loss and hypotension may be of three types:

1. Sustained and profound hypotension in a nonanemic patient without arteriolar sclerosis causes watershed white and gray matter infarction in parietal and occipital lobes. The optic nerves tend to be spared.
2. Brief hypotension in an anemic patient with arteriosclerotic risk factors is mild enough to spare the hemispheric watershed regions, but severe enough to cause juxtalaminar optic nerve infarction that produces a clinical (and pathologic) picture consistent with NAION.
3. Hypotension in an anemic patient without arteriosclerotic risk factors predisposes the patient to PION that is caused by infarction in the posterior orbital portion of the optic nerve, where pial end vessels are subject to compression from hypoxic edema.

The syndrome of AION after hemorrhage occurs in two main settings. Some patients develop visual loss after spontaneous hemorrhage. Others experience visual loss following surgery complicated by hemorrhage, anemia, and hypotension. It also has been postulated that blood loss alone (i.e., without systemic hypotension) can cause an increase in the release of endogenous vasoconstrictor agents that can lead to direct vasoconstriction and occlusion of optic nerve head capillaries, resulting in AION.

Patients in whom visual loss occurs after spontaneous hemorrhage are usually 40 to 60 years old and debilitated. Most of these patients have experienced repeated episodes of bleeding, but cases following a single episode of massive hemorrhage with secondary hypotension have been reported. The visual loss is usually bilateral and symmetric, but it may affect both eyes asymmetrically or be unilateral. The severity of visual loss ranges from mild or transient blurred vision in one eye to irreversible total blindness in both eyes. There may be a time lag between the bleeding and the onset of visual loss, usually less than 10 days, but occasionally as long as 2 to 3 weeks.

About 50% of patients who experience AION after an acute spontaneous hemorrhage experience some recovery of vision, but only 10 to 15% recover completely. The source of bleeding seems to be irrelevant, although the most frequent sites are the gastrointestinal tract in men and the uterus in women. In most documented cases of bilateral blindness related to systemic blood loss, the hemoglobin measures less than 5.0 g/dL at the time of visual loss. However, higher hemoglobin levels have been reported, emphasizing the likely importance of both anemia *and* hypotension in the pathogenesis of optic nerve infarction.

NAION occurs in the setting of various surgical interventions, including cardiopulmonary bypass, aortobifemoral bypass, various abdominal procedures, hip surgery, mitral valvulotomy, cholecystectomy, parathyroidectomy, and, particularly, lumbar spine surgery. It has also been described after hemodialysis and after coronary angiography. In most of these cases, the NAION is an isolated phenomenon; in others, it occurs in conjunction with evidence of retinal and choroidal ischemia, indicating involvement of the ophthalmic artery. Most cases are associated with hypotension, anemia, or both. The distinguishing feature of the cases of AION associated with back surgery is the deliberate reduction of intraoperative blood pressure to reduce bleeding and the admitted reluctance of the operating teams to transfuse the patient because of the fear on the part of the patient, the physician, or both of transmission of human immunodeficiency virus (HIV) type 1, hepatitis B virus, or hepatitis C virus in contaminated blood.

Most patients with perioperative AION are over 40 years of age and have typical vascular risk factors for AION, including hypertension, coronary artery disease, diabetes mellitus, and a history of smoking. Both eyes are affected in about 60% of cases. Visual acuities are worse than 20/100 in over 50%, and substantial recovery of vision is unusual. Optic disc swelling is present at the time of initial visual loss in most cases, but it can be delayed in appearance by several days. In most of these cases, the optic nerve is the *only* site of infarction by both clinical and imaging criteria, underscoring the apparent selective vulnerability of the optic nerve to hypotension and anemia. These patients may be anatomically predisposed to AION in having optic discs that are small with little or no cupping, consistent with a "disc at risk." Orbital or ocular compression may play a role in some cases of both AION and PION in which the patient was face down during surgery.

Although severe anemia alone may not cause AION, even a short episode of hypotension in an already anemic patient may predispose to AION-induced vision loss. Because a low hematocrit in the presence of other factors may predispose more surgical patients to visual loss, the current low level of hemoglobin at which blood transfusion is deemed to be indicated (7–8 g/dL) may not be as safe as previously supposed, especially in the setting of hypotension. During the process of "informed consent," we believe it advisable to indicate to patients that postoperative visual loss is a rare complication, but that it occurs especially in situations of hypotension and low hematocrit. This discussion may be most appropriate for patients who are about to undergo procedures associated with induced hypotension or probable significant blood loss but who are reluctant to receive transfusion.

Early recognition of postoperative AION-induced visual loss is important if intervention and possible salvage of vision are to be successful. In rare situations, rapid, aggressive, and early treatment of hypotension and anemia may benefit patients with postsurgical AION. However, vision may continue to decline despite stabilization of blood pressure and blood transfusions.

Unfortunately, delay in the diagnosis of postoperative AION is quite common. In some instances, patients do not complain of loss of vision, either because they are lethargic or sedated and do not recognize the visual loss, or because they have the mistaken impression that postoperative visual loss is an expected occurrence. In other cases, the patient, the patient's nurses, or the patient's physicians assume that there is some other cause for the visual disturbance. An assessment of visual function by means of brief questions and an examination by the anesthesiologist, a member of the surgical team, or an informed nurse in the critical care unit or on the hospital ward may minimize delays in the diagnosis of visual loss and ensure prompt ophthalmologic consultation and treatment, thus optimizing the patient's chance of regaining vision.

A condition called **uremic optic neuropathy** may, at least in some cases, be a form of AION caused by hypotension and anemia. The early recognition of the optic neuropathy may allow for timely correction of the hypotension and anemia, leading to partial recovery of vision. It would appear that at least in some forms of ischemic optic neuropathy, the optic nerve can survive periods of severe ischemia for several hours.

Cases of AION resulting from rapid correction of malignant hypertension occur. The pathogenesis of AION that occurs in this setting is likely related to impaired autoregulation of the nutrient vessels supplying the optic nerve head and to reduction in perfusion pressure, leading to ischemia.

Probably related to AION associated with systemic blood loss is the "optic neuritis" associated with **favism.** Favism occurs rarely in the United States but is well known in Mediterranean countries, where it occurs after fava beans are eaten. Persons who are sensitive develop an acute hemolytic anemia from loss of reduced glutathione and impaired survival of erythrocytes hereditarily deficient in glucose-6-phosphate dehydrogenase. Sudden visual loss associated with optic disc swelling after eating fava beans likely represents AION in this setting.

Nocturnal hypotension has been implicated as a causative factor in the pathogenesis of AION. In one study, for example, 24-hour ambulatory blood pressure measurements documented a decrease in mean systolic and diastolic blood pressure measurements at night. In another study, there was a significant association of nocturnal hypotension and AION, characterized by progressive visual field loss in patients with arterial hypertension who were taking oral hypotensive therapy. These studies suggest that nocturnal hypotension, particularly when associated with other vascular risk factors, may reduce the optic nerve head blood flow below a critical level and thereby may play a role in the pathogenesis of AION. Not all studies show similar results, however. For example, one study showed that patients with NAION did not differ from control subjects with respect to the nighttime diastolic nadir or daytime peak systolic blood pressure. Patients with NAION did, however, have a lower daytime mean blood pressure and a lag in the usual rise in blood pressure in the morning to meet increasing demands of perfusion. This study suggests that the greatest risk for ischemia may not be during the nocturnal nadir of sleep but rather in the subsequent early daytime hours, when patients with NAION do not mount as steep a rise in blood pressure to achieve normal daytime levels as rapidly as do normal persons. Abnormal vascular autoregulation or overtreated hypertension may lead to chronic hypoperfusion of the nutrient vessels of the optic nerve head that in susceptible optic discs (i.e., discs at risk) predisposes to AION. It is often claimed that patients with NAION usually discover the visual loss upon awakening in the morning, thus suggesting that acute ischemia from severe nocturnal hypotension is the *immediate* preceding cause of NAION. This argument is not supported by data from the IONDT, which reported that 41% of patients *did not* experience visual loss within the first 2 hours of awakening. The fact that 42% of patients with NAION in the IONDT did experience visual loss within 2 hours of awakening may simply reflect a uniform distribution of NAION onset throughout the day; that is, (8 hours sleep + 2 hours awake)/24 hours $\times$ 100% = 42%.

Some investigators have reported an association of **elevated intraocular pressure** (IOP) and glaucoma with NAION. These authors suggest that because perfusion pressure in the optic nerve is a balance between systemic blood pressure and IOP, a transient rise in IOP could result in ischemia to the optic nerve head from a fall in perfusion pressure below some critical level. Several other studies, including the IONDT, have found no association of elevated IOP and NAION, so the role of elevated IOP in the pathogenesis of NAION remains unclear.

NAION may occur in the setting of **migraine.** Vasospasm is the presumed underlying mechanism and also may be responsible for the NAION that has been reported in patients with acute intermittent porphyria and in patients with severe preeclampsia.

Numerous investigators have described AION occurring after uncomplicated **cataract extraction.** In most cases, the interval between cataract extraction and visual loss is 4 to 6 weeks. It is therefore likely that most, if not all, of these cases are examples of spontaneously occurring NAION in patients who have happened to undergo recent eye surgery. However, occasional cases with a more convincing temporal relationship suggest there may indeed be some association. One theory is that the condition occurs from a rise in IOP in the immediate postoperative period.

As noted above, a variety of systemic disorders may be found in patients with otherwise typical NAION. Some of these associations are probably fortuitous. In rare cases, NAION is associated with cavernous sinus thrombosis, presumably from decreased flow through the posterior ciliary arteries as a result of elevated intraorbital and intraocular pressure. Blunt trauma may be another unusual cause of AION.

Although **radiation optic neuropathy** (RON) is almost always a retrobulbar process (see below), rare patients with this condition present with evidence of an *anterior* optic neuropathy that is characterized by optic disc swelling, peripapillary hemorrhages, and retinal exudates. Such cases usually occur in the setting of radiation retinopathy following treatment of orbital or intraocular lesions, rather than intracranial lesions.

Clinical Characteristics

Typically, the first visual symptoms noticed by patients with NAION are blurred central vision, loss of part of the visual field, or both. Some patients lose all vision in the eye. In most patients, there are no symptoms of transient visual loss prior to the development of sudden visual loss; however, some patients complain of spots, a shadow, a veil, or a curtain in a portion of the field of vision just before more complete visual loss. Of patients in the IONDT, 5% reported their initial visual loss as intermittent.

The loss of vision in NAION is usually painless; however, 8 to 12% of patients report discomfort behind or around the eye at the time of visual loss. The pain in patients with NAION is usually mild and almost never associated with eye movement. Thus, although pain or ocular discomfort is more common in patients with anterior optic neuritis (noted by greater than 90% of patients) than in NAION, this complaint does not exclude a diagnosis of NAION.

Variability in initial visual acuity in patients with NAION ranges from 20/20 or better to no light perception. Among those studies providing visual acuity data from the initial appearance of symptoms, 31 to 52% of patients have initial acuity better than 20/64, whereas 34 to 54% have acuity worse than 20/200. In the IONDT, patients with visual acuity better than 20/64 were significantly younger and had a lower incidence of diabetes mellitus and hypertension compared with those with a visual acuity worse than 20/64. Other studies also suggest that patients under 65 years of age present with significantly better initial visual acuity than patients over age 65.

Almost all patients with NAION have diminished color perception on the affected side. The degree of color vision loss, as demonstrated by testing with pseudoisochromatic plates, often appears to be directly related to the amount of visual acuity loss (as opposed to patients with optic neuritis in whom color vision may be significantly impaired despite minimal loss of visual acuity).

Visual field defects develop in almost all eyes with NAION, although they may be difficult to detect in mild cases, particularly when the field is tested by kinetic perimetry instead of static perimetry. Altitudinal defects (Fig. 7.1) comprise the most common pattern of visual field loss, occurring in 55 to 80% of cases. Most of the defects are inferior and in many cases spare fixation. Decreased sensitivity of the ''spared'' altitudinal hemifield, as demonstrated on automated perimetry, suggests more extensive ischemia to the optic nerve head than might be expected from the results of kinetic perimetry. Other types of optic nerve–related visual field defects that occur in NAION include central scotomas, arcuate defects, quadrantic defects, generalized constriction of the field, or a combination of these (see Fig. 7.1).

Almost every eye with NAION has a relative afferent pupillary defect. The only exceptions are patients in whom there is preexisting or concurrent damage to the retina or optic nerve of the opposite eye. In general, the worse the visual acuity or visual field, the more obvious the afferent pupillary defect.

Ophthalmoscopic examination in patients with NAION shows a swollen optic disc, with the swelling being either diffuse (in about 75% of cases) or focal (in about 25% of cases) (Fig. 7.2). When diffuse, the swelling may be massive, thus simulating the choked disc appearance of papilledema, or it may be mild, with only slight blurring of the peripapillary nerve fiber layer. When it is focal, the swelling often corresponds to the visual field defect. Whether diffuse or focal, disc swelling in NAION may be pale or hyperemic, although pale swelling is more

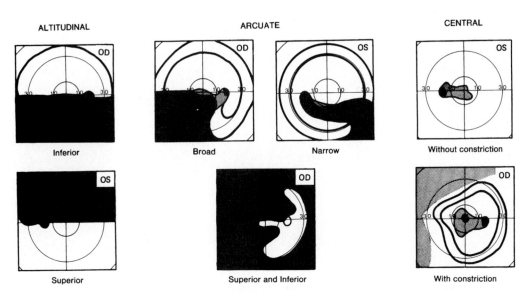

Figure 7.1. Typical visual field defects in anterior ischemic optic neuropathy. Altitudinal and arcuate defects occur in the majority of cases, but central scotomas, peripheral constriction, and combinations of these defects are not uncommon. (Redrawn from Boghen DR, Glaser JS. Ischaemic optic neuropathy: The clinical profile and natural history. Brain 1975;98:689–708.)

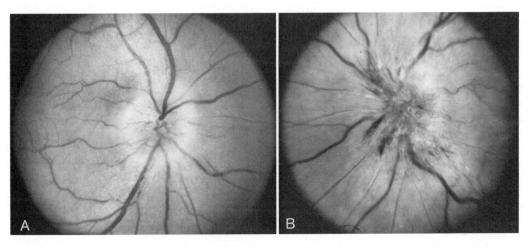

Figure 7.2. Ophthalmoscopic appearance of nonarteritic anterior ischemic optic neuropathy. *A.* Pallid swelling of the optic disc associated with a few small flame-shaped hemorrhages at the disc margin. *B.* Hyperemic swelling of the optic disc associated with numerous hemorrhages and a few soft exudates.

common. In most cases, single or multiple flame-shaped hemorrhages are present at or near the disc margin. Cotton-wool spots are almost never seen (as opposed to arteritic AION—see below), but retinal arteries are often focally or generally narrowed and attenuated. Hard exudates occur in about 7% of cases, resulting in a hemi-star or, rarely, a complete star figure in the macula (Fig. 7.3). Such cases may initially be misdiagnosed as neuroretinitis (see Chapter 6).

Not all ischemic changes that occur at the level of the optic disc produce obvious disc swelling. Infarcts can occur in the prelaminar portion of the optic disc that are unassociated

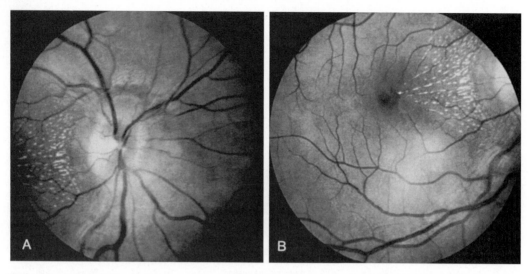

Figure 7.3. Anterior ischemic optic neuropathy with star formation. Note that the macular star is incomplete, being present only in the nasal part of the macula.

with disc swelling. Such patients, some of whom have systemic hypertension, typically have the sudden onset of visual disturbance usually associated with relatively good visual acuity and small arcuate or paracentral field defects. Ophthalmoscopy in the acute stage often reveals a small nerve fiber layer hemorrhage at the disc margin. Within several days, the affected portion of the disc becomes pale and is associated with a shallow increase in the optic cup that may be mistaken for glaucomatous change despite repeatedly normal intraocular pressures. As a rule, patients who develop this syndrome of focal disc infarction do not experience progression of either visual acuity or field loss, although they may develop subsequent similar events in the same eye (as opposed to patients with NAION who rarely develop subsequent attacks in the involved eye).

Fluorescein angiography in NAION demonstrates delayed optic disc filling; however, there is no consistent delay in adjacent peripapillary choroidal filling. In contrast, arteritic AION is characterized by marked delays in choroidal filling (see below).

Course

Deterioration of visual acuity, and occasionally of visual field, may progress over several days or even weeks after onset of NAION. The proportion of patients with worsening vision, as reported in the literature, ranges from a "few"

to 36%. The majority of patients stabilize within 10 days, although up to 10% of patients continue to worsen thereafter. Like visual acuity, visual field defects may change over time, with worsening of defects reported in 3 to 30% of patients.

Focal hyperemic telangiectatic vessels may appear on the optic disc of an eye with NAION within days to weeks after the onset of symptoms (Fig. 7.4). This phenomenon has been interpreted as luxury perfusion, a vascular autoregulatory response to ischemia characterized by dilation of blood vessels and increased perfusion of tissues in a region surrounding an infarct. It is associated with focal early disc hyperfluorescence and corresponds to a spared region of the visual field. In some instances, this vascular response is so impressive that it is misinterpreted as a capillary hemangioma or neovascularization of the disc.

After the acute episode of disc swelling, optic atrophy rapidly develops and is associated with further narrowing and constriction of retinal arteries (especially proximally) and resolution of hemorrhages and exudates (Fig. 7.5). The disc morphology does not markedly change after NAION, as opposed to arteritic AION, in which the disc shows increased cupping mimicking that of glaucoma.

Visual Outcome

Comparing various studies in regard to final visual acuity of patients with NAION is prob-

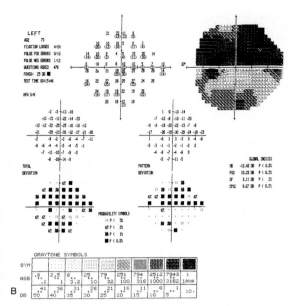

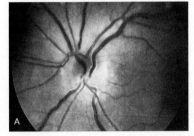

Figure 7.4. Luxury perfusion and its association with anterior ischemic optic neuropathy. *A.* Hyperemic area of luxury perfusion superiorly in an otherwise pale left optic disc after anterior ischemic optic neuropathy. *B.* Static perimetry shows superior altitudinal defect corresponding to inferior disc pallor and spared visual field corresponding to area of disc with luxury perfusion. (Reprinted with permission from Friedland S, Winterkorn JMS, Burde RM. Luxury perfusion following anterior ischemic optic neuropathy. J Neuroophthalmol 1996;16:163–171.)

lematic, because of variable follow-up times, incomplete follow-up, and the fact that final visual acuity is often reported only for a subset of the original patients. In the IONDT, approximately 52% of randomized patients (i.e., those with initial visual acuity of 20/64 or worse) had visual acuities of 20/200 or worse at the 6-month follow-up visit, and this figure increased to 58% at the 30-month follow-up visit. Other studies report that 31 to 41% of patients with NAION have a final visual acuity of 20/200 or worse, and 21 to 53% of patients have a final visual acuity of 20/40 or better. The most unexpected and encouraging finding from the IONDT was the high rate of spontaneous improvement of visual acuity observed in the untreated randomized group. At the 6-month evaluation, 42.7% of patients in this group improved by three or more lines from their baseline evaluation. One reason for this high rate of improvement compared with earlier studies may be that follow-up times in prior studies varied and may have been insufficient in some cases to detect improvement.

Recurrent NAION

NAION rarely affects the same eye more than once, with recurrences reported in less than 5%

of patients. When NAION does recur, it does not indicate any underlying abnormalities other than the general risk factors noted for all patients with NAION. Two theories have been advanced to explain the rarity of recurrence in NAION. Some investigators believe that the blood supply from the infarcted area of the disc may be shunted to the remainder of the disc, thus providing protection from further ischemia. Others suggest that because crowding of nerve fibers in a tight scleral canal may predispose certain optic discs to NAION (see below), subsequent atrophy of infarcted axons may relieve this crowding and reduce the probability of a subsequent attack of NAION.

Disc Swelling Preceding Visual Loss

Patients may develop disc swelling from NAION *before* they have any visual symptoms. In such cases, the patient may be thought to have papilledema or a compressive optic neuropathy from an orbital mass. Often, however, the asymptomatic disc swelling is noted in the fellow eye of a patient with a history of a previous attack of NAION, and the diagnosis is less confusing. Although in most cases the patient eventually becomes visually symptomatic, the swell-

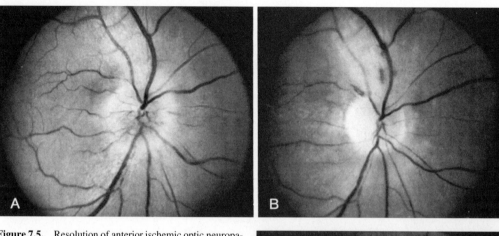

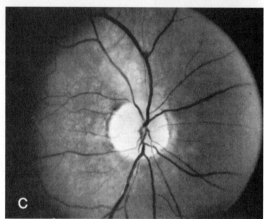

Figure 7.5. Resolution of anterior ischemic optic neuropathy. *A.* In the acute phase of visual loss, the right optic disc is hyperemic and swollen. *B.* Two weeks after the onset of visual loss, the temporal portion of the disc has become pale. The nasal disc is still slightly swollen, and there are a few small, nerve fiber layer hemorrhages. Note the apparent narrowing of retinal arteries and arterioles. *C.* Two months after visual loss, the disc is diffusely pale with loss of the nerve fiber layer and apparent narrowing of retinal arteries and arterioles. Visual acuity remained 20/100 throughout this period.

ing occasionally resolves with no permanent sequelae. This phenomenon seems to occur with increased frequency in patients with diabetes mellitus (see below).

Diabetic Papillopathy

An atypical form of NAION called **diabetic papillopathy** occurs most commonly in young diabetic patients. In most instances, transient unilateral or bilateral disc swelling develops in a juvenile diabetic who has minimal if any visual symptoms, and the swelling resolves spontaneously within several weeks. In some cases, there is a transient arcuate field defect; in others, the field defect persists. In most cases, however, there is only enlargement of the blind spot. When visual acuity is initially affected, it usually recovers as the disc swelling resolves. Eyes with diabetic papillopathy usually show prominent, dilated, telangiectatic vessels over the disc that

mimic optic disc neovascularization (Fig. 7.6) but do not share the same fluorescein angiographic features. This phenomenon is akin to the luxury perfusion phenomenon described after typical NAION. As disc swelling resolves, these vessels usually disappear, although they may occasionally persist. Diabetic papillopathy may develop in eyes with evidence of both preproliferative and proliferative diabetic retinopathy as well as in eyes with no evidence of retinopathy.

It must be emphasized that patients with juvenile diabetes mellitus may also develop typical NAION, with persistent decrease in visual acuity and permanent visual field defects. In some patients, true disc neovascularization develops after resolution of visual symptoms and disc swelling. Although diabetic papillopathy was initially described in juvenile diabetics, the condition also may occur in patients with adult-onset diabetes mellitus.

Patients with diabetic papillopathy, like patients with typical NAION, have a disc at risk. Thus, although the clinical features of diabetic papillopathy are different from those of typical NAION, this condition probably is a variant of NAION with a similar pathogenesis.

Bilateral NAION

NAION in both eyes, occurring simultaneously or nonsimultaneously, has been reported in 10.5 to 73.0% of patients. The majority of patients who experience NAION in both eyes do so **nonsimultaneously.** Retrospective studies suggest that the risk of bilateral sequential NAION is 12% within 2 years and 19% within 5 years. The IONDT continues to prospectively follow patients enrolled in the study. During a follow-up period ranging from 1 to 3 years, 25 of 216 patients (12%) randomized to treatment or nontreatment (i.e., with baseline visual acuity of 20/64 or worse in the affected eye; see below) developed NAION in the second eye. Among patients enrolled in the study but not randomized (i.e., patients with baseline visual acuity better than 20/64 in the better eye), 5 of 136 (4%) developed involvement in the second eye. This latter group, as noted above, was younger and had a lower prevalence of hypertension and diabetes mellitus compared with the randomized group.

Patients with bilateral, nonsimultaneous NAION present to the ophthalmologist with optic disc swelling in one eye and optic atrophy in the other (Fig. 7.7). Although the appearance of the ocular fundi may suggest the Foster Kennedy syndrome, the history and clinical picture are entirely different because the patient has experienced *acute* loss of visual function in the eye with the swollen disc and also has a history of *sudden* visual loss in the opposite eye with the pale disc. These symptoms are inconsistent with papilledema and increased intracranial pressure but are typical of ischemia or inflammation.

Bilateral, **simultaneous** NAION occurs, but it is rare compared with the frequency of occurrence of bilateral simultaneous arteritic AION (see below). Nevertheless, a special type of NAION that occurs in juvenile diabetics presents simultaneously in both eyes in up to 30% of patients (see above).

Few studies compare the visual outcome between affected eyes in patients with bilateral NAION, and those that do provide conflicting results. In some studies, there is a correlation between affected eyes with respect to visual acuity, color vision, and visual fields, whereas in others no such correlation can be demonstrated.

Pathogenesis

NAION is thought to be caused by vascular insufficiency leading to optic nerve head ischemia. This hypothesis is supported by several observations, including the abrupt onset of vision loss typical for vascular disease, the common occurrence of the condition in older patients

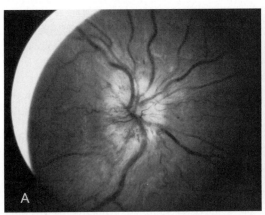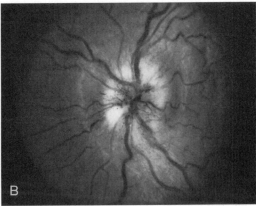

Figure 7.6. Appearance of diabetic papillopathy. The patient was an 18-year-old man with juvenile diabetes mellitus who was noted to have optic disc swelling during a routine eye examination. He had no visual complaints. Note dilated telangiectatic vessels mimicking neovascularization on the surface of both optic discs. *A.* Right optic disc. *B.* Left optic disc.

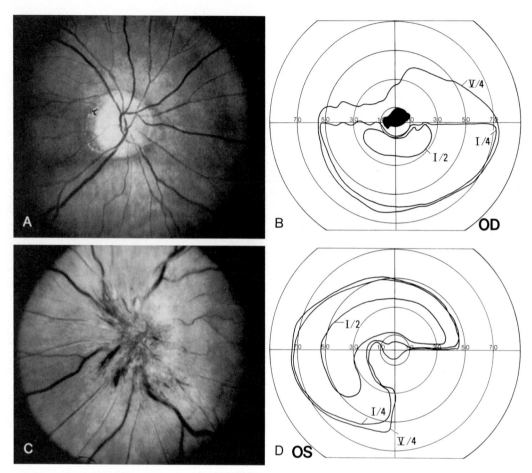

Figure 7.7. Pseudo-Foster Kennedy syndrome in a patient with bilateral, nonsimultaneous anterior ischemic optic neuropathy. *A.* The right optic disc is pale, and the arteries are narrowed. *B.* The right visual field shows a relative, superior altitudinal defect with a central scotoma. *C.* The left optic disc is hyperemic and swollen with numerous superficial retinal hemorrhages and several soft exudates. *D.* The left visual field shows a complete, inferior arcuate defect. The patient gave a history of sudden visual loss in the right eye followed 3 months later by sudden visual loss in the left eye. Visual acuity was 20/400 in the right eye and 20/50 in the left eye.

with underlying systemic vasculopathies, pathologic evidence of closure of small blood vessels in some specimens, lack of clinical or histopathologic evidence of inflammation, and experimental production of an NAION-like picture in monkeys from occlusion of the posterior ciliary arteries.

The critical regions of damage in both nonarteritic and arteritic AION are the prelaminar, laminar, and immediately retrolaminar portions of the optic nerve. Although the most superficial portion of the prelaminar optic nerve head is supplied by branches of the central retinal artery, both the prelaminar and laminar portions of the optic nerve head are supplied primarily by branches of the posterior ciliary arteries (Fig. 7.8). The contribution of the peripapillary choroid to the anterior optic nerve is minimal compared with the direct contribution from the paraoptic branches of the short posterior ciliary arteries. Posterior to the lamina cribrosa, the optic nerve is supplied primarily by the pial plexus, which receives contributions from the posterior ciliary arteries, extraneural branches of the central retinal artery, and small branches from various orbital arteries. The particular vas-

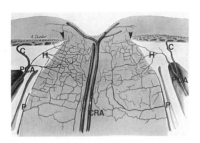

Figure 7.8. Composite illustration to scale of the vascular supply of the optic disc and retrolaminar optic nerve. Venous vessels and superficial central retinal artery (CRA) are not drawn in full. In the retrolaminar portion of the nerve, branches of the central retinal artery and the pial arteries (P) anastomose to supply the nerve tissue. The laminar and immediately prelaminar portions of the nerve are supplied primarily by branches (H) of the posterior ciliary arteries (PCA). Although some arterial branches extend from the choroid to the optic nerve head (*arrowheads*), these are small and inconsequential. C: choroidal branches of the posterior ciliary arteries. (Reprinted with permission from Lieberman MF, Maumenee AE, Green WR. Histologic studies of the vasculature of the anterior optic nerve. Am J Ophthalmol 1976;82:405–423.)

terior ciliary arteries may result in optic disc hypoperfusion and infarction that results in an altitudinal pattern of visual field involvement.

There are many mechanisms by which local and systemic diseases could interfere with the blood supply of the optic nerve head. Blood flow in the optic nerve head is directly proportional to the perfusion pressure (mean blood pressure minus intraocular pressure) and is inversely proportional to the vascular resistance in its blood vessels. Vascular resistance is influenced by the efficiency of autoregulation of blood flow and by blood vessel wall changes, both of which may be affected to a varying degree by disease states such as hypertension, diabetes mellitus, arteriosclerosis, and vasospasm.

Besides vascular anatomic considerations, structural and mechanical factors may render the optic disc more susceptible to vascular damage. The optic discs of patients with NAION are usually small, with little or no physiologic cupping. A small cup-to-disc ratio implies a small optic disc diameter and smaller scleral canal. Thus,

cular anatomy of the laminar and prelaminar portions of the optic nerve head may render these regions especially vulnerable to infarction. Functional properties of the disc vasculature (e.g., the capacity of optic disc vessels to autoregulate) may also play a role in this vulnerability.

The prelaminar and laminar portions of the optic nerve are supplied by an elliptical arterial "circle" (i.e., Zinn's corona or Haller's circle) formed by anastomoses around the optic nerve between medial and lateral paraoptic short posterior ciliary arteries (Fig. 7.9). Branches originating from this arterial circle run anteriorly to the peripapillary choroid, transversely to the optic nerve (prelaminar and laminar region), and posteriorly to the pial plexus system. The location of the circle is approximately 200 to 300 microns posterior to the suprachoroidal space. The arterial circle usually cannot be visualized with fluorescein angiography because of blockage of fluorescence by the sclera. The ellipse is divided into superior and inferior parts by the entry points of the lateral and medial short posterior ciliary arteries, providing an altitudinal blood supply to the anterior optic nerve (see Fig. 7.9). Reduced perfusion pressure within the territory of the paraoptic branches of the short pos-

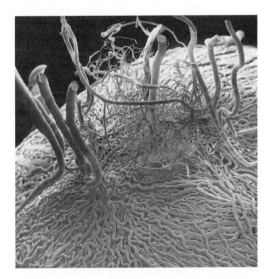

Figure 7.9. Low-power scanning electron micrograph showing the vasculature of the posterior aspect of the globe as viewed from behind the globe. The posterior ciliary arteries (long and short) are visualized as are their branches to the choroid and optic nerve head. Note that the Zinn-Haller arterial circle is really two half circles that are separated at the horizontal meridian. (Reprinted with permission from Risco JM, Grimson BS, Johnson PT. Angioarchitecture of the ciliary artery circulation of the posterior pole. Arch Ophthalmol 1981;99:864–868.)

discs with NAION tend to have small scleral openings and crowding of the nerve fibers as they pass through a restricted space in the lamina cribrosa and optic disc. Axoplasmic flow stasis is responsible for the optic disc swelling in AION, and subclinical ischemia caused by hypoperfusion or loss of autoregulation could lead to axoplasmic stasis. This, in turn, could cause further compression of capillaries located among the nerve fiber bundles in the restricted space of the optic nerve head. Thus, a cycle develops in which ischemia increases the stasis of axoplasmic flow within the axons, the axons swell and compress adjacent capillaries, and further ischemia occurs.

The finding that optic discs with NAION tend to be smaller than discs with arteritic AION also has diagnostic implications. Because the vast majority of both optic discs and cups of the fellow eyes of NAION are small, a large cup in the fellow eye should raise the physician's index of suspicion of giant cell arteritis (see below). A small cup is nondiagnostic, however, because it may be associated with either arteritic or nonarteritic AION.

As noted above, the morphology of the optic disc in patients with NAION probably explains the rarity with which recurrent NAION occurs. It is postulated that the initial optic nerve infarct reduces the number of fibers in the scleral canal, thereby decompressing the remaining fibers and protecting them from further ischemic damage. It has even been speculated that NAION might be prevented in an at-risk second eye by performing panretinal photocoagulation to reduce the number of axons passing through the optic nerve, thus decompressing the scleral canal.

The typical optic disc seen in patients with NAION is called a "disc at risk" and is characterized by a small physiologic cup, elevation of the disc margins by a thick nerve fiber layer, anomalies of blood vessel branching, and the appearance of a crowded and small optic nerve head. One feature of the optic disc that may put it at risk is that the retinal ganglion cell axons make a 90° turn as they penetrate the lamina cribrosa. It may be that high energy demands are placed on the axoplasmic transport system to overcome the mechanical features of this sharp turn. Any process that leads to relative energy deficiency (e.g., hypoperfusion from deficient autoregulation) may produce swelling of axons, thus compressing small vessels and initiating the cycle of ischemia described above. Although speculative, these theories serve as useful conceptual models that suggest possible directions for future research into the pathogenesis and treatment of NAION.

Pathologic material in patients with NAION is rare. Interestingly, although NAION is thought to be caused by occlusion of posterior ciliary arteries supplying the laminar, prelaminar, and immediate retrolaminar portions of the optic disc, pathologic studies generally have shown no evidence of this process. The pathogenesis of NAION is likely multifactorial, and the size and shape of the optic disc and the optic cup may be more important than the mechanism by which ischemia occurs. The available evidence strongly favors abnormal blood flow that may be related to disturbances in autoregulation, decreased perfusion, or thrombus formation.

Treatment

Although both medical and surgical treatment have been proposed for patients with NAION, no therapy is of significant benefit. For example, numerous drugs have been used to treat patients with NAION, including anticoagulants, diphenylhydantoin, sub-Tenon's injections of vasodilators, intravenous norepinephrine, thrombolytic agents, corticosteroids, and aspirin. None of these agents is convincingly beneficial in improving visual outcome, nor is heparin-induced low-density lipoprotein/fibrinogen precipitation. Studies showing some degree of visual improvement in patients with long-standing NAION treated with the combination of levodopa and carbidopa (Sinemet) or hemodilution have not been confirmed.

Attempts to treat acute NAION surgically have also proved ineffective. Stellate ganglion block has been used without success, as has optic nerve sheath fenestration. In particular, the efficacy of optic nerve sheath fenestration in the treatment of eyes with NAION was evaluated in a multicenter randomized clinical trial funded by the National Eye Institute, The Ischemic Optic Neuropathy Decompression Trial. Eligible patients were 50 years of age or older and had best-corrected visual acuity of 20/64 or worse in the affected eye, optic disc swelling, and a relative afferent pupillary defect. A baseline eligibility visit was performed within 14 days of onset of visual symptoms, and eligible patients were randomized to surgery or follow-up. Surgery was performed within 14 days of the onset of symptoms in order to optimize the timing of treatment of NAION.

Patients eligible for randomization by all criteria except that visual acuity was better than 20/64 at the baseline examination were also enrolled in the study but were not randomized unless the visual acuity in their affected eye deteriorated to 20/64 or worse within 30 days from the onset of symptoms. Late-entry patients were defined as having progressive NAION for the purposes of the study.

The IONDT ceased recruitment in 1994, on the recommendation of its Data and Safety Monitoring Committee, because it had become clear that patients assigned to surgery did not have a better outcome than patients assigned to follow-up only. When improvement was defined as improvement in visual acuity of three or more lines at 6 months, 32.6% of the surgery group improved, compared with 42.7% of the group randomized to follow-up. Similarly, there was no difference in the visual outcome with respect to visual field abnormalities in the treated and untreated patients based on initial and final mean deviations. In addition, patients who underwent surgery had a significantly greater risk of losing three or more lines of vision at 6 months—23.9% in the surgery group compared with 12.4% in the follow-up group. No difference in the effect of treatment on either visual acuity or visual field was observed in patients with progressive NAION compared with nonprogressive NAION. Thus, the results from the IONDT indicated that optic nerve decompression surgery for NAION was not only ineffective, but was possibly harmful and should not be used to treat NAION.

Prevention

Two reports have evaluated the role of aspirin in reducing the risk of NAION in the second eye following the occurrence in the first eye. In one retrospective study of 100 patients with NAION, second eye NAION developed within 2 years in 10 of the 57 (17.5%) patients who were aspirin users and in 23 of the 43 (53.5%) who were not aspirin users, thus suggesting a beneficial effect of aspirin in reducing second eye events. However, in a second retrospective cohort study, the rate of second eye involvement in 153 patients with NAION who were aspirin users was compared with 278 patients not taking aspirin for any reason. The 2-year cumulative probability of second eye NAION was 7% in the aspirin user group and 15% in the nonuser group, whereas the 5-year cumulative probabilities in the two groups were 17% and 20%, respectively. These findings suggest a possible short-term (1 to 2 years) benefit, but little or no long-term (5 years) benefit of aspirin in reducing the risk of second eye NAION. The results of these studies must be viewed with caution, however, because standardized controlled protocols were not used.

ARTERITIC ANTERIOR ISCHEMIC OPTIC NEUROPATHY

Although AION can be caused by a variety of different vasculitides (see below), the most common vasculitic process is giant cell arteritis (GCA, or temporal arteritis). Conversely, AION is the most common cause of visual loss in patients with GCA. Arteritic AION has been implicated as the cause of visual loss in GCA in 71 to 83% of cases, with central and branch retinal artery occlusion, choroidal infarction, and PION accounting for the remaining cases. In contrast, only about 5% of patients with AION have GCA.

The average age of patients with arteritic AION is significantly higher than that of patients with NAION. This reflects the fact that the incidence of GCA increases with age, from 2.3 per 100,000 among patients in the sixth decade of life to 44.7 per 100,000 for patients in their ninth decade.

Clinical Characteristics

Visual loss caused by arteritic AION may occur abruptly, or it may be preceded by several episodes of transient monocular loss of vision that occasionally may be induced by activity or changes in posture. The characteristics of the visual loss are identical with those of the transient monocular visual loss encountered in patients with atherosclerotic, cerebrovascular, or cardiovascular disease. The episodes are caused by transient ischemia of the optic nerve, retina, choroid, or a combination of these structures, and they may be followed by central or branch retinal arterial occlusion, choroidal infarction, or ischemic optic neuropathy.

Patients with arteritic AION generally have more severe visual loss than do patients with NAION. Loss of vision is usually profound, with 70% of patients having visual acuity of 20/200 or worse and many patients seeing less than hand motions. The profound visual loss seen in arteritic AION may be related not only to the severe optic nerve ischemia that occurs in GCA but also to the added effects of concurrent retinal or choroidal ischemia.

Visual field defects in patients with arteritic AION tend to be more extensive than those in patients with NAION. The predominant patterns of visual field loss in testable eyes are altitudinal and arcuate defects.

The affected optic disc in arteritic AION usually shows milky or pale swelling, indicating true infarction of nerve tissue, although hyperemic disc swelling is occasionally seen. Cotton-wool spots and flame-shaped intraretinal hemorrhages may be present in the peripapillary region (Figs. 7.10 and 7.11).

Unlike the optic discs of patients with NAION, which are smaller and have a smaller cup-to-disc ratio compared with normal controls (see above), the optic discs of patients with arteritic AION may be of any size. Thus, a small disc and cup or a normal disc with a small cup may be associated with either arteritic or nonarteritic AION, whereas a normal or large cup in a patient with AION should raise the physician's index of suspicion for GCA.

Course

The natural history of arteritic AION is progressive visual loss and involvement of the second eye in 25 to 50% of patients within days or weeks if treatment with corticosteroids is not begun immediately or is stopped while the disease is still active. With time, the disc swelling resolves, the optic disc becomes pale, and the retinal arteries become narrow. Glaucomatous-like optic disc cupping may develop in some eyes after arteritic AION. This is in contrast to the optic disc morphology after NAION, which does not change as the disc becomes atrophic. Specifically, optic disc cupping does not develop in cases of NAION.

Pathogenesis and Pathology

Arteritic AION is caused by inflammatory occlusion of the short posterior ciliary arteries that supply the immediate retrolaminar and laminar portions of the optic disc (Fig. 7.12). The inflammation may also produce sectorial areas of choroidal ischemia (Fig. 7.13). Most of the orbital vessels—including the ophthalmic artery, posterior ciliary arteries, and the intraneural central retinal artery—may be affected by the arteritic process. Arteritis of intraocular vessels is rare, however; this is probably related to the lack of

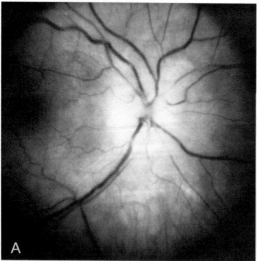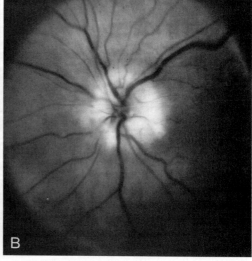

Figure 7.10. Bilateral simultaneous anterior ischemic optic neuropathy in a patient with giant cell arteritis. The patient was an 81-year-old woman with a 4-month history of headaches, malaise, and scalp tenderness who suddenly lost vision in both eyes. When initially examined, she had no light perception in either eye. *A–B.* The right and left optic discs show marked pale swelling. An erythrocyte sedimentation rate was markedly elevated. The patient refused a temporal artery biopsy.

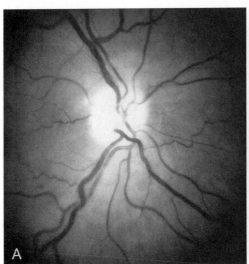 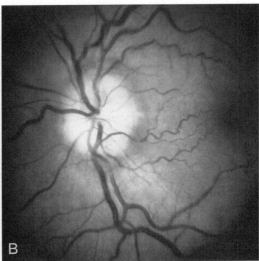

Figure 7.11. Bilateral nonsimultaneous anterior ischemic optic neuropathy in a patient with giant cell arteritis. The patient was a 77-year-old woman with a 2-week history of headache and jaw pain who suddenly lost vision in the right eye. The right optic disc was noted to be swollen. A diagnosis of anterior ischemic optic neuropathy was made, but no evaluation was performed. Six weeks later, the patient lost vision in the left eye. Visual acuity was 20/100 OD and 20/400 OS. *A.* The right optic disc is pale and still slightly swollen. *B.* The left optic disc is moderately swollen and pale. Note that neither disc has a large optic cup. An erythrocyte sedimentation rate was elevated, and a temporal artery biopsy confirmed the diagnosis of giant cell arteritis.

an internal elastic lamina in these vessels. Involvement of the posterior ciliary arteries in arteritic processes results in interruption of the normal blood supply to the laminar and retrolaminar portions of the optic nerve, leading to AION. Presumably, it is the extent of damage that dictates the severity of visual acuity and field loss in such patients.

Diagnosis and Ancillary Tests

In the patient with AION, the following should raise suspicion for GCA:

• Advanced age.
• History of headache, scalp tenderness, jaw claudication, ear pain, muscle aches, fatigue, and weight loss.
• Premonitory visual symptoms, such as transient monocular visual loss or diplopia.

Patients who complain of transient or permanent monocular or binocular loss of vision or diplopia should be questioned *specifically* about systemic symptoms of GCA. Bilateral involvement and concurrent signs of retinal circulation ischemia, such as cotton-wool spots or retinal infarction,

are other features that suggest an arteritic etiology of AION.

Ancillary testing suggestive of temporal arteritis includes an elevated erythrocyte sedimentation rate (ESR). An elevated ESR is found in over 95% of patients with biopsy-proven GCA, although the degree of elevation does not predict which patients are at increased risk for the development of ocular complications of the disease. In addition, between 8 and 22% of patients with clinical symptoms suggesting GCA and a positive temporal artery biopsy have an ESR within the normal range. Thus, the finding of a normal ESR in a patient with symptoms or signs suggesting GCA should not dissuade the physician from proceeding with a temporal artery biopsy.

Most authors recommend that the Westergren method be used to determine the ESR in patients with suspected GCA. Although there have been no definitive studies regarding the range of the ESR in normal persons, we recommend that physicians divide a patient's age by 2 to determine the maximum normal ESR for men and divide the age plus 10 by 2 to determine the maximum normal ESR for women. Thus, the maximum normal ESR for a 70-year-old man is

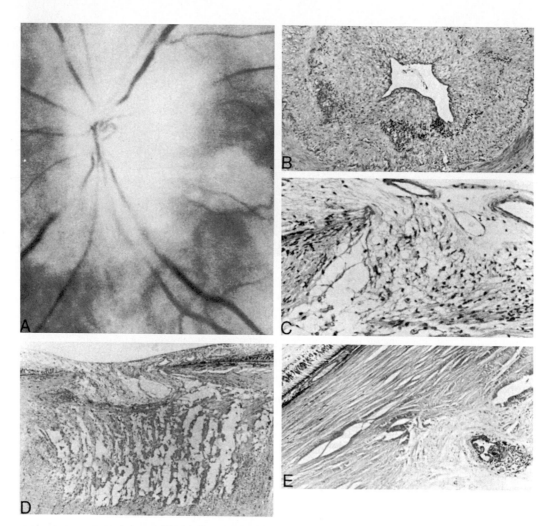

Figure 7.12. Pathology of arteritic anterior ischemic optic neuropathy. The patient was a 68-year-old man with a 4-week history of severe headache, scalp tenderness, and anorexia who suddenly lost vision in the left eye. Visual acuity was 20/50 OD and no light perception OS. The intraocular pressure in the left eye was 7 mm Hg compared with 13 mm Hg in the right eye. *A.* The left optic disc shows marked pale swelling with peripapillary retinal edema. An erythrocyte sedimentation rate was 125 mm/hour. The patient was placed on intravenous methylprednisolone, and a temporal artery biopsy was performed. *B.* The biopsy specimen shows thickening of the intima and necrosis of the media, with infiltration of the entire wall by lymphocytes, epithelioid cells, and giant cells. There is disintegration of the internal elastic lamina and narrowing of the lumen of the vessel. Ten days after starting treatment, the patient developed a right hemiparesis and progressive loss of consciousness. He died 18 days after the onset of visual symptoms. *C.* Longitudinal section through the proximal portion of the affected optic nerve shows persistent swelling of prelaminar, peripheral nerve axons. *D.* Another longitudinal section shows areas of cavernous atrophy in the prelaminar, laminar, and immediate retrolaminar portions of the affected optic nerve. *E.* Section through a short posterior ciliary artery shows obstruction of the vessel by an inflammatory process consisting of lymphocytes and giant cells. Other arteries in the orbit were similarly affected. (Reprinted with permission from Hinzpeter EN, Naumann G. Ischemic papilledema in giant-cell arteritis: mucopolysaccharide deposition with normal intraocular pressure. Arch Ophthalmol 1976;94:624–628.)

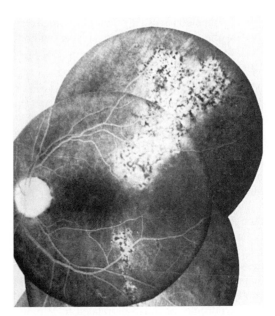

Figure 7.13.   Sectorial choroidal ischemia in a patient with giant cell arteritis. The patient was a 79-year-old woman who suddenly lost vision in the left eye and who had optic disc swelling consistent with an anterior ischemic optic neuropathy. At 2 weeks after the onset of visual loss, the left optic disc is pale, the retinal arteries are narrow, and there is a large, triangular choroidal scar with both hyper- and hypopigmentation in the superotemporal region. A smaller region of scarring is present inferotemporally. (Reprinted with permission from Spolaore R, Gaudric A, Coscas G, et al. Acute sectorial choroidal ischemia. Am J Ophthalmol 1984;98:707–716.)

35 mm/hour and for a 70-year-old woman is 40 mm/hour. Nevertheless, an elevated ESR does not necessarily indicate arteritic AION. The reason for an elevated ESR must be considered for each individual patient, and a temporal artery biopsy should be performed to rule out GCA when it is clinically indicated.

C-reactive protein (CRP) is an acute phase reactant that is present in normal human serum and is increased in a variety of conditions, including GCA. Some authors advocate measuring the concentration of serum CRP in patients with suspected GCA and pursuing the diagnosis further if the CRP is elevated, even if the ESR is not. Indeed, some authors quote a combined sensitivity of diagnosing GCA of 97% when both the ESR and CRP are used as screening tools. We have not been impressed with the usefulness of CRP in diagnosing GCA.

Fluorescein angiography in arteritic AION often demonstrates delayed or absent filling of the choroidal circulation. GCA should be strongly suspected in patients with AION in whom fluorescein dye appearance in the choroid is delayed by more than 15 seconds or in whom choroidal filling is delayed by more than 18 seconds. In patients who present with sudden visual loss and normal optic discs, the finding of delayed choroidal filling on fluorescein angiography suggests PION caused by GCA.

Treatment

AION caused by GCA requires emergency intervention to prevent complete blindness. High doses of corticosteroids must be instituted immediately—prompt initiation of treatment not only may prevent further damage to the affected eye but also may prevent visual loss in the opposite eye. Return of vision following treatment for arteritic AION is rare but occurs in a small percentage (<15%) of patients. There is evidence that early use of high-dose intravenous steroids (at least 1 gram/day of intravenous methylprednisolone) is more effective than low-dose oral steroids in providing improvement in the affected eye and protecting the fellow eye. Unfortunately, further loss of vision in the affected eye and new loss of vision in the previously unaffected fellow eye can occur even during intravenous treatment with high doses of methylprednisolone.

Temporal artery biopsy must be obtained to confirm the diagnosis of GCA, but it should not delay the initiation of treatment. Biopsies are likely to remain positive even after 14 days of steroid therapy. Skip lesions may lead to false-negative biopsy results in 4 to 5% of cases, but such areas are extremely small and unlikely to lead to misdiagnosis as long as a biopsy specimen of several millimeters is obtained. Patients in whom the diagnosis of GCA is strongly suspected but in whom a unilateral temporal artery biopsy is negative should undergo biopsy of the contralateral temporal artery, because this increases the likelihood of a positive biopsy by 8 to 13%.

Vasculitides Other Than Giant Cell Arteritis

Arteritic conditions other than GCA may cause AION, including herpes zoster, relapsing polychondritis, rheumatoid arthritis, Takayasu's arteritis, Behçet's disease, Crohn's disease, and connective tissue disorders such as periarteritis nodosa, systemic lupus erythematosus, and allergic granulomatosis (Churg-Strauss angiitis). The clinical picture is typically that of sudden unilateral or bilateral visual loss, often central and sometimes accompanied by pain, with minimal recovery. Although this clinical picture may suggest a diagnosis of optic neuritis, the etiology is vascular, with fibrinoid necrosis of the arterioles and secondary myelin and axon loss.

VASCULAR OPTIC DISC SWELLING WITHOUT VISUAL LOSS

It is clear that local tissue responses to vascular changes can produce disc swelling that is not associated with visual loss. Such a phenomenon can occur in both systemic hypertension and chronic pulmonary insufficiency, without evidence of raised intracranial pressure or abnormal CSF. Patients with iron deficiency anemia may also develop disc swelling as well as retinal hemorrhages and exudates.

Optic disc swelling without visual loss occurs in patients with rickettsial diseases, including Rocky Mountain spotted fever, scrub typhus, epidemic typhus, and endemic (murine) typhus. In none of the reported cases has there been visual loss, and when tested, the CSF has been normal with respect to pressure and content. It is likely that the disc swelling in such cases, rather than being directly caused by inflammation, results from local vascular changes at the level of the optic disc and retina.

PAPILLOPHLEBITIS

Papillophlebitis, also called "retinal vasculitis," "papillary vasculitis," "benign retinal vasculitis," "optic disc vasculitis," and "the big blind spot syndrome," is characterized by

- Unilateral occurrence in most cases.
- Occurrence in healthy, young adults.
- Vague visual complaints of blurred vision or photopsias with minimal impairment of acuity.
- Marked optic disc swelling with variably engorged retinal veins and occasional retinal hemorrhages.
- Marked enlargement of the blind spot on visual field testing.

- Spontaneous, usually complete, recovery within several months to 1 year without therapy.

Most authors consider this condition a form of central retinal vein occlusion that occurs in healthy, young patients with no underlying systemic disease. Unlike typical central retinal vein occlusion in older patients, which generally has a poor visual outcome, almost all patients with papillophlebitis retain excellent visual function throughout the course of the disorder (Fig. 7.14).

The etiology of this disorder is unknown, although some patients have evidence of an underlying coagulopathy. The histologic findings in one severe case revealed extensive phlebitis of the vessels within the optic nerve. It seems likely that the condition is related to involvement of the central retinal vein and its intraneural tributaries. This syndrome may also be related to vitreous traction.

Although the exact nature of papillophlebitis remains unclear, this syndrome should be considered in young, healthy patients who develop unilateral optic disc swelling and dilated retinal veins with minimal or no visual symptoms once orbital and intracranial pathology have been ruled out using appropriate neuroimaging studies and lumbar puncture, if necessary.

POSTERIOR (RETROBULBAR) ISCHEMIC OPTIC NEUROPATHY

Although the anterior form of ION is far more common than the posterior variety, ischemia of the retrobulbar portions of the optic nerve occurs in many settings, both arteritic and nonarteritic. Ischemia can independently affect the posterior portion of the optic nerve because of the distinct and separate arterial supplies of the anterior and posterior portions of the optic nerve. The retrobulbar orbital portion of the optic nerve is supplied by a pial plexus arising from the first branches of the ophthalmic artery, whereas the intracanalicular optic nerve is supplied by two independent vascular circles derived from the ophthalmic artery, and the intracranial optic nerve is supplied by branches of the ipsilateral internal carotid, anterior cerebral, and anterior communicating arteries. Therefore, ischemia of the retrobulbar portion of the optic nerve can occur with sparing of the blood supply to the

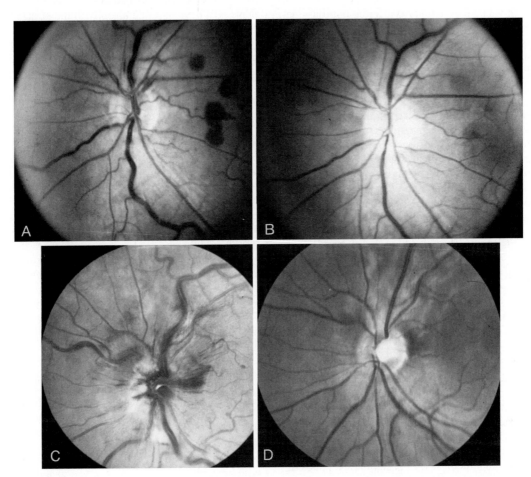

Figure 7.14. Two cases of central retinal vein occlusion in young, healthy patients with retention of good visual acuity. This condition, often called "papillophlebitis," usually resolves spontaneously. *A.* In a 27-year-old man who complained of photopsias in the left eye, the retinal veins are dilated and tortuous. Several peripapillary flame-shaped, intraretinal hemorrhages are seen, as are several blot hemorrhages in the posterior pole. Note that the optic disc is not swollen. The patient underwent a complete systemic evaluation that was unremarkable. His symptoms resolved spontaneously without treatment. *B.* Three months after the onset of visual symptoms, the patient's left ocular fundus appears almost normal. The retinal veins are perhaps minimally dilated, but they are no longer tortuous. The flame-shaped hemorrhages have disappeared, and the blot hemorrhages are almost invisible. The patient had no further visual difficulties over the next 5 years of follow-up, nor did he develop any evidence of systemic vascular disease. *C.* In a 24-year-old woman who complained of photopsias and blurred vision in the left eye, the retinal veins are moderately dilated and tortuous. There are multiple, peripapillary, flame-shaped hemorrhages and several peripapillary soft exudates (cotton-wool spots). The optic disc is moderately swollen. Despite these findings, the patient's visual acuity was 20/20 OU. A systemic evaluation was unremarkable, and no treatment was given. The patient's visual symptoms gradually resolved over several months. *D.* Two months after the onset of visual symptoms, the left ocular fundus is normal. The retinal veins are no longer dilated or tortuous, the intraretinal hemorrhages have disappeared, and the disc swelling has resolved. The patient had no further visual complaints, nor did she develop any systemic diseases over the next 8 years.

optic nerve head. This results in the clinical findings of an ischemic optic neuropathy associated with visual loss, a relative afferent pupillary defect, and visual field loss but a **normal-appearing optic disc.** In such cases, optic disc pallor usually develops within 4 to 6 weeks. Thus, PION is distinguished from AION by evidence of optic nerve dysfunction unassociated with optic disc swelling. PION should, in many cases, be diagnosed only after rigorous exclusion of a compressive, inflammatory, or toxic cause of optic neuropathy; however, in other cases, such as the elderly patient with symptoms of GCA who abruptly loses vision in one eye and who has a relative afferent pupillary defect but a normal ocular fundus, the diagnosis can be made with relative certainty.

ARTERITIC POSTERIOR ISCHEMIC OPTIC NEUROPATHY

PION frequently occurs in GCA and, less frequently, in other systemic vasculitides. GCA thus should be considered in any elderly patient who loses vision acutely and is found to have a normal-appearing fundus in the affected eye. The visual loss need not be profound.

PION occurs in GCA from interruption of blood flow to the retrolaminar portion of the optic nerve. The infarction may affect the orbital, intracanalicular, or intracranial portions of the nerve, or a combination of these.

PION may occur in the setting of systemic vasculitis other than GCA, including herpes zoster ophthalmicus, herpes zoster oticus, relapsing polychondritis, and the connective tissue disorders, particularly systemic lupus erythematosus and polyarteritis nodosa.

NONARTERITIC POSTERIOR ISCHEMIC OPTIC NEUROPATHY

Several investigators have attempted to establish a pathophysiologic basis for nonarteritic PION by examining the optic nerves in autopsy series of cases with cardiovascular and cerebrovascular disease. It would appear that patients with severe arteriosclerosis of large vessels have similar involvement of the arterioles in the pia and within the substance of the optic nerves, suggesting a pathophysiologic basis for the development of retrobulbar optic nerve ischemia.

Carotid artery disease is a causative factor in some cases of PION. Patients with carotid artery disease can develop a hemisphere stroke associated with ipsilateral PION: a retrobulbar form of the **optico-cerebral syndrome.** The patients will develop optic atrophy in the affected eye within 2 months of onset of visual and neurologic manifestations. However, PION caused by carotid artery disease is sometimes an isolated finding.

Patients with **severe diffuse atherosclerosis** can experience an attack of NAION in one eye and then develop progressive PION in the fellow eye. Endarterectomy in such patients may sometimes stabilize or reverse the visual loss in such patients. The finding of iris neovascularization in conjunction with PION, in the absence of diabetic retinopathy or central retinal vein obstruction, strongly suggests concomitant (and causative) carotid occlusive disease. PION can even occur from traumatic or spontaneous carotid artery dissection.

PION can occur after bilateral **radical neck dissection.** The etiology in such cases is multifactorial. In some cases, there is hypotension associated with anemia (see below). In others, there may be reduction of blood flow in the ipsilateral common or internal carotid artery during the surgery.

PION can occur after both **spontaneous and intraoperative blood loss** that results in anemia and hypotension. The diagnosis in such cases may be straightforward or extremely difficult. PION is easily diagnosed in a patient with unilateral loss of vision, a relative afferent pupillary defect, and a normal fundus following acute blood loss. It can also be diagnosed in a patient with bilateral asymmetric loss of vision and normal fundi, when a relative afferent pupillary defect is seen, and in a patient with bilateral complete or nearly complete loss of vision and normal fundi in whom there are sluggish or absent pupillary light reflexes. However, when there is bilateral symmetric loss of vision, normal pupillary reactions to light, and normal fundi, there may be confusion as to whether the site of damage is the occipital lobes or the retrobulbar optic nerves. The confusion may remain despite neuroimaging until optic atrophy eventually develops about 4 to 6 weeks after the visual loss, at which time the diagnosis of PION can be made with assurance.

One histopathologic study of a 59-year-old woman with anemia who became totally blind from PION after repeated gastrointestinal hemorrhage and acute hypotension showed normal neuropathology except for bilateral infarctions

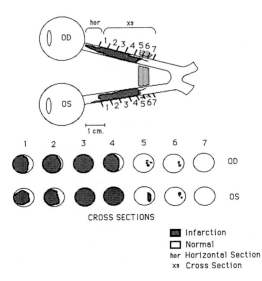

Figure 7.15. Schematic illustration of extent of optic nerve infarction in the patient described in the text. Note that the main region of infarction in both nerves is in the midorbital portion. (Reprinted with permission from Johnson MW, Kincaid MC, Trobe JD. Bilateral retrobulbar optic nerve infarctions after blood loss and hypotension. Ophthalmology 1987; 94:1577–1584.)

of the orbital portion of the optic nerves. Both nerves showed torpedo-shaped infarcts, affecting the full thickness of the nerve in the midorbit, that tapered forward and backward to spare the nerve periphery at its junction with the globe and the optic canal (Fig. 7.15). The principal histopathologic changes were interstitial edema, loss of myelin and astrocytes, and diapedesis of erythrocytes. Axis cylinders were only partially destroyed.

As noted above, visual loss from hypotension may be of three types:

1. Sustained and profound hypotension in a nonanemic patient without arteriolar sclerosis causes watershed white and gray matter infarction in parietal and occipital lobes. The optic nerves tend to be spared.
2. Brief hypotension in an anemic patient with arteriosclerotic risk factors is mild enough to spare the hemispheric watershed regions, but severe enough to cause juxtalaminar optic nerve infarction that produces a clinical (and pathologic) picture of NAION (see above).
3. Hypotension in an anemic patient without

arteriosclerotic risk factors favors PION with infarction in the posterior orbital portion of the optic nerve, where pial end vessels are subject to compression from hypoxic edema. In such cases, the optic discs initially appear normal but eventually develop optic atrophy.

The majority of cases of perioperative PION occur after coronary bypass, lumbar spine, and major abdominal surgery. Among these, intraoperative hypotension is documented in most cases. In cases without evidence of intraoperative hypotension, as well as in many cases in which hypotension has occurred, significant anemia or hypothermia have usually occurred as well. Among such patients whose hemogram is reported, the mean hemoglobin level typically decreases from 40 to 50% in the perioperative period. Thus, hypotension and anemia are thought to be the primary causative factors in almost all cases of perioperative PION.

The distinguishing feature of many of these cases is the deliberate reduction of intraoperative blood pressure to reduce bleeding and the admitted reluctance of the operating team to transfuse because of a fear of transmission of HIV or hepatitis viruses B or C via contaminated blood. Although severe anemia alone may not cause PION, even a short episode of hypotension in an already anemic patient may predispose to PION-induced vision loss. Orbital or ocular compression may also play a role in some cases of both AION and PION after the patient has been face down during surgery.

Because a low hematocrit in the presence of other factors may predispose a surgical patient to permanent visual loss, the current low level of hemoglobin at which blood transfusion is deemed to be indicated (7–8 g/dL) may not be as safe as previously supposed, especially in the setting of hypotension. During the process of informed consent, we believe it advisable to indicate to patients that postoperative visual loss is a rare complication, and that it occurs especially in situations of hypotension and anemia. This discussion may be most appropriate for patients who are about to undergo procedures associated with induced hypotension or probable significant blood loss and who are reluctant to allow transfusion.

Unfortunately, delay in the diagnosis of postoperative PION is quite common. In some instances, patients do not complain, either because they are lethargic or sedated and do not recognize the visual loss, or because they have the mistaken impression that postoperative visual loss is an expected occurrence. In other cases, the patient, the patient's nurses, or the patient's physicians assume that there is some other cause for the visual disturbance. Even when patients with perioperative PION complain of visual loss, the absence of any fundus abnormalities may delay a request for ophthalmologic consultation. An assessment of visual function by means of brief questions and an examination by the anesthesiologist, a member of the surgical team, or an informed nurse in the critical care unit or on the hospital ward may minimize delays in the diagnosis of visual loss and ensure prompt ophthalmologic consultation and treatment, thus optimizing the patient's chance of regaining vision.

PION occasionally occurs in patients with **migraine.** In some patients, it is associated with other evidence of a middle cerebral artery stroke; in others, it occurs as an isolated phenomenon after an attack of otherwise typical migraine with visual aura. The pathophysiology of migraine-associated ION is unclear, but it is presumed that vasospasm is responsible.

Arachnoiditis involving the intracranial optic nerves and chiasm most often occurs in association with basal meningitis, head injury, intracranial tumor, empty sella syndrome, foreign body reaction to muslin wrapping, or systemic disease, but it may occur rarely as an isolated phenomenon. The cause of visual impairment has been attributed to several factors, including constriction of neural tissue by scar and vascular occlusion. It is reasonable to assume that some cases of retrobulbar optic neuropathy associated with arachnoiditis are ischemic in origin and thus constitute a form of PION.

Other reported causes of presumed PION include lymphoma, sepsis, intranasal corticosteroid injection, intranasal epinephrine-containing anesthetic injection, and amyloidosis.

Radiation optic neuropathy (RON) is thought to be an ischemic disorder of the optic nerve that usually results in irreversible severe visual loss months to years after radiation therapy to the brain and orbit. It is most often a retrobulbar process and thus falls into the category of nonarteritic PION. RON occurs most frequently after irradiation of paranasal sinus

and other skull base malignancies, but it may develop after radiation treatment for pituitary adenomas, parasellar meningiomas, craniopharyngiomas, frontal and temporal gliomas, and intraocular tumors. It has also been reported after stereotactic radiosurgery, and after low-dose radiation therapy for dysthyroid orbitopathy, although only in patients with diabetes mellitus.

The pathogenesis of delayed radionecrosis in the central nervous system (CNS) is not fully understood. At one time it was thought to be primarily vascular damage with subsequent neuronal injury; however, it may be that both direct effects on replicating glial tissue and secondary effects from damage to vascular endothelial cells are important in the pathogenesis of this condition. Somatic mutations in the glial cells induced by ionizing radiation are thought to result in genetically incompetent cells that are metabolically deficient. Over time, these cells gradually increase, producing demyelination and neuronal degeneration. A similar process may occur in vascular endothelial cells, eventually resulting in vascular occlusion and necrosis. This model is consistent with the observed long latent period of delayed radionecrosis, because both the glial and endothelial cells have a slow cellular turnover rate. It is also consistent with the observation of direct neuronal demyelination and degeneration prior to the development of any vascular changes. Pathologic specimens of optic nerves with RON show ischemic demyelination, reactive astrocytosis, endothelial hyperplasia, obliterative endarteritis, and fibrinoid necrosis.

Both the total dose of radiation given and the daily fractionation size are important factors in determining the risk of delayed radiation necrosis in the CNS. Most investigators agree that a maximum total dose of 5000 centigray (cGy) in fractions under 200 cGy provides an acceptable low risk, except in patients with diabetes mellitus and in patients receiving chemotherapy. The cumulative doses of radiation therapy reported in patients with RON range from 2400 cGy to 12500 cGy; however, over 75% of the reported cases of RON have received a total dose of more than 5000 cGy. The risk of RON thus appears to increase significantly at doses over 50 Gy. The tolerance level of the optic nerve appears to be 50 to 55 Gy.

In contrast to patients irradiated for paranasal

and oral cavity tumors, patients irradiated for pituitary tumors can develop RON after doses ranging from 42 to 50 Gy. Hence, it has been theorized that optic nerve compression and vascular compromise lower the optic nerve threshold to injury from radiation. Similarly, patients who have received chemotherapy in conjunction with radiation therapy and those with growth hormone–secreting pituitary adenomas are also reportedly at higher risk for RON even at lower cumulative doses. In some cases, the dose actually delivered to the optic nerves is higher than desired because of improper calibration or equipment malfunction. Consequently, RON should be considered even in situations where "safe" doses of radiation therapy have supposedly been administered.

RON is almost always a retrobulbar process that is characterized by rapid and progressive painless visual loss in one or both eyes leading to irreversible blindness. Visual loss in one eye may be rapidly followed by visual loss in the fellow eye. Episodes of transient visual loss may precede the onset of RON by several weeks. The onset of visual symptoms associated with RON may be as short as 3 months or as long as 8 years after radiation therapy, but the majority of cases occur within 3 years after radiation, with a peak at 1.5 years. Progression of visual loss over weeks to months is common. Final vision is no light perception in 45% and worse than 20/200 in an additional 40% of affected eyes. Thus, 85% of eyes with RON have final visual acuity of 20/200 or worse.

Most patients with RON initially have a normal-appearing optic disc that subsequently becomes pale over 4 to 6 weeks. Others already have pallor of the disc when they first present with visual loss, indicating that the process has been going on for 1 month or longer, even though the patient's symptoms have not been present for that length of time. The visual field may show altitudinal loss or central scotoma. A junctional syndrome with an optic neuropathy and contralateral temporal hemianopia may occur in patients with damage to the distal optic nerve. Patients with radionecrosis of the optic chiasm typically develop a bitemporal hemianopia that initially may suggest recurrence of the tumor for which the patient was irradiated.

As noted above, RON may rarely present as an **anterior** optic neuropathy characterized by optic disc swelling, peripapillary hemorrhages,

and retinal exudates. Such cases usually occur in the setting of radiation retinopathy following treatment of orbital or intraocular lesions.

The diagnosis of RON is generally suspected from the clinical setting and may be confirmed in most cases with neuroimaging. The differential diagnosis of RON includes recurrence of the primary tumor, secondary empty sella syndrome with optic nerve and chiasmal prolapse, arachnoiditis, and radiation-induced parasellar tumor. CT scanning in RON is typically normal and shows no abnormal enhancement with contrast media. MRI is the diagnostic procedure of choice to distinguish tumor recurrence from RON (Fig. 7.16). In RON, the unenhanced T1- and T2-weighted images show no abnormality, but on T1-weighted images following intravenous administration of paramagnetic contrast material such as gadolinium-DTPA, there is marked enhancement of the optic nerves, optic chiasm, and, in some cases, the optic tracts (see Fig. 7.16). The enhancement usually resolves in several months, at which time visual function usually stabilizes.

Treatment for RON is controversial. Although delayed radionecrosis in the CNS can be treated with some success with systemic corticosteroids, which are effective in reducing tissue edema and may have some beneficial effect on demyelination, their use in RON, in oral or intravenous form, has produced disappointing results. Among 16 reported cases treated with steroids alone, only two cases improved. Similarly, the use of anticoagulation, which has been reputed to reverse or stabilize CNS radionecrosis, does not appear to provide similar results in patients with RON (see Fig. 7.16).

Hyperbaric oxygen therapy (HBO) is used in the treatment of radionecrosis of bone and following irradiation in poorly healing wounds in oral and maxillofacial surgery. At 2.0 atmospheres, the level of dissolved oxygen in blood may be raised 14-fold, thus extending the oxygen diffusion distance in ischemic tissue, enabling limited correction of local hypoxia. HBO therapy enhances fibroblastic activity, collagen synthesis, and neovascularization in irradiated tissues. To the extent that RON is an ischemic process, HBO has a theoretical basis for effectiveness, but clinical results are not uniform. If HBO is to be tried, it should be commenced as early as possible after onset of visual loss, even if there is a possibility that the visual loss is

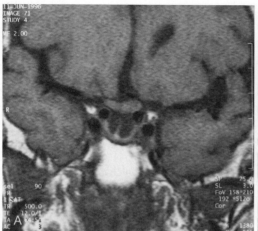

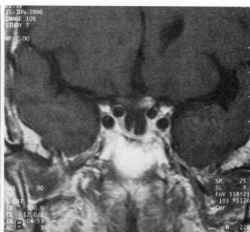

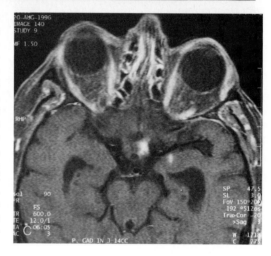

Figure 7.16. Radiation optic neuropathy (RON) in a 65-year-old woman who had undergone transsphenoidal resection of a nonsecreting pituitary macroadenoma followed by radiation therapy totalling 5500 cGy 18 months earlier. While taking Coumadin for cardiac disease, the patient began to experience progressive loss of vision in the left eye and was found to have a right homonymous field defect. *A.* T1-weighted MRI, coronal view, shows enlargement of the left side of the optic chiasm. *B.* T1-weighted MRI, coronal view, after intravenous injection of paramagnetic contrast material, shows enhancement of the enlarged region. *C.* T1-weighted MRI, axial view, after intravenous injection of paramagnetic contrast material, shows enhancement and enlargement of the distal portion of the left optic nerve and the left side of the optic chiasm. A diagnosis of RON was made, and the patient was treated with a 1-week course of heparin without improvement. She subsequently underwent hyperbaric oxygen therapy with stabilization of visual function.

caused by some other process, such as recurrent tumor. The HBO should consist of 30 sessions, of 90 minutes each, breathing 100% oxygen at a minimum pressure of 2.4 atmospheres. Although we have not been impressed with the efficacy of HBO in our own patients, this is currently the only treatment that is associated with any significant visual improvement in patients with RON, and it is the best alternative at this time.

FOR MORE INFORMATION:
See Walsh & Hoyt's *Clinical Neuro-Ophthalmology,* 5th edition, Volume 1, Chapter 11, pages 549–598; Volume 3, Chapter 55, pages 3447–3453; and Chapter 57, pages 3760–3764.

CHAPTER 8

Compressive and Infiltrative Optic Neuropathies

COMPRESSIVE OPTIC NEUROPATHIES
   Compressive Optic Neuropathies with Optic Disc
      Swelling (Anterior Compressive Optic
      Neuropathies)
   Compressive Optic Neuropathies without Optic
      Disc Swelling (Retrobulbar Compressive Optic
      Neuropathies)
	INFILTRATIVE OPTIC NEUROPATHIES
	   Tumors
	   Inflammatory and Infectious Infiltrative Optic
	      Neuropathies

COMPRESSIVE OPTIC NEUROPATHIES

COMPRESSIVE OPTIC NEUROPATHIES WITH OPTIC DISC SWELLING (ANTERIOR COMPRESSIVE OPTIC NEUROPATHIES)

Lesions within the orbit, occasionally within the optic canal, and extremely rarely intracranially, may compress the optic nerve, resulting in optic disc swelling (Fig. 8.1). Such lesions include tumors, infections, inflammations, and even adnexal structures that have become swollen or enlarged by disease.

Within the orbit, lesions that compress the proximal optic nerve and produce optic disc swelling include optic gliomas, meningiomas, hamartomas (e.g., hemangiomas, lymphangiomas), choristomas (e.g., dermoid cysts), and malignancies (e.g., carcinoma, lymphoma, sarcoma, multiple myeloma). Progressive visual loss associated with optic disc swelling caused by an arachnoid cyst of the intraorbital optic nerve has been described, but such lesions are rare, and most patients with visual loss associated with ipsilateral enlargement of the optic nerve sheath harbor an optic nerve sheath meningioma at the apex of the orbit.

In most cases of anterior compressive optic neuropathy, there is progressive visual loss associated with proptosis; however, in many patients, visual acuity remains normal or near nor-

mal, and there is almost no external evidence of orbital disease despite obvious disc swelling. This clinical picture occurs particularly in patients with orbital hemangiomas adjacent to the optic nerve and in patients with primary optic nerve sheath meningiomas. In such patients, careful testing of color vision may reveal subtle defects, and there may occasionally be a relative afferent pupillary defect despite retention of normal acuity. The visual field of the affected eye generally shows only enlargement of the blind spot or minimal reduction in the mean deviation on automated perimetry. When other signs of orbital disease are not present (e.g., proptosis, limitation of ocular motility, orbital congestion), these patients may be thought to have unilateral papilledema from increased intracranial pressure. Although it is obvious that patients with slowly progressive, unilateral visual loss and proptosis associated with disc swelling should undergo evaluation for a possible orbital lesion, patients with unilateral optic disc swelling without signs of intraocular inflammation and *without* visual loss or other evidence of an optic neuropathy should also undergo such an evaluation, particularly when there are no systemic or neurologic symptoms or signs of increased intracranial pressure. Without question, orbital disease is the most common cause of unilateral disc swelling without visual loss.

Transient monocular visual loss can occur in patients with orbital lesions. The visual loss usu-

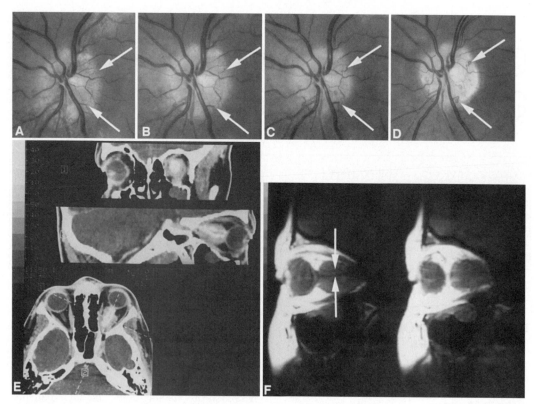

Figure 8.1. Optociliary shunt veins in a patient with optic nerve sheath meningioma. *A–D.* Progressive development of optociliary shunt veins (*arrows*) from the stage of chronic disc swelling (*A*), through intermediate stages of shunt vein formation (*B–C*), to the final stage of optic atrophy with fully formed optociliary shunts (*D*). Neuroimaging with computed tomographic (CT) scanning and magnetic resonance imaging (MRI) provides complementary information. Calcified psammoma bodies in the tumor produce a well-delineated "tram-track" sign in the contrast-enhanced, reconstructed CT images (*E*), whereas MRI with surface coil (T1-weighted, without fat suppression or enhancement) (*F*) clearly defines the nerve surrounded by tumor (*arrows*).

ally occurs only in certain positions of gaze, and vision immediately clears when the direction of gaze is changed. It is assumed that either direct pressure on the optic nerve or interruption of blood supply is responsible for this phenomenon.

Computed tomographic (CT) scanning, magnetic resonance imaging (MRI), and ultrasonography are rapid, safe, and accurate methods of determining the presence of an orbital lesion, its location, and, occasionally, its identity. CT scanning and MRI offer superior topographic depiction (size, shape, and location) of lesions, whereas standardized echography provides supplementary information that often helps in refinement of the differential diagnosis. CT scanning is particularly useful for imaging bone, calcium, and metallic foreign bodies (suspicion of the latter being a contraindication for the use of MRI), whereas MRI excels at defining inflammatory and intrinsic disease of the visual pathway and parasellar area. MRI is particularly suited to imaging the intracanalicular optic nerve, as it is not affected by partial volume averaging from adjacent bone as is CT scanning. With the use of fat-saturation techniques and intravenous injection of paramagnetic substances such as gadolinium-DTPA, demarcation of optic nerve sheath meningiomas can be optimized. Plain skull radiographs should no longer play a role in the evaluation of most patients with unexplained visual loss.

Inflammatory conditions involving the orbit, including abscesses and the nonspecific condition called "idiopathic inflammatory pseudotumor," may also cause compression of the proximal optic nerve and secondary disc swelling. Affected patients usually experience visual loss, pain, proptosis, and congestion associated with the optic disc swelling, and the presence of an orbital process is rarely in question. Infrequently, meningiomas of the orbital apex produce a similar clinical picture.

Patients with thyroid eye disease may develop evidence of a compressive optic neuropathy associated with optic disc swelling (Fig. 8.2). In such patients, congestive symptoms almost always precede visual loss, which is usually bilateral, symmetric, and gradual in onset. Presenting visual acuities are usually 20/60 or worse, with central scotomas often combined with arcuate defects. The compressive etiology of the optic neuropathy in dysthyroid optic neuropathy is attested to by the typical CT findings of moderate to severe enlargement of the extraocular muscles at the orbital apex (see Fig. 8.2).

In addition to proptosis, congestion, and limitation of ocular motility, patients with orbital disease may develop various folds or striae that occur at the posterior pole, adjacent to the optic disc (see Fig. 8.2). These folds may be horizontal or vertical.

Patients with meningiomas confined entirely to the optic canal may occasionally present with blurred vision and optic disc swelling. The mechanism by which disc swelling occurs in such cases is not clear, but it presumably results from direct compression of the optic nerve with blockage of axon transport.

Even more uncommon than optic disc swelling from an intracanalicular lesion is optic disc swelling from compression of the **intracranial portion** of the optic nerve by an aneurysm or tumor. Intracranial lesions, particularly sphenoid wing meningiomas, not infrequently extend through the optic canal, compressing the intracranial, intracanalicular, and intraorbital optic nerve in the process. Optic disc changes, from swelling to pallor, may be minimal in such cases, even when the lesion is quite large (Fig. 8.3).

In many patients with chronic compression of the intracanalicular or intraorbital optic nerve, a specific clinical triad develops. This triad consists of visual loss, optic disc swelling that evolves into optic atrophy, and the appearance of optociliary (retinochoroidal) shunt veins (see

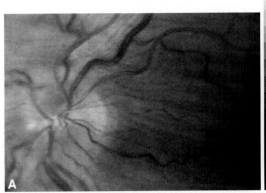

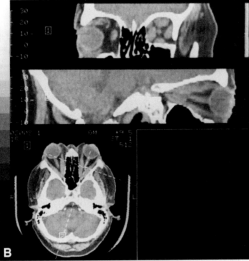

Figure 8.2.   Optic disc swelling and choroidal folds in thyroid eye disease. *A.* The left optic disc shows mild hyperemia, swelling, and blurring of the peripapillary retinal nerve fiber layer at the upper and lower poles. Horizontal chorioretinal folds extend across the posterior pole toward the macula.

B. Coronal and off-axis sagittal reconstructed CT scans show greatly enlarged extraocular muscles surrounding the optic nerve within the orbit. Note that the muscles actually appear to be in contact with the nerve.

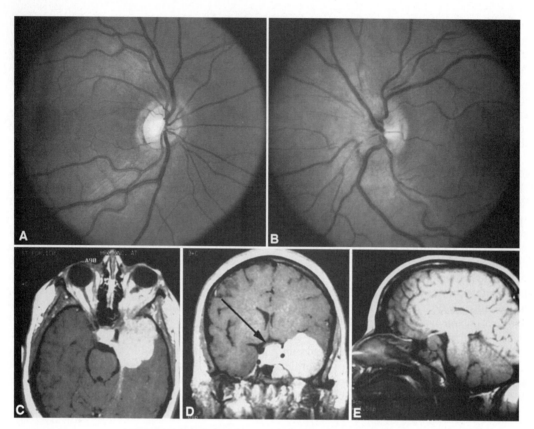

Figure 8.3. Optic disc swelling in a patient with a large meningioma with intraorbital, intracanalicular, and intracranial components. The patient was a 21-year-old woman who experienced reduced vision in the left eye during pregnancy. A. Normal right optic disc. B. Mild swelling of left optic disc. C. T1-weighted MRI, axial view, obtained after intravenous injection with gadolinium-DTPA shows a large mass involving the left sphenoid wing and posterior orbit. Although both coronal (D) and sagittal (E) images clearly show compression of the optic chiasm by the tumor (arrow), the resulting visual field defect was purely unilateral, affecting only the left eye.

Fig. 8.1). The optociliary veins overlie the optic disc and peripapillary region and shunt venous blood between the retinal and choroidal venous circulations. The vessels may occur as congenital anomalies, in which case they are associated with normal visual acuity and shunt blood from the choroid to the retina. When they occur with chronic optic nerve compression, however, they are generally associated with severe visual loss and disc swelling or optic atrophy, and they shunt blood from the retina to the choroid. The common denominator in such cases appears to be prolonged compression of the optic nerve with gradual compression and obstruction of the central retinal vein. The normal route of retinal venous blood flow is through the central retinal vein directly to the cavernous sinus. Chronic obstruction of the central retinal vein presumably results in dilation of a previously existing system that shunts blood to the choroid, allowing it to leave the eye via the vortex veins. These veins drain directly into the superior and inferior ophthalmic veins that anastomose with the facial and angular veins and with the pterygoid venous plexus. Thus, an outlet is provided for retinal venous blood other than via the central retinal vein to the cavernous sinus. This clinical picture is most frequently seen in patients with sphenoorbital meningiomas, but it can also occur in patients with optic nerve gliomas, chronic papilledema, craniopharyngioma, sarcoidosis, and other rare causes of optic nerve compression.

COMPRESSIVE OPTIC NEUROPATHIES
WITHOUT OPTIC DISC SWELLING
(RETROBULBAR COMPRESSIVE
OPTIC NEUROPATHIES)

The importance of early diagnosis of compressive lesions that affect the retrobulbar portions of the optic nerve and do not cause optic disc swelling cannot be overemphasized. Early decompression of the optic nerves or chiasm may result in significant return of visual function, whereas delayed diagnosis may result in progressive visual failure and irreversible visual loss, neurologic dysfunction, or death. Unfortunately, intracranial, intracanalicular, and occasionally posterior orbital compressive lesions usually do not produce disc swelling or significant neurologic or systemic manifestations. Thus, by the time such lesions cause visible optic pallor, significant damage to the optic nerve has often already occurred, preventing return of visual function even with otherwise successful decompression. The physician managing a patient with unexplained unilateral visual loss therefore must be aware of the characteristic history and early findings in patients with a retrobulbar compressive optic neuropathy.

Progressive Visual Dysfunction in Retrobulbar Compressive Optic Neuropathies

In cases of monocular incipient prechiasmal optic nerve compression, progressive dimming of vision is noted at an early stage. Such patients may have normal or near normal visual acuity, but they complain of "foggy," "dim," or "blurred" vision. Although these patients may read the 20/25 or even 20/20 Snellen letters with the affected eye, they do so slowly and with great difficulty compared with the ease with which they read the 20/15 line with the opposite eye. Painless, slowly progressive visual dimming should be the first warning that compression of the visual system might be responsible.

Patients with unilateral visual complaints from compression of the optic nerve usually have some type of visual field defect, particularly when tested with automated perimetry, but the nature of the defect does not, in itself, suggest the etiology of the visual loss. Compression of the optic nerve may produce *any* type of field defect, including an altitudinal, arcuate, hemianopic, central, or cecocentral scotoma. These same defects can be caused not only by other types of optic neuropathies but also by intraocular disorders, including cataract and macular disease.

By far the two most striking abnormalities that are present in a patient with a retrobulbar compressive optic neuropathy are unilateral dyschromatopsia, as detected using pseudoisochromatic color plates or simple red objects, and an ipsilateral relative afferent pupillary defect. The afferent defect is obvious even when visual acuity is minimally reduced and provides the observer with absolute evidence that the visual difficulty is caused by something other than a simple refractive error, incipient cataract, or minimum macular disease. Once a relative afferent pupillary defect is detected in a patient with an apparently normal fundus who is complaining of progressive dimming of vision, compression must be ruled out by whatever neuroimaging studies are available and best suited to the task. CT scanning and MRI are the best screening tests to use in this setting.

Despite the almost universal availability of CT scanning and MRI, it is astonishing that patients with progressive visual loss continue to be diagnosed as having macular degeneration, cataract, glaucoma, or "chronic optic neuritis." As has been stated elsewhere, probably no branch of neuro-ophthalmology has to its discredit the abundance of erroneous diagnoses as has optic neuritis. Certainly, chronic optic neuritis occurs and may produce slowly progressive visual loss in one or both eyes (see Chapter 6); however, *chronic optic neuritis is a diagnosis of exclusion.* This diagnosis should not be made in any patient until neuroimaging studies have been performed and have failed to detect a compressive lesion of the optic nerve. Even then, the diagnosis of chronic optic neuritis must be made with caution. We have seen several patients with unilateral progressive visual loss in whom neuroimaging studies failed to demonstrate a compressive lesion, but who subsequently were found— either by subsequent scanning or during surgical exploration—to have such a lesion.

The optic disc of a patient with a compressive optic neuropathy may appear normal or show a variable degree of pallor. Asymmetric cupping of the optic disc is not usually a prominent feature, but it may occur and be quite prominent in some patients (Fig. 8.4). In such cases, the visual

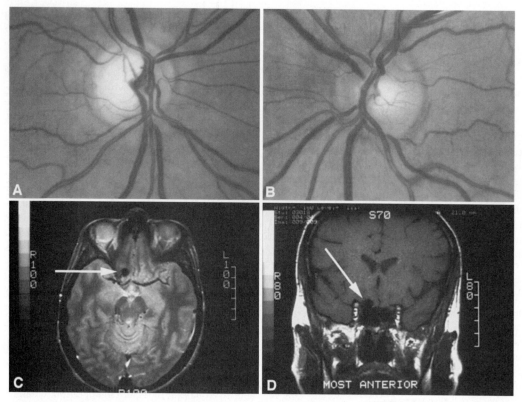

Figure 8.4. Optic disc cupping in a patient with aneurysmal compression. The patient was a 55-year-old woman who suddenly lost the inferior field in the right eye after suffering mild head trauma in a motor vehicle accident 8 days earlier. *A.* Cupped and pale right optic disc. *B.* Normal left optic disc. *C–D.* Magnetic resonance images, axial (*C*) and coronal (*D*) views, revealing flow void (*arrows*) in a carotid-ophthalmic aneurysm that is compressing the right optic nerve.

loss may be thought to have resulted from glaucoma, particularly when there is an arcuate defect. Analysis of the occurrence of optic disc cupping in eyes with compressive optic neuropathy, using highly reproducible planimetric measurement techniques applied to stereoscopic disc photographs, has revealed evidence of acquired enlargement of the ipsilateral cup in patients with unilateral optic nerve compression. Pathologic examination of the optic nerve from one patient with progressive cupping of the optic disc caused by aneurysmal optic nerve compression demonstrated loss of axons and glial tissue in the nerve head. It is unclear how neural compression results in loss of glial tissue in the disc of some patients and why significant cupping is such an uncommon accompaniment of compressive optic neuropathy. Optic atrophy in one eye and disc swelling in the other may result from asymmetric optic nerve compression or from the more traditional explanation of tumor-induced direct optic nerve compression in one eye and papilledema from increased intracranial pressure in the other (Foster Kennedy syndrome).

Almost any field defect may be present in patients with a retrobulbar compressive optic neuropathy. Central, paracentral, cecocentral, arcuate, altitudinal, nasal, or temporal hemianopic defects, as well as uniform depression of the visual field have all been described in patients with compressive lesions. Although a hemianopic field defect, a central scotoma that breaks out into the periphery, or a ''junctional'' scotoma in the superior temporal field of the opposite eye strongly suggest a compressive lesion, it is the **insidious, progressive** nature of the symptoms that is most often the critical feature of the compressive process.

In our experience, most cases of delayed diagnosis of compression of the anterior visual system are caused by what Dr. J. Lawton Smith once called the sins of "omission" and "commission." Sins of omission include failure to (1) perform color vision or visual field testing; (2) carefully examine the opposite, "normal" eye; (3) test for a relative afferent pupillary defect; and (4) obtain appropriate neuroimaging studies. Sins of commission include (1) incorrect performance or interpretation of the various diagnostic tests, (2) ordering inappropriate or inadequate neuroimaging studies, and (3) incorrect interpretation of these studies. Although it is true that in many cases a negative neuroimaging evaluation results from the use of the incorrect study, the incorrect performance of the correct study, or incorrect interpretation of the results of the study, there are still lesions, particularly meningiomas, that remain nearly invisible to all types of neuroimaging investigations in spite of the rapid advances in this field. However, with continuing advances in CT scanning (including thin-section technique and CT angiography), MRI (including the use of paramagnetic substances such as gadolinium-DTPA), special techniques

(e.g., orbital fat suppression, magnetization transfer, fluid-attenuated inversion-recovery), and MR angiography, it is now a rare lesion that escapes detection.

We believe that when modern neuroimaging techniques that have been carefully tailored to the clinical problem at hand, properly performed, and correctly interpreted, are unrevealing, then **observation** rather than neurosurgical intervention is more apt to serve the patient's best interests. Reports supporting the concept of optic nerve compression by adjacent dolichoectatic internal carotid arteries add weight to such an approach. Rarely does a patient require exploratory craniotomy to define the cause of compressive optic neuropathy, although decompression of the optic canal may be therapeutic in selected cases.

Causes of retrobulbar optic nerve compression include intraorbital and intracranial benign and malignant tumors; aneurysms (Fig. 8.5); inflammatory lesions (particularly of the paranasal sinuses); primary bone disease (e.g., os-

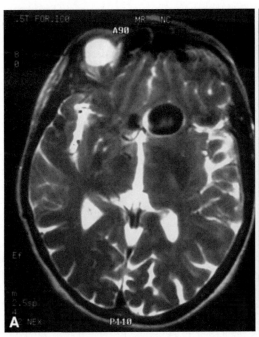
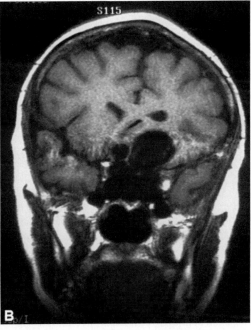
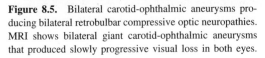

Figure 8.5. Bilateral carotid-ophthalmic aneurysms producing bilateral retrobulbar compressive optic neuropathies. MRI shows bilateral giant carotid-ophthalmic aneurysms that produced slowly progressive visual loss in both eyes. An ophthalmologist, internist, and psychiatrist had all ascribed the patient's loss of vision to conversion-hysteria. *A.* Axial view. *B.* Coronal view.

teopetrosis, fibrous dysplasia, craniometaphyseal dysplasia, Paget's disease); orbital fractures; dolichoectatic intracranial vessels; congenital and acquired hydrocephalus; thyroid eye disease; and orbital hemorrhage, whether spontaneous, traumatic, iatrogenic, or associated with orbital, paranasal sinus, or systemic diseases. Anterior visual system compression has also been reported from such disparate causes as intranasal balloon catheters placed for treatment of severe epistaxis, errant placement of intraventricular catheters, downward displacement of the gyrus rectus in patients with meningiomas of the anterior falx cerebri, basal encephalocele, hypertrophic pachymeningitis, and fat packing after transsphenoidal hypophysectomy for pituitary tumor.

Sudden Visual Loss with Retrobulbar Compressive Lesions

The sudden onset of unilateral visual loss, combined with signs of retrobulbar optic nerve dysfunction, usually suggests a diagnosis of optic neuritis or ischemic optic neuropathy. In rare instances, however, compressive lesions produce acute monocular visual loss, presumably from hemorrhage or from sudden interruption of the vascular supply to the optic nerve. This phenomenon probably occurs most frequently in patients with pituitary apoplexy, but it has also been reported in patients with pituitary tumors and meningiomas during pregnancy and in otherwise healthy patients upon awakening. Sudden onset of monocular visual loss can also occur from a ruptured ophthalmic artery aneurysm, fibrous dysplasia, orbital hemorrhage, subperiosteal abscess, and orbital cellulitis.

With orbital processes, proptosis is usually present and optic nerve traction with dramatic tenting of the posterior globe can often be demonstrated by orbital neuroimaging studies. The combination of ocular pain and unilateral visual loss, simulating retrobulbar neuritis, has been observed in cases of pituitary adenoma, aneurysm, craniopharyngioma, and in patients with mucoceles or pyoceles of the paranasal sinuses, particularly the sphenoid sinus. In other cases, patients with sudden retrobulbar optic neuropathies from compressive lesions have initially improved when treated with systemic corticosteroids. In such cases, visual function invariably worsens as soon as steroids are tapered. Lesions that cause this syndrome include pituitary adenoma, craniopharyngioma, plasmacytoma, and medulloblastoma.

Visual Recovery Following Decompression

Restoration of visual function is not only possible following surgical decompression, but it can begin within hours to days after surgery, sometimes with full recovery. On the other hand, other cases of compressive optic neuropathy have been recorded in which there has been gradual improvement of vision over several years following decompression of the optic nerve. "Medical decompression" of the optic nerve with bromocriptine or cabergoline in patients with prolactin-secreting pituitary tumors has yielded similar improvements in visual function.

Although it is not surprising that prompt decompression may restore visual function in patients rendered suddenly blind by pituitary apoplexy, it is not intuitively obvious that patients who have lost all light perception for days or weeks can occasionally experience dramatic visual recovery following decompression surgery. With increasing use of the transsphenoidal technique for removal of pituitary tumors and the improvements in anesthesia for patients undergoing neurosurgical procedures, it has become possible to evaluate patients several hours after they have undergone decompression of the intracranial optic nerves, optic chiasm, or both. Patients with pituitary adenomas who have normal fundi (as well as many who have mild disc pallor and loss of the nerve fiber layer) invariably experience impressive return of visual acuity and visual field that can be detected almost immediately after they awaken from anesthesia. In most other cases of optic nerve compression in which adequate decompression has been obtained, patients are aware of improvement within several days. Many patients achieve maximum recovery by the time they are discharged from the hospital 5 to 10 days after surgery; others experience improvement during this period but continue to improve over the subsequent weeks to months.

Although there are patients who do not improve dramatically immediately after decompression surgery but do improve gradually several months following surgery, such patients are increasingly rare and consist primarily of those with preoperative hydrocephalus or postoperative cerebral edema. There is no correlation between the rapidity of visual loss and the rapidity of visual return. Tumor volume has also proved to be a poor predictor of the extent of visual recovery, both for pituitary adenomas and suprasellar meningiomas.

In light of the substantial improvement noted after decompression, it is highly unlikely that most of the visual loss in patients with compressive optic neuropathies is caused by vascular insufficiency. Rather, most compressive visual loss is likely caused by demyelination insufficient to cause cell death. It has been theorized that there are three stages of visual recovery after decompression of the anterior visual pathway:

1. Relief of visual pathway compression is initially followed by **rapid recovery** of some vision within minutes to hours. This recovery can be likened to the relief of conduction block after an arm or leg ''goes to sleep.''
2. This initial recovery is followed by **delayed recovery** of additional function over weeks to months. This improvement may be related to progressive remyelination of previously compressed demyelinated axons.
3. Finally, there is an even longer period of improvement, taking many months to years. The mechanism by which this **late recovery** occurs is unknown.

INFILTRATIVE OPTIC NEUROPATHIES

The optic nerve can become infiltrated by a variety of different processes, primarily tumors and inflammatory processes (Table 8.1). Such processes typically produce one of three clinical pictures: (1) optic disc elevation with evidence of an optic neuropathy, (2) optic disc elevation with no evidence of optic nerve dysfunction, and (3) a normal-appearing optic disc associated with evidence of an optic neuropathy.

Infiltration of the proximal portion of the optic nerve, either anterior or just posterior to the lamina cribrosa, produces elevation of the optic disc. When the prelaminar portion of the nerve is infiltrated, the elevation of the disc is caused by the infiltrative process and is not true disc swelling. When the retrolaminar portion of the nerve is infiltrated, the disc elevation is caused by true swelling of the disc, and the appearance is indistinguishable from the disc swelling caused by

Table 8.1
Lesions That Infiltrate the Optic Nerve

Primary Tumors
- Optic Glioma
    Benign
    Malignant
- Ganglioglioma
- Hemangioma
    Capillary
    Cavernous
- Hemangioblastoma
- Other

Secondary Tumors
- Metastatic carcinoma
- Nasopharyngeal carcinoma and other contiguous tumors
- Lymphoreticular tumors
    Lymphoma
    Leukemia
    Other

Infections and Inflammations
- Sarcoidosis
- Idiopathic perioptic neuritis
- Bacteria
- Viruses
- Fungi

such diverse entities as increased intracranial pressure, ischemia, and inflammation.

The disc elevation observed in patients with infiltrative processes of the optic nerve, whether true swelling or an infiltrative process, may be associated with other signs of optic nerve dysfunction. In such cases, there is variable loss of visual acuity and color vision, a visual field defect that can be of any type, and a relative afferent pupillary defect when the infiltration is unilateral or asymmetric. In other cases, the disc elevation is asymptomatic, and there is no clinical evidence of an optic neuropathy, although electrophysiologic testing, such as visual-evoked responses, may be abnormal.

In general, the more distal (posterior) the infiltrative process, the less likely it is that any change will be noted in the optic disc. In such cases, the optic nerve initially appears normal, and the clinical picture is that of a retrobulbar optic neuropathy.

The most common lesions that infiltrate the optic nerve are tumors and inflammatory or infectious processes. Tumors may be primary or secondary. The most common inflammatory disorder is sarcoidosis; the most common infectious agents are opportunistic fungi.

TUMORS

Tumors that can infiltrate the optic nerve may be primary or secondary. Primary tumors are far more common than are secondary ones.

Primary Tumors

Primary tumors that infiltrate the nerve include optic gliomas, astrocytic hamartomas, gangliogliomas, capillary and cavernous hemangiomas, hemangioblastomas, and melanocytomas.

Optic Nerve Glioma

The most common lesion that infiltrates the optic nerve is probably the optic glioma (Fig. 8.6). Optic pathway gliomas represent 1% of all intracranial tumors and 1.5 to 3.5% of all orbital tumors. Gliomas confined to the optic nerve constitute about 25% of all optic pathway gliomas, with the remainder infiltrating the optic chiasm and optic tracts in addition to one or both optic nerves. Seventy percent of patients with optic pathway gliomas develop visual symptoms or

signs in the first decade of life, and 90% of the lesions are detected by the second decade. There seems to be no particular sex predilection for these tumors.

Patients with gliomas confined to the optic nerve have three clinical presentations that are determined in part by the location, size, and extent of the tumor. When the glioma is confined to the orbital portion of the nerve or the bulk of the lesion is within the orbit, the patient typically develops proptosis associated with evidence of an anterior optic neuropathy (loss of visual acuity and color vision, a visual field defect, a relative afferent pupillary defect, and a swollen optic disc). Whether the optic disc swelling that is observed in such patients results from infiltration alone, vascular insufficiency, or compression by the arachnoidal proliferation or extension of the tumor outside the pia-arachnoid of the nerve that may accompany such lesions is unclear.

Another mechanism that may be responsible for disc swelling in such patients is secondary obstruction of the cerebrospinal fluid (CSF) space surrounding the orbital portion of the optic nerve by the tumor. Patients with gliomas that

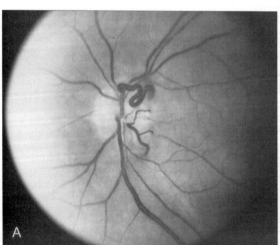
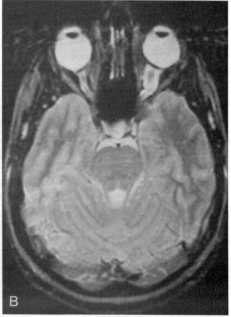

Figure 8.6. Optociliary shunt vessels in a patient with an optic nerve glioma. *A.* The left optic disc is pale and mildly swollen. There are optociliary shunt vessels on its surface. *B.* T2-weighted MRI, axial view, shows diffuse enlargement of orbital portion of left optic nerve. The patient was initially thought to have an optic nerve sheath meningioma. Note "pseudo-CSF sign" caused by extension of tumor into subdural space around intraorbital optic nerve.

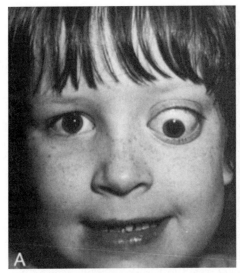
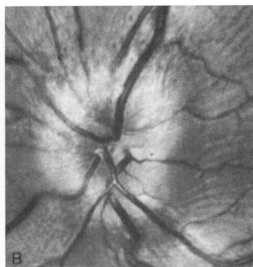

Figure 8.7.   Optic nerve glioma producing proptosis, optic disc swelling, and chorioretinal striae in a 7-year-old girl.   *A.* The left eye is proptotic and displaced inferiorly. *B.* The left optic disc is swollen, and chorioretinal striae are present.

both infiltrate and compress the optic nerve can eventually develop optociliary shunt vessels—congenital venous channels that enlarge in the setting of chronic compression of the optic nerve and that shunt blood from the retinal to the choroidal circulations. This allows the blood to bypass the central retinal venous drainage and to exit the eye and orbit via the vortex veins that drain into the superior and inferior ophthalmic veins (see Fig. 8.6). Hyperopia may be induced by the increased volume of the optic nerve pressing on the globe. In such a case, retinal striae may be seen (Fig. 8.7).

When the tumor is located posteriorly in the orbit, and especially when the process begins in, or is limited to, the intracanalicular or intracranial portions of the nerve, the presentation is that of a slowly progressive or relatively stable retrobulbar optic neuropathy. In most of these cases, the optic disc on the affected side is pale when the patient is first assessed, and the disc does not appear to have been previously swollen. Such patients do not typically have proptosis; if they do, it is usually less than 3 mm.

With the increasing availability of neuroimaging, particularly MRI and the increasing tendency of physicians to screen patients with neurofibromatosis type 1 (NF-1) radiologically, an increasing number of patients with asymptomatic presumed optic gliomas are being identified.

Such patients have no visual complaints and may or may not have evidence of visual dysfunction (e.g., an asymptomatic visual field defect or a relative afferent pupillary defect) on careful testing, although most have abnormal visual-evoked responses to pattern stimuli.

Many patients first come to medical attention because they develop a sensory strabismus. In other patients, the tumor displaces the globe, producing a primary strabismus. Such patients may have variable visual loss that is caused not by the tumor per se but by strabismic amblyopia. The diagnosis in such cases may be suspected when color vision is normal or is less severely affected than is visual acuity. Pain is not a feature of the clinical presentation of optic nerve gliomas, unless they suddenly hemorrhage.

Patients with optic nerve gliomas may have stable and even normal visual acuity for many years. In some cases, however, there is slowly progressive visual loss, and in rare cases, there is sudden and profound visual loss that simulates the clinical picture of acute optic neuritis and that is caused by intratumoral hemorrhage.

The diagnosis of an optic nerve glioma should be suspected in any young child who develops or is found to have decreased vision with evidence of an anterior or retrobulbar optic neuropathy or who has asymptomatic optic disc swelling or pallor, particularly if the child has stigmata of NF-1. Both CT scanning and MRI can be used to identify the lesion, which typically appears as a fusiform enlargement of the orbital portion of the optic nerve, with or without concomitant enlargement of the optic canal (Figs. 8.6*B* and 8.8). In other cases, the nerve is diffusely enlarged, thus mimicking a meningioma.

MRI is generally better at defining the extent of an optic nerve glioma than is CT scanning. On MRI, optic gliomas typically have normal to slightly prolonged T1 relaxation times and are isointense or hypointense to normal brain on T1-weighted images. Many of these tumors also have a prolongation of the T2 relaxation times. The T2-weighted images are better at assessing the extent of the tumor than are T1-weighted images. Although gliomas of the optic nerve may show minimal enhancement after intravenous injection of a paramagnetic contrast mate-

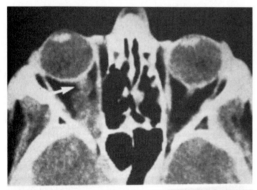

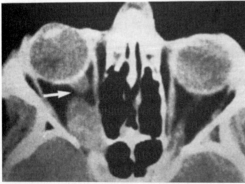

Figure 8.8. Kinking of the optic nerve in a patient with neurofibromatosis type 1 and an optic nerve glioma. CT scan, two adjacent axial views, shows "kinking" (*arrow*) of an enlarged optic nerve within the right orbit. This sign is pathognomonic of an optic nerve glioma.

rial, the enhancement is not nearly as pronounced as is typically seen with a meningioma.

Two important signs help differentiate optic nerve gliomas from other lesions. One is an unusual "kinking" of the optic nerve within the orbit (see Fig. 8.8). This is seen exclusively in patients with NF-1. The other is a double-intensity tubular thickening of the nerve, best seen on MRI. This sign is called the "pseudo-CSF" signal because the increase in T2 signal surrounding the nerve may be misinterpreted as a CSF signal (Fig. 8.9). The genesis of this signal is perineural arachnoidal gliomatosis that occurs in optic nerve gliomas in patients with NF-1. Kinking of the nerve and the pseudo-CSF signal are often seen together.

Approximately 29% of optic pathway gliomas occur in the setting of NF-1. Therefore, any patient found to harbor an optic pathway glioma should be assessed for evidence of NF-1, and patients with cutaneous lesions consistent with NF-1 should be screened for optic pathway gliomas and other intracranial lesions that occur in patients with neurofibromatosis. Among visually asymptomatic children with NF-1, neuroimaging reveals optic pathway gliomas in about 15% of cases.

Gliomas that affect the optic nerve may occasionally be confined to the optic disc. Most of these rare lesions occur in patients with NF-1. They may cause a change in the appearance of the optic disc that simulates true swelling, or, as in most cases, the normal features of the optic disc are obscured by a mass of whitish, gray, or yellow tissue that projects from and above the disc surface. Visual acuity in patients with gliomas of the optic disc is variably affected.

Optic nerve gliomas are not hamartomas but rather are true neoplasms with a potential for significant visual morbidity and a small but significant mortality. Most of these tumors, regardless of their localization or extent within the nerve, are of the juvenile pilocytic variety and have a benign appearance on microscopy. Less common features include capillary proliferation, tissue necrosis with hemorrhage, glial giant cells, and even mitotic figures. A reactive leptomeningeal hyperplasia occurs around some of these lesions, both within the orbit and within the optic canal. This can lead to the erroneous diagnosis of optic nerve meningioma if only the superficial aspect of the nerve is biopsied. Gliomas that occur in patients with NF-1 show the

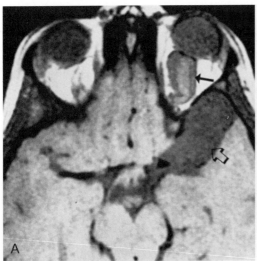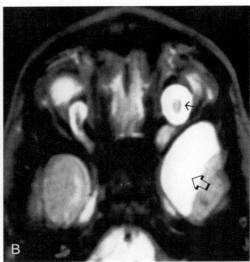

Figure 8.9.   The pseudo-CSF sign in a patient with neurofibromatosis type 1 and bilateral optic nerve gliomas. *A.* T1-weighted MRI, axial view, shows that the orbital portion of the left optic nerve consists of a fusiform area of low intensity (*solid arrow*) surrounding a core of high signal intensity. An arachnoid cyst (*hollow arrow*) occupies the left anterior cranial fossa. Note that the peripheral (outer) tumor signal is isointense to the CSF in the cyst. The tumor is kinked posteriorly. The right optic nerve glioma cannot be seen on this image. *B.* T2-weighted MRI, axial view, shows a donut-shaped signal of high intensity (*black arrow*) surrounding an inner circle of low signal intensity in the left orbit. This image represents a tangential cut through the superior aspect of the upwardly kinked tumor. In the right orbit, a linear area of high signal intensity surrounds a central core of low signal intensity. Note that the outer signal within both tumors is isointense to CSF within the arachnoid cyst (*hollow arrow*). (Reprinted with permission from Brodsky MC. The ''pseudo-CSF'' signal of orbital optic glioma on magnetic resonance imaging: a signature of neurofibromatosis. Surv Ophthalmol 1993;36:213–218.)

unique feature of extension of tumor into the subarachnoid and dural spaces surrounding the nerve, whereas gliomas that occur in patients without neurofibromatosis produce diffuse enlargement of the nerve without extension into the subdural or subarachnoid space.

Most optic nerve gliomas do not change substantially in size or shape over many years. Some, however, rapidly enlarge and extend along the nerve to the chiasm and even into the 3rd ventricle. Others suddenly expand from intraneural hemorrhage. Conversely, rare lesions exhibit spontaneous regression.

The potential for gliomas apparently confined to one optic nerve to extend to the optic chiasm, the opposite optic nerve, or both is unclear. Most authors consider such extension to be extremely rare; however, in one study of 106 patients with unilateral gliomas initially confined to the orbit at study entry, local progression occurred in 20% of untreated patients, in 29% following incomplete surgical resection, and in 2.3% following

apparent complete excision. Thus, it is important to follow patients with optic nerve gliomas both clinically and with neuroimaging, regardless of whether or not they are treated.

The optimum treatment of optic nerve gliomas is also unclear. The natural history of these benign lesions is generally good, with long-term useful visual function and few, if any, neurologic complications. Indeed, some gliomas appear to regress spontaneously, resulting in gradual improvement in vision in the affected eye. Some gliomas, however, enlarge and cause progressive visual loss in one or both eyes. Such lesions may even extend into the hypothalamus and 3rd ventricle. For this reason, consideration is often given to treating patients with gliomas confined to one optic nerve with surgical resection, radiation therapy, chemotherapy, or a combination of these modalities. We generally reserve surgical resection for those patients who are already blind when we first see them, for patients with severe proptosis, and for patients whose lesions seem

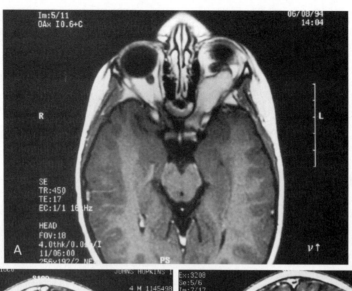

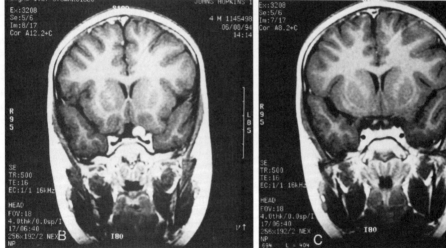

Figure 8.10. Left optic glioma near the optic chiasm in a 6-year-old boy without neurofibromatosis type 1. *A.* T1-weighted MRI, axial view, after intravenous injection of paramagnetic contrast material, shows that the glioma extends through the optic canal up to the optic chiasm. *B.* T1-weighted enhanced MRI, coronal view, shows enlargement and enhancement of the intracranial portion of the left optic nerve. *C.* T1-weighted enhanced MRI, coronal view, 3 mm posterior to the view seen in *B* shows that the left optic nerve just anterior to the optic chiasm is normal in size and does not enhance, suggesting that the tumor has not yet reached this site. This is the type of patient who might be considered a candidate for excision of the tumor.

to be threatening the optic chiasm but that have not yet reached it (Fig. 8.10). No clinical trials have been performed to indicate if removal of an apparently unilateral optic nerve glioma is associated with a better visual and neurologic prognosis than no treatment.

We rarely treat patients with optic nerve glio-
mas with either chemotherapy or radiation therapy unless or until the lesion extends into the optic chiasm, opposite optic nerve, or hypothalamus. It must be remembered that radiation therapy can have significant side effects, particularly in children. These include developmental delay, vasculitis, moyamoya disease, leukoencepha-

lopathy, radionecrosis of the temporal lobes, endocrinopathies, behavior disturbances, and the induction of secondary malignancies.

The efficacy of chemotherapeutic agents in the treatment of optic nerve gliomas is unclear. Most investigators agree that the drugs are never curative; however, they may stabilize or reduce the growth rate and progression of visual manifestations of the tumor and thus delay the need for radiation therapy, particularly in young children.

Most gliomas that infiltrate the optic nerve or chiasm are, as noted above, benign juvenile pilocytic astrocytomas; however, some are malignant. Malignant optic gliomas almost always occur in adults and produce one of two clinical pictures. When the tumor initially affects the intracranial optic nerves or chiasm, there is rapidly progressive visual loss associated with optic discs that initially appear normal but that rapidly become atrophic. The visual loss in these cases is often bilateral and simultaneous, but it may initially begin in one eye and thus may be mistaken for retrobulbar optic neuritis, particularly when there is associated pain. When the malignant glioma initially affects the proximal portion of the intraorbital optic nerve, there is acute loss of vision associated with optic disc swelling and the ophthalmoscopic appearance of a central retinal vein occlusion. The prognosis in almost all cases of malignant optic glioma is poor, regardless of treatment with radiotherapy or chemotherapy. Most patients become completely blind within several months after the onset of symptoms, and most die within 6 to 12 months.

Ganglioglioma

Tumors primarily composed of mature ganglion cells may occur in both the peripheral nervous system and the central nervous system (CNS). Ganglion cell tumors of the CNS are less common than their peripheral counterparts. Such tumors nevertheless do exist and appear to be of two main types.

- **Ganglioneuromas** (also called gangliocytomas) are composed predominantly of mature ganglion cells supported by a stroma of spindle cells and containing calcospherites.
- **Gangliogliomas** are composed of a mixture of mature ganglion cells and mature

glial cells and are thus true mixed neurogliogenic tumors.

These two types of tumor represent extremes of the spectrum of tumors containing mature ganglion cells, and there are many tumors that must be considered transition forms between them.

Ganglion cell tumors occur most frequently in children and young adults. Nevertheless, the age range is broad, from several months to 80 years of age. They occur with equal frequency in males and females.

The most common location of ganglion cell tumors is the floor of the 3rd ventricle, where they produce symptoms and signs related to dysfunction of the hypothalamus or pituitary gland, including precocious puberty, diabetes insipidus, acromegaly, and panhypopituitarism. In rare instances, the gangliogliomas originate within the substance of the optic chiasm or intracranial portion of the optic nerves, and thus may be mistaken for a typical "optic glioma." The MRI findings have no distinguishing features, showing only a fusiform dilation of the optic nerve with enhancement after intravenous injection of paramagnetic contrast material. Chiasmatic infiltration by a ganglioglioma can also occur, either from extension from adjacent brain or originating within the chiasm.

The microscopic appearance of the ganglion cell tumors varies according to the extent to which neuronal and glial elements participate in the neoplastic process. The pure ganglioneuroma is a poorly or moderately cellular tumor in which the cells are clearly neuronal in origin but are often abnormal in appearance. Although some of the cells are well differentiated, others are extremely bizarre, varying greatly in size and shape from tiny mononuclear cells to giant multinucleated forms. Mitoses are almost never observed. The distribution of nerve cells varies throughout the tumor. The cells may form closely packed clusters, especially near blood vessels, or be fairly evenly interspersed among glial cells. In pure ganglioneuromas, the glial element consists of a scanty stroma of spindle cells; but in gangliogliomas there is clear evidence of neoplastic astrocytic proliferation. Gangliogliomas thus contain glial cells that show histologic differentiation that parallels that of neurons. The degree of differentiation may be so great that such tumors may initially be thought to be pleomorphic fibrillary astrocytomas until careful examination reveals their true composition.

Most ganglion cell tumors, whether ganglioneuromas or gangliogliomas, have a good prognosis because they behave biologically as low-grade astrocytomas; however, the survival rates may be somewhat lower for patients with chiasmatic infiltration. In addition, some of these tumors do have malignant features. In these tumors, the malignant elements are usually glial, rather than neuronal, and metastases may occur.

Astrocytic Hamartoma

Astrocytic hamartomas can infiltrate the optic disc. In most cases, they protrude above or overlie the surface of the affected disc. They initially have a grayish or grayish-pink appearance, but they later develop a glistening, yellow, mulberry appearance (Fig. 8.11). Although this latter appearance is similar to that of optic disc drusen, drusen are located within the substance of the disc, whereas astrocytic hamartomas overlie the disc (Fig. 8.12).

The appearance of an astrocytic hamartoma is also similar to that of an endophytic or regressing retinoblastoma; however, astrocytic hamartomas do not exhibit the same rapid growth characteristics as a retinoblastoma. They also tend to be more yellow and glistening than retinoblastomas.

The visual function in an eye with an astrocytic hamartoma of the optic disc is usually normal. Some eyes, however, develop a serous detachment of the retina or vitreous hemorrhage, resulting in variable loss of vision.

Astrocytic hamartomas are composed almost entirely of acellular laminated calcific concretions. In many specimens, these concretions are interspersed among areas composed of large glial cells.

Most astrocytic hamartomas occur in patients with tuberous sclerosis or NF-1. In about 30% of cases, however, the patient has no evidence of any of the phacomatoses or of any other systemic disorder.

Capillary and Cavernous Hemangiomas

Both capillary and cavernous hemangiomas can occur within the substance of the optic disc. In addition, cavernous hemangiomas can develop at any location in the optic nerve and in the optic chiasm.

Capillary hemangiomas may be endophytic or exophytic. The *endophytic* type appears as a circular, reddish, slightly elevated mass internal to the disc vasculature and is represented histologically by a capillary hemangioma lying im-

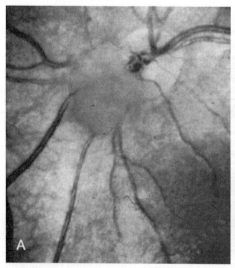 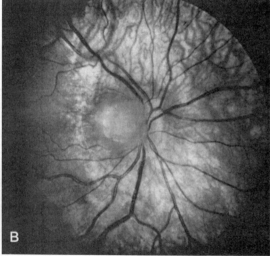

Figure 8.11. Astrocytic hamartoma of the optic disc. *A.* Before significant calcification, lesion appears as a pinkish gray mass rising above the disc. *B.* When calcification occurs, small globular clusters can be observed within the mass. Eventually, the entire mass may become calcified.

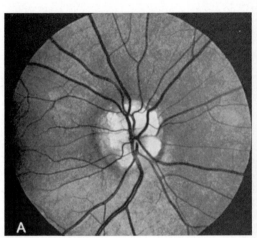
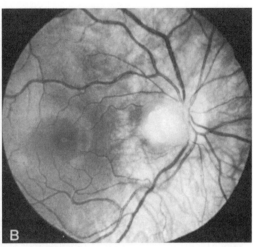

Figure 8.12.   Difference in ophthalmoscopic appearance of optic disc drusen and astrocytic hamartoma of the optic disc. *A.* Optic disc drusen are located within the substance of the disc **beneath** the vessels. *B.* Astrocytic hamartomas are located **above** the optic disc, thus obscuring the vessels.

mediately beneath the internal limiting membrane (Fig. 8.13). These lesions may be a manifestation of von Hippel-Lindau disease, or they may occur as an isolated phenomenon. The *exophytic* type of capillary hemangioma is typically seen as blurring and elevation of the disc margin, often associated with a variable degree of serous detachment of the peripapillary sensory retina and a ring of lipid deposition (Fig. 8.14). This lesion is often misdiagnosed as unilateral papilledema or papillitis, but fluorescein angiography clearly demonstrates the vascular anomaly, as does ultrasonography. These tumors may also occur as part of von Hippel-Lindau disease. Rarely, exophytic capillary angiomas are bilateral. In such instances, they are often misdiagnosed as papilledema; but again, fluorescein angiography and ultrasonography are invaluable in making the correct diagnosis. Capillary angiomas do not occur within the substance of the optic nerve or chiasm.

Cavernous hemangiomas consist of large-caliber vascular channels. When these lesions occur as isolated masses within the orbit, they are well circumscribed and encapsulated. Within the eye, however, their appearance is that of a cluster of small purple blobs located within and above the substance of the optic disc (Fig. 8.15). The blood flow within the vessels in cavernous hemangiomas is extremely slow, indicating that

this lesion is more isolated from the general circulation than its capillary counterpart.

Cavernous hemangiomas of the optic disc are usually unilateral. They occur more commonly in females than in males, with an irregularly autosomal-dominant inheritance pattern. The lesion is almost always asymptomatic, with visual acuity being normal and visual fields showing only a variably enlarged blind spot; however, rare cases have been reported in which there has been vitreous hemorrhage. Usually these lesions do not grow, although there are rare exceptions.

Cavernous hemangiomas, unlike capillary hemangiomas, can occur within the retrolaminar, intracanalicular, and intracranial optic nerves, the optic chiasm, or the optic tracts. In some cases, the lesion itself causes slowly progressive loss of vision. In most cases, however, visual loss is rapidly progressive and occurs because of hemorrhage into the surrounding tissue. Factors such as alcohol abuse, the hormonal effects of pregnancy, and the Valsalva maneuver have been associated with the onset of visual loss in patients with these lesions, which typically occur in the third or fourth decade of life; the triad of symtoms are (1) sudden headache, (2) an acute change in visual acuity, and (3) a significant defect in the visual field. Interestingly, up to one-third of patients have episodes

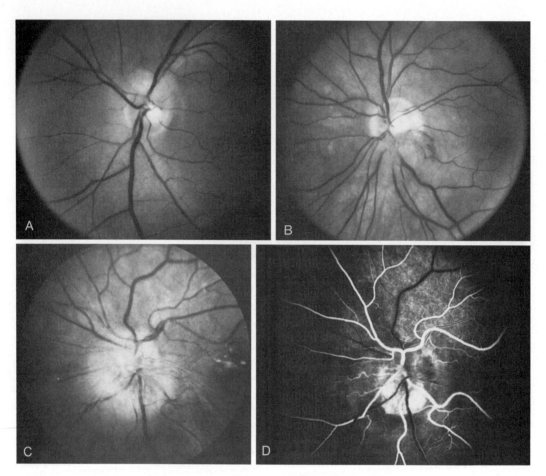

Figure 8.13. Endophytic capillary angioma. *A–C.* The lesions appear as a circular, reddish, slightly elevated mass internal to the disc vasculature. *D.* Fluorescein angiography of lesion seen in *C* shows intense staining and leakage from vessels at inferior aspect of disc.

of transient visual loss that are erroneously diagnosed as optic neuritis.

Cavernous hemangiomas are not associated with von Hippel-Lindau disease, but they are often associated with similar lesions of the skin and brain and may also be associated with anomalies of extracranial and intracranial arteries. In contrast to the benign nature of the ocular lesion, associated CNS vascular hamartomas may produce convulsions, intracranial hemorrhage, cranial nerve palsies, and multiple neurologic deficits.

Optic Nerve Hemangioblastoma

Not all vascular lesions within the substance of the optic nerve are benign. Both the orbital and intracranial portions of the nerve can be infiltrated by a malignant hemangioblastoma. Only 30% of these lesions are associated with the von Hippel-Lindau disease; however, partial expression of genetic disorders is being documented with increasing frequency, and many of the other lesions associated with von Hippel-Lindau disease may not become apparent for a number of years, especially because the previously documented cases were reported in individuals ranging in age from 15 to 44 years. Furthermore, the investigation of family members in some of these cases may have been incomplete, leading to the erroneous conclusion that the disorder was not familial.

The typical patient with an optic nerve heman-

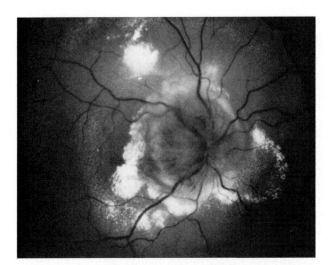

Figure 8.14. Exophytic capillary angioma of the optic disc. This lesion appears as diffuse blurring and elevation of the disc, associated with a variable degree of serous detachment of the peripapillary sensory retina and a ring of lipid deposition. (Courtesy of Dr. Andrew Schachat.)

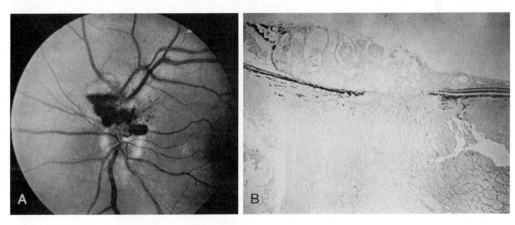

Figure 8.15. Cavernous angioma of the optic disc. *A.* Note "cluster of grapes" appearance of lesion. *B.* Histologic appearance of a cavernous angioma showing multiple dilated vessels above and adjacent to the disc surface. (Reprinted with permission from Davies WS, Thumin M. Cavernous hemangioma of the optic disc and retina. Trans Am Acad Ophthalmol Otolaryngol 1956;60:217–218. AFIP Acc. 219953.)

gioblastoma presents with progressive visual loss and evidence of an optic neuropathy that may be anterior or retrobulbar, depending on the location of the lesion. The degree of visual loss is variable, and any type of visual field defect may be present. There is always a relative afferent pupillary defect. The affected portion of the optic nerve is enlarged and has a fusiform appearance that mimics an optic nerve glioma on neuroimaging (Fig. 8.16).

Hemangioblastomas of the optic nerve, like their counterparts elsewhere in the CNS, usually have a plane of section that permits surgical re-

moval without sacrificing the entire optic nerve. However, some of these lesions envelop the nerve and cannot be removed without producing permanent and complete visual loss in the affected eye.

Melanocytomas

Melanocytomas are intraocular tumors that typically occur within the substance of the optic disc. Clinically, these lesions are elevated masses that are gray to dark black in color and are located eccentrically on the disc (Fig. 8.17). About 90% are 2 disc diameters or less in diame-

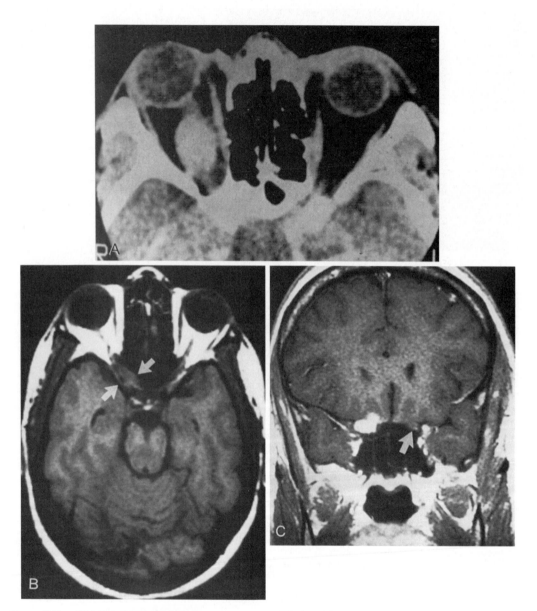

Figure 8.16. Neuroimaging appearance of hemangioblastomas of the optic nerve. *A.* In a 37-year-old man with von Hippel-Lindau disease. CT scan, axial view, after intravenous injection of iodinated contrast material shows that the right optic nerve has an enhancing fusiform appearance similar to that of an optic nerve glioma. The diagnosis was established at surgery. (Reprinted with permission from Tanaka E, Kimura C, Inoue H, et al. A case of intraorbital hemangioblastoma of the optic nerve. Folia Ophthalmol Jpn 1984;35: 1390–1395.) *B.* In a 40-year-old woman, T1-weighted MRI, axial view, shows enlargement of the intracanalicular portion of the right optic nerve (*arrows*). *C.* In the same patient as *B*, T1-weighted MRI, coronal view, after intravenous injection of paramagnetic contrast material shows enlarged, enhancing right optic nerve within the optic canal. Note normal sized optic nerve on left (*arrow*). (*B–C:* Reprinted with permission from Kerr J, Scheithauer BW, Miller GM, et al. Hemangioblastoma of the optic nerve: case report. Neurosurgery 1995;36:573–579.)

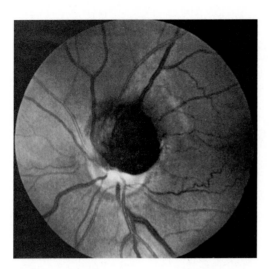

Figure 8.17. Melanocytoma of the optic disc. The optic disc is almost completely obscured by an elevated, black mass. The mass is much darker than a malignant melanoma.

ter, and the majority are less than 2 mm in height. Swelling of the disc occurs in about 25% of cases and is thought to be caused by a disturbance of axoplasmic flow secondary to chronic compression. Vascular sheathing may be seen in 30% of eyes, and subretinal fluid is observed in approximately 10% of patients. A nevus may be seen adjacent to a melanocytoma in up to 50% of cases. Visual acuity remains 20/20 or better in the majority of patients, and nearly all patients retain visual acuity of 20/50 or better. Although few patients are aware of any visual distortion, most have abnormal visual fields, especially blind spot enlargement, arcuate scotomas, and even generalized constriction.

Not all patients with a melanocytoma have good visual acuity. Some patients develop an associated central retinal artery occlusion, and others develop ischemic necrosis of the tumor and surrounding neural tissue. The underlying mechanism in both settings is believed to be compression of large and small vessels of the disc. Rarely, spontaneous recovery of vision occurs.

Histologically, melanocytomas are composed of two types of cells. The predominant cells are plump polyhedral nevus cells containing numerous giant melanosomes. These cells show advanced differentiation and appear to be metabolically inactive. The second cell type is a smaller, lightly pigmented, spindle-shaped cell that is more metabolically active.

Melanocytomas are benign tumors that do not require therapy. Slight growth may occur over many years in a minority of patients, and malignant transformation is not characteristic. The deep black appearance of melanocytomas generally allows them to be differentiated not only from optic disc swelling but also from other lesions that infiltrate the optic disc, particularly malignant melanomas. Nevertheless, the distinction can be difficult in rare cases, particularly when the lesion is not changing in size or shape (Fig. 8.18).

Secondary Tumors

The most common secondary tumors that infiltrate the optic nerve are metastatic and locally invasive carcinomas and various lymphoreticular malignancies, particularly lymphoma and leukemia.

Metastatic and Locally Invasive Tumors

The optic nerve may be the site of metastasis from distant tumors or of spread of tumor from a contiguous structure. Metastases can reach the optic nerve by one of four routes: (1) from the choroid, (2) by vascular dissemination, (3) by invasion from the orbit, or (4) from the CNS. Regardless of the mode of spread, the substance of the nerve is affected more often than the sheath. Bilateral involvement occurs in approximately 18% of patients.

Patients with metastases to the optic nerve usually have evidence of an optic neuropathy. The visual loss is usually severe, but relatively normal vision may be present in the early stages. Any type of field defect may be present. A relative afferent pupillary defect is usually present unless the patient has bilateral optic nerve metastases or the opposite retina or optic nerve has previously been damaged by some other condition. When the metastasis is located in the prelaminar or immediately retrolaminar portion of the optic nerve, the optic disc is usually swollen; a yellow-white mass can be seen to protrude from the surface of the nerve (Fig. 8.19); and clumps of tumor cells can occasionally be seen in the vitreous overlying the disc. A central retinal vein occlusion occurs in up to 50% of eyes. When the metastasis is to the posterior aspect of the orbital portion of the optic nerve or to the intracanalicular or intracranial portions of the nerve, the optic disc initially appears normal.

The most common metastatic tumors to the optic nerve are adenocarcinomas, primarily be-

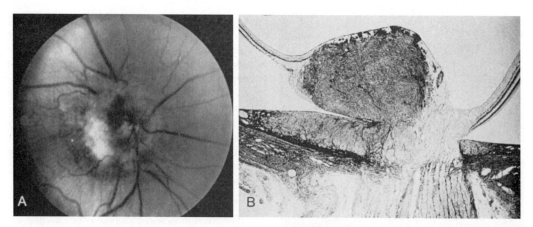

Figure 8.18. Malignant melanoma of the choroid invading the optic disc. *A.* The disc tissue is elevated and shows areas of pigmentation with partial obscuration of vessels and blur- ring of disc margins. *B.* Histologic appearance of a juxtapapillary malignant melanoma invading the optic nerve.

cause these are the most common metastatic tumors to all parts of the body. In women, carcinomas of the breast and lung are the most common tumors, whereas carcinomas of the lung and bowel are most common in men. Other tumors that can metastasize to the optic nerve include carcinomas of the stomach, pancreas, uterus, ovary, prostate, kidney, and tonsillar fossa. Skin cancers, malignant melanoma, and mediastinal tumors also may metastasize to one or both optic nerves. Isolated metastases to the optic nerve of intracranial tumors, such as medulloblastomas, may rarely occur.

Contiguous spread of primary tumors from the paranasal sinuses, brain, and adjacent intraocular structures to the optic nerve occurs much less often than does metastasis to the nerve. Because of its close anatomic association with the paranasal sinuses, the optic nerve can be infiltrated or compressed by cancer that arises in the sinuses or the nasopharynx. In most cases, the tumor invades the posterior orbit or cavernous sinus, producing a syndrome that is characterized by loss of vision, diplopia, ophthalmoparesis, and trigeminal sensory neuropathy. Rarely, a Foster Kennedy syndrome occurs.

Most patients with metastatic tumor to the optic nerve already have a known diagnosis of a primary carcinoma with other evidence of metastases at the time that visual loss occurs. This makes the diagnosis relatively straightforward, whereas most patients with a tumor that spreads

contiguously to the optic nerve are not known to harbor a tumor when they first experience loss of vision. Nevertheless, any person with known cancer in another part of the body, with or without other evidence of metastases, who develops an optic neuropathy should be suspected of having cancer as the cause until proven otherwise. Similarly, any patient with a basal skull tumor who develops an optic neuropathy should be assumed to have spread of tumor to the optic nerve, unless there has been previous radiation therapy to the region, in which case the possibility of radiation-induced optic neuropathy must also be considered.

Neuroimaging should be performed in all patients suspected of having infiltration of the optic nerve by cancer. CT scanning typically shows an enhancing nerve that may or may not be enlarged (Fig. 8.20). On MRI, the nerve is usually enlarged and shows varying T1 and T2 values that are presumed to be related to associated hemorrhage or exudate.

Most metastatic optic nerve tumors show at least a temporary response to radiation therapy. Tumors that spread contiguously to the optic nerve from the base of the skull or paranasal sinuses are typically less radiosensitive than metastatic tumors and also tend to be less responsive to chemotherapy.

Rarer than cases of metastatic or locally invasive tumors of the optic nerve are cases of "tumor within a tumor" or so-called "collision

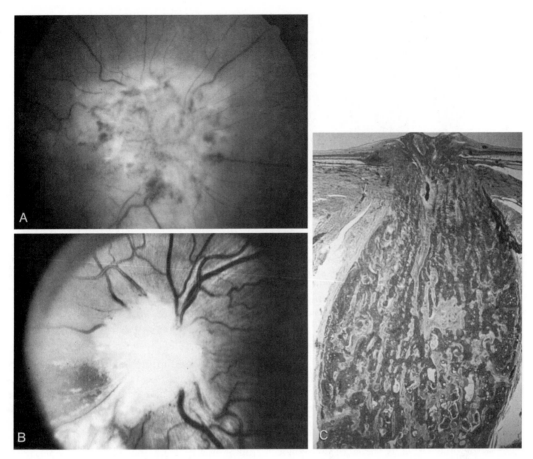

Figure 8.19.   Metastatic adenocarcinoma to the optic disc. *A.* Breast carcinoma in a 47-year-old woman. The entire optic disc is infiltrated by a large mass of yellow-white tissue. Note loss of normal disc architecture. There were nu- merous malignant cells in the vitreous. *B.* Lung carcinoma in a 56-year-old man. Note the white mass protruding from disc surface. *C.* Appearance at autopsy of optic nerve infiltra- tion by adenocarcinoma of the lung.

tumors.'' In these cases, one tumor is metastatic to another tumor. Renal cell carcinoma seems to be the best recipient or host tumor to ''attract'' other cancers, with lung carcinoma being the most common primary tumor to metastasize to the site. In the cases of metastasis to benign optic nerve tumors, the host tumor is usually a benign optic nerve meningioma.

Meningeal Carcinomatosis (Carcinomatous Meningitis)

Meningeal tumor cuffing or direct infiltration of the optic nerve can cause loss of vision in the setting of meningeal spread of carcinoma. This phenomenon is called **carcinomatous meningitis** or **meningeal carcinomatosis.**

The frequency of optic nerve involvement in patients with carcinomatosis of the meninges ranges from 15 to 40%. Patients who develop meningeal carcinomatosis with visual loss may do so after the primary lesion, usually lung or breast, has already been diagnosed. In other cases, visual loss may occur coincident with other signs of chronic meningitis or as an iso- lated finding as the first sign of disease.

Although blindness may begin in one eye, both eyes are usually affected within a short pe- riod of time. In rare instances, visual loss re- mains strictly unilateral. The optic neuropathy that occurs in the setting of meningeal carcino- matosis is usually associated with a ''diagnostic quartet'' that consists of (1) headaches typical

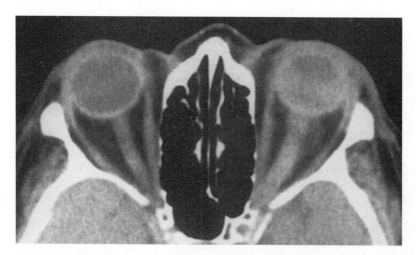

Figure 8.20. Neuroimaging appearance of infiltration of optic nerve by metastatic carcinoma. CT scan, axial view, in a 56-year-old woman with small-cell carcinoma of the lung and progressive loss of vision in the left eye associated with a massive retinal infiltrate with nasal retinal detachment reveals that the orbital portion of the left optic nerve is diffusely enlarged. (Reprinted with permission from Allaire GS, Corriveau C, Arbour J-D. Metastasis to the optic nerve: clinicopathological correlations. Can J Ophthalmol 1995;30: 306–311.)

of raised intracranial pressure, (2) blindness, (3) sluggish or absent pupillary reflexes, and (4) normal-appearing optic discs.

Histopathologic examination of cases with meningeal carcinomatosis and blindness generally shows marked cuffing of the subarachnoid space of the optic nerve by sheets of malignant cells, with little invasion of the nerves themselves. Thus, in some cases, there is true infiltration; in other cases, the lesion is more compressive than infiltrative.

Lymphoreticular Malignancies

Hematopoiesis is the orderly process of cell proliferation and maturation that maintains the normal concentration of cellular elements in the peripheral blood. Any cell involved in hematopoiesis, regardless of its degree of differentiation, may proliferate excessively, producing a hematologic proliferative disorder. Some of these disorders, particularly leukemia and lymphoma, can infiltrate the optic nerve.

LYMPHOMA

CNS involvement in non-Hodgkin's lymphoma (NHL) is unusual, but it occurs in about 10% of cases. Of these, 5% (or a total of 0.5% of patients with NHL) will have infiltration of the optic nerve at some time during the course

of their disease. Infiltration of the optic nerve in Hodgkin's disease is even less common. Nevertheless, infiltration of the retrobulbar optic nerve and optic chiasm occurs in patients with both Hodgkin's disease and NHL. In most of these cases, the infiltration occurs from spread of CNS tumor, rarely from the adjacent paranasal sinuses.

In many cases of lymphomatous infiltration of the anterior visual sensory pathway, the patient is known to have NHL or Hodgkin's disease at the time visual signs and symptoms develop, and the diagnosis is not in doubt. In other cases, the visual loss is the presenting sign of the disease.

The symptoms and signs of patients with lymphomatous infiltration of the anterior visual system depend on the location and extent of the lesion. In some cases, the visual loss is insidious in onset and slowly progressive, whereas in other cases the visual loss is acute and mimics optic neuritis or ischemic optic neuropathy.

The appearance of optic nerve or chiasm infiltration by lymphoma is nonspecific. The infiltrated structure is enlarged and reveals increased density on CT scanning; it enhances after intravenous injection of iodinated contrast material. The same structure can be iso-, hyper-, or hypo-intense on T1-weighted MRI; it is hyperintense on T2-weighted MRI, and enhances after intravenous injection of paramagnetic contrast material (Fig. 8.21).

LEUKEMIA

About 4% of children with acute leukemia have evidence of optic nerve infiltration. In some of the patients, visual acuity is lost abruptly; in others, there is a gradual progression of visual loss over days, weeks, or months. In still others, the disc appears swollen, but there is no evidence of visual dysfunction.

Most patients with leukemic infiltration of the optic nerve are known to have leukemia at the time the visual loss occurs or the patient is found to have asymptomatic disc swelling; however, in some cases, the optic neuropathy is the first evidence of the disease. Patients can have acute lymphocytic leukemia, acute myelogenous leukemia, monocytic leukemia, erythroleukemia, or chronic lymphocytic leukemia. Two distinct clinical patterns of infiltration can occur: (1) infiltration of the optic disc, and (2) infiltration of the immediate retrolaminar portion of the proximal optic nerve.

In **leukemic infiltration of the optic disc,** the features of the disc are obscured by a whitish fluffy infiltrate that is often associated with true disc swelling and peripapillary hemorrhage (Fig. 8.22). The visual acuity in such patients is mini-

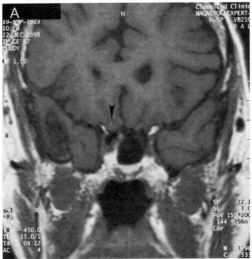

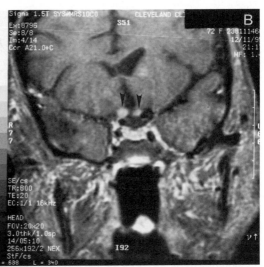

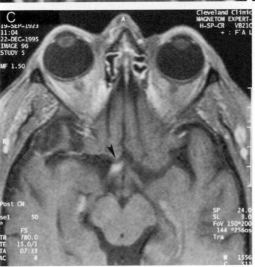

Figure 8.21. Neuroimaging appearance of infiltration of the right optic nerve, chiasm, and tract by a lymphoma. *A.* T1-weighted MRI, coronal view, shows enlarged right optic nerve (*arrowhead*). *B.* T1-weighted MRI, coronal view, after intravenous injection of paramagnetic contrast material shows enhancement of the right optic nerve and, to a lesser extent, the left optic nerve (*arrowheads*) just anterior to the optic chiasm. *C.* T1-weighted MRI, axial view, after intravenous injection of paramagnetic contrast material shows enhancement of anterior portion of the right optic tract (*arrowhead*).

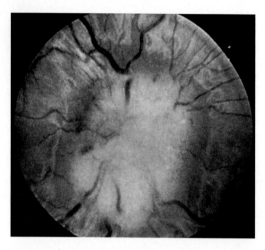

Figure 8.22. Leukemic infiltration of the optic disc mimicking optic disc swelling in a child with acute lymphocytic leukemia. The child was thought to be in remission at the time the abnormality was discovered. The disc is whitish gray and markedly elevated with obscuration of vessels. Visual acuity is 20/25.

mally affected, unless the infiltration or associated edema and hemorrhage extend into the macula.

Infiltration of the proximal optic nerve just posterior to the lamina cribrosa usually produces markedly decreased visual acuity associated with true optic disc swelling. Such patients have a variety of visual field defects, and a relative afferent pupillary defect is invariably present unless the infiltration is bilateral and symmetric. In addition, there are often peripapillary and peripheral retinal hemorrhages. Neuroimaging in such cases typically reveals a diffusely enlarged optic nerve that usually enhances after intravenous injection of contrast material.

The response of leukemic infiltration of the optic nerve to radiation therapy is usually rapid and dramatic. In almost all cases, visual function returns to normal or near normal, and the disc elevation, if present, resolves.

It must be emphasized that swelling of the optic disc can occur in patients with acute leukemia when CNS involvement by the disease results in increased intracranial pressure. Optic disc swelling and neovascularization also occur as a local phenomenon in the setting of the diffuse retinopathy of acute leukemia. Thus, one must consider a number of pathologic mechanisms in addition to infiltration in any patient

with acute leukemia and apparent optic disc swelling.

The acute leukemias are responsible for most of the reported cases of infiltrative optic neuropathies caused by lymphoreticular disorders; however, patients with chronic forms of leukemia may also develop optic nerve infiltration. Autopsy studies reveal a high percentage of asymptomatic CNS involvement in patients with chronic lymphocytic leukemia. Patients with optic nerve infiltration in the setting of chronic lymphocytic leukemia and other chronic leukemias have a more indolent clinical course than patients with the acute leukemias. Visual loss is less severe, and retinal changes of the type seen in acute leukemia are rare. Optic disc swelling, however, is indistinguishable from that which occurs in patients with infiltration in the setting of acute leukemia.

OTHER LYMPHORETICULAR TUMORS

Multiple myeloma, lymphomatoid granulomatosis, and Langerhans cell histiocytosis can all produce an optic neuropathy. In some of these cases, the optic neuropathy, which may be of the anterior or retrobulbar variety, appears to be produced by infiltration of the nerve, rather than from compression.

INFLAMMATORY AND INFECTIOUS INFILTRATIVE OPTIC NEUROPATHIES

The intraocular, intraorbital, intracanalicular, and intracranial segments of the optic nerve can all be infiltrated by inflammatory and infectious processes. The most common inflammatory process that produces an infiltrative optic neuropathy is sarcoidosis. The most common infectious processes that produce an infiltrative optic neuropathy are syphilis, tuberculosis, and opportunistic fungal infections such as cryptococcosis.

Inflammatory Disorders
Sarcoidosis

Optic nerve dysfunction probably is the most common neuro-ophthalmologic manifestation of sarcoidosis. The optic nerve may be affected at any time during the course of the disease and may be the site of its initial presentation. Sarcoidosis may affect the optic nerve in several different ways. It may produce papilledema, a compressive anterior or retrobulbar optic neuropathy, an ischemic optic neuropathy, or anterior or retrobulbar optic neuritis. The optic neuritis results from granulomatous infiltration of the optic disc, anterior orbital, posterior orbital, intracanalicular, or intracranial portions of the nerve, or a combination of these. In some cases, more than one process is responsible.

Granulomatous infiltration of the optic disc may or may not be associated with evidence by neuroimaging or ultrasonography of diffuse enlargement of the orbital portion of the optic nerve. The optic disc in such cases usually is markedly elevated, either diffusely or sectorially (Fig. 8.23), and it often has a solid or nodular appearance that can best be demonstrated using ultrasonography. There may be dilated vessels resembling neovascularization on the surface of the disc.

The appearance of optic disc infiltration by sarcoid granulomas may mimic that of papilledema, except that the former condition is more often unilateral than bilateral, and it is usually associated with decreased vision, slit-lamp biomicroscopic and ophthalmoscopic evidence of intraocular inflammation, neuroimaging evidence of an intracranial process affecting the base of the skull, or a combination of these. When the process is bilateral, however, the disc swelling may easily be mistaken for papilledema.

When the proximal portion of the intraorbital optic nerve is infiltrated by granulomatous inflammation in patients with sarcoidosis, the condition typically presents as an acute, subacute, or rarely chronic optic neuritis. The patient typi-

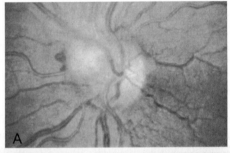

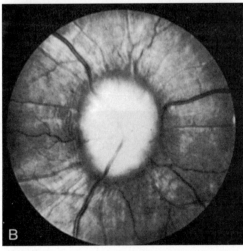

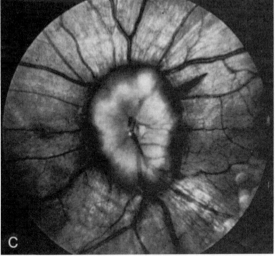

Figure 8.23. Sarcoid granulomas infiltrating the optic disc. *A.* In a 25-year-old woman with visual acuity of 20/20 OU. There is a small elevated yellow-white mass overlying the nasal portion of the left optic disc. A small hemorrhage is just nasal to the mass. (Reprinted with permission from Laties AM, Scheie HG. Evolution of multiple small tumors in sarcoid granuloma of the optic disk. Am J Ophthalmol 1972; 74:60–66.) *B.* In another patient, the entire disc is infiltrated by granulomas. Note diffuse symmetric elevation of the disc substance. *C.* In a third patient, a multinodular granuloma has infiltrated the left optic disc. (Reprinted with permission from Jampol LM, Woodfin W, McLean EB. Optic nerve sarcoidosis. Arch Ophthalmol 1972;87:355–360.)

cally experiences progressive loss of vision, decreased color vision, and a worsening visual field defect. A relative afferent pupillary defect is present unless there is also a contralateral optic neuropathy. The optic disc is swollen. This condition may be impossible to differentiate clinically from demyelinating optic neuritis and even from certain causes of compressive optic neuropathy, particularly optic nerve sheath meningioma. Even ultrasonography, which reveals enlargement of the orbital portion of the nerve in almost all cases, and neuroimaging, which shows enlargement and enhancement of the orbital portion of the optic nerve (Fig. 8.24), cannot establish the diagnosis with certainty. In some cases, the diagnosis is made by finding clinical, radiographic, or laboratory evidence of sarcoidosis elsewhere. In other cases, the diagnosis is not confirmed until a biopsy of the nerve is performed.

The posterior retrobulbar or intracanalicular portion of the optic nerve can also be affected by sarcoid. In such cases, the patient develops acute or, more often, progressive loss of vision associated with evidence of an optic neuropathy. The optic disc in such cases is normal but gradually becomes pale if no treatment is given. The neuroimaging appearance is variable. The posterior orbital portion of the optic nerve may be enlarged and may enhance after contrast injection on both CT scanning and MRI (Fig. 8.25). The optic foramen may be enlarged.

Because of the predilection of neurosarcoidosis to affect the basal meninges, the intracranial portion of one or both optic nerves and the optic chiasm may occasionally be affected by the disease, producing a variety of patterns of visual loss. In some patients, loss of vision occurs as an isolated phenomenon, either simultaneously in both eyes or in one eye followed within days to weeks by loss of vision in the other eye. In other patients, visual loss is associated with evidence of hypothalamic dysfunction, hypothalamic hypopituitarism (particularly gonadotropin failure), or both.

The diagnosis of sarcoidosis depends on a compatible clinical picture combined with appropriate imaging studies and, in some cases, serologic evaluation for elevated levels of angiotensin-converting enzyme (ACE) and histologic evidence of the disease by biopsy of involved tissues. A standard chest radiograph is an essential part of the evaluation, and chest CT and MRI may prove useful. Abnormal uptake on gallium scanning, although not specific for sarcoidosis, may represent areas accessible for biopsy. Conjunctival or lacrimal gland biopsy can establish the diagnosis, especially if the biopsied tissues are clinically affected.

The primary treatment of sarcoidosis is with corticosteroids. Most of the neurologic manifestations, including optic neuropathy, respond promptly to treatment; however, many patients require chronic therapy. Other agents reported beneficial in the treatment of sarcoid optic neuropathy, either separately or in combination with steroids, include immunosuppressive drugs such as cyclosporine, azathioprine, methotrexate, and cyclophosphamide, and radiation therapy.

Idiopathic Nongranulomatous Optic and Perioptic Neuritis

Some patients with otherwise typical acute optic neuritis associated with orbital or ocular pain, decreased vision, and visual field defects develop generalized enlargement of the orbital portion of the optic nerve that can be appreciated with both CT scanning and MRI. The enlarged portion of the nerve typically shows enhancement after intravenous injection of either iodinated contrast material (for CT scanning) or paramagnetic contrast material (for MRI). In the rare patients in whom a biopsy has been performed, the optic nerve sheath is found to be thickened and gray, and the optic nerve is found to be enlarged and of abnormal consistency. Histopathologic evaluation of the sheath shows a nongranulomatous inflammatory process without evidence of an infectious agent. The nerve contains a similar process.

Infectious Disorders

Tuberculosis can infiltrate the optic nerve. In some cases, the tuberculoma is adjacent to the optic nerve and is part of a dense adhesive arachnoiditis that may or may not be separable from the surrounding structures. In other cases, however, the inflammatory tissue actually invades the nerve, making removal impossible. Rarely, a tuberculoma is completely contained within the optic nerve.

Syphilitic gummas may act in a similar fashion. Retrobulbar optic neuritis occurs in patients with syphilis, and gummas within the optic disc also have been described.

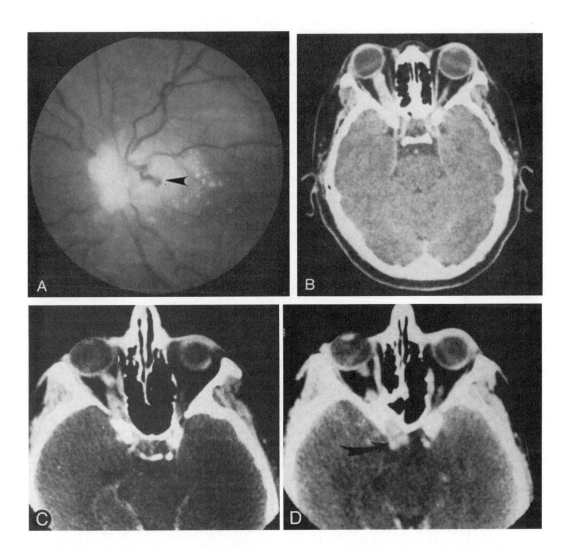

Figure 8.24. CT scanning of optic nerve sarcoidosis. *A.* Bilobed mass projecting from the medial aspect of the left optic disc in a patient with sarcoidosis. Note optociliary shunt vessel (*arrowhead*). *B.* CT scan, axial view, after intravenous injection of contrast material shows diffuse thickening and enhancement of the orbital portion of the left optic nerve. (Reprinted with permission from Lustgarden JS, Mindel JS, Yablonski ME, et al. An unusual presentation of isolated optic nerve sarcoidosis. J Clin Neuroophthalmol 1983;3:13–18.) *C.* CT scan, axial view, after intravenous injection of contrast in another patient with painless progressive loss of vision in the right eye and biopsy-proven sarcoid- osis shows diffuse enlargement and enhancement of the orbital portion of the right optic nerve. Note the "kinking" of the nerve, similar to that seen in patients with optic nerve glioma in the setting of neurofibromatosis type 1. *D.* CT scan, axial view, after intravenous contrast enhancement at a slightly higher plane in the same patient as *C* shows intracranial extension of the optic nerve lesion (*arrow*). (Reprinted with permission from Jordan DR, Anderson RL, Nerad JA, et al. Optic nerve involvement as the initial manifestation of sarcoidosis. Can J Ophthalmol 1988;23: 232–237.)

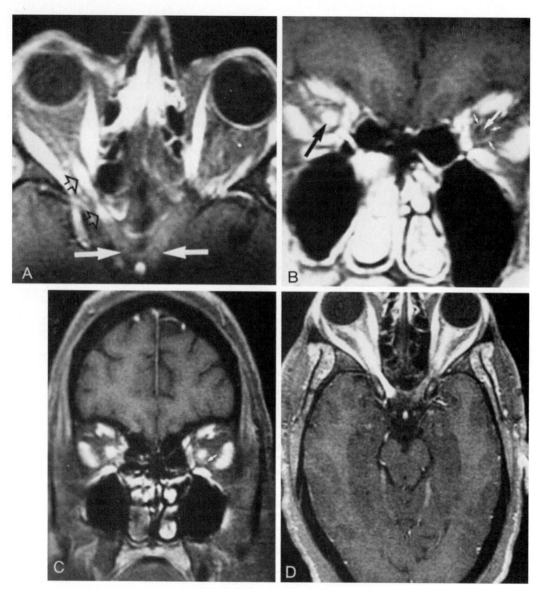

Figure 8.25. MRI in patients with sarcoidosis of the optic nerves. *A.* T1-weighted fat-suppressed MRI, axial view, after intravenous injection of paramagnetic contrast material in a 52-year-old woman with progressive loss of vision in the right eye shows irregular enhancement of the right optic nerve near the apex of the orbit and within the optic canal (*hollow arrows*). The intracranial portions of the optic nerves and the optic chiasm do not enhance and appear normal in size and shape (*solid arrows*). *B.* Enhanced T1-weighted fat-suppressed MRI, coronal view, in the same patient shows enlargement and abnormal enhancement of the orbital portion of the right optic nerve (*black arrow*). The left optic nerve is normal in size and does not enhance (*large white arrow*); however, there is mild enhancement of its leptomeningeal sheath (*small white arrows*). A biopsy of the nerve revealed noncaseating granulomas. *C.* Enhanced T1-weighted fat-suppressed MRI, coronal view, in another patient with sarcoidosis and progressive bilateral loss of vision with evidence of bilateral optic neuropathies reveals enlargement and abnormal enhancement of the orbital portions of both optic nerves. The right optic nerve is slightly larger than the left. Note mild enhancement of the leptomeningeal sheath of the left optic nerve (*arrow*). *D.* Enhanced T1-weighted fat-suppressed MRI, axial view, in the same patient shows enlargement and abnormal enhancement of both optic nerves throughout the orbits, with extension through the optic canal on the right side. (Reprinted with permission from Engelken JD, Yuh WTC, Carter KD, et al. Optic nerve sarcoidosis: MR findings. AJNR Am J Neuroradiol 1992; 13:228–230.)

Viral diseases such as cytomegalovirus and some of the herpes viruses can produce an infiltrative process of the optic nerve (see Chapter 6).

Invasion of the anterior visual system by cryptococcal organisms in the setting of cryptococcal meningitis is not uncommon, especially in patients with the acquired immune deficiency syndrome (AIDS). Visual loss in such instances may reflect direct optic nerve or chiasmal invasion by the organisms, adhesive constricting arachnoiditis, increased intracranial pressure with papilledema, or a combination of these processes. Visual loss can be sudden, subacute over days, or chronic over a period of months. Presumably, other organisms causing both acute and chronic meningitis cause visual loss in a similar manner.

FOR MORE INFORMATION:

See Walsh & Hoyt's *Clinical Neuro-Ophthalmology,* 5th edition, Volume 1, Chapter 13, pages 649–662; Chapter 15, pages 681–714; Volume 2, Chapter 39, pages 1941–1957; Chapter 40, pages 2044–2051; and Volume 5, Chapter 70, pages 5465–5529.

CHAPTER 9

Traumatic Optic Neuropathies

EPIDEMIOLOGY	PATHOLOGY
CLASSIFICATION	PATHOGENESIS
CLINICAL ASSESSMENT	Primary Mechanisms of Optic Nerve Injury
History	Secondary Mechanisms of Optic Nerve Injury
Examination	PHARMACOLOGY
Visual-Evoked Potentials	MANAGEMENT
Imaging Studies	

Traumatic optic neuropathy is classically separated into two types of injury: direct and indirect. *Direct* optic nerve injuries result from orbital or cerebral trauma that transgresses normal tissue planes to disrupt the anatomic and functional integrity of the optic nerve, such as a bullet penetrating the orbit or an endoscopic forceps avulsing the optic nerve. *Indirect* injuries are caused by forces transmitted at a distance from the optic nerve. Normal tissue planes are not transgressed in indirect optic nerve injuries. Instead, the anatomy and function of the optic nerve are compromised by energy absorbed by the nerve at the moment of impact. The classic example of an indirect injury to the optic nerve is that which occurs when blunt trauma to the forehead results in a transmission of force through the cranium to the confined intracanalicular portion of the nerve.

The prognosis of an optic nerve injury depends in part on whether it is direct or indirect. Direct injuries tend to produce severe and immediate visual loss with little likelihood of recovery. Indirect optic neuropathies, on the other hand, are not infrequently associated with visual recovery and may also produce delayed visual loss that occurs several hours to days after the injury.

Although the concept of direct and indirect optic nerve injury is helpful in some respects, the distinction between a direct and indirect injury does not necessarily illuminate the pathobiology of the injury, because both types of damage share certain common pathways following the initial injury. In addition, it is not always possible to determine which of the mechanisms is responsible or if both mechanisms have played a role in the visual loss.

EPIDEMIOLOGY

Optic nerve injury may be associated with little or no evidence of significant head trauma; however, in many cases, there is multisystem trauma or serious brain injury. Indeed, loss of consciousness occurs in 40 to 72% of patients with traumatic optic neuropathy. Traumatic optic neuropathy occurs in about 1.6% of head trauma cases and in 2.5% of patients with maxillofacial trauma and midface fractures.

The severity of initial visual loss in patients with traumatic optic neuropathy varies dramatically, from no light perception to 20/20 with an associated field defect. Although early studies reported visual acuities of light perception or worse in 67 to 100% of patients, the true prevalence of severe initial visual loss from traumatic optic neuropathy probably ranges from 43 to 56%. Visual loss is more likely to be severe in patients with neuroimaging evidence of a fracture of the optic canal.

The type of trauma that produces a traumatic optic neuropathy is usually a deceleration injury of significant momentum. In cases of isolated traumatic optic neuropathy, the force of the impact is typically directed to the ipsilateral forehead or to the midface region. Motor vehicle and bicycle accidents are the most frequent causes, accounting for 17 to 63% of cases. Motorcycle accident victims may be particularly vulnerable to traumatic optic neuropathy, with up to 18% of such accidents resulting in optic nerve dysfunction. Falls are the next most common cause, producing 14 to 50% of cases. Traumatic optic neuropathy can also occur in such diverse settings as frontal impact caused by falling debris, assault, stab wounds, gunshot wounds, skateboarding, and following seemingly trivial head trauma. It may also occur from iatrogenic injury, particularly after endoscopic sinus surgery and orbital surgery.

Traumatic optic neuropathy that occurs in the setting of orbital hemorrhage defines an important subset of optic nerve injury that does not fit well into the classic delineation of direct and indirect optic nerve injuries. For example, orbital hemorrhage after retrobulbar block occurs in 0.44 to 3% of patients. In most cases, the hemorrhage is quickly recognized and readily managed, with little impact on visual outcome unless a direct optic nerve injury has occurred from perforation of the nerve by the retrobulbar needle. Thus, the incidence of traumatic optic neuropathy in the setting of iatrogenic orbital hemorrhage is extremely low.

When retrobulbar hemorrhage occurs in association with blunt trauma to the orbit, the risk of visual loss is much greater. In this setting, blood may be dispersed throughout the orbit, in the subperiosteal space, and in the optic nerve sheath. In other cases, a hematic cyst may form, resulting in optic neuropathy from compression of the nerve by the cyst. Imaging studies can help to localize the hemorrhage in such cases.

Orbital emphysema is also a rare cause of optic nerve injury. It can follow orbital fractures, usually after vomiting or nose blowing force air into the orbit, compromising the optic nerve. Orbital emphysema with visual loss was reported in a patient following the use of a high-speed air-cooled drill during a dental procedure.

CLASSIFICATION

There are several different ways of classifying traumatic optic neuropathies. As noted above, optic nerve injuries can be divided into direct or indirect injuries. Optic nerve injuries can also be classified anatomically as optic disc trauma (avulsion), anterior optic neuropathy, or posterior optic neuropathy.

An avulsion of the optic nerve as it enters the globe produces a distinct ophthalmoscopic appearance, consisting of a partial ring of hemor-

rhage at the optic nerve head. In some cases, the site of the avulsion can be identified (Fig. 9.1).

Injuries to the proximal portion of the optic nerve within 10 mm of the globe, anterior to where the central retinal artery enters and the central retinal vein leaves the nerve, produce a variety of disturbances that are immediately apparent in the ocular fundus, including an ophthalmoscopic picture of a central retinal or branch artery occlusion, central retinal vein occlusion, or anterior ischemic optic neuropathy (Fig. 9.2).

In contrast, injuries to the optic nerve posterior to the entrance and exit of the central retinal artery and vein, respectively, produce no immediate change in the appearance of the ocular fundus. Specifically, the optic disc remains normal in appearance for at least 3 to 5 weeks, following which it becomes pale. The most common site of posterior indirect optic nerve injury is the optic canal.

The intracranial optic nerve is the next most common site of injury. When the intracranial portion of the optic nerve is injured, the field defect is likely to be hemianopic, and bilateral injury is common, as is associated injury to the optic chiasm.

It is important to distinguish among injuries to the orbital, intracanalicular, and intracranial portions of the optic nerve, because the treatment of injuries to these different areas is quite different (see below). Neuroimaging studies, particularly computed tomographic (CT) scan-

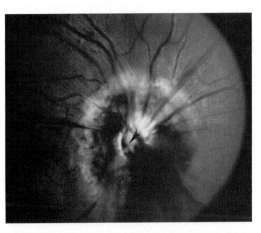

Figure 9.1. Traumatic avulsion of the optic disc. Note ring of hemorrhage around the optic disc. The site of avulsion is clearly visible as a crescentic dark area at the temporal portion of the disc (*arrowhead*).

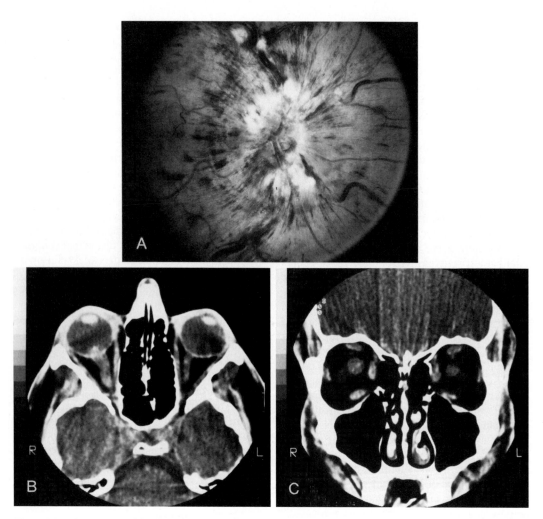

Figure 9.2. Central retinal vein occlusion in a case of anterior (proximal) optic neuropathy. The patient was a 24-year-old man who was struck in the left eye while playing basketball and who immediately noted loss of vision in the eye. Visual acuity was light perception OD and 20/15 OS. *A.* Ophthalmoscopic appearance of right ocular fundus reveals moderate swelling of the optic disc. The disc is surrounded by hemorrhage and soft exudates. The retinal veins are dilated and tortuous. *B.* Computed tomographic (CT) scan, axial view, shows moderate enlargement of the orbital portion of the right optic nerve. *C.* CT scan, coronal view, shows enlargement of right optic nerve compared with left nerve. Note small areas of increased density, consistent with hemorrhage, within the enlarged nerve.

ning and magnetic resonance imaging (MRI), are often sufficient to make this distinction.

CLINICAL ASSESSMENT

Traumatic optic neuropathy is a clinical diagnosis typically made when there is evidence of an optic neuropathy that is temporally related to blunt or penetrating head trauma. The head trauma may have been severe, in which case the patient may be unconscious. There may be a history of transient loss of consciousness, or the trauma may have seemed trivial, and the patient is neurologically intact. In some cases, there is no other evidence of orbital or ocular trauma; in other cases, there is obvious evidence of injury to the eye or orbit, such as periorbital or ocular hemorrhage, ecchymosis, or lacerations.

Respiratory and cardiovascular resuscitation and stabilization are the first priority in all cases of trauma, regardless of the severity of ocular injury. Thus, care of the patient with a traumatic optic neuropathy often requires a team approach, involving emergency medicine physicians, trauma surgeons, head and neck surgeons, neurosurgeons, and ophthalmologists.

HISTORY

The clinical evaluation of a patient with visual loss following trauma should begin with a complete history. The history should be obtained from family, friends, or witnesses to the trauma if the patient is unconscious or otherwise incapable of providing it. It is particularly important, for both medical and legal purposes, to determine if the patient with evidence of visual loss had any visual deficits before the injury. A detailed medical, drug, and drug allergy history is also necessary. For example, an open injury creates a risk for tetanus, and the patient's tetanus immunization status should be assessed in this setting.

EXAMINATION

The examination of a patient with a possible traumatic optic neuropathy is limited by numerous patient factors, including the presence or absence of other injuries, the patient's level of consciousness, and the patient's ability or willingness to cooperate with the examiner. Nevertheless, the examiner should attempt to obtain as much information as possible about the patient's visual status as soon as possible after the injury.

Whenever possible, the **visual acuity** should first be determined using a Snellen chart or a hand-held near card, using the patient's refraction. The physician must remember that injured patients may not have their glasses with them, and an attempt should be made to determine if the patient has worn glasses in the past. It may even be appropriate to try to determine if the glasses were ''thick,'' indicating a significant refractive error. Patients over 40 years of age invariably have some degree of presbyopia. Thus, the physician testing visual acuity at the bedside should have at least a $+3.00$ sphere available to neutralize the presbyopia.

Color vision is an excellent test of optic nerve function. The simplest method of checking color vision is with a red test object. The alert patient is asked whether there is a difference in the color of the object when viewed with one eye compared with the other. An eye with an optic neu-

ropathy may see the red object as black, brown, or orange. The color may also be described as ''faded.'' In some cases, the color cannot be identified at all. Color vision can also be tested using some type of pseudoisochromatic color plates.

Whenever possible, some type of **visual field** testing should be performed in the awake cooperative patient with possible traumatic optic neuropathy. The visual field, by virtue of the retinotopic organization of the optic nerve, can provide limited information regarding the possible location of optic nerve damage. Within the optic canal, for example, the pial penetrating vessels that provide blood to the optic nerve are subject to shearing forces at the moment of injury. Because the superior portion of the optic nerve is most tightly bound within the canal, these pial vessels are thought to be the most susceptible to shearing forces. If this concept is correct, patients with injuries to the intracanalicular portion of the optic nerve that spare some vision should have a visual field defect that is worse inferiorly than superiorly. It must be emphasized, however, that there is no pathognomonic visual field defect that is diagnostic of optic nerve trauma. Altitudinal, central, paracentral, cecocentral, and hemianopic defects can all occur, as can generalized field constriction. Initial visual field testing is important not only for localization of optic nerve injury but also for establishing a baseline to assist in documenting either the return or the loss of visual function following injury.

As is the case with testing of visual acuity and color vision, the method by which visual field testing is performed on a patient with a known or presumed traumatic optic neuropathy depends to a large extent on the systemic, neurologic, and visual status of the patient. The most basic and often the most useful test is a confrontation visual field. In patients with vision that is insufficient to count fingers, the detection of hand movements or light in various regions of the visual field may be all that can be obtained. Patients who are ambulatory and cooperative can undergo formal visual field testing. Both the peripheral and central fields should be tested using kinetic perimetry, static perimetry, or both.

The diagnosis of a unilateral optic neuropathy should not be made unless a **relative afferent pupillary defect** (RAPD) is present on the side of the presumed optic nerve injury. A patient with a presumed traumatic optic neuropathy who does not have an RAPD either does not have an optic neuropathy at all or has a bilateral optic neuropathy. It must also be emphasized that because patients with 20/20 vision in the setting of an optic neuropathy can have an RAPD, the presence of an RAPD in a comatose or semicomatose patient whose visual acuity cannot be measured cannot be taken as evidence that there is little or no vision in the eye. Only when the pupil does not react at all to direct light but reacts consensually (indicating intact efferent function) can one be certain that the patient has no light perception. An RAPD can be quantified using calibrated neutral density filters and the swinging flashlight test (see Chapter 14). The severity of the RAPD in log units of filter required to neutralize it is roughly equivalent to the severity of visual loss and thus can be used in comatose, semicomatose, or uncooperative patients to detect improvement or worsening in visual function.

A thorough examination of the eye and ocular adnexa is essential in a patient who has suffered trauma to the eye or orbit. The examiner should look for areas of hemorrhage, ecchymosis, or lacerations. Palpation of the orbital rim can identify a fracture. An exophthalmometer should be used to determine if enophthalmos or proptosis is present, particularly when there is periorbital swelling that may mask displacement of the globe. Both retropulsion of the globe and tonometry should be performed in intact globes, because both can identify an orbit that is tense from a retrobulbar hemorrhage. Lid swelling can increase the difficulty in performing the ocular examination, and an assistant may be needed to retract the eyelids.

Patients with blunt or penetrating trauma to the orbit should be assessed using a slit lamp biomicroscope for evidence of a penetrating or perforating injury to the eye. The observation of uveal prolapse, a focal area of chemosis, or a shallow anterior chamber are all signs of a ruptured or penetrated globe. The examiner should also evaluate the patient for an anterior chamber hyphema, angle recession, damaged iris, dislocated lens, and vitreous hemorrhage.

An attempt should be made to assess the appearance of the ocular fundus in any patient with ocular or orbital trauma, particularly a patient with visual dysfunction; however, if the patient is neurologically unstable, the ophthalmologist should consult the attending physician before dilating the eyes to prevent confusion regarding possible intracranial herniation. If a dilated examination is performed, the time of dilation and the type of agents used should be documented both in the nursing and physician notes, and this information should also be posted prominently at the bedside. Only short-acting mydriatic solutions should be used to dilate the pupils in this setting.

An adequate fundus examination includes assessment of the optic disc, retina, and choroid. Partial and complete avulsion of the optic nerve head produces a ring of hemorrhage at the site of injury, often associated with a dark crescentic area indicating the avulsion (see Fig. 9.1). Injuries to the portion of the orbital optic nerve anterior to the point at which the central retinal artery enters and the central retinal vein exits that nerve produce disturbances in the retinal circulation, including arterial and venous obstruction and disc swelling (see Fig. 9.2). Hemorrhages in the optic nerve sheath posterior to the origin of the central retinal vessels may leave the circulation of the retina intact but produce optic nerve head swelling. Disc swelling may also occur in the absence of direct or indirect trauma to the orbital portion of the optic nerve when head trauma produces increased intracranial pressure. In this case, the disc swelling is actually papilledema (see Chapter 5). Damage to the distal optic nerve in the orbit, optic canal, or intracranial cavity does not cause any change in the appearance of the optic disc for 3 to 5 weeks, after which the disc becomes progressively pale and atrophic. The observation of optic atrophy in a patient with acute head trauma and evidence of an optic neuropathy absolutely indicates that at least some disturbance of the optic nerve was present *before* the trauma and was not caused by it, although patients with a mild asymptomatic compressive optic neuropathy from a slowly expanding intracranial mass can occasionally experience acute loss of vision after seemingly trivial trauma from the effects of the trauma on an already compromised optic nerve.

Visual loss in a patient with ocular or orbital trauma is not necessarily caused by damage to the optic nerve. Corneal, anterior chamber, lens, and vitreous disturbances can all be responsible. A choroidal rupture, commotio retinae, or a macular hemorrhage may also cause loss of vision;

however, unless large areas of the retina are involved, none of these conditions should result in a RAPD. Thus, the finding of decreased visual acuity and a RAPD in the absence of intraocular pathology or in the presence of minor localized ophthalmoscopic abnormalities should suggest a posterior orbital, intracanalicular, or intracranial injury to the optic nerve.

VISUAL-EVOKED POTENTIALS

The visual-evoked potential (VEP) may be helpful in the assessment of optic nerve function in an unresponsive patient suspected of having a traumatic optic neuropathy. This is especially true in possible bilateral cases where a RAPD may not be present. The usefulness of the VEP is limited in such patients, however, because most VEPs are measured in a laboratory that is distant from the hospital ward or intensive care unit where the patient is located, and transporting the patient to the laboratory may not be possible because of the patient's neurologic or systemic injuries. Like the RAPD, the VEP is useful only when it is not recordable, in which case it may be assumed that there is complete loss of vision in the affected eye and that the chance of visual recovery is low.

IMAGING STUDIES

CT scanning permits visualization not only of the optic nerve and adjacent soft tissue in the orbit and neural and vascular structures in the brain, but also of the bony anatomy of the optic canals and paranasal sinuses. CT evidence of a fracture through the optic canal on the side of a traumatic optic neuropathy occurs in about 36 to 67% of cases. The frequency of optic canal fracture and adjacent sphenoid fractures may be much higher than was once suspected by plain radiographs. The fracture in such cases may injure the optic nerve directly, or it may serve as a marker of the severity of force transferred into the optic nerve. Regardless, a fracture through the optic canal in a patient with a traumatic optic neuropathy is dramatic evidence of the forces that are applied to the sphenoid and through the sphenoid to the optic nerve within the optic canal (Fig. 9.3). Individual case reports also demonstrate the value of CT scanning in the serial management of traumatic optic neuropathy.

Although CT scanning is clearly superior to MRI in delineating fractures of bone, MRI is superior to CT scanning in its ability to image soft tissue. The role of MRI in traumatic optic neuropathy has yet to be fully defined. Certainly, MRI is more sensitive in the detection and the evaluation of associated intracranial abnormalities, and it may indeed prove useful in the detection of subtle hemorrhage of the optic nerve or

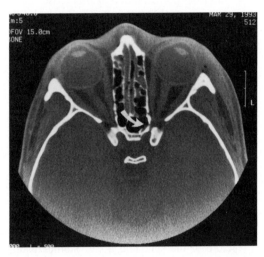

Figure 9.3. CT scan appearance (axial view) of an optic canal fracture (*arrow*) in a patient with a traumatic left optic neuropathy.

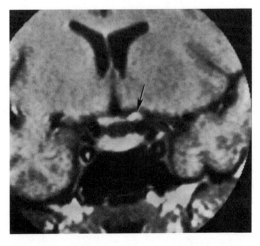

Figure 9.4. MRI of intrasheath hemorrhage in a patient with a traumatic optic neuropathy. MRI, coronal view, shows hemorrhage in the optic nerve sheaths (*arrow*). (Reprinted with permission from Crowe NW, Nickles TP, Troost T, et al. Intrachiasmal hemorrhage: a cause of delayed posttraumatic blindness. Neurology 1989;39:863–865.)

sheath, especially within the optic canal (Fig. 9.4). In general, MRI should be performed only after a metallic intracranial, intraorbital, or intraocular foreign body has been ruled out by CT scanning or conventional radiographs.

PATHOLOGY

Pathologic examination of the optic nerves from autopsies performed soon after closed head trauma has revealed optic nerve dural sheath hemorrhages in 83% of cases, interstitial optic nerve hemorrhages in 36% of cases (with the hemorrhage being present in the optic canal in two-thirds of these cases), and shearing lesions and ischemic necrosis in 44% of cases (with the intracanalicular optic nerve and the intracranial optic nerves affected 81% and 54% of the time, respectively).

The not uncommon finding of fractures of the sphenoid bone in patients with traumatic optic neuropathy after blunt head trauma is one indication of the substantial force that is transmitted to the optic nerve in such cases. Studies using CT scanning suggest that over 50% of cases of traumatic optic neuropathy are associated with a fracture of the sphenoid bone. Studies using laser interferometry suggest that, whether or not there is a fracture of the optic canal, the forces applied to the frontal bone during a deceleration injury are transmitted to and concentrated in the region of the optic canal. Indeed, the entire force of deceleration is applied to the facial bones over several milliseconds, whereupon elastic deformation of the sphenoid bone results in the direct transfer of force into the intracanalicular portion of the optic nerve. Because the nerve sheath is tightly adherent to the bony canal, the forces cause immediate contusion necrosis of the nerve by disrupting axons and vasculature. The development and location of a fracture in such cases is determined by the elastic limits of the affected bone. Thin bone is more likely to deform, whereas thick bone is inelastic and more likely to fracture. It must be emphasized that, although fractures of the optic canal are not uncommon in patients with traumatic optic neuropathy, direct injury to the nerve by displaced bone fragments is infrequent.

It has been hypothesized that swelling of the optic nerve within the bony canal may make the intracanalicular portion of the nerve especially susceptible to the delayed effects of trauma through the effects of progressive ischemia. An initial injury to the intracanalicular portion of the nerve causes it to swell within the bony confines of the optic canal. Compression of the swollen nerve by the bony canal produces further ischemia, thus inducing more swelling and more ischemia. This hypothesis forms the rationale for opening the optic canal along its length in patients with posterior traumatic optic neuropathy, in the hope of decompressing the optic nerve and thus breaking the cycle of swelling and ischemia.

In fact, there is little evidence that optic nerve swelling within the optic canal plays a significant role in traumatic posterior optic neuropathy. Instead, reactive vascular changes in and around the optic nerve may be more important than primary swelling of the nerve itself. Following brain injury, there is profound loss of autoregulation of blood flow within the central nervous system (CNS), resulting in a direct relationship between intracranial pressure and cerebral perfusion pressure. Patients with intracranial pressure above 400 mm of water tend to have a significant reduction in perfusion pressure and a poor prognosis. Even a brief rise in intracranial pressure may reduce perfusion pressure to the optic nerve within the optic canal, and the resultant reduction in blood flow to the nerve may be the major factor in permanent loss of vision in such cases.

The intracranial portion of the optic nerve can be injured by forces that are produced during blunt head trauma. Forces delivered by a shifting brain at the moment of impact can injure the intracranial optic nerve by displacing it upward against the falciform dural fold that overlies the intracranial end of the optic canal, resulting in direct or indirect injury (Fig. 9.5).

Partial and complete avulsions of the optic nerve from the globe can result from violent rotations of the globe; however, the transfer of damaging force to the optic nerve following direct injury does not necessarily sever the nerve, nor does it preclude visual recovery. A direct optic nerve injury may irreversibly injure a portion of the nerve but leave other areas with the potential for visual recovery.

PATHOGENESIS

Whether direct or indirect, optic nerve injury results in both mechanical and ischemic damage. This damage can result from both primary and secondary mechanisms. **Primary mechanisms**

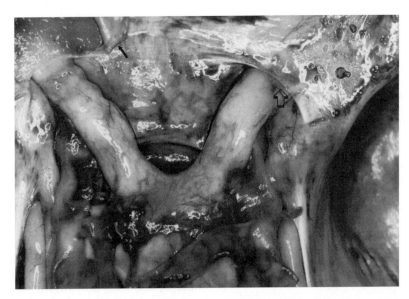

Figure 9.5. Relationship of the optic nerves and the falciform dural folds. *Hollow arrow:* The falciform dural fold in close association to the optic nerve as it enters the optic canal. *Solid arrow:* The falciform dural fold has been reflected, exposing the underlying sphenoid bone. (Reprinted with permission from Gossman MD, Roberts DM, Barr CC. Ophthalmic aspects of orbital injury. Clin Plast Surg 1992; 19:71–85.)

cause permanent injury to the optic nerve axons at the moment of impact. Thus, the primary injury may be caused by laceration of the optic nerve or by shearing forces of deceleration that are transferred to the nerve, particularly within the optic canal, where the nerve is tightly bound.

Secondary mechanisms cause damage to the optic nerve subsequent to the force of impact. These mechanisms include vasoconstriction and swelling of the optic nerve within the confines of the nonexpansile optic canal, leading to worsening ischemia and irreversible damage to axons that may have been spared at the time of the initial injury or that were injured but possessed the potential for recovery immediately following impact. The implication in this concept is that immediate and appropriate intervention after an initial optic nerve injury has the potential to stop secondary injury and preserve vision by salvaging the axons that survived the initial insult.

PRIMARY MECHANISMS OF OPTIC NERVE INJURY

Shearing injury, a mechanism by which blunt trauma to the head produces an indirect optic nerve injury, is a primary mechanism of optic nerve trauma. Autopsy studies demonstrating

hemorrhage in the optic nerve and its sheaths are consistent with tearing injuries to the microvasculature, and shearing of optic nerve axons themselves may also be responsible for visual loss in such patients. However, shearing of other CNS axons is no longer considered a common cause of neurologic dysfunction in patients with head trauma. Rather than directly shearing brain axons, trauma induces a focal axon abnormality characterized in part by impaired axon transport. This, in turn, produces a functional separation of the nerve into a proximal and distal segment, usually within 6 to 24 hours of injury. The distal segment that is separated from the soma undergoes Wallerian degeneration, whereas the proximal segment that is still in contact with the soma swells to produce a retraction ball. There is evidence that the somas of injured neurons may subsequently undergo *apoptosis,* a type of programmed cell death. This type of degeneration has been documented in optic nerves after ischemic optic neuropathy, with experimental glaucoma, and after trauma.

SECONDARY MECHANISMS OF OPTIC NERVE INJURY

Adjacent to areas of irreversible optic nerve damage, cellular homeostasis is also disturbed.

If this disturbance is sufficiently great, neurons that survive the initial insult can be lost from a number of processes referred to as secondary injury mechanisms. These mechanisms are diverse and interrelated; however, *ischemia* is perhaps the most important feature of secondary injury following trauma. The mechanism of injury is not simply cessation of blood flow. Partial ischemia and reperfusion of transiently ischemic regions generate **oxygen free radicals** resulting in reperfusion damage.

The cell membranes of axons are composed of high concentrations of polyunsaturated lipids. The release of oxygen free radicals that follows trauma or ischemia is thought to result in the peroxidation of these lipids, thus damaging the neural membrane. Oxygen free radicals and **lipid peroxidation** thus may play a central role in cell death following ischemia or traumatic injury.

Bradykinin and kallidin are substances that are activated following injury and play an important role in cerebral dysfunction following trauma and ischemia. Bradykinin initiates the release of arachidonic acid from neurons, and the resulting prostaglandins, oxygen free radicals, and lipid peroxides produce a loss of cerebrovascular autoregulation. In the case of optic nerve trauma, the resulting edema in the confines of the optic canal may produce a compartment syndrome causing increased ischemia.

Based on the action of bradykinin, specific bradykinin antagonists should be of benefit clinically in treating CNS injury. Bradykinin antagonists are likely to have their greatest application in combination with 21-amino steroids, because treatment of cerebral (and optic nerve) ischemia and edema begins after the initial binding of bradykinin. Consequently, treatment must be aimed at blocking further bradykinin binding and controlling the effects of prostaglandins and oxygen free radicals that have already been formed.

Calcium ions (Ca^{2+}) play an essential role in mediating intracellular metabolism. Excess intracellular calcium leads to cell death. Consequently, mechanisms normally exist to regulate carefully intracellular calcium concentration. Following cerebral ischemia, optic nerve ischemia, and spinal cord injury, calcium shifts from the extracellular space to the intracellular space by several mechanisms, including both voltage-gated and receptor-gated calcium chan-nels. Increased intracellular calcium acts as a metabolic toxin that leads to cell death.

The early phases of CNS injury are characterized in part by the release of mediators of **inflammation** that are chemoattractive for polymorphonuclear leukocytes (PMNs) and macrophages. In CNS trauma, the blood-brain barrier is significantly disrupted, permitting the passage of these cells. It thus is not surprising that inflammatory cells are a prominent feature in experimental animal models of optic nerve injury. PMNs release a broad array of enzymes and damaging free radical compounds, but the role of activated PMNs in destroying already compromised axons is undefined.

In the first 1 to 2 days after injury, PMNs predominate but are then replaced by macrophages, which reach peak numbers at 5 to 7 days after injury. Whereas PMNs are thought to contribute to immediate tissue damage, macrophages are implicated in delayed tissue damage in experimental spinal cord injury models. Macrophage activity appears to correlate with delayed post-injury demyelination and plays an important role in post-ischemic CNS damage. Macrophages also release glial promoting factors, and inhibition of the macrophage response is associated with a reduction in reactive gliosis. This phenomenon is important because the astroglial response that occurs following spinal cord injury may limit the opportunity for axon regeneration, and reduction of the response could result in improved outcome.

PHARMACOLOGY

Research in acute spinal cord trauma demonstrates that the pharmacologic actions of very high doses of corticosteroids in this setting are separate and distinct from the actions of steroids in the doses more typically encountered in clinical practice (1–2 mg/kg/day). Experimental studies have demonstrated a biphasic dose response to methylprednisolone in a range of doses much higher than the usual clinical usage. Specifically, in animals with experimental CNS injury and ischemia, there appears to be a distinct pharmacologic benefit of doses of methylprednisolone in the range of 30 mg/kg—15 to 30 times the standard clinical dose. The most important of these effects appears to be as an antioxidant that limits tissue damage caused by oxygen free radicals.

The second National Acute Spinal Cord Injury Study (NASCIS-2) was a multicenter, randomized, double-blind, placebo-controlled study. Patients enrolled in the study were randomized to one of three treatment arms within 12 hours of injury. The treatment arms consisted of placebo, naloxone, and methylprednisolone. Naloxone, an opiate receptor partial agonist that is effective in limiting neurologic injury in animals, was administered in an initial bolus of 5.4 mg/kg and then at a continuous infusion rate of 4.0 mg/kg/hour for 24 hours. Methylprednisolone was administered as an initial dose of 30 mg/kg followed by a continuous infusion of 5.4 mg/kg/hour for 24 hours (i.e., about 160 mg/kg or 10 grams total over 24 hours). This study showed that treatment with methylprednisolone within 8 hours of injury at the dose described above resulted in a significant improvement in motor and sensory function compared with either patients who received the placebo or patients treated with naloxone. Patients treated with methylprednisolone more than 8 hours after injury did not demonstrate an improvement in neurologic scores when compared with patients given the placebo. Indeed, subsequent analysis of the NASCIS-2 data suggests that methylprednisolone treatment given in the manner and dose described above and begun more than 8 hours after injury not only may not be beneficial but actually may be detrimental.

Although high doses of steroids in the range used by the NASCIS-2 study are usually tolerated well without significant side effects, clinicians should be aware that adverse effects do occur. Gastrointestinal side effects can occur with steroids at any dosage, and concomitant treatment with histamine$_2$ antagonists, antacids, or both is prudent. Steroid lethargy and psychosis, seizures, and steroid-induced cardiac conduction abnormalities can occur even after short-term steroid therapy, whereas aseptic necrosis of the joints, impaired wound healing, and immunosuppression generally occur only after prolonged administration. Serum glucose should be monitored even in patients without diabetes mellitus because of the risk of glucose intolerance.

Aminosteroids (lazaroids), GM$_1$ gangliosides, thromboxane receptor antagonists, and drugs such as apolipoprotein E may induce nerve regeneration and are under investigation for possible utility in spinal cord and brain trauma. These drugs may eventually turn out to play a role in traumatic optic neuropathy.

MANAGEMENT

The management of traumatic optic neuropathy should be guided by the Hippocratic adage to do no harm. There is very little help from the published literature on this subject. For example, it is very difficult to use the retrospective data in the literature to characterize the natural history of traumatic optic neuropathy, in part because older series tend to report cases with severe visual loss, whereas contemporary studies contain larger numbers of patients with mild visual loss. In addition, traumatic optic neuropathy is a complex injury that often has both direct and indirect components and both primary and secondary intracellular and extracellular mechanisms of damage. Without an accurate knowledge of the natural history of traumatic optic neuropathy, determining the beneficial effect of a medical, surgical, or combined approach is very difficult.

At present, no studies validate a particular approach to the management of traumatic optic neuropathy other than suggesting that some form of treatment is better than no treatment at all; however, the use of systemic corticosteroids in the management of this condition has become commonplace. The beneficial clinical effect of these agents in the treatment of spinal cord injury provides a rationale for the use of these agents in traumatic optic neuropathy, although the doses used by most authors do not approach those used in the NASCIS-2 study. In addition, there are fundamental differences between the spinal cord and the optic nerve, so the successful application of high-dose corticosteroids in the treatment of spinal cord injury may not fully generalize to the treatment of optic nerve trauma. To date, no clinical studies have considered the possibility that corticosteroids may actually have a harmful effect on a traumatized optic nerve.

Until a prospective, randomized, double-blind, placebo-controlled study is performed, treatment with systemic corticosteroids must be considered empiric. We believe that clinicians should inform their patients with traumatic optic neuropathy that there is little evidence that high-dose steroids are beneficial, and it is also not known if they are harmful. One approach is to treat optic nerve trauma with methylprednisolone in the doses given in the NASCIS-2 (30 mg/kg as a loading dose and 5.4 mg/kg/hour thereafter) as soon as the diagnosis is made, and continue treatment for 48 hours. Another approach is to not treat optic nerve trauma with systemic steroids at all because of experimental evidence that methylprednisolone may be harmful to a traumatized optic nerve.

If there is no visual improvement within 48 hours of injury, regardless of whether or not the patient has been placed on steroids, surgical decompression of the optic canal can be offered. If vision is improving without treatment, we continue to monitor the patient's vision; if vision is improving on steroid treatment, the patient is placed on oral prednisone in a tapering dose. If the vision deteriorates on the taper, high-dose intravenous methylprednisolone is reinstituted, diagnostic imaging is performed, and surgical decompression is considered.

Surgical intervention for traumatic optic neuropathy is also empiric. The reduction of bone fragments impinging on the optic nerve is a compelling reason for surgical intervention, especially in cases of delayed visual loss, although such cases are rare, and visual loss in such cases is likely to be irreversible. Individual case reports and series demonstrate visual improvement following evacuation of an intraoptic nerve sheath hematoma or subperiosteal hematoma with optic nerve compression. These examples provide case experience on which to base recommendations for surgery for individual patients.

Because injury to the intracanalicular portion of the optic nerve is the most common form of traumatic optic neuropathy, decompression of the optic canal is the most commonly reported surgical intervention. In considering the value of this procedure, one must carefully weigh its potential risks and benefits. Theoretically, opening the canal to reduce compression of a swollen optic nerve and to provide room for the optic nerve to swell should be beneficial. However, there is no information about the time course in which intervention must take place. If swelling within the optic canal occurs, it may produce a compartment syndrome. Increased tissue pressure within the canal could then reduce tissue perfusion, thus worsening post-injury ischemia. This is likely to diminish the prospect for visual recovery.

If optic canal decompression is to be performed, the appropriate technique must be used.

Criteria for adequate decompression of the optic canal include:

1. Removal of at least 50% of the circumference of the osseous canal.
2. Removal of bone along the entire length of the canal.
3. Total longitudinal incision of the dural sheath, including the annulus of Zinn.

All of these objectives can be met through a transcranial, external ethmoidectomy, transantral/transethmoidal, or transnasal approach, but only a transcranial approach permits decompression when the anterior clinoid is fractured and allows unroofing of the canal with removal of the falciform dural fold.

Either a medial or lateral orbitotomy can be used to evacuate an optic nerve sheath hematoma. A medial approach is more appropriate if there is a medial subperiosteal hematoma causing posterior compression of the optic nerve. A lateral approach permits reduction of a depressed lateral orbital wall fracture that compromises the nerve. Thus, an accurate anatomic and pathophysiologic diagnosis must be made to plan appropriate surgical intervention.

Avoidance of surgical intervention on the unconscious patient continues to be a reasonable recommendation until such time as clear evidence establishing the value of this procedure exists, particularly given the difficulty in determining visual function in such a patient unless the pupil is nonreactive to direct but not consensual light. Given the uncertainty associated with the benefits of these procedures, the patient and those involved in making decisions concerning his or her care need to be thoughtfully counseled in the processes of an informed consent.

The management of orbital hemorrhage that creates a compressive orbitopathy and optic neuropathy is well defined and relatively uncontroversial. The initial diagnosis is clinical. Patients present with a history of trauma. Vision may be extremely poor from optic nerve compression or ischemia or from compromise of retinal perfusion. Proptosis is invariably present, and the intraocular pressure is usually substantially elevated. Initial treatment is lateral canthotomy and cantholysis to permit expansion of the orbital contents. These initial maneuvers should be followed immediately by orbital imaging to determine if there is a subperiosteal hemorrhage or other pathology that may explain the basis of visual compromise.

If initial treatment does not provide sufficient visual improvement, orbital decompression may be necessary to provide sufficient space for orbital soft tissue expansion. There is little or no role for anterior chamber paracentesis in the treatment of orbital hemorrhage, and there are no data to support the use of systemic corticosteroids in this setting.

The considerations used to determine treatment of direct injuries of the optic nerve should follow the approach for indirect optic nerve injuries. Although the prospects for visual recovery are worse for direct optic nerve injuries, recovery of vision can occur with and without treatment. The rationale for the empiric use of high-dose corticosteroids applies in these settings, whereas the empiric use of surgery should be approached on an individual basis.

There is reason to believe that traumatic optic neuropathy is a true emergency. In patients with spinal cord trauma, treatment with high-dose methylprednisolone must be initiated within 8 hours to have a discernible effect. It is quite possible that the window of opportunity for successful intervention in the treatment of many cases of traumatic optic neuropathy is similar. If this is correct, medical or surgical treatment initiated days after the injury is likely to be no more successful than natural history. Therefore, the initial goal in treating traumatic optic neuropathy must be early recognition of the condition. This means educating emergency room staff and providing appropriate ophthalmic coverage in trauma centers. It may be that the visual outcome in patients with no light perception immediately following injury could be significantly improved by early intervention. Because these approaches are empiric, definitive recommendations must await the results of collaborative, prospective studies.

FOR MORE INFORMATION:

See Walsh & Hoyt's *Clinical Neuro-Ophthalmology,* 5th edition, Volume 1, Chapter 16, pages 715–739.

Toxic and Deficiency Optic Neuropathies

Physicians have known for centuries that the anterior visual pathway is vulnerable to damage from nutritional deficiency and chemicals. The resulting disorders share many signs and symptoms, and several appear to have a multifactorial etiology in which both undernutrition and toxicity play a role. In light of these facts, it is reasonable to group them together. Although evidence for the localization of the primary lesions is lacking in many of the so-called toxic and nutritional "amblyopias," they are generally assumed to be optic neuropathies and that is the rubric under which they are considered here.

ETIOLOGIC CRITERIA

Although certain optic neuropathies have an obvious toxic or nutritional etiology, the toxic or nutritional basis of others is merely presumptive, and the attribution may ultimately prove false. It is also likely that a few of the optic neuropathies now considered idiopathic or ascribed to some other etiology actually result from toxicity or nutritional deficiency. The proliferation of drugs and the introduction of new chemicals into the workplace and environment guarantees that additional toxic optic neuropathies will be identified. For medical and legal reasons, physicians

must be alert to the possibility, both in sporadic cases of visual loss and in epidemics of visual loss, that intoxication or nutritional deficiency are factors.

NUTRITIONAL OPTIC NEUROPATHIES

Proving a nutritional basis for an optic neuropathy is by no means a simple task. The first criterion is that the patient be nutritionally deficient and has been so sufficiently long to deplete nutrients. Evidence from epidemics indicates that this requires months (see below). The reports of large numbers of cases of visual loss after economic and political upheavals suggests the possibility of a nutritional etiology. The patient should show evidence of undernutrition, usually manifested in such obvious forms as weight loss and wasting. Victims of nutritional optic neuropathy, however, are not necessarily emaciated. Other signs such as peripheral neuropathy, keratitis, or the cutaneous and mucous membrane stigmata of the avitaminoses are useful, when present.

There is an important exception to the foregoing statements. The optic neuropathy of pernicious anemia or dietary vitamin B_{12} deficiency can occur in seemingly healthy individuals without obvious symptoms or signs of nutritional deficiency (see below).

Supporting laboratory evidence for the diagnosis of nutritional optic neuropathy can be obtained in the form of direct or indirect vitamin assays, serum protein concentrations, and antioxidant levels. The symptoms and signs should be those typical of nutritional optic neuropathy, and other disorders should be considered and eliminated by appropriate investigations. Both in individual cases and in epidemics it is especially important to establish if the patient has been exposed to substances toxic to the visual pathway. In such cases, intoxication may be the alternative explanation or be a cofactor. The absence of an optic neuropathy in well-nourished individuals in the same environment, and recovery of vision in patients with restitution of an improved diet strongly support, but do not prove, a nutritional basis.

Identifying the specific nutritional deficiency responsible for an optic neuropathy is very difficult. Undernourished individuals are rarely deficient in only one nutrient; multiple deficiencies are the rule. Even if a specific deficiency is identified in a patient with loss of vision, it does not prove that the deficiency caused the visual loss. Nor does recovery when the deficient nutrient is resupplied establish that the resupplied nutrient effected the cure. With the exception of vitamin B_{12} (which only rarely becomes deficient for dietary reasons), no specific nutrient deficiency has been conclusively proved to cause amblyopia in humans. There are few good animal models of nutritional deficiency optic neuropathy. At the present state of knowledge, one can only speculate about which specific deficiencies can cause or contribute to nutritional amblyopia.

TOXIC OPTIC NEUROPATHIES

The primary issue in patients suspected of having a toxic amblyopia is whether they were exposed to a substance that has been proved to damage the optic nerve by the same route of exposure. Visual loss may occur from either acute or chronic intoxication depending upon the agent, but there should not be a long interval between the cessation of the exposure and the onset of symptoms. The patient must have symptoms and signs that are compatible with a toxic optic neuropathy and typical of those in other patients proved to have suffered loss of vision from the same agent. Of course, the symptoms cannot have preceded the exposure.

The response of patients to rechallenge is helpful in evaluating the validity of presumed intoxications and in helping to establish the cause of the patient's optic neuropathy. If a patient who has recovered vision following cessation of exposure to a drug or chemical loses vision again when reexposed, the recurrent loss of vision tends to verify the neurotoxic nature of the agent and the toxic etiology of the visual loss. Epidemiologic data, especially those showing correlation of changing disease incidence when and where specific drugs or chemicals are introduced or withdrawn, can also prove quite useful.

Confirmatory evidence of exposure from laboratory tests or from associated nonvisual symptoms is desirable. Nontoxic disorders must be considered in the diagnosis of these patients and should be ruled out with appropriate investigations.

Animal models can help to validate the optic nerve toxicity of putative intoxicants. Despite such problems as species variation in susceptibility and difficulty in measuring visual function in animals, some useful models are available.

CLINICAL CHARACTERISTICS OF NUTRITIONAL AND TOXIC OPTIC NEUROPATHIES

Persons of all ages, races, places, and economic strata are vulnerable to the toxic and deficiency optic neuropathies. Certain groups are at higher risk because they are under treatment with drugs, have occupational exposure, or practice habits such as smoking and alcohol consumption. Nutritional optic neuropathy is more likely to occur in the economically disadvantaged and during times of war and famine. The value of taking a thorough history—including dietary intake, exposure to drugs, use of tobacco, and social and occupational background—is obvious.

The symptoms and signs of nutritional and toxic optic neuropathy are similar and resemble those of most of the other optic neuropathies, primarily those that occur bilaterally and simultaneously. No single characteristic or combination of characteristics is pathognomonic.

Toxic and nutritional amblyopias are not painful. Thus, one should inquire carefully about this symptom because associated ocular or orbital pain suggests some other diagnosis.

Dyschromatopsia is present early and may be the initial symptom in observant patients. Some patients notice that certain colors, such as red, are no longer as bright and vivid as previously. Others experience a general loss of color perception.

Patients with nutritional or toxic optic neuropathies often initially notice a blur, fog, or cloud at the point of fixation, following which the visual acuity progressively declines. The rate of decline can be quite rapid. Although vision can decrease to any level, total blindness or vision limited to light perception is unusual in cases of nutritional optic neuropathy even if the patient is neglected. With the exception of methanol, which typically produces complete or nearly complete blindness, visual loss less than 20/400 is unusual in the toxic optic neuropathies. Bilaterality is the rule, although in the early stages one eye may be affected before the other becomes symptomatic. Profound loss of vision in one eye with completely normal findings in the other eye should cast doubt on the diagnosis of a toxic or nutritional optic neuropathy.

Visual field defects are usually present in patients with toxic or nutritional optic neuropathies. Much has been made of the significance of the cecocentral scotoma in these disorders. Some perimetrists claimed that cecocentral scotomas with "nuclei" between fixation and the physiologic blind-spot were the hallmark of toxic optic neuropathy, especially the variety blamed on tobacco. There were and are many who doubt this, and most authorities now recognize that both central and cecocentral scotomas may be encountered in either disorder. Some patients have a central scotoma in one eye and a cecocentral scotoma in the fellow eye. However, what is incontestable is that these visual field defects are the most prevalent among patients with toxic and deficiency optic neuropathies (Fig. 10.1). The anatomic basis of the cecocentral scotoma has yet to be established. Peripheral constriction and altitudinal visual field loss are rare.

Because of the symmetric and bilateral visual impairment in toxic and nutritional optic neuropathies, a relative afferent pupillary defect is not a common finding in affected patients. When the patient is blind or nearly so—for example, as a consequence of methanol poisoning—the pupillary light response will be absent or weak and the pupils will be dilated. Otherwise the pupils are likely to have relatively normal responses to light and near stimulation.

In the early stages of nutritional optic neuropathy, the disc is normal or slightly hyperemic. Disc hemorrhages may be present in eyes with hyperemic discs, but they are usually small. Optic atrophy supervenes rather late. Most patients in the acute stages of toxic amblyopia also have normal discs, but disc swelling may be seen in some intoxications (Fig. 10.2). Optic atrophy develops after a variable interval (Fig. 10.3).

Electrophysiologic examinations of patients with toxic or nutritional optic neuropathies may

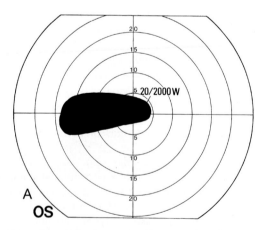

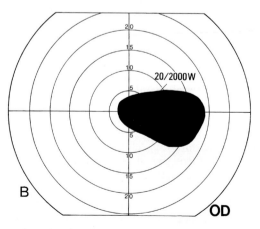

Figure 10.1. Visual fields of a patient with a bilateral toxic optic neuropathy caused by chloramphenicol. Note cecocentral scotomas in the visual fields of the left (*A*) and right (*B*) eyes. The peripheral fields were normal.

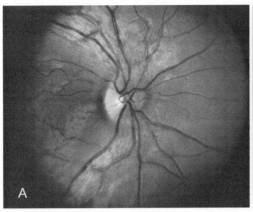
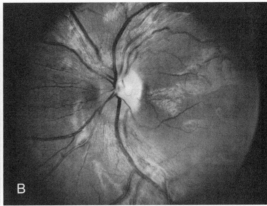

Figure 10.2.   Appearance of optic discs in a patient with bilateral toxic optic neuropathy from chloramphenicol. Note that right (*A*) and left (*B*) discs are hyperemic and somewhat swollen nasally. There is already mild pallor of the temporal portions of both optic discs, associated with early loss of the nerve fiber layer in the papillomacular bundle of both eyes.

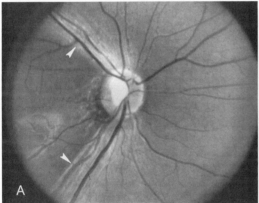
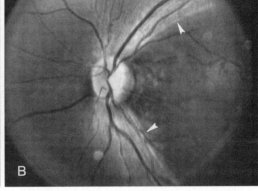

Figure 10.3.   Appearance of optic discs in a patient with bilateral optic neuropathy in the setting of poor nutrition and alcohol abuse. Note extent of loss of nerve fiber layer from the papillomacular bundle (*arrowheads*) and marked temporal disc pallor. Visual acuity was 20/400 in both eyes, and there were bilateral central scotomas.

reveal changes in the electroretinogram (ERG), visual-evoked potential (VEP), or both. A reduced amplitude of the VEP is common, and cone function in the ERG may be abnormal if there are also retinal effects. There is no tendency for the P100 wave of the VEP to be delayed, however, except in pernicious anemia.

In most cases, analysis of the symptoms and signs obtained from a detailed history and physical examination will establish the diagnosis of a toxic or nutritional optic neuropathy. It is prudent to obtain neuroimaging unless one is absolutely confident of the diagnosis. Magnetic resonance imaging (MRI), before and after intravenous injection of gadolinium-DTPA or a similar paramagnetic contrast material with special attention to the optic nerves and optic chiasm, is the optimum investigation in most cases. A vitamin B_{12} level should be determined to identify pernicious anemia, and red blood cell folate levels provide one marker of general nutritional status.

When a specific intoxicant is suspected, one should try to identify the toxin or its metabolites in the patient's tissues or fluids. The advice of a toxicologist is invaluable in such instances. In cases of suspected intoxication, one should attempt to evaluate or obtain information about other persons who have had similar exposure. The resulting information has potential public health implications and can help to validate the toxicity of chemicals not previously recognized as dangerous to the human optic nerve.

DIFFERENTIAL DIAGNOSIS

When an individual complains of bilateral visual loss that refraction cannot correct and has an otherwise normal examination, there are many diagnostic possibilities in addition to the toxic and nutritional optic neuropathies. Certain maculopathies can present in this guise. With time, the fundus will show abnormalities, but until then fluorescein angiography or focal electroretinography may be the only means of establishing the nature of the lesion. Full-field electroretinography may not reveal the defect.

One should be alert to the possibility of a conversion disorder or malingering in cases of bilateral visual loss. The absence of optic atrophy is an important clue when the visual loss is longstanding. In the acute phase, the characteristics of the visual field defects may help the clinician recognize that the loss of vision is nonorganic. The visual field defects in the toxic and nutritional optic neuropathies are typically central or cecocentral. Such defects are exceptional in patients with a conversion reaction or who are malingering. In conversion reaction and malingering, the visual fields are usually constricted and may show spiraling or have a tubular configuration (see Chapter 23).

Dominantly-inherited (Kjer's) and mitochondrially-inherited (Leber's) optic neuropathies can be confused with nutritional optic neuropathy if no other family members are known to be affected. The confusion is most likely to occur in patients who are first evaluated late in their course. Kjer's disease progresses more slowly than the nutritional and toxic optic neuropathies, and optic atrophy is an early finding. In Leber's optic neuropathy, the onset of visual loss is not infrequently symmetric or nearly so, and this disorder must therefore be considered in any patient in whom a toxic or nutritional optic neuropathy is thought to be present. Appropriate testing for the various mitochondrial mutations may be required in some cases (see Chapter 11).

It can be tragic to mistake a compressive or infiltrative lesion of the optic chiasm for nutritional or toxic optic neuropathy. There are few instances in which one should be so confident of the diagnosis of toxic or nutritional amblyopia that neuroimaging is omitted. Cecocentral scotomas and the bitemporal visual field defects of chiasmal disease resemble each other, and there are many examples of bilateral central and even cecocentral scotomas from tumors.

If a demyelinating, inflammatory, or infectious optic neuritis begins simultaneously in both eyes, there may be confusion with the toxic and nutritional optic neuropathies. The visual field defects are similar, but there is pain or disc swelling in greater than 90% of cases of optic neuritis (see Chapter 6). In some cases, MRI will indicate the nature of the lesion. In others, it may be necessary to examine the cerebrospinal fluid (CSF); perform specific tests for syphilis, sarcoidosis, or systemic vasculitis; and perform a complete neurologic examination.

SPECIFIC NUTRITIONAL OPTIC NEUROPATHIES

EPIDEMIC NUTRITIONAL OPTIC NEUROPATHY

The most useful observations regarding nutritional amblyopia have come not from sporadic cases encountered in practice, but rather from epidemics during war and famine. Two well-documented epidemics afflicted Allied prisoners of war of the Japanese during World War II and Cubans in the early 1990s. The characteristics of the disorder in those two populations are reasonably consistent.

The symptoms developed in an undernourished population after 4 or more months of food deprivation. Among the prisoners of war, vision loss occurred sooner in those who were undernourished at the time they were first incarcerated. Only a minority of people at risk developed loss of vision, and the occurrence of visual loss did not appear to correlate very well with the severity of malnutrition. In some cases, a superficial keratopathy was a prelude to the visual loss, but visual loss developed both with and without a preceding keratopathy. The visual loss was symmetric and often appeared suddenly. In up to one-quarter of cases the visual nadir was reached in 1 day. Vision plateaued after 1 month in the remainder. At the time of visual loss, many victims also had pain or sensory loss in their extremities. There was a high incidence of bilateral sensorineural hearing loss. The fundi were usually normal at first, but a minority had peripapillary hemorrhages associated with mild optic disc hyperemia and swelling. Optic atrophy was a late development. The visual field defects were central or cecocentral. Most abnormalities could be reversed with improved nutrition.

Pathologic information on nutritional optic neuropathies is scarce. Postmortem examinations on repatriated Allied prisoners found atrophy of the papillomacular bundle and lesions in the fasciculus gracilis of the spinal cord. In a review of the records of civilian patients in whom atrophy in the papillomacular bundle was found at autopsy, investigators concluded that malnutrition associated with alcoholism was common.

In 1992 and 1993, an epidemic of optic neuropathy and peripheral neuropathy similar to that reported among the WW II prisoners of war occurred in Cuba. The epidemic began in the province of Pinar del Río, located at the northwestern tip of Cuba, and gradually spread southeast. More than 50,000 persons were affected with bilateral optic neuropathy, sensory and dysautonomic peripheral neuropathy, sensory myelopathy, spastic paraparesis, or sensorineural deafness in various combinations. Slightly more than half of the affected persons had evidence of optic neuropathy, which occurred as a painless rapid loss of vision in both eyes associated with marked dyschromatopsia, central or cecocentral scotomas, and normal appearing optic discs. Patients who did not recover vision developed temporal pallor of the optic discs, associated with marked loss of the nerve fiber layer in the papillomacular bundle (Fig. 10.4). The majority of

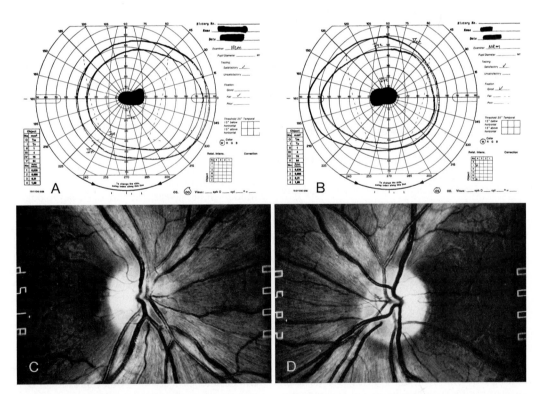

Figure 10.4.   Visual fields and appearance of ocular fundi in a patient with Cuban epidemic optic neuropathy. The patient was a 23-year-old Cuban man who developed progressive loss of vision in both eyes associated with a peripheral neuropathy in 1993. Examination revealed visual acuity of 20/200 OU. Visual fields performed by kinetic perimetry reveal a cecocentral scotoma in the field of both the right (A) and left (B) eyes. Photographs of the right (C) and left (D) optic fundi show temporal pallor of the optic discs associated with marked loss of the retinal nerve fiber layer in the papillomacular bundle.

cases occurred in people between 25 to 64 years old, with a predominance of males being among those with optic nerve disease. Partial and complete recovery occurred following treatment with parenteral and oral vitamins. In addition, subsequent supplementation of the general population with B-complex vitamins and vitamin A coincided with a dramatic decrease in new cases of the condition.

Although the loss of vision in the epidemic cases was undoubtedly caused by malnutrition, it is impossible to identify a specific deficient nutrient that caused either of the epidemics. Malnourished individuals have multiple deficiencies. Clinical and laboratory data make it unlikely that vitamin deficiency was the sole factor. Systematic investigation of Cuban epidemic optic neuropathy and controls showed an increased risk associated with cassava consumption and a decreased risk associated with high serum levels of antioxidant carotenoids, ingestion of B vitamins, and ingestion of animal products.

Factors other than malnutrition must explain the visual loss in these cases and in similar cases in other countries such as Tanzania. Tobacco use, especially cigar use, was a risk factor in Cuba. Physical labor also seemed to be a risk factor among the prisoners of war. In any case, the conclusion that epidemic cases of nutritional optic neuropathy (and probably sporadic cases as well) are the result of some multifactorial etiology is inescapable.

The treatment of nutritional optic neuropathy is improved nutrition. Unless the vision loss is extensive, there is an excellent prospect for recovery or at least improvement with such treatment.

VITAMIN B_{12} DEFICIENCY

Although the role of vitamin B_{12} in the maintenance and function of the nervous system has yet to be explained, depletion of this nutrient almost invariably leads to neurologic dysfunction. The body's nutritional requirements must be met entirely by food (particularly meat and dairy products). The abundant stores, particularly in the liver, are redistributed so gradually that it takes years for poor intake to cause disease. However, a poor diet is rarely the cause of vitamin B_{12} deficiency, and when it is, it is found only in strict vegans. Impaired absorption because of diphyllobothriasis, intestinal disease, or

gastrointestinal surgery accounts for only a few cases. Pernicious anemia is by far the most common condition in which vitamin B_{12} deficiency and its complications are encountered. This presumably autoimmune disorder results from impaired absorption of the vitamin from the ileum, because the patient lacks the intrinsic factor elaborated by the parietal cells of the gastric mucosa.

Pernicious anemia is most often found in, but is not limited to, middle-aged and elderly whites of northern European extraction. The anemia is megaloblastic. It develops slowly and can be severe. Unless treatment is instituted early, most patients with pernicious anemia develop neurologic manifestations. The pathologic substrate is a white-matter lesion that affects both myelin and axons initially in the posterior columns of the upper thoracic and lower cervical portions of the spinal cord ("subacute combined degeneration"). The process subsequently affects other white-matter tracts and other levels of the spinal cord. Paresthesias and weakness in the extremities are heralding symptoms. With time, vibration sense is lost, and the patient develops spasticity, with hyperactive knee and ankle jerks, and extensor plantar responses. Dementia may also develop.

Deficiency of vitamin B_{12}, whether from inadequate diet or interference with absorption, can cause an optic neuropathy. Lesions in the optic nerves and optic chiasm have been demonstrated in some postmortem examinations of patients with pernicious anemia. There are also primate models of the disease. Severe optic nerve degeneration is found in experimental vitamin B_{12} deficiency in monkeys even before there is anemia or a spinal cord lesion. In light of this finding, it is not surprising that in humans, an optic neuropathy may be the first symptom of pernicious anemia and may precede the hematologic disturbance. Indeed, abnormal VEPs can be recorded in patients with pernicious anemia who have no visual symptoms, suggesting that there may also be subclinical damage to the visual pathway in this disease.

The optic neuropathy that results from vitamin B_{12} deficiency resembles other nutritional optic neuropathies. The visual loss is symmetric, painless, and progressive. Central and cecocentral scotomas are the rule, and the optic disc appears normal in the early stages of the condition. Unless optic atrophy becomes well established, one can expect recovery of vision with intramuscular injections of hydroxycobalamin. The optic neuropathy of pernicious anemia, unlike the other deficiency optic neuropathies, does not usually respond to an improved diet.

The optic neuropathy of vitamin B_{12} deficiency is essentially indistinguishable from many other toxic and nutritional deficiency optic neuropathies. It can present before there is anemia or myelopathy, and it requires parenteral treatment, so it is important to obtain a serum vitamin B_{12} level in all cases of unexplained bilateral amblyopia.

OTHER VITAMIN DEFICIENCIES

The association of visual loss with beriberi, known for centuries, focused attention on vitamin B_1 (thiamine) deficiency as a cause of nutritional optic neuropathy. This vitamin has received more attention in this regard than any other nutrient and, despite contrary evidence summarized in the following paragraphs, many authorities still consider thiamine deficiency an important factor in the causation of nutritional deficiency amblyopia.

There are experimental, biochemical, and clinical data that suggest that thiamine deficiency may cause an optic neuropathy. Some studies of thiamine deprivation in rats have shown that an optic neuropathy may occur. However, the results of these experiments are not conclusive, because the animals may have had other deficiencies and few animals were affected. In another study, when chronic thiamine deficiency was produced in human volunteers, their vision did not suffer. The prisoner-of-war studies also present strong evidence against a primary role for thiamine deficiency in nutritional optic neuropathy. One study showed that vision loss developed just as the incidence of beriberi was declining. In fact, beriberi was as prevalent among prisoners of war with normal vision as it was among those who had loss of vision. Finally, among civilians in a Japanese prison camp, nutritional optic neuropathy could not be cured with injections of thiamine, and some prisoners developed visual loss while being treated with thiamine for beriberi.

The disorder consequent to thiamine depletion is Wernicke's encephalopathy. There is an excellent primate model of this disorder, and in this model there are no pathologic changes in the optic nerves. Indeed, loss of vision is uncommon among patients with Wernicke's disease. These observations cast further doubt on a role for thiamine deficiency in human nutritional amblyopia.

There can be no doubt that many prisoners of war who experienced loss of vision were thiamine deficient, and there is good biochemical evidence that many of the patients with nutritional optic neuropathy encountered sporadically in civilian populations are thiamine deficient. There is, however, no basis to conclude that thiamine deficiency is a primary cause of an optic neuropathy.

The roles of pyridoxine, niacin, folic acid, and riboflavin deficiency in causing an optic neuropathy are also controversial. As with thiamine, these vitamins are apt to be depleted in patients who are generally malnourished, but there is no definitive evidence indicating that such deficiencies play a primary etiological role in nutritional amblyopia. For example, low folate levels have been documented in the red blood cells and occasionally in the serum of patients with nutritional optic neuropathy, and some malnourished patients with optic neuropathy recover when treated with folic acid supplements. As discussed above, however, this does not prove that the folate deficiency caused the loss of vision or that the folic acid supplements effected the recovery.

Despite the lack of convincing evidence, it remains possible that there are some patients who develop loss of vision from damage to optic nerves consequent to dietary deficiency of thiamine and these other vitamins. It thus makes sense to enrich the diet of patients with loss of vision and evidence of poor nutrition with all of the water-soluble vitamins in which they might be deficient.

TROPICAL OPTIC NEUROPATHY

There are optic neuropathies endemic to tropical regions for which a nutritional etiology has been invoked. An early report by Strachan from Jamaica appeared in 1897. The clinical features of his patients resemble in some ways those of the epidemic cases described above. There was numbness and cramps in the hands and feet. The visual loss was bilateral and was sometimes accompanied by hearing loss. However, other features were unusual. Muscle wasting often developed. The pain was so severe that patients were kept awake. A dermatopathy was a constant finding. In any case, Strachan made no claim for a nutritional etiology. When the disorder was subsequently reevaluated by others, they concluded that this was not a nutritional disease. Despite that, some authors inappropriately use "Strachan's syndrome" to designate nutritional optic neuropathy.

It should be noted that there is an otherwise unexplained bilateral optic neuropathy called "West Indian amblyopia" found in black expatriates from the West Indies. Examples of this condition have been reported from Great Britain and the United States. The history is typically that of bilateral, painless progressive visual decline in a well-nourished adult. The visual field defects tend to be central or cecocentral, but annular scotomas and peripheral constriction have been reported. Optic atrophy develops. Deafness is also present in some of the patients. No treatment, including various vitamin regimens, is effective in reversing either the visual or the nonvisual manifestations of the disorder. Although a toxic basis ("bush tea") has been postulated, there is no good evidence for either a toxic or nutritional etiology.

A disorder similar to so-called Strachan's syndrome has been described in Nigerians. It differs from the West Indian cases (and the epidemic and sporadic nutritional amblyopias) in that the majority of patients have constricted visual fields and that total blindness can occur. Poor diet is said to be the common denominator in the African cases, but investigators have also suggested that exogenous cyanide from an excess of cassava in the diet is an etiologic factor. However, the manner in which cassava is prepared in this population would probably make for minimal exposure to cyanide. Indeed, the evidence that cyanide plays a role in causing any optic neuropathy is tenuous at best and is discussed further in the section on tobacco optic neuropathy. The endemic tropical neuropathy in Nigeria might result from nutritional deficiency, but this has not been proved.

SPECIFIC TOXIC OPTIC NEUROPATHIES

Table 10.1 lists substances that are suggested or presumed to be toxic to the human optic nerve. It is not always clear if the association of ingestion of, or exposure to, a particular substance and the subsequent visual loss is fortuitous or cause and effect. The literature is uneven in this regard, and several of the agents are of academic interest only because they are no

Table 10.1

Substances Known or Believed to Cause Toxic Optic Neuropathy

Amantadine hydrochloride	Ethambutol
Amiodarone	Ethchlorvynol
Amoproxan	Ethylene glycol
Arsenicals	5-Fluorouracil
Aspidium (male fern)	Halogenated
Cafergot	hydroxyquinolines
Carbon disulfide	Hexachlorophene
Carbon tetrachloride	Interferon-alpha
Catha edulis	Iodoform
Chlorambucil	Iodoquinol
Chloramphenicol	Isoniazid
Chlorodinitrobenzene and	Lead
dinitrobenzene	Methanol (methyl alcohol)
Chlorpromazine	Methyl acetate
Chlorpropamide	Methyl bromide
Cisplatin	Octamoxin
Clioquinol	Organic solvents
Clomiphene	Penicillamine
Cobalt chloride	Pheniprazine
Cyclosporine	Plasmocid
Dapsone	Quinine
Desferrioxamine	Streptomycin
(desferroxamine;	Styrene (vinyl benzene)
deferoxamine)	Sulfonamides
Dinitrobenzene	Tamoxifen
Dinitrochlorobenzene	Thallium
Disulfiram	Tobacco
Elcatonin (synthetic	Toluene
analog of calcitonin)	Triethyl tin
Emetine	Trichloroethylene
Ergot	Vincristine

longer in use. A recurrent dilemma in patients who develop loss of vision or a clear-cut optic neuropathy is deciding whether the disease or the treatment is responsible for the visual loss. In some cases, it is impossible to decide. In addition, the suspected toxin may not be the only agent to which the patient has been exposed, further confounding the issue of causation. Several toxic-induced optic neuropathies are discussed below in detail.

METHANOL

Methanol ingestion is the most widely recognized cause of a toxic optic neuropathy, and methanol toxic neuropathy is also the best characterized pathogenetically and clinically. Unlike some of the intoxicants mentioned in this chapter which are medications and therefore apt to be supplanted in time, methanol is likely to remain a permanent threat. Hence, it deserves special attention in this chapter. However, it must be noted that methanol intoxication is not an ideal paradigm for the toxic neuropathies. The combination of acute onset, life-threatening systemic symptoms, and severe irreversible visual loss is atypical.

Cases are encountered in both epidemic and sporadic form. The victim almost always has consumed the poison accidentally because it was mistaken for, substituted for, or added to ethyl alcohol, the taste and smell of which it closely resembles. Although blindness can result from drinking an ounce or less of pure methanol, the toxic effect is ameliorated if it is ingested together with ethyl alcohol.

In the primate model of methanol intoxication, there is optic disc swelling, but the lesion is retrobulbar. The evidence from human postmortem examinations also favors a retrobulbar locus. The early lesion is demyelinating; the later lesion is necrotic.

Initially, the patient has nausea and vomiting, but these symptoms may seem so insignificant that the physician falsely concludes that the patient has not been seriously intoxicated. After 18 to 48 hours, however, the patient begins to experience respiratory distress, headache, and visual loss. Abdominal pain, generalized weakness, confusion, and drowsiness are commonly present at this stage. Coma and death from respiratory failure may follow. Metabolic acidosis is one of the hallmarks of methanol intoxication, and it is consequent to the accumulation of formate. The severity of the acidosis is a rough guide to the severity of the intoxication, but the visual complications are not consequent to the acidosis per se.

Methanol intoxication can reduce vision to any level, including total irrevocable blindness. Central and cecocentral scotomas predominate in cases of partial visual loss. The optic disc is often hyperemic, with blurred margins in the acute stage, and there may be some edema of the peripapillary retina. The reaction of the pupils to light is reduced in cases of severe, but not complete loss of vision; however, when the patient is blind, the pupils are dilated and nonreactive to light. The lack of a pupillary reaction to light likely signifies a poor prognosis.

Patients may regain vision, usually within a week, but occasionally later. In some cases, vision fails again weeks after first improving. The optic discs gradually become pale, and there is often cupping of the optic disc that may be indistinguishable from that in glaucoma. There may also be thinning of retinal arteries.

The diagnosis of methanol poisoning can be substantiated by demonstrating a serum methanol level of greater than 20 mg/dL. Other biochemical findings include a large anion gap, a high serum formate level, and a reduced serum bicarbonate level.

Treatment of methanol poisoning must be instituted promptly. In patients seen relatively early, who have ingested methanol but have not yet developed visual symptoms, there is the potential for preventing loss of vision. Even patients who have already lost vision may experience some degree of recovery if prompt treatment is instituted. Ethanol should be given, because it interferes with the metabolism of methanol. The metabolic acidosis responds to bicarbonate, and hemodialysis can help eliminate the toxin.

ETHYLENE GLYCOL

Ethylene glycol is the active ingredient in automobile antifreeze and may be consumed accidentally or in a suicide attempt. This poison is toxic to the optic nerve, and the metabolic consequences resemble those of methanol poisoning, with which it could easily be confused.

As in methanol intoxication, the victim initially has nausea, vomiting, and abdominal pain. Stupor and coma follow, and there is cardiac failure within a few days. Unlike the situation in methanol intoxication, however, there is a high incidence of renal failure. The outcome can be fatal, or recovery can occur. Patients who survive may have permanent residual neurologic and ophthalmologic deficits.

Despite the metabolic similarities to methanol intoxication, the frequency of visual loss seems to be much lower in patients poisoned by ethylene glycol. Nevertheless, profound visual loss can occur, with dilated pupils that do not react to light. True papilledema, caused by cerebral edema, may occur, or the optic discs can initially appear normal, only to become pale with time. Unlike the situation in methanol intoxication, patients with ethylene glycol intoxication may develop nystagmus and ophthalmoplegia.

One clue to the cause of the intoxication is the presence of oxalate crystals in the urine. The accumulation of glycolate causes a metabolic acidosis and a large anion gap. Treatment is essentially the same as the treatment of methanol intoxication. Bicarbonate is used to combat the acidosis, ethanol is administered to retard the metabolism of the ethylene glycol, and hemodialysis is employed to promote elimination of the poison.

ETHAMBUTOL

Of all the drugs used throughout the world, ethambutol is undoubtedly the one most often implicated in toxic optic neuropathy. Experiments in monkeys and rats show that ethambutol intoxication causes an axonal neuropathy with a special predilection for the optic chiasm. The biochemical basis of ethambutol toxicity has yet to be elucidated. Ethambutol is metabolized to a chelating agent, and this has been suggested as somehow responsible for the optic neuropathy. It is interesting in this regard that two other chelators—disulfiram and DL-penicillamine—have been implicated in toxic optic neuropathies. Reduced serum zinc levels are found in several toxic optic neuropathies.

Human ethambutol intoxication is dose-related, with loss of vision most likely to occur in patients receiving 25 mg/kg/day or more. However, vision loss may occur in patients receiving much lower doses. Visual loss rarely occurs until the patient has been receiving the drug for at least 2 months, with 7 months being the average. There is evidence that there is greater susceptibility to intoxication and more severe visual impairment in patients with renal tuberculosis, perhaps because ethambutol depends on the kidneys for excretion.

Some authors claim that dyschromatopsia is the earliest symptom of the toxic optic neuropathy produced by ethambutol, with blue-yellow color changes being the most common. In any case, the loss of vision is bilaterally symmetric and begins insidiously. Central scotomas are the rule, but patients may also develop bitemporal defects or peripheral constriction. The fundi are initially normal, but if the drug is not stopped vision continues to worsen and optic atrophy develops. Visual acuity, color vision, and visual field usually improve slowly once ethambutol is discontinued; however, some patients, particularly but not exclusively those in whom optic atrophy has already developed, do not experience an improvement in visual function.

Beyond stopping the drug, there is no specific therapy for the toxic optic neuropathy caused by ethambutol. Patients receiving ethambutol should have a baseline (pretreatment) ophthalmologic examination that includes assessment of visual acuity, color vision, and visual fields, and these parameters should be monitored periodically for the duration of treatment. Some authors suggest that VEPs be monitored in patients taking ethambutol to detect the earliest evidence of a toxic effect on the optic nerves.

HALOGENATED HYDROXYQUINOLINES

The halogenated hydroxyquinolines are amebacidal drugs. One of these (iodochlorhydroxyquin) was promoted in some parts of the world for preventing or treating travelers' diarrhea and chronic diarrheas. In that setting, it caused a syndrome of optic neuropathy, myelopathy, and peripheral neuropathy (subacute myelo-optic neuropathy or SMON). The irony is that there is no evidence that the halogenated hydroxyquinolines actually prevent traveler's diarrhea. The impact on public health was significant, with over 10,000 cases documented in Japan between 1956 and 1970. SMON virtually disappeared in Japan when the use of these drugs was stopped.

Although Japanese investigators were the first to call attention to the problem, the disorder is not limited to geographic or ethnic boundaries. Cases have been described in Australia, Europe, and the United States.

The neurotoxicity of the halogenated hydroxyquinolines is dose-related. Patients with gastrointestinal disease, who constitute a high proportion of those taking these drugs, are especially vulnerable.

Symptoms can appear as early as 5 days after beginning treatment. Initially, there is abdominal discomfort that is followed by paresthesias and dysesthesias in the legs. This may progress to paraparesis or paraplegia. One quarter of the patients experience visual impairment in one form or another. Dyschromatopsia is an early symptom and occasionally is the only deficit; however, central acuity is usually affected, and about 5% of patients become effectively blind.

Children with acrodermatitis enteropathica, a rare hereditary disease in which there is malabsorption of zinc, appear to have a low threshold for loss of vision from halogenated hydroxyquinolines. Interestingly, they often experience the visual loss without developing the other neurologic deficits.

DISULFIRAM

Disulfiram is a drug with a role, albeit a small one, in the treatment of chronic alcoholism. Disulfiram interferes with the metabolism of acetaldehyde, a metabolic product of ethanol. The concurrent ingestion of alcohol and disulfiram causes uncomfortable symptoms, including flushing, nausea, and vomiting as a result of the accumulation of acetaldehyde.

Disulfiram can cause an optic neuropathy, and because the optic neuropathy can occur in patients who have remained abstemious, alcohol toxicity presumably does not play a role in such cases. The mechanism of this toxicity is unknown, but disulfiram, like several other optic nerve toxins, is a chelating agent.

The symptoms and signs in patients with toxic optic neuropathy caused by disulfiram are quite typical of those of other toxic and nutritional optic neuropathies. The visual loss is subacute or chronic, affecting both eyes symmetrically. Pain is not a feature. The visual field defects are central or cecocentral. The optic discs are usually initially normal in appearance, but they can become pale late in the course. Some affected persons also develop a sensorimotor peripheral neuropathy. The prognosis for complete recovery is good if the disulfiram therapy is discontinued.

TOBACCO

The mechanism, nature, nosology, semiology, and existence of a toxic optic neuropathy caused by tobacco has been debated for many years. For much of this time, the designation "tobacco-alcohol amblyopia" has obfuscated these issues. It is our opinion that although tobacco probably can cause or contribute to a toxic optic neuropathy, alcohol is not a primary or contributing factor, and the two do not exert any toxic effect in concert. If ever a medical term deserved to be expunged, it is "tobacco-alcohol amblyopia."

The frequency with which tobacco-induced optic neuropathy is encountered varies from time to time and place to place. This remarkable variability may reflect nothing more than the lack of good criteria for proving the diagnosis. In the mid-19th century in Scotland, chronic cases were allegedly seen every day at one eye infirmary. One hundred years later, physicians in the

United States were not even seeing one case a year, and investigators in Australia had also not seen a single case. In the 1970s, most authorities agreed that this was a disease whose incidence was declining—an apparent paradox because the consumption of tobacco products actually *increased* during the same period. A shift away from pipe and cigar smoking (which carries a higher risk) to cigarette smoking (which carries a lower risk) might explain the paradox. In any case, convincing cases of tobacco amblyopia are still encountered. Indeed, the field investigation of Cuban patients with epidemic optic neuropathy (see above) provided further validation of a role for tobacco in optic nerve disease.

The mechanism by which tobacco damages the optic nerves is unclear. One possibility relates to concurrent malnutrition. The Cuban experience suggests that tobacco may be a secondary factor in patients predisposed to an optic neuropathy by malnutrition. In Belgium prior to World War II, tobacco "amblyopia" was rarely encountered. However, during the Nazi occupation of Belgium when there was widespread malnutrition, the incidence of the disease increased dramatically. Vitamin B_{12} deficiency may also play a role in some cases of tobacco amblyopia. Tobacco itself may actually interfere with the absorption of the vitamin. In most cases of tobacco amblyopia, however, there is no defect in vitamin B_{12} metabolism, and blood levels of the vitamin are within normal limits.

Cyanide is present in tobacco smoke, and this has led to a suspicion that tobacco amblyopia is a limited form of cyanide poisoning. It has been theorized that there is a defect in sulfur metabolism and of cyanide detoxification in patients with visual loss associated with smoking tobacco. However, attempts to produce a cyanide optic neuropathy in nonhuman primates have failed on numerous occasions. Chronic cyanide injections caused an optic neuropathy in rats, but the characteristics were not those of human tobacco amblyopia. The onset was sudden. More importantly, the optic neuropathy only occurred when extensive brain lesions were already present. Thus, the role of cyanide in tobacco amblyopia has yet to be proved. As with the nutritional amblyopias, it seems likely that the etiology of tobacco amblyopia in many cases is multifactorial.

Tobacco amblyopia occurs primarily in middle-aged or elderly persons. It is overwhelmingly a disease of men, perhaps because the victims are overwhelmingly pipe and cigar smokers. Why cigarette smokers should be less vulnerable is unknown. The disorder is painless and characterized by slowly progressive, bilateral dyschromatopsia and visual loss. The characteristic visual field defect is a cecocentral scotoma. The optic discs initially appear normal, with pallor being a late feature. Patients with tobacco amblyopia slowly improve if they stop smoking, or if they are treated with injections of hydroxycobalamin.

FOR MORE INFORMATION:
See Walsh & Hoyt's *Clinical Neuro-Ophthalmology,* 5th edition, Volume 1, Chapter 14, pages 663–679.

Hereditary Optic Neuropathies

The hereditary optic neuropathies comprise a group of disorders in which the cause of optic nerve dysfunction appears to be hereditable as demonstrated or suggested by familial expression or genetic analysis. Clinical variability, both within and among families with the same disease, often makes recognition and classification difficult. Traditionally, classification has relied on the recognition of similar characteristics and similar patterns of transmission, but genetic analysis now permits diagnosis of the hereditary optic neuropathies in the absence of family history or in the setting of unusual clinical presentations. As a result, the clinical phenotypes of each disease are broader, and it is easier to recognize unusual cases.

The inherited optic neuropathies typically manifest as symmetric, bilateral, central visual loss. In many of these disorders, the papillomacular nerve fiber bundle is affected, with resultant central or cecocentral scotomas. The exact location of initial pathology along the ganglion cell and its axon, and the pathophysiologic mechanisms of optic nerve injury remain unknown. Optic nerve damage is usually permanent and, in many diseases, may be progressive. Once optic atrophy is observed, substantial nerve injury has already occurred.

In classifying the hereditary optic neuropathies, it is important to exclude the primary retinal degenerations that may masquerade as primary optic neuropathies because of the common finding of optic disc pallor (see Chapter 2). Retinal findings may be subtle, especially among the cone dystrophies, where optic disc pallor may be an early finding. The possibility of a primary retinal process should be considered in patients with temporal optic atrophy, even when the retina itself is not obviously abnormal. Retinal arterial attenuation and an abnormal electroretinogram (ERG) should help distinguish these diseases from the primary optic neuropathies. However, optic nerve disease and retinal pathology may also coexist. Among the multisystem disorders (see below), primary retinal degeneration with secondary optic disc pallor is a frequent occurrence and may be difficult to distinguish from primary optic nerve involvement. At times, there may be coexistent pathology.

Customary classification of the inherited optic neuropathies is by pattern of transmission. The most common patterns of inheritance are autosomal dominant, autosomal recessive, and maternal (i.e., mitochondrial). The same genetic defect may not be responsible for all pedigrees with optic neuropathy inherited in a similar fashion. Similarly, different genetic defects may cause identical or similar phenotypes—some inherited in the same manner, others not. Alternatively, the same genetic defect may result in different clinical expression, although the pattern of inheritance should be consistent. To complicate matters further, single cases are often presumed or proven to be caused by inherited genetic defects, making the pattern of familial transmission unavailable as an aid in classification.

In some of the hereditary optic neuropathies, optic nerve dysfunction is the only manifestation of the disease. In others, various neurologic and systemic abnormalities are regularly observed. Furthermore, inherited diseases with primarily neurologic or systemic manifestations, such as the multisystem degenerations, can include optic atrophy. This chapter classifies the hereditary optic neuropathies into three major groups:

1. Optic neuropathies that occur primarily without associated neurologic or systemic signs.
2. Optic neuropathies that frequently have associated neurologic or systemic signs.
3. Optic neuropathies that are secondary in the overall disease process.

The hereditary optic neuropathies reflect a number of different inheritance patterns and can be caused by defects in either the nuclear or mitochondrial genomes. As more specific genetic defects are discovered, our concept of the phenotypes of these disorders will likely change, as will our classification. More accurate definition of the underlying genetic abnormalities will also aid genetic counseling. Furthermore, identification of the gene defect, elucidation of the gene product and its normal function, and clarification of the abnormality caused by the mutation should improve our understanding of the pathophysiologic mechanisms of optic nerve dysfunction and allow for the development of directed therapies.

MONOSYMPTOMATIC HEREDITARY OPTIC NEUROPATHIES

LEBER'S OPTIC NEUROPATHY

Numerous pedigrees of **Leber's hereditary optic neuropathy** (LHON) have been reported from Europe, North America, Australia, and Asia since the mid-19th century. In the late 1980s and early 1990s, LHON received significant notoriety as a maternally inherited disease linked to abnormalities in mitochondrial deoxyribonucleic acid (mtDNA). Genetic analysis subsequently broadened our view of what constitutes the clinical presentation of LHON.

Clinical Features

Men become symptomatic more frequently than women, with a male predominance of 80 to 90% in most pedigrees. The prevalence of the disease has not been adequately studied, but LHON accounts for about 2% of legal blindness in persons under 65 years of age in Australia. Approximately 20 to 60% of men at risk for LHON experience visual loss. Among women at risk, the occurrence rate ranges from 4 to 32%. Affected females are more likely to have affected children, especially daughters, than unaffected female carriers. Over the past century, there appears to have been a decline in the risk of visual loss among pedigrees with LHON and a decrease in disease penetrance.

The onset of visual loss typically occurs between the ages of 15 and 35 years, but otherwise classic LHON occurs in many individuals both younger and older, with a range of onset as broad as 1 to 80 years. This age variability occurs even among members of the same pedigree.

Visual loss typically begins painlessly in one eye. Indeed, the absence of pain is a major feature that differentiates LHON from other optic neuropathies, particularly optic neuritis, which occurs in the same general age group. Some patients complain of a sensation of mist or fog obscuring their vision, whereas others first experience a mild central fading of colors. The second eye is usually affected weeks to months later. Reports of simultaneous onset are numerous and likely reflect both instances of true simultaneous bilateral visual loss and cases in which initial involvement of the first eye went unrecognized. Rarely, loss of vision in the second eye occurs after a prolonged interval (8 years or longer). Even more infrequently, involvement remains monocular (up to 16 years) or subclinical.

The onset of visual loss is usually not associated with other symptoms. Uhthoff's symptom (a transient worsening of vision with exercise or warming) may occur in patients with LHON, as it does in patients with other optic neuropathies. Other reported symptoms at the time of visual loss are usually minor and nonspecific.

The duration of progression of visual loss in each eye also varies and may be difficult to document accurately. Usually, the course is characterized as acute or subacute, with deterioration of visual function stabilizing after about 3 to 4 months. However, sudden and complete visual loss or slowly progressive disease over years can occur.

Visual acuities at the point of maximum visual loss range from no light perception to 20/20, but most patients deteriorate to acuities worse than 20/200. Color vision is severely affected, often early in the course, but rarely before there is significant visual loss. Pupillary light responses may be relatively preserved when compared with the responses in patients with optic neuropathies from other causes. Visual field defects are typically central or cecocentral. The scotomas may be relative during the early stages of visual loss but rapidly become large and absolute. Rarely, field abnormalities mimicking the bitemporal configuration of chiasmal defects occur.

Even the earliest descriptions of this disease noted funduscopic abnormalities other than optic atrophy. Hyperemia of the optic disc, dilation and tortuosity of vessels, rare retinal and disc hemorrhages, macular edema, exudates, retinal striations, and obscuration of the disc margins may be seen, especially during the acute phase of visual loss. A "classic triad" of signs is seen in many cases of LHON: (1) circumpapillary telangiectatic microangiopathy, (2) swelling of the nerve fiber layer around the disc (pseudoedema), and (3) absence of leakage from the disc or papillary region on fluorescein angiography (distinguishing the LHON optic disc from truly swollen optic discs) (Fig. 11.1). These funduscopic changes may be seen in symptomatic patients, some "presymptomatic" cases, and in asymptomatic maternal relatives. However, having abnormalities of the peripapillary nerve fiber layer does not necessarily predict visual loss. Furthermore, many patients with LHON never exhibit the characteristic ophthalmoscopic appearance, even if examined at the time of acute visual loss. The "classic" LHON ophthalmoscopic appearance may be helpful in suggesting the diagnosis if it is recognized in patients or their maternal relatives, but its absence—even during the period of acute visual loss—does not exclude the diagnosis of LHON. Indeed, some patients with LHON have absolutely normal appearing optic discs at the time they become symptomatic, and it is for this reason that many of these patients are initially thought to have nonorganic visual loss.

As visual loss progresses in patients with LHON who have the typical fundus appearance described above, the telangiectatic vessels disappear, and the pseudoedema of the disc resolves. Perhaps because of the initial hyperemia, the optic discs of patients with LHON may not appear pale for some time. This feature, coupled with the relatively preserved pupillary responses and the lack of pain, can also result in the misdiagnosis of nonorganic visual loss in some LHON patients. Eventually, however, optic atrophy—with nerve fiber layer dropout most pronounced in the papillomacular bundle—supervenes (Fig. 11.2). Nonglaucomatous cupping of the optic discs or arteriolar attenuation may also be seen.

In most patients, visual loss remains profound and permanent. However, not uncommonly, recovery of central vision occurs years after visual deterioration. Spontaneous improvement of some degree has been reported in as many as 85% of affected family members within a pedigree. The recovery may occur gradually over 6 months to 1 year after initial visual loss, or it may suddenly occur 2 to 10 years after onset. It may take the form of a gradual clearing of central vision or be restricted to a few central degrees, resulting in a small island of vision within a large central or cecocentral scotoma. Recovery is usually bilateral and symmetric, but it may be bilateral and asymmetric or occur only in one eye. Patients in whom vision improves substantially have a lower mean age at the time of initial

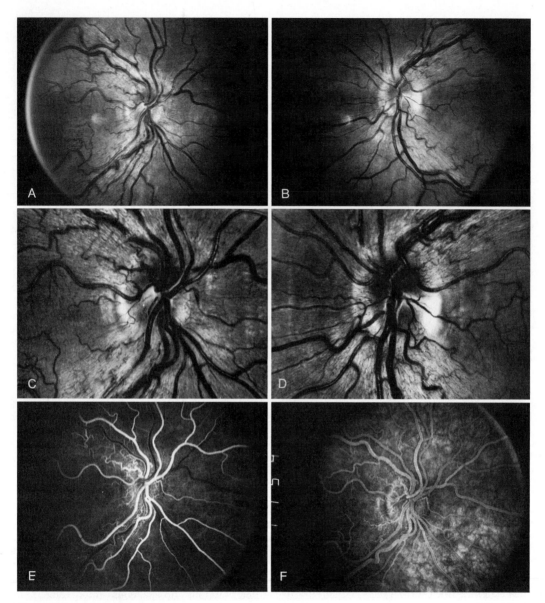

Figure 11.1. Leber's optic neuropathy. *A–B.* Both optic discs in the acute phase of the disorder. Note hyperemic appearance of discs. Peripapillary telangiectatic vessels are present. *C–D.* Both optic discs photographed with red-free (540 nm) light. Note marked hyperemia of the discs with dilation of small vessels both on the surface of the disc and in the peripapillary region. *E–F.* Fluorescein angiogram in arteriovenous (*E*) and late (*F*) phases shows dilation of right disc and peripapillary vessels but no leakage of fluorescein dye.

visual loss, usually less than 20 years. Furthermore, the particular mtDNA mutation also influences prognosis, with the 11778 mutation carrying the worst prognosis for vision, and the 14484 mutation the best (see below). Once visual recovery occurs, recurrent visual loss is extremely rare.

Associated Findings

In the majority of patients with LHON, visual dysfunction is the only significant manifestation of the disease. However, some pedigrees have members with associated cardiac conduction ab-

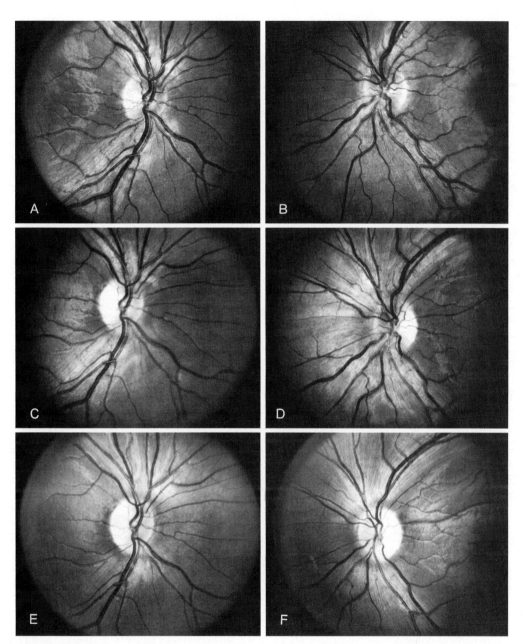

Figure 11.2.   Progression to optic atrophy in a patient with Leber's optic neuropathy. *A–B.* Both discs in acute phase of the disease. Visual acuity is 20/100 in both eyes with large cecocentral scotomas. Telangiectatic vessels are evident adjacent to the inferior margin of both discs. The right disc is already pale temporally, and there is atrophy of the papillomacular nerve fiber layer. *C–D.* Two months after onset of visual loss, visual acuity is 5/200 in the right eye and 8/200 in the left eye. Both discs show moderate pallor, particularly temporally, with loss of nerve fiber layer that is especially evident in the papillomacular region. Previously seen telangiectatic vessels are disappearing. *E–F.* Six months after onset of visual loss, visual acuity remains 5/200 in the right eye and 8/200 in the left eye. Both discs are pale, particularly temporally. The telangiectatic vessels have completely disappeared. One year after these photographs were obtained, the patient noted gradual, partial return of visual acuity in both eyes to 20/50. Subsequent genetic testing showed evidence of a mutation in the mitochondrial DNA at position 14484.

normalities, such as the preexcitation syndromes (specifically Wolff-Parkinson-White and Lown-Ganong-Levine) and prolongation of the corrected QT interval. Rarely, patients experience palpitations, syncope, or sudden death. Familial skeletal abnormalities also occur in pedigrees with LHON.

Minor neurologic abnormalities, such as exaggerated or pathologic reflexes, mild cerebellar ataxia, tremor, movement disorders, muscle wasting, or distal sensory neuropathy, are present in some patients with LHON. In addition, some patients with molecularly confirmed LHON, predominantly women, exhibit symptoms and signs consistent with multiple sclerosis (MS) at the time they begin to experience the progressive, nonremitting visual loss typical of LHON. Cerebrospinal fluid (CSF) and magnetic resonance imaging (MRI) findings are also characteristic of MS in these patients. Population surveys do not demonstrate an increased prevalence of the mtDNA mutations associated with LHON among patients with MS. It is possible that this apparent association of LHON and MS is no greater than the prevalence of the two diseases. An underlying LHON mutation, however, may worsen the prognosis of optic neuritis in patients with MS.

Some pedigrees have been described in which multiple members exhibit the clinical features of LHON in addition to more severe neurologic abnormalities, the so-called ''Leber's plus'' syndromes. These syndromes include:

- Optic neuropathy, movement disorders, spasticity, psychiatric disturbances, skeletal abnormalities, and acute infantile encephalopathic episodes.
- Optic neuropathy, dystonia, and lesions of the basal ganglia by neuroimaging.
- Optic neuropathy and myelopathy.
- Optic neuropathy and fatal encephalopathy in early childhood.

Ancillary Testing

Ancillary tests other than genetic analysis (see below) are generally of limited usefulness in the evaluation of LHON. Fluorescein angiography is helpful in its illustration and confirmation of LHON funduscopic features, particularly the lack of leakage of dye from the optic disc. An electrocardiogram may reveal cardiac conduction abnormalities. Pattern-reversal visual-evoked potentials (VEPs) may be absent or show prolonged latencies and decreased amplitudes, usually in eyes with diminished acuity. The standard flash ERG is typically normal, although occasional attenuation of the b-wave may be noted. Cerebrospinal fluid analysis is usually normal, except in those cases with a MS-like syndrome. Electroencephalograms are unremarkable. Brain computed tomographic (CT) scanning and MRI are normal, except in patients with additional symptoms suggestive of MS and pedigrees with childhood encephalopathy or dystonia and basal ganglia lesions. Optic nerve abnormalities on MRI may be seen in LHON patients, even after the acute phase of visual loss. The results of phosphorus-31 MR spectroscopy indicate impaired mitochondrial metabolism within limb muscle and in occipital lobes in some patients with LHON, as well as in some unaffected carriers. MR spectroscopy may thus prove to be a useful noninvasive way of following patients at risk for LHON. Although morphologic abnormalities of mitochondria on skeletal muscle biopsy are rare in LHON, patients and carriers may exhibit abnormal lactate production with exercise.

The pathologic findings in acute LHON are unknown; thus, the location and nature of the initial damage remain uncertain. Studies performed years after visual loss demonstrate only marked atrophy of retinal nerve fibers, retinal ganglion cells, and the optic nerves. Some atrophic tissues show intramitochondrial calcification, although morphologic changes of mitochondria are rarely seen on muscle biopsy. Deficiency in respiratory chain complex I activity has been demonstrated in muscle and blood samples of LHON patients with the 11778 and 3460 mutations and in leukocytes of LHON patients with the 14484 mutation.

Inheritance and Genetics

All pedigrees clinically designated as LHON have a maternal inheritance pattern. In maternal inheritance, all offspring of a woman carrying the trait will inherit the trait, but only the females can pass the trait on to the subsequent generation. Both the father and the mother contribute to the nuclear portion of the zygote, but the mother's egg is essentially the sole provider of the cytoplasmic contents of the zygote. Therefore, a cytoplasmic determinant is necessary for maternal inheritance. The only source of extra-nuclear DNA in the cell is the intracytoplasmic mitochondria.

Every cell contains several hundred intracytoplasmic mitochondria that generate the cellular energy necessary for normal cellular function and maintenance. Those cells in tissues particularly reliant on mitochondrial energy production, such as the central nervous system (CNS), contain more mitochondria than cells with low energy requirements. Each mitochondrion contains 2 to 10 double-stranded circles of DNA. Each circle of mtDNA contains only 16,500 base pairs compared with the 3×10^9 base pairs contained within the nuclear genome. However, given that there are several mtDNAs in each mitochondrion and hundreds of mitochondria per cell, the mtDNA comprises approximately 0.3% of the cell's total DNA. Its relative small size makes the mtDNA accessible to study, and the entire gene sequence has been determined. Mitochondrial DNA codes for all the transfer ribonucleic acids (RNAs) and ribosomal RNAs required for intramitochondrial protein production, and for 13 proteins essential to the oxidative phosphorylation system. The majority of proteins crucial to normal oxidative phosphorylation function are encoded on nuclear genes, manufactured in the cytoplasm, and transported into the mitochondria. Hence ''mitochondrial disease'' can theoretically result from genetic defects in either the nuclear or mitochondrial genomes. Over 30 mtDNA point mutations and over 100 mtDNA rearrangements have been proposed as etiologic factors in human disease. Expression of these diseases reflects complex genotypic-phenotypic interactions that likely involve nuclear modifying or susceptibility factors.

If a new mutation occurs in the mtDNA, there will be a period of coexistence of mutant and normal mtDNA within the same cell (**heteroplasmy**). At each cell division, the mitochondrial genotype may drift toward pure normal or pure mutant, or it may remain mixed (**replicative segregation**). The phenotype of the cell (and the tissue the cells comprise) depends on the proportional mixture of mtDNA genotypes and the intrinsic energy needs of the cell. The mutant phenotype may only become apparent when the amount of normal mtDNA can no longer provide sufficient mitochondrial function for cell and tissue maintenance (**threshold effect**). Because of the cytoplasmic location of mtDNA, mitochondrial diseases secondary to point mutations in the mtDNA follow a pattern of maternal inheritance.

The first point mutation in mtDNA to be linked to LHON was a single nucleotide substitution (adenine for guanine) at position 11778 in the mtDNA (Fig. 11.3). This region codes for subunit 4 (designated ND4) of complex I (NADH dehydrogenase) in the respiratory chain. The mutation at position 11778 changes an amino acid from arginine to histidine, probably a crucial substitution because arginine is found in this position in the ND4 protein in many other species (i.e., it is **evolutionarily conserved**). The presence of adenine instead of guanine at position 11778 eliminates a site where the restriction endonuclease SfaNI would normally cut the mitochondrial genome, and it creates a site where a different restriction endonuclease, MaeIII, will cut the genome. This provides a simple method for detecting the 11778 mutation on any tissue sample that contains mitochondria, including whole blood. The 11778 mutation is present in many racially divergent pedigrees with LHON, suggesting that the 11778 mutation has arisen independently on multiple occasions. from 31 to 89% of European, North American, and Australian LHON pedigrees have the 11778 mutation. In Japan, the prevalence of the 11778 mutation among LHON families is higher, being greater than 90%.

Mutations at several sites other than 11778 are believed to cause LHON. The majority of these sites are located within genes that also code for proteins comprising complex 1, but all are within subunits other than ND4 (see Fig. 11.3). For example, a point mutation at mtDNA position 3460 within the gene coding for subunit 1 of complex I accounts for 8 to 15% of LHON worldwide, and a point mutation at position 14484 in the gene coding for the sixth subunit of complex I accounts for 10 to 15% of LHON pedigrees. The mutations at sites 11778, 3460, and 14484 are designated ''primary'' mutations for Leber's disease in that they (1) confer a genetic risk for LHON expression individually; (2) change the coding for evolutionarily conserved amino acids in essential proteins; (3) are found in multiple, different, ethnically divergent pedigrees; and (4) are absent or rare among control pedigrees. In total, they account for 85 to 90% of LHON worldwide. Other mtDNA point mutations have been associated with LHON (e.g., at site 15257) (see Fig. 11.3), but their pathoge-

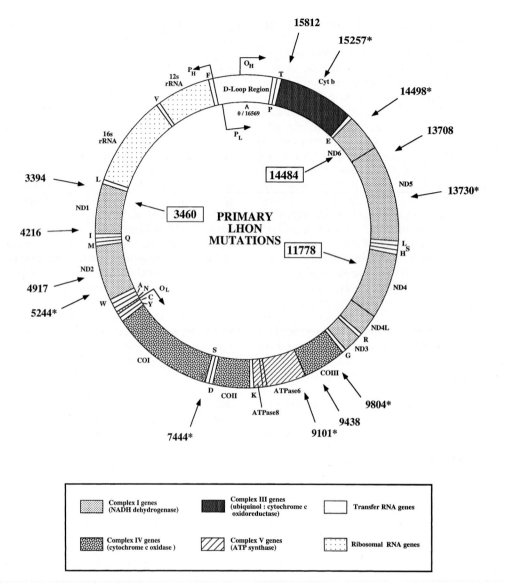

Figure 11.3. Mitochondrial genome showing the point mutations associated with Leber's optic neuropathy. The primary mutations are located inside the genome (circle) and the other mutations are shown outside the genome. Mutations noted with an asterisk may be primary mutations, but when found in the absence of one of the three confirmed primary mutations, they each account for only one or a few probands worldwide. (Courtesy of Marie T. Lott and Douglas C. Wallace. Center for Genetics and Molecular Medicine, Emory University School of Medicine, Atlanta, Georgia.)

netic significance remains less clear. They are considered "secondary" mutations because, although they are found with greater frequency among LHON patients than controls, they do occur in control pedigrees and thus may not in and of themselves confer a risk of blindness. They vary markedly in their prevalence, degree of evolutionary conservation of the encoded amino acids altered, and frequency among controls. Many of these secondary mutations occur in combination with each other and with the primary LHON mutations. Caution must thus be used in assuming a primary causal role for these mutations.

The pedigrees with "LHON plus" and severe neurologic abnormalities in multiple family members may be genetically distinct from those families with more typical, isolated Leber's-type visual loss. The maternal members of an Australian pedigree with optic neuropathies, movement disorders, spasticity, and acute encephalopathic episodes harbor a mutation at mtDNA position 4160 (ND1) in addition to the 14484 primary LHON mutation. An American pedigree with optic neuropathy and fatal childhood encephalopathy has two primary mtDNA point mutations at sites 11778 and 14484. Among the families with optic neuropathy and basal ganglia lesions, some harbor a unique mutation at position 14459 in ND6.

Determinants of Expression

Genetic analysis allows a broad view of what constitutes the clinical profile of LHON. Most striking are the number of patients without a family history of visual loss. Although there is undoubtedly a referral bias for the unusual cases, singleton patients constitute more than 50% of molecularly confirmed LHON in some studies. Some of these singleton cases are women, some are outside the typical age range for LHON, and some do not have the classic ophthalmoscopic appearance. Clearly, the diagnosis of LHON should be considered in any case of unexplained bilateral optic neuropathy, regardless of age of onset, sex, family history, or funduscopic appearance.

Many questions remain unanswered regarding the determinants of phenotypic expression of LHON. For example, does the specific mtDNA mutation dictate particular clinical features? Although pedigrees with the "Leber's plus" syndromes demonstrate that certain mtDNA mutations may result in specific disease patterns of Leber-like optic neuropathies with other neurologic abnormalities, few significant clinical differences can be demonstrated among patients positive for the 11778 mutation, patients with other mtDNA mutations, and patients as yet genetically unspecified. One major exception is the difference in spontaneous recovery rates among patients with the 11778 mutation and those with the 14484 mutation. Among patients with the 11778 mutation, only about 4% experience spontaneous recovery, compared with 37% to 65% of 14484 patients. Furthermore, the ultimate visual acuities in pa-

tients with the 14484 mutation are significantly better than those with the 11778 and 3460 mutations. Cardiac conduction abnormalities occur in 11778 pedigrees, but the 3460 mutation appears to have the highest association with the preexcitation syndromes.

A mtDNA mutation is present in all maternally related family members of patients with LHON, even though most will never become symptomatic. Thus, a mtDNA mutation may be necessary for phenotypic expression, but it may not be sufficient. Does heteroplasmy among individuals in a pedigree play a role in phenotypic expression? In some families, the mutant mtDNA content enriches from one generation to the next and may be at least partially responsible for phenotypic expression of the disease. However, in most large reviews of molecularly confirmed LHON patients, heteroplasmy is documented in the blood of a minority of affected individuals, and once a person becomes symptomatic, there does not appear to be any clinical difference in disease expression among those who are heteroplasmic and those who are homoplasmic.

Assuming that some persons are 100% homoplasmic in all tissues for the causative mtDNA mutation, there is no convincing explanation as to why visual loss should be the sole manifestation of the disease. Varying tissue energy needs may play some role. The CNS is most reliant on mitochondrial adenosine triphosphate (ATP). Histochemical studies of optic nerve in the monkey and rat show a high degree of mitochondrial respiratory activity within the unmyelinated portion of optic nerve fibers located in the most anterior portion of the optic nerve. Ganglion cells and their projections may be especially vulnerable to the energy deficiencies created by mtDNA mutations.

Genetic factors other than the specific mtDNA mutation and the presence and degree of heteroplasmy may play a role in expression. Other mtDNA mutations may be present that modify the expression of the LHON causative mutation or that result in other abnormal proteins involved in mitochondrial function. Nuclear-encoded factors modifying mtDNA expression, mtDNA products, or mitochondrial metabolism may be necessary for phenotypic expression of LHON. The male predominance of visual loss in LHON may be explained by a modifying factor on the X-chromosome, although most studies have failed to confirm X-linkage in this disease. Tissue energy utilization and reserve may also determine the timing and extent of visual loss. Mitochondrial energy production decreases with age, and the timing of visual loss in patients at risk for LHON may reflect the threshold at which already reduced mitochondrial function deteriorates to a critical level.

Environmental factors may also play a role. Both the internal and external environment of the organism must be considered. Systemic illnesses, nutritional deficiencies, and toxins that stress or directly inhibit the body's mitochondrial respiratory capacity may initiate or increase phenotypic expression of the disease. Anecdotal reports suggest a possible role for tobacco and excessive alcohol use in the expression of visual loss, but large studies on the effects of these agents on patients at risk for LHON have yet to be performed.

Treatment

In light of the possibility for spontaneous recovery in some patients with LHON, any anecdotal reports of treatment efficacy must be considered with caution. Attempts to treat or prevent the acute phase of visual loss with systemic steroids, hydroxycobalamin, or cyanide antagonists are ineffective. Similarly, craniotomy with lysis of chiasmal arachnoid adhesions cannot be supported. Some of the manifestations of other mitochondrial diseases, specifically the mitochondrial cytopathies, may respond to therapies designed to increase mitochondrial energy production. Most of the agents used are naturally occurring cofactors involved in mitochondrial metabolism, whereas others have antioxidant capabilities. Therapies tried include coenzyme Q_{10}, idebenone (an analog of coenzyme Q), succinate, vitamin K_1, vitamin K_3, vitamin C, thiamine, and vitamin B_2. Use of coenzyme Q_{10} in patients with LHON and visual loss has been limited, but our preliminary results are not particularly encouraging. It remains to be seen if any of these agents alone or in combination will prove consistently useful in the treatment of acute visual loss in LHON or in the prophylactic therapy of asymptomatic family members at risk.

Nonspecific recommendations to avoid agents that might stress mitochondrial energy production have no proven benefit but are certainly reasonable. We advise our patients at risk for LHON to avoid tobacco use, excessive alcohol intake, and environmental toxins. An electrocardiogram should be obtained and any cardiac abnormalities treated accordingly. Considering the degree of visual acuity loss, it is remarkable that up to 82% of LHON patients are gainfully employed despite their visual handicap. An assessment by a low-vision specialist may be helpful, especially because much peripheral vision may remain intact.

The importance of genetic counseling of patients with this disease and their families cannot be overemphasized. It should be explained to males with an LHON mutation, whether or not they are visually symptomatic, that they **will not** pass the mutation or the disease to their children. On the other hand, women with one of the LHON mutations **will** pass the mutation to all of their children, both male and female, although not all persons with the mutation will become symptomatic (see above). Furthermore, as noted above, symptomatic patients with the 11778 mutation have a very small chance of experiencing spontaneous improvement in vision, whereas patients with the 14484 mutation have a significant chance of visual improvement.

DOMINANT OPTIC ATROPHY

Autosomal-dominant optic atrophy, also called Kjer's or juvenile optic atrophy, is the most common of the hereditary optic neuropathies, with an estimated disease prevalence in the range of 1:50,000 or as high as 1:10,000 in Denmark. Some authors separate the disorder into an infantile and a juvenile form, but we believe that such a distinction is unwarranted because the disorder has substantial interfamilial and intrafamilial clinical variability (see below).

Clinical Features

Dominant optic atrophy is an abiotrophy with onset in the first decade in life. Although it is difficult for patients or their families to identify a precise onset of reduced vision, no congenital case has been documented at birth or even shortly thereafter. The majority of patients appear to become affected between 4 and 6 years of age. Although some severely affected children develop nystagmus and are found to have decreased vision prior to beginning schooling, the majority of persons with autosomal-dominant optic atrophy are unaware of a visual problem. These persons are discovered to have optic atrophy (1) because there is a family history of the condition, (2) as a direct consequence of examination of another affected family member, (3) because they fail a school vision screening examination, or (4) during a "routine" eye examination. These phenomena attest to the usually insidious onset in childhood, mild degree of visual dysfunction, absence of night blindness, and absence of substantial or dramatic progression.

Visual acuity is usually symmetrically reduced in both eyes. Vision ranges from 20/20 to 20/800, with only about 15% of patients eventually developing vision of 20/200 or worse; hand motion or light perception vision is extremely rare. Rare patients have a mild or striking asymmetry between the acuities of the two eyes.

Patients with autosomal-dominant optic atrophy nearly always have a disturbance of color perception. Many patients have a tritanopic defect that is most easily detected using a Farnsworth-Munsell 100-Hues test. A generalized dyschromatopsia, with both blue-yellow and red-green defects, is found in others. There is no correlation between the severity of the dyschromatopsia and the visual acuity.

Visual fields in patients with dominant optic atrophy characteristically show central, paracentral, or cecocentral scotomas. The peripheral fields are usually normal in these patients except for a characteristic chromatic inversion of the peripheral field, with the field of tritanopes being more contracted to blue isopters than to red. Rarely, a visual field pattern consisting of bitemporal depression and thus mimicking the field defects of chiasmal compression is found. It should be remembered, however, that true bitemporal hemianopic scotomas do not normally reduce visual acuity nor are they associated with tritanopic color vision defects.

The optic atrophy in patients with dominantly inherited optic neuropathy may be subtle, temporal only, or may involve the entire disc (Fig. 11.4). The most characteristic change is a translucent pallor with absence of fine superficial capillaries of the temporal aspect of the disc, and a peculiar triangular (wedge) excavation of the temporal portion of the disc. Other ophthalmo-scopic findings reported in these patients include peripapillary atrophy, absent foveal reflex, mild macular pigmentary changes, arterial attenuation, and nonglaucomatous cupping. VEPs are characterized by diminished amplitudes and variable prolongation of latencies.

Although there are a number of dominantly inherited syndromes in which optic atrophy is associated with neurologic dysfunction (see below), most patients with autosomal-dominant optic atrophy have no additional neurologic deficits. Nystagmus in some patients likely reflects early visual deprivation rather than central neurologic involvement. Mild hearing loss has been reported in some families, but severe hearing loss associated with familial optic atrophy is probably a genetically distinct syndrome (see below).

Prognosis

A mild, slow, insidious progression of visual dysfunction occurs in up to 50% of patients with autosomal-dominant optic atrophy. For example, one study found that, on average, the visual acuity decreases about one line per decade of life. There appears to be no correlation between the rate of visual loss and initial visual acuity nor do members of individual pedigrees experience identical rates of progression. Rarely, relatively rapid deterioration of vision occurs after years of stable visual function. Spontaneous recovery of vision is not a feature of this disorder.

Etiology

Autosomal-dominant optic atrophy is believed to be a primary degeneration of the retinal ganglion cells. Genetic linkage studies have mapped the dominant optic atrophy gene to the telomeric part of the long arm of chromosome 3 in almost all pedigrees, but further studies are required to determine if there is any genetic heterogeneity among pedigrees with this condition.

AUTOSOMAL-RECESSIVE OPTIC ATROPHY

Autosomal-recessive optic atrophy is present at birth or develops at an early age and is usually discovered before the patient is 3 or 4 years of age. There is often consanguinity between parents.

The clinical picture is that of visual acuity so severely affected that the patient may be completely blind with searching nystagmus. The vis-

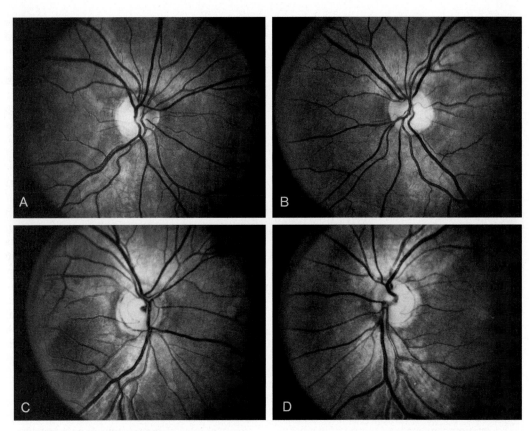

Figure 11.4. Dominant optic atrophy. *A–B*. Right and left optic discs in a patient with 20/40 visual acuity in both eyes, a tritanopic color vision defect, and bilateral, small central scotomas. Note minimal temporal pallor. *C–D*. Right and left discs of the above patient's father. Visual acuity is 20/100 in the right eye and 20/80 in the left eye with severe dyschromatopsia and bilateral central scotomas. The pallor is extensive and is primarily temporal in a "wedge" shape.

ual fields, when they can be tested, show variable constriction, and there are often paracentral scotomas. The optic discs are completely atrophic and often deeply cupped. It is difficult to differentiate this entity from infantile tapetoretinal degeneration by funduscopic appearance alone, because patients with both disorders may have optic disc pallor and vascular narrowing. However, the ERG is normal or supranormal in primary optic atrophy, whereas it is flat in tapetoretinal degeneration.

Autosomal-recessive optic atrophy is stationary and unassociated with other symptoms or signs of systemic or neurologic disease. It is, in our experience, extremely rare, and its very existence as a distinct identity is questionable.

SEX-LINKED OPTIC ATROPHY

Pedigrees with well-documented **sex-linked optic atrophy** are extremely rare. The most con-

vincing are those in which it can be shown that the disease is transmitted from an affected grandfather to his grandson through an unaffected daughter. In the few cases reported, however, neurologic and even retinal abnormalities have often been present, making the designation of this disorder as an isolated, distinct sex-linked optic atrophy problematic.

HEREDITARY OPTIC ATROPHY WITH OTHER NEUROLOGIC OR SYSTEMIC SIGNS

In some pedigrees, hereditary optic atrophy is always associated with specific neurologic or systemic deficits rather than being an isolated finding. Some of these syndromes have been reported in numerous pedigrees; others in only one or two families.

AUTOSOMAL-DOMINANT OPTIC ATROPHY WITH CONGENITAL DEAFNESS

Some pedigrees with presumed autosomal-dominant optic atrophy also have congenital hearing loss. In these cases, there are no systemic or neurologic abnormalities except for congenital sensorineural hearing loss. The hearing loss is usually severe at birth, so without intervention few patients develop speech. Hearing evaluation in some affected individuals, however, reveals that they can hear amplified speech; thus, they may develop adequate speech if they are provided amplification in early childhood and training in oral as well as in manual language.

Although visual dysfunction may be present at an early age, most of the patients have normal acuity until at least 24 years of age. There is great interfamilial and intrafamilial variability in the age of onset of the visual loss, however. In most cases, visual acuity remains better than 20/200.

It is unclear if pedigrees with autosomal-dominant optic atrophy and hearing loss represent a phenotypic variant of isolated autosomal-dominant optic atrophy, a genetically distinct disorder, or a genetically heterogeneous group of disorders with a similar phenotype.

AUTOSOMAL-DOMINANT OPTIC ATROPHY WITH PROGRESSIVE HEARING LOSS AND ATAXIA

In a rare syndrome of autosomal-dominant optic atrophy, bilateral optic atrophy and hearing loss are associated with ataxia and limb weakness. The onset of visual loss is between 2.5 and 9 years of age. The hearing loss is only moderate and, like the optic atrophy, is slowly progressive. The ataxia in these patients primarily involves the legs; weakness and muscle wasting primarily affects the shoulder girdle and hands. This syndrome may be related to Friedreich's ataxia (see below).

HEREDITARY OPTIC ATROPHY WITH PROGRESSIVE HEARING LOSS AND POLYNEUROPATHY

Several pedigrees have been described in which progressive optic atrophy is accompanied by sensorineural deafness and symptomatic or asymptomatic polyneuropathy. The affected individuals vary in the extent of visual and neurologic impairment, and different modes of inheritance—including autosomal-dominant, autosomal-recessive, and X-linked-recessive—have been proposed. These disorders can be included in the spectrum of hereditary polyneuropathies that includes Charcot-Marie-Tooth (CMT) disease (see below).

AUTOSOMAL-DOMINANT OPTIC ATROPHY, DEAFNESS, OPHTHALMOPLEGIA, AND MYOPATHY

A syndrome characterized by optic atrophy, deafness, ptosis, ophthalmoplegia, dystaxia, and myopathy affected 23 members of five generations in one family. The visual loss was first noted between the ages of 6 and 19 years, with an average age of onset of 11 years. Visual loss was occasionally sudden in onset but always progressive to the 20/30 to 20/400 range. ERGs were abnormal, although retinal pigmentary changes were absent. Hearing loss was sensorineural and progressive, with onset in the first or second decades. Ophthalmoplegia, dystaxia, and myopathy occurred in midlife. A muscle biopsy in one affected family member showed ragged-red fibers consistent with a mitochondrial disorder, but the pedigree showed clear-cut male-to-male transmission consistent with an autosomal-dominant inheritance. This disorder may thus represent a mitochondrial disease secondary to a nuclear genetic abnormality.

AUTOSOMAL-RECESSIVE OPTIC ATROPHY WITH PROGRESSIVE HEARING LOSS, SPASTIC QUADRIPLEGIA, MENTAL DETERIORATION, AND DEATH (OPTICOCOCHLEODENTATE DEGENERATION)

An autosomal-recessive syndrome characterized by severe optic atrophy with onset of visual loss in infancy, progressive hearing loss resulting in severe deafness, and progressive spastic quadriplegia beginning in infancy with progressive mental deterioration and death in childhood has been described by several authors. The common denominator in all patients is a selective, systematized degeneration of the optic, cochlear, dentate, and medial lemniscal systems. The basal ganglia are unaffected in this condition. The diagnosis is made clinically. There are no pathognomonic histochemical, cytochemical, or electron-microscopic characteristics found on brain biopsy, nor is the CSF abnormal.

OPTICOACOUSTIC NERVE ATROPHY WITH DEMENTIA

A single family has been described in which a 3-year-old boy and his two maternal uncles had a syndrome characterized by severe sensorineural hearing loss with onset in infancy, followed by progressive optic atrophy in the second or third decades and progressive dementia in adulthood. On autopsy, there was generalized degeneration of the CNS with extensive calcification. Diffuse wasting of skeletal muscles was also found. An X-linked recessive inheritance has been proposed, but mitochondrial inheritance cannot be dismissed as a possibility.

SEX-LINKED RECESSIVE OPTIC ATROPHY, ATAXIA, DEAFNESS, TETRAPLEGIA, AND AREFLEXIA

In a single Dutch family, a unique clinical syndrome affected five generations in an X-linked recessive inheritance pattern. Affected family members demonstrated optic atrophy, ataxia, deafness, flaccid tetraplegia, and areflexia. The course was generally progressive to death. No specific biochemical, immunologic, or genetic defects were identified, although pathologic examination showed almost complete absence of myelin in the posterior columns. This suggests a possible link to the spinocerebellar degenerations.

PROGRESSIVE ENCEPHALOPATHY WITH EDEMA, HYPSARRHYTHMIA, AND OPTIC ATROPHY (PEHO SYNDROME)

Several families have been described with a progressive encephalopathy with onset in the first 6 months of life, followed by severe hypotonia, convulsions with hypsarrhythmia, profound mental deterioration, hyperreflexia, transient or persistent facial and body edema, and optic atrophy. Optic atrophy is usually noted by the first or second year of life, and nystagmus is common. Microcephaly and brain atrophy develop, especially in the cerebellum and brainstem. A metabolic defect has yet to be determined, and an autosomal-recessive mode of inheritance is likely. This could be a form of Behr's syndrome, which probably represents a heterogeneous group of disorders (see below).

PROGRESSIVE OPTIC ATROPHY WITH JUVENILE DIABETES MELLITUS, DIABETES INSIPIDUS, AND HEARING LOSS (WOLFRAM'S SYNDROME, DIDMOAD)

The hallmark of Wolfram's syndrome is the association of juvenile diabetes mellitus and progressive visual loss with optic atrophy, almost always associated with diabetes insipidus, neurosensory hearing loss, or both; hence, the eponym "DIDMOAD," for *d*iabetes *i*nsipidus, *d*iabetes *m*ellitus, *o*ptic *a*trophy, and *d*eafness. Over 250 cases have been reported. The progression and development of this syndrome is variable. Symptoms and signs of diabetes mellitus usually occur within the first or second decade of life and usually precede the development of optic atrophy. In some cases, visual loss associated with optic atrophy is the first evidence of the syndrome. In the early stages, visual acuity may be normal despite mild dyschromatopsia and optic atrophy. In later stages, visual loss becomes severe. Visual fields show generalized constriction, central scotomas, or both. Optic atrophy is uniformly severe, and there may be mild to moderate cupping of the disc.

The onsets of hearing loss and diabetes insipidus in this syndrome are, as with the onset of visual loss, quite variable. Both begin in the first or second decade of life and may be severe. Atonia of the efferent urinary tract is present in 46 to 58% of patients and is associated with recurrent urinary tract infections, sometimes with fatal complications. Other systemic and neurologic abnormalities include ataxia, axial rigidity, seizures, startle myoclonus, tremor, vestibular malfunction, central apnea, neurogenic upper airway collapse, anosmia, and gastrointestinal dysmotility. Endocrine manifestations include, but are not limited to, short stature and primary gonadal atrophy. Ophthalmologic and other neuro-ophthalmologic disturbances include ptosis, cataracts, pigmentary retinopathy, iritis, lacrimal hyposecretion, tonic pupils, ophthalmoplegia, convergence insufficiency, vertical gaze palsy, and nystagmus. Mental retardation may occur, as may psychiatric manifestations, which are also seen at an increased frequency among heterozygous carriers. Laboratory abnormalities include a megaloblastic and sideroblastic anemia, an abnormal ERG, and elevated CSF protein. Neuroimaging studies and pathologic examinations in some patients with Wolfram's syndrome reveal widespread atrophic changes and suggest a diffuse neurodegenerative disorder, with particular involvement of the midbrain and pons.

Many of the associated abnormalities reported in Wolfram's syndrome are commonly encountered in patients with presumed mitochondrial diseases, especially those patients with the chronic progressive external ophthalmoplegia (CPEO) syndromes. This has led to speculation that patients with Wolfram's syndrome may have a unifying pathogenesis in underlying mitochondrial dysfunction. Abnormalities of mitochondrial function can result from nuclear or mitochondrial DNA defects, because both genomes code for proteins essential for normal mitochondrial function. Inheritance patterns should help distinguish the location of the underlying genetic defect. Nuclear mutations are transmitted in a mendelian fashion, and primary mtDNA defects are inherited maternally. However, most cases of Wolfram's syndrome have been classified as sporadic or recessively inherited, the latter usually concluded from sibling expression which we now know could also occur from maternal transmission. Human leukocyte antigen (HLA) typing reveals an association with the HLA-DR2 antigen in some patients, suggesting an influence of HLA on susceptibility to the disease. Linkage analysis in several families suggests localization of a Wolfram's gene to the short arm of chromosome 4. The Wolfram's phenotype may be nonspecific and may reflect a wide variety of underlying genetic defects in either the nuclear or mitochondrial genomes. When the syndrome is accompanied by anemia, treatment with thiamine may ameliorate the anemia and decrease the insulin requirement.

COMPLICATED HEREDITARY INFANTILE OPTIC ATROPHY (BEHR'S SYNDROME)

In this heredofamilial syndrome, commonly referred to as **Behr's syndrome**, optic atrophy beginning in early childhood is associated with variable pyramidal tract signs, ataxia, mental retardation, urinary incontinence, and pes cavus. Both sexes are affected and the syndrome is usually inherited as an autosomal-recessive trait. Visual loss usually manifests before age 10 years, is moderate to severe, and is frequently accompanied by nystagmus. In most cases, the

abnormalities do not progress after childhood. Neuroimaging may demonstrate diffuse, symmetric white-matter abnormalities. In several Iraqi Jewish pedigrees of Behr's syndrome, 3-methylglutaconic aciduria was identified, although the basic enzymatic defect in these families is as yet unknown. These patients have infantile optic atrophy and an early-onset extrapyramidal movement disorder dominated by chorea. Approximately half of the patients developed spastic paraparesis by the second decade. The majority of affected individuals are female. Clinical findings in some patients with Behr's syndrome are similar to those in cases of hereditary ataxia; in fact, Behr's syndrome may be a transitional form between simple heredofamilial optic atrophy and the hereditary ataxias. Behr's syndrome is likely heterogeneous, reflecting different etiologic and genetic factors.

OPTIC NEUROPATHY AS A MANIFESTATION OF HEREDITARY DEGENERATIVE OR DEVELOPMENTAL DISEASES

HEREDITARY ATAXIAS

The hereditary spinocerebellar ataxias (SCAs) comprise a group of chronic progressive neurodegenerative conditions involving the cerebellum and its connections. These diseases are traditionally classified into two main categories: the predominantly spinal forms and the predominantly cerebellar forms. Advances in biochemical and genetic analysis suggest that this phenotypic classification may be misleading. The wide variability of clinical signs and neuropathology—even within families—and the overlap of clinical and pathological phenotypes in disorders now known to be caused by different genetic defects make diagnostic classification by phenotype often inaccurate. A genomic classification by chromosomal location is available for many of these disorders and the abnormal gene products involved are under investigation. Optic atrophy is not uncommon among individuals with the hereditary ataxias.

The prototype of all forms of progressive ataxia is **Friedreich's ataxia.** The onset of the disease is usually between the ages of 8 and 15 years, almost always before age 25. Characteristic clinical features include progressive ataxia of gait and clumsiness in walking and using the hands, dysarthria, loss of joint position and vibratory sensation, absent lower-extremity deep-tendon reflexes, and extensor plantar responses. Common findings include scoliosis, foot deformity, diabetes mellitus, and cardiac involvement. Other manifestations include pes cavus, distal wasting, deafness, nystagmus, eye movement abnormalities consistent with abnormal cerebellar function, and optic atrophy. The course is relentlessly progressive, with most patients unable to walk within 15 years of onset; death from infectious or cardiac causes usually occurs in the fourth or fifth decades. A later onset, more slowly progressive form has also been described.

Friedreich's ataxia is inherited in an autosomal-recessive manner, with the gene defect being localized to the proximal long arm of chromosome 9 (9q13-q21). The majority of cases are homozygous for an intronic, unstable, GAA trinucleotide expansion.

A condition resembling Friedreich's ataxia associated with decreased vitamin E levels has been localized to chromosome 8. Vitamin E supplementation of patients with this condition may be efficacious early in the course of the disease.

Optic atrophy is present in up to 50% of cases of Friedreich's ataxia, although severe visual loss is uncommon. With electrophysiologic testing, most patients show evidence of visual sensory dysfunction, although visual acuity of less than 20/80 is unusual.

Different from Friedreich's ataxia is a group of hereditary ataxic disorders in which the ataxia is related more to degeneration of the cerebellum than to the spinal cord. These diseases are now generally termed the **spinocerebellar ataxias,** although previous eponyms include olivopontocerebellar atrophy (OPCA) and autosomal-dominant cerebellar ataxia (ADCA). They are differentiated from Friedreich's ataxia by their later age of onset, their autosomal-dominant inheritance (although sporadic cases can occur), the persistence or hyperactivity of deep-tendon reflexes, the paucity of skeletal abnormalities, and the more frequent occurrence of ophthalmoplegia.

Genomic classification of the most common of the SCAs is now possible:

1.　Most pedigrees of spinocerebellar ataxia type 1 (SCA1) map to the short arm of chromosome 6, where there is an expansion of a CAG trinucleotide repeat.

2.　Spinocerebellar ataxia type 2 (SCA2) maps to the long arm of chromosome 12 and probably also reflects an expanded trinucleotide repeat.

3.　Machado-Joseph disease is caused by an unstable CAG repeat on the long arm of chromosome 14, and spinocerebellar ataxia type 3 (SCA3) is allelic with the Machado-Joseph locus.

4.　Spinocerebellar ataxia type 4 (SCA4) localizes to the long arm of chromosome 16.

5.　Spinocerebellar ataxia type 5 (SCA5) maps to the centromeric region of chromosome 11.

6.　Dentato-rubro-pallidoluysian atrophy results from unstable CAG repeats on the short arm of chromosome 12.

7.　Autosomal-dominant spinocerebellar atrophy with retinal degeneration maps to the short arm of chromosome 3, with anticipation of clinical findings suggesting that a trinucleotide repeat expansion may also underlie this disorder.

In addition to the above conditions, some spinocerebellar syndromes appear to result from mutations in mtDNA, including the point mutation at position 8993 that is also associated with Leigh's syndrome (see below).

Loss of vision in patients with the SCAs is usually mild but may be a prominent symptom, occurring in association with constricted visual fields and diffuse optic atrophy. In some of these cases, the optic atrophy appears to be primary; in others, however, it is secondary to retinal degeneration. Detailed analysis of the prevalence of optic atrophy among the different genotypes now associated with the spinocerebellar syndromes has yet to be performed.

Prior to genetic analysis, the so-called autosomal-dominant cerebellar ataxias were categorized into four types, with only the first type including persons with primary optic atrophy (approximately 30% of cases). We now know that ADCA type 1 encompasses multiple genetic loci, including those pedigrees now classified genetically as SCA1, SCA2, SCA3, and probably SCA4 and SCA5. Initial studies suggest that patients with the SCA2 genotype do not exhibit optic atrophy, whereas patients with SCA3 may have optic atrophy, especially if their ataxia is severe.

HEREDITARY POLYNEUROPATHIES

Charcot-Marie-Tooth disease encompasses a group of heredofamilial disorders characterized by progressive muscular weakness and atrophy that begins during the first two decades of life. This group of hereditary polyneuropathies accounts for 90% of all hereditary neuropathies, with the prevalence in the United States being about 40 per 100,000. Most forms of CMT begin between the ages of 2 and 15 years, with the first signs being pes cavus, foot deformities, or scoliosis. Affected individuals subsequently experience slowly progressive weakness and wasting, first of the feet and legs and then of the hands. Motor symptoms predominate over sensory abnormalities.

The most common form of CMT is type 1, a demyelinating neuropathy with autosomal-dominant inheritance, mapped most commonly to the short arm of chromosome 17 (type 1A), although a few pedigrees with this phenotype are linked to the long arm of chromosome 1 (type 1B).

CMT type 2 is clinically similar to type 1, but nerve conductions are of normal velocity, suggesting that the process is neuronal rather than demyelinating. Type 2 can be inherited in an autosomal-dominant fashion (linked to the short arm of chromosome 1) or autosomal recessively (linked to the long arm of chromosome 8).

CMT type 3 is the most severe form. When type 3 is inherited in an autosomal-dominant pattern, the linkage is to the same region on chromosome 1 associated with type 1B; when autosomal recessive, the linkage is to the same region on chromosome 17 associated with type 1A.

There are also X-linked forms of CMT, both X-linked dominant (linked to defects on the long arm) and X-linked recessive (linked to regions on either the long arm or the short arm).

Many patients with CMT have optic atrophy. Associated visual loss is usually mild, and many patients are asymptomatic. In fact, taking into account both electrophysiologic and clinical data, up to 75% of patients with CMT have some afferent visual pathway dysfunction, demonstrating that subclinical optic neuropathy occurs in a high proportion of patients with CMT. Pedigrees specifically designated CMT type 6 show a regular association of CMT and optic atrophy. This type of CMT is as yet genetically unspecified and may prove genetically heterogeneous.

Familial dysautonomia (Riley-Day syndrome) is an autosomal-recessive disease that almost exclusively affects Ashkenazi Jews. Abnormalities of the peripheral nervous system cause the clinical manifestations of sensory and autonomic dysfunction. Optic atrophy is very common in patients with familial dysautonomia and is usually noted after the first decade of life. Older patients have more severe deficits than younger patients, suggesting progression. In some cases of familial dysautonomia, optic atrophy may go unrecognized because coincident corneal scarring prevents adequate fundus examination. In most cases, early mortality from the disease probably precludes the later development of large myelinated fiber deterioration and optic atrophy. Nevertheless, in those who survive beyond early childhood, optic atrophy is an important sign of CNS dysfunction in this disorder.

STORAGE DISEASES AND CEREBRAL DEGENERATIONS OF CHILDHOOD

About 100 inherited metabolic diseases with ocular manifestations have been described. The inheritance pattern in these diseases is almost always recessive, usually autosomal recessive but occasionally X-linked. Of the inborn lysosomal disorders with ocular manifestations, the major diseases that include optic neuropathy are the **mucopolysaccharidoses** (MPS) and the **lipidoses.**

Optic atrophy may occur in patients with MPS IH (Hurler), MPS IS (Scheie), MPS IHS (Hurler-Scheie), MPS IIA and IIB (Hunter), MPS IIIA and IIIB (Sanfilippo), MPS IV (Morquio), and MPS VI (Maroteaux-Lamy). In many cases, optic atrophy is caused by hydrocephalus that presumably occurs from meningeal mucopolysaccharide deposition, leading to delayed CSF absorption. Meningeal or scleral mucopolysaccharide accumulation may also cause local compression of the optic nerve, resulting in disc swelling, optic atrophy, or both. In other cases, however, optic atrophy occurs in association with the deposition of mucopolysaccharides within glial cells of the optic nerve.

Among the lipidoses, optic atrophy has been observed in infantile and juvenile GM_1-gangliosidoses (GM_1-1 and GM_1-2), the GM_2-gangliosidoses (Tay-Sachs disease; Sandhoff disease; and late infantile, juvenile, and adult GM_2-gangliosides), and the infantile form of Niemann-

Pick disease. Although reported in the neuronal ceroid lipofuscinoses, optic atrophy is most frequently a secondary feature of the severe retinal degeneration that occurs in these disorders.

Other storage diseases in which optic atrophy figures prominently include the hereditary leukodystrophies, including the infantile and juvenile forms of Krabbe's disease; the Austin variant of sulfatidosis (mucosulfatidosis); and the infantile, juvenile, and adult forms of metachromatic leukodystrophy (MLD).

Metachromatic leukodystrophy is an autosomal-recessive, degenerative disorder of central and peripheral myelin, secondary to arylsulfatase A deficiency. The genetic defect is localized to the long arm of chromosome 22. Optic atrophy is recognized in up to 50% of cases, especially in the juvenile and adult forms.

Pathologic findings similar to those found in MLD are seen in the optic nerves of patients with **Krabbe's disease** who have optic atrophy. Krabbe's disease usually occurs in infancy, although a few cases with juvenile and even adult onset have been reported, some presenting with optic atrophy and visual loss. Like MLD, Krabbe's is a disease of both central and peripheral myelin. It results from a deficiency of the enzyme galactocerebrosidase.

Adrenoleukodystrophy is an X-chromosome–linked recessive disorder characterized by primary atrophy of the adrenal glands—with or without Addison's disease and low plasma cortisol levels—and a severe degeneration of white matter in the CNS with blindness. Changes in behavior signal the onset of the disease toward the end of the first decade of life, followed by relentlessly progressive dementia, pyramidal tract dysfunction, visual loss with optic atrophy, and neuroimaging evidence of demyelination of the entire visual pathway. Visual loss may thus be of both anterior and retrochiasmal origin, although there appears to be an early predilection for the more posterior cerebral white matter. The basic defect in this disorder is accumulation of very long chain fatty acids secondary to a defective enzyme within the peroxisomes, subcellular organelles that contain enzymes necessary for normal cellular function. The defective gene in adrenoleukodystrophy is located at the distal end of the long arm of the X chromosome.

Variants of adrenoleukodystrophy include **adrenomyeloneuropathy**—a disorder clinically similar to adrenoleukodystrophy except for later onset and slower progression—and a syndrome similar to adrenomyeloneuropathy but that occurs in 15% of women heterozygous for the gene. Clinical examination, electrophysiologic studies, and MRI demonstrate visual pathway abnormalities in both variants, even those who are visually asymptomatic.

Zellweger syndrome (cerebrohepatorenal syndrome) is another peroxisomal disorder associated with optic atrophy. Persons with this autosomal-recessive disease, which is characterized biochemically by dysfunction of multiple peroxisomal enzymes, have severe manifestations at birth, including floppiness, dysmorphic facial characteristics, cirrhosis, genital anomalies, skeletal anomalies, pigmentary retinopathy, and optic atrophy.

Pelizaeus-Merzbacher disease, another leukodystrophy, is genetically heterogeneous. It is usually transmitted in an X-linked-recessive fashion, but some cases appear to be autosomal recessive. Clinical manifestations of the disorder are present either at birth or within the first year of life. They include microcephaly, nystagmus, head tremor, ataxia, spasticity, and ultimately seizures, athetoid movements, and failure to thrive. There is a frequent association with pes cavus and scoliosis. The course is progressive for several years, followed by slowing and some degree of stability. Pathology reveals severe patchy absence of myelin in the central, but not the peripheral, nervous system, suggesting that this is a disorder of the oligodendrocytes. The disease is linked to a gene on the long arm of the X chromosome that codes for myelin proteolipid protein and proteins involved in oligodendrocyte maturation. Pallor of the optic discs occurs in some patients with Pelizaeus-Merzbacher disease, although it is usually not severe, and visual acuity may not be significantly reduced.

Infantile neuroaxonal dystrophy (INAD) is an autosomal-recessive neurologic disease characterized by severe, progressive motor disturbance, arrested mental development, and blindness with optic atrophy, beginning within the first year of life. Seizures and myoclonus may be severe, and most patients succumb within the first decade of life. Histopathologically, patients with this disorder have eosinophilic spheroids in the central, peripheral, and autonomic nervous systems; cerebellar degeneration; and degeneration of various neuronal, myelin, and glial elements.

Pathologic findings similar to those seen in INAD occur in **Hallervorden-Spatz disease,** an autosomal-recessive disorder that is of later onset and is more insidiously progressive. The clinical syndrome is dominated by motor findings, both extrapyramidal and pyramidal. Patients with Hallervorden-Spatz disease also have spheroids, but this pathology preferentially occurs in the basal ganglia. The brown discoloration of the globus pallidus secondary to iron-containing pigment deposition serves to distinguish this disease. MRI shows T2-hypointensities in the globus pallidus—the so-called "eye of the tiger" sign; increased uptake of the iron isotope ^{59}Fe in the basal ganglia occurs. Visual loss, when present, may reflect retinal degeneration or primary optic atrophy.

Menkes syndrome, also called "kinky hair disease," is an X-linked-recessive disorder with maldistribution of body copper and resultant cerebral copper deficiency. This degenerative disorder of gray matter manifests in the neonatal period with progressive psychomotor retardation, spasticity, seizures, and colorless, friable hair. Retinal abnormalities are not uncommon, and optic atrophy can also occur.

Canavan's disease (*N*-acetylaspartic aciduria) is an autosomal-recessive cerebral degeneration that occurs during the first year of life. It is characterized by megalencephaly, poor head control, severe floppiness, spasticity, lack of psychomotor development, and optic atrophy. Neuroimaging shows increased lucency of the white matter, poor demarcation of gray and white matter, and eventually severe brain atrophy. Pathology is notable for "sponginess" with extensive demyelination from intramyelinic vacuolation and large abnormal mitochondria. Deficiency of aspartoacylase in skin fibroblasts is diagnostic of the disease. The abnormal gene is localized to the short arm of chromosome 17.

Alexander disease, another cause of macrocephaly, is believed to be a disorder primarily of the astrocytes, although marked cerebral demyelination with frontal predominance is characteristic of both the infantile and juvenile forms. Despite the severe demyelination, optic atrophy is not characteristic of this disease; the optic radiations are classically spared, and VEPs are usually normal. However, patients with an adult-onset form of the disease have been reported with optic disc pallor and homonymous hemianopia.

Cockayne syndrome is an autosomal-recessive multisystem disease with both developmental anomalies and progressive degenerative changes. It is characterized clinically by severe dwarfism, failure to thrive, facial dysmorphisms (including enophthalmos), skin changes, and neurologic deterioration with mental retardation and spasticity. Vision is usually impaired from corneal opacities, cataracts, retinal degeneration, optic atrophy, or a combination of these complications. The disease is probably genetically heterogeneous and in some cases may be related to dysfunctional RNA and DNA repair mechanisms.

The **Smith-Lemli-Opitz syndrome** remains a clinical cluster of somatic abnormalities without a known error of metabolism, specific physiologic defect, or characteristic findings on diagnostic tests. This autosomal-recessive disorder is characterized by microcephaly, ambiguous male genitalia, anteverted nostrils, broad maxillary ridges, syndactyly of the second and third toes, failure to thrive, and death occurring in early childhood. In addition to congenital, bilateral cataracts, there may be extensive loss of peripheral retinal axons and bilateral optic atrophy.

Sibships with osteogenesis imperfecta, infantile blindness, optic atrophy, retinal abnormalities, severe developmental delay, growth retardation, paraplegia, abnormal electroencephalograms, and generalized atrophy on brain CT have been described. This syndrome has overlapping features with the osteoporosis-pseudoglioma syndrome. In other pedigrees, skeletal dysplasia (dysosteosclerosis), intracerebral calcifications, hearing impairment, and mental retardation are associated with optic atrophy. The optic atrophy appears to be primary and not from compression of the optic nerves within the optic canals. The combination of growth retardation, alopecia, pseudoanodontia, and optic atrophy—GAPO syndrome—is probably inherited in an autosomal-recessive fashion. It may result from either ectodermal dysplasia or accumulation of extracellular connective tissue matrix.

Optic atrophy may be a manifestation of quantitative **chromosomal abnormalities.** Karyotyping may reveal variegated mosaicism indicative of chromosomal instability.

Children with **cerebral palsy** have a higher prevalence of ocular defects than normal children. In one study, optic atrophy was found in 10% of children with cerebral palsy. The etiology for the atrophy in these patients was not explained, nor were the clinical characteristics of the patients elucidated.

The **subacute necrotizing encephalomyelopathy of Leigh** (Leigh's syndrome) is a degenerative syndrome that can result from multiple different biochemical defects that all impair cerebral oxidative metabolism. This disorder may be inherited in an autosomal-recessive, X-linked, or maternal pattern, depending on the genetic defect. The clinical manifestations of Leigh's syndrome typically begin between the ages of 2 months and 6 years. They consist of progressive deterioration of brainstem functions, ataxia, seizures, peripheral neuropathy, intellectual deterioration, impaired hearing, and poor vision. Visual loss may be secondary to optic atrophy or retinal degeneration. In infants, the onset of the syndrome is insidious, with initial symptoms being failure to thrive, generalized weakness, and hypotonia. Rarely, patients with a familial, adult form of Leigh's syndrome present with bilateral visual loss, dyschromatopsia, central scotomas, and optic atrophy prior to the development of other neurologic symptoms and signs. Typical pathologic alterations consist of spongy necrotizing degeneration of the neuropil, capillary and glial proliferation, and loss of myelin with relative sparing of neurons. The most commonly affected areas are the tegmentum of the brainstem, the optic nerves, basal ganglia, substantia nigra, tectum of the midbrain, cerebellar cortex, dentate nucleus, and inferior olives. A predisposition for the periaqueductal and periventricular regions of the midbrain, pons, and medulla mimics the findings in Wernicke's encephalopathy, but Wernicke's encephalopathy affects the lower brainstem less frequently, and Leigh's syndrome tends to spare the hypothalamus and mammillary bodies. MRI demonstrates the distinctive pathologic localization, and MR proton spectroscopy may reveal pathologic lactate production. In many of the reported cases, the optic nerves show extensive atrophy with varying degrees of demyelination of the optic nerves, tracts, and chiasm.

Enzyme defects associated with Leigh's syndrome include abnormalities of cytochrome c oxidase, the pyruvate dehydrogenase complex, biotinidase, and the NADH dehydrogenase complex. Leigh's syndrome appears to be a nonspecific phenotypic response to certain abnormalities of mitochondrial energy production. Most of the genetic defects that result in Leigh's syndrome probably occur in nuclear genes encoding proteins essential to mitochondrial oxidative phosphorylation. However, about one-third of Leigh's syndrome cases are associated with a point mutation in the mtDNA at position 8993 within the gene for ATPase 6. This same genetic defect can cause a syndrome of neuropathy, ataxia, and retinitis pigmentosa (NARP) or a condition in which mild pigmentary degeneration of the retina is associated with migraine-like headaches. Visual loss may be caused by retinal or optic nerve degeneration in such cases. The Leigh's phenotype can also occur in patients with the mtDNA point mutations at positions 8344 and 3243—mutations usually associated with the conditions known as myoclonic epilepsy with ragged-red fibers (MERRF) and mitochondrial encephalopathy, lactic acidosis, and stroke-like episodes (MELAS), respectively.

Other presumed mitochondrial disorders of both nuclear and mitochondrial genomic origins may manifest optic atrophy as a secondary clinical feature, often a variable manifestation of the disease. Examples include cases of MERRF, MELAS, and CPEO, both with and without the full Kearns-Sayre phenotype. The other, more constant, phenotypic characteristics of all of these mitochondrial disorders distinguish them from diseases such as LHON in which visual loss from optic nerve dysfunction is the primary manifestation of the disorder.

FOR MORE INFORMATION:
See Walsh & Hoyt's *Clinical Neuro-Ophthalmology,* 5th edition, Volume 1, Chapters 17, pp. 741–773, Volume 2, Chapter 51, pp. 2811–2866.

CHAPTER 12

Topical Diagnosis of Chiasmal and Retrochiasmal Lesions

TOPICAL DIAGNOSIS OF OPTIC CHIASMAL LESIONS

The optic chiasm is one of the most important structures in neuro-ophthalmologic diagnosis (Figs. 12.1 and 12.2). The arrangement of visual fibers in the chiasm accounts for characteristic defects in the visual fields caused by such diverse processes as compression, inflammation, demyelination, ischemia, and infiltration. In addition, damage to neurologic and vascular structures adjacent to the chiasm produces typical additional symptoms. Knowledge regarding the neuro-ophthalmologic and other manifestations of chiasmal lesions is essential to diagnosis.

VISUAL FIELD DEFECTS

Although there are many variations in the visual field defects caused by damage to the optic chiasm, the essential feature is some type of bitemporal defect, the hallmark of damage to fibers that cross within the chiasm. The bitemporal defects may be superior, inferior, or complete, and they may be peripheral, central, or both.

Visual field defects caused by lesions of the optic chiasm are often classified according to the general site of the damage. In many cases, this is an oversimplification, because most lesions that arise in the region of the chiasm affect not only the entire chiasm but also the intracranial optic nerves. Nevertheless, it remains reasonable to continue this approach, because it is often important in determining the precise management of the lesion and in predicting the visual outcome following treatment. Most visual field defects produced by lesions that damage the optic chiasm seem to result from damage at one of three locations: (1) the anterior angle of the chiasm, (2) the body of the chiasm, or (3) the posterior angle of the chiasm. In addition, a very small number of lesions damage nerve fibers at the lateral aspects of the chiasm.

Lesions That Damage the Distal Portion of One Optic Nerve at the Anterior Angle of the Optic Chiasm

It is at the anterior angle of the optic chiasm that the ''junction'' scotoma occurs because of

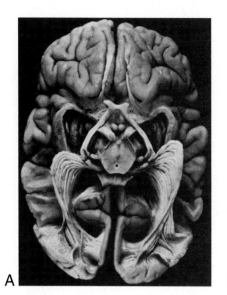

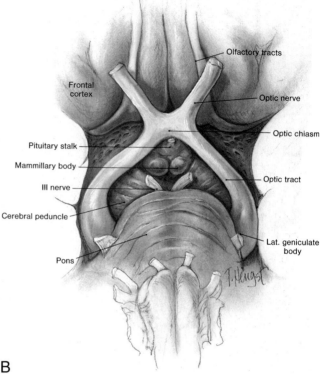

Figure 12.1. Anatomy of the chiasm and postchiasmal visual sensory system. *A.* Appearance of the visual sensory pathway in axial section, viewed from below. Note position of the optic tracts as they originate from the optic chiasm and diverge to end at the lateral geniculate nuclei. (Reprinted with permission from Ghuhbegovic N, Williams TH. The

Human Brain: A Photographic Guide. Hagerstown, MD, Harper & Row, 1980.) *B.* Artist's drawing of the optic chiasm and optic tracts viewed from below. (Redrawn from Pernkopf E. Atlas of Topographical and Applied Human Anatomy. Vol. 1. Ferner H, ed. Philadelphia: WB Saunders, 1963.)

the separation of nasal crossed and temporal uncrossed fibers. When a small lesion damages only the crossing fibers of the homolateral eye, the field defect is monocular, temporal, and has a midline hemianopic character that extends to the periphery of the field. When only the macular crossed fibers from one eye are damaged, the resultant field defect is still monocular and temporal, but it is scotomatous and located in the paracentral region. If there is extensive damage to the visual fibers in an optic nerve, there develops an extensive field defect or total blindness of the homolateral eye. In such cases, but also in less severe cases, the crossed ventral fibers that originate from ganglion cells inferior and nasal to the fovea of the contralateral eye

and that may extend anteriorly a short distance (1 to 2 mm at most) into the affected ipsilateral optic nerve to form the structure called "Wilbrand's knee" may be damaged, producing a defect in the superior temporal field of the contralateral eye (Fig. 12.3). This contralateral field defect, **which occurs in an eye without other evidence of visual dysfunction,** may be overlooked when kinetic perimetry is performed, unless the superior temporal region of the "normal" eye is carefully tested by the examiner, but it is almost always detected when automated static perimetry is used (see Fig. 12.3). There is evidence to suggest that Wilbrand's knee is not a normal anatomic structure, but instead is an artifact that develops during atrophy of the ipsi-

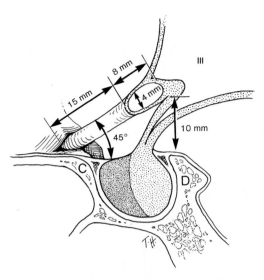

Figure 12.2. Relationships of the optic nerves and optic chiasm to the sellar structures and 3rd ventricle (III). *C,* anterior clinoid. *D,* dorsum sellae. (Redrawn from Glaser JS. Neuro-ophthalmology. 1st ed. Hagerstown, MD: Harper & Row, 1978.)

lateral optic nerve. Nevertheless, the importance of identifying this usually asymptomatic field defect cannot be overemphasized, because it is at this stage that the examiner can make an absolute diagnosis of an anterior optic chiasmal (distal optic nerve) syndrome, and it is at this stage that treatment of the underlying lesion is most likely to result in improvement in visual function.

Lesions That Damage the Body of the Optic Chiasm

Lesions that damage the body of the optic chiasm characteristically produce an bitemporal defect that may be quadrantic or hemianopic and that may be peripheral, central, or both, with or without so-called "splitting of the macula" (Fig. 12.4). In most cases, visual acuity is normal. In some patients, however, visual acuity is diminished, even though no field defect other than a bitemporal hemianopia is present. When the lesion compresses the chiasm from below, such as occurs with a pituitary adenoma, the field defects are typical. When the peripheral fibers are principally affected, the field defects usually commence in the outer upper quadrants

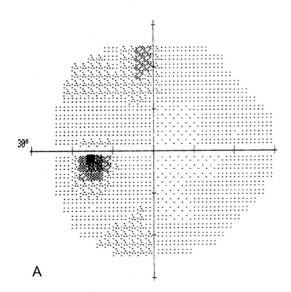

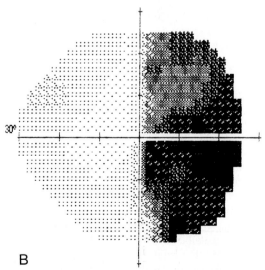

A

B

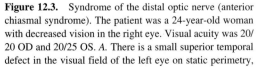

Figure 12.3. Syndrome of the distal optic nerve (anterior chiasmal syndrome). The patient was a 24-year-old woman with decreased vision in the right eye. Visual acuity was 20/20 OD and 20/25 OS. *A.* There is a small superior temporal defect in the visual field of the left eye on static perimetry, using a Humphrey 24–2 Threshold Test. This defect was not detected with kinetic perimetry. *B.* There is a dense temporal hemianopic defect in the visual field of the symptomatic right eye. The patient had a pituitary adenoma.

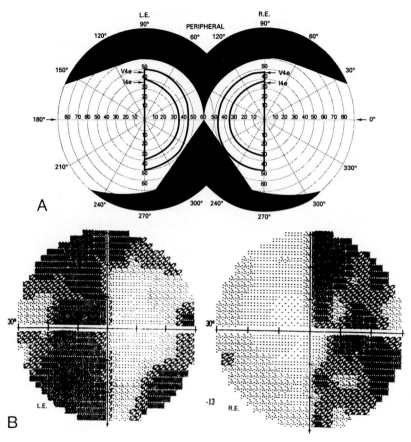

Figure 12.4. Optic chiasmal syndrome. *A.* Kinetic perimetry in a patient with a large pituitary adenoma reveals a complete bitemporal hemianopia. *B.* Static perimetry, using a Humphrey 24–2 Threshold Test, in another patient with a pituitary adenoma, reveals an incomplete bitemporal hemianopia.

of both eyes (Fig. 12.5). In the field of the right eye, the defect usually progresses in a clockwise direction and in the left eye in a counterclockwise direction. The field defects are often unequal in the two eyes; thus, one eye may become almost or completely blind, whereas the defect in the field of the other eye remains rather mild. In the charting of visual field defects resulting from pituitary adenomas and other tumors, scotomas in the peripheral parts of the visual fields are usually dense and not likely to be overlooked, but small relative paracentral scotomas are frequently missed when only kinetic perimetry is performed.

Pituitary adenomas are not, of course, the only compressive lesions that can produce bitemporal field defects that are denser above. Suprasellar but infrachiasmal lesions, such as tuberculum sellae and medial sphenoid ridge meningiomas, craniopharyngiomas, and aneurysms can also produce such defects. The field defects caused by such lesions are indistinguishable from those caused by pituitary adenomas.

Suprasellar, suprachiasmal compressive lesions—such as tuberculum sellae meningiomas, craniopharyngiomas, aneurysms, and dolichoectatic anterior cerebral arteries—may damage the superior fibers of the optic chiasm, as may infiltrating lesions such as germinomas, benign and malignant gliomas, and cavernous angiomas. The defects in the visual fields in such cases are still bitemporal, but are located in the inferior rather than the superior fields of both eyes (Fig. 12.6). Papilledema, which is quite unusual in patients with suprasellar, infrachiasmal lesions, is somewhat more common in suprachiasmal le-

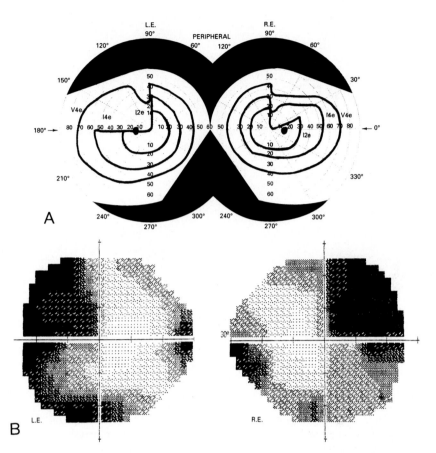

Figure 12.5. Bilateral superior temporal defects in patients with a pituitary adenoma. *A.* Kinetic perimetry in one patient demonstrates defects that are restricted to the superior temporal quadrants of the visual fields of both eyes (a bitemporal superior quadrantanopia). *B.* Static perimetry, using a Humphrey 24–2 Threshold Test, in another patient with a pituitary adenoma demonstrates bitemporal hemianopic defects that are much denser superiorly.

sions because such lesions can extend into and occlude the 3rd ventricle.

Infiltrating tumors, such as gliomas and germinomas, as well as inflammatory and demyelinating lesions that affect the optic chiasm, may produce typical bitemporal field defects (Fig. 12.7). However, such lesions may also produce other types of field defects, such as arcuate defects and nonspecific reduction in sensitivity, that do not necessarily correlate with the location, size, or extent of the lesion.

When trauma damages the optic chiasm, the most common field defect is a complete bitemporal hemianopia. The most common mechanism responsible for a traumatic optic chiasmal syndrome is contusion necrosis.

Although most compressive, infiltrative, or in-

flammatory lesions that damage the body of the chiasm produce defects that are incomplete and that usually have a relative component, we have seen patients in whom a tumor produced a complete bitemporal hemianopia (Fig. 12.8). Successful decompression of the chiasm in such cases not infrequently results in improvement in the visual field, an outcome that might not have been expected from the severity of the visual field defect.

Lesions That Damage the Posterior Angle of the Optic Chiasm

Lesions that damage the posterior aspect of the optic chiasm produce characteristic defects in the visual fields: bitemporal hemianopic sco-

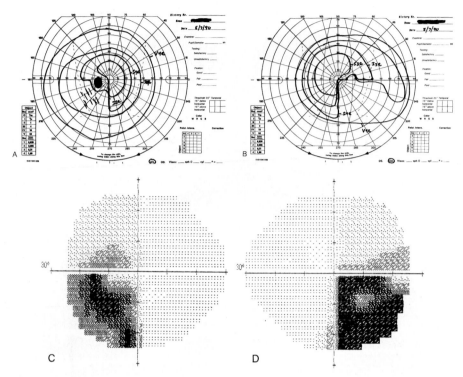

Figure 12.6. Bilateral inferior temporal field defects in a 32-year-old man with a suprasellar mass. *A–B*. Kinetic perimetry reveals inferior temporal quadrantic defects in the visual fields of the left (*A*) and right (*B*) eyes. Note that the defects are scotomatous. Static perimetry, using a Humphrey 24–2 Threshold Test, in the same patient confirms the inferior temporal quadrantic nature of the defects. *C*. Visual field of left eye. *D*. Visual field of right eye. The patient underwent a craniotomy and was found to have a suprasellar suprachiasmatic germinoma.

tomas (Fig. 12.9). Such defects occasionally may be mistaken for cecocentral scotomas and attributed to a toxic, metabolic, or even hereditary process rather than to a tumor; however, true bitemporal hemianopic scotomas are almost always associated with normal visual acuity and color perception, whereas cecocentral scotomas are invariably associated with reduced visual acuity and dyschromatopsia.

Lesions that damage the posterior aspect of the optic chiasm may also damage one of the optic tracts, thus producing an homonymous field defect that is combined with whatever field defect has occurred from damage to the optic chiasm.

Bitemporal homonymous scotomas are particularly important in localizing a lesion, or at least the effects of such a lesion, to the posterior aspect of the optic chiasm. Lesions that produce such defects may be more difficult to treat suc-

cessfully and are, in our experience, more likely to be associated with permanent residual field defects after surgical therapy, radiotherapy, or both. Indeed, we have been impressed that in many patients who undergo otherwise successful removal of a lesion that has produced a posterior chiasmal field defect, the chiasmal field defect is replaced by a field defect consistent with damage to the adjacent optic tract (i.e., an incomplete, incongruous homonymous hemianopia or quadrantanopia; see below).

Lesions That Damage the Lateral Aspects of the Optic Chiasm

The lateral aspect of the optic chiasm occasionally is damaged by various tumors and, according to some authors, by pressure from the supraclinoid portion of sclerotic internal carotid arteries. When such damage occurs, both the uncrossed temporal fibers from the ipsilateral eye

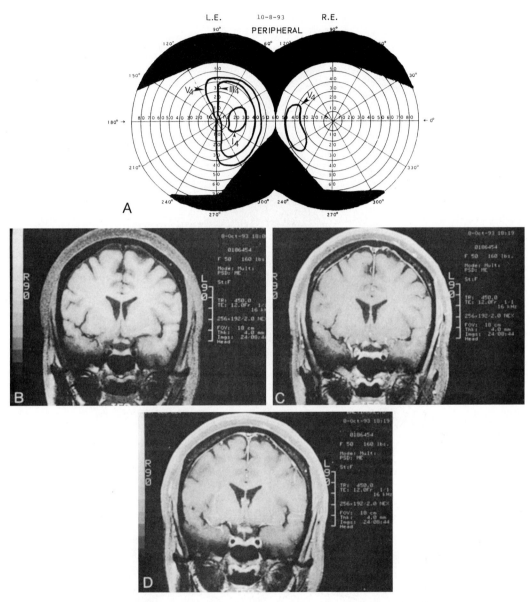

Figure 12.7. Optic chiasmal syndrome in multiple sclerosis. The patient was a 50-year-old woman with a previous history of transient lower extremity weakness who developed progressive loss of vision in both eyes. The patient reported that her vision would worsen considerably whenever she took a steam bath. Visual acuity was counting fingers at 3 feet OD and 20/100 OS. Color vision was diminished in both eyes, and there was a right relative afferent pupillary defect. *A.* Kinetic perimetry at presentation shows a complete temporal hemianopia in the field of vision of the left eye and only a small nasal island in the field of vision of the right eye. *B.* Unenhanced T1-weighted coronal MRI shows an apparently normal optic chiasm. *C–D.* T1-weighted coronal MRI after intravenous injection of contrast material shows enhancement of the intracranial portions of the optic nerves (*C*) and the optic chiasm (*D*). The patient was treated with intravenous corticosteroids. *E–G.* Kinetic perimetry shows progressive improvement in visual fields over the subsequent 10 weeks. (Courtesy of Dr. John B. Kerrison.)

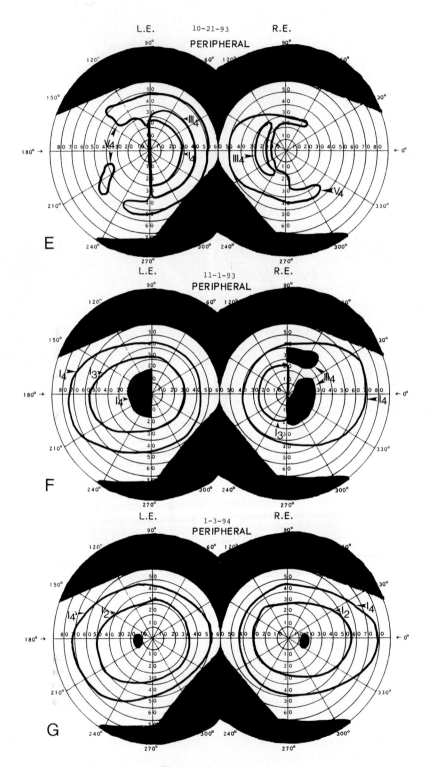

Figure 12.7. *(continued)*

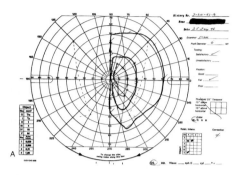 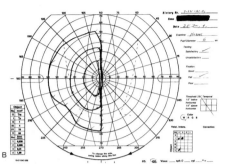

Figure 12.8. Complete bitemporal hemianopia in a 53-year-old woman who developed severe headache, nausea, and vomiting. She then noted difficulty reading. *A.* The visual field of the left eye shows a complete temporal hemi-

anopia. *B.* The visual field of the right eye shows a complete temporal hemianopia. MRI revealed a large pituitary adenoma.

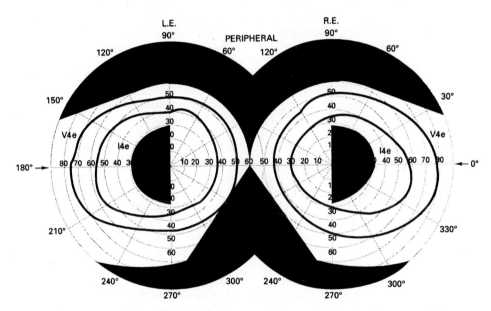

Figure 12.9. Bitemporal hemianopic scotomas in a patient with a pituitary adenoma. Such field defects result from dam-

age to macular fibers in the posterior portion of the optic chiasm.

and crossed nasal fibers from the contralateral eye are affected, producing a contralateral homonymous quadrantanopic or hemianopic defect that cannot be differentiated from that produced by damage to the ipsilateral optic tract. A binasal hemianopia may originate from pressure or other pathologic processes affecting the lateral aspects of the optic nerves, but it probably never originates from damage to the lateral aspects of the optic chiasm.

Visual Field Defects Caused by Lesions That Damage the Optic Chiasm after Initially Damaging the Optic Nerve or Optic Tract

If there is extension of a lesion from the optic nerve or the optic tract to the optic chiasm, the blind eye usually is on the side of the lesion. If, for example, a patient with a blind right eye exhibits a defect in the temporal field of the left eye, the lesion obviously is on the right. Similarly, if there has been a left homonymous hemianopia from a right optic tract lesion and if there is extension of the lesion to affect the optic chiasm, blindness develops in the right eye, or if not blindness, an extensive field defect. Conversely, if a lesion of the optic chiasm that has produced a bitemporal hemianopia extends to the right optic nerve, it will eventually produce blindness or near-blindness of the right eye. Similarly, if a chiasmal lesion extends into the right optic tract, there is again blindness or near-blindness of the right eye. In other words, when there is extension of a lesion from an optic nerve or optic tract to the optic chiasm, the blind (or near-blind) eye is always on the side of the original lesion, and when there is extension of a lesion from the optic chiasm to the optic nerve or to the optic tract, the blind (or near-blind) eye is always on the side of the extension of the lesion.

ETIOLOGIES OF THE OPTIC CHIASMAL SYNDROME

Damage to the optic chiasm can occur from the direct or indirect effects of a variety of lesions. The most common causes of an optic chiasmal syndrome are pituitary adenomas, suprasellar meningiomas, craniopharyngiomas, gliomas, and aneurysms originating from the internal carotid artery. In addition, numerous unusual causes of the optic chiasmal syndrome have been reported, including (in alphabetical order) aneurysm of the basilar artery, arachnoid cyst, arteriovenous malformations, cavernous angioma, choristoma, choroid plexus papilloma, cysticercosis, demyelinating disease, dolichoectatic sclerotic intracranial internal carotid arteries, ependymoma, ethchlorvynol abuse, fibrous dysplasia, ganglioglioma, germinoma, glioblastoma multiforme, granular cell tumor of the neurohypophysis, inflammation (presumed) from Epstein-Barr viral infection, ischemia from small vessel occlusive disease, Langerhans cell histiocytosis, lymphocytic adenohypophysitis, lymphoma, malignant melanoma, medulloblastoma, metastatic carcinoma, multiple myeloma, nasopharyngeal carcinoma, optochiasmatic arachnoiditis, pachymeningitis associated with rheumatoid arthritis, pituitary abscess, plasmacytoma, radiation necrosis, Rathke's cleft cyst, sarcoid granuloma, septum pellucidum cyst, sinus histiocytosis with lymphadenopathy (Rosai-Dorfman), sphenoid sinus mucocele, syphilitic gumma, toxoplasmosis, tuberculoma, varix, vasculitis, venous angioma, and vitamin B_{12} deficiency.

Most authors seem to support the concept that ischemia is the primary explanation for the visual acuity and visual field loss that accompanies mass lesions that compress the optic nerves and chiasm. Nevertheless, the role of axon transport and its disruption from compression has yet to be examined in detail.

During pregnancy, preexisting intrasellar and suprasellar tumors, most commonly pituitary adenomas, may become symptomatic. In most cases, visual symptoms regress after abortion or delivery. In addition, the pituitary gland itself enlarges during the third trimester of pregnancy and may become sufficiently enlarged that it compresses the chiasm, producing visual manifestations. In such cases, visual symptoms resolve spontaneously following delivery. Another cause of an optic chiasmal syndrome that occurs most often during or shortly after pregnancy is lymphocytic adenohypophysitis, an autoimmune disorder of unknown etiology.

Extension of the subarachnoid space into the sella turcica through a deficient diaphragma sellae results in the "empty sella syndrome." A primary empty sella syndrome occurs spontaneously and may be associated with an arachnoid cyst. It is only rarely associated with any significant visual acuity loss or visual field defects; however, a secondary empty sella syndrome follows surgery or radiation therapy in the sellar region. Patients in whom this syndrome occurs may develop any of the chiasmal syndromes described above.

Clinical cases are occasionally observed in which bitemporal field defects occur from damage to the optic chiasm, not from a tumor adjacent to this structure but rather from a posterior fossa lesion that has caused increased intracranial pressure with compression of the chiasm by an enlarged 3rd ventricle. Most of these cases are also associated with papilledema.

An optic chiasmal syndrome can be produced iatrogenically. Most often, the condition occurs after attempted removal of a lesion compressing or infiltrating the chiasm. In our experience, chiasmal damage occurs most often during surgery to remove a suprasellar meningioma or craniopharyngioma and least often after surgery to remove a pituitary adenoma or to clip an intracranial aneurysm. Catheters placed to relieve hydrocephalus can inadvertently damage the chiasm, and a chiasmal syndrome can also occur from exuberant packing of the sphenoid sinus with fat following transsphenoidal resection of a pituitary adenoma.

NEURO-OPHTHALMOLOGIC SIGNS AND SYMPTOMS ASSOCIATED WITH THE OPTIC CHIASMAL SYNDROME

The most frequent complaints of patients with lesions that damage the optic chiasm are progressive loss of central acuity and dimming of the visual field, particularly in its temporal portion. In addition, bitemporal field defects, whether complete or scotomatous, may produce two other types of visual symptoms. One type consists of a **disturbance of depth perception.** Patients with this symptom complain of difficulties with near tasks, such as threading needles, sewing, and using precision tools. In such patients, convergence results in crossing of the two blind temporal hemifields. This produces a completely blind triangular area of field with its apex at fixation (Fig. 12.10). The image of an object posterior to fixation falls on blind nasal retinas and thus disappears.

Patients with bitemporal field defects may also experience diplopia or difficulty reading caused by a horizontal or vertical deviation of images unassociated with an ocular motor nerve paresis, the **hemifield slide phenomenon.** Such patients have difficulty reading because of doubling or loss of printed letters or words. The problems encountered by these patients result from loss of the normal partial overlap of the temporal field of one eye and the nasal field of the contralateral eye. This overlap permits fusion of images and helps stabilize ocular alignment in patients with vertical or horizontal phorias. Because their remaining visual fields represent only the temporal projection from each eye, patients with bitemporal hemianopia do not have a physiologic linkage between the two remaining hemifields. In such patients, a preexisting minor phoria becomes a tropia because of vertical or horizontal separation or overlap of the two nonoverlapping hemifields, thus causing intermittent sensory difficulties (Fig. 12.11). Theoretically, patients with binasal hemianopias should experience similar phenomena, but we have never encountered such patients.

Patients with chiasmal syndromes may or may

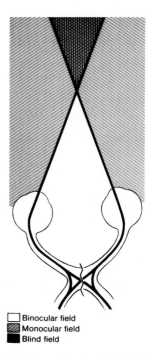

Binocular field
Monocular field
Blind field

Figure 12.10.   Diagram showing the blind triangular area of the binocular visual field that occurs just beyond fixation in patients with complete bitemporal hemianopia. Such patients have intact binocular vision in the triangular area up to fixation and intact uniocular vision temporal and anterior to the triangular blind region. (Redrawn from Kirkham TH. The ocular symptomatology of pituitary tumors. Proc R Soc Med 1972;65:517–518.)

not have ophthalmoscopically apparent nerve fiber layer or optic disc atrophy when first examined. However, when atrophy is present in patients with bitemporal hemianopia, the pattern of atrophy is quite specific. In such cases, degeneration occurs in fibers from peripheral and macular ganglion cells located nasal to the fovea. Axons from peripheral ganglion cells located nasal to the disc (and, thus, nasal to the fovea) attain the disc directly, entering its nasal aspect. Fibers from nasal macular ganglion cells (i.e., about half the fibers that comprise the papillomacular bundle) also attain the optic disc directly, entering its temporal aspect. Finally, fibers from peripheral ganglion cells located nasal to the fovea but temporal to the optic disc—which make up a small portion of the superior and inferior arcuate bundles along with a larger number of fibers from peripheral temporal ganglion cells—enter the superior and inferior

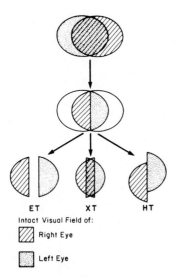

ET   XT   HT

Intact Visual Field of:

[hatched] Right Eye

[stippled] Left Eye

Figure 12.11. Diagram showing the "hemifield slide phenomena" experienced by patients with bitemporal hemianopias. Patients with a preexisting exophoria or intermittent exotropia will have overlapping of the intact nasal fields, whereas patients with a preexisting esophoria or intermittent esotropia will have separation of the nasal hemifields, causing a blind area in the center of the field. Patients with preexisting hyperdeviations will complain of vertical separation of images crossing the vertical meridian. (Redrawn from Kirkham TH. The ocular symptomatology of pituitary tumors. Proc R Soc Med 1972;65:517–518.)

aspects of the disc. Thus, when there is atrophy of nasal fibers, the normal striations of the nerve fiber layer are lost both nasal to the disc and in the papillomacular region. The optic disc shows corresponding atrophy at its nasal and temporal regions with relative sparing of the superior and inferior portions where the majority of spared temporal fibers (subserving nasal field) enter (Fig. 12.12). Thus, the optic atrophy occupies a more or less horizontal band across the disc, wider nasally than temporally, so-called "band" or "bow-tie" atrophy.

It is perhaps clinically more useful when atrophy is *absent* in patients with chiasmal (or optic nerve) compression than when it is present. Although patients with significant nerve fiber bundle defects and optic atrophy can still have impressive return of both acuity and field when successful decompression is obtained, patients with normal appearing fundi should have complete return of visual function with successful

decompression. Thus, it is crucial that decompression be carried out as soon as possible in these patients.

As noted above, papilledema is more frequently associated with suprachiasmal tumors than with infrachiasmal tumors, because the former lesions can invade or compress the 3rd ventricle, ultimately obstructing the flow of cerebrospinal fluid in that structure. In such cases, optic atrophy may result not only from compression of the visual axons in the optic nerves or chiasm but also from the effects of chronic or severe papilledema (i.e., postpapilledema optic atrophy).

Most patients with lesions that affect the optic chiasm have no disturbances of ocular alignment or motility except for the hemifield slide phenomenon. However, patients with lesions that damage the optic chiasm as well as one or more of the ocular motor nerves in the subarachnoid space or within the cavernous sinus on one or both sides almost always complain of double vision. When the ocular motor nerves are damaged within the cavernous sinus, there may also be pain, evidence of a trigeminal sensory neuropathy, or both, in the territory of the first and/or second divisions of the trigeminal nerve. The third division of the nerve, which does not pass through the cavernous sinus, is not affected by such lesions, and a motor neuropathy thus is never present unless the lesion extends posteriorly. The oculosympathetic fibers may also be damaged by a lesion in the chiasmal or parasellar regions, resulting in a postganglionic Horner's syndrome characterized by ipsilateral ptosis and a small reactive pupil (see Chapter 15). Horner's syndrome is often associated with an ipsilateral abducens nerve palsy, because the postganglionic oculosympathetic fibers briefly join the abducens nerve within the cavernous sinus. When both the oculomotor nerve and oculosympathetic fibers are affected, the clinical picture is one of an oculomotor nerve paresis with a small pupil that is normally reactive if the paresis is pupil-sparing or poorly or nonreactive if the paresis involves the pupillomotor fibers. Single or multiple ocular motor nerve pareses in a patient with a bitemporal field defect suggests a process extrinsic to the chiasm rather than an infiltrative intrinsic lesion.

The unusual phenomenon of **seesaw nystagmus** may occur in patients with tumors of the diencephalon and chiasmal regions. This condi-

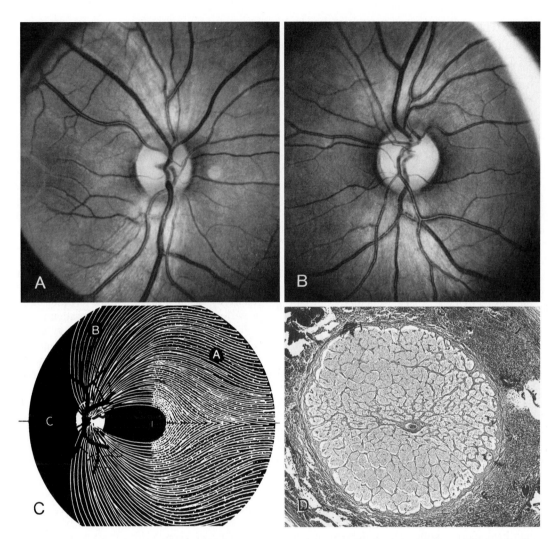

Figure 12.12. Optic chiasmal syndrome. *A–B*. Both right and left optic discs show "band" atrophy with corresponding loss of nerve fibers from ganglion cells located nasal to the fovea. *C*. Diagram of nerve fiber loss in patients with temporal hemianopia. Regions marked *A, B,* and *C* in diagram denote areas of nerve fiber layer preservation, partial loss, and complete loss, respectively. (Reprinted with permission from Hoyt WF, Kommerell G. Der Fundus oculi bei Homonyer Hemianopia. Klin Monatsbl Augenheilkd 162;1973:456–464.) *D*. Transverse section of orbital optic nerve in a patient with a temporal hemianopia shows "band" or "bow-tie" pattern of atrophy with relative sparing of the superior and inferior portions of the nerve. (Reprinted with permission from Unsöld R, Hoyt WF. Band atrophy of the optic nerve. Arch Ophthalmol 1980;98:1637–1638.)

tion is characterized by synchronous alternating elevation and intorsion of one eye and depression and extorsion of the opposite eye. The cause of seesaw nystagmus is unknown, but it may be related to damage to the interstitial nucleus of Cajal or adjacent structures by the tumor.

Lesions causing a chiasmal syndrome may arise from or extend to the hypothalamus. Patients with this presentation may develop diabetes insipidus and hypothalamic hypopituitarism. Prepubertal children may also suffer from both growth retardation and delayed sexual development, and young children and infants may have severe failure to thrive (Russell's syndrome).

TOPICAL DIAGNOSIS OF RETROCHIASMAL VISUAL FIELD DEFECTS

With few exceptions, lesions of the visual sensory pathway beyond the optic chiasm—the optic tract, lateral geniculate body (LGB), optic radiation, or striate cortex (see Fig. 12.1A)—produce homonymous visual field defects without loss of visual acuity. When such defects are complete, they do not, in themselves, allow topical diagnosis. In such instances, the clinician must rely on other symptoms and signs of neurologic disease or on neuroimaging to define both the area of damage and the etiology of the lesion.

Homonymous defects in the visual fields characteristically develop slowly when they are caused by compression and rapidly when they are caused by hemorrhage, ischemia, or inflammation. Compressive lesions generally cause progressive loss of visual field from the periphery of the field to the center. With decompression of the visual system, improvement typically first occurs in the central region and continues toward the periphery. Defects for colored objects invariably appear before disturbances either for form or for black and white objects, a reason to use colored stimuli routinely in the examination of visual fields.

When homonymous visual field defects arise from vascular lesions, the onset of the field defects is sudden. Such defects include complete homonymous quadrantanopias and hemianopias, incomplete homonymous quadrantanopias and hemianopias with varying degrees of congruity, and homonymous paracentral scotomas. When and if improvement occurs, the central field clears first and may be followed by gradual enlargement of the peripheral fields if they have been affected.

The location and causes of homonymous hemianopia depend on the age of the patient and the presence or absence of other neurologic findings. In nonisolated cases of homonymous hemianopic defects, 40 to 51% of patients have occipital lobe pathology, 29 to 57% have lesions of the optic radiations, and 3 to 21% have lesions in the region of the optic tract and the LGB (Fig. 12.13). Vascular causes, including infarction, hemorrhage, and arteriovenous malformations, account for 42 to 71% of cases; mass lesions account for 19 to 38%. On the other hand, almost

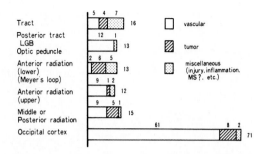

Figure 12.13. Location and causes of homonymous hemianopia in 140 patients. (Reprinted with permission from Fujino T, Kigazawa K, Yamada R. Homonymous hemianopia: a retrospective study of 140 cases. Neuro-ophthalmology 6; 1986:17–21.)

90% of patients with isolated homonymous hemianopia have occipital lobe lesions, usually caused by vascular disease in the territory of the posterior cerebral arteries. Older patients with isolated homonymous hemianopia have an exceedingly high probability of vascular lesions, whereas younger patients may have congenital or acquired nonvascular etiologies, such as neoplasm, abscess, or demyelinating disease. Neuroimaging, preferably MRI, should be the first diagnostic procedure used to determine the location and etiology of an homonymous hemianopia.

TOPICAL DIAGNOSIS OF OPTIC TRACT LESIONS

Although lesions affecting the optic tracts are infrequent, they are of great importance because they are located in the first region beyond the optic chiasm where lesions produce an homonymous visual field defect (Fig. 12.14). Lesions of the optic tract account for about 3 to 11% of cases of homonymous hemianopia. The causes are varied and include tumors, vascular processes, demyelinating disease, and trauma (Figs. 12.15 and 12.16).

Patients with optic tract lesions often have specific findings that permit the recognition of the location of the lesion on clinical grounds alone. All patients with a complete homonymous hemianopia caused by an isolated optic tract lesion have a relative afferent pupillary defect in the eye contralateral to the side of the lesion (i.e., the eye with the temporal field loss). This occurs because (1) the temporal visual field is considerably larger than the nasal field (therefore, there are more crossing nasal fibers than

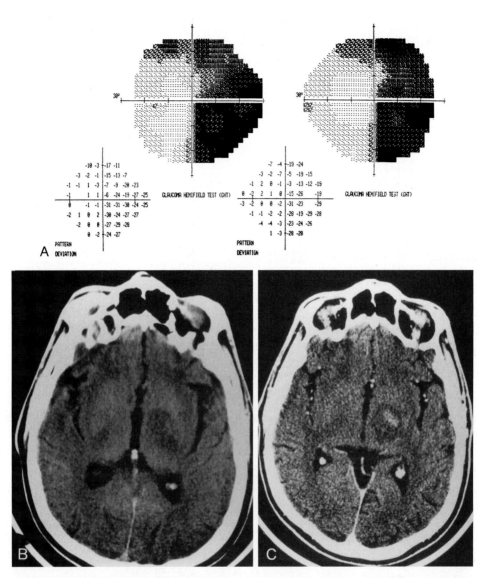

Figure 12.14. A 65-year-old man developed headache, sleepiness, personality changes, memory difficulties, right hemiparesis, and difficulty seeing to the right. *A.* Visual fields reveal an incongruous right homonymous hemi- anopia. *B–C.* CT scans, axial views, before (*B*) and after (*C*) the administration of intravenous contrast reveal an en- hancing lesion with surrounding edema in the region of the left optic tract, diagnosed ultimately as lymphoma.

noncrossing temporal fibers); (2) the pupillomo- tor fibers within the visual sensory pathway hemidecussate in the optic chiasm along with or as part of the visual axons; and (3) the pupillo- motor fibers are present within the optic tract for most of its extent. Because the temporal vis- ual field is 60 to 70% larger than the nasal field, there is a disparity with respect to light input from the two eyes to the mesencephalic pupillary

center. A complete lesion of one optic tract thus preferentially reduces input from the contralat- eral eye.

Another pupillary phenomenon that is some- times associated with lesions of the optic tract that produce a complete or nearly complete hom- onymous hemianopia is pupillary hemiakinesia (hemianopic pupillary reaction or Wernicke's pupil). Because the pupillary afferents are pres-

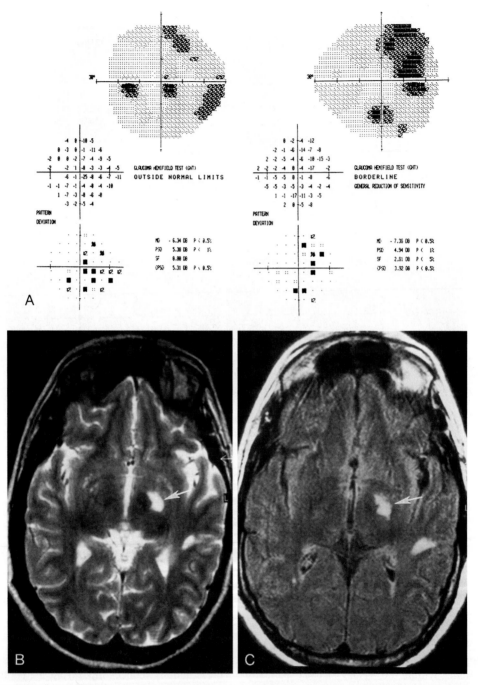

Figure 12.15. A 40-year-old man noted a "black spot" in front of both eyes that gradually worsened over 2 weeks. Visual acuities were normal but there was a trace right relative afferent pupillary defect. *A.* Visual fields show a highly incongruous right homonymous defect. *B–C.* MRI (*B:* T2-weighted; *C:* fluid-attenuated inversion-recovery) reveals multiple white-matter lesions consistent with demyelinating disease, including a large plaque in the left optic tract (*arrows*).

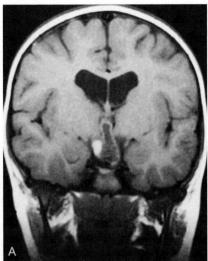

Figure 12.16. A 7-year-old girl presented with precocious puberty and was found to have a suprasellar mass with hydrocephalus. *A.* Coronal, T1-weighted MRI without gadolinium. *B.* Axial, T1-weighted MRI without gadolinium. *C.* Axial, T1-weighted MRI with gadolinium. *D.* Visual field testing reveals an incomplete, incongruous, right homonymous inferior quadrantanopia, consistent with damage to the left optic tract. Biopsy showed findings diagnostic of craniopharyngioma.

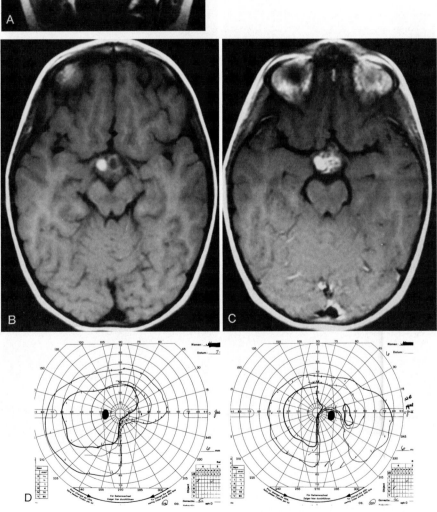

ent in this section of the visual system, when light is projected onto the "blind" retinal elements (subserving the nasal visual field in the ipsilateral eye and the temporal visual field in the contralateral eye), either no pupillary reaction occurs or the reaction is markedly reduced. However, when light is projected onto the intact retinal elements (subserving the temporal visual field in the ipsilateral eye and the nasal visual field in the contralateral eye), a normal pupillary reaction is observed. This phenomenon is best observed with a bright, focused beam of light, such as that from a slit lamp biomicroscope or a hand-held transilluminator.

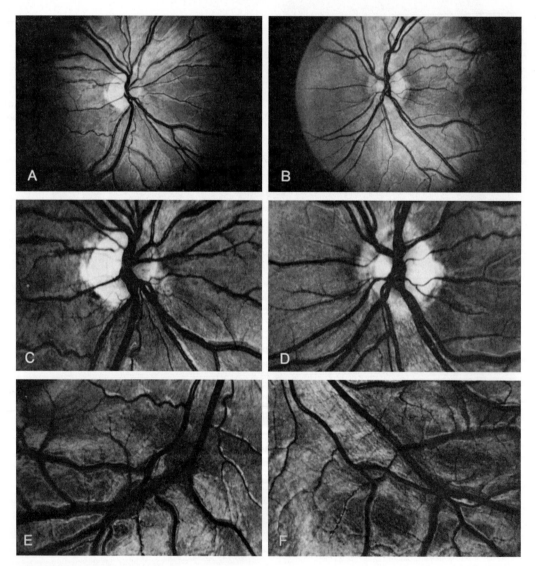

Figure 12.17. Hemianopic optic atrophy in a patient with a left homonymous hemianopia from a right optic tract lesion. *A.* The right optic disc has somewhat diffuse, temporal atrophy from loss of nerve fibers from ganglion cells temporal to the fovea. *B.* The left optic disc shows band atrophy from loss of nerve fibers from ganglion cells nasal to the fovea. *C–D.* Red-free (540 nm) photographs showing atrophy of right and left optic discs. Note band pattern of atrophy of the left disc. *E.* Inferior temporal peripapillary retina of right eye showing relative absence of visible arcuate bundle. *F.* Inferior temporal peripapillary retina of left eye showing relative preservation of arcuate bundle.

Optic tract lesions do not cause loss of visual acuity nor do they affect color vision unless they also damage the optic chiasm or the intracranial portions of one or both optic nerves. Thus, patients with lesions confined to an optic tract have normal visual acuity and color vision, and they have no sensation of reduced light brightness in the eye with the relative afferent pupillary defect. On the other hand, when lesions of the optic tract also damage the ipsilateral optic nerve or chiasm, reduced visual acuity, abnormal color vision, and a relative afferent pupillary defect occur on the side of the lesion.

Patients with a complete or nearly complete homonymous hemianopia from an optic tract lesion eventually develop a characteristic pattern of optic atrophy. There is a "band" of horizontal pallor of the optic disc in the eye contralateral to the lesion (with temporal field loss) (i.e., "bow-tie atrophy"). This pattern of optic nerve atrophy is caused by atrophy of retinal nerve fibers originating from ganglion cells nasal to the fovea and is identical with that seen in both eyes of patients with bitemporal field loss from chiasmal syndromes. At the same time, there is generalized pallor of the optic disc in the eye on the side of the lesion, associated with significant loss of nerve fiber layer details in the superior and inferior arcuate regions that comprise the majority of fibers subserving the nasal visual field and originating from ganglion cells temporal to the fovea (Fig. 12.17).

Not all patients with optic tract lesions have a complete homonymous hemianopia. Many patients have a complete or incomplete homonymous quadrantanopia or an incomplete hemianopia. Such field defects are quite incongruous and may also be scotomatous (see Fig. 12.15). Indeed, the optic tract is one of only two locations in the postchiasmal pathway in which homonymous scotomas routinely occur; the occipital lobe is the other.

Patients with optic tract lesions often have manifestations in addition to homonymous visual field defects, because lesions that damage the optic tract may also damage adjacent neural structures. Neurologic deficits that may occur in patients with lesions of the optic tract include hypothalamic symptoms and signs and contralateral hemiparesis.

In summary, a relative afferent pupillary defect in the eye on the side of a complete homonymous hemianopia in a patient with normal visual acuity and color vision in both eyes indicates a lesion of the contralateral optic tract. In addition, a diagnosis of optic tract syndrome can be made in the setting of a significantly incongruous homonymous visual field defect, with or without associated bilateral nerve fiber layer atrophy, particularly when, despite normal visual acuity and color vision, there is a relative afferent pupillary defect on the side opposite the lesion.

TOPICAL DIAGNOSIS OF LESIONS OF THE LATERAL GENICULATE BODY

Lesions affecting the lateral geniculate body are less commonly diagnosed than those of the optic tract but can be caused by a number of different processes, including vascular disease, neoplasms, inflammation, demyelination, and trauma.

Lesions of the LGB may cause incongruous or congruous homonymous field defects. The dorsal region of the LGB subserves macular function, the lateral aspect of the LGB subserves the superior visual field, and the medial aspect subserves the inferior field (Fig. 12.18). Although the intricate retinotopic organization of the LGB may result in the production of relative defects, incongruous defects, and even (theoretically) monocular defects, vascular lesions are more likely to respect specific anatomic boundaries within the LGB and produce homonymous

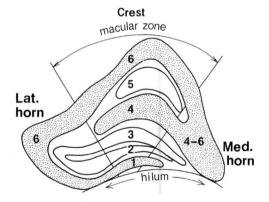

Figure 12.18. Artist's drawing of a coronal section through the lateral geniculate nucleus, viewed from its posterior aspect. Three laminae (white areas, layers 2, 3, and 5) receive input from ipsilateral retinal ganglion cells, and three laminae (stippled layers, 1, 4, and 6) receive input from contralateral retinal ganglion cells.

Figure 12.19. Visual field defects in patients with lesions of the lateral geniculate body (LGB). *A–B.* Homonymous horizontal sectoranopia from damage to the LGB in the territory of the lateral choroidal artery. *A.* In a patient with a small arteriovenous malformation. *B.* In a patient with presumed thrombosis of the lateral choroidal artery. Note the relative congruity of the field defect in both cases. (Reprinted with permission from Frisén L, Holmegaard L, Rosencrantz M. Sectorial optic atrophy and homonymous, horizontal sectoranopia: a lateral choroidal artery syndrome? J Neurol Neurosurg Psychiatry 1978; 41:374–380.) *C–D.* Homonymous quadruple sectoranopia from damage to the LGB in the territory of the distal anterior choroidal artery. *C.* In a patient with occlusion of the distal anterior choroidal artery. (Reprinted with permission from Frisén L. Quadruple sectoranopia and sectorial optic atrophy: A syndrome of the distal anterior choroidal artery. J Neurol Neurosurg Psychiatry 1979;42:590–594.) *D.* In another patient with occlusion of the distal anterior choroidal artery. (Reprinted with permission from Helgason C, Caplan LR, Goodwin J, et al. Anterior choroidal artery-territory infarction. Report of cases and review. Arch Neurol 1986;43:681–686.)

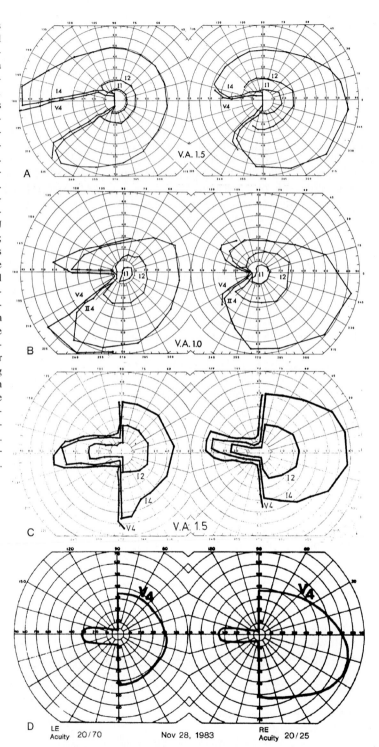

sector defects that are, in fact, quite congruous, with abruptly sloping borders (Figs. 12.19 and 12.20). Two specific patterns of relatively congruous homonymous field defects can occur, most often attributable to focal disease of the LGB caused by infarction in the territory of two specific arteries. Ischemia or other damage in the territory of the lateral choroidal artery typically causes a **congruous homonymous horizontal sectoranopia** (see Fig. 12.19A and B). Ischemia in the region of the LGB supplied by the distal portion of the anterior choroidal artery results in loss of the upper and lower homonymous sectors in the visual fields of the two eyes, producing a **congruous homonymous quadruple sectoranopia** (see Figs. 12.19C, 12.19D, and 12.20).

The specificity of homonymous sectoranopic visual field defects for lesions of the LGB is challenged by neuroimaging evidence of retrogeniculate lesions in some cases. Occasional lesions in both the optic radiations and the occipital lobe have been implicated. Nevertheless, in our experience, both the congruous homonymous horizontal sectoranopia and the homonymous quadruple sectoranopia are almost always caused by a lesion of the contralateral LGB.

Because the pupillomotor fibers leave the optic tract to ascend in the brachium of the supe-

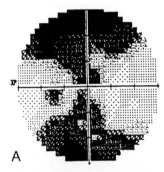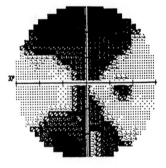

A

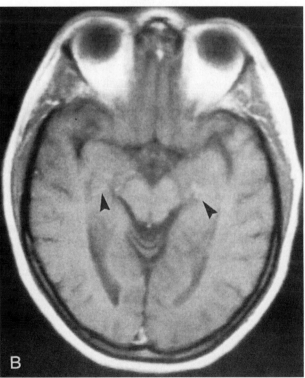

B

Figure 12.20. A 37-year-old woman had central pontine myelinolysis and complained of bilateral visual loss. Visual acuity was 20/25 OD and 20/30 OS. *A.* Automated static perimetry demonstrates fairly congruous defects having an hourglass configuration, with near total depression superior and inferior to fixation. *B.* T1-weighted, axial MRI reveals bilateral enhancement in the region of the lateral geniculate bodies. The visual field defects were similar to those reported after anterior choroidal artery infarction, prompting the authors to propose that the cells supplied by the anterior choroidal artery in the lateral geniculate might be particularly susceptible to metabolic insult, such as rapid changes in serum sodium level. (Reprinted with permission from Donahue SP, Kardon RH, Thompson HS. Hourglass-shaped visual fields as a sign of bilateral lateral geniculate myelinolysis. Am J Ophthalmol 1995;119:378–380.)

rior colliculus, the pupillary reactions in patients with LGB lesions are normal (unless the lesion also damages the optic tract or the brachium)—there is neither a contralateral relative afferent pupillary defect nor a hemianopic pupillary phenomenon. However, the visual axons from retinal ganglion cells first synapse in the LGB. Thus, sectorial or hemianopic atrophy of the retinal nerve fiber layer and optic disc occurs in patients with lesions of the LGB that damage the incoming axons. Such defects, when associated with acquired homonymous field defects, whether congruous or incongruous, must be taken as evidence of optic tract or LGB damage in all cases.

Patients with lesions of the LGB frequently have neurologic symptoms and signs consistent with damage to the ipsilateral thalamus or pyramidal tract. Thalamic damage may result in gross impairment of sensation on the side of the body opposite the lesion, or there may be a complaint of pain of central origin that is referred to the opposite side of the body. Damage to the pyramidal tract causes contralateral hemibody weakness.

TOPICAL DIAGNOSIS OF LESIONS OF THE OPTIC RADIATION

The optic radiation is that part of the postchiasmal visual sensory pathway that begins in the LGB and transmits visual information to the striate cortex. It may be damaged by lesions in several different locations, including the internal capsule, temporal lobe, and parietal lobe.

LESIONS OF THE INTERNAL CAPSULE

Efferent projection fibers from and afferent projection fibers to the cerebral cortex traverse the subcortical white matter where they form a radiating mass of fibers, the corona radiata, which converges toward the brainstem (Fig. 12.21). In the rostral brainstem, the fibers form a broad but compact fiber band, the **internal capsule,** that is bordered medially by the thalamus and caudate nucleus and laterally by the lenticular nucleus. The afferent fibers comprise the thalamocortical radiations in the posterior limb of the internal capsule. The efferent bundles include:

- The corticospinal and corticobulbar tracts in the anterior limb.
- The frontopontine tract from the prefrontal and precentral regions of the cerebral cortex in the anterior limb.
- The temporoparietopontine tract from the temporal and parietal lobes in the posterior limb.
- The optic radiation, which begins in the LGB and occupies only a small region of the capsule because it does not proceed to the brainstem.

The internal capsule is thus composed of all fibers, afferent and efferent, that go to, or come from, the cerebral cortex. The most posterior component of the internal capsule is the optic radiation.

Interruption of the optic radiation is characterized by a contralateral, usually complete, homonymous hemianopia that is typically associated with contralateral hemianesthesia from damage to the adjacent thalamocortical fibers in the posterior limb of the internal capsule. Other ocular findings in lesions of the internal capsule include a transient deviation of the eyes to the side of the lesion in many instances and weakness of the frontalis and orbicularis oculi on the contralateral hemiplegic side in a minority of cases. Vascular causes predominate.

LESIONS OF THE TEMPORAL LOBE

Temporal lobe lesions may damage the optic radiation. Such lesions account for about 13 to 24% of homonymous visual field defects, with tumors and abscesses causing the majority of cases. Temporal lobe surgery for epilepsy may also cause such defects, which are often asymptomatic.

The disposition of the visual fibers in the temporal lobe is controversial, and there may be considerable individual variability in the spatial distribution of optic radiation fibers within the temporal lobe. Clearly, the most anterior portion of the temporal lobe may be damaged or removed without the production of any visual field defect. The amount of temporal lobe that may be removed without a resulting field defect is disputed, however. It would appear that up to 4 cm of anterior temporal lobe can be removed in most patients without interruption of visual fibers to the extent that a field defect is produced. Once the lobe is sectioned 4 cm or more poste-

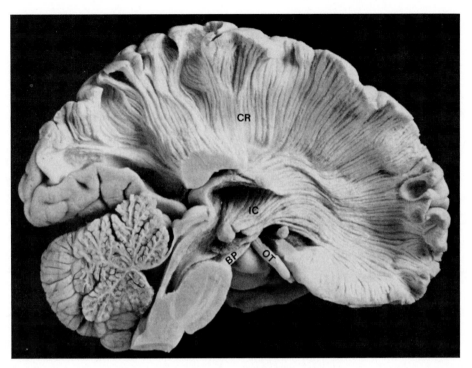

Figure 12.21.   Specimen showing the corona radiata and internal capsule, and their relationship to the optic tract. The internal capsule and corona radiata have been exposed by removal of the corpus callosum, caudate nucleus, and diencephalon. Note that the fibers of the basis pedunculi pass adjacent to the optic tract. *CR*, corona radiata. *IC*, internal capsule. *BP*, basis pedunculi. *OT*, optic tract. (Reprinted with permission from Ghuhbegovic N, Williams TH. The Human Brain. A Photographic Guide. Hagerstown, MD: Harper & Row, 1980.)

rior to the tip, however, most patients will develop an homonymous field defect. In most cases, the homonymous defect is incomplete and is either confined to the superior quadrants or is denser above, reflecting the anatomy of Meyer's loop—the portion of the optic radiation that courses anteriorly in the temporal lobe around the temporal horn of the lateral ventricle and that consists entirely of axons subserving the superior visual fields of the two eyes. These field defects have other characteristics:

1. They do not affect visual acuity.
2. They do not alter the size of the blind spot.
3. They tend to have sloping inferior margins unless they occur after a temporal lobectomy, in which case they may have sloping superior margins.
4. They may cross the horizontal midline.
5. They are usually incongruous but may be congruous (Fig. 12.22).

Most series report a tendency for macular sparing in patients with partial or complete quadrantic defects from temporal lobe damage. However, the peripheral field, including the monocular crescent, is never spared in these field defects. With temporal lobectomies beyond 8 cm, almost all patients have a complete homonymous hemianopia.

A few further comments can be made regarding the visual field defects associated with temporal lobe lesions. First, an incongruous homonymous wedge-shaped defect in the upper visual fields, often called a "pie-in-the-sky" defect to emphasize its superior location and wedge shape, almost always indicates damage to the optic radiation in the temporal lobe. Second, most visual field defects resulting from temporal lobe lesions are incongruous, but the incongruity

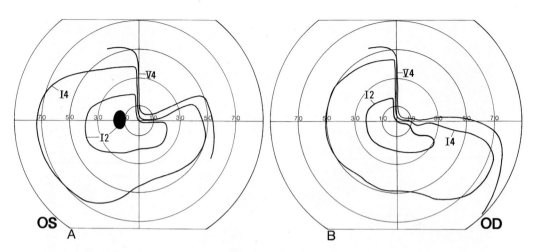

Figure 12.22. Homonymous quadrantanopia in a patient with a glioblastoma of the left temporal lobe. The defects are primarily superior and are moderately incongruous. Note that the greater defect is on the side opposite the lesion.

is usually not as severe as that seen with optic tract and some LGB lesions. Third, a superior homonymous quadrantic defect suggests damage to the inferior fibers of the optic tract, the optic radiation in the temporal lobe, or the inferior occipital cortex. When the defect is congruous, an occipital lobe location is most likely, but the lesion may still be in the temporal lobe (Fig. 12.23). When the defect is incongruous, the lesion is either in the optic tract or the temporal lobe, not in the occipital lobe.

Nonvisual manifestations of lesions of the temporal lobe are common. If there is a mass lesion of the temporal lobe, headache may be a prominent accompaniment. Bilateral lesions of the transverse gyri of Heschl can cause cortical deafness, usually associated with aphasia; unilateral lesions may cause a disturbance of hearing and sound discrimination contralateral to the lesion. If the lesion is in the dominant temporal lobe, the patient may have difficulty memorizing a series of spoken words, whereas if the lesion is in the nondominant temporal lobe, the patient may exhibit various forms of auditory agnosia. Auditory hallucinations or illusions may occur with lesions of either temporal lobe. Severe disturbances of language can result from lesions in the dominant, usually left, temporal lobe. Disturbances of memory are common in patients with such lesions.

Tumors of the temporal lobe frequently cause seizures. These seizures are typically characterized by transient changes in emotions, mood, and behavior and are associated with motor automatisms—so-called complex partial seizures or psychomotor epilepsy. If the lesion is situated anteriorly and affects the uncinate gyrus, either directly or through pressure, so-called "uncinate fits" occur that are characterized by an aura of unusual taste or smell, followed by abnormal motor activity of the mouth and lips, during which the patient is not in contact with his or her surroundings.

Patients with temporal lobe lesions that produce an homonymous visual field defect may also experience visual hallucinations. The hallucinations are typically of the formed type and consist of both animate (e.g., people, animals) and inanimate (e.g., flowers, trees, buildings) objects. They are often seen in color and are always in the affected homonymous hemifield on the side contralateral to the lesion. Visual hallucinations caused by temporal lobe lesions may be pleasurable or frightening to the patient and may be accompanied by auditory hallucinations.

LESIONS OF THE PARIETAL LOBE

Lesions in the parietal lobe may produce ocular symptoms that have value in topical diagnosis. Homonymous hemianopia affecting primarily the lower fields is caused by damage to the optic radiation in the superior parietal lobe (Fig. 12.24). Such defects are usually more congruous than those produced by lesions of the temporal lobe. Because the entire optic radiation passes

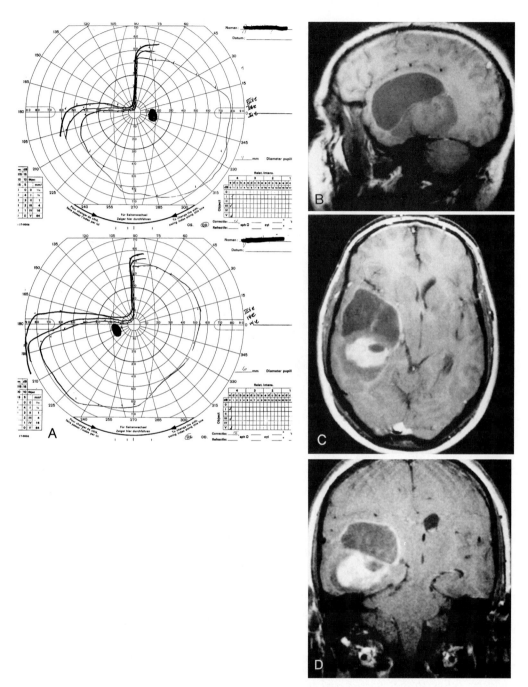

Figure 12.23. A 29-year-old man presented with 2 months of headaches with mood swings and mania, and 3 days of intermittent greenish-blue lines appearing in his superior left visual field. Examination was normal except for papilledema and a left homonymous superior quadrantanopia (*A*). *B–D.*

T1-weighted MRI (*B:* sagittal pregadolinium; *C:* axial postgadolinium; *D:* coronal postgadolinium) show an inhomogenously enhancing, cystic mass in the right temporal lobe. Biopsy was diagnostic of glioblastoma multiforme.

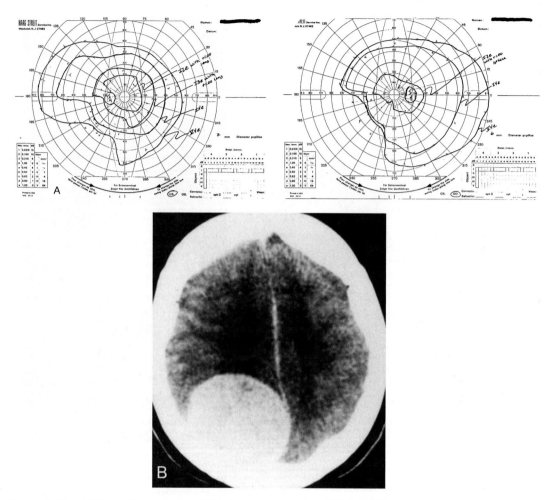

Figure 12.24. A 37-year-old woman complained of intermittent headaches associated with visual hallucinations of "a swirling black circle in the left eye." *A.* Examination was normal except for left homonymous inferior quadrantic visual field defects. *B.* CT scan, axial view, after intravenous injection of iodinated contrast material reveals a large, dural-based homogenously enhancing right parietal lobe tumor with little mass effect, confirmed at surgery to be a meningioma.

through the parietal lobe, large lesions may produce complete homonymous hemianopia with macular splitting.

The optic radiation is a continuous sheet of fibers with no separation of fibers into those ultimately projecting to the superior and inferior visual cortices. Thus, most field defects in patients with lesions of the optic radiation have sloping borders that do not precisely respect the horizontal meridian (Fig. 12.25). Exceptions occur, however, especially when the causative lesion is in the posterior optic radiation where the fascicles approach the calcarine cortex.

Neuro-ophthalmologic features suggesting a lesion in the parietal lobe include an incomplete and relatively congruous (or mildly incongruous) homonymous hemianopia that is denser below than above, conjugate movements of the eyes to the side opposite the lesion on forced lid closure (Cogan's sign), and an abnormal optokinetic response when the target is moved toward the side of the lesion. A disturbance of fixation reflexes sufficient to interfere with reading ability may develop before the appearance of other symptoms. This disturbance is sometimes manifest during visual field testing, during which the

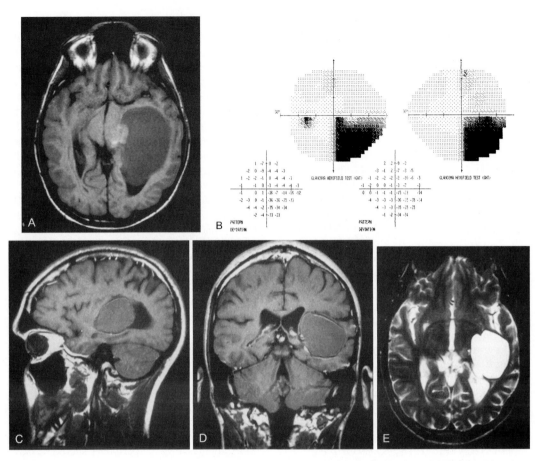

Figure 12.25. A 17-year-old man had a complex partial seizure and was found to have a left temporal lobe cystic fibrillary astrocytoma. *A.* T1-weighted axial MRI shows location of the tumor. The tumor was partially resected and then irradiated. *B.* Visual fields performed 6 years later show a left homonymous inferior quadrantanopia. *C–E.* Repeat MRI (*C:* T1-weighted sagittal image after gadolinium; *D:* T1-weighted axial image after gadolinium; *E:* T2-weighted axial image) now reveals a smaller cystic lesion in the region of the optic radiation. Note that the lesion does not extend into the occipital lobe.

patient cannot maintain central fixation despite repeated instructions to do so, an apparent understanding of the instructions, and an apparent willingness to comply. Other types of visual disturbances caused by lesions in the parietal lobe include visual neglect, visual agnosia, and difficulties with word recognition.

Patients with parietal lobe lesions and homonymous visual field defects are often unaware of their visual deficits. This phenomenon is more likely to occur when the underlying abnormality is in the nondominant cerebral hemisphere (usually the right parietal lobe), but it can also occur in patients with dominant parietal lobe lesions. In other patients, the primary visual pathways may be unaffected or minimally affected, but the patient neglects the contralateral visual field.

The parietal lobe is the principal sensory area of the cerebral cortex, and its postcentral convolution is of particular importance. The patient may complain of numbness but more commonly has complex problems of sensory integration that can be demonstrated using tests of tactile discrimination, position sense, stereognosis, and visual-spatial coordination. Irritative lesions of the postcentral convolution cause sensory Jacksonian seizures that begin contralateral to the lesion at the part of the body that corresponds to the focus of excitation. Tingling or numbness spreads to other adjacent parts of the body according to the order of their representation in the cortex. Lesions in the dominant parietal lobe can cause aphasia (usually fluent), apraxia, agnosia, acalculia, and agraphia. A lesion in the dominant parietal lobe involving the angular gyrus may produce Gerstmann's syndrome (finger agnosia, right-left disorientation, agraphia, and acalculia) in association with a right homonymous hemianopia. Lesions in the nondominant parietal lobe may cause impaired constructional ability, dyscalculia, and, most commonly, inattention or neglect. Indeed, left spatial neglect after a right hemisphere lesion may accentuate the left hemianopia, hemianesthesia, and hemiplegia, and thus contribute to poor recovery.

LESIONS OF THE OCCIPITAL LOBE AND VISUAL CORTEX

Most lesions affecting the occipital lobe are vascular or traumatic in origin, with tumors, abscesses, demyelinating, and toxic disorders of white matter occurring much less frequently. Because of the close anatomic relationship of fibers from corresponding portions of the two retinas, lesions of the occipital lobe cause defects that are almost exclusively homonymous and are also increasingly congruous the more posteriorly situated the lesion.

UNILATERAL LESIONS OF THE POSTERIOR OCCIPITAL LOBE

Defects seen with these lesions are always homonymous. Lesions of the tip of the occipital lobe (occipital pole) produce central homonymous scotomas that are exquisitely congruous. The central 10° of visual field are represented by at least 50 to 60% of the posterior striate cortex, and the central 30° by about 80% of the cortex (Figs. 12.26 and 12.27). Lesions located more anteriorly may produce primarily central field defects that break out into the periphery (Fig. 12.28). Impressive congruity is a feature of such field defects, and the phenomenon of sparing of the macula is often seen in such cases (see below).

UNILATERAL LESIONS OF THE ANTERIOR OCCIPITAL LOBE

Because the temporal field in each eye is larger than the nasal field, the fibers subserving that portion of the peripheral temporal field that has no nasal correlate must be unpaired through-

out the postchiasmal portion of the visual sensory pathway. Damage to these unpaired peripheral fibers produces a monocular defect in the extreme temporal visual field. This field defect is crescentic in shape, and its widest extent is in the horizontal meridian, where it extends from 60° out to approximately 90°. Because of the peculiar shape of the defect, patients with the defect are said to have the **temporal crescent (or half-moon) syndrome** (Fig. 12.29). The most anterior portion of the striate cortex harbors the projected monocular temporal crescent of the contralateral eye. Therefore, lesions of the posterior striate cortex tend to spare the temporal crescent, whereas lesions of the anterior striate cortex may selectively produce a defect in the temporal crescent or eliminate it entirely. Both upper and lower temporal crescents may be scotomatous in the field of one eye, or only the upper or lower temporal crescent may be affected. Alternatively, the temporal crescent may be spared when the remainder of the temporal visual field is involved in a homonymous hemianopia (Fig. 12.30).

Two important, if basic, facts should be kept in mind when considering the temporal crescent syndrome. First, monocular peripheral temporal visual field defects are probably caused most often by *retinal* lesions, not by intracranial ones. Thus, the nasal retinal periphery should be carefully examined ophthalmoscopically in patients with a presumed temporal crescent syndrome. Second, because these defects begin approximately 60° from fixation, central field testing (i.e., that performed using a tangent screen or most automated static perimetry programs) gives normal results and will not detect such defects (see Fig. 12.29).

SPARING OF THE MACULA

In homonymous hemianopia, when a portion of the central field of each eye is preserved as a result of deviation of the vertical meridian between the functioning and nonfunctioning halves of the visual fields, there is said to be "sparing of the macula" or "macular sparing." In a majority of such cases, visual acuity is normal, with the zone of preserved visual field ranging from 1° or 2° to almost 10° in width (Fig. 12.31). Macular sparing is seen in patients with postgeniculate—usually occipital—lesions, but absence of sparing does not necessar-

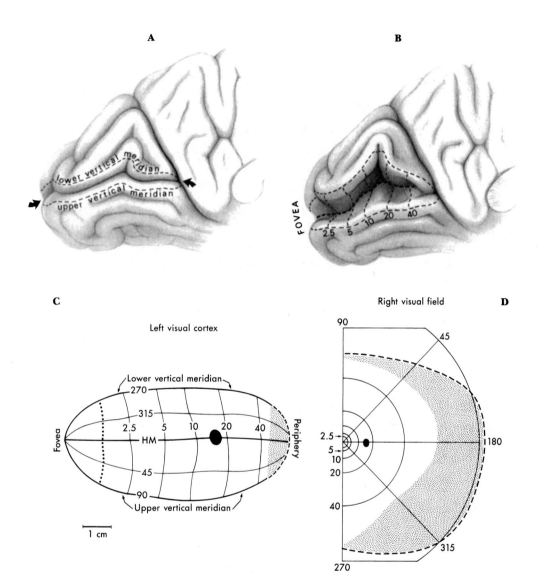

Figure 12.26.   The representation of the visual field in the human striate cortex. *A.* Left occipital lobe showing location of striate cortex within the calcarine fissure (between arrows). The boundary (dashed line) between the striate cortex (area V1) and extrastriate cortex contains the representation of the vertical meridian. *B.* View of striate cortex after opening the lips of the calcarine fissure. The dashed lines indicate the coordinates of the visual field map. The representation of the horizontal meridian runs approximately along the base of the calcarine fissure. The vertical dashed lines mark the iso-eccentricity contours from 2.5° to 40°. Striate cortex wraps around the occipital pole to extend about 1 cm onto the lateral convexity where the fovea is represented. *C.* Schematic map showing the projection of the right visual hemi-

field upon the left visual cortex by transposing the map illustrated in *B* onto a flat surface. The row of dots indicates approximately where striate cortex folds around the tip of the occipital lobe. The black oval marks the region of the striate cortex corresponding to the blind spot of the contralateral eye. *HM,* horizontal meridian. *D.* Right visual hemifield plotted with a Goldmann perimeter. The stippled region corresponds to the monocular temporal crescent, which is mapped within the most anterior 8 to 10% of the striate cortex. (Reprinted with permission from Horton JC, Hoyt WF. The representation of the visual field in human striate cortex. A revision of the classic Holmes map. Arch Ophthalmol 1991;109:816–824.)

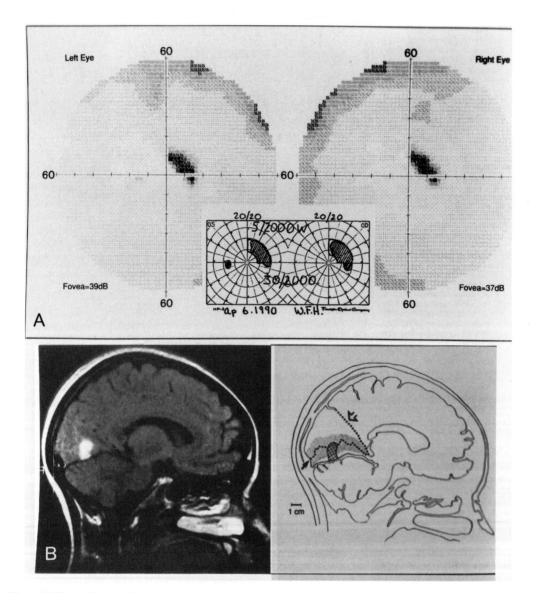

Figure 12.27. A 30-year-old woman reported several episodes of flashing, colored lights in her right upper quadrant of vision. *A.* Merged 30–2 and 60–2 full-threshold visual field tests using a Humphrey Field Analyzer. A homonymous, congruous scotoma was present in the right upper quadrant. In the inset, the visual fields are mapped at the tangent screen. The scotoma extended from 6° to 18°. *B.* Parasagittal magnetic resonance image of the left occipital lobe. The lesion (cross-hatched area in the diagram on the right) is within the visual cortex (stippled area in the diagram on the right). The calcarine sulcus (*solid arrow*) and the parieto-occipital sulcus (*hollow arrow*) are marked by dots. On biopsy, the lesion was a presumed tuberculoma. (Reprinted with permission from Horton JC, Hoyt WF. The representation of the visual field in human striate cortex. Arch Ophthalmol 109;1991:816–824.)

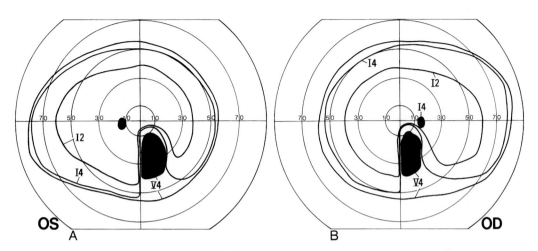

Figure 12.28.   Inferior homonymous hemianopic scotomas that break out to the periphery in a patient with an infarct of the left superior occipital cortex.

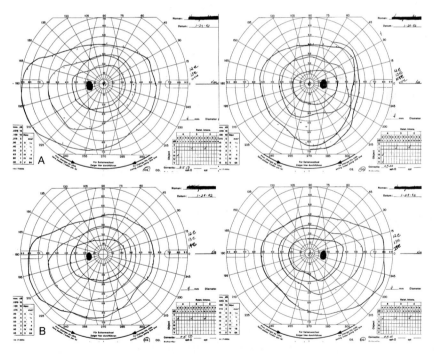

Figure 12.29.   Migrainous loss of the temporal crescent. A 31-year-old woman with a history of migraine without aura had the sudden onset of a bright light in the temporal field of vision of the right eye, followed by loss of vision in this same region and subsequent headache. *A.* Kinetic perimetry performed at the time of visual symptoms shows loss of the temporal crescent in the right eye. The field deficit persisted for a few days and then resolved. *B.* Visual fields performed 5 days later are full in both eyes. MRI performed at the time of the initial deficit was completely normal.

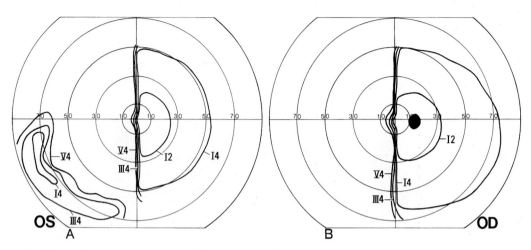

Figure 12.30. Visual field defects in a 56-year-old woman with a right occipital lobe infarction. There is a left homonymous hemianopia with sparing of the inferior portion of the left temporal crescent.

ily indicate that the lesion is either noncortical or pregeniculate.

The etiology of macular sparing is controversial. Three theories have been proposed to explain the phenomenon:

1. An artifact of testing.
2. Bilateral representation of the macula.
3. Incomplete damage of the visual sensory pathway.

As far as the first theory is concerned, there is no doubt that some cases of ''macular sparing'' are caused by inaccurate fixation. It is impossible for even otherwise normal persons to obtain perfect fixation, and physiologic movements of the fixing eye, so slight that they cannot be detected by ordinary means, probably account for at least 1° to 2° of deviation of the vertical meridian about the central area.

As far as the second theory is concerned, histochemical studies demonstrate that, to some extent, a small portion of each macula probably has representation in each occipital lobe. There is a small area of nasotemporal overlap on either side of the vertical meridian in which some axons from ganglion cells temporal to the fovea cross within the chiasm, whereas some axons from ganglion cells nasal to the fovea remain uncrossed. However, the mere presence of an overlap does not necessarily have any major visual consequences.

In fact, most clinically obvious cases of homonymous hemianopia with macular sparing occur in the setting of incomplete damage to the visual sensory pathway, usually the occipital lobe, and appear to be related to a residual intact area of the pathway. The unique dual blood supply of the occipital cortex from the posterior cerebral and middle cerebral arteries provides a mechanism for this partial damage. Thus, in patients with homonymous hemianopia and substantial macular sparing, not only is the location of the lesion almost always the occipital lobe, but the pathogenesis is almost always posterior cerebral artery territory infarction.

BILATERAL OCCIPITAL LOBE LESIONS

Bilateral lesions of the occipital lobes may occur simultaneously or consecutively. In addition, because such lesions are neurologically asymptomatic except as regards the visual system, patients with unilateral lesions that cause an homonymous field defect may not be aware of the defect until it is called to their attention (e.g., during a routine ocular examination or after the patient is involved in a motor vehicle accident) or until they experience a similar event on the opposite side, producing a more extensive visual deficit.

A double homonymous hemianopia may occur from a single event. In a majority of these cases, there is complete visual loss at the onset (i.e., cortical blindness) that is usually transient,

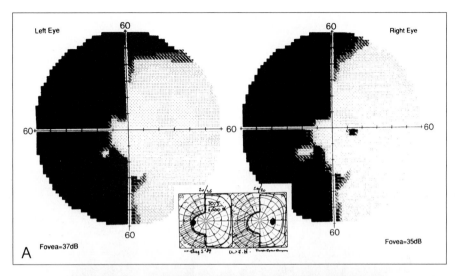

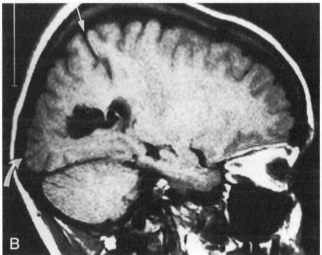

Figure 12.31. A 28-year-old woman suffered a persistent visual field defect after an unusually severe migraine attack. *A.* Full-threshold 60° visual fields using a Humphrey Field Analyzer shows that the central 15° of the left hemifield are intact. In the inset, the visual fields mapped at the tangent screen show that the field defect bisects the blind spot representation of the left eye. *B.* T1-weighted parasagittal MRI through the right occipital lobe shows an arteriovenous mal-formation involving the anterior portion of the right calcarine cortex. The posterior margin of the lesion is situated 31 mm from the occipital tip, marking the approximate location of the representation of the left eye's blind spot. The calcarine (*curved arrow*) and parieto-occipital (*straight arrow*) sulci are indicated. (Reprinted with permission from Horton JC, Hoyt WF. The representation of the visual field in human striate cortex. Arch Ophthalmol 1991;109:816–824.)

lasting from minutes to days, followed by some degree of clearing in one or both homonymous hemifields. Affected patients have similarly shaped visual field defects on corresponding sides of the vertical midline for each eye, equal visual acuity for each eye that is usually normal, normal pupils and fundi, and full ocular motility unless there is a coexisting brainstem lesion. The majority of these patients have vascular causes of their visual loss.

Much more commonly, bilateral homony-mous hemianopia occurs from consecutive events, invariably vascular in nature (Fig. 12.32). In such cases, the patient experiences an

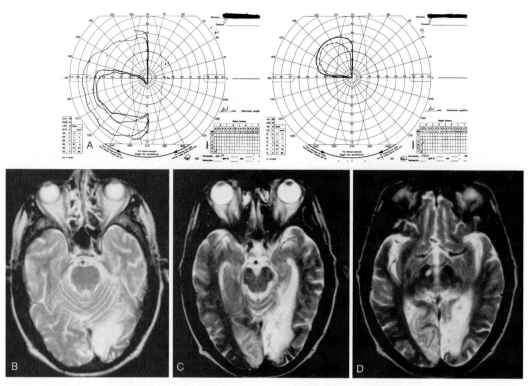

Figure 12.32.   Bilateral homonymous hemianopic defects secondary to bilateral posterior cerebral artery infarction. *A.* Kinetic perimetry reveals a dense right homonymous hemianopia combined with a left inferior homonymous quadrantanopia with sparing of the left temporal crescent. *B–D.*

Three T2-weighted, axial MRIs demonstrate bilateral posterior cerebral artery infarctions, worse on the left than the right, and extending less inferiorly and less anteriorly on the right.

acute homonymous hemianopia with retention of normal vision with or without sparing of the macula. At a later time, varying from weeks to years, the patient develops a sudden homonymous hemianopia on the opposite side, again with or without macular sparing. After this second event, the patient is either blind or has only a small central field around the point of fixation.

Whether simultaneous or consecutive, bilateral lesions of the occipital lobes produce bilateral homonymous field defects that are characteristic and vary only in their extent. They may be complete or scotomatous, and they may or may not be accompanied by macular sparing (Figs. 12.33 and 12.34). Occasionally, such scotomas have enough central sparing to produce a "ring" scotoma (see Fig. 12.33).

Bilateral occipital lobe disease—whether from infarction, compression, inflammation, infection, or trauma—may result in various types of bilateral homonymous visual field defects (see Fig. 12.34). First, there may be complete (cortical or cerebral) blindness. Second, there may be a complete hemianopia on one side and an incomplete, congruous hemianopia on the other. Third, there may be an homonymous hemianopia on one side and a quadrantanopia on the other (Figs. 12.32 and 12.35). Fourth, there may be a bilateral homonymous hemianopia with bilateral macular sparing of a different degree on each side. The remaining visual field thus appears to be severely constricted, and such patients may be thought to have bilateral optic nerve or retinal disease or may even be thought to have nonorganic visual field loss. As with bilateral homonymous hemianopic scotomas, however, careful testing along the vertical midline will establish the bilateral nature of the field defect and its correct origin (see Fig. 12.33). Finally, a crossed-quadrant homonymous defect

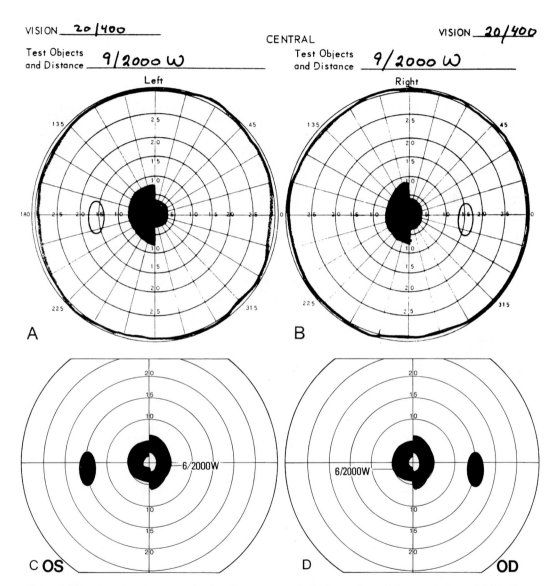

Figure 12.33. Bilateral homonymous hemianopic scotomas. *A* and *B*. In a patient with bilateral nonsimultaneous occipital lobe strokes. Note vertical step that differentiates these defects from a true central scotoma. *C* and *D*. with macular sparing in a patient who suffered trauma to the occipital region. The tractor on which he was riding overturned, pinning him underneath for several minutes. Initially, he was completely blind, but vision returned within several minutes. He subsequently realized that he had a "ring" of blurred vision around fixation. Note that the homonymous scotomas "respect" the vertical midline.

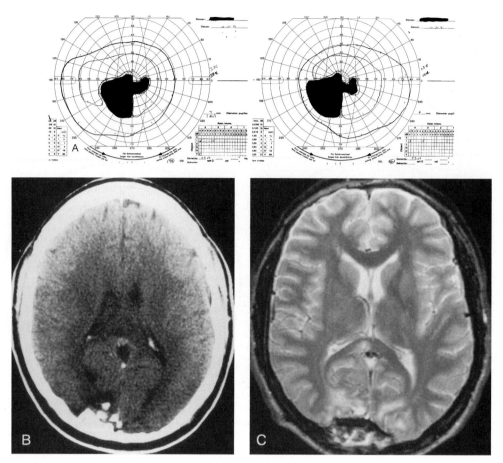

Figure 12.34. A 40-year-old man suffered occipital head trauma with a depressed skull fracture and visual complaints. Visual acuity was 20/20 in both eyes. *A.* Kinetic perimetry reveals exquisitely congruous bilateral homonymous scoto- mas. *B.* CT scan, axial view, reveals a right occipital pole lesion, but axial MRI (*C*) confirms bilateral occipital pole involvement.

results when patients develop bilateral quadrantic defects that affect the superior occipital lobe above the calcarine fissure on one side and the inferior occipital lobe below the fissure on the other side. Such defects are sometimes called ''checkerboard'' fields and occur quite infrequently, almost always after consecutive rather than simultaneous infarctions (Fig. 12.36).

In addition to the homonymous defects described above, trauma, infarction, and, rarely, tumors affecting both occipital lobes may produce bilateral superior or inferior **altitudinal** field defects (Fig. 12.37). Although vascular damage can produce either superior or inferior defects, traumatic injury (most commonly from bullet wounds) usually causes only bilateral in-

ferior altitudinal defects. This is probably because damage to the lower portions of the occipital lobes, which would produce bilateral superior altitudinal defects, often results in laceration of the dural sinuses or torcular herophili, with almost uniformly fatal results.

CORTICAL BLINDNESS AND CEREBRAL BLINDNESS

The term *cortical blindness* indicates loss of vision in both eyes from damage to the striate cortex. *Cerebral blindness* is a more general term indicating blindness from damage to any portion of both visual pathways posterior to the LGBs. Thus, cortical blindness is a form of cerebral blindness.

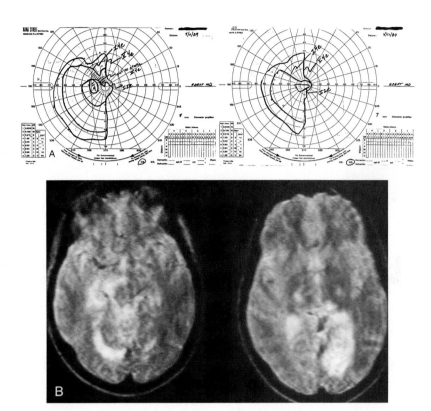

Figure 12.35. After strenuous exercise, a 33-year-old man experienced intermittent confusion, gait disturbances, and right facial weakness, followed by permanent left hemiparesis and difficulties with vision. *A.* Visual fields reveal a right homonymous hemianopia with macular sparing and a left superior homonymous quadrantanopia. *B.* Axial MRIs reveal corresponding infarctions in the occipital lobes bilaterally. Note the involvement of the inferior occipital lobe on the right and the entire calcarine cortex on the left with sparing of the most posterior pole. The patient also had cerebellar and brainstem infarctions, all secondary to artery-to-artery emboli from a vertebral artery dissection.

The essential features of cerebral (and thus also cortical) blindness are:

1. Loss of vision in both eyes.
2. Retention of the reflex constriction of the pupils to illumination and to convergence movements (the near response).
3. Integrity of the normal structure of the retinas as verified with the ophthalmoscope (except for patients who are blind from prenatal or perinatal injury).
4. Retention of full extraocular movements, unless there is also damage to ocular motor structures.

Some authors stipulate that patients with bilateral postgeniculate visual loss should be said to have cerebral or cortical blindness only if visual acuity is light perception or no light perception. Others modify this definition to add that any level of visual acuity is possible with cerebral blindness, as long as the visual acuity is equal in the two eyes (assuming there is no superimposed abnormality of the anterior visual pathways).

Hypoxia or anoxia involving the occipital lobes is the main etiologic factor producing cerebral blindness. Such damage is, of course, bilateral. Most commonly, an infarction in the posterior cerebral artery territory is initially unrecognized, but this previously silent hemianopia contributes to complete cortical blindness when a contralateral lesion occurs (see above). The most common mechanism for the infarction is cerebral embolism from either the heart or

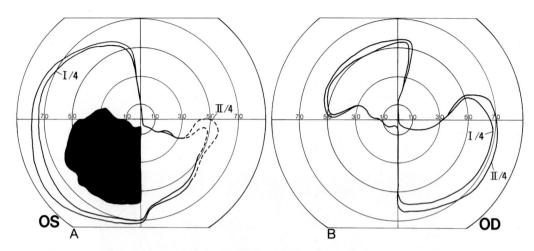

Figure 12.36. Crossed-quadrant (checkerboard) hemianopia. These field defects occurred suddenly in a 70-year-old woman with basilar artery disease. Note the quadrantic defects in the right upper field and the left lower field with the narrow congruous isthmus near fixation. Also note the sparing of the left temporal crescent and the incongruity of the field defects along the upper vertical meridian and the right horizontal meridian. (Courtesy of University of California Hospital, San Francisco.)

the more proximal vessels of the vertebrobasilar system (Fig. 12.38). Prolonged hypotension can cause cerebral blindness from bilateral watershed infarctions at the parieto-occipital junctions.

Cerebral blindness is observed under many circumstances other than infarction, as shown in Table 12.1. The mechanism of injury underlying the cerebral blindness caused by these events or substances is not always known, but vascular insufficiency plays a role in many of them.

In certain situations, cerebral blindness is transient. This is particularly true in patients who experience temporary vascular insufficiency in the vertebrobasilar system, in hypertensive syndromes following restoration of normal blood pressure, after removal of many of the toxic agents listed in Table 12.1, and after trauma. Children are more likely to experience recovery from cerebral blindness than adults, regardless of the underlying cause. On rare occasions, transient cerebral blindness may follow seizures or be an ictal manifestation. Because focal lesions may be responsible for ictal amaurosis, we believe that MRI should be performed in all cases. We would also emphasize that complete recovery from ictal or postictal blindness can occur even if the blindness lasts for several days.

The relationship between cerebral blindness and the visual-evoked potential (VEP) remains confusing. At least in adults, VEPs do not appear to be useful in establishing the diagnosis or prognosis in patients with cortical or cerebral blindness. The usefulness of VEPs in children with cerebral visual dysfunction also remains controversial, with some studies demonstrating correlation and others not. The variable results from these studies may reflect the many different underlying etiologies of cerebral blindness in children and the many other associated neurologic factors that may contribute to poor recovery.

It is not unusual for patients with cortical blindness to be unaware of their defect. This denial of blindness is called *anosognosia* or **Anton's syndrome.** The syndrome also occurs rarely in patients with blindness from causes other than occipital lobe disease, such as cataracts, retinopathies, or optic atrophy. The explanation for Anton's syndrome is unclear and may be different in different cases. It is probable that in many patients with cerebral or cortical blindness there are lesions in various areas of the brain responsible for the recognition and interpretation of visual images. In such patients, denial of blindness is caused not by the lesion in the primary visual pathway but by another lesion in another region of the brain. In other patients, denial of visual loss may reflect an emotional or psychiatric response, or it may represent a memory disorder.

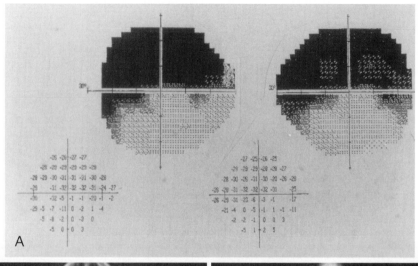

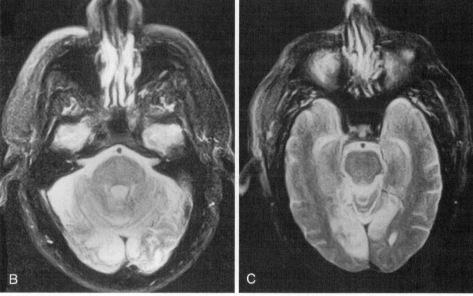

Figure 12.37.   A 71-year-old man had the acute onset of complete visual loss, followed by clearing inferiorly. Examination was normal except for visual fields (*A*), which show bilateral superior altitudinal visual field defects (bilateral superior homonymous quadrantanopias). *B–F*. T2-weighted MRI (*B–D:* axial views; *E–F:* coronal views to the right and left of midline, respectively) demonstrates bilateral posterior cerebral artery infarctions involving primarily the inferior occipital lobes.

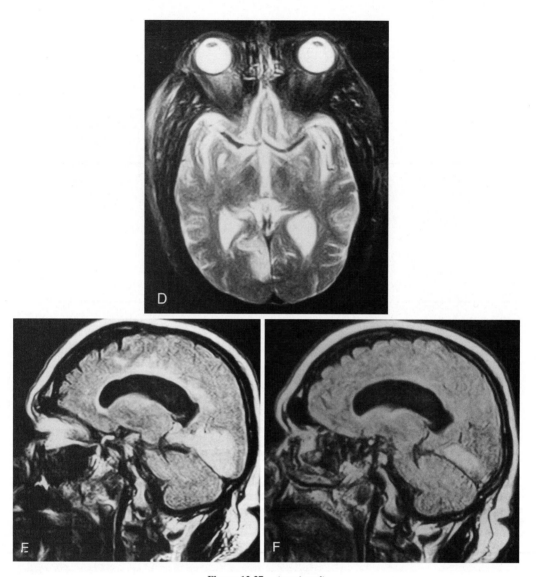

Figure 12.37. *(continued)*

OTHER VISUAL FEATURES OF OCCIPITAL LOBE DAMAGE

Although most patients with unilateral lesions of the occipital lobe have visual deficits totally restricted to the contralateral visual field, lesions of the occipital lobe may disrupt not only the striate and extrastriate cortex, but also adjacent underlying white matter. Such damage may alter interhemispheric connections along their presplenial course and disturb the synthesis of visual information from both hemifields. Clini-

cally, these disturbances are subtle compared with the homonymous visual field defect, but they may be responsible for various unexplained complaints of reduced performance in some of these patients, particularly for tasks with high visual information-processing demands such as reading and driving.

Some patients with homonymous hemianopia, especially those with a vascular occlusion in the occipital lobe, report phosphenes in the blind visual field, particularly early in the course of

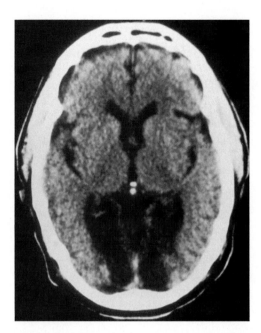

Figure 12.38.   Bilateral simultaneous posterior cerebral artery occlusion secondary to embolic infarction from a cardiac arrhythmia. The patient was initially cortically blind with no light perception vision. Over the course of a few weeks, his vision improved to 20/30 vision in each eye because of 5° of macular sparing.

Table 12.1
Circumstances of Cerebral Blindness

Acute intermittent porphyria
Bacterial endocarditis
Blood transfusions
Cardiac arrest
Cerebral angiography
Correction of hyponatremia
Creutzfeldt-Jakob disease
Diseases of white matter
   Adrenoleukodystrophy
   Metachromatic leukodystrophy
   Pelizaeus-Merzbacher disease
   Progressive multifocal leukoencephalopathy
   Schilder's disease
Electroshock
Epilepsy
Exposure to or ingestion of toxins
   Carbon monoxide
   Cisplatin
   Cyclosporin
   Ethanol
   Interferon
   Lead
   Mercury
   Methamphetamine
   Methotrexate
   Nitrous oxide
   Tacrolimus (FK506)
   Vincristine
   Vindesine
Hypoglycemia
Infectious and neoplastic meningitis
Mitochondrial encephalopathy, lactic acidosis, and stroke-like episodes (MELAS)
Neoplasm
Malignant hypertension
Subacute sclerosing panencephalitis
Sudden elevation or reduction in intracranial pressure
Syphilis
Toxemia of pregnancy
Trauma
Uremia
Ventriculography

their disorder. Many of the visual field defects in these patients resolve substantially, suggesting that the phosphenes may be viewed as a prognostically favorable symptom. Visual association areas bordering damaged primary cortex may be the source of these visual symptoms when they are released from normal inhibitory inputs from primary visual cortex.

LESIONS OF THE EXTRASTRIATE CORTEX WITH DEFECTS IN THE VISUAL FIELD

The striate cortex (Brodmann's area 17) is the primary visual cortex and the principal recipient of output from the LGB (Fig. 12.39). Surrounding the striate cortex within the occipital lobe are two visual association areas, Brodmann areas 18 and 19, also referred to as the "extrastriate visual cortex." Areas 18 and 19 together comprise at least five distinct cortical areas devoted to visual processing. These visual areas—designated V2, V3, V3a, V4, and V5 in the monkey—can be mapped with precision, and corresponding regions are thought to be present in the human occipital cortex. Regions V2 and V3 are the major recipient areas for projections from both the magnocellular and parvocellular systems from the primary striate cortex (Fig. 12.40). However, V1 (primary striate cortex) also projects directly to areas V4 and V5, bypassing V2.

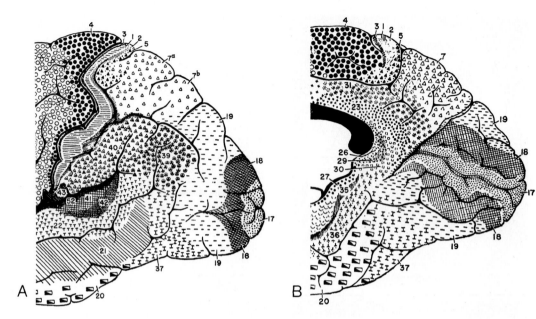

Figure 12.39. The areas occupied by the primary visual cortex and the extrastriate areas, according to Brodmann's classification. *A.* Mesial surface. *B.* Lateral surface. (Reprinted with permission from R Lindenberg, FB Walsh, JG Sacks. Neuropathology of Vision: An Atlas. Philadelphia: Lea & Febiger, 1973.)

It has been proposed that a lesion in extrastriate cortex alone can cause an homonymous defect in the visual field. Indeed, not only may a lesion of V2/V3 be sufficient to create a visual field defect, but such lesions may be the principle cause of quadrantic defects that strictly respect the horizontal meridian (Fig. 12.41).

DISSOCIATION OF VISUAL PERCEPTIONS

In Chapter 13 of this text, we discuss the topographic diagnosis of disorders of visual processing distal to the primary visual cortex. Because many of these disorders result from lesions in the extrastriate cortex of the occipital lobes, it is worth mentioning a few of the more prominent syndromes in this chapter.

The human visual cortex is specialized with respect to specific functions. For example, an area in the lingual and fusiform gyri of the prestriate cortex corresponds to area V4 in the monkey and subserves the perception of color. Lesions in this region may spare the visual field but produce acquired dyschromatopsia in the contralateral hemifield. The area of functional specialization for visual motion is localized to the temporoparieto-occipital junction, a region corresponding to area V5 in the monkey. Lesions in this region, especially when bilateral, may cause a selective deficit in the perception of visual movement without a visual field defect and without impairment of nonvisual movement perception (i.e., movement perceived by acoustic or tactile stimulation).

In some patients, damage to an occipital lobe can cause a complete homonymous hemianopia to nonmoving objects with retention of the ability to detect moving objects within the blind hemifield—this is static-kinetic dissociation, also called the **Riddoch phenomenon.** Such dissociation may have prognostic significance, because it usually means that some degree of recovery can be expected to occur. Static-kinetic dissociation is not a pathologic phenomenon that is purely limited to the occipital lobe. In fact, even normal individuals perceive moving objects better than static objects of the same size, shape, and luminance. The Riddoch phenomenon may occur in patients with lesions of the optic nerves and chiasm, as well as in patients with retrochiasmal visual pathway damage that spares the occipital lobes.

The Riddoch phenomenon is one form of a general category of visual phenomena desig-

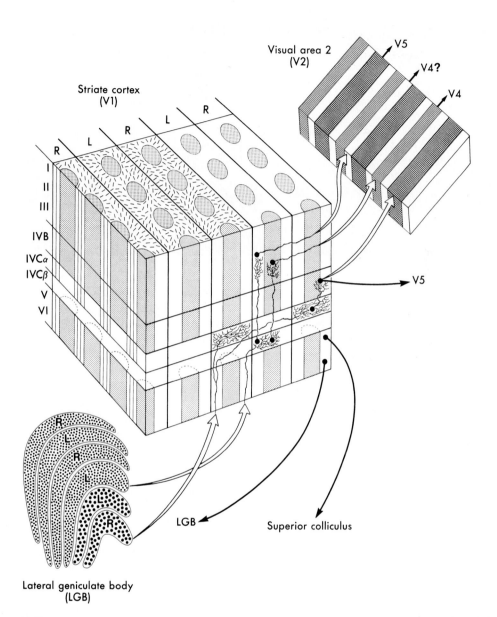

Figure 12.40. Schematic diagram showing the magnocellular (originating from large dots) and parvocellular (originating from small dots) pathways from the lateral geniculate body through areas V1 and V2 to areas V4 and V5. Each module of striate cortex contains a few complete sets of ocular dominance columns (R and L), orientation columns, and about a dozen cytochrome oxidase-positive blobs (stippled cylinders). The orientation columns, depicted with hash marks on the cortical surface, extend through all layers except $4C_\alpha$. Their borders are not discrete. The magnocellular stream courses through layer $4C_\alpha$ to layer 4B and then to dark thick stripes in area V2 and to area V5. The parvocellu-

lar stream courses through layer $4C_\beta$ to layers 2 and 3. Cells within the cytochrome oxidase blobs project to dark thin stripes in area V2, whereas cells within interblob regions project to pale thin stripes in V2. Both dark and pale thin stripes in area V2 probably project to area V4 and other regions. Note that layers 5 and 6 in area V1 send projections to the superior colliculus and the lateral geniculate body, respectively. (Reprinted with permission from Horton JC. The central visual pathways. In: Hart WM Jr, ed. Adler's Physiology of the Eye. 9th ed. St Louis: CV Mosby, 1992: 751.)

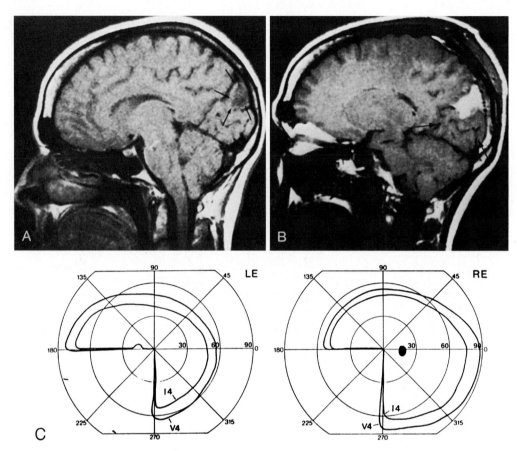

Figure 12.41. A 39-year-old woman had experienced multicolored visual hallucinations in her left lower quadrant since childhood. *A.* T1-weighted sagittal MRI reveals a lesion within the cuneus of the right occipital lobe which on en bloc resection was found to be a grade I astrocytoma. *B.* Postoperative T1-weighted sagittal MRI reveals the area of resection. *C.* Postoperative visual fields demonstrate a left inferior homonymous quadrantanopia with precise respect of the horizontal and vertical meridia. The patient could detect gross hand motion within the quadrantic defect. (Reprinted with permission from Horton JC, Hoyt WF. Quadrantic visual field defects: a hallmark of lesions in extrastriate (V2/V3) cortex. Brain 1991;114:1703–1718.)

nated as "blindsight." Some patients with extensive damage to the occipital lobes appear to retain a rudimentary form of vision involving the perception of visual stimuli other than just moving objects. Most patients are not consciously aware of this ability to look, point, detect, and discriminate without truly "seeing." In many cases, blindsight is most likely a result of islands of preserved area 17. However, in some cases, blindsight is a genuine phenomenon that reflects nonstriate visual pathways, such as a direct geniculoextrastriate cortical projection and a retinocollicular projection that reaches extrastriate cortical visual areas via the pulvinar nucleus.

Another way in which visual perceptions may be dissociated is in the syndrome of unilateral inattention or neglect. Patients with this defect may appear to have normal visual function if tested in routine fashion, because they are able to correctly perceive objects in each hemifield with either eye. However, when two test objects are presented in the right and left hemifields of each eye simultaneously, the patient perceives only the test object in the hemifield ipsilateral to the lesion. This phenomenon, called **visual extinction,** can occur following damage to the parietal or occipitoparietal cortex as well as to several different regions of the brain, reflecting the complex integrated network that exists for the modulation of directed attention within extrapersonal space.

NONVISUAL SYMPTOMS AND SIGNS OF OCCIPITAL LOBE DISEASE

As might be expected, vascular lesions of the occipital lobe are asymptomatic, except with regard to the visual system. Many patients with occipital infarctions experience acute pain of the head, brow, or eye ipsilateral to the lesion. This presumably reflects the dual trigeminal innervation of the posterior dural structures and the periorbital region. Patients with homonymous hemianopia may also complain of disturbances of equilibrium, a sense that their body is swaying toward the side of the hemianopia. This so-called "visual ataxia" may reflect unopposed tonic input of vision from the intact hemifield rather than any true vestibular impairment or neglect.

If the posterior cerebral artery is occluded proximally, patients with an infarct in the occipital lobe may also have hemiplegia from damage to the posterior internal capsule or cerebral peduncle, language dysfunction from damage to posterior parietal and temporal structures, and symptoms indicating damage to the ipsilateral thalamus. In addition, because the condition is ordinarily seen in patients with severe atherosclerosis, there may be other evidence of vertebrobasilar insufficiency, including ocular motor abnormalities referable to the rostral brainstem. Patients who develop a bilateral homonymous hemianopia in this setting may be more severely impaired than patients with blindness from bilateral retinal or optic nerve disease. Such patients present major problems as regards rehabilitation.

Tumors of the occipital lobe may cause non-visual manifestations by virtue of their mass effect. Headache is the most common symptom, occurring in up to 90% of patients. Other symptoms and signs include nausea and vomiting, ataxia, hallucinations that are usually unformed (e.g., flashing lights, geometric shapes), seizures, and mental status changes. Many of these symptoms are nonlocalizing and related to increased intracranial pressure.

TREATMENT AND REHABILITATION FOR HOMONYMOUS HEMIANOPIA

Some spontaneous recovery of homonymous visual field defects occurs in no more than 20% of patients within the first several months after brain injury. Despite a certain amount of plasticity even in the adult cerebral cortex, patients with visual field defects have a consistently poor rehabilitation outcome. The exact anatomic location of the lesion causing the homonymous hemianopia does not appear to affect the functional outcome; however, the more associated neurologic deficits present, the more difficult the rehabilitation and the poorer the functional performance. Contributing further to poor functional improvement is the relatively advanced age of most of these patients, a factor associated even in normal individuals with progressive cognitive, sensory, and motor deficits. Finally, the presence of neglect, especially in patients with nondominant hemisphere lesions, also interferes with the rehabilitation process.

Several techniques may assist in the treatment and rehabilitation of patients with homonymous hemianopia. A mirror attachment can be used to project the mirror image of the blind field into the seeing half-field. The mirror is attached to the nasal side of the spectacle frame behind the lens. For many patients, however, such mirrors do not prove satisfactory; the patient has to turn the head toward the mirror, the mirror produces a scotoma that blocks a portion of the seeing field, and spatial disorientation is common (images seen in the mirror are reversed and projected to the opposite side of the midline).

Fresnel prisms can be placed on glasses for use in the rehabilitation of patients with homonymous hemianopias. One option is to place the prism on the outside half of the spectacle lens ipsilateral to the hemianopia with the base oriented toward that side. For example, for a patient with a left homonymous hemianopia, a 30-prism diopter prism is placed base-out on the left half of the left lens, thus displacing the image of an object in the patient's left hemifield 15° to the right. Alternatively, 20-prism diopter Fresnel prisms can be placed on both spectacle lenses, allowing for a 5° movement of the eyes before they encounter the prism edge. The power and placement of the prisms can then be modified, depending on patient adaptation. The goal is to increase the patient's scanning skills over time, although the effects on activities of daily living are likely minimal.

Patients with hemianopia commonly experience reading difficulties. Patients with right hemianopias cannot see which letters or words follow those that they have already deciphered.

Patients with left hemianopias may read without difficulty until they come to the end of the line, but in attempting to return to the beginning of the next line, they move into their blind hemifield and lose their place, often beginning again on an unrelated line. Simple maneuvers to help improve reading include the use of a ruler placed under the line of text, maintaining the left index finger or thumb at the beginning of each line, or even turning the material 90° and reading vertically within the intact hemifield.

Another strategy that may help rehabilitate patients with homonymous hemianopia who have difficulty reading is assessment of the saccadic strategy that the patient uses during attempted reading, followed by systematic retraining of saccadic eye movements and ocular scanning techniques. Many hemianopic patients exhibit a restricted field of ocular motor visual exploration, so practice with spatially organized visual searching can improve functional outcome for these patients.

FOR MORE INFORMATION:
See Walsh & Hoyt's *Clinical Neuro-Ophthalmology,* 5th edition, Volume 1, Chapter 8, pp. 307–376, 1835–1837, and 1844–1848.

Central Disorders of Visual Function

This chapter addresses aspects of behavior disorders caused by damage to the visual cortex and white matter connections. These conditions are often referred to as "central disorders of vision," "cerebral disorders of vision," or "higher disorders of vision." The understanding of these disorders continues to improve with the development of new techniques for measuring visual dysfunction, imaging the behaving brain, rehabilitating visual dysfunction in patients with brain damage, and even creating visual sensations in the blind with prostheses to stimulate visual cortex.

Vision was once thought to be primarily a serial (or hierarchic) process in which visual signals were altered or enhanced at successive way stations from retina to brain until an image of the physical world somehow emerged at the level of conscious experience. It has subsequently be-

come clear that serial processing is only one of several mechanisms used by the brain to process visual signals. The primate visual system also uses parallel processing, beginning in the retina. Different types of retinal ganglion cells are specialized to transduce different types of physical signals and give rise to different channels. There is cross-talk between these channels at several levels from the retina to the cortex, and there also are feed-forward and feed-back connections between early and late stages of the visual sensory system. Instead of just serial processing, visual functions are explained in terms of multiple interactions among specialized brain regions in the same hemisphere and across the corpus callosum. Central disorders of vision thus can be interpreted as a consequence of disturbing the processing in different sectors or pathways in a complex interconnecting network.

SEGREGATION OF VISUAL INPUTS

The functional segregation of visual inputs in the primate visual system is well documented (Figs. 13.1 and 13.2). Retinal information is communicated to cortical neurons through a set of pathways that appear specialized to convey a particular class of visual information. For example, the **parvocellular** or P-pathway, named for its connections to simian striate cortex (area V1) via parvocellular layers 3 to 6 of the lateral geniculate body (LGB), is characterized by color opponency and slow-conducting axons that convey sustained signals. This pathway has strong projections to secondary areas such as V4 and inferior temporal (IT) cortex, located in the inferior occipital lobe and adjacent temporo-occipital regions. These regions, along the ventral or temporal cortical pathway (the "what" pathway), are presumed to play a role in the perception of color, luminance, stereopsis, and pattern recognition. In contrast, the **magnocellular** or M-pathway is characterized by large, fast-conducting axons that convey information about more transient visual signals. This pathway connects to areas in visual association cortex, including the middle temporal (MT) and medial superior temporal (MST) areas. These regions, located along the dorsal or parietal cortical pathway (the "where" pathway), are thought to analyze the spatial location and movement of objects in the panorama (Fig. 13.3).

The notion of two separate visual systems is a useful and fruitful paradigm in the macaque animal model, and it is also applicable to human vision. Analyses of data from a large number of patients with focal lesions of the visual cortex and its connections, as defined by computed tomographic (CT) scanning and magnetic resonance imaging (MRI), support the general concept of separate dorsal and ventral processing pathways as a framework for interpreting human clinical disorders. For example, damage to the inferior visual cortex and adjoining temporal regions impairs pattern recognition and learning, producing agnosia for objects and faces (prosopagnosia) or inability to read despite previous literacy (alexia). It can also reduce color perception in the contralateral field—cerebral achromatopsia. By contrast, damage to the superior visual cortex and the adjacent parietal cortex produces disorders of spatial-temporal analysis—inability to judge location, distance, orientation, size, or motion of objects, as well as marked disturbances of visually guided eye and hand control. Balint's syndrome is a striking example.

Each of these major divisions probably has functional subdivisions. Furthermore, although the dorsal and ventral visual cortex are associated with different, behaviorally separable functions, there is growing evidence that these two major divisions also have overlapping functions.

Explaining visual phenomena in humans on the basis of a neural substrate requires caution. There is a natural tendency to formalize the relationship of perceptual states to physiologic states. As we learn more about the neural organization of the visual system, it becomes increasingly tempting to assign particular visual functions to particular stages. This issue can be addressed by using proper tests in a precise manner; the characteristics of the input stimulus must be precisely defined (by mathematical techniques and physical measurements), and the perceptual and behavioral output must be properly recorded. In this way, inferences can be made regarding the intervening stages of vision in normal healthy observers, and these strategies can also be applied in patients with focal brain lesions to obtain information on the anatomic constraints for different processing stages. Lesions of the visual cortex produce relative dissociations of function, such as color versus motion, that reveal the independence of certain perceptual properties. Thus, one can assess how certain types of information are condensed or dispersed and which stages of visual processing precede others. This can contribute to a flow diagram of perceptual processing with potential cross-referencing with human neuroanatomy at the level of MRI analyses. Unique evidence from human lesion studies of vision can also be complemented by functional imaging and by anatomic studies.

Behavior studies in patients with brain damage provide much of the critical data that underlie our understanding of vision. It is therefore important to understand the perspective and limitations of these studies, including the nature of the information they provide and the factors that affect their interpretation. For example, some patients cannot describe their perceptual experience because of an acquired damage in language processing areas of the left hemisphere. Other

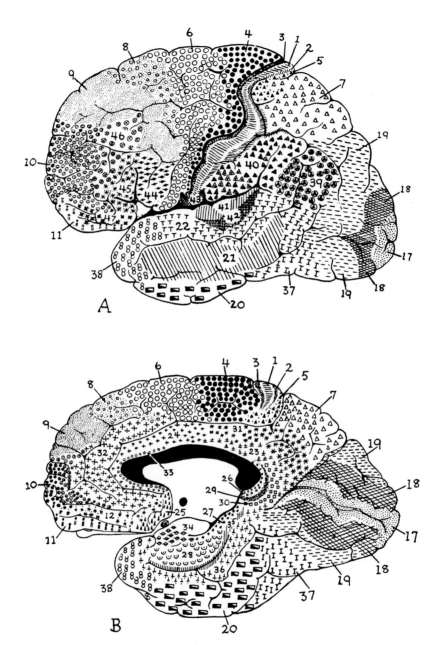

Figure 13.1. Brodmann's cytoarchitectonic areas are depicted on lateral (*A*) and mesial (*B*) views of the hemisphere of a human brain. The primary visual cortex area 17, also called area V1, lies above and below the calcarine fissure and is seen mainly in the mesial aspect of the hemisphere. Areas 18 and 19 of the occipital lobe extend onto the lateral surface of the hemisphere. These areas contain secondary visual maps homologous to those identified in nonhuman primates. A dorsal pathway includes V1, V2, a portion of V3, the middle temporal (MT) area, and adjacent parieto-occipital areas. It is thought to process visuospatial information including motion. A ventral, temporo-occipital pathway includes V1, V2, portions of V3, V4, and the inferior temporal (IT) cortex and is thought to process sustained signals, including color and static shape (see text). (Reprinted with permission from Brodmann K. Vergleichende localisation-slehre der grosshirnrinde in ihren Prinzipien dargestellt auf Grund des Zellenbaues. Leipzig: JA Barth, 1909.)

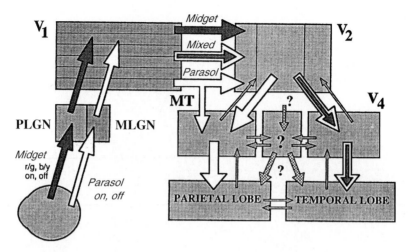

Figure 13.2. Diagram of the major connections in the primate visual system. Note parallel processing beginning at the level of the retina. Midget ganglion cells connect to striate cortex (V1) via parvocellular layers of the lateral geniculate nucleus (PLGN). The larger parasol cells connect to striate cortex via the magnocellular layers of the lateral geniculate nucleus (MLGN), which send connections from there to the middle temporal area (MT) and the parietal lobe. These latter structures comprise the dorsal visual pathway. Connections via areas V2 and V4 (located in areas 18 and 19) to the temporal lobe (including area IT) comprise the ventral visual pathway. Higher disturbances of vision such as cerebral akinetopsia and cerebral achromatopsia can be interpreted in terms of damage to these areas and connections. *r/g,* red/green. *b/y,* blue/yellow. (Reprinted with permission from Schiller PH. Visual processing in the primate extrastriate cortex. In: Papathomas TV, Chubb C, Gorea A, Knowler E, eds. Early Vision and Beyond. Cambridge, MA: MIT Press, 1995.)

patients may not be aware of their perceptual defect and therefore do not report it, a condition known as **anosognosia.**

BLINDSIGHT AND RESIDUAL VISION

Some patients with lesions of area V1 causing an homonymous field defect perform better than chance on simple forced-choice detection tasks or on localization tasks measuring the accuracy of finger pointing or eye movements toward targets presented in the defective field of vision. Some of these patients deny any conscious experience of the objects they reportedly localize or detect and are thus said to have **blindsight**.

Precise anatomic analyses are critical to the interpretation of cases of presumed blindsight. For example, it would be highly undesirable to mistake residual vision from sparing of the cortical representation of the monocular temporal crescent with blindsight. In addition, a distinction should be made between blindsight and residual vision. Some studies describing patients with blindsight indicate that the patients are aware of visual stimuli within an homonymous scotoma from damage to the striate cortex. This "residual vision" differs from the nonconscious visual abilities in patients with true blindsight.

The dominant hypothesis in blindsight research is that the phenomenon represents residual function in a visual pathway parallel to the retino-geniculo-calcarine system. The initial candidate was a second system involving the superior colliculus, and indeed this remains so for investigators who report blindsight in hemidecorticate patients. However, remnant perception of pattern and motion are not easily explained on the basis of known tectal response properties, and these findings led to suggestions that tectal projections to the pulvinar may provide an indirect visual input to extrastriate cortex. This would require a pathologic adaptation of pulvinar function, because the visual responses in this thalamic nucleus normally derive solely from visual cortex. Moreover, the retino-tecto-pulvino-cortical relay can also be challenged because some patients with blindsight demonstrate perception of color in their blind hemifields, and tectal neurons lack color opponency. Another theory is that blindsight results from a projection

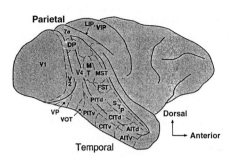

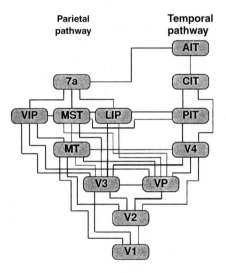

Figure 13.3. Parallel pathways for visual function in the cerebral cortex of the nonhuman primate. Borders between visual areas are indicated by fine dashed lines. The superior temporal sulcus has been opened to show areas that are normally out of sight. The medial hemisphere is not shown. The lower panel shows a flow diagram from area V1 (primary visual cortex) to the parietal pathway that includes area MT and the temporal pathway that includes area V4. The visual information encoded by neurons varies greatly among these different areas. The human brain is likely to respect a similar organization. *7a*, Brodmann's area 7a. *AIT*, anterior inferotemporal area (*d*, dorsal subdivision; *v*, ventral subdivision). *CIT*, central inferotemporal area (*d*, dorsal subdivision; *v*, ventral subdivision). *DP*, dorsal parietal area. *FST*, fundus of the superior temporal area. *LIP*, lateral intraparietal area. *MST*, medial superior temporal area. *MT*, middle temporal area. *PIT*, posterior inferotemporal area (*d*, dorsal subdivision; *v*, ventral subdivision). *STP*, superior temporal polysensory area. *V1*, visual area 1 (striate cortex). *V2*, visual area 2. *V4*, visual area 4. *VIP*, ventral intraparietal area. *VOT*, ventral occipitotemporal area. *VP*, ventral posterior area. (Reprinted with permission from Maunsell JHR. The brain's visual world: representation of visual targets in cerebral cortex. Science 1995;270:765–769.)

to extrastriate cortex from a few remnant lateral geniculate neurons that survive the retrograde degeneration after a striate lesion.

There are also explanations of blindsight that do not invoke parallel pathways. Remnant striate cortex is one possibility, especially given the difficulty of proving complete destruction without an autopsy. Of course, blindsight may simply reflect a testing phenomenon known as **criterion shift,** in which patients tend to use fairly conservative criteria when asked to respond Yes or No during a detection task but use more relaxed criteria when forced to choose an alternative (i.e., guess) in a discriminatory paradigm.

In conclusion, the existence of blindsight in both humans and nonhuman primates remains controversial. Demonstrations of blindsight require circumventing the need for a subject to assert that a stimulus is present, usually by means of forced-choice methods or by measuring localization accuracy for eye or hand movements. In addition, for the results to be meaningful, studies that attempt to determine if hemianopic patients have blindsight must eliminate all potential testing artifacts, including inadequate fixation, light scatter, nonvisual cues, and nonrandom presentation of targets.

Assuming these criticisms can be answered, an overview of blindsight studies offers three general points. First, visual discriminations in blind hemifields are less accurate and more variable than those in normal hemifields. Although there are some exceptional results in which blindsight is reported to equal that of normal vision, usually the residual ability does not appear to confer any benefit to affected individuals.

Second, the range of visual function demonstrated in patients with either blindsight or residual vision is impressive, including perception of spatial location and discrimination of form, orientation, color, and motion. No clear pattern of visual abilities that are preserved or destroyed has emerged in such patients. The variability in blindsight profiles may have an anatomic basis in the inevitable variability of naturally occurring human lesions. Most lesions of striate cortex also involve some extrastriate regions, but the degree and the areas affected differ from one patient to the next. Thus, the patterns of residual ability mirror the pattern of extrastriate sparing. In general, studies have not found a correlation between blindsight and lesion extent.

Third, not all patients with cortical field defects have blindsight. Why some patients have blindsight and others do not is unclear. Its presence or absence may reflect differences in lesion anatomy, but this is not proven. Unfortunately, this anatomy is too often incompletely documented. Another possibility is age at onset. Some studies have found that blindsight was present only in patients with hemianopia occurring in childhood, a period of presumably greater neural plasticity, but other studies have not confirmed this impression. A requirement for childhood onset is inconsistent with reports that training in older patients can lead to blindsight.

The existence of blindsight probably will be difficult to disprove without more detailed testing. It is not logically possible to conclusively prove a negative assertion (e.g., prove that elephants don't fly). Nevertheless, if blindsight exists, it is uncommon.

CEREBRAL ACHROMATOPSIA

Cerebral achromatopsia, also called central achromatopsia, is an uncommon defect of color perception caused by damage to the visual cortex. Some patients with this condition complain that colors look dull, wrong, or less bright, whereas others report that their world is completely colorless and that objects appear only in shades of gray, like in old black and white movies. Although the term "cerebral achromatopsia" is sometimes used to include all degrees of cerebral color deficits, we believe that this term is best reserved for the most severe cases and that the term **cerebral dyschromatopsia** should be used in cases where there is residual color sensation.

Either cerebral achromatopsia or cerebral dyschromatopsia may be a presenting symptom or may evolve during recovery from cortical blindness. The most common setting is vertebrobasilar ischemia affecting the posterior cerebral arterial blood supply to the occipital lobes. Other causes of achromatopsia include herpes simplex encephalitis, cerebral metastases, recurrent focal seizures, and dementia with visual cortical involvement. Transient achromatopsia may also occur as part of the aura of migraine.

ANATOMY

Anatomic and functional imaging studies indicate that color is processed by a large network of structures, including V1, V2, V3, V4 (the most emphasized), and IT. Nevertheless, the lesions causing cerebral achromatopsia are rather restricted and usually affect the ventromedial sectors of the occipital lobe in the lingual and fusiform gyri (Fig. 13.4). These findings are consistent with the results of positron emission tomographic (PET) scanning and functional MRIs, which show increased activity in these cerebral regions in normal individuals viewing color stimuli. Studies using three-dimensional MR localization show a strong association of cerebral achromatopsia with lesions in the middle third of the lingual gyrus, the white matter immediately behind the posterior tip of the lateral ventricle, or both. Neither lesions more anteriorly in areas 37, 20, or 21, nor lesions superior (dorsal) to the calcarine fissure in area 19 of the occipital lobe or in areas 5 and 7 of the superior parietal lobule appear to cause cerebral achromatopsia.

Both cerebral hemispheres possess the capacity to process color. Thus, full-field color loss requires bilateral lesions, either simultaneously or sequentially. Unilateral lesions of the left or right hemispheres can produce loss of color vision in the contralateral homonymous hemifields, a condition called **hemiachromatopsia** (or hemidyschromatopsia) (see Fig. 13.4). Suggestions of a right hemispheric dominance for color are unsupported.

ASSOCIATED DEFICITS

Common accompaniments of cerebral achromatopsia include superior homonymous quadrantanopia, visual agnosia, and acquired alexia. The **quadrantanopia** may be complete or incomplete; but in either case, the achromatopsia affects the remaining inferior quadrants of the visual fields on the side opposite the lesion (i.e., on the same side as the visual field defect). **Visual agnosia**—the inability to recognize previously familiar objects or to learn the identity of new objects by sight alone despite adequate visual sensory abilities—is also seen in patients with cerebral achromatopsia, particularly in patients with bilateral lesions. The syndrome in such patients includes **prosopagnosia,** in which the agnosic defect is most striking for faces; and **topographagnosia** or topographic disorientation, in which patients tend to get lost in familiar visual surroundings, partly because of an inability to recognize previously familiar local landmarks. Some patients have **pure alexia,** also known as

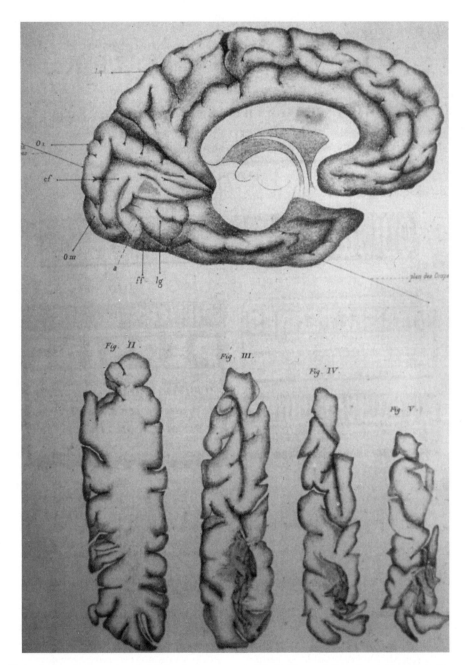

Figure 13.4. Lesions in a woman with right hemiachromatopsia. The lesions are located in areas 18 and 19 of the left ventromesial visual association cortex, in the middle portion of the fusiform and lingual gyri. (Reprinted with permission from Verrey, D. Hemiachromatopsie droite absolue. Arch Ophtalmol (Paris) 1988;8:289–301.)

alexia without agraphia, the acquired inability to read in previously literate individuals (see below). Defects of visual memory and even generalized amnesia can accompany cerebral achromatopsia, depending on the extent of the lesion into more anterior and mesial structures in the temporal lobes.

None of the aforementioned deficits—quadrantanopia, alexia, agnosia, or memory loss—is necessary or sufficient for the development of cerebral achromatopsia. Cerebral achromatopsia can occur without quadrantanopia and vice versa; color perception can be normal in patients with pure alexia; and dissociations of color perception and visual recognition occur in some cases of carbon monoxide poisoning.

COLOR PERCEPTION AND COLOR TESTING

What is the nature of color perception in cerebral achromatopsia? Color is not an inherent property of an object but rather a subjective sensation that depends on the reflectance of surfaces. The psychologic experience of color is synthesized in the brain from basic photoreceptor inputs and can be characterized along three main axes:

1. The first direction in chromatic space is the so-called **tritan axis,** along which the level of short-wavelength-sensitive (S or "blue") cone excitation varies with an unvarying ratio of long-wavelength–sensitive (L or "red") cone excitation to middle-wavelength–sensitive (M or "green") cone excitation.
2. The second direction in chromaticity space is the **red-green axis,** along which the ratio of L- and M-cone excitation varies at a fixed level of S-cone excitation.
3. The third direction is the **achromatic axis** along which the ratio of stimulation of the three cone types remains constant and the total flux varies.

By testing the residual vision of achromatopsic patients along S-cone, L-M, and achromatic axes, it should be possible to characterize the psychophysical impairments associated with the abnormal color experience in achromatopsic individuals.

Patients with full-field achromatopsia are rare, but their color deficits can be analyzed using the same standardized tests (e.g., color plate and arrangement tests) used to assess patients with hereditary impairments of retinal origin (see Chapter 1). The American Optical Hardy-Rand-Rittler pseudoisochromatic plates and the Standard Pseudoisochromatic Plates, part 2, employ plates made of colored circles of different size, hue, and lightness. Consistent differences from background by color alone define a target figure such as a letter, number, or shape. Their advantage over the Ishihara test is that they screen for blue-yellow (tritan) defects as well as red-green (deutan or protan) defects. Patients are asked to report the target figure in each plate. If they are unable to do so, they should be instructed to trace any perceived pattern with their finger to avoid mistaking an abnormal performance related to alexia or aphasia with a true color vision defect.

Color arrangement tests can also be performed in patients with suspected cerebral color vision deficits. These tests consist of color chips mounted on caps that can be arranged in a unique sequence. They vary in the number of chips, the degree of discrimination ability needed, and the sector of color space they probe. These tests include the Farnsworth D-15 Test, the Lanthony New Color Test, the Lightness Discrimination Test, and the Sahlgren Saturation Test. Another instrument designed to detect and diagnose color vision defects is the Nagel anomaloscope, which provides a matching test.

Hemifield color deficits can result from unilateral lesions of the right or left occipital lobes. Patients with such lesions may be asymptomatic unless the defect is demonstrated to them. When hemiachromatopsia is associated with a superior quadrantanopia, the color defect in that hemifield can only be demonstrated in the remaining inferior quadrants of the two eyes. These quadrantic color deficits may evolve during recovery from a dense homonymous hemianopia. Quantitative assessment of color processing in patients with partial field color deficits is a challenge, because the standard color tests used are designed for viewing within the central few degrees of vision. Tests have been developed using color patch matching off fixation.

Central achromatopsia encompasses a range of color processing impairments with varied psychophysical characteristics. In addition, color is only one of several surface and light source effects processed by the central nervous system. Other effects include transparency, specularity, iridescence, and fluorescence. The neural basis of these effects and whether they are processed in common or separately from hue is largely unexplored.

COLOR AND SHAPE

Not all color processing is necessarily lost in patients with cerebral achromatopsia, even in patients who report a world without hue. Photopic spectral sensitivity curves can show preserved trichromacy and color opponency, indicating function of the three cones and the retinal ganglion cells of the parvocellular pathway. Testing in patients who report the world in shades of gray, as a monochromat would, can instead suggest extremely anomalous trichromacy. Furthermore, severely affected achromatopsic observers who fail to identify colors or who order them incorrectly by hue, may still detect differences between isoluminant color patches, allowing them to resolve the chromatic borders in an image. Such ability may reflect residual opponent color processing in striate cortex.

The finding that perception of chromatic boundaries can be dissociated from the sensation of color suggests that chromatic information is processed in separate functional subdivisions. Whether or not shape-from-color is preserved in cerebral achromatopsia requires further study, as does the question of whether or not shape from color can be impaired in the absence of achromatopsia.

COLOR PERCEPTION, LANGUAGE, AND MEMORY

One should be cautious in interpreting the verbal report of a patient with cerebral achromatopsia, and also be wary of the results of tests that rely on verbal responses, such as color naming. Color naming can be a useful index of color processing in patients with normal perception and language; however, during tests of color sorting, matching, and on pseudo-isochromatic plates, brain-damaged patients with aphasia or color anomia may accurately discriminate, match, and recognize colors that they cannot name. They do not complain of impaired color perception and may not even be aware of naming difficulties. Conversely, color naming may actually remain normal in a color aberrant field because the million or so colors discriminable by

the visual system subtend no more than about a dozen categoric names in any language. Shifts of spectral sensitivity may alter color sensitivity but not enough to shift color percepts across the boundaries of differently named categories.

Assessment of color naming and associations can and should be conducted independently of color perception testing. This allows the best opportunity to distinguish cerebral achromatopsia and dyschromatopsia from color anomia, agnosia, and related defects of language and memory. First, color naming ability can be tested by asking patients to name saturated color objects, such as Munsell tokens. All patients with complete achromatopsia and color anomia should have difficulty performing this task, whereas patients with dyschromatopsia are sometimes able to perceive the hues in highly saturated colors and to name them appropriately.

Second, it is helpful to have patients attempt matching colors to objects. One such task requires patients to choose from among four different color patches which one is best suited to color a line-drawing of a familiar object (e.g., choosing among yellow, blue, pink, and green to color a drawing of a frog). Patients with anomia or aphasia should still be able to perform this task, but patients with achromatopsia and patients with visual agnosia should not be able to do so: achromatopsics will not perceive the proper color patch, and agnosics may not recognize the frog.

Third, having patients attempt to recall the color names of objects can be helpful. Patients can be asked to state the usual color names by completing short sentences spoken to them by the examiner, such as ''apples are ————,'' or ''grass is ————.'' Patients with cerebral achromatopsia or dyschromatopsia can perform this task, but not patients with color anomia, aphasia, or verbal memory impairments.

Note that the sentence ''apples are ————,'' can be completed using different strategies, depending on the patient's visual and verbal abilities. A congenitally blind person knows that an apple is red because of the frequent verbal associations in the language. This is a verbal-verbal response. A sighted person might conceivably resort to visual imagery to answer such a question, mentally picturing the named object and its color before producing the appropriate color name. This response is both visual and verbal.

On the other hand, the naming of colors in visually presented target objects can use a verbal-verbal strategy that relies neither upon color perception nor upon naming of colors. In this way, a patient with cerebral achromatopsia or color anomia may recognize a picture (or uncolored line drawing) of an apple and then give the appropriate color name, "red," through verbal association. Asking a patient to give the color name associated with a nonpicturable abstraction, such as cowardice (yellow) or envy (green), can maximize the chance of observing the operation of a verbal-verbal mechanism. Here, the responses may be quite variable, depending on the culture and experience of the individual.

A patient's visual imagery capacity also can be challenged by verbal means by asking patients to recall and name the colors of individual objects with which they are visually familiar, such as their own car, house, or cat. Such items are unlikely to have strong cultural verbal-verbal associations for color naming, in contrast to items like fire engines and bananas. To score the performance, the examiner must have access to a reliable external source, such as the patient's spouse.

Color anomia is often part of a more general anomia in aphasic patients, but there are instances in which color naming is disproportionately affected. These cases tend to occur with left occipital lesions and are associated with a complete right homonymous hemianopia, rather than just the upper quadrantanopia seen with cerebral achromatopsia. One possible mechanism in such cases is an interhemispheric disconnection syndrome associated with right homonymous hemianopia and pure alexia. Because of the complete right homonymous hemianopia, visual input to language areas in the left hemisphere must arise from the right visual cortex. However, a concurrent lesion of the splenium of the corpus callosum interrupts this process. Affected patients can perceive colors yet not name them (color anomia) and may also see letters but not be able to read them (pure alexia). Preserved tactile naming in such patients suggests preservation of callosal fibers anterior to those required for reading and color naming. Color anomia, together with pure alexia, can also occur without a callosal lesion when there is damage near the posterior aspect of the occipital

horn on the left, interrupting connections from both visual fields to language areas.

Color dysphasia is a syndrome related to color anomia. Affected patients not only fail to name the colors of visual objects, but they are also unable to produce the names of colors associated with the names of familiar objects spoken aloud to them, which might represent a dysphasic defect of the color lexicon.

PROSOPAGNOSIA AND RELATED DISTURBANCES OF OBJECT RECOGNITION

Visual agnosia is an inability to recognize familiar objects, despite adequate visual perception. In this condition, a patient cannot arrive at the meaning of some or all categories of previously known nonverbal stimuli, despite being alert, attentive, and having adequate intellect and language abilities.

Prosopagnosia is a restricted form of visual agnosia characterized by the impaired ability to recognize familiar faces or to learn to recognize new faces. It is a specific functional disorder with a specific neuroanatomic basis. Debate about its nature has centered on whether it is a disturbance of perception or memory. Prosopagnosia may actually cover a spectrum of deficits, with individual patients varying in the degree of perceptual versus memory dysfunction or even having disconnections between the two processes. Furthermore, abnormal face recognition may be part of more generalized perceptual, cognitive, or memory problems. We and others reserve the term "prosopagnosia" for cases in which the facial recognition deficit is disproportionately more severe than other associated deficits (Fig. 13.5).

SYMPTOMS

Patients with prosopagnosia are usually aware of their difficulty and complain of the social embarrassment of not recognizing acquaintances. When they do recognize others, it is often by reliance on specific facial features or paraphernalia (e.g., a hairstyle, glasses, beards and mustaches, a missing tooth, or a particular scar) that bypass the need for an overall analysis of the shape of the face. They may also use nonfacial visual cues, such as gait and posture, or nonvisual cues, such as voice. The context of the encounter is also important. For example, patients with

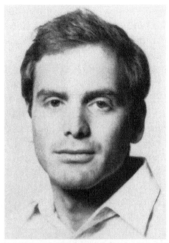
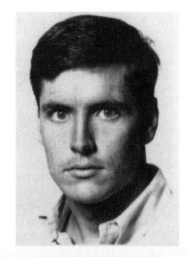
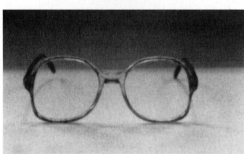
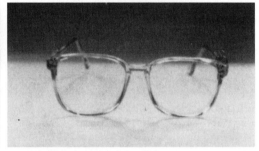

Figure 13.5. Matching the complexity of face and object recognition. Most tests of object recognition use stimuli that are much easier to distinguish from each other than are faces. To increase the level of difficulty in object recognition, one study asked patients to match pairs of glasses that differed in subtle individual details. Patients with prosopagnosia still had more trouble matching faces (*top*) than matching glasses (*bottom*), suggesting that the recognition defect is specific for faces. (Reprinted with permission from Farah MJ, Levinson KL, Klein KL. Face perception and within-category discrimination in prosopagnosia. Neuropsychologia 1995; 33:661–674.)

prosopagnosia may be able to recognize hospital staff but are unable to recognize the same persons when they meet them later on the street. Persons with childhood onset of prosopagnosia and, occasionally, persons with onset in adulthood may be ignorant of their deficit. The ability to use nonfacial cues to identify people distinguishes prosopagnosia from a bizarre person-specific amnesia, in which recognition is reportedly impaired, irrespective of the sensory cue.

Despite abnormal recognition of familiar faces, many patients with prosopagnosia can accurately discriminate among unfamiliar faces, even with varying lighting conditions or facial views (i.e., Benton Facial Recognition Test). However, patients with prosopagnosia may require much more time than normal to arrive at correct judgments, suggesting that they use an inefficient and abnormal route for processing face information.

Some individuals with prosopagnosia can judge the age, gender, and emotional expression of faces they cannot recognize, and some even lip-read. Again, prosopagnosics may use different perceptual processes from those used by normal individuals to make such judgments. For example, a patient with prosopagnosia might rely on wrinkles to tell age, whereas normal individuals can still make age judgments in the absence of such local features. Other prosopagnosic patients, usually those with more pervasive perceptual dysfunction, are impaired with respect to judgments about facial age, sex, emotional expression, and the direction of the person's gaze, the last item being an important social signal.

An important theoretical issue is whether the prosopagnosic defect is specific for faces or also affects perception of other objects. Some patients have difficulty distinguishing types of objects, such as makes of cars, flowers, food, and coins. They also have trouble identifying previously familiar items, such as buildings, handwriting, and personal belongings or clothing. These cases imply that in prosopagnosia, impaired facial recognition may simply be the most prominent manifestation of a more general recognition or perceptual problem. On the other hand, some patients can distinguish nonface objects relatively well despite severe prosopagnosia. Specific tests of face versus object recognition appear to confirm this dissociation (see Fig. 13.5).

Although patients with prosopagnosia deny familiarity with and cannot identify known faces, some patients retain covert (i.e., nonconscious) recognition of these faces at a variety of levels. Investigators have shown two main phenomena: **covert familiarity,** in which the patient is able to distinguish previously familiar but unrecognized faces from completely unknown faces, and **covert semantic knowledge,** in which the patient retains information about name, occupation, and other facts associated with a face.

Patients with prosopagnosia usually have difficulty recognizing faces of people with whom they were familiar before the start of the illness (retrograde prosopagnosia) as well as people whom they meet after the onset of the condition (anterograde prosopagnosia). Some patients have slightly better recognition of people long known to them, whereas others have only anterograde prosopagnosia.

FORMS OF PROSOPAGNOSIA

Prosopagnosia historically has been segregated into two main forms: apperceptive and associative (dysmnesic).

Apperceptive prosopagnosia may be caused by a generalized defect in configurational analysis, manifest most strikingly in the structural encoding of faces. These patients have abnormal perception of facial expression, sex, and age, and they also perform poorly on tests of facial matching. The apperceptive trouble extends to other categories of objects like cars, animals, and inanimate objects and is marked for unusual perspectives. The faulty perception does not allow partial activation of personal memories, so covert processing is not expected.

Patients with **associative prosopagnosia** have normal configural processing and face perception, allowing normal judgment of expression, sex, and age, lip-reading, and normal matching performance on the Benton Facial Recognition Test. Covert processing is possible if the activation of memories by the facial recognition units is only partly damaged. Although the defect may not be face-specific, it can appear more so than in the apperceptive form.

The distinctions between apperceptive and associative forms of prosopagnosia described above require caution. There is overlap in these syndromes, and perceptual testing must be accurately controlled. Furthermore, there are as yet no clear anatomic distinctions between the lesions of apperceptive and amnestic forms of prosopagnosia. Indeed, current concepts hold that perception, mental imagery, and modality-specific memory rely on the same neural structures. Pure apperceptive and pure dysmnesic types of prosopagnosia would be unlikely, although elements of one type may predominate.

ASSOCIATED DEFICITS

Almost all patients with prosopagnosia have other visual deficits. Visual field defects are frequent, the most common being left homonymous hemianopia, left superior homonymous quadrantanopia, bilateral superior quadrantanopia, or combinations of these. Visual acuity is uncommonly reduced, and spatial contrast sensitivity may be impaired. The visual field defect, achromatopsia or hemiachromatopsia, and topographagnosia often form a common tetrad with prosopagnosia. Nevertheless, cases of prosopagnosia associated with normal color vision exist, showing that prosopagnosia and achromatopsia are dissociable. Visual object agnosia is said to be absent in some patients with prosopagnosia and present though proportionately milder in others.

A frequent finding in patients with prosopagnosia is impaired visual memory. In some of these patients, the memory deficit also affects verbal material. Other patients with prosopagnosia also have simultanagnosia, palinopsia, visual hallucinations, constructional difficulties, and left hemineglect. Hemisensory deficits or hemiparesis occur in some patients with unilateral right-sided lesions, although in some of these cases, the motor and sensory findings are related to other lesions. Pure alexia (see below) can occur in some patients with prosopagnosia.

ANATOMY AND ETIOLOGIES

In most cases of prosopagnosia, the lesion is in the inferior temporo-occipital cortex, usually in the lingual and fusiform gyri (Fig. 13.6). In occasional cases, the lesion appears to be located in the more anterior temporal cortex.

All autopsied cases of prosopagnosia have **bilateral** lesions. Indeed, studies of split-brain patients suggest the existence of mechanisms for facial recognition in each hemisphere. Lack of prosopagnosia following right hemispherectomy has the same implications. Neuroimaging has confirmed bilateral lesions in many cases with CT scanning, MRI, and PET scanning. The bilateral lesions in prosopagnosia are often symmetric, presumably affecting homologous regions of both hemispheres (see Fig. 13.6). However, the position of the left-sided lesion can be more variable. A left-sided hemisphere lesion or a lesion of the splenium of the corpus callosum might disconnect a right hemispheric locus for facial recognition from visual input of the right hemifield, with critical effects in cases with left homonymous hemianopia. Furthermore, reports of neuroimaging showing apparently unilateral right temporo-occipital lesions have accumu-

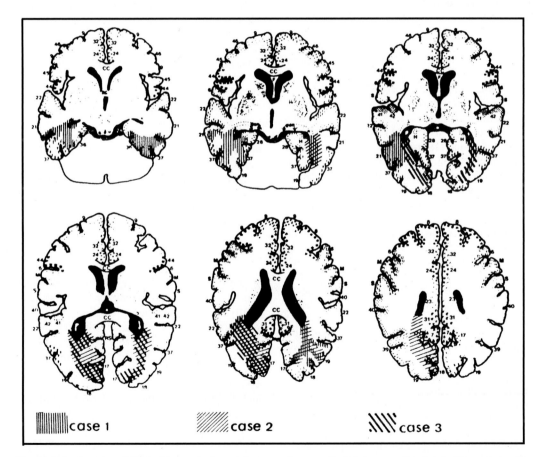

Figure 13.6.   Location of bilateral lesions in three patients with prosopagnosia. Axial template drawings with shaded areas representing the lesions of three patients with prosopagnosia. Bilateral damage, greater on the left than the right, is present in all three cases. (Reprinted with permission from Damasio AR, Damasio H, van Hoesen GW. Prosopagnosia: anatomic basis and behavioral mechanisms. Neurology 1982;32:331–341.)

lated. Indeed, there is mounting evidence that prosopagnosia can occur from a right-sided lesion of the fusiform gyrus.

The type of face perception deficits caused by unilateral as opposed to bilateral cerebral lesions may differ. It has been suggested that apperceptive types of prosopagnosia occur with damage to right ventral and dorsal temporo-occipital areas, whereas bilateral ventral temporo-occipital lesions result in an associative or dysmnesic form. Given the role of the right hemisphere in face perception, it is puzzling why prosopagnosia is not more commonly seen with right posterior cerebral artery infarcts. Possible compensation by the left hemisphere may occur.

The most common lesions causing prosopagnosia are posterior cerebral artery infarctions and, less often, viral encephalitis. The predominance of these conditions may be related to their potential to inflict bilateral damage, although the neuroimaging in some cases shows only a unilateral lesion. Other unilateral lesions, such as tumors, hematomas, abscesses, and surgical resections, are less frequently reported to cause prosopagnosia.

Impaired facial recognition can occur as part of the generalized dementia in Alzheimer's disease, in Parkinson's disease, and rarely in elderly patients with bilateral or unilateral right temporal lobar degeneration. The last disorder is one of the focal progressive atrophies, others of which affect the frontal, parietal, or left temporal lobes. These degenerative conditions have an uncertain relation to Alzheimer's and Pick's diseases.

Developmental prosopagnosia also has been described. Patients with this condition usually are not aware that they have problems with face recognition until they experience social difficulties related to the impairment. In addition to problems with facial recognition, these patients have difficulty judging facial age, sex, and expressions. They also perform facial matching tasks very slowly, suggesting a perceptual process differing from normal. In some cases, developmental prosopagnosia is present in other family members, possibly as an autosomal-dominant trait, and coexists with the Asperger syndrome of autism. The prevalence of prosopagnosia among all autistic individuals is unknown, as are the effects of the face perception disorder on other aspects of psychosocial development.

ACQUIRED ALEXIA

Acquired alexia is the loss of efficient reading for comprehension, despite adequate visual acuity. Reading is a complex behavior involving perception of form, spatial attention, ocular fixation, scanning saccadic eye movements, and linguistic processing. Not surprisingly, many types of cerebral or visual dysfunction can disrupt the reading process. Although other clinical signs may overshadow the difficulty, impaired reading is sometimes the chief complaint. The severity of reading difficulty can range from a mild defect with slow reading and occasional errors, which may only be identified by comparison with normal controls matched for educational level, to a complete inability to read even numbers and letters. Analysis of not only the severity but also the type of reading errors can help differentiate among the various forms of reading impairment and their causes.

Note that the term ''alexia'' implies a complete inability to read. The term ''dyslexia'' is more appropriate in persons who have preservation of aspects of reading. Unfortunately, dyslexia is also used to describe developmental reading impairments, creating potential confusion. In this chapter, we use the term ''dyslexia'' only when describing *acquired* reading impairments of cerebral origin.

Most syndromes of alexia can be explained by the disconnectionist theories. The left angular gyrus stores the visual representation of words necessary for reading and writing. Therefore, disconnecting the visual inputs of both hemispheres from the left angular gyrus could disrupt reading but leave writing intact—that is, pure alexia.

PURE ALEXIA (WORD BLINDNESS, ALEXIA WITHOUT AGRAPHIA)

The key feature of **pure alexia** is a dramatic dissociation between the ability to read and the ability to write. Patients with this condition can write fluently and spontaneously, but having done so are unable to read what they have just written. The severity varies from a slow, laborious reading of words one letter at a time (letter-by-letter reading; spelling alexia) to complete inability to read words or letters (global alexia) and sometimes even numbers or other symbols. In the milder version of spelling alexia, the letter-by-letter reading strategy is revealed by a word-length effect, in which the time to read a word characteristically increases with the number of letters in the word. In Japanese, which has two different writing systems, a phonetically based form (kana) and a nonphonetic ideographic form (kanji), alexia is manifest as impaired reading of kanji but preserved reading of kana, presumably representing the equivalent of letter-by-letter reading with European languages.

Associated signs with pure alexia are common. There is often a right homonymous field defect, usually a complete homonymous hemianopia but sometimes only a superior quadrantanopia, in which case there may also be a right hemiachromatopsia. Pure alexia cannot be attributed to the field defect, however, because pure alexia can occur without a field defect, and many patients with a right homonymous hemianopia that splits (i.e., does not spare) the macula do not have pure alexia. Although associated dyschromatopsia is generally restricted to the right homonymous hemifield, naming of colors in the whole field may be abnormal. Naming problems can also extend to other visual objects and photographs. Anomia is not necessarily restricted to the visual modality but can include objects perceived by touch, implying some nonvisual language disturbance from extension of the lesion outside the visual association cortex. Verbal memory deficits and visual agnosia can occur. Some authors describe a form of optic ataxia (see below) in which the dominant right hand has difficulty with purposeful movements to objects in the nondominant left visual field.

Covert reading ability can be detected in at least some patients with pure alexia. These patients have aspects of preserved reading ability of which they are not aware. Some patients can indicate whether a string of letters forms a word (lexical decision task). This ability varies with linguistic features, such as the frequency of the word in daily usage, the amount of visual imagery evoked by the word, and the grammatic category of the word, with better performance for nouns. Covert comprehension of word meaning also occurs in some patients with pure alexia. Such patients can categorize words semantically (e.g., indicate which are animals or foods) or match words to objects or pictures.

Lesions causing pure alexia are almost always located in the left hemisphere, most commonly in the medial and inferior temporo-occipital region (Fig. 13.7). The majority are caused by infarction within the vascular territory of the left posterior cerebral artery, but other causes include primary and metastatic tumors, arteriovenous malformations, hemorrhage, herpes sim-

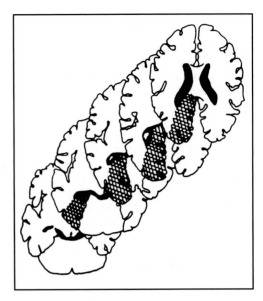

Figure 13.7. Location of lesions causing pure alexia, right homonymous hemianopia, and color dysnomia. Template drawings of axial CT images, combined from five patients, show lesions affecting the left medial and lateral occipital lobes, medial temporo-occipital lobe and paraventricular white matter, and forceps major, sometimes extending into the splenium proper. (Reprinted with permission from Damasio AR, Damasio H. The anatomic basis of pure alexia. Neurology 1983;33:1573–1583.)

plex, encephalitis, and a rare focal posterior cortical dementia.

One popular explanation of pure alexia is that it is a disconnection of visual information from linguistic processing centers (see Fig. 13.7). Visual information from the right hemifield is either absent in cases with right hemianopia, or it is interrupted in its course through left extrastriate centers to the reading center in the left angular gyrus. Callosal pathways transmitting visual information from visual association cortex of the right hemisphere to homologous regions in the left hemisphere are interrupted by a lesion in the splenium, forceps major, or periventricular white matter surrounding the occipital horn of the lateral ventricle. Thus, words in the left hemifield also cannot access the left angular gyrus. Similarly, other visual information is isolated, causing the associated anomia for colors and objects.

Pure alexia without an homonymous hemianopia occurs in some patients with lesions of the white matter underlying the angular gyrus. Such "subangular" lesions presumably disconnect the input from both hemispheres to the angular gyrus very distally. This phenomenon suggests to some authors that the right hemispheric callosal fibers travel in the white matter ventral to the occipital horn. Others speculate that some callosal fibers travel dorsal to the occipital horn, and that these are preserved in letter-by-letter or spelling alexia, which they consider a partial form of pure alexia, but are destroyed in global alexia, which they consider the complete form.

Although some cases of pure alexia may be a visual agnosia from left extrastriate damage, at least some cases do represent a true visual-verbal disconnection. The best evidence for disconnection comes from cases of pure alexia with atypical lesions. For example, pure alexia can occur with the combination of a splenial lesion and a left geniculate nuclear lesion causing a right homonymous hemianopia; there is no damage to striate or extrastriate cortex in such patients. These cases demonstrate that disconnection is sufficient to cause pure alexia.

The disconnection hypothesis involves two deafferentations of the left angular gyrus: the disconnection of right-hemisphere vision and the disconnection or destruction of left-hemisphere vision. Each of these can occur independently and is called a **hemi-alexia.** In left hemi-alexia, reading is impaired in the left hemifield only, because of isolated damage to the posterior corpus callosum or callosal fibers elsewhere. Right hemi-alexia occurs when a lesion of the left medial and ventral occipital lobe spares other visual functions in the right field.

Left **hemiparalexia** is a rare syndrome attributed to damage to the splenium of the corpus callosum. The reading pattern in patients with this condition is similar to that in patients with left hemineglect, in that substitution and omission errors occur for the first letter of words. However, these patients do not have evidence of hemineglect, and although patients with left hemineglect usually have a right hemispheric lesion and an associated left homonymous hemianopia, some of the patients with left hemiparalexia have left occipital lesions and a right homonymous hemianopia (Fig. 13.8). Patients with left hemiparalexia may have other signs of callosal disconnection, such as inability to name objects felt by the nondominant (left) hand, left-hand agraphia, and inability to duplicate the unseen movements of one hand by the other.

ALEXIA WITH AGRAPHIA

A combination of impaired reading and writing constitutes **alexia with agraphia.** This syn-

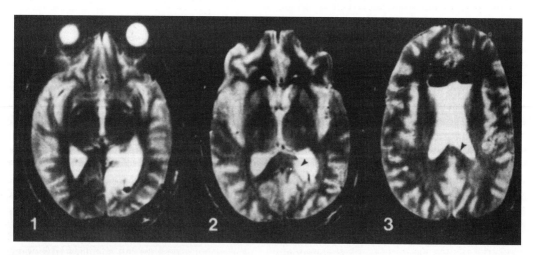

Figure 13.8. Neuroimaging in a patient with left hemiparalexia. *1–3.* Axial T2-weighted MRI at three successive levels from a 40-year-old woman who underwent embolization of a left medial parieto-occipital arteriovenous malformation. After the procedure, she had a right homonymous hemianopia, left unilateral tactile dysnomia, and alien hand syndrome on the left. During reading, she missed the letters on the left side of words, even though she had an intact left homonymous hemifield and no left hemineglect. The images show changes consistent with infarction in the left ventral-caudal splenium (*arrowhead,* level 2) and medial occipital lobe (levels 1 and 2), with sparing of the rostral splenium (*arrowhead,* level 3). (Reprinted with permission from Binder JR, Lazar RM, Tatemichi TK, et al. Left hemiparalexia. Neurology 1992;42:562–569.)

drome usually is associated with lesions of the left angular gyrus, although lesions of the adjacent temporoparietal junction have also been implicated. In patients with left parietal lesions, alexia with agraphia may be accompanied by acalculia, right-left disorientation, and finger agnosia, the other elements of **Gerstmann's syndrome.** In some rare cases, there is relative preservation of oral and auditory language functions, although more often there are other elements of aphasia.

Another form of alexia and agraphia is described as an accompaniment of Broca's aphasia (nonfluent aphasia), which is caused by lesions of the dominant (left) inferior frontal lobe. These patients have difficulty reading aloud and writing, attributable to their problems with all forms of expressive language output. However, comprehension of text is also often impaired in such patients, despite relatively preserved comprehension of auditory language. In contrast with the letter-by-letter reading in pure alexia, these patients are better at occasionally grasping a whole word, even though they are unable to name the letters of the word. Thus, this type of alexia with agraphia sometimes is called **literal alexia** or ''letter blindness.'' These patients also have impaired comprehension of syntactic structure, just as their speech output often demonstrates a significant impairment of syntax called **agrammatism.** The underlying mechanism is unknown. Gaze paresis and difficulty in maintaining verbal sequences have been proposed but not proven. It may be that this frontal alexia is a variant of deep dyslexia, a type of central dyslexia (see below).

DYSLEXIA RELATED TO ABNORMAL VISION, ATTENTION, OR EYE MOVEMENT

Some patients with visual field defects have reading problems despite normal or near normal visual acuity. In particular, patients with complete homonymous hemianopia may have significant difficulty reading. Such patients are said to have **hemianopic dyslexia.** This condition mainly occurs when the field defect affects parafoveal vision and is more often evident in the acute aftermath of the hemianopia. With languages written from left to right, patients with a left homonymous hemianopia may encounter trouble when they reach the end of one line and try to find the beginning of the next line, because the left margin disappears into the scotoma as

they scan rightward. Marking their place with an L-shaped ruler can reduce this frustrating difficulty. A right homonymous hemianopia prolongs reading times, causing prolonged fixation and reduced amplitude of reading saccades to the right. A complete bitemporal hemianopia or a dense bitemporal hemianopic scotoma from damage to the optic chiasm can cause the **hemifield slide phenomenon.** With only nasal hemifields left, there is no region of the visual field that has binocular representation. Patients with a preexisting heterophoria thus have no opportunity for binocular fusion, and the heterophoria becomes a heterotropia (see Chapter 12). A similar phenomenon can occur in patients who develop a complete superior altitudinal defect in the visual field of one eye and a complete inferior altitudinal defect in the other from a bilateral retinopathy or, more often, a bilateral optic neuropathy. Patients with the hemifield slide phenomenon experience double vision. During reading, they may note duplication or disappearance of letters at the vertical meridian because of transient eso- or exodeviation, or lines of text may merge erroneously across the vertical meridian when there is a vertical tropia, causing confusion.

Disturbances of attention can also cause a number of so-called peripheral dyslexias. Simultanagnosia, in which perception of single items is adequate but perception of several objects simultaneously is impaired, has been implicated in **attentional dyslexia.** Patients with this condition read single words normally but not several words together. They also identify single letters but not the letters in a word. Their reading may show literal migration errors, in which a letter from one word is substituted at the same place in an adjacent word (e.g., LONG TURN becomes TONG TURN or LONG LURN), and letters of similar appearance are more likely to be confused (e.g.,. G for C or E for F). Attentional dyslexia occurs from lesions in the left temporooccipital junction and the left parietal lobe. Its diagnosis rests upon the difference between reading of single versus multiple words and the presence of simultanagnosia for other visual items besides words.

Left hemineglect is an attentional deficit that causes **neglect dyslexia,** a condition characterized by left-sided reading errors. This can occur for a whole text, so that the reader misses the left side of an entire line or page, or with individual words, so that the reader makes omissions (FLAME becomes LAME), additions (ACT becomes TACT), or substitutions (TONE becomes BONE) at the beginning. These defects are specific for left hemispace rather than word beginnings; such errors do not occur for vertically printed words. Many patients with left hemineglect also have a left homonymous hemianopia. The underlying lesion is often in the right parietal lobe, although right frontal and subcortical lesions can also cause hemineglect. The diagnosis of left hemineglect is made by the recognition that mistakes are restricted to the left side of words or text. Associated hemineglect for nonverbal material is usually present, but neglect dyslexia dissociated from other manifestations of hemineglect can occur.

Abnormalities of ocular fixation and scanning saccades may impair reading. Most cortical lesions are single and unilateral and tend to cause fairly subtle saccadic abnormalities if any; however, bilateral frontal or parietal lesions can cause an acquired ocular apraxia, in which the ability to make voluntary saccades to targets is disrupted. As a result, the scanning of a scene is abnormal, and reading is consequently impaired. Although the saccadic abnormality is blamed for the dyslexia by some authors, simultanagnosia may contribute to the saccadic abnormality in patients with biparietal lesions, and the reading disturbance may be an attentional dyslexia (see below). Severe and enduring saccadic and fixation dysfunction can also occur with brainstem lesions. Reading difficulties from such lesions have not been well studied, but it has been reported, for example, that progressive supranuclear palsy causes difficulty reading, a problem that some authors attribute to the disruption of fixation by square-wave jerks and the disruption of scanning by hypometric and slow saccades. Our own experience is that convergence insufficiency is responsible for most of the problems with reading experienced by patients with progressive supranuclear palsy as well as by patients with Parkinson's disease.

CENTRAL DYSLEXIAS

Subtle acquired dyslexic deficits occur in addition to the more overt disturbances described above. Many of these deficits occur in association with other aphasic features and thus could be classified as aphasic alexias; however, they can occasionally occur as isolated deficits. The reading defects are sometimes labeled **central dyslexias,** because they reflect dysfunction of central reading processes rather than "peripheral" attention or visual deficits.

Central dyslexias are defined in terms of reading models derived from cognitive neuropsychology. One of the main concepts involved is that of parallel information processing in reading. The perception of visual features and the abstraction of letter identity are controlled by at least two distinct modes of processing. One route is a direct phonologic process, in which the units of a letter string are converted into units of sound (grapheme-phoneme correspondence) using the generic pronunciation rules of a given language. These components are then assembled into the pronounced whole word, identified in an internal dictionary of word sounds (phonologic lexicon), and linked to information about word meaning in a semantic lexicon. Another route is an indirect lexical process, in which the whole word is perceived and identified in an internal dictionary of written words (orthographic lexicon). When the correct word-form is activated, a corresponding entry in the semantic lexicon is also activated, leading in turn to access to the phonologic lexicon and the pronunciation of the word.

Surface dyslexia occurs from disruption of the indirect lexical reading process. Word recognition is critical for pronunciation of words with irregular spelling (e.g., LOSE vs. HOSE). Because they lack the ability to access an internal semantic dictionary, patients with surface dyslexia are dependent on the grapheme-phoneme rules that usually apply but that fail with irregularly spelled words. Thus, these patients correctly read regularly spelled words but consistently mispronounce irregular words. Anatomic data suggest that surface dyslexia can be caused by focal lesions of the posterior superior or middle temporal gyri of the left hemisphere. Surface dyslexia also occurs in patients with Alzheimer's disease.

The converse of surface dyslexia is **phonologic dyslexia.** Patients with this condition do not have access to grapheme-phoneme correspondence rules for pronunciation. Thus, they can only pronounce words that already have entries in their internal semantic dictionary. They easily pronounce real words, whether regular or irregular in spelling, but their ability to read nonwords or pseudowords is severely impaired.

Their reliance on whole-word processing rather than component or letter processing is revealed by good performance in reading handwriting but an inability to read words printed backwards.

Deep dyslexia resembles phonologic dyslexia in that it is characterized by an inability to pronounce nonwords because of damage to the phonologic route; however, patients with deep dyslexia also make semantic paralexic errors with familiar words, characteristically substituting words with a similar meaning for the correct one (e.g., JET for PLANE). Errors are more likely with function words (e.g., AND or WHETHER) than with verbs or nouns, and with abstract words as opposed to concrete words. Thus, it is thought that deep dyslexia may represent damage to both the direct and indirect reading routes. The association of deep dyslexia with extensive left hemisphere damage supports the concept that deep dyslexia represents remnant reading ability of the right hemisphere.

ASSESSMENT

Reading can be assessed in the office or clinic by having the patient scan any readily available material, such as a magazine or book. It is also important to have patients write a sentence spontaneously. Inability to write a sentence (not explained by paresis or incoordination) precludes a diagnosis of pure alexia and suggests the possibility of a more pervasive language disturbance. For example, patients with aphasia may have alexia with agraphia.

There are also standardized tools available for formal assessment of reading. The Chapman-Cook Speed of Reading Test requires the reading of brief paragraphs. The patient must cross out the word that spoils the meaning of the paragraph. The Wide Range Achievement Test (Wilmington, DE) requires reading aloud words of increasing difficulty until the patient makes a string of errors, at which time the test is halted.

Premorbid intellectual ability and intellect must always be considered in determinations of alexia. Most Americans can read, but they vary widely in this ability. Pure alexia can easily be distinguished from more pervasive language deficits by neuropsychologic testing (e.g., on the Boston Diagnostic Aphasia Examination [BDAE] or the Multilingual Aphasia Examination).

Evaluation of alexia should include a reading comprehension test, independent of verbal response (e.g., BDAE Reading Sentences and Paragraphs with a pointing response). A common error in the diagnosis of alexia is using only an oral reading test and confusing an impairment in verbal output with a defect in reading comprehension. Just because a person is mute does not mean he or she cannot read. Conversely, a patient may read aloud quite well and yet understand very little of what is read. The development and selection of appropriate tools for assessing the pattern of errors in central dyslexia requires linguistic expertise.

Finally, caution should be used in administering certain standardized tests of visual function to patients with alexia, because the results can be misleading. For example, testing visual acuity in patients with alexia who cannot read single letters should rely on simplified test forms (e.g., the directional "E's" of the Snellen Chart). Similarly, the diagnosis of color impairment in an alexic should not be based only upon failure to read the symbols on color plate tests. Such a patient should be asked to trace the symbols with a finger or to try to match colors in a nonverbal manner (e.g., using Farnsworth Panel D-15 or Farnsworth-Munsell 100-Hues tests).

DISORDERS OF MOTION PERCEPTION (CEREBRAL AKINETOPSIA)

Akinetopsia (cerebral akinetopsia) is the term used to describe complete loss of movement perception from an acquired cerebral lesion. Although akinetopsia requires bilateral cerebral lesions, subtle and generally asymptomatic disturbances of motion perception can occur with unilateral cerebral lesions.

Motion perception plays many roles in vision. One is the perception of moving objects in the environment. Because objects usually occupy only a small part of the visual field, their perception is facilitated by comparing their motion with that of the background. Object motion guides limb-reaching movements and smooth-pursuit eye movements, and it influences saccadic accuracy. In addition to object motion, information about self-motion can be obtained from motion perception. As the observer moves or turns the head or eyes, the image of the entire visual environment moves in the opposite direction. Thus, motion of large portions of the visual field usually implies self-motion rather than motion of an external object. This large-field motion generates optokinetic responses that complement the vestibulo-ocular reflex in stabilizing sight during head- or self-motion. Information about object identity is also available from visual motion. For example, the difference in motion between a figure and its background reveals two-dimensional shape, and the pattern of velocity gradients within a moving object encodes its three-dimensional form.

There are few clinical tests of motion perception. Smooth pursuit and optokinetic nystagmus can be observed and measured, but only indirect conclusions about the underlying state of motion perception can be made from these. More definitive tests of motion perception—such as animated displays of moving dots (random-dot cinematograms) or moving gratings—can be designed to probe discrimination of motion direction, motion speed, the presence of a motion boundary, and forms defined by motion, but

these are still experimental tools and are not widely used in the clinical setting.

MANIFESTATIONS

Cerebral akinetopsia appears to require bilateral lesions affecting the lateral temporo-occipital cortex. Only two cases of cerebral akinetopsia have been well described. One patient complained of no sensation of motion in depth or of rapid motion. Rapidly moving objects appeared to "jump" rather than move. On testing, predictions of target trajectories were impaired at faster speeds, as was smooth pursuit, although a moving tactile target could be pursued. The perception of differences in temporal frequency or speed of gratings was also impaired, and the minimum and maximum displacements needed to distinguish motion direction were abnormal. This patient could still distinguish moving from stationary stimuli, but her reaction times were

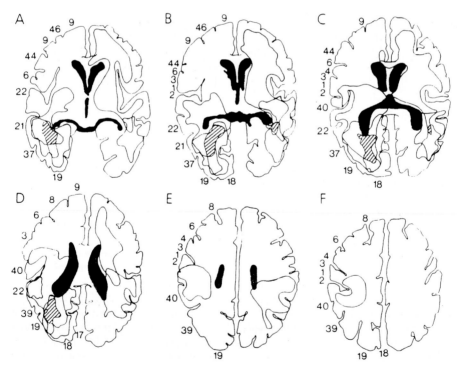

Figure 13.9. Impaired central perception of motion-defined form. *A–F.* Axial template drawings from CT scans, showing the outlines of the lesions of seven patients who had abnormal speed thresholds for recognizing letters whose boundaries were defined by differences in motion from the background. Ventricles are black, and hatched areas indicate overlap between three or more patients. Numbers indicate Brodmann areas of the right hemisphere. (Reprinted with permission from Regan D, Giaschi D, Sharpe JA, et al. Visual processing of motion-defined form: selective failure in patients with parietotemporal lesions. J Neurosci 1992;12: 2198–2210.)

slow. During testing with random-dot cinematograms, small amounts of random motion (noise) or even stationary dots degraded performance. The use of motion cues for other tasks was also impaired in this patient.

The other patient had somewhat similar deficits. His ability to discriminate differences in speed was severely impaired, and discrimination of direction in random dot cinematograms with background noise was abnormal. Smooth pursuit appeared impaired. This patient could not use relative speed differences to perceive two-dimensional forms. In contrast to the first patient, he could use motion cues to discern three-dimensional forms, and he also recognized shapes from biologic motion.

Unilateral lesions of extrastriate cortex cause more subtle abnormalities of motion perception than cerebral akinetopsia. There are reports of contralateral hemifield defects for speed dis-

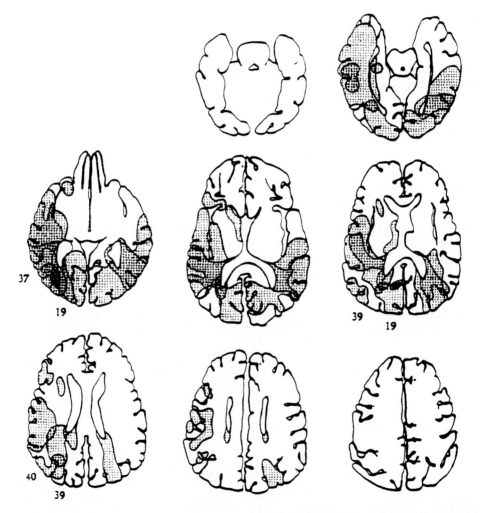

Figure 13.10. Abnormal central motion direction discrimination. Axial template drawings from CT or MRI scans, showing lesions (stippled areas) of six patients with abnormal signal-to-noise thresholds for the discrimination of motion direction in foveally presented displays. In most, the defect affected motion primarily toward the side of the lesion. Numbers indicate Brodmann areas. Areas of denser stippling indicate greater overlap, with the highest density at the junction of Brodmann areas 19 and 37. (Reprinted with permission from Barton JJS, Raymond J, Sharpe JA. Retinotopic and directional defects in motion direction discrimination after human cerebral lesions. Ann Neurol 1995; 37:665–675.)

crimination, for detection of boundaries between regions with different motion, and for discrimination of direction from backgrounds of motion noise (Figs. 13.9 and 13.10). As is the case in patients with cerebral akinetopsia, patients with these deficits have normal motion detection and contrast thresholds for motion direction, and their lesions are also located in lateral temporo-occipital cortex or the inferior parietal lobule, but only on one side of the brain. **Hemiakinetopsia** may not be commonly detected because of masking of the motion-perception deficits by an homonymous hemianopia caused by damage to the optic radiations or striate cortex.

Abnormalities in central motion perception also occur with unilateral lesions. Patients with right- or left-sided lesions may have defects in detecting or recognizing two-dimensional structures from motion cues and may have abnormal direction discrimination, especially for motion toward the side of the lesion (see Fig. 13.10).

ASSOCIATED DEFICITS

Patients with motion perception deficits may have other abnormalities caused by lesions of the lateral temporo-occipital area. The first patient with cerebral akinetopsia described above had remarkably normal psychophysical testing, including extensive perimetry, but her perception of form was abnormal, and she had an impaired ability to use cues from texture, dynamic

stereopsis, or static density to determine form. The other patient had a left incomplete homonymous hemianopia with some sparing in the superior quadrant. He was poor at recognizing objects in noncanonic (unusual) views and in incomplete outline drawings. Tests of spatial vision, such as hyperacuity, line orientation, line bisection, and spatial location, also gave abnormal results, as did tests of stereopsis.

ANATOMY

The first patient described above had experienced a superior sagittal sinus thrombosis that caused bilateral infarctions involving the lateral aspects of Brodmann areas 18, 19, and 39 (lateral occipital, middle temporal, and angular gyri) (Figs. 13.11 and 13.12). The second patient had experienced an acute hypertensive hemorrhage and also had bilateral lesions in the lateral temporo-occipital regions (Fig. 13.13). Most of the patients with more subtle abnormalities of motion perception caused by unilateral lesions have predominantly vascular lesions in the right more than left temporo-occipital or parieto-occipital regions. There is also some evidence that lesions of the cerebellum adversely affect the perception of motion.

PET scanning studies performed in normal humans during motion perception show activation in the lateral occipital gyri at the junction of Brodmann areas 19 and 37. This motion-selec-

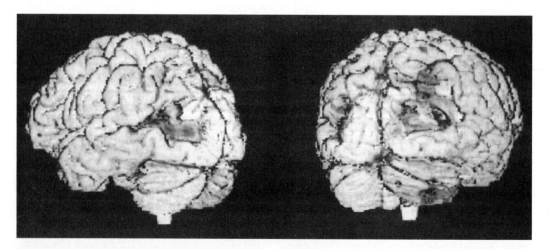

Figure 13.11. Three-dimensional MRI reconstruction of bilateral temporo-occipital lesions of patient L.M., who developed cerebral akinetopsia associated with a sagittal sinus thrombosis. *Left:* View of left posterior brain. *Right:* View of right posterior brain. (Reprinted with permission from Shipp S, de Jong BM, Zihl J, et al. The brain activity related to residual motion vision in a patient with bilateral lesions of V5. Brain 1994;117:1023–1038.)

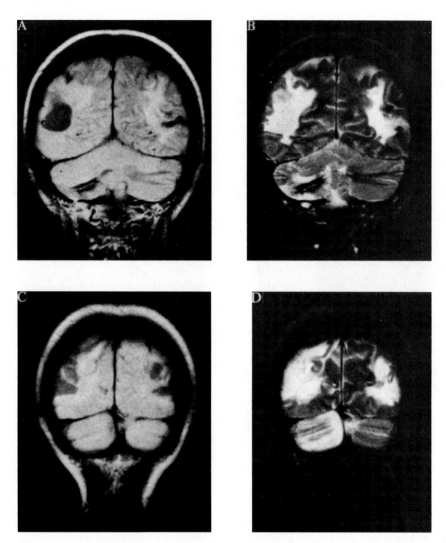

Figure 13.12.   Conventional coronal MRI through the occipital lobes in same patient whose three-dimensional MRI is seen in Figure 13.11. *A.* T1-weighted image through mid-occipital region shows hypointense areas, right greater than left, consistent with infarcts, surrounded by mild hyperintense areas consistent with edema. *B.* T2-weighted image at same location, showing large hyperintense areas with minimal mass effect on both sides. Note similar areas in cerebellum, primarily in right hemisphere and in the midline. *C.* T1-weighted image through posterior occipital lobes shows persistent bilateral hypointense areas with surrounding minimal hyperintensity. *D.* T2-weighted image at same location shows large areas of hyperintensity in both occipital lobes. (Reprinted with permission from Zihl J, von Cramon D, Mai N, et al. Disturbance of movement vision after bilateral posterior brain damage: further evidence and follow-up observations. Brain 1991;114:2235–2252.)

tive area is most consistently related to the conjunction of the anterior limb of the inferior temporal sulcus with the lateral occipital sulcus. Other areas activated during motion perception include V1, V2, and the dorsal cuneus, which may correspond to V3 in nonhuman primates (Fig. 13.14). Viewing of optic flow increases blood flow in the dorsal cuneus, superior parietal lobe, and the fusiform gyrus.

Studies with functional MRI show motion-selective responses in the lateral temporo-occipital cortex as well as in V2 and the superior and

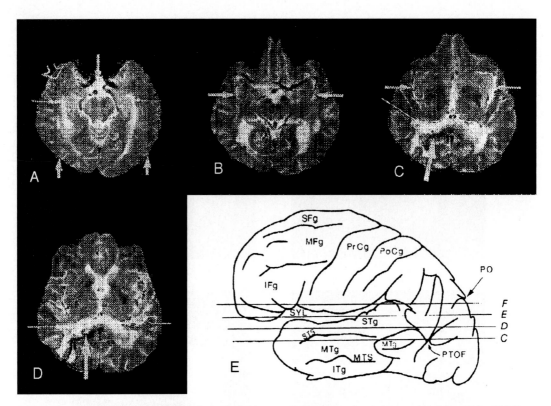

Figure 13.13. MRI in a patient with cerebral akinetopsia. The patient, A.F., had previous hypertensive hemorrhages that affected the temporo-parieto-occipital junctions bilaterally. *A–D.* Axial MRI. *E.* Drawing shows the location of the axial slices on a lateral view of the cortical surface of the brain. (Reprinted with permission from Vaina LM. Functional segregation of color and motion processing in the human visual cortex: clinical evidence. Cereb Cortex 1994; 5:555–572.)

inferior parietal lobules. Signal changes in lateral temporo-occipital cortex also correlate with motion after-effects. Both motion perception and pursuit-related signals are present in lateral temporo-occipital cortex.

Magnetic stimulation can be used to create temporary dysfunction within specific cortical areas. Stimulation over lateral temporo-occipital cortex impairs motion direction discrimination but not form discrimination in the contralateral hemifield and, to a lesser degree, in the ipsilateral hemifield.

These findings suggest that the human lateral temporo-occipital cortex participates in a variety of complex motion tasks, including speed discrimination, motion integration over a display to discern average direction and three-dimensional structure, and separation of regions with differ-

ent motion to discern two-dimensional structure. Elementary spatial and temporal aspects of motion perception and simpler tasks such as detection of motion and discrimination of direction in the absence of noise are not impaired, however. Thus, motion perception is not completely abolished but is impaired in its more interpretative functions; the more elementary motion signals are processed at other cortical sites, probably at a lower level. The role of lateral temporo-occipital cortex may be to use elementary motion signals to derive a higher order representation of motion, much as a color region may use elementary striate wavelength responses to derive a higher order perception of color. It is for this reason that the destruction of lateral temporo-occipital cortex does not leave a patient completely motion-blind.

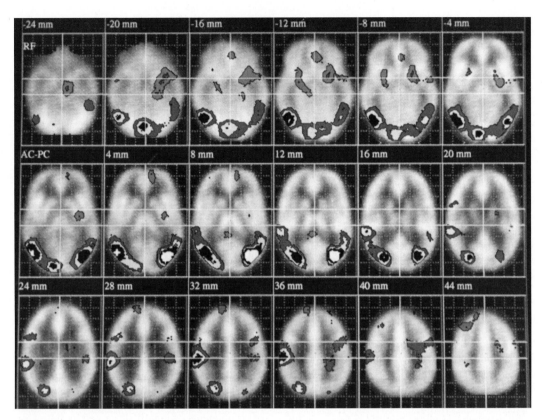

Figure 13.14. Positron emission tomographic (PET) study of motion perception. Areas with changing regional cerebral blood flow during motion perception, averaged over all normal subjects. Results are shown in axial section, with numbers indicating distance from a line joining the anterior and posterior commissures (negative values are inferior). Pixels indicate changes in blood flow, with black and white pixels indicating areas with highly significant increases in blood flow. Several areas of activation are seen, including the lateral temporo-occipital cortex. (Reprinted with permission from Dupont P, Orban GA, de Bruyn B, et al. Many areas in the human brain respond to visual motion. J Neurophysiol 1994;72:1420–1424.)

BALINT'S SYNDROME AND RELATED VISUOSPATIAL DISORDERS

BALINT'S SYNDROME

In 1909, Balint described a triad of visual defects in a man with bilateral parieto-occipital lesions (Fig. 13.15). The most significant deficit was an inability to perceive together at any one time the several items of a visual scene, which Balint interpreted as a "spatial disorder of attention." Other terms used to describe this deficit subsequently included "visual disorientation" and "simultanagnosia" (an inability to interpret the totality of a picture scene despite preservation of ability to apprehend individual portions of the whole). The patient described by Balint also had an inability to move the eyes voluntarily to objects of interest despite unrestricted eye rotations, so-called "psychic paralysis of gaze," "spasm of fixation," or "acquired ocular apraxia." The third deficit present in the patient described by Balint was a defect of hand movements under visual guidance despite normal limb strength and position sense, termed "optic ataxia."

Among the many reported causes of so-called **Balint's syndrome** are cerebrovascular disease (especially watershed infarctions as in Balint's original case), tumor, trauma, prion diseases

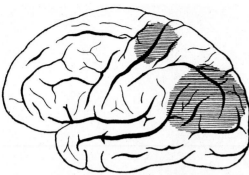 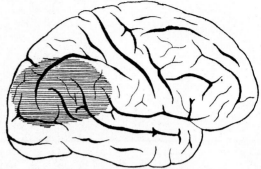

Schema I. Linke Hemisphäre.   Schema II. Rechte Hemisphäre.

Figure 13.15. Drawing of the locations of the major lesions in the case described by Balint in 1909, as pictured on lateral views of the hemispheres. The views are idealized and do not convey the full extent of the pathology. The surface of the brain was actually atrophic. Not seen in this view are several lesions of potential importance to the patient's behavior presentation. These included lesions of the posterior white matter in which optic radiations travel on both sides, and of the pulvinar, a critical structure for visuospatial integration in primates. (Reprinted with permission from Balint R. Seelenlahmung des "Schauens," optische Ataxie, räumliche Störung der Aufmerksamkeit. Monatschr Psychiatr Neurol 1909;25:51–181.)

such as Creutzfeldt-Jakob disease, infection by human immunodeficiency virus (HIV) type 1, and degenerative conditions such as Alzheimer's disease.

The definition of simultanagnosia can be operationalized as an inability to report all the items and relationships in a complex visual display despite unrestricted head and eye movements. A suitable screening tool is the Cookie Theft Picture from the Boston Diagnostic Aphasia Examination or any similar picture containing a balance of information among the four quadrants (Fig 13.16). The patient's report can be correlated with a checklist of the items in the picture. Exclusion criteria should include aphasia severe enough to impair the verbal descriptions of a display, so as to avoid confusing a defect of language with one of visual perception. It is also crucial to exclude or at least be aware of defective visual acuity or visual fields. For example, objects may seem to vanish into a central scotoma, paracentral scotoma, or a hemianopia, causing complaints that mimic simultanagnosia. Extensive peripheral scotomata or marked constriction of the visual fields, such as occurs in patients with retinitis pigmentosa or chronic atrophic papilledema, may hinder visual search and "simultaneous perception" despite unrestricted viewing, thus also producing an incoherent report.

Significant scientific concerns surround the lapidary reports upon which Balint's syndrome is based. Indeed, Balint's syndrome may not exist as a sufficiently autonomous complex. Affected patients often have a number of other devastating defects in behavior, and the classic triad of components originally described by Balint are not as closely bound as is often assumed. Moreover, individual components of the syndrome appear to represent relatively broad categories comprising other more specific defects. Furthermore, Balint's syndrome does not appear to have a specific neuroanatomic significance, because bilateral damage to the parieto-occipital regions can cause other defects, and damage elsewhere in the brain can cause similar clinical disorders.

The wide variety of perceptual phenomena reported in cases such as Balint's (including "vanishing" objects, tilted vision, metamorphopsia, palinopsia, and "positive" phenomena) are not likely to represent the behavioral expression of a single underlying neurophysiologic mechanism. Rather, Balint's syndrome may be considered a variety of combined deficits from lesions of the dorsolateral visual association cortices, which include the putative human area MT complex and its projections to the parieto-occipital cortex. Damage to these areas and to the cortices surrounding the angular gyrus and parietal insular cortex can disturb multiple aspects of spatial and temporal processing, including the perception of visual motion, perceptions of structure

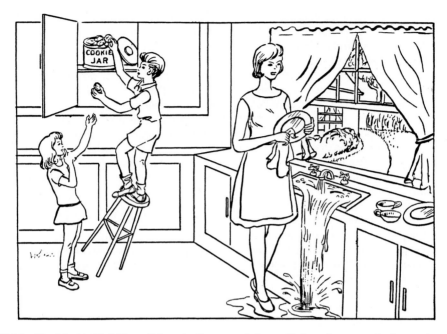

Figure 13.16.   The ''Cookie Theft Picture'' from the Boston Diagnostic Aphasia Examination. This picture contains a balance of information among the four quadrants. The patient is asked to describe the events depicted in the picture.

from motion and dynamic stereopsis, the perception of egomotion, and coordination of visual (eye-centered) and vestibular (gravity-centered) coordinate systems that orient us in the physical world. Bilateral lower quadrantanopias may co-occur from damage to the primary visual cortex lining the dorsal banks of the calcarine fissure (human area V1), thus adding to a patient's overall problem.

The clinical observations made by Balint provided preliminary evidence of a neural substrate for limb control, gaze control, and visual attention. They supported the idea that attention is not a single entity but comprises several abilities that operate in and among modalities and can be dissociated by different brain lesions. His report foreshadowed current concepts that view human behavior using information processing models and posit varieties of attention. The neuroanatomic underpinnings of these different abilities remain an important research issue that can be better understood by experimental neuroanatomic investigations, cerebral activation studies, and the use of specialized techniques for assessing eye movements, reaching and grasping, and attention in patients with focal brain lesions. Thus, the observations of Balint are historically

important and relevant, but there is probably little to be gained clinically or scientifically by perpetuating the diagnostic category of ''Balint's syndrome.''

DISORDERS OF VISUALLY GUIDED REACHING AND GRASPING

Reaching and grasping external objects is a fundamental activity that demands the coordination of several different nervous system functions. To accomplish this task, the brain transforms a target's visual coordinates to body-centered space, plans a hand path and trajectory (the sequence of hand position and velocity to target), and computes multiple joint torques, especially about the shoulder and elbow. It also specifies the necessary limb segment orientations from among many possibilities, activates appropriate muscle groups, and inhibits others to meet those specifications. The sensory feedback, frames of reference, and neural mechanisms used to solve these complex motor control problems are active research topics.

Reaching can be separated into two different phases. In the **transport phase** of reaching, the hand is moved toward an object whose position is determined by vision or memory. In the **acqui-**

sition phase, grasp formation depends on somatosensory and visual information on the limb and target, familiarity with the target, and perhaps on predetermined motor programs. These two phases mature at different rates, may be controlled independently before becoming coordinated, and can be dissociated by focal brain lesions. Posterior parietal damage may affect neurons coding eye position in the head and stimulus location on the retina that, together with neurons in motor and premotor cortex, permit hand movements to visual targets in a body-centered coordinate system.

The observations of Balint on what he called optic ataxia sparked interest in the neural basis of visually guided reaching and grasping. In this condition, patients reportedly reach as if blind toward targets they nevertheless can see and describe. Limb strength and position sense are normal; however, there is severe visual sensory loss and poor visuospatial perception, and patients may even appear demented because of their extensive bilateral lesions. Inability to reach and grasp targets in these cases is often multifactorial, including V1-type visual field defects, defective visual attention, and inability to locate targets with the eyes. Indeed, in screening for optic ataxia, the examiner should verify that the patient has foveated the target for a reach before making any observations on limb movement control. Another possible cause of defective reaching is abnormal sensorimotor transformation, an inability to transform the visual coordinates of external objects to appropriate limb coordinates for generating accurate reaches.

Lesions in the right inferior and superior parietal lobules, as in Balint's original case, are likely to produce visuomotor difficulty in reaches conducted with the left hand to both visual fields (hand effects) and with both hands to the left visual fields (field effects). Subsequent studies of patients with defective reaching have demonstrated lesions in the inferior parietal lobule, the occipitotemporal region, or both. Distance and direction errors may be dissociable, especially with lesions of the inferior posterior parietal cortex, suggesting that localization of a target with reaching movements depends on a network of structures in the visual association cortex.

POSITIVE VISUAL PHENOMENA

Cerebral lesions that affect vision usually create deficits in the visual fields—that is, **negative phenomena.** On occasion, however, they create **positive phenomena,** in which false visual images are seen by the patient. These false visual images can be classified as visual perseverations, hallucinations, and distortions (dysmetropsia). They occur in the absence of defects of the ocular surface, ocular media, or retina. They may occur with diverse pathologies, including stroke, migraine, epilepsy, neurodegenerative disease, infections such as HIV, and drug effects at specific receptor sites, and they probably reflect specific patterns of activation or damage within visual cortex.

VISUAL PERSEVERATION

Visual perseveration is the persistence, recurrence, or duplication of a visual image. It is a rare complaint in patients with cerebral lesions. Several varieties exist, including palinopsia, polyopia, and illusory visual spread:

Palinopsia (or paliopsia)—the perseveration of a visual image in time.

Cerebral diplopia or **polyopia**—the perseveration of a visual image in space.

Illusory visual spread—the contents or surface appearance of an object spread beyond the spatial boundaries of the object.

Both spatial and temporal perseveration can occur in the same patient, as in palinopsic polyopia. Some patients report that as an object moves, they see multiple copies of the object in its trail. Although this may be considered an example of cerebral polyopia, it also is clearly a form of palinopsia. Palinopsic images may be larger than the original images, suggesting illusory visual spread combined with palinopsia.

Palinopsia

The content of visual hallucinations is often imagery created de novo, or sometimes from the distant past (experiential hallucinations), but the palinopsic illusion contains elements of a more recently viewed scene or even one that is still being viewed. Nevertheless, the difference is not always clear, and patients can have both perseverative and hallucinatory phenomena concurrently.

There are at least two forms of palinopsia, an immediate and a delayed type. With the *immediate type* of palinopsia, an image persists after the disappearance of the actual scene, usually fading after a period of several minutes. This type of palinopsia bears some similarity to the normal phenomenon of an afterimage experienced after prolonged viewing of a bright object. With the *delayed type* of palinopsia, an image of a previously seen object reappears after an interval of minutes to hours, sometimes repeatedly for days or even weeks. Some patients have both immediate and delayed types of palinopsia.

A perseverated image can assume almost any location in the visual field. It may persist in the same retinal location as the original image, which is usually at the fovea, and thus move as the eyes move, much as a normal afterimage does. Sometimes, the image is translocated into a coexistent visual field defect and indeed can be a transient feature in the evolution of cerebral homonymous field defects. In other cases, the image is multiplied across otherwise intact visual fields. On rare occasions, the location of palinopsic images is contextually specific, as when patients report that after viewing a face on television, everyone else in the room has the same face as the person on television, or that the sign over one shop reappears on the boarding over other shops. Although some of these cases may represent a complex form of palinopsic polyopia, others may also be consistent with a constant foveal or perifoveal perseverative image that repeatedly manifests itself when the context is appropriate.

A wide range of other symptoms can accompany palinopsia. An associated homonymous visual field defect is almost always present and may be a complete hemianopia, incomplete hemianopia, superior quadrantanopia, or inferior quadrantanopia. There may be other spatial illusions, such as metamorphopsia, macropsia, and micropsia. Less frequently, ventral stream deficits occur, such as topographagnosia, prosopagnosia, and achromatopsia.

The natural history of palinopsia is variable. In some patients, palinopsia is a transient phase in either the resolution or progression of a visual field defect and lasts from days to months, eventually resolving. Other cases of palinopsia persist for months or even years. Anticonvulsant medication may prove helpful in prolonged cases.

The pathophysiologic mechanisms of palinopsia are unclear. The main hypotheses include:

1. A pathologic exaggeration of the normal afterimage.

2. A seizure disorder.
3. Hallucinations.
4. Psychogenic.

It is likely that different mechanisms account for similar palinopic phenomena in different patients.

In etiologic investigations, drug-induced palinopsia must first be considered. Intoxication with hallucinogens such as mescaline, lysergic acid diethylamide (LSD), and 3,4-methylenedioxymethamphetamine (Ecstasy) can cause palinopsia, sometimes permanently. Isolated reports assert that palinopsia and other visual illusions may occur with prescribed medication, such as clomiphene, interleukin 2, and trazodone, or with abnormal metabolic states such as nonketotic hyperglycemia. Palinopsia can also occur in psychiatric conditions, such as schizophrenia and psychotic depression, but it is always accompanied by other signs of mental illness. Once intoxication and psychiatric conditions are excluded, visual perseveration almost always indicates a cerebral lesion.

The localizing value of palinopsia is not clear. Most studies find a predominance of right parieto-occipital lesions in patients with palinopsia, although left hemispheric lesions may be under-represented because of aphasia. There are also reports of medial occipital and temporo-occipital lesions verified by neuroimaging, autopsy results, or both.

Cerebral Polyopia

Patients with cerebral polyopia see two or more copies of a single object simultaneously. This form of visual perseveration is described much less frequently than is palinopsia. It occurs with monocular viewing, distinguishing it from the binocular diplopia caused by misalignment of the eyes. Cerebral polyopia can generally be differentiated from monocular polyopia caused by such ocular abnormalities as uncorrected or miscorrected refractive errors, corneal opacities, and cataract because the images of cerebral polyopia are all seen with equal clarity, do not resolve during viewing with a pinhole, and are unchanged in appearance whether the patient is viewing binocularly or monocularly with either eye. Some patients experience cerebral polyopia only in certain positions of gaze, causing confusion with tropic diplopia until the monocular nature of the polyopia is recognized. Some patients see only two images; others see dozens.

Associated clinical manifestations are usually present in patients with cerebral polyopia. These include homonymous visual field defects, difficulties with visually guided reaching, cerebral achromatopsia or dyschromatopsia, object agnosia, fluctuations in the visual image, and abnormal visual afterimages.

Cerebral polyopia can occur as a transient phase in the recovery from cortical blindness secondary to traumatic injury. Other reported causes of cerebral polyopia include encephalitis, multiple sclerosis, and tumors. We have encountered this condition most often after parietal lobe or parieto-occipital region strokes.

Illusory Visual Spread

Patients with illusory visual spread, as noted above, see the contents or surface appearance of an object spread beyond the spatial boundaries of the object. Thus, wallpaper patterns spread beyond the surface of the wall, and cloth patterns spread from a shirt to the wearer's face. Illusory visual spread may occur in isolation or may be a feature of palinopsic images.

VISUAL HALLUCINATIONS

Hallucinations are perceptions without external stimulation of the relevant sensory organ. They are common in patients with dementia or confusional states secondary to metabolic insults, including alcohol withdrawal, where they form the predominant type of hallucination. Drugs reported to cause hallucinations include digoxin, bupropion, ganciclovir, vincristine, cyclosporine, lithium, lidocaine, itraconazole, and dopaminergic agonists. Baclofen withdrawal may also induce visual hallucinations.

Visual hallucinations can occur in patients with a variety of psychiatric disorders. In such cases, they are usually accompanied by hallucinations in other sensory modalities (especially auditory) and by other signs of mental illness.

Isolated visual hallucinations in persons with intact cognition and mental function are often a sign of underlying neurologic or ophthalmologic disease. Isolated visual hallucinations can be separated into three main pathophysiologic groups: (1) release hallucinations, (2) visual seizures, and (3) migraine.

Release Hallucinations (Charles Bonnet Syndrome)

Bilateral simultaneous or sequential visual loss from any cause can result in visual hallucinations. These are often called **release hallucinations,** because it is thought that they arise from, or are "released" in, visual cortex that is no longer receiving the incoming visual sensory impulses that usually filter out nonvisual stimuli. Release visual hallucinations usually occur in patients with visual acuity in the better eye of 20/60 or worse. Any type of visual loss, whether ocular or cerebral in origin, can lead to release hallucinations. When the disease causing visual loss is ocular and occurs first in one eye and then in the other, hallucinations usually do not develop until the second eye loses vision.

Some series report that up to 57% of patients with a variety of causes of visual loss have release hallucinations. In fact, the true incidence of release hallucinations may be much higher because of a reluctance on the part of affected patients to tell their physicians that they are experiencing hallucinations, for fear of being labeled "crazy." Patients with release hallucinations are mentally lucid; the majority are aware that the visions are not real; and, in general, they are not distressed by them. Notable is the absence of other sensory hallucinations.

Release hallucinations can be classified as simple (unformed) or complex (formed) (Fig. 13.17). Simple hallucinations consist of brief flashes or points of light, colored lines, shapes, or patterns (phosphenes). Complex hallucinations contain recognizable objects and figures, such as flowers, animals, and humans, with a potential for bizarre, dreamlike imagery of considerable detail and clarity, including dragons, angels, and miniature policemen. Sometimes the vision is a recognizable image from the patient's past, such as a deceased friend or relative. Simple hallucinations are at least twice as common as complex ones. Indeed, in most series, complex hallucinations account for 10 to 30% of release hallucinations.

Some authors reserve the term "Charles Bonnet syndrome" for the association of visual loss with complex formed hallucinations. However, some patients have simple hallucinations initially and later experience complex ones. A similar progression in visual hallucinatory content is reported in normal people subjected to sensory

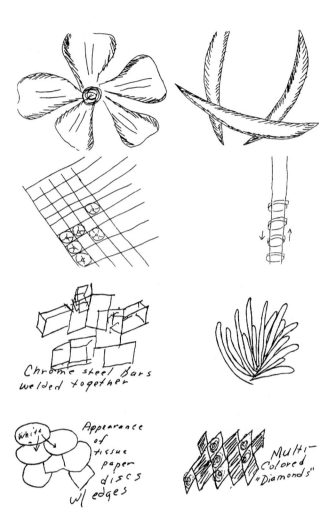

Chrome steel bars welded together

Appearance of tissue paper discs w/ edges

White

Multi-colored "Diamonds"

Figure 13.17. Appearance of both simple and complex hallucinations. Drawing by a patient with occipital lobe damage showing his most frequent hallucinations. Note that some are complex (*above*), whereas others are simple (*middle and below*). (Reprinted with permission from Anderson SW, Rizzo M. Hallucinations following occipital lobe damage: the pathological activation of visual representations. J Clin Exp Neurol 1994;16:651–663.)

deprivation. Also, because the type of release hallucination does not correlate with the site of visual loss, the distinction between complex and simple release hallucinations lacks diagnostic value.

There must be other contributing factors besides visual loss in the development of release hallucinations, because they do not develop in all patients with visual loss. Older age may be one risk factor, but even patients as young as 10 years can have release hallucinations. Social isolation is another potential factor, thought to act by accentuating the sensory deprivation of visual loss. There may be an increased incidence of posterior periventricular white matter lesions on MRI in patients with visual hallucinations from ocular disease, although this finding remains unverified.

There are several theories regarding the pathogenesis of release hallucinations, but most authorities believe that all release hallucinations have a similar origin. In the brain, visual experience is represented by patterns of coordinated impulses within the visual cortex. These patterns are generated by sensory stimuli and represent the current experience of the individual; however, the brain can generate these neural patterns spontaneously and, in fact, does so during sensory deprivation from either imposed isolation or pathologic denervation. These spontaneous neural patterns then correspond to hallucinations. A similar explanation has been invoked for the phantom-limb phenomenon after amputation and presumably also underlies other release phenomena, such as musical hallucinations in cases of deafness. Supporting evidence for the analogy with sensory deprivation includes the fact that these hallucinations tend to occur when patients are alone or inactive, and in the evening or night when the lighting is poor.

Hallucinations often begin close to the time of visual loss. They most often follow the onset of visual loss by several days or weeks, but the delay can be even longer. That loss of vision triggers the hallucinations is supported by the observation that release hallucinations disappear in patients whose vision subsequently improves (e.g., patients whose cataracts are removed or patients whose cortical blindness is transient).

Release hallucinations may be brief, with each episode lasting a few seconds or minutes, or nearly continuous. When the hallucinations are episodic, their frequency varies from several per day to twice a year. In many patients, release hallucinations last for a few days to a few months and then spontaneously disappear even though visual function remains stable. In others, however, the hallucinations persist for years or even decades.

Release hallucinations do not bother most patients, and some persons even enjoy them. Treatment of the visual disturbance in such patients, other than reassurance concerning the significance of the hallucinations, is not indicated. However, some patients find the hallucinations annoying, upsetting, or distracting. Unfortunately, there is no agreement on effective treatment for such patients. Moving socially isolated patients into a more stimulating environment may lessen the hallucinations, and anticonvulsant drugs may improve the hallucinations but not consistently. Mixed results also occur with haloperidol and tiapride.

Visual Seizures

Visual seizures are not common in patients with epilepsy. When they do occur, they can be confused with migraine and release hallucinations. Indeed, much of the confusion related to the localizing value of the visual content of hallucinations stems from failure to distinguish between release hallucinations and true visual seizures. Clearly, the content of release hallucinations is highly variable and independent of the site of pathology. Rather, it is the nature of the associated field defect that has localizing value in this setting. However, the same conclusion may not be valid for visual seizures. Older human stimulation experiments found that simple flashes of light and colors resulted from electric activity in striate cortex, whereas stimulation of visual association cortex in areas 19 and temporal regions resulted in complex formed images. A similar distinction probably holds for epileptic visual hallucinations (Fig. 13.18). Nevertheless, temporal lobe lesions can produce simple unformed hallucinations, and occipital lesions can produce complex hallucinations. In the latter setting, spread of ictal activity into extrastriate cortex probably is responsible for the complex character of the hallucinations. As a result, the content at the onset of a visual seizure has the most localizing value.

The distinction between visual seizures and release hallucinations can be difficult in patients with cerebral lesions. The association with other ictal phenomena or an homonymous visual field defect may be helpful. Accompanying head or eye deviation (usually but not always contralateral) and rapid blinking are common accompaniments of occipital seizures. Other features that also strongly support ictal origin are signs of more distant spread of seizure activity, such as confusion, dysphasia, tonic-clonic limb movements, and the automatisms of complex partial seizures. The diagnostic uncertainty between release hallucinations and visual seizures may be resolved by seizure monitoring, although the routine scalp electroencephalographic leads often do not localize the occipital focus accurately; suspicion of such a focus usually requires intracranial electrodes for confirmation.

Although a variety of pathologies in the visual cortex may be associated with visual seizures, one syndrome requiring emphasis is **benign childhood epilepsy with occipital spike-waves.** This idiopathic epilepsy syndrome begins between 5 and 9 years of age and ceases spontaneously in the teenage years. Seizures are characterized by blindness and/or hallucinations of both simple and complex types, and it may progress to motor or partial complex seizures. Some children develop nausea and headache following the visual seizure, leading to an erroneous diagnosis of migraine. The diagnosis is established by occipital spike-waves occurring during eye closure on electroencephalography.

Migrainous Hallucinations

A variety of visual phenomena can occur in migraine. In migraine with visual aura (classic migraine), the visual phenomena generally pre-

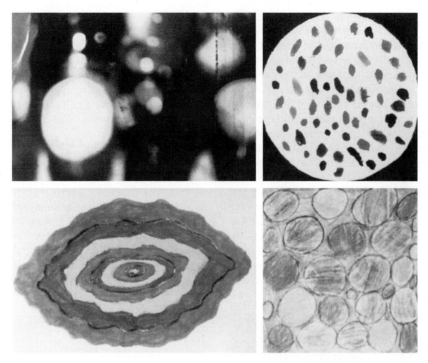

Figure 13.18. Visual illusions of occipital lobe epilepsy as perceived by four different patients. (Reprinted with permission from Panayiotopoulos CP. Elementary visual hallu-cinations in migraine and epilepsy. J Neurol Neurosurg Psychiatry 1994;57:1371–1374.)

cede the headache, whereas in migraine aura without headache (acephalic migraine), visual phenomena occur alone. Photopic images are most common in both settings and are described as spots, wavy lines, or shimmering of the environment similar to heat waves over a road on a hot day. The scintillating scotoma is a blind region surrounded by a margin of sparkling lights, which often slowly enlarges over time and which may move across the visual field or expand concentrically from a small point to distort some or all of the field of vision of both eyes. In some patients, the sparkling margin can be discerned as a zig-zag pattern of lines oriented at 60° to each other, usually in one hemifield and on the leading edge of a C-shaped scotoma (Fig. 13.19). This is the fortification spectrum or teichopsia (from the Greek word *teichos,* meaning "town wall"), which is so-named because of the resemblance of the zig-zag margin to the ground plan of town fortifications in Europe. There may be several sets of zig-zag lines in parallel, often shimmering or oscillating in brightness. They may be black and white or viv-

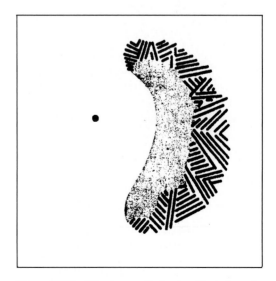

Figure 13.19. Visual aura of migraine. Illustration of a typical fortification scotoma. The gray area represents a transient region of blindness that moves outward, roughly parallel to the expanding arc. (Reprinted with permission from Richards W. The fortification illusions of migraine. Sci Am 1971;224:89–96.)

idly colored. These zig-zag lines begin near the center of the field and expand toward the periphery with increasing speed over a period of about 20 minutes, with both the speed and the size of the lines increasing with retinal eccentricity (Fig. 13.20). The relation of speed and size to eccentricity is predicted by the cortical magnification factor, which is a measure of the area of visual field represented in a given amount of striate cortex as a function of retinal eccentricity. This suggests that migrainous hallucinations are generated by a wave of neuronal excitation spreading from posterior to anterior striate cortex at a constant speed, leaving a transient neuronal depression that causes the temporary scotoma in its wake. It is also hypothesized that the zig-zag nature of the lines reflects the sensitivity to line orientation of striate cortex and the pattern of inhibitory interconnections within and

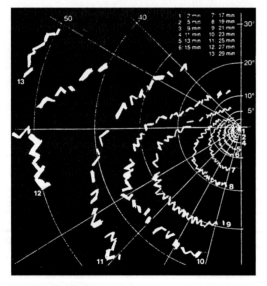

Figure 13.20. Photographic negative of a migraine phosphene protocol. The scintillating phosphene was progressing through the lower quadrant and part of the upper quadrant of the left visual hemifield. Thirteen drawings were made between 2 and 29 minutes after the phosphene first appeared near the center of the visual field. To evaluate the distance between the phosphene and the center of the visual field, several radii were drawn across the protocol. The angular distance from the fovea center, computed in degrees of visual angle, is indicated by circles. Circles and radii were added to the sheet after the observations were made. Observation distance = 34 cm. (Reprinted with permission from Grüsser O-J. Migraine phosphenes and the retino-cortical magnification factor. Vision Res 1995;35:1125–1134.)

among striate columns. Although both migraine and visual seizures can feature abnormal hallucinations followed by headache and vomiting, the two disorders can sometimes be distinguished by their visual imagery, with black and white zig-zag lines being more suggestive of migrainous hallucinations and colored circular patterns being more common in ictal hallucinations.

Other Types of Hallucinations

Hallucinations other than those described above can occur in patients with a variety of intracranial diseases. These hallucinations include peduncular hallucinations and hallucinations that are present only during eye closure.

Hallucinations associated with lesions of the mesencephalon, so-called **peduncular hallucinations** (or peduncular hallucinosis), are rare. They have many similarities to the complex release hallucinations associated with visual loss described above. They can be continuous or episodic, with detailed formed imagery, such as flying birds, dogs, roaring lions, crawling snakes, gangsters with knife wounds, and men herding cattle. These hallucinations are not stereotyped. Instead, they vary from one episode to the next. In some cases with thalamic rather than midbrain infarcts, the hallucinations are from events in the patient's past. Like patients with release hallucinations associated with loss of vision, many patients with peduncular hallucinations realize that the hallucinations are not real. Other patients do not possess this insight, however, and may even attempt to interact with the hallucinations. Similar hallucinations occur for sounds, and some patients have multimodality hallucinations, involving vision, touch, sound, and even the sense of body posture.

Unlike release hallucinations, peduncular hallucinations are almost invariably associated with inversion of the sleep-wake cycle—that is, diurnal somnolence and nocturnal insomnia. Other associated signs from damage to adjacent structures in the midbrain include unilateral or bilateral oculomotor nerve palsy, hemiparkinsonism, hemiparesis, and gait ataxia.

The most frequently described etiology of peduncular hallucinations is infarction involving the substantia nigra pars reticulata and its connections to the pedunculo-pontine nucleus, and/or the reticular formation and the ascending reticular activating system. Peduncular hallucinosis can occur in patients with the "top-of-the-basilar'' syndrome. It may also occur as a vascular complication of cerebral angiography and transiently after microvascular decompression surgery for trigeminal neuralgia. Compression of the midbrain by an extrinsic tumor can also cause these hallucinations. In cases caused by infarction, the hallucinations can resolve, but they usually persist indefinitely, although the episodes may become shorter.

Rare patients experience **hallucinations with eye closure.** Causative settings include drug toxicity from atropine and probably lidocaine, infection with high fever, and after major surgery. It has been proposed that they are similar to hypnagogic hallucinations, suggesting a disturbance in sleep-wake cycle mechanisms.

VISUAL DISTORTIONS (DYSMETROPSIA)

Illusions about the spatial aspect of visual stimuli can be separated into three main categories:

Micropsia—the illusion that objects are smaller than in reality.

Macropsia—the illusion that objects are larger than in reality.

Metamorphopsia—the illusion that objects are distorted.

Of these, micropsia is probably the most common and has the largest variety of possible etiologies.

Micropsia

Etiologically, several types of micropsia exist. **Convergence-accommodative micropsia** is a normal and physiologic phenomenon in which an object at a set distance appears smaller when the observer focuses at near rather than far, even though there is no change in the retinal angle covered by the object and no change in its spatial relations to the surround. Investigations of this induced micropsia at near (or alternatively, macropsia at far) have concluded that vergence rather than accommodation is responsible. Convergence micropsia may play a role in preserving size constancy at small distances. Its origins remain unclear, although it is theorized that the sizes of visual receptive fields are modified during convergence. It is unusual for accommodative micropsia to be a source of complaints.

Psychogenic micropsia occurs in psychiatric patients. It is the subject of extensive psychoanalytic interpretations, with the most prevailing

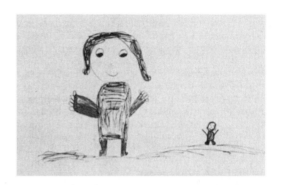

Figure 13.21. Drawing of cerebral micropsia by a child with migraine. The child stated that during some of her attacks, other children (*right*) appeared unusually small to her (*left*). (Reprinted with permission from Hachinski VC, Porchawka J, Steele JC. Visual symptoms in the migraine syndrome. Neurology 1973;23:570–579.)

theory being that it occurs in patients who are literally trying to ''distance'' themselves from environments fraught with conflict.

Retinal micropsia occurs when the distance between photoreceptors is increased. The micropsia usually occurs in foveal vision and is caused by macular edema. There may be associated metamorphopsia if the receptor separation is irregular. Visual acuity is also reduced in such cases. Causes of macular edema and micropsia include central serous chorioretinopathy, diabetic retinopathy, severe papilledema, and retinal detachment. The condition may resolve or persist for years. Retinal micropsia is often monocular, but it can be binocular, depending on the type of ocular pathology.

Cerebral micropsia, in contrast to retinal micropsia, is always binocular. Unusual variants include **hemimicropsia,** which occurs in the hemifield contralateral to the cerebral lesion. Given the small number of cases, the localization value of cerebral micropsia is uncertain. Temporo-occipital lesions are present in some cases, with either medial or lateral involvement. One survey of over 3000 adolescent students revealed that complaints of episodic micropsia or macropsia were not rare, occurring in 9%. Some occurred in the hypnagogic state or during fever, and there was a correlation with a history of migraine. Indeed, micropsia occurs not infrequently in migraine, particularly in childhood, and migraine is probably the most common setting in which cerebral micropsia is encountered (Fig. 13.21).

Macropsia

Macropsia is much less frequently described than micropsia. Retinal macropsia can occur in the late scarring stage of macular edema, and it can be a side effect of the drug zolpidem. Cerebral macropsia can rarely occur during seizures. Cerebral hemimacropsia was reported in a patient with a left occipital tumor and also in a patient with a right occipital infarct. As noted above, both micropsia and macropsia occur episodically in children and seem to correlate with childhood migraine.

Metamorphopsia

Ocular causes of metamorphopsia are far more common than cerebral causes. Most often, the metamorphopsia occurs from retinal pathology, such as macular edema, and in such cases, it often coexists with micropsia. Disorders that cause traction and distortion of the macula, such as an epiretinal membrane, may also cause metamorphopsia. As with retinal micropsia, metamorphopsia from ocular disease is usually monocular. In those rare cases in which it is binocular, the distortions are almost never identical in the two eyes. Thus, as in patients with micropsia, patients with symmetric monocular bilateral metamorphopsia are more likely to have a cerebral lesion than an ocular one. Although metamorphopsia is most often tested using an Amsler grid, psychophysical tests of hyperacuity that require the alignment of dots or comparison of dot spacing in a dot bisection task can also be used to quantitate metamorphopsia.

Cerebral metamorphopsia occurs in some patients during seizures. Other reported causes include a right parietal glioma, a right parietal arteriovenous malformation, posterior cerebral artery infarction, a transient stage in the development of cortical blindness, and even brainstem lesions. The lesions with posterior cerebral infarcts are medial, with one lesion being said to have involved only the left cingulate gyrus and retrosplenial area.

TESTS OF HIGHER VISUAL FUNCTION

Chapter 1 of this text contains detailed descriptions of the standard vision tests used by ophthalmologists, neurologists, and neuro-ophthalmologists to measure the visual abilities

and track the deficits in their patients. However, as indicated above, standard vision and screening tools generally do not provide a measure of higher order visual functions, nor are they meant to do so. Basic categories of higher visual function tests include tests of

1. *Reading,* such as the reading subtest of the Wide Range Achievement Test and Chapman-Cook Speed of Reading Test.
2. *Visual recognition,* such as the recognition of famous faces, the Boston Naming Test, and the Visual Naming Test from the Multilingual Aphasia Examination.
3. *Mental imagery,* such as the Hooper Visual Organization Test (Fig. 13.22).
4. *Visual perception,* such as the Facial Recognition Test (Fig. 13.23) and Judgment of Line Orientation.
5. *Visual attention,* such as the Cookie Theft Picture (see Fig. 13.16), and the line bisection task.
6. *Visuoconstruction,* such as drawing to dictation and copy (Fig. 13.24), writing to dictation copy and spontaneously, and the 3-D Block Construction Test.
7. *Visual memory,* such as the Benton Visual Retention Test, BVRT (Fig. 13.25).

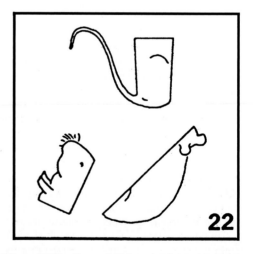

Figure 13.22. Tests of higher visual function. A plate (number 22/30) from the Hooper Visual Organization Test (HVOT). The patient is required to identify each of the 30 items on the plate from their cut-up rearranged line drawings. This test is memory dependent, in that it depends on the history of exposure of the patient to the items on the plate.

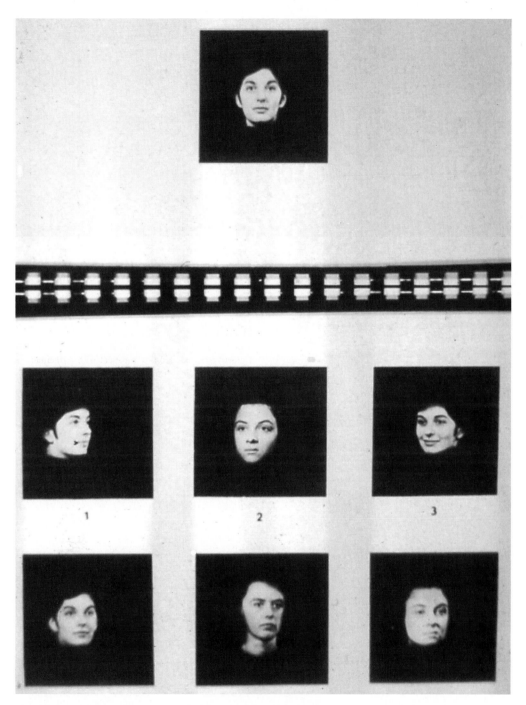

Figure 13.23.   An item from the Benton Facial Recognition Test is shown. This test measures visuoperceptual capacity. The patient is asked to choose which three of six face pictures below match the unfamiliar face pictured above (Courtesy of Arthur Benton).

Rey-O Complex Figure Test

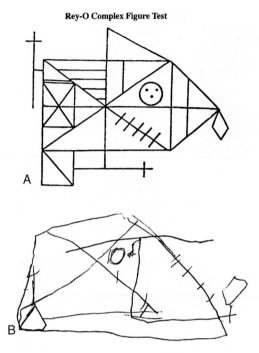

Benton Visual Retention Test
Form C, Design 5

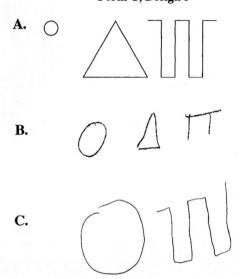

Figure 13.24. Tests of higher visual function. *A*. The Rey-Osterreith Complex Figure. *B*. Defective copy of this figure by a 74-year-old woman with Alzheimer's disease.

Figure 13.25. Tests of higher visual function. *A*. Plate (design 5) from the Benton Visual Retention Test (BVRT). *B*. Defective reproduction by a patient with Alzheimer's disease. *C*. Omission of the one of the left figures in a patient with a right hemisphere lesion causing left hemineglect.

GLOSSARY OF CEREBRAL VISUAL DEFICITS

Achromatopsia. Loss of color vision.

Agnosia (also known as associative agnosia). The inability to recognize previously familiar objects despite adequate perception. Objects are effectively stripped of their meanings.

Alexia without agraphia (also known as pure alexia or acquired dyslexia). The acquired inability to read in previously literate individuals. Should not be confused with developmental dyslexia.

Anosognosia. Failure to recognize one's own impairment (see Anton's syndrome).

Anton's Syndrome. The denial of cerebral blindness.

Apperceptive agnosia. Failure to identify previously familiar objects due to impaired perception.

Balint's syndrome. A condition characterized by the triad of simultanagnosia, ocular apraxia, and optic ataxia.

Blindsight. Residual vision in the fields of a putative striate scotoma; later redefined more broadly as a "visual capacity in a field defect in the absence of acknowledged awareness."

Central (paracentral) scotoma. A visual field defect at (near) the fixation point.

Cerebral achromatopsia (also known as central achromatopsia). An uncommon defect of color perception caused by damage to the visual cortex and connections. The term achromatopsia implies complete color loss. The term dyschromatopsia should be used when there is some sparing of color sensation.

Cerebral akinetopsia. Defective processing of visual motion cues due to cerebral lesions. The ability to perceive motion direction, shape from motion, and other "higher order" motion processes may be impaired.

Cerebral blindness. Bilateral loss of vision from bilateral damage to the optic radiations or striate cortex. Cortical blindness (see below) is a form of cerebral blindness.

Charles Bonnet syndrome. A condition in which hallucinations, usually of the complex (formed) type, are associated with visual deprivation.

Color agnosia. Inability to identify colors despite preserved ability to discriminate among colors.

Color anomia. Inability to name colors despite adequate color perception and recognition.

Cortical blindness. Inability to see following bilateral damage to the visual cortex. Affected patients generally have considerable damage that extends well beyond V1. Cortical blindness is a specific form of cerebral blindness (see above).

Foveal (macular) sparing. An homonymous hemianopia in which 2° to 10° of the central vision are preserved on the affected side.

Foveal (macular) splitting. An homonymous hemianopia that includes the entire foveal representation on the affected side.

Hemianopia (or hemianopsia, or homonymous hemianopia). A visual field defect that occupies both the upper and lower visual portions of the same hemifield of both eyes.

Keyhole vision (cerebral tunnel vision). Homonymous hemianopias may be bilateral (double homonymous hemianopia) leading to a severe loss of peripheral vision; if there is bilateral foveal sparing, a tunnel or keyhole of vision remains around fixation.

Macropsia. The illusion that objects are larger than in reality.

Metamorphopsia. The illusion that objects are distorted.

Micropsia. The illusion that objects are smaller than in reality.

Monocular temporal crescent. A crescentic portion of the extreme peripheral temporal field of vision in each eye that has no nasal counterpart in the opposite eye (i.e., it is purely monocular). It is represented in the most anterior aspect of the striate cortex.

Ocular apraxia (also called psychic paralysis of gaze or spasm of fixation). An inability to move the eyes to objects of interest despite unrestricted ocular rotations. This phenomenon may occur as part of Balint's syndrome.

Optic ataxia. A defect of hand movements under visual guidance despite adequate limb strength, position sense, and coordination. This phenomenon may occur as part of Balint's syndrome.

Palinopsia. Persistence of visual after-images of an object despite looking away.

Prosopagnosia. Inability to recognize previously familiar faces or to learn new faces despite adequate perception. This is a restricted form of (associative) agnosia.

Quadrantanopia. A visual field defect that is restricted to the upper or lower quadrant of a hemifield.

Scotoma. An area of blindness surrounded by intact vision. The physiologic blind spot is a scotoma.

Simultanagnosia (simultagnosia). This is often equated with Balint's "spatial disorder of attention." An inability to interpret the totality of a picture scene despite preservation of ability to apprehend individual portions of the whole.

FOR MORE INFORMATION:
See Walsh & Hoyt's *Clinical Neuro-Ophthalmology,* 5th edition, Volume 1, Chapter 9, pp. 387–483.

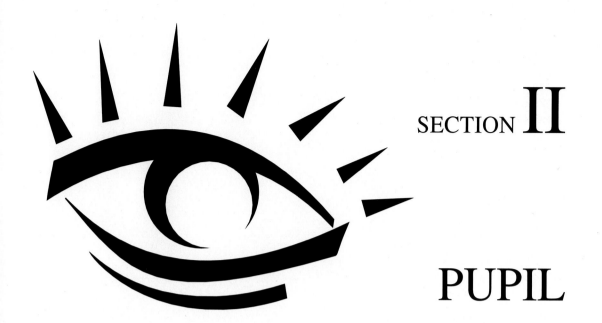

SECTION II

PUPIL

CHAPTER 14

Examination of the Pupils, Accommodation, and Lacrimation

ASSESSMENT OF PUPILLARY SIZE, SHAPE, AND FUNCTION

As is the case with any assessment, assessment of the pupils requires a meticulous history and a rigorous examination. This is followed in some instances by pharmacologic testing of the pupil using a variety of topical agents.

HISTORY

Patients with disturbances of pupillary size or shape are frequently unaware that any abnormality is present. Most often, their spouse, a friend, or a physician brings the abnormality to their attention. The disturbance may appear suddenly, or it may develop gradually over time. It may be present at all times, or it may be episodic.

In obtaining a history from a patient with a disturbance in pupillary size or shape, particularly anisocoria, dating the onset of the abnormality may be important. The easiest and most reliable method is to view a driver's license or credit card with the patient's photograph on it, which the patient is likely to have available at the time of the evaluation. The examination of family album photographs that have been taken over time (sometimes jokingly called "family album tomography" or "FAT scanning") can be performed with the naked eye or with a magnifying lens and may save both time and money in attempting to determine the onset of a pupillary disturbance.

Symptoms that may be elicited in a patient with disturbances of pupillary size and shape include light sensitivity or photophobia, difficulty focusing when going from dark to light or light to dark, and blurring of vision. The blurred vision is typically a nonspecific and poorly defined complaint; however, if one pupil is abnormally small, images of objects observed with that eye may appear slightly dimmer than those observed with the opposite eye.

The past medical history may also be helpful. A history of previous infections (e.g., herpes zoster), trauma, operations (especially in the neck), or migraine may suggest the etiology of the pupillary disturbance. The patient's occupation may also be important. A farmer or gardener may be exposed to plants or pesticides that can produce pupillary dilation or constriction by topical contamination. A physician, nurse, or other health professional may work with or have access to topical dilating or constricting substances that may produce changes in pupillary size by design or chance.

EXAMINATION

Simple inspection of the anterior segment of the eyes at the slit lamp is helpful in determining if a pupillary abnormality is present. For example, examination of the cornea may reveal an abrasion or injury that could affect the pupillary size, whereas examination of the anterior chamber may reveal inflammation that explains a small pupil in the setting of ciliary spasm. It may also be important to perform gonioscopy to assess the anterior chamber angle in a patient with a dilated pupil, particularly when there is a history of pain or redness in the eye. Assessment of the iris should include not only inspection of the integrity of the sphincter muscle but also transillumination of the iris to determine if there is evidence of iris damage from previous ocular trauma. In addition, by placing a wide beam at an angle to the iris and turning the light off and on, the light reflex can be assessed for segmental defects, such as occur in eyes with tonic pupils or aberrant regeneration of the oculomotor nerve.

Pupil measurements can be performed in several ways. A simple hand-held pupil gauge can be used to determine pupil size in both light and darkness. Pupil gauges may be circular or linear. They consist of a series of solid or open circles or half-circles with diameters that increase by 0.2 mm in steps (Fig. 14.1). They can be held next to the eye to estimate the size of the pupil.

An accurate method of measuring pupillary size and comparing pupils before and after pharmacologic testing is with a hand-held pupil camera. With this device, the pupils can be photographed in various illuminations, although not in darkness (Fig. 14.2).

Infrared video pupillometry is perhaps the most accurate method of assessing the size of the pupil. An infrared video pupillometer permits observation of pupils not only in lighted conditions but also in total darkness. Some computer programs associated with these pupillometers allow the examiner to measure not only the diameter and area of the pupil but also the latency and velocity of the pupillary response to both light and near stimulation.

During the clinical evaluation of the pupils, it is helpful to determine the answers to certain questions. For example, because the diameter of the pupil typically decreases with age (Fig. 14.3), the examiner should determine if the pu-

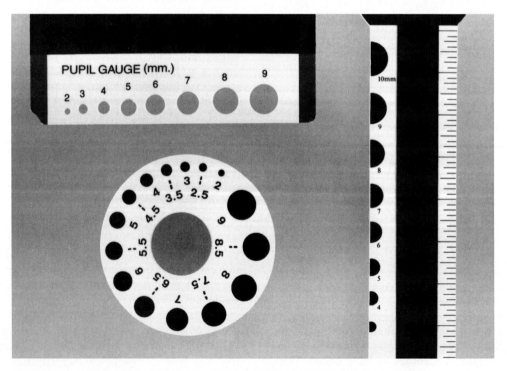

Figure 14.1. Pupil gauges. The best gauges measure in 0.5 millimeter steps.

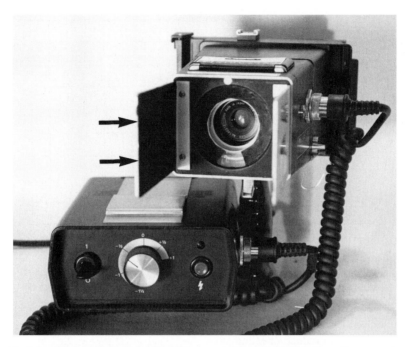

Figure 14.2.   The Polaroid hand-held camera is indispensable in recording pupil sizes. It is particularly good at comparing sizes in darkness and light, looking for light-near dissociation or dilation lag. Recording pre- and post-drop size is also helpful. This particular model has its own light power pack. The guide (*arrows*) allows for focused pictures.

pillary size is appropriate for the patient's age (see Fig. 14.3). Other important questions to answer include the following: Are the pupils equal? If not, which setting makes the difference in size greater: light or darkness? Do the pupils constrict to light equally and with the same velocity? Do they redilate equally and with the same velocity? Is the pupillary reaction to light stimulation equal to the pupillary reaction to near stimulation? Is there reflex dilation to psychosensory stimulation? Is there a relative afferent pupillary defect (RAPD)?

Assessing Pupillary Size

The diameter of both pupils should be estimated or measured in light, using either normal room light or a hand-held transilluminator or other light source. The diameter of the pupils should then be assessed in darkness, using the dimmest room light in which the examiner can still see the edge of the pupil. Finally, the pupillary size should be assessed during near stimulation using an accommodative target to achieve maximum constriction of the pupils.

The measurements of the two pupils in light and darkness should also be compared to determine if there is **anisocoria:** a difference between the two pupils of 0.4 mm or more. A substantial percentage of the normal population has clinically detectable anisocoria of 0.4 mm or more, with the percentage increasing with increasing age. Whereas 20% of the general population aged 17 years and under have this so-called "physiologic anisocoria," the prevalence rises to 33% in otherwise normal persons over 60 years of age. In addition, anisocoria may be produced by damage to the iris sphincter or dilator muscles or to their nerve supply. The amount of anisocoria may be affected by illumination. For instance, a greater degree of anisocoria is present in darkness than in light in patients with physiologic anisocoria or Horner's syndrome. Anisocoria can also be affected by the degree of accommodation, by fatigue, and by sympathetic drive (anxiety).

Testing the Pupillary Reaction to Light

When testing the reaction of a pupil to light shined in the eye—the **direct pupillary light reaction**—it is important to have a dimly lit

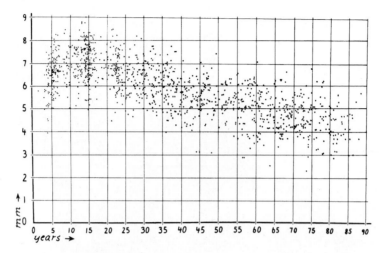

Figure 14.3. Graph showing relationship of age to pupil size in normal individuals. Note that, in general, pupillary size decreases with age. (Reprinted with permission from IE Loewenfeld. Pupillary changes related to age. In: Thompson HS, ed. Topics in Neuro-ophthalmology. Baltimore: Williams & Wilkins, 1979:124–150.)

room that is quiet so as to reduce or eliminate emotional effects on the pupil. Furthermore, one must be certain that the patient is fixating on a distance target to eliminate any effect of accommodation on pupillary size. The examiner must be certain that the patient is not attempting to close the eyelids during the test, because this produces a variable degree of pupillary constriction.

A bright light source should be used to illuminate the pupil and produce pupillary constriction, because increased stimulus intensity is associated with an increased light reflex amplitude and a maximum rate of constriction and redilation. If the light source is too bright, however, a prolonged contraction lasting several seconds (''spastic miosis'') will occur and make determination of the normal light reflex difficult or impossible. A fully charged transilluminator or ophthalmoscope light is the optimum light source. In addition, it is helpful to use a dim secondary light source to provide oblique illumination of the pupil in some cases, because this technique increases visualization of darkly pigmented irides (Fig. 14.4).

The light source should be shined straight into the eye for a few seconds and then moved downward away from the eye to eliminate the stimulation. The pupil response should be assessed during this maneuver, which should be repeated several times. The normal response to a bright

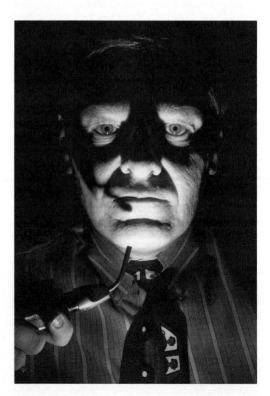

Figure 14.4. Use of indirect lighting to view pupils in darkness.

light is a contraction called "pupillary capture." "Pupillary escape," on the other hand, is a phenomenon in which the pupil initially constricts and then slowly redilates and returns to its original size. Pupillary escape most often occurs on the side of a diseased optic nerve or retina and in normal persons tested with a low-intensity light source. The initial size of the pupil is important in assessing both pupillary capture and pupillary escape; a larger pupil is more likely to show pupillary escape, whereas a smaller pupil is more likely to show pupillary capture.

The latency and speed with which a pupil constricts to light and redilates after light stimulation can be assessed using pupillography. This technique reveals that normal persons have pupillary waveforms with a latency of 0.20 to 0.28 seconds and a duration of contraction of 0.45 seconds. The use of pupillography to record waveforms of pupillary constriction and dilation is generally limited to research.

When light is shined in one eye, the contralateral pupil should also constrict. This is the **consensual light response.** The consensual response to light is best assessed using a light source for illumination of the pupil of one eye and a dimmer light source that can be held obliquely to the side of the contralateral eye to be observed. The consensual pupillary response should be approximately equal in both velocity and extent to the direct response, because the pupillary decussation in the midbrain is about 50% to each eye. In fact, the consensual reaction to light in normal humans is slightly less than the direct reaction, producing about 0.1 mm or less of what has been called "alternating contraction anisocoria."

Testing the Pupillary Near Response

The near response, a co-movement of the near triad that also includes accommodation and convergence (see below), should be tested in a room with light that is adequate for the patient to fixate an accommodative target. A nonaccommodative target, such as a pencil, pen, or the patient's own thumb, may not be a sufficient stimulus to produce a normal near response even in a normal person, and these targets should be avoided (except in a patient who is blind, in which case one must stimulate the pupillary near response using proprioception from one of the patient's own fingers or thumb). Similarly, the near response should not be induced by having the patient look

at a bright light stimulus, because the light itself may produce pupillary constriction. The examiner should attempt to test the pupillary near response several times to give the patient practice. One can document the light and near response with photographs or pupillometry (Fig. 14.5).

If a patient is unable to cooperate for a near effort, some authors advocate using the "lid-closure reflex," in which the patient attempts to squeeze the eyes shut while the physician tries to open them. This maneuver typically causes the pupils to constrict.

Assessment of Pupillary Dilation

Dilation of the pupils occurs in a variety of settings. Most often, the pupils dilate after they have constricted to light or near stimulation. In patients with certain retinal and, less often, optic nerve disease, they may actually dilate when light is shined in one eye (paradoxical pupillary response). Reflex pupillary dilation can also be elicited by sudden noise or by pinching the back of the neck.

When assessing pupillary dilation, the examiner should look specifically for dilation lag. This phenomenon is present when there is more anisocoria 4 to 5 seconds after pupillary constriction to light than there is 15 seconds after pupillary constriction. Dilation lag typically occurs in patients with a defect in the sympathetic innervation of the pupil (i.e., Horner's pupil), although it also occurs in some normal subjects.

Dilation lag is usually easy to detect. One method is simply to observe both pupils simultaneously in very dim light after a bright room light has been turned off. Normal pupils return to their widest size within 12 to 15 seconds, with most of the dilation occurring in the first 5 seconds. Pupils that show dilation lag may take up to 25 seconds to return to maximum size in darkness, with most of the dilation occurring about 10 to 12 seconds after the light goes out. A second way to determine if dilation lag is present is to take flash photographs at 5 and 15 seconds after the lights are turned off.

Testing for Light-Near Dissociation

A dissociation between the pupillary response to light stimulation and the pupillary response to near stimulation (light-near dissociaton) occurs in patients with a variety of disorders (see Chapter 15). In almost all cases, the pupillary reaction to light is impaired, whereas the pupil-

Figure 14.5. Use of a hand-held camera to document size of the pupils in light and darkness in a normal subject. *A.* In room light without any other stimulation. *B.* In room light during stimulation with a bright light. *C.* In room light during stimulation with an accommodative target. Note associated convergence.

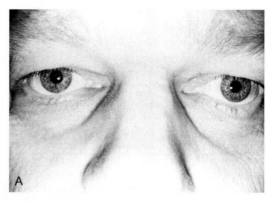

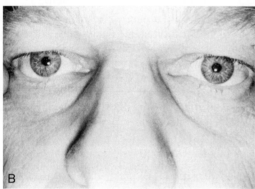

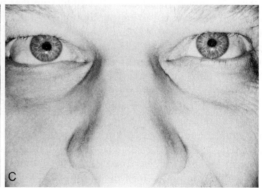

lary response to near is normal or near normal. Thus, light-near dissociation should be considered in any patient with an impaired pupillary light reaction. Essentially all cases of light-near dissociation in which there is a normal pupillary reaction to light and a poor pupillary response to near are caused by lack of effort on the part of the patient during attempted near viewing.

Testing for a Relative Afferent Pupillary Defect

When a patient has an optic neuropathy in one eye or an asymmetric bilateral optic neuropathy, covering one eye and then the other reveals that the pupil of the normal eye constricts when it is uncovered and the abnormal eye is covered, whereas the pupil of the abnormal eye dilates when it is uncovered and the pupil of the normal eye is covered (Fig. 14.6). This is known as the "Marcus Gunn" or "Gunn" phenomenon, and the abnormal pupil is often called a "Marcus Gunn pupil." We prefer the term "relative afferent pupillary defect," because this term describes the nature of the pupillary abnormality.

With the **swinging flashlight test** (Fig. 14.7) the differences in pupillary response to light are accentuated. The patient focuses on a distant target in a darkened room, and a light is swung back and forth multiple times to bring out the best response. The swinging flashlight test is probably the most valuable clinical test of optic nerve dysfunction available to the general physician.

It is important to perform the swinging flashlight test in the correct manner. First, a bright handlight and a darkened room are essential. The more contrast there is between the light beam and the darkened room, the greater will be the amplitude of the pupillary movement, and the easier it will be to see a small RAPD. It is possible, however, to use too much light. In such cases, a bright afterimage is produced that may keep the pupils small for several seconds, thus obscuring the pupillary dilation in the abnormal eye. Second, the patient must fixate on a distant target during the test. This prevents the miosis that occurs during the near response. Third, in patients with ocular misalignment (i.e., strabis-

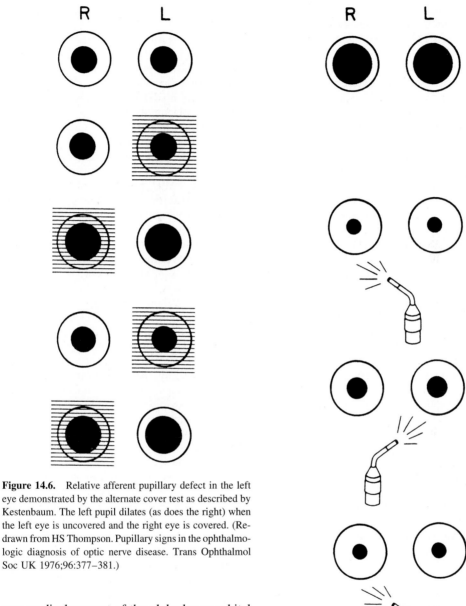

Figure 14.6. Relative afferent pupillary defect in the left eye demonstrated by the alternate cover test as described by Kestenbaum. The left pupil dilates (as does the right) when the left eye is uncovered and the right eye is covered. (Redrawn from HS Thompson. Pupillary signs in the ophthalmologic diagnosis of optic nerve disease. Trans Ophthalmol Soc UK 1976;96:377–381.)

mus or displacement of the globe by an orbital or intracranial process), care must be taken to shine the light along the visual axis. Fourth, the light should cross from one eye to the other fairly rapidly but should remain on each eye for 3 to 5 seconds to allow pupillary stabilization. Thus, there are really two parts of the pupillary response that must be observed during the swinging flashlight test: (1) the initial pupillary constriction response and (2) the pupillary escape that is observed for 2 to 5 seconds after the light meets the pupil. Most examiners vary the rate

Figure 14.7. Relative afferent pupillary defect in the left eye demonstrated using the swinging flashlight test. The pupils constrict when the light is shined directly into the right eye; however, when the flashlight is swung back to the left eye, both pupils dilate. (Redrawn from HS Thompson. Pupillary signs in the ophthalmologic diagnosis of optic nerve disease. Trans Ophthalmol Soc UK 1976;96:377–381.)

at which they move the light from eye to eye, and there is often an optimum swing rate that brings out an RAPD and that varies among patients.

Some authors recommend moving the light from one pupil to the other before the latter can escape from the consensual response to bring out an afferent defect. However, **the light should never be left longer on one eye than on the other.** This might tend to create a RAPD in the eye with the longer light exposure, because the longer the light is kept on the eye, the more pupillary dilation occurs as the eye adapts to the light.

In addition, if the retina becomes bleached in one eye and not in the other, a small RAPD will be produced. Special care must be taken to keep retina bleach equal, especially when measuring with neutral density filters greater than 1.2 log units in density (see below).

Finally, the swinging flashlight test can be performed as long as there are two pupils, even when one pupil is nonreactive and dilated or constricted from neurologic disease, iris trauma, or topical drugs. Recall that as the light is shifted from the normal to the abnormal eye, the total pupillomotor input is reduced. Thus, the efferent stimulus for pupillary constriction is reduced in *both* eyes so that both pupils dilate. In performing the swinging flashlight test, one tends to observe only the pupil that is being illuminated; however, the opposite pupil is responding *in an identical fashion.* Thus, if one pupil is mechanically or pharmacologically nonreactive, one can simply perform a swinging flashlight test observing only the reactive pupil. If the abnormal eye is the eye with a fixed pupil, the pupil of the normal eye will constrict briskly when light is shined directly in it and will dilate when the light is shined in the opposite eye. If the abnormal eye is the eye with the reactive pupil, the pupil will constrict when light is shined in the opposite eye and dilate when the light is shined directly in it. This is extremely helpful in attempting to determine if a patient with an oculomotor nerve paresis or traumatic iridoplegia also has an optic neuropathy or retinal dysfunction.

The swinging flashlight test can be further refined in patients in whom a unilateral optic neuropathy is suspected but who do not seem to have a RAPD when a standard swinging flashlight test is performed. In such patients, the use of a neutral density filter with a transmission of 0.3 logarithmic units often permits the detection of the defect (Fig. 14.8). The test is performed as follows. The filter is first placed over one eye, and the swinging flashlight test is performed. The filter is then placed over the opposite eye, and the swinging flashlight test is repeated. If there is truly no defect in the afferent system in either eye, placing the filter over either eye will simply induce a slight but symmetric RAPD in the eye covered by the filter, from reduction in the amount of light entering the system through that eye. On the other hand, if one eye already has a mild RAPD, placement of the filter over that eye will further reduce the amount of light entering the system through that eye, thus increasing the previously inapparent defect and causing it to become recognizable; placement of the filter over the opposite (normal) eye will simply balance the afferent defect in the opposite eye, and there will be no significant asymmetry in pupillary responses to light.

One can quantify the RAPD using graded neutral density filters that are calibrated in percent transmittance. After determining that a RAPD is present, the examiner balances the defect by adding successive neutral density filters in 0.3 logarithmic steps over the **normal** eye while performing the swinging flashlight test until the defect disappears (Fig. 14.9). The most useful neutral density filters are those ranging in transmission from 80% (0.1 log unit) to 1% (2.0 log units) (Fig. 14.10).

A decision as to whether or not a RAPD is present should be made within 2 to 3 swings after the filter is placed in front of the normal eye. If more swings are needed, the examiner must rebleach the retina of the covered eye and resume measuring. The neutral density filters should be held near the nose so that stray light does not affect the measurement. Filters more than 1.2 log units in density are so dark that it is hard to see the pupil through them, even when light is shined on the eye. The examiner thus may need to peek around the filter to make a judgment.

To reach the endpoint of the test, the examiner should "overshoot the endpoint"—that is, produce a RAPD in the normal (covered) eye. The examiner should then rebleach the retina of that eye and perform the swinging flashlight test with another filter at the next lower amount. Several "rules of thumb" in measuring the RAPD for various conditions are found in Table 14.1.

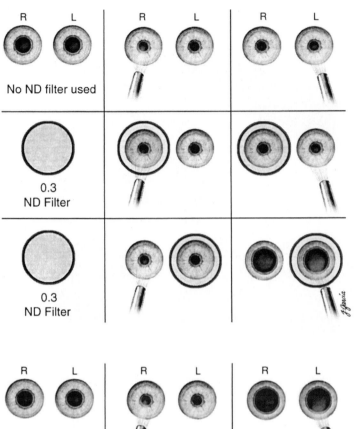

Figure 14.8. The use of neutral density filters to bring out a relative afferent pupillary defect (RAPD). A previous swinging flashlight test has failed to demonstrate a convincing RAPD. A 0.3 log unit neutral density filter is placed over the right eye and a swinging flashlight test is performed. The filter is then placed over the left eye, and the test is repeated. If there is a subtle optic neuropathy in the left eye, placing the filter in front of that eye will reduce the light stimulation even further, and there will now be a RAPD during the swinging flashlight test. When the filter is placed in front of the right eye, however, the reduced brightness in the right eye will tend to balance the reduced brightness in the left eye (from the optic neuropathy), and no RAPD will be seen.

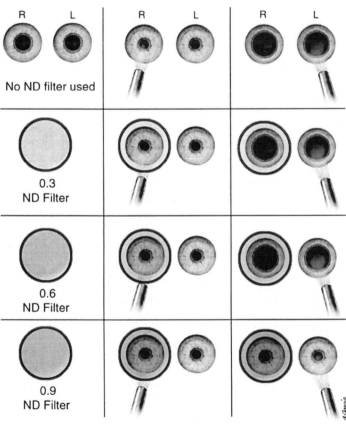

Figure 14.9. Quantification of the relative afferent pupillary defect (RAPD) using neutral density filters and the swinging flashlight test. Neutral density filters of increasing density are placed in front of the normal eye in a patient with a contralateral RAPD, and a swinging flashlight test is performed until the RAPD disappears. In this case, the RAPD is balanced with a 0.9 log unit filter.

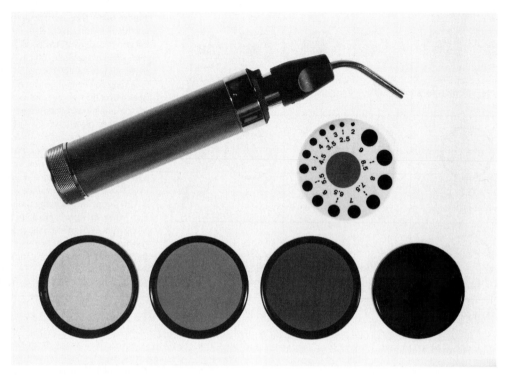

Figure 14.10. The equipment needed to quantify or bring out a relative afferent pupillary defect includes a bright hand-held light source, a pupil gauge, and a set of photographic neutral density filters in 0.3, 0.6, 0.9, and 1.2 steps.

Table 14.1
Expected RAPD in Various Situations—"Rules of Thumb"

CONDITION	EXPECTED RAPD IN LOG UNITS	COMMENT
Optic neuritis	0.3 to over 3 log units	If no RAPD, suspect bilateral disease
Optic tract	0.4–0.6 contralateral eye	Look for temporal visual field defect
Pretectal lesion	Contralateral RAPD without VF loss	
Visual field defect	Correlates with Goldmann/Humphrey	
Amblyopia	Less than 0.5 log units	If greater than 1.0 log unit, look for other disease
Anisocoria	0.1 log unit for every 1 mm	Test in light
Macular disease	Better than 20/200, no more than 0.5	Worst macular disease less than 1.0 log unit
Central serous	Less than 0.3 log units	
Central retinal vein occlusion	Ischemic 0.9–1.2 log units	
	Nonischemic <0.6 log units	
Retinal detachment	1 Quad 0.3; 2 Quad 0.6; macular 0.9; complete 2.0	
Retinitis pigmentosa	0.3 log units or less	
Cataract	None	If dense, expect RAPD in opposite eye
Patching; dark adaptation	Up to 1.5 log units in unoccluded eye	Maximum RAPD in 30 min; reverses in 10 min
Glaucoma	Varies	Corresponds with retinal rim
Nonorganic visual loss	None	

There is some correlation between the severity of an RAPD and the size of the peripheral field defects detected with kinetic perimetry using a Goldmann perimeter. There is less convincing evidence of a correlation between the pupillary response and field defects in the central field detected using static perimetry.

If there is still doubt about the existence of a small RAPD after a complete clinical examination, pupillography can be used to record specific features of the light response. Pupillary reactions that occur during stimulation of an eye that has a damaged retina or optic nerve have a prolonged latent period, a shortened duration, and a diminished amplitude of constriction. For example, inflammatory diseases of the optic nerve and optic atrophy are associated with significant prolongation of the latent period; ischemic optic neuropathy produces a lesser prolongation; and acute papilledema unassociated with clinical evidence of an optic neuropathy does not affect latency at all.

Tests used to detect a RAPD, particularly the swinging flashlight test, are sensitive tests for optic nerve dysfunction; however, they represent only one type of test used to determine whether a patient has an optic neuropathy, and, if so, what the degree of severity of the optic nerve dysfunction is (see Chapter 1).

Other Clinical Tests of Pupillary Function

The swinging flashlight test provides only relative information regarding the visual sensory system of the two eyes, because the pupillary light response of one eye is compared with that of the other eye. To assess the pupillary light reflex of each eye separately, one can evaluate the number of pupillary oscillations that occur over a fixed amount of time or determine the time it takes for a pupil to oscillate a specific number of times when stimulated by light.

In this test, a thin beam of light (0.5 mm wide) is placed horizontally across the inferior aspect of the pupillary margin (Fig. 14.11). The light induces pupillary constriction that moves the light out of the pupil. The pupil then redilates until the beam is once again at the edge of the pupillary margin, whereupon the pupil again constricts, creating a cycle. A set number of cycles (usually 10, 20, or 30) are then timed by a stopwatch to the nearest 0.1 second, and the time of the cycle—**the edge-light pupil cycle time**—is calculated as msec/cycle. Alterna-

tively, the number of cycles that occur during a fixed period of time, usually 1 minute, are counted. In both cases, the results are compared with results from normal control subjects. Normal pupils generally cycle at a rate of 900 msec/cycle.

Unfortunately, the edge-light pupil cycle time is not a particularly sensitive indicator of optic nerve disease compared with the swinging flashlight test or visual-evoked potentials (VEPs). In addition, it may be difficult or impossible to induce regular oscillations in some patients; and as with other tests of pupillary constriction, the edge-light pupil cycle time is affected by disease of the efferent arm of the pupillary light reflex, such as oculomotor nerve dysfunction. Nevertheless, it is a potentially useful initial diagnostic test in one-eyed patients or in patients with presumed bilateral symmetric retinal or optic nerve disease.

The **pupil cycle induction test** is a variation of the edge-light pupil cycle time. It is used to assess the difficulty in producing regular and sustained light-induced pupillary oscillations. A beam with a thickness of 0.45 mm or less is placed horizontally at the lower edge of the pupillary margin in much the same way as in testing the edge-light pupil cycle time. The pupils of almost all eyes with normal optic nerve function can generally be induced to cycle at regular intervals, whereas the pupils of almost all eyes with optic nerve disease show altered responses, such as complete failure to cycle or prolonged pauses in the cycle. We find both the edge-light pupil cycle time and the pupil cycle induction tests to be difficult to interpret and not as sensitive as the results of a simple swinging flashlight test. We use them only when assessing monocular patients.

PHARMACOLOGIC TESTING

A few cautionary comments should be made regarding the interpretation of pupillary responses to topically instilled drugs. If a judgment is to be made about the dilation or constriction of the pupil in response to a drop of some drug in the conjunctival sac, then whenever possible one pupil should be used as an internal control. Thus, if the condition is unilateral, the drug should be placed in both eyes so that the responses of the two eyes can be compared. When the condition is bilateral, no such comparison is possible, but an attempt should be made

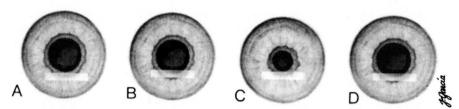

Figure 14.11. Testing the edge-light pupil cycle time. The pupil can be induced to cycle at the slit lamp by placing a horizontally oriented slit beam on the lower pupil margin. The beam is then moved slightly upward, inducing pupillary constriction that moves the light out of the pupil. The pupil then redilates until the beam is once again at the edge of the pupillary margin, whereupon the pupil again constricts, creating a cycle.

Table 14.2
Pharmacologic Testing in Diagnosing Common Pupil Conditions

AGENT	PURPOSE	DOSE	TIME	LIGHTING	MEASURE
Dilute Pilocarpine	Supersensitivity testing	0.625%	30 min	Dim light or darkness	Change in pupil diameter
Pilocarpine 2%	Pharmacologic pupil blockade	2%	40 min	Darkness	Change in pupil diameter
Cocaine	To demonstrate sympathetic defect	10%	60 min	Light	Post-cocaine anisocoria
Hydroxyamphetamine	To detect postganglionic sympathetic defect		50–60 min	Light	Absolute dil. OU or anis. >1 mm or change in anis. >1 mm

to make certain that the observed response is indeed caused by the instilled drug. In such cases, the drug may be placed in one eye only so that the responses of the medicated and unmedicated eyes can be compared. Occasionally, in patients with presumed bilateral disease, we place drops in both of the patient's eyes and in one of our own, to serve as a type of external control.

Other problems can occur when performing pharmacologic testing of the pupil using topical drugs. The drug may be outdated and thus more or less potent; the patient may develop sufficient tearing that the strength of the drug is altered by dilution or washed out of the inferior conjunctival sac before it can be absorbed; the patient may squeeze the eyes tightly during instillation of the drug, thus preventing a sufficient amount of drug from being placed in the inferior conjunctival sac. Penetration of the drug through the cornea may be altered, especially if other topical medications such as anesthetics have been used, or if the integrity of the corneal epithelium has been altered by manipulation of the cornea during tonometry or testing of corneal sensation. One must also consider individual variations in the action of the drug on patients of different ages or with different-colored irides. Even the psychic state of the individual must be considered, because the pupils tend to be miotic in persons who are tired or listless and mydriatic in patients who are upset or anxious.

Determining the results of pupillary testing can also be difficult depending on the initial size of the pupil. Differences in pupillary diameter or area can have profound results on the ultimate outcome in pharmacologic testing.

Finally, it is important to remember why a particular test is being performed in the first place (Table 14.2). The correct drug must be used and placed in the eyes in the proper fashion. For instance, we always place the drug in the eye of concern first and then place the drug in the contralateral eye so that if there is no response in the first eye, we cannot blame squeezing or tearing as the cause.

ASSESSMENT OF ACCOMMODATION, CONVERGENCE, AND THE NEAR RESPONSE

Most visual problems associated with accommodation occur because accommodation is too great, too little, or too slow. Disturbances of the other two components of the near response—convergence and pupillary miosis—can also be of importance if they are too active, or if they have insufficient activity.

HISTORY

The symptoms of patients with disturbances of accommodation tend to be nonspecific, but some aspects of the history may be important. Patients with accommodative insufficiency, for instance, usually complain of blurred vision at near and not in the distance. Patients with the most common problem with accommodation, presbyopia, may report that the farther away they hold an object, the better they can see it. Some patients with accommodative insufficiency report monocular diplopia; others complain of discomfort during attempted reading, a noticeable delay in focusing when changing fixation from a distant to a near object, or binocular diplopia. Some patients report headache, light intolerance, or other asthenopic symptoms. Frequently, presbyopia and other accommodative insufficient states can be precipitated with medications having anticholinergic effects.

Accommodative excess or spasm is typically associated with clear vision at near but poor distance vision. Objects may look larger or smaller (macropsia or micropsia) than normal in this setting. In addition, these patients often complain of brow ache. When convergence is affected in addition to accommodation, other symptoms may be present. Convergence excess is often associated with diplopia in the distance, blurring of vision, oscillopsia, or pain. On the other hand, convergence insufficiency is associated with trouble reading, diplopia at near, blurred vision that clears when either eye is covered, and pain or discomfort during near tasks.

In patients with spasm of the near reflex, symptoms are related to dysfunction of all three components. Such patients have accommodative spasm (up to 8 to 10 diopters), extreme miosis, and strabismus caused by convergence. These patients tend to complain of blurred or dim vision, binocular horizontal diplopia at both distance and near, temple pain or diffuse headache, pain in the eyes, and even trouble walking.

EXAMINATION
General Principles

Accommodation is the ability of the lens to change its refractive power in order to keep the image of an object clear on the retina. The primary stimulus for accommodation is blur, and most tests of accommodation depend on producing or eliminating blur. There are, however, other stimuli for accommodation besides blur, including chromatic aberration and perceived nearness, and these can also be used to test accommodation.

Accommodation is part of a complex triad that maintains clear near vision: the **near response** (also called the *near reflex*). Even though the components of the near response—accommodation, convergence, and pupillary miosis—normally work in concert during near viewing, each component can be tested separately. For example, one can weaken the stimulus to accommodation with plus lenses or strengthen the stimulus to accommodation with weak minus lenses without stimulating convergence or miosis. One can use weak base-out prisms to stimulate convergence without changing accommodation. Under certain conditions, one can test accommodation without inducing pupillary constriction. In addition, even in presbyopia, in which accommodation fails, convergence and miosis continue. Furthermore, if one paralyzes accommodation with drugs, convergence remains intact. **Relative accommodation** is the term used to describe the amount of accommodation that is free from convergence; **relative convergence** describes the amount of convergence free from accommodation.

The **near point of accommodation** (NPA) is the point closest to the eye at which a target is sharply focused on the retina. The **far point** is the distance at which light rays strike the retina in focus without invoking any accommodative effort. An *emmetrope* has a far point of infinity. A *myope* has a far point located a measurable distance in front of the eye. A *hyperope* has a far point located a measurable distance behind the eye.

Accommodation is measured by the **accommodative amplitude**—the power that the lens can vary from the nonaccommodative state to full accommodation. This power is measured in units called **diopters.** A diopter (D) is the reciprocal of the fixation distance. For example, 1 meter is 1 D; 0.5 m is 2 D; 0.33 m is 3 D; etc. The **range of accommodation** is the distance between the farthest point an object is in clear sight and the nearest point at which the eye can maintain clear vision.

Convergence is a vergence adduction movement that increases the visual angle to permit single binocular vision during near viewing. Convergence can be voluntary but need not be; that is, no stimulus needs to be present to elicit it. It is also reflexive and a co-movement in the near response. Accommodation and convergence are related; a unit change in one normally causes a unit change in the other. Convergence may be separated into four subtypes:

1. tonic convergence
2. accommodative convergence
3. fusional convergence
4. voluntary convergence

The eyes normally tend to diverge. Keeping the eyes straight thus requires increased tone in the medial rectus muscles. This tone is **tonic convergence.**

Accommodative convergence is the amount of convergence elicited for a given amount of accommodation. The relationship between accommodation and convergence is usually expressed as the ratio of accommodative convergence in prism diopters to accommodation in diopters: the AC/A ratio. Because accommodation decreases with age, the AC/A ratio increases with age. Just as convergence can be stimulated by accommodation, so accommodation can be stimulated by convergence. The ratio of convergence accommodation in diopters to convergence in prism diopters is called the CA/C ratio.

Fusional convergence is convergence that is stimulated not by changes in accommodation but by disparate retinal images. It is thus thought to be used to "fine tune" normal convergence. Pupillary constriction can occur with fusional vergence, but the amplitude of this form of convergence is not as great as that of accommodative convergence.

Voluntary convergence is measured by determining the near point of convergence (NPC)—the nearest point to which the eye can converge. It is closer to the eyes than the near point of accommodation and, in general, does not deteriorate with age as the NPA does. The NPC is usually 10 cm or less.

The pupil constricts when changing fixation from distance to near—this is **miosis.** This movement can occur in darkness, is slower than the light reflex, and is maintained as long as the near reaction is maintained. Miosis improves the range through which an object is seen clearly without any change in accommodation, called the **depth of field.** In patients with presbyopia, pupil size continues to decrease even when accommodation has reached its maximum. This probably occurs because aging changes limit alterations in the lens or ciliary muscles, whereas the pupillary sphincter is still functional and responsive to stimulation. On the other hand, artificially induced (i.e., pharmacologic) miosis reduces the amplitude of accommodation.

In testing accommodation and the near vision response, the above relationships must be remembered. Furthermore, one must remember that accommodation is never measured or tested in an absolute sense, but rather in response to how it changes under certain testing conditions.

Accommodation

The principal handicaps in the clinical application of adequate tests of accommodation are the subjective nature of the end points and the number of variables that must be controlled. The first step in any testing of components of accommodation or the near response is to perform an adequate refraction in the distance and at near. In children and some adults, a cycloplegic refraction with an agent like cyclopentolate (Cyclogyl) is mandatory. This accurately determines the far point. Pseudomyopia may be the first clue to accommodative spasm. Excellent distance vision and poor near vision may indicate accommodative insufficiency or presbyopia.

The NPA is the most frequent measure of accommodation. It is best measured using a scale device such as the Prince, Krimsky, or Behrens Rules—rulers with markings in both centimeters and diopters on which there is a small sliding chart containing Snellen letters (Fig. 14.12). The technique of testing accommodation is called the "push-up method." One eye is tested at a time. Wearing an optimum distance refraction and with the opposite eye occluded, the patient fixes on small (usually 5-point) type on a card that is attached to the rule and that can be slid forward and backward. The zero point of the rule should be 11 to 14 mm in front of the cornea. This corresponds to the approximate position of the spectacle correction. The size of the type is also important, because the smallest type will evoke the strongest accommodative response. The card is moved from a distance to the closest point at which the patient can see the print before it starts

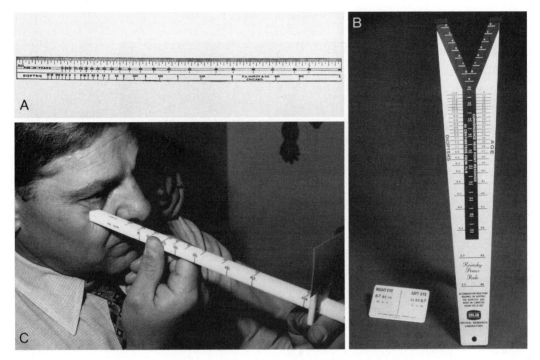

Figure 14.12. Photographs of accommodative rules. *A.* The Prince Rule. (Reprinted with permission from CA Wood. The American Encyclopedia and Dictionary of Oph-thalmology. Chicago: Cleveland Press, 1919:10961.) *B.* The Krimsky-Prince rule. (Photo courtesy of Paul Montague, CRP.) *C.* The Behrens rule.

to blur. This is the NPA. The maneuver should be repeated several times until the test gives reproducible results.

Once the measurement is made in centimeters, the accommodative amplitude can be calculated by dividing 100 by the NPA in centimeters. For example, in a person with an NPA of 10 cm, the accommodative amplitude is 10 D; if the NPA is 25 cm, the amplitude is 4 D. This means that the accommodative power of the eyes in these two examples corresponds to a lens with a focal distance of 10 or 4 diopters, respectively.

Using the push-up method, age-related normative data for accommodation have been developed (Fig. 14.13). When interpreting these results, however, the examiner must be sure that the patient fully cooperated with the testing. If, on repeated testing, the NPA or range of accommodation is consistently out of the range considered to be normal for age, the results should be considered truly abnormal. Adequate room lighting obviously should be available, and it is usually recommended that light be directed over the right shoulder when testing the right eye and

over the left shoulder when testing the left eye. Indeed, illumination is a critical factor in performing the test. By increasing illumination from 1 to 25 foot candles, the accommodative range can be increased by 28% in nonpresbyopes and by 73% in presbyopes.

The range of accommodation can be tested in a fashion similar to that used to test the accommodative amplitude. The patient should be instructed to indicate when the object blurs at near (the near point) and when it blurs in the distance (the far point). The range of accommodation is then calculated by determining the far point and near point in diopters and by subtracting the far point from the near point. For an emmetrope, the near point is the range of accommodation, because the far point is at infinity. For a myope whose far point is 50 cm or 2 diopter in front of the eye and whose near point is 10 cm or 10 D, the range of accommodation is $10 - 2 = 8D$. For a hyperopic eye with a far point of 25 cm or 4 diopters *behind* the eye and a near point of 10 cm or 10 D, the range of accommodation is $10 - (-4) = 14$ D.

Numerical Values of Limits for Each Age

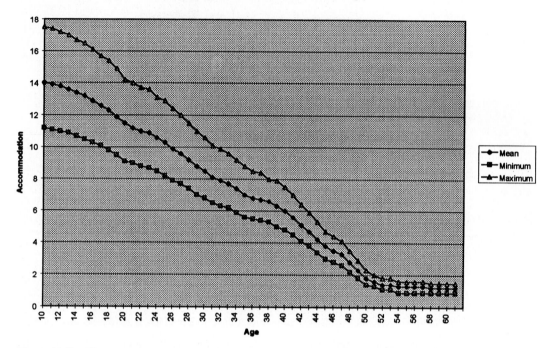

Figure 14.13. The relationship between accommodation and age. Note the relatively linear decrease in accommodation with age until about age 52, when almost all accommodation has been lost. (Graph obtained using data from A. Duane. The accommodation and Donders curve and the need of revising our ideas regarding them. J Am Med Assoc 1909; 52:1992–1996.)

If the patient is too presbyopic or myopic to do the test, corrective lenses should be used. One must then adjust the results to reflect the correction. If a minus lens has been used, the dioptric power of the lens is added to the result; if a plus lens has been used, the dioptric power of the lens is subtracted.

A second method of measuring accommodative amplitude is the "method of the spheres." The patient fixates on a reading target at 40 cm, and accommodation is stimulated by adding minus (concave) lenses until the print blurs. Accommodation is subsequently relaxed by adding stronger plus (convex) lenses until the print blurs. The sum of the lenses is the measure of the accommodative amplitude.

Convergence

Total convergence is usually measured by testing the NPC. This is usually done by asking the patient to fixate on an accommodative target held 33 cm from the eyes. The target is then moved toward the nose, with the patient being instructed to try to keep the target in focus. The end point of the test is when the patient reports horizontal diplopia, and the distance at which this occurs can be determined with a millimeter ruler placed alongside the patient's nose.

The NPC can be determined more objectively by performing the above test and noting the distance from the nose at which one of the inward turning eyes is observed to turn suddenly outward. In normal persons, the NPC is usually between 5 and 10 cm. An NPC greater than 30 cm indicates convergence insufficiency.

Another way to determine whether or not convergence is normal is to perform a cover-uncover test while the patient is reading. This is helpful only if the patient has full versions and no previous strabismus.

A way of determining if convergence is sufficient for the amount of accommodation is measuring the AC/A ratio. There are two different methods for measuring the AC/A ratio. The **gra-**

dient method determines the AC/A ratio by the change in deviation in prism diopters that occurs when a lens of varied power is placed over both eyes to stimulate or relax accommodation. An accommodative target must be used, and the working distance is held constant. Plus or minus lenses ($+1$, $+2$, -1, -2, etc.) are used to vary the accommodative requirement. The difference between the ocular alignment with and without the lens, divided by the power of the lens, is the AC/A ratio. The **heterophoria method** uses the distance-near relationship to determine the AC/A ratio. A similar ocular alignment should be present for both distance and near viewing. If a patient is more exotropic or less esotropic at near, this indicates less convergence—that is, a low AC/A ratio; if more esotropic or less exotropic at near, this indicates a high AC/A ratio.

The normal AC/A ratio is between 3 and 6, regardless of the method of testing that is used. Values above 6 indicate an excess of convergence per unit of accommodation, whereas values below 3 suggest convergence insufficiency. The AC/A ratio varies from person to person and from day to day or hour to hour in an individual, depending on that person's level of fatigue or alertness. The AC/A ratio may be genetically determined.

Testing convergence accommodation—that is, the CA/A ratio—requires that the patient experience no blur during the test. This can be accomplished by the use of a pin-hole device, dim illumination, or a Gaussian target. Measurements of accommodation are made as convergence is produced using base-out prisms. The CA/C ratio decreases with decreasing accommodation amplitude and therefore with age, and, of course, with cycloplegics.

ASSESSMENT OF LACRIMATION

The tear film is a trilaminar structure having a superficial oil layer, an aqueous middle component, and a mucin component. In order to discern a problem of the tear secretion, one should attempt to determine if only one layer is affected or all the layers are affected.

The main function of the **oil layer** is to retard evaporation of the tear film. Removal of the oil layer causes a 19-fold increase in evaporation, and abnormalities in the oil layer are often present with blepharitis and ocular rosacea.

The **aqueous layer** is the thickest component of the tears. It contributes the most to the volume of the tear film, and most of the tests that measure the quantity of the tear film test the aqueous layer. This layer is produced by the primary lacrimal gland and also by the accessory lacrimal glands of Krause and Wolfring. These small glands are similar in structure to the main lacrimal gland but are much smaller in size. The glands of Krause are located in the upper fornix, whereas the glands of Wolfring are situated farther down on the eyelid, above the tarsus. The relative importance of the main and accessory lacrimal glands in the maintenance of normal tear secretion is controversial. It is generally accepted that the main lacrimal gland, having an efferent parasympathetic innervation, functions primarily during reflex tear secretion, whereas the accessory lacrimal glands provide nonreflex basal tear secretion.

The **mucin layer** is a biphasic layer that allows the aqueous component to adhere to the hydrophobic cornea epithelium. This layer thus helps to maintain the integrity of the aqueous component of tears and the quality of the tear film. Abnormalities in this layer (and also in the oil layer) can create tear film disturbances despite good aqueous tear production. The mucin layer is produced by goblet cells located in the conjunctiva.

The normal basal tear volume is 5 to 9 microliters, and the normal flow rate averages 0.5 to 2.2 microliters per minute. In general, neither basal tear volume nor flow changes with increasing age, but reflex tearing does decrease with age.

The main disturbances of lacrimation relate to excess or insufficient tear production and to obstruction of the normal passage of tears through the lacrimal drainage apparatus. Thus, the assessment of patients with difficulties should be oriented to an evaluation of tear production and drainage.

HISTORY

Excessive drying of the eyes occurs in several settings. It may result from reduced production, increased evaporation, or excessive drainage of tears. **Epiphora**—excessive tearing—also occurs under several different circumstances. An increased production of tears may be present; the lacrimal drainage system may be obstructed; or the excess tearing may actually be reflexive in nature and related to a *deficiency* of normal basal tearing.

Patients with dry eyes often complain of a scratchy sensation in or around the eyes, as if there is a foreign body present. The sensation may be minimal when the patient awakens in the morning but worsens throughout the day as the eyes are used. The patient may also complain of blurred vision that seems to improve with blinking or prolonged closure of the eyes.

Epiphora may also be associated with blurred vision that is present during both distance and near viewing. Patients with epiphora should be asked about recent trauma to the eyelids or nose and about previous surgery in this area. They should also be queried about any symptoms or signs of recent infections or inflammations.

Episodic epiphora may, in fact, be a symptom of dryness of the eyes. As noted above, tears are produced by two main structures, the accessory lacrimal glands of Krause and Wolfring and the main lacrimal gland. Baseline tear secretion is produced by the accessory tear glands, whereas reflex tearing is produced by the main lacrimal gland. Patients with dry eyes from a variety of causes related to dysfunction of the glands of Krause and Wolfring may nevertheless have a functioning lacrimal gland. Irritation from a dry cornea may stimulate excess tearing from the lacrimal gland, thus creating the paradoxical situation of a patient with dry eyes who complains of excess tearing.

EXAMINATION

The examination of a patient with a disturbance of lacrimation is directed toward the three potential abnormalities described above: decreased tear production, increased tear production, and partial or complete obstruction of the lacrimal drainage apparatus.

Lid function is critical to spreading the tear film and should be assessed in any patient suspected of having an abnormality of tear function. Disturbances of eyelid structure and function can be detected both by simple external examination and by slit lamp biomicroscopy. Slit lamp examination can also detect punctate staining of the inferior cornea related to dry eyes, exposure (lagophthalmos), or a lid abnormality.

Tests of the tear film may be separated into those that test a particular part of the tear film or a particular function of the tears, those that measure the amount of tear secretion, and those that detect obstruction of tear drainage.

Specific tests of the mucin layer of the tears include a conjunctival biopsy to determine whether goblet cells are present, and if so in what number. A qualitative test for mucin can also be performed. In this test, a cotton strip (3 × 10 mm) is placed in the inferior cul de sac of an unanesthetized eye for 5 minutes. The strip is then placed on a glass slide and stained with the periodic acid-Schiff (PAS) stain. If the stain is positive, mucin is present. Impression cytology can also be used to determine if goblet cells are present and in what numbers. In this simple technique, cellulose acetate filter strips are placed on the conjunctival epithelium and then transferred to a glass slide, where they are stained with hematoxylin and PAS. This procedure can be used to diagnose not only dry eye conditions but also vitamin A deficiency.

An examination of the aqueous layer should begin with an assessment of the tear meniscus, which should be observed for evidence of protein precipitates and debris. At the same time, the relation of the tear meniscus to the lower eyelid can be assessed. The eyelids and lashes should be observed for evidence of entropion, ectropion, and stray lashes and for the position and integrity of the lower lacrimal punctum, because such abnormalities may cause disturbances that simulate those caused by abnormal tear production.

Other qualities of the tear film can be tested individually. For example, the tear film contains various proteins, including albumin, immunoglobulins, and lysozyme. Lysozyme, an enzyme that lyses bacterial walls and is reduced in dry eye syndromes, can be detected using the lysozyme lysis test. This test is said to be more reliable and sensitive than the Schirmer test (see below); however, the lysozyme lysis test requires gels, broth cultures, and measurements after incubating tear-soaked filter papers in the gel for 24 hours, whereas the Schirmer test requires only a strip of filter paper and a topical anesthetic. Other assays, such as an assay for tear lactoferrin, may also be useful in diagnosing such conditions as keratoconjunctivitis sicca.

The osmolarity of the tear film can be measured. An increasing osmolarity may be diagnostic of keratoconjunctivitis sicca.

Nonspecific tests of tear secretion are usually performed in patients with symptoms that suggest insufficient tear production. The sensitivity and specificity of these tests vary greatly, depending on the specific test used and the reference criteria for normal values.

Judging the height of the tear meniscus may predict the amount of tear production and secretion, as may assessment of radius of curvature, height, width, and cross-sectional area; however, there is little correlation between the results of this technique and the results of "quantitative" tests of tear production (e.g., the Schirmer test) unless quantitative measurements of the meniscus are performed.

The "noninvasive tear film break-up time" is perhaps the simplest test used to determine the adequacy of the tear film. The examiner touches the conjunctiva of an unanesthetized eye with a fluorescein strip. The fluorescein stains the mucin layer of the tear film, which is then assessed using the cobalt-blue filter of the slit lamp. The patient is asked to look straight ahead without blinking. A normal test is characterized by the persistence of the fluorescein over the cornea for 10 seconds or longer. A break up and disappearance of the fluorescein in less than 10 seconds is abnormal and indicates an abnormality in one of the layers of the tear film. The test has relatively good sensitivity (82%) and specificity (86%).

Another test of tear function is the "rose bengal test." The eye is first anesthetized with a 5% solution of proparacaine, and a small drop of a 1% solution of rose bengal is placed either directly on the cornea or just superior to it. Rose bengal solution stains dead and degenerating cells. An elaborate scoring method of judging staining in the medial and lateral aspects of the conjunctiva and the cornea has been proposed. Staining is judged from 0 to 3 in these three positions, giving scores from 0 to 9. Normal patients have little if any staining, whereas patients with a dry eye or a poor mucin layer will have mild to severe staining.

As noted above, tear secretion may be classified as basal, reflex, or total. Tests of tear secretion can thus be separated into those that test basal tear production (from the glands of Krause and Wolfring) and those that test reflex tear production (from the primary lacrimal gland). The Schirmer test, first described in 1903, is a simple and practical clinical way of measuring both reflex secretion and basal secretion. Total tear secretion is usually tested first, because no anes-

thetic drop is applied to the eye in this test (often called the Schirmer 1 test). The patient sits in a quiet, dimly lit room. After drying the inferior conjunctival fornices on both sides with soft cotton, the examiner places a strip of special absorbent filter paper in the lower conjunctival sac on both sides, with care being taken to keep the strip from touching the cornea by placing it either medially or laterally (Fig. 14.14). The strips are stabilized by folding the indented end over the lid margin. The patient is then advised to look straight ahead or slightly upward for 5 minutes, during which time he or she can blink normally. After 5 minutes, the strip is removed, and the amount of wetting is measured from the folded end. This wetting is the result of both basal tear secretion and reflex secretion.

A variant of the Schirmer 1 test can be performed by anesthetizing the eyes with a topical drug such as proparacaine 0.5%. (Topical cocaine should not be used as an anesthetic, because it irritates the cornea and inflames the eye.) Once the eye has been anesthetized, the paper strips are placed as indicated above, and the nasal mucosa is stimulated using a cotton-tipped applicator or with a tissue or piece of cotton that has been soaked with benzene or a similar trigeminal stimulant. Regardless of the technique used, normal persons wet 10 to 30 mm in 5 minutes. By multiplying the millimeters of wetting in 1 minute by a factor of three, the standard 5-minute Schirmer 1 test could be shortened by 4 minutes.

Basal tear secretion is determined using the Schirmer 2 test. A topical anesthetic is placed in the lower fornix of both eyes. After a minute or so, the examiner uses a small piece of cotton or filter paper to dry the inferior fornices. The paper strips are then placed in the manner of the Schirmer 1 test, and the patient is given instructions identical with those given for the Schirmer 1 test. After 5 minutes, the strips are removed, and the amount of wetting is measured. The wetting in this test should represent only the basal tear secretion, as the topical anesthetic should prevent stimulation of the main lacrimal gland. In addition, by subtracting the amount of basal tear secretion obtained from the Schirmer 2 test from the total secretion measured in the Schirmer 1 test, one should obtain the amount of reflex tearing (see below, however).

A variation of the Schirmer test is the "cotton thread test." In this test, a white cotton thread

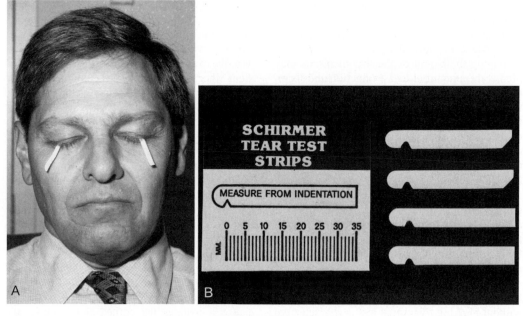

Figure 14.14. *A.* Patient with Schirmer strips properly placed laterally in inferior fornix of both eyes. *B.* Schirmer filter strips and measuring scale on packet of strips.

measuring 0.5 mm in diameter and 70 mm in length that has been soaked in alcohol or ether to remove any lipid residue is placed in the lateral upper conjunctival sac of each eye after 2 mm of one end of the thread has been stained with 10% fluorescein dye and dried. The thread is removed from the fornix after 5 minutes, and the length of the fluorescein stain is measured. A modification of this variation uses different colored threads.

All of the above tests can be criticized for providing inexact and highly variable results; however, there seems to be a linear relationship between the length of wetting during the Schirmer test and the increase in weight of the filter paper, and we agree with others that the Schirmer test *does,* in fact, give a reproducible and fairly precise estimation of tear flow, even in cases with markedly reduced tearing. A review that compared Schirmer testing, rose bengal staining, tear film break-up time, and lactoferrin levels in patients with Sjögren's syndrome reported that the best balance between specificity and sensitivity was achieved by performing both a rose bengal test and a Schirmer 1 test.

Fluorophotometric methods can be used to measure both tear volume and flow. These tech-

niques are not clinically applicable and are best used as research tools.

Patients who have epiphora should be evaluated not only for excess tear production but also for possible blockage of the tear drainage system. The punctae should be examined to see if they are patent, and the examiner should gently press on the lacrimal sac to see if there is regurgitation of contents through the punctae, indicating a block at the nasolacrimal duct.

The patency of the drainage system can next be tested by instillation of one drop of 2% fluorescein dye into the inferior conjunctival sac of both eyes, followed by observation of the difference at the end of 5 minutes between the two eyes in the residual fluorescein in the conjunctival sac and on the sclera, graded in terms of color intensity. A slightly more quantitative version of this test is to instill the dye in both inferior conjunctival sacs and to place a small cotton pledget or cotton-tipped applicator in the nose just below both inferior turbinates within 1 to 5 minutes. The pledgets or applicators are then examined to see if they are stained with dye that should have passed through the lacrimal punctae into the lacrimal canaliculi and then to the lacrimal sac, eventually exiting the lacrimal duct just below the inferior turbinate. If no dye is present, a secondary dye test is performed. The lacrimal system is flushed with clear saline, and the fluid emanating from the nose is checked for fluorescein staining. If there is still no dye, the nasolacrimal apparatus can be probed. If, after probing, dye is present at the inferior turbinate, then incomplete blockage exists and the lacrimal pump is functioning. If, however, there is clear fluid at the inferior turbinate, then a nonfunctioning pump exists and a complete block is present.

Lacrimal scintillography has also been proposed to test lacrimal flow. This technique uses Technetium-99 combined with specific scanning techniques to identify abnormal secretion and abnormal tear flow patterns.

Taste tests in which a specific substance, such as saccharin or Chloromycetin, is placed in the conjunctival sac can be used to determine if there is an intact lacrimal drainage system. These tests, however, give poorly reproducible results and have not been standardized.

Dacryocystography is a radiologic evaluation of the lacrimal drainage system in which contrast is placed into the lower fornix on the side of the presumed obstruction, and radiographs, computed tomographic (CT) scans, magnetic resonance images (MRI), or angiographic images are obtained to determine if and where the contrast material stops, thus localizing the obstruction.

FOR MORE INFORMATION:
See Walsh & Hoyt's *Clinical Neuro-Ophthalmology,* 5th edition, Volume 1, Chapter 23, pp. 933–960.

CHAPTER 15

Disorders of Pupillary Function, Accommodation, and Lacrimation

DISORDERS OF PUPILLARY FUNCTION	DISORDERS OF ACCOMMODATION
Efferent Abnormalities: Anisocoria	Accommodation Insufficiency and Paralysis
Afferent Abnormalities	Accommodation Spasm and Spasm of the Near
Light-Near Dissociation	Reflex
Disturbances during Seizures	DISORDERS OF LACRIMATION
Disturbances in Coma	Topical Diagnosis
Disturbances in Disorders of the Neuromuscular	Denervation Supersensitivity
Junction	Paradoxic Gustolacrimal Reflexes: Crocodile Tears
Drug Effects	Drug Effects
Structural Defects of the Iris	GENERALIZED DISTURBANCES OF
	AUTONOMIC FUNCTION

DISORDERS OF PUPILLARY FUNCTION

The value of observation of pupillary size and motility in the evaluation of patients with neurologic disease cannot be overemphasized. In many patients with visual loss, an abnormal pupillary response is the only objective sign of organic visual dysfunction.

EFFERENT ABNORMALITIES: ANISOCORIA

Efferent disturbances of the pupil are usually unilateral and thus produce a difference in the size of the pupils called **anisocoria** (Fig. 15.1). Thus, when assessing the pupils, one should always attempt to determine if anisocoria is present. If anisocoria is present, there is often something wrong with one or both irises or with the innervation of the iris muscles.

Once it is determined that anisocoria is present, the physician should determine if the degree of anisocoria is greater in light or darkness. This is best tested by illuminating the eyes from below with a hand light and turning the room lights off and on. If there is more anisocoria in darkness, the anisocoria may be caused by weakness of the dilator muscle in the eye with the smaller pupil (as in Horner's syndrome), or it may be a physiologic (simple) anisocoria. If there is more anisocoria in light (assuming that the condition is recent), the iris sphincter can be presumed to be weak in the eye with the bigger pupil. This could be due to anticholinergic medication, to a tonic pupil (e.g., Adie's syndrome from postganglionic denervation of the sphincter), to an oculomotor nerve palsy (i.e., preganglionic denervation of the sphincter), or to a spasm of the dilator muscle (adrenergic medication). Causes of anisocoria are described below and are outlined in Table 15.1.

More Anisocoria in Darkness

Physiologic Anisocoria (Simple Anisocoria, Central Anisocoria, Benign Anisocoria)

In dim light, almost 20% of the normal population has an anisocoria of 0.4 mm or more at

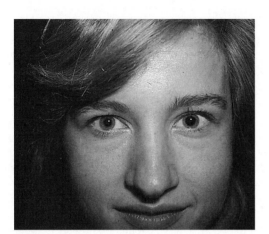

Figure 15.1. Anisocoria. The left pupil is larger than the right.

Table 15.1
Causes of Anisocoria

MORE ANISOCORIA IN DARKNESS
Simple (physiologic) anisocoria
Inhibition of the sympathetic pathway
• Horner's syndrome
• Pharmacologic (dapiprazole, thymoxamine)
Stimulation of the sympathetic pathway
• Tadpole pupils
• Intermittent dilation of one pupil caused by sympathetic
 hyperactivity
• Pharmacologic (cocaine, eye-whitening drops, adrenergic
 drugs)
Pharmacologic stimulation of the parasympathetic pathway
 (eserine, organophosphate esters, pilocarpine, methacho-
 line, arecoline)

MORE ANISOCORIA IN LIGHT
Damage to the parasympathetic outflow to the iris sphincter
 muscle
• Oculomotor nerve paresis
• Tonic pupil syndromes (including Adie's)
• Intermittent dilation of one pupil caused by inhibition of
 the parasympathetic pathway
Trauma to the iris sphincter
Acute glaucoma siderosis
Pharmacologic inhibition of the parasympathetic pathway
 (atropine, scopolamine)

the same in light and in dark, but there is a tendency for it to decrease in light, perhaps because the smaller pupil reaches the zone of mechanical resistance first, giving the larger pupil a chance to catch up.

Physiologic anisocoria is not caused by damage to the peripheral nerves that innervate the sphincter and dilator muscles of the iris, which is why it is sometimes called "central anisocoria." It is presumed to occur because the inhibition of the sphincter nuclei in the midbrain is not balanced with any more precision than is necessary for clear, binocular vision. Other terms for physiologic anisocoria are "simple anisocoria," "central anisocoria," and "benign anisocoria."

In a patient with physiologic anisocoria, the

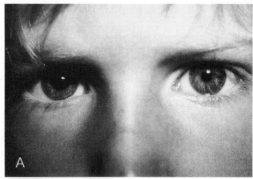

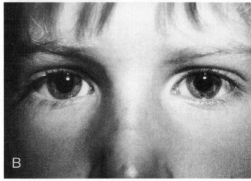

Figure 15.2. Physiologic (simple) anisocoria. The patient was a 5-year-old boy whose parents noted that the right pupil was larger than the other. The anisocoria was more obvious in dark than in light, and both pupils reacted normally to light stimulation. *A.* Appearance of the patient. Note anisocoria, with right pupil larger than left. *B.* Both pupils are dilated 45 minutes after instillation of a 10% solution of cocaine into both inferior conjunctival sacs, indicating that anisocoria is not caused by sympathetic denervation.

the moment of the examination. In room light, this number drops to about 10%. This form of anisocoria, called **physiologic anisocoria,** is rarely more than 0.6 mm, but it may be as much as 1.0 mm (Fig. 15.2) The anisocoria is almost

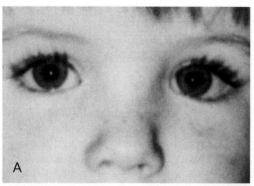

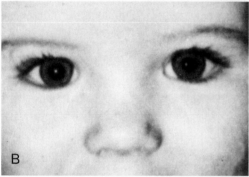

Figure 15.3. Value of old photographs in the assessment of anisocoria. *A*. This 3-year-old boy was noted by his parents to have intermittent anisocoria, with the right pupil larger than the left. *A*. The anisocoria was greater in darkness than in light, and both pupils reacted normally to light stimulation. *B*. Photograph of patient at age 7 months shows obvious anisocoria. A diagnosis of physiologic anisocoria was made.

amount of pupillary inequality may change from day to day or even from hour to hour. It is unrelated to refractive error. When physiologic anisocoria is suspected, reviewing old photographs, such as a driver's license, photo identification card, or a family album, may be more valuable than any neuroimaging studies (Fig. 15.3). Physiologic anisocoria will usually be seen in many of the pictures, all the way back to infancy or early childhood. The anisocoria seldom reverses. If the right pupil is larger than the left pupil when the patient is examined, the right pupil is likely to be larger than the left in most of the previous photographs.

Horner's Syndrome

When the sympathetic innervation to the eye is interrupted, the retractor muscles in the eye-

lids are weakened, allowing the upper lid to droop and the lower lid to rise. The dilator muscle of the iris is also weakened, allowing the pupil to become smaller, and vasomotor and sudomotor control of parts of the face may be lost. This combination of ptosis, miosis, and anhidrosis is called **Horner's syndrome** (Fig. 15.4).

CLINICAL FEATURES

The affected eye often looks small or sunken in patients with Horner's syndrome. The upper eyelid is slightly drooped because of paralysis of the sympathetically innervated smooth muscle (Müller's muscle) that contributes to the position of the opened upper eyelid. This **ptosis** is sometimes so slight or so variable that it escapes attention. Similar smooth muscle fibers in the lower eyelid also lose their nerve supply in Horner's syndrome; thus, the lower lid is usually slightly elevated, producing an "upside-down ptosis," further narrowing of the palpebral fissure, and an **apparent enophthalmos.**

The palsy of the iris dilator muscle in Horner's syndrome allows the iris sphincter to constrict, producing **miosis.** Interestingly, if the dilator muscle is stimulated (e.g., after an adrenergic eye drop is used), the pupil will dilate widely. Endogenous catecholamines can produce a similar phenomenon if the iris dilator muscle is supersensitive because of denervation. In some patients in the setting of intense emotional excitement, the pupil on the side of the sympathetic lesion becomes larger than the normal pupil. This "paradoxical pupillary dilation" is caused by denervation supersensitivity of the dilator muscle to circulating adrenergic substances.

In Horner's syndrome, the weakness of the dilator muscle is most apparent in darkness. The anisocoria is greater in the dark and almost disappears in light. The anisocoria of Horner's syndrome is diminished in bright light because the normal action of both sphincters tends to make the two pupils more nearly equal. In bright light, the pupils become very small, and it becomes physically difficult to constrict the iris sphincter muscle any more than it already is. Thus, the larger pupil "catches up" with the smaller pupil, diminishing the difference in size between the two pupils.

Anisocoria in Horner's syndrome also varies with the alertness of the patient. When the patient is awake and alert, the normal pupil is di-

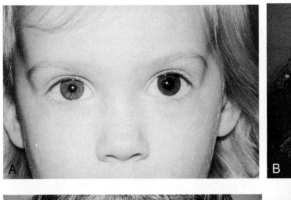
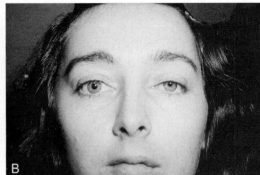
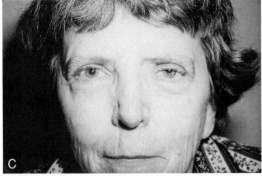
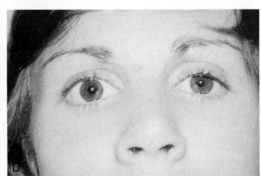

Figure 15.4. Horner's syndrome in four patients. *A.* Congenital right Horner's syndrome. Note associated heterochromia iridis and minimal ptosis. *B.* Left Horner's syndrome after neck trauma. *C.* Left Horner's syndrome associated with apical lung (Pancoast) tumor. *D.* Left Horner's syndrome in a patient with Raeder's paratrigeminal neuralgia.

lated, whereas the pupil of Horner's syndrome is less so. When the patient is fatigued or drowsy, the amount of anisocoria diminishes as the hypothalamic sympathetic outflow to both eyes subsides.

Thus, the actual amount of anisocoria in Horner's syndrome varies with:

1. The resting size of the pupils.
2. The completeness of the injury.
3. The alertness of the patient.
4. The extent of reinnervation of the dilator muscle.
5. The brightness of the examiner's light or the ambient light in the room.
6. The degree of denervation supersensitivity.
7. The fixation of the patient at distance or near.
8. The concentration of circulating adrenergic substances in the blood.

Paresis of the dilator muscle in Horner's syndrome can be detected in several ways. When the lights are turned out, the Horner's pupil dilates more slowly than the normal pupil, so-called **dilation lag** (Fig. 15.5, and see Chapter 14). A psychosensory stimulus such as a sudden noise will cause a normal pupil to dilate. Part of this dilation results from inhibition of the Edinger-Westphal nucleus, but the other major component is a sympathetic discharge to the dilator muscle. This component is absent in Horner's syndrome. Thus, a sudden noise will produce a transient increase in anisocoria. Hence, when looking for dilation lag in a patient with anisocoria that may be caused by Horner's syndrome, it is helpful to interject a sudden noise just after the lights go out.

Depigmentation of the ipsilateral iris is not usually seen in patients with an acquired Horner's syndrome, but it is a typical feature of congenital Horner's syndrome (see below). Never-

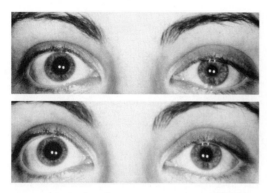

Figure 15.5. Dilation lag in a patient with a left Horner's syndrome, observed using infrared pupillary videography. *Top:* Photo taken 5 seconds after room lights turned off. *Bottom:* Photo taken after 15 seconds of darkness. Note that the right pupil is already maximally dilated within 5 seconds of turning the room lights off; however, the left pupil still has not dilated maximally after 15 seconds of darkness.

theless, it rarely can occur after injury to the sympathetic nervous system in adults.

Characteristic vasomotor and sudomotor changes of the facial skin occur on the affected side in some patients with Horner's syndrome. The best known of these is loss of sweating (**anhidrosis**). In a warm environment, the skin on the affected side will feel dry whereas the skin on the normal side will be so damp that a smooth object, such as a plastic prism, will not slide easily on the skin but will stick. Because most persons live and work in temperature-controlled spaces, patients with Horner's syndrome rarely complain of disturbances of sweating; however, occasionally, a patient with Horner's syndrome will offer, as a primary complaint, ''When I exercise, half my face gets red'' or ''The left side of my face stays completely dry, but on the right side my hair is wet and the sweat pours off my face.''

The postganglionic sympathetic sudomotor fibers for the face, after synapsing at the superior cervical ganglion, follow the external carotid artery to the face, whereas the sympathetic fibers to the eye travel via the carotid plexus of the internal carotid artery, carrying only a few sweat fibers for the skin of the forehead (Fig. 15.6). Thus, anhidrosis occurs only in patients with a central or preganglionic Horner's syndrome, never with a postganglionic Horner's syndrome.

After acute, preganglionic sympathetic denervation, the temperature of the skin rises on the side of the lesion because of loss of vasomotor control and consequent dilation of blood vessels. Acutely, there may be some flushing and some conjunctival hyperemia, epiphora, and nasal stuffiness. Some time after the injury, however, the skin of the ipsilateral face and neck may have a lower temperature and be more pale than that of the normal side. This occurs from supersensitivity of the denervated blood vessels to circulating adrenergic substances with resultant vasoconstriction.

Paradoxic ipsilateral sweating with flushing of the face, neck, and sometimes the shoulder and arm can be a late development in patients with a surgically induced Horner's syndrome following cervical sympathectomy, and the same syndrome may develop following a cervical injury. Apparently, some axons in the vagus nerve normally pass into the superior cervical ganglion. These parasympathetic axons can establish, by collateral sprouting, anomalous vagal connections with postganglionic sympathetic neurons to the head and neck. Affected patients may experience bizarre sudomotor and pilomotor (gooseflesh) activity and vasomotor flushing geared reflexly to certain functions of the vagus nerve. The patterns of anomalous sweating vary but often involve the central portions of the face and forehead.

There is an increase in **accommodative amplitude** on the side affected by Horner's syndrome. An intact sympathetic innervation of the ciliary muscle helps that muscle loosen and tighten the zonules with alacrity. This is a minor effect and is clinically insignificant.

DIAGNOSIS

Not all patients with unilateral ptosis and ipsilateral miosis have Horner's syndrome. As noted above, the prevalence of physiologic anisocoria in the normal population is about 20%. If a patient with physiologic anisocoria develops a ptosis (e.g., from levator dehiscence) on the side of the smaller pupil, the appearance will mimic a Horner's syndrome. It is therefore important to differentiate a Horner's syndrome from physiologic anisocoria.

Fortunately, the diagnosis of Horner's syndrome can be made by pharmacologic testing. The **cocaine test** is most commonly used and is based on the failure of cocaine to dilate a sympathetically denervated eye. Cocaine blocks the reuptake of norepinephrine into the sympathetic

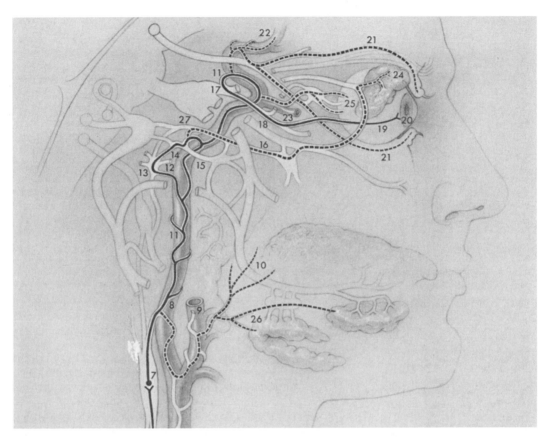

Figure 15.6. Sympathetic pathways to the face and eye. The solid line indicates the pathway of the pupillary dilator fibers, while the dashed lines show some of the other sympathetic pathways to the orbit and face. *7,* superior cervical ganglion; *8,* internal carotid artery; *10,* sudomotor fibers to the face; *11,* carotid plexus; *12,* caroticotympanic nerve; *13,* tympanic plexus; *14,* deep petrosal nerve; *15,* lesser superficial petrosal nerve; *16,* sympathetic contribution to vidian nerve; *17,* ophthalmic division of the trigeminal nerve; *18,* nasociliary nerve; *19,* long ciliary nerve; *20,* ciliary muscle and iris dilator muscle; *21,* probable pathway of sympathetic contribution to retractor muscles of the eyelids; *22,* vasomotor and some sudomotor fibers; *23,* ophthalmic artery; *24,* lacrimal gland; *25,* short ciliary nerves; *26,* sympathetic contribution to salivary glands; *27,* greater superificial petrosal nerve. (Chart prepared by Dr. H.S. Thompson and drawn by J. Esperson.)

nerve endings. Thus, in a normal eye, a 10% solution of cocaine causes dilation of the pupil, often to 8 mm or more, within about 45 minutes. However, a sufficient quantity of norepinephrine does not accumulate at the receptors of effector cells unless norepinephrine is continually being released by action potentials within the sympathetic nerves to those cells, which does not occur when there is sympathetic denervation of the pupillary dilator muscle (Fig. 15.7).

The first drop of topical cocaine stings briefly until the anesthetic effect occurs. We never use more than two drops in each eye, and we have not yet damaged the corneal epithelium. Peak effect is attained in 40 to 60 minutes. There are no apparent psychoactive effects from a 10% solution of cocaine, but metabolites of the drug can be found in the urine in 100% of patients after 24 hours and in 50% at 36 hours.

It is important to remember that cocaine affects only the sympathetic system, not the parasympathetic system. If the patient is simply observed while seated in a lighted room or in a hallway, the pupils may appear not to have responded to the cocaine because the light tends to produce pupillary constriction. The patient

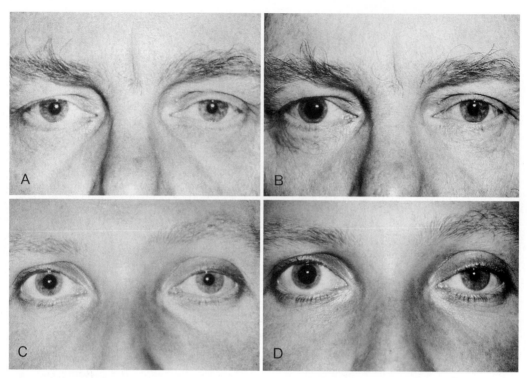

Figure 15.7. Response of Horner's pupils to cocaine. *A.* Left Horner's syndrome associated with Raeder's paratrigeminal neuralgia in a 55-year-old man. *B.* Photo taken 45 minutes after conjunctival instillation of 2 drops of a 10% cocaine solution in each eye. The right pupil is dilated, whereas the left pupil remains unchanged. *C.* Left Horner's syndrome in a 25-year-old man following trauma. *D.* At 45 minutes after conjunctival instillation of 2 drops of 10% cocaine in each eye, the right pupil is dilated, whereas the left pupil is unchanged.

must be brought into the examination room and the lights dimmed, at which time the pharmacologic dilation of one or both pupils can easily be appreciated.

The odds of an anisocoria being caused by an oculosympathetic palsy increase with the amount of anisocoria measured 45 minutes after the instillation of 10% cocaine into both eyes. It is not necessary to compare the before and after measurements; a post-cocaine anisocoria of 0.8 mm is sufficient to diagnose a Horner's syndrome.

LOCALIZATION

Regardless of the site of the lesion in the long sympathetic pathway, all patients with Horner's syndrome have a similar ptosis and miosis. It is, however, clinically important to separate the pathway into three major divisions: the central (first-order), the preganglionic (second-order), and the postganglionic (third-order) neurons.

Central Horner's Syndromes The **central** (first-order) neuron begins in the ipsilateral hypothalamus and extends to the ciliospinal center of Budge and Waller in the intermediolateral gray column of the spinal cord at C8-T1 (Fig. 15.8). The path may actually be polysynaptic, but it seems to stay lateral in the brainstem and cervical cord. Thus, Horner's syndrome caused by damage to the central neuron is almost always unilateral. A lesion in this neuron often produces a hemihypohidrosis of the entire body. There is no pharmacologic test that identifies a central-neuron Horner's syndrome, so the clinician must put localizing weight on the associated clinical signs. For example, lesions of the hypothalamus that cause an ipsilateral Horner's syndrome are often associated with a contralateral hemiparesis, and some of these patients also have a contralateral hypesthesia.

Another neurologic syndrome characterized in part by a central Horner's syndrome is **Wal-**

lenberg's syndrome. This condition, which is caused by damage to the lateral medulla, is also characterized by ipsilateral impairment of pain and temperature sensation over the face, limb ataxia, and a bulbar disturbance causing dysarthria and dysphagia. Contralaterally, pain and temperature sensation are impaired over the trunk and limbs. Lateropulsion, a compelling sensation of being pulled toward the side of the lesion, is often a prominent complaint of patients with Wallenberg's syndrome and is also evident in the ocular motor findings.

The occurrence of a unilateral Horner's syndrome and a contralateral trochlear nerve paresis indicates involvement either of the trochlear nucleus on the side of the Horner's syndrome or of the ipsilateral fascicle before its decussation. However, not all patients with a first-order neuron Horner's syndrome have other neurologic manifestations. Patients with cervical spondylosis, for example, may have no symptoms or signs of spinal cord disease. Such patients may present only with a Horner's syndrome and perhaps some neck pain.

What appears to be an **alternating Horner's syndrome** can be seen in association with cervical cord lesions and in some patients with systemic dysautonomias. It would be reasonable to

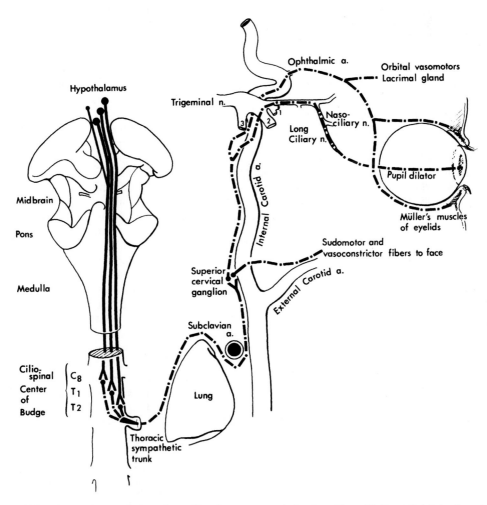

Figure 15.8.   The oculosympathetic pathway. Note location of central (first-order), preganglionic (second-order), and postganglionic (third-order) neurons. (Reprinted with permission from Glaser JS. Neuro-Ophthalmology. 1st ed. Hagerstown, MD: Harper & Row, 1978:173.)

expect a true alternating Horner's syndrome to be the result of an abnormality within the central nervous system (CNS), because to insist on a peripheral defect would require postulating a transient dysfunction that switched sides. It is possible that some patients with a presumed alternating Horner's syndrome actually have a permanent central Horner's syndrome on one side, but that intermittently they have an attack of "autonomic dysreflexia," exciting the ciliospinal center of Budge on the affected side (the C8-T1 intermediolateral gray column may, in fact, be supersensitive as a result of its disconnection). This firing would widen the pupil on the affected side, lift the eyelid, blanch the conjunctiva, and increase sweating on that side of the face—a pattern that would be difficult to distinguish from a Horner's syndrome on the other side. The cocaine test is of no help in this setting.

Preganglionic Horner's Syndromes   The **preganglionic** (second-order) neuron exits from the ciliospinal center of Budge and passes across the pulmonary apex (see Fig. 15.8). It then turns upward, passes through the stellate ganglion, and goes up the carotid sheath to the superior cervical ganglion, near the bifurcation of the common carotid artery.

The ptosis and miosis of a preganglionic Horner's syndrome are nonspecific, but the distribution of anhidrosis is characteristic. The entire side of the head, the face, and the neck down to the clavicle are usually involved.

Malignancy is a common cause of a preganglionic Horner's syndrome. The most common tumors, not surprisingly, are lung and breast cancer, but Horner's syndrome is usually not an early sign of these tumors. Tumors that spread behind the carotid sheath at the C6 level may produce a preganglionic Horner's syndrome associated with paralysis of the phrenic, vagus, and recurrent laryngeal nerves: the "Rowland Payne syndrome." Just 3 inches lower, at the thoracic outlet, these nerves are more widely separated and are less likely to be involved together. Thus, if a patient is newly hoarse and has a preganglionic Horner's syndrome, a chest radiograph, computed tomographic (CT) scan, or magnetic resonance imaging (MRI) may be warranted to see if the hemidiaphragm ipsilateral to the Horner's syndrome is elevated. Benign tumors in this region, such as a schwannoma of the sympa-

thetic chain, can also produce a preganglionic Horner's syndrome.

A preganglionic Horner's syndrome can be caused by accidental or surgical injury (e.g., disc herniation at C8 or T1, trauma to the brachial plexus, pneumothorax, coronary artery bypass surgery, or insertion of a pacemaker). The preganglionic neuron can also be transiently blocked by an epidural anesthetic that flows the wrong way or by an interpleural anesthetic that soaks through the pleura at the pulmonary apex to reach the stellate ganglion. Chest tubes, vascular catheters, and stray bullets can directly injure the preganglionic sympathetic nerves.

A preganglionic Horner's syndrome occasionally occurs after tonsillectomy or penetrating intraoral trauma. The Horner's syndrome in these and similar cases is probably caused by inadvertent damage to the superior cervical ganglion, which is located about 1.5 cm behind the palatine tonsil.

Postganglionic Horner's Syndromes   The **postganglionic** (third-order) neuron of the sympathetic pathway to the iris dilator muscle extends from the superior cervical ganglion behind the angle of the mandible and up along the internal carotid artery, where it is called the "carotid plexus" or the "carotid nerve" (see Figs. 15.6 and 15.8). Within the cavernous sinus, the sympathetic fibers leave the internal carotid artery, join briefly with the abducens nerve, and then leave it to join the ophthalmic division of the trigeminal nerve, entering the orbit with its nasociliary branch (Fig. 15.9). The sympathetic fibers in the nasociliary nerve divide into the two long ciliary nerves that travel with the lateral and medial suprachoroidal vascular bundles to reach the anterior segment of the eye and innervate the iris dilator muscle.

Lesions that affect the postganglionic third-order sympathetic neuron may be extracranial or intracranial. Extracranial lesions damage the cervical sympathetics in the neck, whereas intracranial lesions damage the sympathetic chain at the base of the skull, in the carotid canal and middle ear, or in the region of the cavernous sinus. It is very unusual for an orbital lesion to produce an isolated Horner's syndrome.

Lesions of or along the internal carotid artery are a common cause of a postganglionic Horner's syndrome. Both traumatic and spontaneous **dissections of the internal carotid artery** can

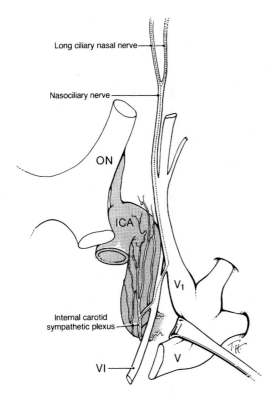

Figure 15.9.   Diagram showing the course of the sympathetic, postganglionic fibers from the internal carotid plexus. Note that they join briefly with the abducens nerve (VI) before entering the orbit with the nasociliary nerve, a branch of the ophthalmic division (VI) of the trigeminal nerve. After reaching the nasociliary nerve, the sympathetic fibers reach the iris dilator muscle as the long ciliary nerves. *ICA*, internal carotid artery. *ON*, optic nerve. (Modified from Solnitzky O. Horner's syndrome: its diagnostic significance. Georgetown Univ Med Cent Bull 1961;14:204–222.)

produce sudden ipsilateral face and neck pain associated with a postganglionic Horner's syndrome. This condition is easily diagnosed using MRI and is probably more common than previously realized. Indeed, Raeder's paratrigeminal neuralgia, the name given to a headache syndrome characterized by persistent trigeminal pain associated with a postganglionic Horner's syndrome, likely represents unrecognized carotid dissection in many patients.

Atherosclerosis of the internal and external carotid arteries can apparently produce a postganglionic Horner's syndrome, as can lesions of the jugular vein in the neck. Similarly, a postganglionic Horner's syndrome may be caused by tumors, inflammatory lesions, and other masses in the neck. Indeed, any neoplasm that extends or metastasizes to the cervical lymph nodes may also damage the cervical sympathetic chain. A postganglionic Horner's syndrome, paralysis of the tongue, anesthesia of the pharynx, and dysphagia, all on the same side, may indicate a tumor of the nasopharynx or jugular foramen.

Tumors, aneurysms, infections, and other lesions in the cavernous sinus may produce a postganglionic Horner's syndrome. In many of these cases, there is associated ipsilateral ophthalmoplegia as well as pain or dysesthesia of the ipsilateral side of the face caused by involvement of one or more ocular motor nerves and the trigeminal nerve within the sinus. Because the abducens nerve and oculosympathetic nerves are briefly joined in the cavernous sinus, an abducens palsy and a postganglionic Horner's syndrome occurring together without other neurologic signs should immediately suggest a cavernous sinus lesion.

Cluster headaches often occur at night and usually last 30 to 120 minutes. The patient is completely preoccupied with a very severe lancinating or dysesthetic pain. In addition, the eye is red and half closed from an associated sympathetic palsy, and there is ipsilateral nasal stuffiness. Typically, the Horner's syndrome persists after the headache resolves. Other ischemic conditions, such as giant cell arteritis, can cause a postganglionic Horner's syndrome.

A middle fossa mass encroaching on Meckel's cave and on the internal carotid artery at the foramen lacerum can also produce a postganglionic Horner's syndrome associated with pain. Other lesions at the base of the skull, including a basal skull fracture, can produce a similar clinical picture.

Differentiating Localizations   The **hydroxyamphetamine test** can be used to differentiate between a postganglionic and a preganglionic or central Horner's syndrome (Fig. 15.10). This test should be performed only after a cocaine test has established the diagnosis of a Horner's syndrome or in a setting in which the diagnosis of Horner's syndrome is clear cut. If a cocaine test has been performed, the hydroxyamphetamine test should not be performed for 24 to 48 hours, to allow the corneas and pupils to recover from the effects of the cocaine. The hydroxyamphetamine test is performed as follows. Two

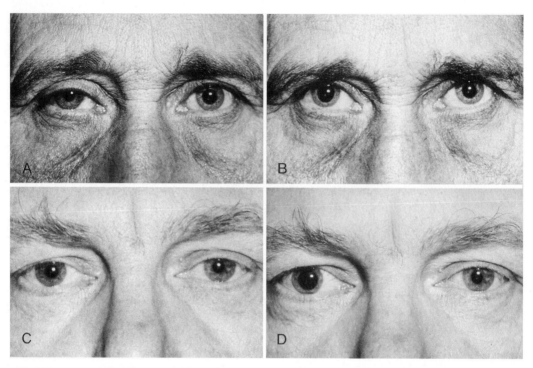

Figure 15.10. Response of Horner's pupils to hydroxyamphetamine. *A.* Right Horner's syndrome in a 45-year-old man with an apical lung tumor. *B.* At 45 minutes after conjunctival instillation of 2 drops of 1% hydroxyamphetamine solution (Paredrine) in each eye, both pupils are dilated, indicating an intact postganglionic neuron (i.e., a preganglionic Horner's syndrome). *C.* Left Horner's syndrome associated with cluster headaches in a 55-year-old man. *D.* At 45 minutes after conjunctival instillation of 2 drops of 1% hydroxyamphetamine solution in each eye, only the right (normal) pupil is dilated. The left pupil is unchanged, indicating damage to the postganglionic neuron (i.e., a postganglionic Horner's syndrome).

drops of hydroxyamphetamine hydrobromide 1% (Paredrine) are placed in the lower cul-de-sac of each eye, and the pupils are assessed in a dim light about 45 minutes later. Hydroxyamphetamine releases norepinephrine from the stores in the adrenergic nerve ending, producing variable but usually significant mydriasis in normal subjects. When the lesion causing a Horner's syndrome is in the postganglionic neuron, the nerve endings themselves are destroyed, there are no stores of norepinephrine to release, and hydroxyamphetamine thus has no mydriatic effect. If the lesion is in the preganglionic or central neuron, however, the pupil will dilate fully and may even become larger than the opposite pupil, presumably because of up-regulation of the postsynaptic receptors on the dilator muscle. Although there are occasional false-negative responses to the hydroxyamphetamine test, such responses usually occur only in patients who are

tested within the first week after the Horner's syndrome has developed, presumably before the stores of norepinephrine at the presynaptic terminals have been depleted. Paredrine is available in the United States through the services of licensed compounding pharmacists (e.g., Leiter's Park Ave Pharmacy, San Jose, CA, 408–292–6772, or Thayer's Colonial Pharmacy, Orlando, FL, 407–896–7001).

A smaller pupil that fails to dilate to cocaine and subsequently does not dilate after topical administration of hydroxyamphetamine or a similar substance is likely to be caused by a lesion of the postganglionic sympathetic neuron. Such a pupil should show evidence of denervation supersensitivity to adrenergic substances and should dilate to a weak, direct-acting topical adrenergic drug such as a 1% solution of phenylephrine hydrochloride or a 2% solution of epinephrine. Indeed, such a pupil not only will dilate but will become larger than the opposite pupil. Denervation supersensitivity of the iris to adrenergic drugs apparently does not occur immediately after damage to the postganglionic sympathetic nerve but may take as long as 17 days to develop. Although denervation supersensitivity to weak solutions of adrenergic drugs can be used to localize a Horner's syndrome, localization is likely to be more accurate when hydroxyamphetamine or a similar topical agent is used.

ACQUIRED HORNER'S SYNDROME IN CHILDREN

An acquired Horner's syndrome in childhood is always worrisome, because it is sometimes associated with neoplasia, including spinal cord tumors, embryonal cell carcinoma, neuroblastoma, and rhabdomyosarcoma. However, this association is quite rare. In our experience, a Horner's syndrome in childhood is usually *not* associated with a tumor and is often an isolated finding of no significance. Other causes of an acquired Horner's syndrome in childhood include traumatic brachial plexus palsy, intrathoracic aneurysm, and thrombosis of the internal carotid artery. If old photographs clearly indicate that a Horner's syndrome in a child is acquired, we are more likely to pursue an evaluation, beginning with CT scanning or MRI of the chest.

CONGENITAL HORNER'S SYNDROME

Congenital Horner's syndrome is an uncommon disorder. In its fully developed form, the syndrome consists of ptosis, miosis, facial anhidrosis, and hypochromia of the affected iris. Injury to the brachial plexus at birth is responsible for many of these cases (Fig. 15.11), but some cases occur in association with congenital tumors, and others occur after viral infections.

Most patients with congenital Horner's syndrome can be separated into one of three groups:

- Those with evidence of obstetric trauma to the internal carotid artery sympathetic plexus.
- Those without a history of birth trauma but with a lesion that is clinically and pharmacologically localized to the superior cervical ganglion.
- Those with evidence of surgical or obstetric injury to the preganglionic sympathetic pathway.

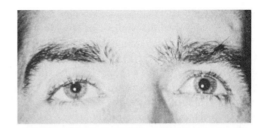

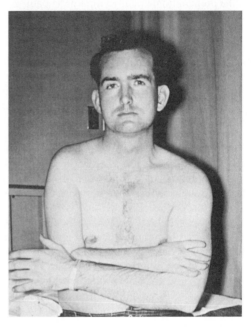

Figure 15.11.   Horner's syndrome (*top*) associated with injury of the right brachial plexus at birth. Note the underdeveloped right arm and forearm (*bottom*).

The first group of patients tends to have had substantial perinatal head trauma as a result of difficult forceps deliveries. In all cases, the trauma is significant and includes the use of high forceps and rotation for fetal malposition. Clinically, such patients have obvious ptosis and miosis with generally intact facial sweating. Pharmacologic testing is consistent with a postganglionic lesion.

In the second group of patients, pharmacologic testing also is consistent with a postganglionic lesion but such patients have facial anhidrosis, indicating a lesion proximal to the separation of the sudomotor fibers with the external carotid artery. This combination of postganglionic oculosympathetic paralysis and complete loss of facial sweating localizes the lesion to the superior cervical ganglion. The causes of such a lesion could include an embryopathy directly involving the superior cervical ganglion, damage to the vascular supply of the superior cervical ganglion, or transsynaptic dysgenesis of the superior cervical ganglion following a defect located more proximally in the sympathetic pathway.

The third group of patients has suffered trauma to the preganglionic oculosympathetic pathway. Injuries include trauma to the brachial plexus and surgery in the thoracic region. Although patients in this group should have a preganglionic Horner's syndrome, some have pharmacologic testing consistent with a postganglionic lesion, presumably indicating transsynaptic degeneration occurring in the postganglionic neuron following preganglionic injury.

Parents of infants with congenital Horner's syndrome sometimes report that the baby develops a hemifacial flush when it is nursing or crying. Although it is often hard to tell from these accounts if it is the side with the ptosis and miosis or the opposite side that becomes flushed, we believe it likely that the hemifacial flushing seen in infants is on the side opposite the Horner's syndrome and is simply the normal response, which appears more obvious because of the impaired facial vasodilation on the side of a congenital Horner's syndrome.

Children whose hair is naturally curly and who have a congenital Horner's syndrome have straight hair on the side of the Horner's syndrome. The reason for this abnormality is unclear, but it probably relates to lack of sympathetic innervation to the hair shafts on the affected side of the head.

When a child has unilateral ptosis and ipsilateral miosis, and there is doubt as to whether or not a sympathetic defect is present, a cycloplegic refraction can sometimes unexpectedly solve the problem by producing an atropinic flush. This reaction only occurs when there is an intact sympathetic innervation to the skin and thus is absent on the side of the Horner's syndrome (Fig. 15.12).

A child with Horner's syndrome and very blue eyes will not develop visible iris heterochromia, but most children with Horner's syndrome have the more pale iris on the affected side. This occurs whether the lesion is preganglionic or postganglionic because of anterograde transsynaptic dysgenesis. When the sympathetic pathway is interrupted in the preganglionic neuron (e.g., at

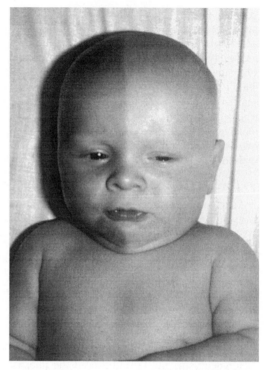

Figure 15.12. Lack of atropinic flushing in a child with a congenital left Horner's syndrome. Note that the atropinic flush is present only on the side of the face opposite the Horner's syndrome.

the stellate ganglion at the apex of the lung), the next distal ganglion—the superior cervical ganglion—does not develop normally. There are fewer cells in the ganglion, and their axons have fewer arborizations, so there are fewer nerve endings at the dilator muscle and less norepinephrine stores to release with hydroxyamphetamine. This, in turn, results in impaired development of iris melanophores, causing hypochromia of the iris stroma.

Sympathetic Hyperactivity

Sympathetic hyperactivity occurs in a number of settings in which the pupils are affected. In such cases, there may be anisocoria that is more obvious in darkness than in light.

An occasional patient, more often a woman than a man, will report that the pupil of one eye becomes distorted for a minute or two. In most cases, the eye feels "funny," and the vision in the eye becomes slightly blurred. Looking in the mirror reveals that the pupil is pulled in one direction like the tail of a tadpole (Fig. 15.13).

This phenomenon, called **tadpole pupil,** may occur many times a day for a week or two and then stop, only to recur several months later. It is both temporary and benign. The etiology of tadpole pupils is unclear; however, because many patients with this condition have a partial postganglionic Horner's syndrome on the affected side, it may be that repeated bursts of sympathetic innervation pull one segment of the iris toward the limbus. This irritation eventually causes loss of fibers and a Horner's syndrome.

We believe that this condition is different from the **episodic unilateral mydriasis** that occurs in some young patients during a typical migraine attack, although there is some similarity. For example, many patients with unilateral mydriasis in the setting of migraine do not have an associated unilateral accommodative paresis, suggesting that their mydriasis is related to sympathetic discharge rather than to parasympathetic blockade.

Some patients who sustain trauma (e.g., whiplash injury) to the low cervical or high thoracic spinal cord experience episodes of unilateral pupillary dilation associated with unilateral sweating. Pharmacologic testing in such patients suggests that the mydriasis is caused by episodic sympathetic irritation.

This regional sympathetic response is similar to that seen in spinally transected animals and is thought to provide a clinically useful sign of a painful condition that is located below the analgesic level in patients with spinal cord injuries.

Pharmacologic Stimulation of the Iris Sphincter

Almost all cases of acute anisocoria in which one pupil is nonreactive are caused by pharmacologic blockade of the iris sphincter muscle. In such cases, the anisocoria is worse in light than in darkness because the affected pupil cannot constrict. In rare instances, however, a pharmacologic agent, such as an organophosphate, may produce anisocoria by stimulating rather than blocking the parasympathetic system, thus producing a nonreactive, **miotic** pupil. Anisocoria caused by parasympathetic stimulation can occur after handling one of the many organophosphate pesticides used in gardening or a pet's flea collar containing an anticholinesterase agent. In such cases and in other cases of pharmacologic stimulation of the ocular parasympathetic pathway, a 1% solution of tropicamide will dilate the larger, reactive pupil but will fail to dilate the small, nonreactive pupil.

Pharmacologic Stimulation of the Iris Dilator

Topical cocaine placed in the nose for medical or for other reasons can back up the lacrimal duct into the conjunctival sac. Most eye-whitening drops that contain sympathomimetic components are too weak to dilate the pupil, but if the cornea is abraded (e.g., by a contact lens), enough of the oxymetazoline or the phenylephrine may get into the aqueous humor to dilate the pupil. Other adrenergic drugs given in a mist for pulmonary therapy may escape around the edge of the face mask and condense in the conjunctival sac, causing pupillary dilation that is more evident in darkness than in light.

More Anisocoria in Light

Damage to the Parasympathetic Outflow to the Iris Sphincter Muscle

The final common pathway for pupillary reactivity to light and near stimulation begins in the mesencephalon with the visceral oculomotor nuclei, continues via the oculomotor nerve to the

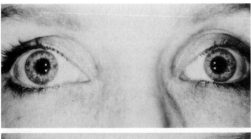
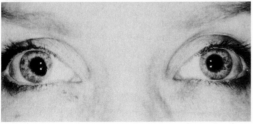

Figure 15.13. Tadpole pupil. *A.* Before the episode, the pupils are normal in size and shape. *B.* During the episode, the right pupil develops an eccentric shape, with the 5 o'clock portion of the pupil being displaced outward. (Reprinted with permission from Thompson HS, Zackon DH, Czarnecki JSC. Tadpole-shaped pupils caused by segmental spasm of the iris dilator muscle. Am J Ophthalmol 1983;96: 467–477.)

ciliary ganglion, and reaches the iris sphincter through the short ciliary nerves. Lesions that affect this parasympathetic pathway can produce absolute paralysis of pupillary constriction. The pupil is then dilated and nonreactive, and all constrictor reflexes are absent. In many cases, all parasympathetic input to the eye is damaged simultaneously so that accommodation is also lost. This combination of iridoplegia and cycloplegia is often called **internal ophthalmoplegia** to distinguish it from the external ophthalmoplegia that occurs when the extraocular muscles are paralyzed in the setting of normal pupillary responses.

Topical diagnosis of paralysis of the iris sphincter is simplified when signs of an oculomotor nerve palsy are present. In the setting of ptosis and paralysis of the superior, inferior, and medial rectus muscles, as well as the inferior oblique muscle, a nonreactive, dilated pupil is but a part of the classic picture of a lesion of the oculomotor nerve. However, isolated iris paralysis can be a difficult diagnostic problem. One must consider lesions of the mesencephalon, the oculomotor nerve, the ciliary ganglion, the short ciliary nerves, and the eye itself.

DAMAGE TO THE EDINGER-WESTPHAL NUCLEI

Lesions of the rostral mesencephalon almost never produce an isolated unilateral, nonreactive, dilated pupil. When there is isolated damage to the Edinger-Westphal nuclei, bilateral pupillary abnormalities are the rule. In addition, most lesions in this region that produce pupillary abnormalities also affect other parts of the oculomotor nucleus, causing ptosis, ophthalmoparesis, or both.

DAMAGE TO PUPILLOMOTOR FIBERS IN THE OCULOMOTOR NERVE FASCICLE

The fascicle of the oculomotor nerve can be damaged within the mesencephalon by a variety of processes, including ischemia, inflammation, and infiltration. Such processes can produce a complete or incomplete isolated oculomotor nerve paresis or a syndrome in which an oculomotor nerve paresis is associated with other neurologic signs, such as contralateral hemiparesis or tremor. Because the fibers emerging from the Edinger-Westphal nucleus are among the most rostral in the oculomotor group (Fig. 15.14), it is possible for a lesion to damage just the fibers serving pupillary function, thus producing a unilateral, dilated, nonreactive pupil. In other patients, a lesion affecting the oculomotor fascicle may damage only the fibers destined for the extraocular muscles, levator palpebrae superioris, or both, sparing the bundle headed for the iris sphincter and thus producing a pupil-sparing complete or incomplete oculomotor nerve palsy.

DAMAGE TO PUPILLOMOTOR FIBERS IN THE SUBARACHNOID PORTION OF THE OCULOMOTOR NERVE

The separate bundles of the oculomotor nerve that leave the mesencephalon merge to form the oculomotor nerve in the subarachnoid space. The nerve takes a short course between the posterior cerebral and superior cerebellar arteries and then enters the cavernous sinus. In this part of the preganglionic path, the pupillary fibers are superficial and migrate from a superior medial position to the inferior part of the nerve (Fig. 15.15).

Noxious influences carried by the cerebrospinal fluid (CSF) are a hazard to the oculomotor nerve within the subarachnoid space. In basal meningitis, for example, the nerve is surrounded by pus, and the superficially located pupillary fibers are particularly at risk; hence, the axiom that any meningitis that seems disproportionately to impair the pupillary light reflex while sparing the extraocular muscles should be promptly treated as tuberculosis, even before that diagnosis is confirmed. In fact, basal meningitis from a variety of organisms, including bacteria, viruses, and spirochetes, can produce unilateral or bilateral poorly reactive pupils.

Although intracranial aneurysms, particularly those at the junction of the internal carotid artery and the posterior communicating artery, may produce a dilated, nonreactive pupil, this is nearly always associated with other evidence of oculomotor nerve dysfunction. Cases of aneurysmal oculomotor nerve palsies characterized only by a dilated, nonreactive pupil are extremely unusual. Nevertheless, such cases do occur. In our experience, aneurysms of the tip of the basilar artery are more likely to produce isolated pupillary dilation than are aneurysms of the internal carotid artery. Such lesions can be readily diagnosed using standard MR imaging,

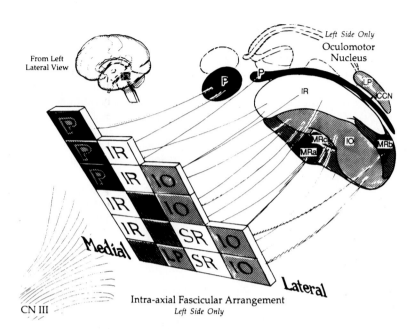

Figure 15.14. Position of the pupillomotor fibers in the fascicle of the human oculomotor nerve. Note that the fibers destined to innervate the iris sphincter muscle (*P*) are located rostral and medial to the fibers that innervate the extraocular muscles and the levator palpebrae superioris (*LP*). *IO*, inferior oblique. *IR*, inferior rectus. *MR*, medial rectus. *SR*, superior rectus. *MRa*, *MRb*, and *MRc*, subnuclei serving medial rectus function in the oculomotor nuclear complex. *CCN*, central caudal nucleus. (Reprinted with permission from Ksiazek SM, Slamovits TL, Rosen CE, et al. Fascicular arrangement in partial oculomotor paresis. Am J Ophthalmol 1994; 118:97–103.)

MR angiography, CT angiography, or a combination of these noninvasive imaging techniques.

Intrinsic lesions of the oculomotor nerve in the subarachnoid space can produce an oculomotor nerve paresis that begins with a dilated pupil. Such lesions include schwannomas and angiomas.

DAMAGE TO THE CAVERNOUS PORTION OF THE OCULOMOTOR NERVE

The pupillomotor fibers are located inferiorly and superficially in the portion of the oculomotor nerve located within the cavernous sinus. Damage to the intrinsic aspect of the nerve, particularly ischemia in the setting of diabetes mellitus, not uncommonly produces a pupil-sparing oculomotor nerve palsy; however, it is exceptionally rare to observe an isolated, dilated, nonreactive pupil from damage to the pupillomotor fibers in this region.

DAMAGE TO THE CILIARY GANGLION AND ITS ROOTS IN THE ORBIT: TONIC PUPIL

Damage to the postganglionic parasympathetic innervation of the intraocular muscles produces a characteristic syndrome. Initially, there may be an isolated internal ophthalmoplegia. Later, one or more of the following abnormalities may be observed:

- A poor pupillary reaction to light that can be seen to be a regional palsy of the iris sphincter by slit lamp biomicroscopy.
- Paresis of accommodation.
- Cholinergic supersensitivity of the denervated muscles.
- A pupillary response to near stimuli that is unusually strong and tonic.
- A slow and tonic redilation after constriction to near stimuli.

Pupils that react in this manner are called **tonic pupils** (Fig. 15.16). The lesions that produce them damage the ciliary ganglion or the short ciliary nerves in the retrobulbar space or in the intraocular, suprachoroidal space (Figs. 15.17 and 15.18). The slowness and tonicity of the pupillary movement is caused by aberrant regeneration of ciliary nerves into the iris sphincter.

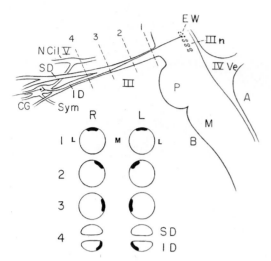

Figure 15.15. Course of preganglionic autonomic nerve fibers from the brainstem to the ciliary ganglion in humans. A sagittal reconstruction of the brainstem with the course of the oculomotor nerve is shown at top. The corresponding locations of the preganglionic autonomic fibers for pupillo-constriction and accommodation within the right (R) and left (L) oculomotor nerves are shown in black in coronal sections through slices at 1 (emergence from the brainstem), 2 (mid-point in the subarachnoid space), 3 (at the point where the third nerve enters the dura), and 4 (in the anterior cavernous sinus where the fibers have entered the anatomical inferior division of the third nerve). The autonomic fibers are located superiorly as the oculomotor nerve exits the brainstem and then come to lie more medially as the oculomotor nerve passes toward the orbit. *A,* dorsal, and *B,* ventral side of brainstem; *P,* pons; *M,* medulla; *EW,* Edinger-Westphal nucleus; *IIIn,* somatic portion of 3rd nerve nucleus; *III,* 3rd nerve; *ID,* inferior division of 3rd nerve; *SD,* superior division of 3rd nerve; *NCilV,* nasociliary branch of the 5th nerve; *CG,* ciliary ganglion; *Sym,* sympathetic route; *m,* medial; *l,* lateral. (Reprinted with permission from Kerr FWL, Hallowell OW. Location of pupillomotor and accommodation fibers in the oculomotor nerve: experimental observations on paralytic mydriasis. J Neurol Neurosurg Psychiatry 1964; 27:473–481.)

Tonic pupils can be separated into three categories: local, neuropathic, and the Holmes-Adie (Adie's) syndrome.

Local Tonic Pupil   Acute internal ophthalmoplegia followed by the development of a tonic pupil occurs from a variety of inflammations, infections, and infiltrative processes that affect the ciliary ganglion in isolation or as part of a systemic process. Disorders that can cause this

type of **local** tonic pupil include herpes zoster, chickenpox, measles, diphtheria, syphilis (both congenital and acquired), sarcoidosis, scarlet fever, pertussis, smallpox, influenza, sinusitis, Vogt-Koyanagi-Harada syndrome, rheumatoid arthritis, viral hepatitis, choroiditis, primary and metastatic choroidal and orbital tumors, blunt injury to the globe, and penetrating orbital injury. Siderosis from an intraocular iron foreign body apparently damages the nerves more than the sphincter muscle and may produce an iron mydriasis. Various ocular or orbital surgical procedures, including retinal reattachment surgery, inferior oblique muscle surgery, orbital surgery, optic nerve sheath fenestration, photocoagulation, transconjunctival cryotherapy, transscleral

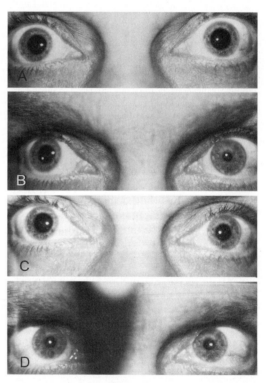

Figure 15.16. Tonic pupil syndrome. About 4 months earlier, this 38-year-old man noted that his right pupil was larger than this left pupil. *A.* In the dark looking in the distance, both pupils are dilated and relatively equal in size. *B.* In bright light, the right pupil does not constrict, whereas the left pupil constricts normally, producing a marked anisocoria. *C.* In room light looking in the distance, there is a moderate anisocoria. *D.* During near viewing, however, both pupils constrict. The right pupil constricted much slower than the left and redilated slowly.

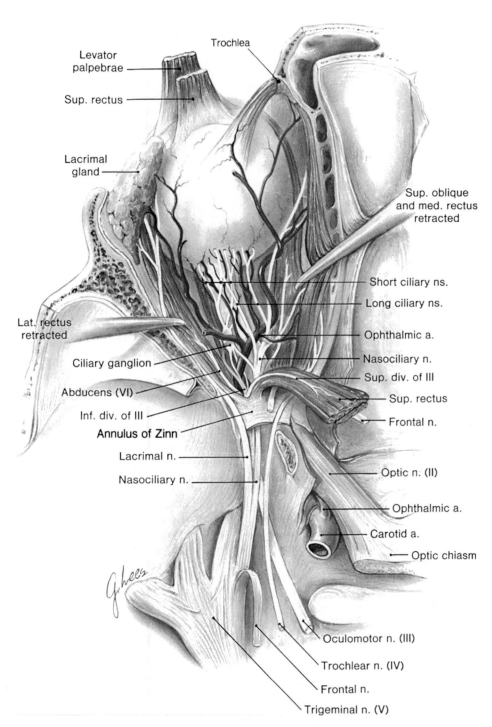

Figure 15.17.   Superior view of the orbit. Note that the inferior division of the oculomotor nerve supplies branches to the ciliary ganglion that in turn gives off numerous short posterior ciliary nerves. (Redrawn from Wolff E. Anatomy of the Eye and Orbit. 6th ed. Philadelphia: WB Saunders, 1968.)

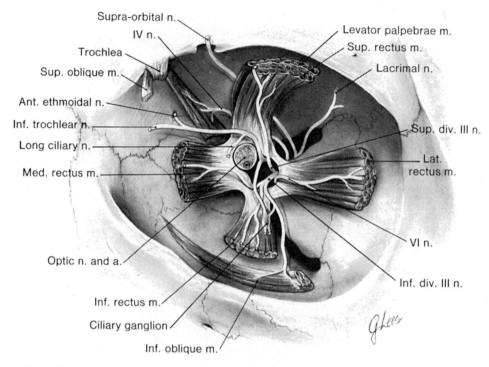

Supra-orbital n.
IV n.
Trochlea
Sup. oblique m.
Ant. ethmoidal n.
Inf. trochlear n.
Long ciliary n.
Med. rectus m.
Optic n. and a.
Inf. rectus m.
Ciliary ganglion
Inf. oblique m.

Levator palpebrae m.
Sup. rectus m.
Lacrimal n.
Sup. div. III n.
Lat. rectus m.
VI n.
Inf. div. III n.

Figure 15.18. View of the posterior orbit showing the relationship of the optic nerve to the ocular motor nerves and extraocular muscles. Note the location of the ciliary ganglion. (Redrawn from Wolff E. Anatomy of the Eye and Orbit. 6th ed. Philadelphia: WB Saunders, 1968.)

diathermy, and retrobulbar injections of alcohol can cause a local tonic pupil, as can inferior dental blocks with local anesthesia. Ischemia of the coats of the eye from quinine toxicity and ischemia of the ciliary ganglion or short ciliary nerves from migraine, giant cell arteritis, and other vasculitides also can cause a tonic pupil.

Neuropathic Tonic Pupil **Neuropathic tonic pupils** occur in patients in whom a tonic pupil is part of a generalized, widespread, peripheral or autonomic neuropathy that also involves the ciliary ganglion, the short ciliary nerves, or both. In some cases, there is evidence of both a sympathetic and a parasympathetic disturbance. Diseases that produce this syndrome include syphilis, chronic alcoholism, diabetes mellitus, some of the spinocerebellar ataxias, Guillain-Barré syndrome (GBS), and the Miller Fisher variant of GBS. Other systemic diseases involving autonomic nervous system dysfunction that may be associated with a tonic pupil are acute pandysautonomia, Shy-Drager syndrome,

and Ross syndrome (hyporeflexia, progressive segmental hypohidrosis, and tonic pupil). Patients with systemic lupus erythematosus may develop tonic pupils in association with a more generalized autonomic neuropathy, as may patients with Sjögren's syndrome, in whom the pupillary disturbance may even be the first sign of the disorder. Tonic pupils can also develop in patients with systemic amyloidosis and hereditary sensory neuropathy, they may be a distant effect of cancer, occurring either as an isolated phenomenon or as part of a more extensive autonomic polyneuropathy, and they appear to occur with increased frequency in patients with hereditary motor-sensory neuropathy (Charcot-Marie-Tooth disease). They have been described in patients with trichloroethylene intoxication.

Holmes-Adie Tonic Pupil Syndrome The **Holmes-Adie tonic pupil syndrome** (also called Adie's syndrome) consists of unilateral or bilateral tonically reacting pupils developing in otherwise healthy persons and in patients with unrelated conditions. Most of these patients also have a disturbance in deep-tendon reflexes, but they have no evidence of local ocular or orbital disease or of generalized peripheral or autonomic nervous system dysfunction.

Adie's syndrome is not common. It nearly always occurs as a sporadic entity, although it can be familial. It is uncommon before age 15, and most patients are between 20 and 50 years of age when the condition is noticed. Although Adie's syndrome occurs in both sexes, there is a clear predilection for women, with about 70% of cases being in women and only 30% in men. The age of onset is not significantly different for men and women. Adie's syndrome is unilateral in about 80% of cases. When the condition is bilateral, the onset is occasionally simultaneous but usually occurs in separate episodes months or even years apart.

Most patients with Adie's syndrome have visual complaints. Symptoms include photophobia, blurred near vision, an enlarged pupil, and headaches. Over time, the dilated pupil becomes smaller, and accommodation improves; however, many patients continue to have difficulty focusing. Such patients can see clearly at both distance and near, but they experience a noticeable lag period when shifting fixation from distance to near or vice versa. As might be expected, this is particularly troublesome if their work involves constant shifting from far to near and back again, especially if the unaffected eye is amblyopic, or if the patient is prone to overaccommodation. If, some years later, the other eye is similarly affected, as occurs in about 4% of cases per year, it seems to produce far fewer symptoms, and may in fact pass unnoticed.

A balanced bifocal add will usually relieve the irritating symptoms induced by tonicity of accommodation. Indeed, we find that many patients with Adie's syndrome can comfortably wear bifocals of a strength that is not yet needed by the unaffected eye.

Adie's syndrome usually occurs acutely as an internal ophthalmoplegia. It may initially be mistaken for an oculomotor nerve palsy, even though there is no ptosis and no ophthalmoparesis. It may also be confused with a pharmacologically induced mydriasis and cycloplegia until a slit lamp examination is performed, at which time segmental contractions of the iris sphincter are observed (Fig. 15.19). These segmental contractions are observed in all forms of

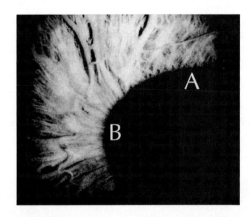

Figure 15.19. Segmental palsy of the iris sphincter in Adie's tonic pupil syndrome. *A.* This part of the iris sphincter is denervated and does not react to light. *B.* This sphincter segment constricts to light.

tonic pupil, including Adie's syndrome, whereas a pharmacologic anticholinergic blockade always paralyzes the *entire* sphincter and does not leave any segments still responding to light.

"Vermiform" movements of the iris often occur in patients with Adie's syndrome. These movements probably represent physiologic pupillary unrest or hippus that occurs only in portions of the iris in which the sphincter still reacts and are the same as segmental contractions of the iris. Segmental palsy of the iris sphincter is a critical diagnostic observation. Almost every Adie's pupil that has any reaction to light (about 90%) has such a segmental palsy of the sphincter.

In most patients with Adie's syndrome, the accommodative paresis resolves over several months. In some patients, however, aberrant regeneration within the ciliary muscle produces an accommodative paresis that may persist until presbyopia develops and diminishes the symptoms.

A regional decrease in corneal sensation occurs in some patients with Adie's syndrome. This phenomenon supports the contention that the lesion in Adie's syndrome is located in the ciliary ganglion or short ciliary nerves.

Hyporeflexia or areflexia is present in a substantial number of patients with Adie's syndrome. It is difficult to explain the association of such abnormal deep-tendon reflexes with a unilateral or bilateral peripheral lesion of the pupilloconstrictor pathway, but the most likely explanation is that the responsible lesion is located centrally within the spinal cord. Indeed, pathologic studies in a few patients with Adie's syndrome report atrophic changes in the dorsal columns. It thus seems most likely that degeneration of cell bodies in the dorsal columns similar to that which occurs in the ciliary ganglion is responsible for the loss of deep-tendon reflexes that occur in the majority of patients with Adie's syndrome.

The tonic pupil of patients with Adie's syndrome is supersensitive to acetylcholine and similar substances, including pilocarpine. For example, conjunctival administration of 2 drops of a 2.5% solution of methacholine chloride (Mecholyl) or a 0.1% solution of pilocarpine causes intense miosis in most tonic pupils (Fig. 15.20), whereas such solutions do not generally cause any change in the size of normal pupils.

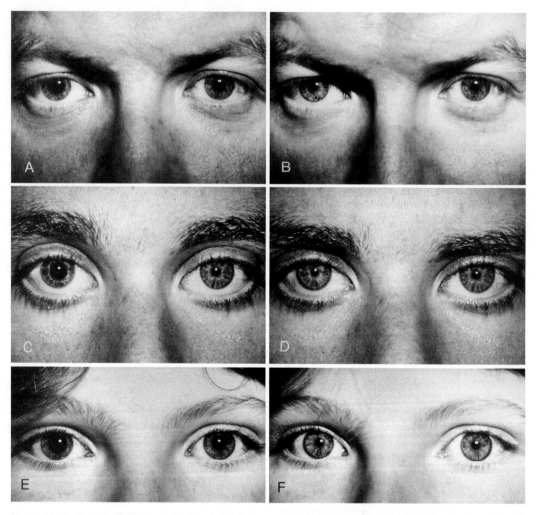

Figure 15.20. Postganglionic supersensitivity in the tonic pupil syndrome. *A.* A right tonic pupil in a 28-year-old man. *B.* At 45 minutes after conjunctival instillation of 2 drops of 2.5% methacholine (Mecholyl) in each eye, the right pupil is constricted and nonreactive. The left pupil is unchanged in size and reacts normally. *C.* A right tonic pupil in a 36-year-old woman. *D.* At 45 minutes after conjunctival instillation of 2 drops of 0.1% pilocarpine solution in each eye, the right pupil is constricted and nonreactive. The left pupil remains unchanged and normally reactive. *E.* Bilateral tonic pupils in a 14-year-old girl. *F.* At 45 minutes after conjunctival instillation of 2 drops of 0.1% pilocarpine solution in each eye, both pupils are constricted and nonreactive. The same solution in the author's eye did not produce any pupillary constriction.

Unfortunately, the clinical usefulness of the **denervation supersensitivity test** for a tonic pupil is limited because the pupils of many patients with oculomotor nerve palsies constrict about as much as Adie's pupils to weak solutions of both methacholine and pilocarpine. We believe that too much emphasis is placed on the importance of denervation supersensitivity of the iris sphincter to cholinergic substances. It is at best an uncertain diagnostic test, and it seldom provides useful clinical information.

The basic pharmacologic principles are unchallenged: an effector cell *does* become more sensitive to a transmitter substance or its analogs after the nerves have been severed. This increased sensitivity occurs whether the preganglionic or the postganglionic neuron is damaged, although the degree of supersensitivity is generally somewhat greater after a postganglionic denervation than after a preganglionic denervation. However, variability in corneal penetration of topically applied medications frequently causes variability in the interpretation of all such tests. If one is going to perform one of these tests, one should use a fairly stringent criterion for supersensitivity. For example, rather than using the amplitude of constriction, the sphincter should not be considered supersensitive unless it becomes the smaller of the two medicated pupils. If the diagnosis of a tonic pupil is uncertain, it is certainly appropriate to test for cholinergic supersensitivity. We use a 0.1% pilocarpine solution, prepared in a syringe from 1 part commercially available 1% pilocarpine and 9 parts normal saline, although bacteriostatic water can also be used and may have less constricting effect on a normal iris sphincter muscle.

Five features of Adie's syndrome change over time:

1. The accommodation paresis seems to recover.
2. The pupillary light reaction does not recover and may become even weaker. At least one-third of patients with Adie's syndrome show further loss of light reaction in additional segments of the iris sphincter in their affected eye.
3. Deep-tendon reflexes tend to become increasingly hyporeflexic.
4. The affected pupil gradually becomes smaller.
5. There is a tendency for patients with uni-

lateral Adie's syndrome to develop a tonic pupil in the opposite eye with time.

The etiology of Adie's syndrome remains obscure. Attempts to identify viral or other antibodies in the serum of patients with Adie's syndrome have been unsuccessful. Both pharmacologic studies and pathologic studies indicate that the ciliary ganglion, short ciliary nerves, or both are the location of the lesion that produces Adie's syndrome.

The explanation for why the light reflex is so much more severely impaired than the near vision constriction is that the near vision reaction is not so much **spared** as it is **restored.** Fibers originally destined for the ciliary muscle resprout randomly, with some of the fibers reaching the iris sphincter and causing a miosis every time the ciliary muscle is stimulated.

In addition, pupillomotor fibers to the iris sphincter muscle constitute only about 3% of the total number of postganglionic neurons that leave the ciliary ganglion; the remainder innervate the ciliary muscle. Thus, when the ciliary ganglion is injured, there is a greater chance of survival for cells or fibers that serve accommodation than for those that innervate the iris. When the new collateral fibers sprout, the probability is much greater that these new fibers arise from accommodative elements than from those that originally innervated the iris. These new fibers now innervate both the ciliary muscle and the iris, and the pupil once again constricts when the patient looks at a near object (Fig 15.21).

Because of damage to the postganglionic fibers, the iris sphincter and ciliary muscle become supersensitive to acetylcholine. Thus, when stimulated, their response is strong and tonic, and their relaxation is slow and sustained.

Very dilute solutions of eserine provide symptomatic relief for some patients with Adie's syndrome who complain of photophobia and anisocoria. Pilocarpine can also be used, but the duration of action of eserine is longer than that of pilocarpine. Weak solutions of either drug can also be used to constrict both pupils for cosmetic purposes (especially in patients with light-colored irides). Most patients do not need this treatment for very long, because within about 1 year the affected pupil usually becomes smaller; in dim light, it soon becomes the smaller of the two pupils. We generally offer a miotic only to patients who are significantly bothered by pho-

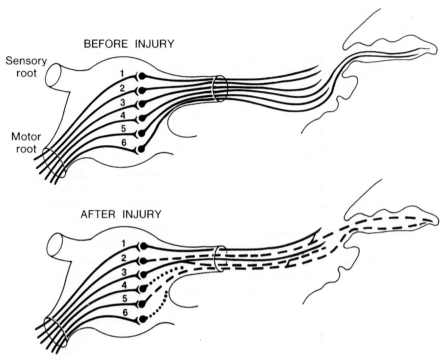

Figure 15.21. Misregeneration theory as it pertains to the findings in the tonic pupil syndrome. *Above:* Before injury, most of the fibers in the ciliary ganglion are destined for the ciliary muscle to produce accommodation. *Below:* Following injury, it is more likely that a regenerating postganglionic fiber will be one for accommodation; however, many of these fibers send branches or collaterals to the iris, producing pupillary constriction during attempted accommodation-convergence. In this drawing, postganglionic fiber 1, for ac- commodation, has not been injured; fibers 2 and 5, also ac- commodative, have regenerated, sending sprouts to both the ciliary muscle and the iris sphincter; fiber 3, for pupillary constriction, has sent a sprout to the ciliary muscle via the remaining nerve sheath of fiber 4, which has been damaged; fiber 6, for pupillary constriction, has been destroyed and has not regenerated. Thus, accommodation and pupillary constriction will occur primarily on attempted accommoda- tion-convergence.

tophobia or are concerned about their appear- ance. Most patients do, however, need reassur- ance about the benign nature of the syndrome.

Damage to the Iris Sphincter

Tears in the iris sphincter or in the iris base may occur from blunt trauma to the eye. Such damage may produce a nonreactive or poorly reactive irregularly dilated pupil that may be mistaken for the dilated pupil of an oculomotor nerve palsy, particularly if the patient is lethargic or comatose from the injury. In most cases, care- ful examination of the dilated pupil with a hand light reveals subtle irregularities in its normally smooth contour, and the iris tears or dialysis are easily observed using a standard or portable slit

lamp (Fig. 15.22). Other signs suggesting dam- age to the eye, which may be present in a patient with iris sphincter damage, include scattered pigment on the anterior iris stroma, pigment on the anterior lens capsule (Vossius' ring), focal cataract, choroidal rupture, commotio retinae, and retinal hemorrhages.

Pharmacologic Blockade with Parasympatholytic Agents

A dilated, nonreactive pupil can be caused by topical administration of one of several para- sympatholytic agents, many of which are de- scribed below in the section on drug effects. It suffices here to emphasize that such agents block the action of acetylcholine on the iris sphincter and ciliary muscles, that they produce both mydriasis and cycloplegia, and that the mydriasis produced by such drugs is extreme, usually more than 8 mm. Because an acute tonic pupil may have a somewhat similar appearance, it is necessary to be able to distinguish between these two entities. In addition, although a dilated pupil from oculomotor nerve involvement is rarely widely dilated and is nearly always associated with other signs of oculomotor nerve dysfunction, clinicians occasionally become concerned that a dilated, nonreactive pupil may be the earliest sign of an acute oculomotor nerve palsy. Fortunately, a 1% solution of pilocarpine can be used to differentiate a pupil that is dilated from pharmacologic blockade of the iris sphincter cells from a pupil that is dilated from neurologic damage to the parasympathetic pathway from the brainstem to the iris sphincter. A pupil that is dilated from pharmacologic blockade will be unchanged or poorly constricted by a topical so-

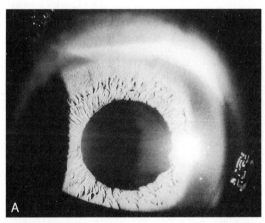

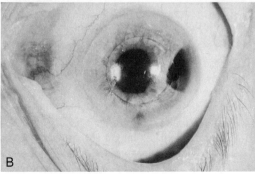

Figure 15.22.   Pupillary changes after direct iris trauma. *A.* Tears in iris sphincter causing dilated pupil. *B.* Iris dialysis producing pseudopolycoria. (Courtesy of Dr. Walter J Stark.)

lution of pilocarpine strong enough to maximally constrict the opposite pupil (Fig. 15.23), and a tonic pupil will constrict to even weaker solutions of pilocarpine because of denervation supersensitivity (see above) and should certainly constrict to 1% pilocarpine. A pupil that is dilated from oculomotor nerve dysfunction will also constrict maximally after instillation of pilocarpine. Thus, there should never be any confusion between a pupil that is pharmacologically dilated and one that is neurologically dilated.

Anisocoria That May Be More Obvious in Darkness or in Light

When some normal persons look in extreme lateral gaze, the pupil on that side becomes larger than the pupil on the opposite side, which becomes smaller. This phenomenon is called **Tournay's phenomenon.** It is likely that Tournay's phenomenon results from "straying" of impulses that were meant for the medial rectus subnucleus to the nearby Edinger-Westphal nucleus. This would cause slight constriction of the pupil when the eye adducts and relative dilation of the pupil when the medial rectus subnucleus is inhibited (during abduction). The prevalence of Tournay's phenomenon is low and its extent small. It is of no clinical significance.

Transient unilateral dilation of the pupil occurs in otherwise healthy young adults in association with blurred vision and headaches (Fig. 15.24). No other signs of oculomotor nerve palsy are present in these patients, and neuroimaging studies, including cerebral arteriography, show no intracranial abnormalities. Such patients were once thought to have a variant of ophthalmoplegic migraine, and it was believed that damage to efferent pupillomotor fibers along the oculomotor nerve or in the orbit were responsible; however, some patients demonstrate sympathetic hyperactivity of the iris rather than parasympathetic weakness.

Thus, the first step in determining the management of a patient with a headache and a unilateral dilated pupil is to determine, by assessing the reactivity of the pupils to light and the amount of accommodative amplitude if the anisocoria is caused by parasympathetic or sympathetic dysfunction. If sympathetic hyperactivity is present, no further assessment is necessary. Although some patients with parasympathetic insufficiency may require angiography to exclude an aneurysm, the availability of increas-

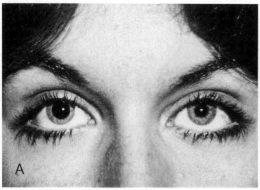

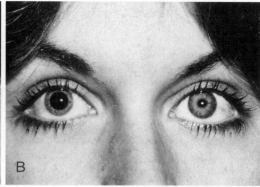

Figure 15.23. Pharmacologically dilated pupil. *A.* Non-reactive, dilated right pupil in an 18-year-old woman complaining of headache and blurred vision. *B.* At 45 minutes after conjunctival instillation of 2 drops of 1% pilocarpine in each eye, the right pupil is unchanged, whereas the left pupil is markedly constricted. The patient subsequently admitted having placed topical scopolamine in the right eye.

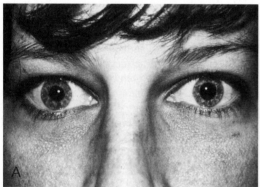

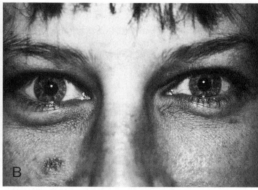

Figure 15.24. Intermittent unilateral pupillary dilation in a young woman during a severe migraine headache. *A.* During the migraine attack, the left pupil is dilated and poorly reactive. Accommodation is normal, however, suggesting that the dilation is caused by sympathetic hyperactivity rather than parasympathetic hypoactivity. *B.* Between attacks, the pupils are isocoric.

ingly sensitive neuroimaging tests, such as standard MRI, MR angiography, and CT angiography, allows such patients to be evaluated in a noninvasive manner, and, if the studies are negative, to be followed for either resolution of pupillary dilation or development of other signs of oculomotor nerve dysfunction.

Transient unilateral pupillary dilation occurs in some healthy persons unassociated with headache, and this phenomenon may also be caused by parasympathetic interruption or sympathetic irritation (Fig. 15.25). Such episodes may last minutes, hours, or even weeks, and they may recur for several years. In some patients, the pupillary dilation is associated with evidence of loss of accommodation in the affected eye, thus implicating a parasympathetic process; however, in others, there is other evidence of autonomic dysfunction, including labile blood pressure and erythromelalgia of the neck and thorax. These features, along with normal accommodation, suggest hyperactivity of the sympathetic

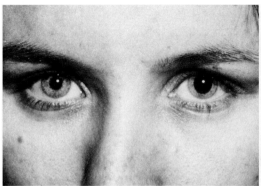 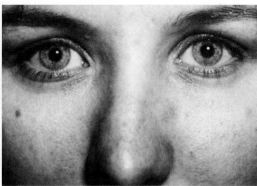

Figure 15.25. Intermittent unilateral pupillary dilation unassociated with migraine. This operating room nurse was noted to have a dilated left pupil while she was assisting at surgery. She had no headache at the time, nor did she have any visual symptoms other than a vague sense of blurred vision. A. During the episode, the left pupil is markedly dilated. Visual acuity at this time was 20/20 OU at both distance and near. The right pupil constricted normally to light stimulation; the left pupil constricted minimally under the same conditions. B. Two hours later, the pupils are isocoric. Both pupils now reacted normally to light stimulation.

system. Thus, episodic unilateral pupillary mydriasis, whether or not it is associated with headache, may be caused by parasympathetic hypofunction or sympathetic hyperfunction.

Differentiation of Anisocoria

From a practical standpoint, anisocoria that is more evident in darkness than in light indicates that the iris sphincter muscles and the parasympathetic pathway that constricts them are intact; that is, there is more dilation in darkness of one pupil than the other, because both pupils constrict to light stimulation, but one pupil dilates more in darkness than the other. Anisocoria that is more evident in light than in darkness indicates a defect of the ocular parasympathetic pathway, the iris sphincter muscles, or both (i.e., both pupils dilate maximally in the dark, but one pupil does not constrict to light stimulation). This permits a relatively straightforward approach to the patient with anisocoria, using the reaction of the pupils to light stimulation as the initial differentiating feature (Fig. 15.26).

If there is a good light reaction in both eyes, the patient almost always has either physiologic anisocoria or a Horner's syndrome. These two entities are then differentiated using the cocaine test (see above). If the cocaine test indicates that the patient has a Horner's syndrome, the hydroxyamphetamine test is performed on another occasion at least 24 hours later to differentiate a central or preganglionic Horner's syndrome from a postganglionic Horner's syndrome. We do not routinely test for sympathetic denervation sensitivity; however, this can be done using a 1% solution of phenylephrine or a similarly weak solution of epinephrine.

If there is a poor light reaction in one or both eyes, the patient has a defect of the parasympathetic system or the iris sphincter muscle. The iris should be examined using a slit lamp biomicroscope to determine if there is a sphincter tear or other iris damage and to see if there is any evidence of a segmental palsy of the iris sphincter or vermiform movements. If there is no evidence of iris damage, a 1% solution of pilocarpine can be used to distinguish between a pharmacologically blockaded pupil and a neurogenic cause. If the results of the test indicate neurogenic anisocoria, but there is no other evidence of an oculomotor nerve paresis (e.g., ipsilateral ptosis, diplopia, or ophthalmoparesis), a 0.1% solution of pilocarpine can be used at another time to detect denervation supersensitivity of the parasympathetic system that most often occurs in association with a tonic pupil syndrome. Alternatively, one can begin with a 0.1% solution of pilocarpine to test for denervation supersensitivity. If neither pupil constricts, a 1% solution of pilocarpine can then be used at the same sitting.

ANISOCORIA

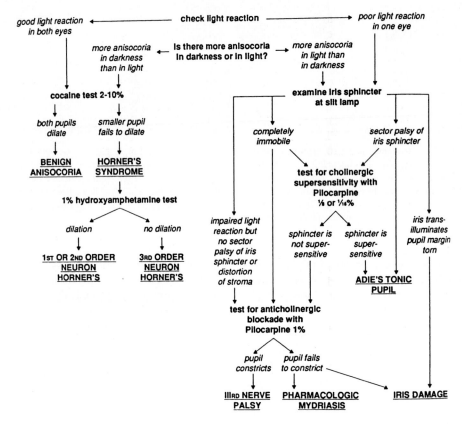

Figure 15.26. Flow chart indicating steps that should be taken to differentiate among causes of anisocoria.

AFFERENT ABNORMALITIES

The Relative Afferent Pupillary Defect

The relative afferent pupil defect (RAPD) is one of the most important objective signs in ophthalmology. It may be the only evidence of organic afferent visual sensory system dysfunction in a patient who complains of visual loss in one or both eyes but who has a normal ocular fundus; and it is much more sensitive in detecting optic nerve or retinal disease than the observation of redilation of the pupil during continuous illumination (i.e., pupillary escape) (see Chapters 1 and 14).

Most patients with a unilateral or pathologically asymmetric bilateral **optic neuropathy,** regardless of the cause, have a RAPD (Fig. 15.27). Patients with **glaucoma** have a RAPD only if

the glaucoma is unilateral or asymmetric, and patients with **optic disc drusen** have a RAPD only when there is associated visual field loss in one eye only or asymmetrically in both eyes. If visual acuity is 20/200 or better and is caused by **macular disease,** such as macular degeneration, any RAPD will usually be 0.5 log units or less. Indeed, it is difficult to produce a RAPD greater than 1.0 log units with a lesion confined to the macula. Central serous maculopathy, which can occasionally mimic an optic neuropathy, produces a minimal RAPD, usually 0.3 log units or less. A RAPD can occur in a patient with a **retinal detachment.** Each quadrant of a fresh, bullous retinal detachment produces about 0.3 log of RAPD, and when the macula detaches, the RAPD increases by about another 0.7 log units. A RAPD can be produced by a **central**

retinal vein occlusion (CRVO), particularly when the occlusion is of the ischemic variety. About 90% of nonischemic CRVOs are associated with a RAPD that is 0.3 log units or less, and none have a RAPD larger than 0.9 log units. In contrast, over 90% of ischemic CRVOs are associated with a RAPD of 1.2 log units or more, and none have a RAPD smaller than 0.6 log units.

In **anisocoria,** the eye with the smaller pupil has a relatively shaded retina, and when less light strikes one retina during the swinging flashlight test it can look like a RAPD. This asymmetry only becomes clinically significant when one pupil is very small or when the anisocoria is large (2 mm or more). In suppression **amblyopia,** a small RAPD can often be seen in an amblyopic eye. It is generally less than 0.5 log units, and the number does not correlate well with the visual acuity nor does it predict the effect of occlusion therapy. An eye that is **occluded** by a ptotic lid or eye patch becomes increasingly dark-adapted and light-sensitive during the first 30 minutes of occlusion. This can produce up to 1.5 log units of a false RAPD in the unpatched eye. Thus, if a patient is examined because of an injured eye, and prior to the examination the injured eye has been covered with a protective patch, the retina in that eye has become more sensitive to light and, in the first few minutes of the examination, it will be difficult to judge from the pupil reactions if the retina or optic nerve has also been damaged in the injured eye. After 10 to 15 minutes in room light, however, both retinas should have roughly equal light sensitivity, and any RAPD that is observed should be considered as indicating damage to the retina or optic nerve.

A unilateral **cataract**, even one that is very dense and brunescent, produces little or no RAPD. This may be partly because of the dark-adapted retina behind the cataract and partly because the beam of light coming through the pupil is caught by the cataract and lights up the crystalline lens like an intraocular Chinese lantern. The light then shines in all directions, causing excess retinal stimulation. Indeed, a unilateral, white, opaque cataract routinely seems to produce a small RAPD in the opposite eye.

A complete or nearly complete lesion of the **optic tract** not only produces a contralateral homonymous hemianopia, it also produces a

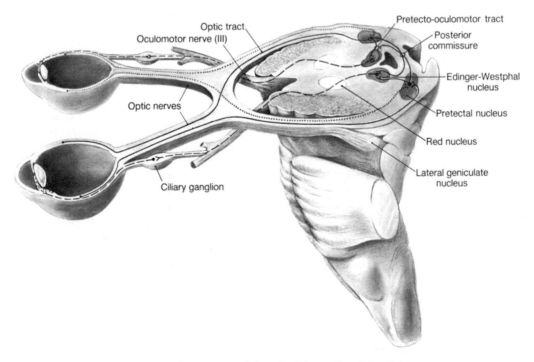

Figure 15.27.   Diagram of the path of the pupillary light reflex.

definite RAPD (0.3 to 1.8 log units) in the contralateral eye—the eye with the temporal field loss. This is partly because there are more crossed than uncrossed fibers in the chiasm and also because there are more crossed than uncrossed fibers in the midbrain hemidecussation of the pupillary pathways.

Most patients with homonymous hemianopias do not have a RAPD unless the lesion affects the contralateral optic tract. An exception is the patient with a **postgeniculate congenital homonymous hemianopia.** In such cases, the RAPD is on the side opposite the lesion (on the side of the hemianopia) and results from transsynaptic degeneration of the optic tract ipsilateral to the lesion. Such patients also have bilateral, hemianopic retinal and optic nerve atrophy.

A unilateral lesion in the **pretectal nucleus or in the brachium of the superior colliculus** will damage the pupillary fibers coming from the ipsilateral optic tract. This can produce a contralateral RAPD without any loss of visual acuity or color vision and without any visual field defect, although the RAPD may occasionally be associated with an ipsilateral or contralateral trochlear nerve paresis if the lesion affects the ipsilateral trochlear nerve nucleus, the predecussation portion of the ipsilateral trochlear nerve fascicle, or the postdecussation portion of the contralateral trochlear nerve fascicle. In addition, lesions that involve the lateral geniculate body or the proximal portion of the retrogeniculate pathway may be associated with a contralateral RAPD not from involvement of that pathway but from involvement of the adjacent intercalated neurons between the visual pathway and the pupillomotor centers in the pretectum. **Neither nonorganic loss of visual acuity nor nonorganic constriction of the visual field in one eye ever produces a RAPD.** In contrast, the vast majority of patients with monocular neurogenic loss of the visual field do have a RAPD. Thus, the absence of this sign in a patient with monocular loss of vision and no evidence of a refractive error, opacified media, or small macular lesion should suggest a nonorganic process. If a patient with a suspected unilateral optic neuropathy, regardless of the cause, has no RAPD, either the patient does not have an optic neuropathy or the patient has a bilateral optic neuropathy.

Some normal subjects show a persistent but small RAPD in the absence of any detectable pathologic disease. The RAPD in such cases is quite small, usually 0.3 log units or less, and variable in degree. It also may vary from side to side. Although it is tempting to suggest that this finding indicates that a RAPD is not a sensitive indicator of organic visual loss, it is likely that in some cases it is such an exquisitely sensitive indicator of visual sensory system dysfunction that it may be observed in patients without subjective or other objective evidence of visual pathway dysfunction but who nevertheless have pathologic damage.

Wernicke's Pupil

When the optic chiasm is bisected sagittally, the nasal halves of each retina become insensitive to light so that there is not only a bitemporal hemianopia but also a bitemporal pupillary hemiakinesia; that is, light falling on the nasal retina of either eye will fail to produce pupillary constriction. If the pupil is examined carefully with a very dim light in eyes with clear media, it is possible to form the impression that such a pupil reacts better when the light comes from one side than when it comes from the other. The results of this test when performed at the bedside are, however, often inconclusive and unreliable.

Poorly Reacting Pupils
from Midbrain Disease

Dilated, nonreactive pupils and pupils that react poorly to both light and near stimuli may be produced by damage to the afferent input to the visceral oculomotor nuclei or by damage to the nuclei and their efferent fiber tracts. The precise location of such lesions is almost impossible to determine unless there is associated evidence of ocular motor nerve dysfunction. A variety of pupillary abnormalities can be detected in patients with tumors in the pineal region. Some patients have markedly impaired light reactions but relatively intact responses to near stimuli (classic light-near dissociation), whereas others have impairment of both light and near reactions, and rare patients have relatively intact light reactions but impaired responses to near stimuli (inverse Argyll Robertson pupils).

Dilated, nonreactive or poorly reactive pupils that occur in patients with pinealomas and other tumors that damage the dorsal mesencephalon are usually bilateral and may precede the development of supranuclear paralysis of conjugate upward gaze. In some cases, there may initially be pupillary paralysis to light stimuli with relative sparing of the pupillary reaction during accommodation-convergence (light-near dissociation).

Bilateral, dilated, nonreactive pupils rarely occur in isolation when caused by damage to the rostral oculomotor nuclear complex. Lesions that produce these changes must be located in the periaqueductal gray matter near the rostral end of the aqueduct. Vascular, inflammatory, neoplastic, and demyelinating diseases that affect this area almost always produce associated signs, including nuclear ophthalmoplegia, paralysis of vertical gaze, loss of convergence, exotropia, ptosis, and other defects of ocular movement.

Paradoxical Reaction of the Pupils to Light and Darkness

Patients with congenital stationary night blindness, congenital achromatopsia, blue-cone monochromatism, and Leber's congenital amaurosis often exhibit a ''paradoxical'' pupillary response characterized by constriction in darkness. In a lighted room, such patients often have moderately dilated pupils; however, when the room lights are extinguished, the patients' pupils briskly constrict and then slowly redilate. Such responses occasionally occur in patients with optic disc hypoplasia, autosomal-dominant optic atrophy, and bilateral optic neuritis. These pupillary responses probably occur not from abnormalities in the CNS but from selective delays in afferent signals from the retinal photoreceptors to the pupillomotor center.

LIGHT-NEAR DISSOCIATION

Normal pupils constrict not only from light stimulation but also during near viewing as part of the **near response** of convergence, accommodation, and miosis. Any time it seems that the pupillary reaction to light is a little slow or weak, the near response should be tested. A constriction of the pupils during near viewing that is stronger than the light response—**light-near dissociation**—may be caused by a defect in the afferent or the efferent system subserving pupillary function. For example, this is the primary feature of the Argyll Robertson pupils that occur from efferent dysfunction, mainly in patients with neurosyphilis, but it is also seen in patients with pregeniculate blindness, compressive and infiltrative mesencephalic lesions, and damage

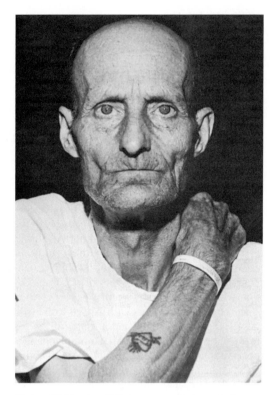

Figure 15.28. Argyll Robertson pupils in a tabetic merchant seaman. Even in the semidarkness that preceded the photographer's flash, the pupils are so small as to be hidden behind the corneal reflection.

to the parasympathetic innervation of the iris sphincter.

Argyll Robertson Pupils

The characteristic features of this syndrome as first described are (1) retinas sensitive to light, (2) pupils unresponsive to light, (3) normal pupillary constriction during accommodation and convergence for near objects, and (4) very small pupils (Fig. 15.28). The Argyll Robertson pupil is widely accepted as being almost pathognomonic of neurosyphilis.

Argyll Robertson pupils are typically small and dilate poorly in darkness. An additional important feature is irregularity of the pupil, and many shapes have been described, including horizontally or vertically ovoid, egg-shaped, teardrop-shaped, irregularly polygonal, serrated, or eccentric. In the fully developed Argyll Robertson pupil, there is complete loss of pupillary constriction, both to direct and consensual light stimulation; however, because the lesion usually does not develop acutely, impairment of the light reflex precedes its final abolition. Furthermore, although constriction of the pupils to near stimulation often appears normal, the reaction usually is slightly impaired. Argyll Robertson pupils are usually bilateral and symmetric. Nevertheless, the pupils can be asymmetric in both size and degree of light-near dissociation. Rarely, the condition is strictly unilateral.

Argyll Robertson pupils usually develop over the course of months or years. They may stabilize at any stage and remain stable for many years, but the usual picture is one of progression. Although improvement and even recovery of the light reaction are occasionally reported, this is certainly very rare. In patients with Argyll Robertson pupils who later develop syphilitic ophthalmoplegia, a complete loss of accommodation with mydriasis may occur.

In some luetic patients with Argyll Robertson pupils, there is an associated atrophy of the iris that can be easily recognized. Common changes observable in such irides include loss of radial folds in the middle portion of the iris, disappearance of iris crypts, and sector-shaped areas of atrophy that produce an irregular shape and uneven movements of the pupil. Various other iris abnormalities, including heterochromia, irregular pigment deposition, ovoid depressions in the superficial layers of the iris, and eccentricity of the minor circle of the iris in relation to the pupillary margin, may also occur. It is also important to note that iris atrophy may develop in patients with syphilis but without typical Argyll Robertson pupils. Most Argyll Robertson pupils dilate well to both atropine and cocaine as long as there is no associated iris atrophy. Similarly, in the absence of iris damage, Argyll Robertson pupils constrict well to miotics.

The site of the lesion responsible for the production of Argyll Robertson pupils is the region of the sylvian aqueduct in the rostral midbrain. In this location, the damage interferes with the light reflex fibers and the supranuclear inhibitory fibers as they approach the visceral oculomotor nuclei, but it spares the fibers subserving pupillary constriction for near viewing.

The "complete" Argyll Robertson syndrome may be observed in patients with diabetes mellitus, chronic alcoholism, encephalitis, multiple sclerosis, age-related and degenerative diseases of the CNS, some rare midbrain tumors, and,

rarely, in systemic inflammatory diseases, including sarcoidosis and neuroborreliosis. However, a patient with Argyll Robertson pupils should still be assumed to have neurosyphilis until proven otherwise. Such a patient should undergo appropriate testing of both serum and CSF in an attempt to diagnose this treatable disease.

Mesencephalic Lesions

Pressure on the dorsal mesencephalon may produce Parinaud's syndrome (also called the sylvian aqueduct syndrome or dorsal midbrain syndrome). This syndrome of the rostral midbrain in the region of the posterior commissure consists of supranuclear paralysis of upward gaze (often worse for saccades than pursuit), lid retraction, accommodation difficulties, convergence-retraction nystagmus on attempted upward gaze, and disturbances of pupillary function. The pupils in such patients are typically large, fail to constrict to light or do so very poorly, and yet react well to near stimuli (Fig 15.29). Such pupils may be the first sign of a pineal or other tumor that compresses or infiltrates the doral midbrain or of hydrocephalus, particularly that caused by aqueductal stenosis or a blocked shunt.

In rare cases, the pupils of patients with midbrain lesions are small and fail to react to light, yet they constrict vigorously with a near-vision effort. Such cases may be confused with Argyll Robertson pupils.

Lesions of the Afferent Pathway

Lesions of the visual sensory pathway from the retina to the point at which the pupillomotor fibers exit impair the light reaction but spare the near response. If the patient is blind from optic nerve disease, for example, there will be no reaction of the pupil in the blind eye to direct light stimulation, but the near reaction may be well preserved when tested using proprioception as a stimulus. In our experience, blindness from retinal, optic nerve, or optic chiasmal disease is the most common setting in which pupillary light-near dissociation occurs in standard clinical ophthalmologic, neurologic, and neurosurgical practice.

Aberrant Regeneration after Damage to the Innervation of the Iris Sphincter

In some patients who have had damage to the innervation of the iris sphincter, the light reac-

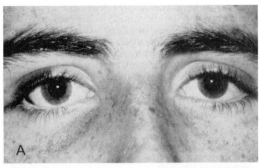

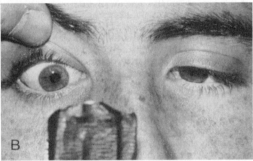

Figure 15.29.   Pupillary light-near dissociation in a patient with a dysgerminoma producing a dorsal midbrain syndrome. In a dimly lighted room, both pupils were large and slightly anisocoric. *A.* When a bright light is shined in either eye, both pupils constrict sluggishly and incompletely. *B.* When the patient is asked to look at an accommodative target, both pupils constrict briskly and extensively. The patient also had difficulty with upward gaze.

tion is not truly "spared," rather it is restored by aberrant regeneration of damaged fibers. In Adie's syndrome (see above), for example, the light reaction is lost because of damage to the ciliary ganglion or the short ciliary nerves. Nerve impulses originally destined for the ciliary muscle grow randomly into the iris sphincter muscle, producing a light-near dissociation every time an effort is made to focus the lens.

A similar phenomenon occurs in the setting of aberrant regeneration after structural damage to the **preganglionic** oculomotor nerve; fibers headed for extraocular muscles or the ciliary muscle may be diverted into the iris sphincter, which is such a small muscle that only a few of these fibers are sufficient to make the iris sphincter contract. Although such pupils are often called "tonic" pupils, two cardinal features of the tonic pupil—a slow sustained contraction to near effort and a slow redilation after constric-

tion—are absent. In general, pupils that show light-near dissociation in the setting of aberrant regeneration of the oculomotor nerve constrict briskly to near stimulation and also redilate briskly when near effort ceases.

DISTURBANCES DURING SEIZURES

Some patients, most of them children, experience unilateral, transient pupillary mydriasis during and after seizures. In most instances, the seizures are of the petit mal type, but they may be of other types, including adversive seizures. The mechanism of the pupillary dilation that occurs during and following seizure activity appears to be a combination of interruption of parasympathetic impulses and irritation of the sympathetic system. That the sympathetic system is involved in some cases is suggested by the finding that in such patients the pupillary dilation is accompanied by facial pallor and perspiration and is followed by miosis and facial flushing.

Not all patients with pupillary disturbances during a seizure have dilation of the pupils. Some experience ictal unilateral or bilateral pupillary constriction, with and without ptosis.

DISTURBANCES IN COMA

Coma is a state of unarousable psychologic unresponsiveness in which the patient lies with eyes closed. Patients in coma show no psychologically understandable response to external stimuli or inner needs. Causes of coma include supratentorial lesions, infratentorial lesions, and diffuse brain dysfunction from a variety of inflammatory, infectious, degenerative, and metabolic processes. The prevalence of pupillary abnormalities in comatose patients is high and may, in some instances, help in the initial understanding and localization of the process. One should carefully examine the pupillary size, shape, and reactivity in any patient who appears to be in a comatose state.

Cerebral lesions that cause coma may produce primary abnormalities of pupillary size and reactivity. For example, damage to the **hypothalamus,** especially in the posterior and ventrolateral regions, may produce an ipsilateral central Horner's syndrome. Downward displacement of the hypothalamus with unilateral Horner's syndrome is often the first clear sign of incipient transtentorial herniation. Damage to the **diencephalon,** particularly during rostral-caudal brainstem deterioration caused by supratentorial lesions, produces symmetrically small but briskly reactive pupils.

Lesions of the dorsal tectal or pretectal regions of the **mesencephalon** interrupt the pupillary light reflex but may spare the response to near stimuli (light-near dissociation). The pupils are either in midposition or slightly dilated and are round. They do not react to light, but their size may fluctuate spontaneously. Mesencephalic lesions in the region of the oculomotor nerve nucleus nearly always damage both sympathetic and parasympathetic pathways to the eye. The resulting pupils are usually slightly irregular and unequal. They are midposition and nonreactive to light stimuli. Lesions that affect the pupillary fibers in the fascicle of the oculomotor nerve can produce a complete or incomplete oculomotor nerve palsy with a dilated, nonreactive pupil. Such parenchymal lesions are frequently bilateral. **Midbrain corectopia** is an upward, inward movement of the pupils in a comatose patient with mesencephalic disease. This phenomenon is presumably caused by incomplete damage to the parasympathetic pupillary fibers in the mesencephalon. Midbrain corectopia is not limited to patients in coma, however. Some patients are fully alert at a time when one or both pupils are obviously oval and displaced.

Lesions of the tegmental portion of the **pons** may interrupt descending sympathetic pathways and produce bilaterally small pupils. In many cases, especially those with pontine hemorrhage, the pupils are pinpoint, presumably from a combination of sympathetic interruption and parasympathetic disinhibition. Despite the size of such pupils, a pupillary light reflex is usually present and can be observed with the aid of magnification within several hours after the onset of the primary intracranial event.

The pupillary fibers within the **peripheral oculomotor nerve** are particularly susceptible when uncal herniation compresses the nerve against the posterior cerebral artery or the edge of the cerebellar tentorium. In these instances, pupillary dilation may precede other signs of ocular motor nerve paralysis, and such patients may present with nonreactive, dilated or oval pupils.

The nature of pupillary dysfunction in a comatose patient often reflects the level and degree of brainstem dysfunction. In addition, once coma occurs, the state of consciousness per se becomes less useful as a localizing sign and has little value as an immediate index to whether patients are improving, stable, or worsening. Thus, when consciousness is lost, careful attention to respiratory, pupillary, and ocular motor signs is helpful not only in diagnosing causes of coma but also in determining the direction of the disease process. This is particularly true when brainstem dysfunction is produced by an expanding supratentorial lesion.

Supratentorial lesions produce neurologic dysfunction by two mechanisms: primary cerebral damage and secondary brainstem dysfunction from displacement, tissue compression, swelling, and vascular stasis. Of the two processes, secondary brainstem dysfunction is the more threatening to life. It usually presents as one of two main patterns. Most patients develop signs of bilateral diencephalic impairment: **the central syndrome.** In this syndrome, pupillary, ocular motor, and respiratory signs develop that indicate that diencephalic, mesencephalic, pontine, and, finally, medullary function are being lost in an orderly rostral-caudal fashion. Other patients develop signs of uncal herniation with oculomotor nerve and lateral mesencephalic compression, either ipsilaterally or contralaterally: **the uncal syndrome.**

In patients in deep coma, the state of the pupils may become the single most important criterion that clinically distinguishes between metabolic and structural disease. Pupillary pathways are relatively resistant to metabolic insults. Thus, the presence of preserved pupillary light reflexes despite concomitant respiratory depression, caloric unresponsiveness, decerebrate rigidity, or motor flaccidity suggests **metabolic coma.** Conversely, if asphyxia, drug ingestion, or preexisting pupillary disease can be eliminated as a cause of coma, the absence of pupillary light reflexes in a comatose patient strongly implicates a structural lesion rather than a metabolic process.

Cheyne-Stokes respiration (CSR) is a pattern of periodic breathing in which phases of hyperpnea regularly alternate with apnea. CSR is a neurogenic alteration in respiratory control that usually results from intracranial causes and implies bilateral dysfunction of neurologic structures usually lying deep in the cerebral hemispheres or diencephalon. During CSR, the size of the pupils fluctuates. They dilate in the hyperpneic phase unless there is a concomitant sympathetic nerve paralysis, and they constrict during the apneic phase unless there is a concomitant oculomotor nerve paralysis. This form of cyclic breathing and pupillary movement is also associated with cyclic changes in the level of consciousness.

DISTURBANCES IN DISORDERS OF THE NEUROMUSCULAR JUNCTION

Despite being of neuroectodermal origin, the iris musculature may be affected by systemic myopathies and by generalized disorders of the neuromuscular junction. Although most investigators describe no pupillary abnormalities in patients with **myasthenia gravis,** rare patients with ocular myasthenia gravis have anisocoria, sluggishly reactive pupils, or both that show fatigue on prolonged light stimulation. These pupillary abnormalities resolve when the myasthenia is successfully treated. However, in the vast majority of patients, this dysfunction **is not clinically significant** and should not confuse the diagnosis.

Botulism is a life-threatening disease that occurs from the effects of the toxin produced by one of several strains of the organism, *Clostridium botulinum.* In most instances, the source of the botulism is oral ingestion of the toxin in spoiled foods; however, in rare cases, the infection begins in a wound. The toxin that produces botulism interferes with calcium metabolism at cholinergic nerve terminals and blocks the release of acetylcholine. Nearly all patients who develop botulism have multiple symptoms and signs of cholinergic dysfunction, including dilated, poorly reactive or nonreactive pupils, paresis of accommodation, ptosis, and ophthalmoplegia. In type E botulism, the pupillary findings (as well as ptosis) are often the initial neurologic manifestations of the disease, whereas in types A and B, systemic symptoms tend to occur simultaneously with the onset of ocular symptoms.

DRUG EFFECTS

Drugs That Dilate the Pupils

Parasympatholytic (Anticholinergic) Drugs

The pharmacology of the parasympathetic innervation of the iris is illustrated in Figure 15.30.

The **belladonna alkaloids** occur naturally. They can be found in various proportions in deadly nightshade (*Atropa belladonna*), hen-

bane (*Hyoscyamus niger*), and jimson weed (*Datura stramonium*). The beautiful flowering plant called "angel's trumpet" (*Datura suaveolens*) and the "blue nightshade" plant (*Solanum dulcamara*) are sometimes found in home gardens. Inadvertent topical ocular application with the juice from these plants can produce a dilated nonreactive pupil that gradually returns to normal in 1 to 6 days.

Atropine and **scopolamine** block parasympathetic activity by competing with acetylcholine at the effector cells of the iris sphincter and ciliary muscle, thus preventing depolarization. Accidental mydriasis and anisocoria can be caused by topical absorption after ocular contact with these drugs in their natural form, but the most frequent way the drug reaches the eye is by a finger from a scopolamine patch (used for vertigo, seasickness, or postoperative pain) to the conjunctival sac or by the deliberate instillation of the drug into one or both eyes by a person attempting to feign a neurologic disorder. **Tropicamide** (Mydriacyl) and **cyclopentolate** (Cyclogyl) are synthetic parasympatholytics with a relatively short duration of action.

Botulinum toxin blocks the release of acetylcholine, and **hemicholinium** interferes with the synthesis of acetylcholine both at the preganglionic and at the postganglionic nerve endings, thus interrupting the parasympathetic pathway in two places. Topical **gentamycin** may produce a similar effect. The outflow of sympathetic impulses is also interrupted by systemic doses of these drugs, because the chemical mediator in sympathetic ganglia is also acetylcholine.

Lidocaine and similar anesthetic agents produce a dilated pupil when injected into the orbit. In most cases, the anesthetic agent is injected to produce both anesthesia and akinesia for intraocular or strabismus surgery, and the dilation is expected. In other cases, however, the anesthetic is injected anteriorly but diffuses posteriorly. In most of these cases, the pupil returns to normal within 24 hours. A dilated, nonreactive pupil may also result from anesthesia that enters the orbit by other means, such as dental anesthesia.

As noted above, a widely dilated, nonreactive pupil caused by pharmacologic blockade of the iris sphincter by atropine may be hard to distinguish from a denervated iris sphincter. The first clue is that an atropinized sphincter is always weakened all the way around—the full

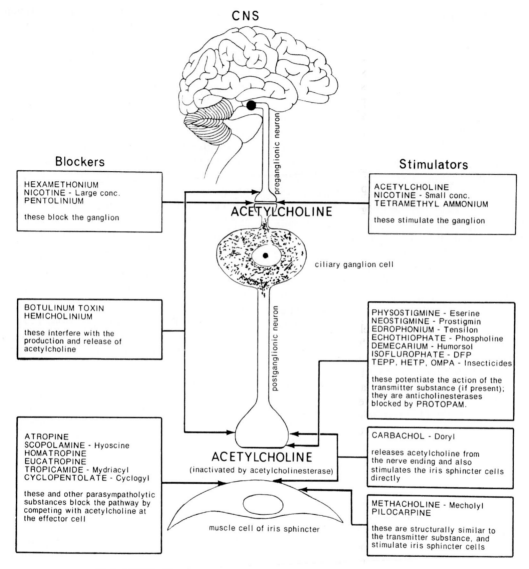

Figure 15.30. The pharmacology of the parasympathetic innervation of the iris.

360°—because the drug is carried to all parts of the sphincter muscle by the convective circulation of the aqueous humor. If, at the slit lamp, there is still a sector of the sphincter that constricts to light, the pupil is not pharmacologically dilated and must therefore be denervated. Even though preganglionic denervation of the iris sphincter (i.e., proximal to the ciliary ganglion) is almost always associated with other signs of oculomotor nerve dysfunction, and even though a minority (about 10%) of postganglionic iris sphincter denervations (i.e., tonic pupils) involve 100% of the muscle, it is sometimes useful to establish that the iris sphincter is not pharmacologically blockaded. This can be accomplished by pharmacologic testing with 1% pilocarpine, which will not displace an anticholinergic drug from the receptors of the iris sphincter muscle but will produce a definite constriction of the contralateral normal pupil; it will also constrict a denervated pupil (oculomotor nerve or tonic pupil). It is important to note that even a **partial response** to 1% pilocarpine indicates pharmacologic blockade, because a denervated pupil should constrict at least as well as the normal pupil and perhaps even more, given possible denervation supersensitivity.

A pupil that is dilated because of blunt ocular trauma also tends to constrict poorly to pilocarpine because the sphincter muscle itself is damaged; however, iron mydriasis, which is usually caused by an intraocular iron foreign body, is apparently mostly caused by toxic damage to the iris nerves rather than to the iris muscle. These pupils constrict to 1% pilocarpine.

Sympathomimetic (Adrenergic) Drugs

The pharmacology of the sympathetic innervation of the iris is illustrated in Figure 15.31.

Epinephrine (Adrenalin) stimulates the receptor sites of the dilator muscle cells directly. A 10% solution of **phenylephrine** (Neo-Synephrine) also has a powerful mydriatic effect. Its action is almost exclusively a direct alpha-stimulation of the effector cell. The pupil recovers in 8 hours and shows a "rebound miosis" that lasts several days. Pupils dilated with this drug should still react to light stimulation. **Ephedrine** acts chiefly by releasing endogenous norepinephrine from the nerve ending. It also has a definite direct stimulating effect on iris dilator muscle cells and can produce significant mydriasis, depending on the concentration used.

Tyramine hydrochloride (5%) and **hydroxyamphetamine hydrobromide** (1%) have an indirect adrenergic action on the pupillary dilator muscle, releasing norepinephrine from the stores in the postganglionic nerve endings. **Cocaine** is applied to the conjunctiva as a topical anesthetic, a mydriatic, and a test for Horner's syndrome (see above). Its mydriatic effect is the result of an accumulation of norepinephrine at the receptor sites of the dilator cells because cocaine prevents the reuptake of the norepinephrine back into the cytoplasm of the nerve ending.

Tetrahydrozoline hydrochloride, pheniramine maleate, and **chlorpheniramine maleate** are sympathomimetic agents often used in topical ocular decongestants. Instillation of eye drops containing these substances may produce mydriasis, particularly when the drops contain more than one of the drugs.

Muscle Relaxants

Papaverine hydrochloride belongs to the benzylisoquinoline group of alkaloids. The most characteristic effect of this drug is the relaxation of the tonus of smooth muscle, especially muscle that is spasmodically contracted. Thus, patients who are given the drug may develop bilaterally dilated, poorly reactive pupils.

Drugs That Constrict the Pupils

Parasympathomimetic (Cholinergic) Drugs

The pharmacology of the parasympathetic innervation of the iris is illustrated in Figure 15.30.

Pilocarpine and **methacholine** (Mecholyl) are structurally similar to acetylcholine and are capable of depolarizing the effector cell, thus causing miosis and spasm of accommodation. Pilocarpine solutions of 0.5% to 2% are usually required to produce miosis of a normal pupil. **Arecoline** is a naturally occurring substance with an action similar to that of pilocarpine and methacholine. Its chief clinical advantage is that it acts quickly. A 1% solution produces a full miosis in 10 to 15 minutes (compared with 20 to 30 minutes for 1% pilocarpine). **Carbachol** (carbamylcholine, Doryl) acts chiefly at the postganglionic cholinergic nerve ending to release the stores of acetylcholine. There is also some direct action of carbachol on the effector cell. It can thus produce mild pupillary constriction.

Acetylcholine is liberated at the cholinergic nerve endings by the neural action potential and is promptly hydrolyzed and inactivated by cholinesterase. Cholinesterase, in turn, can be inactivated by any one of many **anticholinesterase drugs,** which either block the action of cholinesterase or deplete the stores of the enzyme in the tissue. These drugs lose their cholinergic activity once the innervation is completely destroyed.

Physostigmine (eserine) is an anticholinesterase agent that causes marked pupillary constriction. The synthetic organic phosphate esters (echothiophate [phospholine], isofluorphate [diisopropyl fluorophosphate, DFP], tetraethyl pyrophosphate, hexaethyltetraphosphate, parathion), many of which are in widespread use as **insecticides,** cause a much longer-lasting miosis than the other anticholinesterases, but this potent effect can be reversed by pralidoxime chloride (2-PAM).

Sympatholytic (Antiadrenergic) Drugs

The pharmacology of the sympathetic innervation of the iris is illustrated in Figure 15.31.

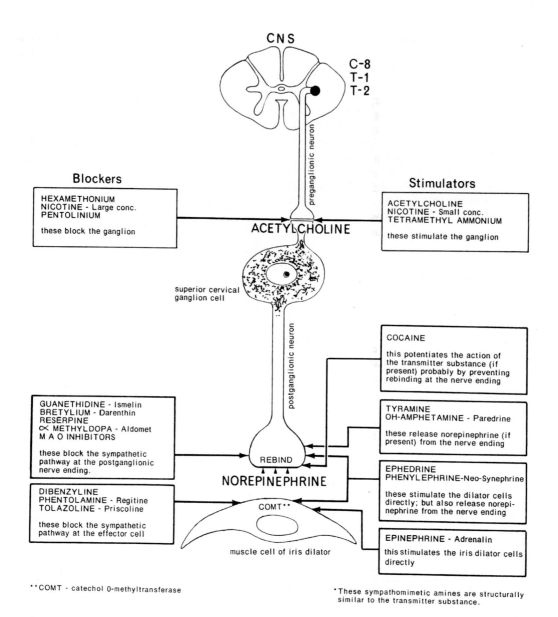

CNS

C-8
T-1
T-2

preganglionic neuron

Blockers

HEXAMETHONIUM
NICOTINE - Large conc.
PENTOLINIUM

these block the ganglion

Stimulators

ACETYLCHOLINE
NICOTINE - Small conc.
TETRAMETHYL AMMONIUM

these stimulate the ganglion

ACETYLCHOLINE

superior cervical
ganglion cell

postganglionic neuron

COCAINE

this potentiates the action of
the transmitter substance (if
present) probably by preventing
rebinding at the nerve ending

GUANETHIDINE - Ismelin
BRETYLIUM - Darenthin
RESERPINE
∝ METHYLDOPA - Aldomet
M A O INHIBITORS

these block the sympathetic
pathway at the postganglionic
nerve ending.

TYRAMINE
OH-AMPHETAMINE - Paredrine

these release norepinephrine (if
present) from the nerve ending

REBIND

NOREPINEPHRINE

EPHEDRINE
PHENYLEPHRINE-Neo-Synephrine

these stimulate the dilator cells
directly; but also release norepinephrine from the nerve ending

DIBENZYLINE
PHENTOLAMINE - Regitine
TOLAZOLINE - Priscoline

these block the sympathetic
pathway at the effector cell

COMT**

muscle cell of iris dilator

EPINEPHRINE - Adrenalin

this stimulates the iris dilator cells
directly

**COMT - catechol 0-methyltransferase

*These sympathomimetic amines are structurally
similar to the transmitter substance.

Figure 15.31. The pharmacology of the sympathetic innervation of the iris.

Thymoxamine hydrochloride (0.5%) and **dapiprazole hydrochloride** 0.5% ("Rev-Eyes") are α-adrenergic blocking agents that can reverse phenylephrine mydriasis by binding the α-receptor sites on the iris dilator muscle. Other drugs that block α-receptors are less precise in their modes of action and are rarely used in clinical ophthalmology. These include dibenzyline (phenoxybenzamine), phentolamine (Regitine), and tolazoline (Priscoline).

Guanethidine (Ismelin) and **Reserpine** interfere with the normal release of norepinephrine from the nerve ending and deplete the norepinephrine stores. When applied to the eye, they produce a Horner's syndrome.

Other Drugs That Affect the Pupil

Substance P affects the sphincter fibers directly, stimulating constriction. The chief pupillary action of the opiate alkaloid **morphine** is to interrupt cortical inhibition of the iris sphincter nucleus in the midbrain, causing significant miosis. **Nalorphine** and **levallorphan** are antinarcotic drugs that, when given parenterally, reverse the miotic action of morphine. **Naloxone hydrochloride,** a similar drug, also dilates the pupils of opiate addicts but not the pupils of healthy unmedicated subjects. Intravenous **heroin** seems to produce miosis in proportion to its euphoric effect. Habituated heroin users require larger doses than nonhabituated users to produce the same amount of pupillary constriction.

During the induction of **anesthesia,** a patient may be in an excited state, and the pupils are often dilated. As the anesthesia deepens, supranuclear inhibition of the sphincter nuclei is interrupted, and the pupils become small. If the anesthesia becomes dangerously deep and begins to shut down the midbrain, the pupils become dilated and fail to react to light.

The concentration of **calcium** and **magnesium** ions in the blood may affect the pupil. Calcium facilitates the release of acetylcholine, and when calcium levels are abnormally low, the pupils may be relatively dilated. Magnesium has an opposite effect: a high concentration of magnesium can block transmission, and this may weaken the sphincter and dilate the pupils.

Iris Pigment and Pupillary Responses to Drugs

In general, the more pigment in the iris, the more slowly the drug takes effect and the longer its action lingers. This is probably because the drug is bound to iris melanin and then slowly released. It should be noted that there are wide individual differences in pupillary responses to topical drugs. Some of these individual differences are due to corneal penetration of the drug.

STRUCTURAL DEFECTS OF THE IRIS

Congenital

Aniridia is a congenital abnormality in which the iris appears clinically to be absent (Fig. 15.32A). In fact, true aniridia is exceedingly rare. In almost all cases, histologic or gonioscopic examination reveals small remnants of iris tissue. **Square pupils** are thought to be caused by incomplete aniridia. Patients with aniridia often have poor visual acuity, nystagmus, and photophobia. The condition is usually bilateral and may occur as a hereditary condition or as a

sporadic phenomenon. When the condition is hereditary, it is usually transmitted in an autosomal-dominant fashion; however, rare cases of recessive transmission occur in children of consanguineous parents. Patients with aniridia usually have other ocular abnormalities, including nystagmus, glaucoma, cataracts, ectopia lentis, corneal degeneration, and optic nerve or macular hypoplasia or aplasia. Systemic abnormalities found in patients with aniridia include polydactyly, oligophrenia, cranial dysostosis, malformations of the extremities and external ears, hydrocephalus, cerebellar ataxia, and mental retardation. The most important association, however, is with the childhood cancer Wilms' tumor.

A **coloboma** is a full-thickness defect that may be limited to the iris tissue or that may be part of a larger defect that involves the ciliary body, choroid, and optic disc (see Fig. 15.32B). Coloboma of the iris may be transmitted either as a dominant or a recessive trait.

Elliptic pupils, such as those seen in cats, occasionally occur in humans. They are most apparent under conditions of strong illumination. Irregular, cup-shaped indentations in the pupillary margins occur as a congenital anomaly in some irides. However, most **scalloped pupils** are acquired from familial amyloidosis, trauma to the sphincter muscle, or uveitis complicated by posterior synechiae. An unusual form of congenital partial iris sphincter atrophy, **peninsula pupils,** results in oval pupils, usually bilaterally.

Misplaced or **ectopic pupils** (corectopia, ectopia pupillae) are usually bilateral and symmetric. Although the pupils may be displaced in any direction, they are often up and out from the center of the cornea. Such displacement of the pupils may be isolated but is frequently associated with ectopia lentis, congenital glaucoma, microcornea, ocular coloboma, albinism, external ophthalmoplegia, and high myopia. Although acquired corectopia may occur in patients with severe midbrain damage (see above), the clinical setting and the variability of the acquired defect usually allow the physician to distinguish easily between the congenital and acquired forms. Similarly, the corectopia that occurs during the course of purely ocular disorders, such as the iridocorneal-endothelial (ICE) adhesion syndromes and posterior polymorphous corneal dystrophy, should be easily differentiated from congenital and neurologic corec-

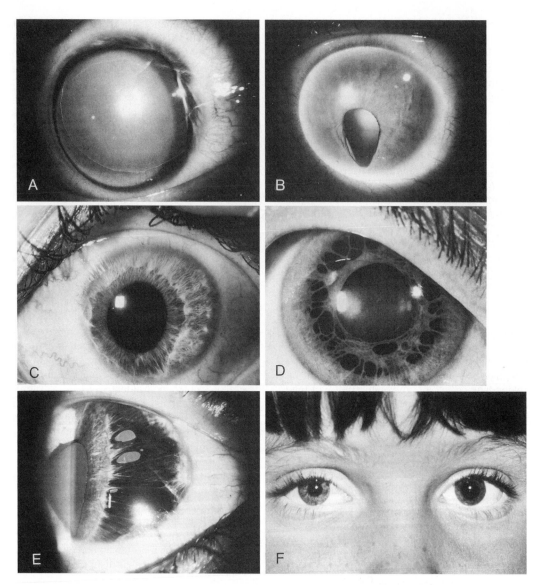

Figure 15.32. Iris anomalies that may simulate neurologic pupillary abnormalities. *A.* Aniridia. Note associated upward lens dislocation. (Courtesy of Dr. Irene H. Maumenee.) *B.* Typical iris coloboma. (Courtesy of Dr. Irene H. Maumenee.) *C.* Acquired corectopia in iridocorneal-endothelial adhesion syndrome. (Courtesy of Dr. Harry A. Quigley.) *D.* Persistent pupillary membrane. (Reprinted with permission from Gutman ED, Goldberg MF. Persistent pupillary membrane and other ocular abnormalities. Arch Ophthalmol 1976;94:156–157.) *E.* Pseudopolycoria from iridocorneal-endothelial adhesion syndrome. (Courtesy of Dr. Harry A. Quigley.) *F.* Heterochromia iridis in a patient with congenital Horner's syndrome. Note that the lighter iris is the abnormal iris.

topia by the clinical setting and the associated ocular signs (see Fig. 15.32*C*).

Persistent pupillary membrane remnants are vestiges of the embryonic pupillary membrane that can be seen as thread-like bands running across the pupillary space and attaching to the lesser circle of the iris (see Fig. 15.32*D*). These remnants do not interfere with pupillary movements, and they rarely have clinical significance.

In true **polycoria**, the extra pupil or pupils are equipped with a sphincter muscle that contracts on exposure to light. In fact, most additional pupils are actually just holes in the iris without a separate sphincter muscle. This **pseudopolycoria** may be a congenital disorder, such as an iris coloboma or persistent pupillary membrane, or it may be part of one of several syndromes characterized by mesodermal dysgenesis. More commonly, pseudopolycoria occurs as an acquired disorder from direct iris trauma, including surgery, photocoagulation, ischemia, and glaucoma, or as part of a degenerative process such as the ICE syndrome (see Fig. 15.32E).

Congenital miosis, which is usually bilateral, is characterized by extremely small pupils that react slightly to light stimuli and dilate poorly after instillation of sympathomimetic agents. The anomaly appears to result from congenital absence of the iris dilator muscle. Congenital miosis may be an isolated phenomenon, or it may be associated with other ocular abnormalities, including microcornea, iris atrophy, myopia, heterochromia iridis, and anterior chamber angle deformities. Patients with congenital miosis may also have albinism, the congenital rubella syndrome, the oculocerebrorenal syndrome of Lowe, Marfan's syndrome, skeletal anomalies, hereditary spastic ataxia, or Stormorken syndrome.

Congenital mydriasis is a unilateral or bilateral disorder that may be difficult to distinguish from aniridia unless a careful ocular examination is performed. There appear to be numerous causes of congenital mydriasis. It may occur as an isolated phenomenon or in association with developmental delay and has been reported in a patient with Waardenburg syndrome.

The color of the iris depends upon the pigment in the iris stroma. In albinism, there is failure of mesodermal and ectodermal pigmentation. Consequently, the iris has a transparent, grayish-red color and transilluminates readily. In a number of congenital and acquired conditions, the iris of one eye differs in color from the iris of the other eye. In other instances, one iris is entirely normal, and a part of the iris in the opposite eye has a different color than the rest of the iris surrounding it ("iris bicolor"). These abnormalities, collectively called **heterochromia iridis,** may occur as: (1) an isolated congenital anomaly; (2) in association with other ocular abnor-malities, such as iris or optic disc coloboma; (3) in association with systemic congenital abnormalities, as in patients with Waardenburg's syndrome, congenital Horner's syndrome, or incontinentia pigmenti; or (4) from an acquired ocular condition (see Fig. 15.32F). When iris heterochromia is part of a pathologic condition, it is necessary to determine which is the abnormal eye. For example, the darker eye is abnormal in patients with a diffuse iris and ciliary body melanoma and in siderosis from an intraocular foreign body or vitreous hemorrhage. The lighter iris is pathologic in congenital Horner's syndrome, in Fuch's heterochromic iridocyclitis, and after iris atrophy following unilateral iritis or acute glaucoma.

Acquired

Iritis or **iridocyclitis** in its acute stages produces swelling of the iris, miosis, and slight reddening of the circumcorneal tissues. The miosis of iritis results from the release of a neurohumor, substance P, that produces miosis through interaction with a specific receptor in the iris sphincter muscle. In patients with intraocular inflammation, dilation of the pupil with mydriatics may be difficult because of adhesions between the iris and the lens (posterior synechiae). These adhesions in chronic iritis may distort the shape of the pupil. They may also fix the pupil in a dilated position. Occasionally, the adhesions are not evident until the pupil is further dilated by a mydriatic.

Ischemia of the anterior segment of the globe can produce iridoplegia. Transient dilation of the pupil may occur during an episode of monocular amaurosis associated with carotid occlusive disease, migraine, giant cell asteritis, or Raynaud's disease. This unilateral pupillary change is *not* caused by the blindness but by the hypoxic process that affects the entire eye, including the iris sphincter. If the whole globe is ischemic (as in angle-closure glaucoma), iris ischemia will relax the iris sphincter and dilate the pupil. Chronic ischemia of the anterior segment of the globe results in neovascularization of the chamber angle and the surface of the iris (rubeosis iridis), producing iris atrophy, ectropion of the pigment layer at the pupillary margin (ectropion uveae), glaucoma, and immobility of the iris. Severe, generalized atherosclerosis may also result in vascular insufficiency of both irides, producing oval pupils from bitemporal palsy of the pupillary sphincters.

Very few **tumors** affect the iris, but those that do can cause irregularity of the iris border, anisocoria, and an abnormally reactive pupil. Leiomyoma, malignant melanoma, and lymphoma can all present in this fashion.

Spastic miosis is a constant and immediate result of **trauma** to the globe and occurs immediately after blunt trauma to the cornea or perforating injury to the eye. The constriction of the pupil is profound but usually transient and often followed by iridoplegia. Transient spasm of accommodation also often occurs in this setting. Dilation of the pupil frequently occurs after concussion of the globe and is often followed by paralysis of accommodation after the initial intense miosis has resolved. Because both the iris sphincter and dilator muscles are involved, the term "traumatic mydriasis" is misleading, as it suggests injury to the sphincter alone. The clinical picture is that of a moderately dilated pupil with both the direct and consensual reactions to light and near stimuli being diminished or absent. The deformity may resolve in a few weeks, but it is usually permanent. This abnormality may have several causes. The frequent absence of detectable pathologic change suggests that the effect may occur from injury of the fine nerves of the ciliary plexus. In other cases, contusion necrosis directly produces a lesion in the iris and ciliary body. Finally, tears in the iris or rupture of the iris sphincter may be identified using slit lamp biomicroscopy with transillumination (see Fig. 15.22A), and a traumatic, peripheral iridodialysis may be present, with resultant distortion of the normally round pupil (see Fig. 15.22B).

An acute attack of **angle-closure glaucoma** usually presents no problem in diagnosis, but, occasionally, the pain is minimal or nonexistent. Redness of the eye is common. The pupil is usually mid-dilated and nonreactive (Fig. 15.33), but it may be oval. If the acute rise in intraocular pressure abates in an hour or two, the patient may never complain about the pain but instead may seek medical attention for the subsequent iridoplegia.

Iris **atrophy** may be caused by inflammation, ischemia, or trauma (Fig. 15.34). It may be circumscribed or diffuse and may involve the anterior border layer, the stroma and sphincter muscle, the anterior epithelium and dilator muscle, the posterior pigmented epithelium, or a combination of these structures. Patients with unilateral iris atrophy that involves the dilator muscle often develop anisocoria, with the smaller pupil on the side of the atrophy. Patients in whom iris atrophy involves the sphincter muscle develop anisocoria with the larger pupil on the side of the atrophy. With age, the iris may become gray and of a more uniform color. Its stroma becomes thin, and the sphincter appears as a gray-brown ring. Stromal fibers may be partly torn and may float in the anterior chamber (iridoschisis). Typical of the aged iris are changes on the edge of the pupil, which becomes thin and loses its pigment so that it resembles a fine lacework.

Some patients experience an irreversible mydriasis and pupillary immobility after an otherwise uncomplicated keratoplasty or uneventful

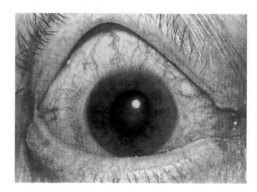

Figure 15.33. Appearance of the eye during an attack of acute angle closure glaucoma. The pupil is dilated and nonreactive. Note the slightly opaque cornea and dilation of the conjunctival vessels.

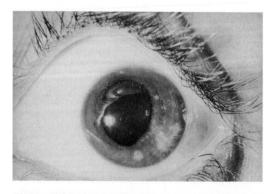

Figure 15.34. Iris atrophy following several attacks of herpes zoster ophthalmicus. (Courtesy of Dr. David L. Knox.)

cataract extraction. This **postoperative mydriasis** or "atonic pupil" probably results from direct damage to the iris sphincter muscle during surgery.

DISORDERS OF ACCOMMODATION

Abnormalities of accommodation are usually acquired, although congenital anomalies do occur. Acquired disturbances of accommodation occur most frequently as part of the normal aging process (presbyopia); however, disturbances of accommodation may also occur in otherwise healthy persons, in persons with generalized systemic and neurologic disorders, and in persons with lesions that produce a focal interruption of the parasympathetic (and, rarely, the sympathetic) innervation of the ciliary body. Finally, accommodation may be voluntarily disrupted.

ACCOMMODATION INSUFFICIENCY AND PARALYSIS

Congenital and Hereditary Accommodation Insufficiency and Paralysis

Congenital defects are a rare cause of isolated lack of accommodation. The ciliary body is, however, defective in a number of congenital ocular anomalies. In most cases, vision is so defective that the inability to accommodate is never noted by either the patient or the physician. Aniridia and choroidal coloboma cause obvious defects of the ciliary body, but ciliary aplasia also occurs in well-formed eyes in which the iris is intact and reacts normally to light. This defect is present in infancy and is nonprogressive. Defective accommodation is found in some dyslexic children, suggesting that there may be an association between the two disorders.

Acquired Accommodation Paresis

Isolated Accommodation Insufficiency

Accommodation insufficiency may be separated into two groups: static insufficiency and dynamic insufficiency.

Patients with **static insufficiency** of accommodation have normal ciliary body innervation and normal innervational impulses, but there is an inadequate response of either the lens or the ciliary muscle. A majority of patients in this group suffer from presbyopia. Static accommodation insufficiency usually occurs gradually as changes occur in either the lens or the ciliary body. In some cases, however, there is sudden loss of accommodation that does not recover. Patients with static accommodation insufficiency require appropriate spectacle correction.

Patients with **dynamic insufficiency** have inadequate parasympathetic impulses required to stimulate the ciliary musculature. Patients with isolated dynamic accommodation insufficiency have normal pupillary size and reactivity. The diagnosis of dynamic accommodation insufficiency is made by measurements of accommodation that are found to be below the minimum for the age of the patient. Such patients often have associated convergence insufficiency, although this may simply be a secondary manifestation of the primary accommodation weakness. The symptoms of dynamic accommodation insufficiency are asthenopia, tiring of the eyes sometimes associated with brow ache, irritation and burning of the eyes, blurred vision particularly for near work, inability to concentrate, and photophobia. Dynamic insufficiency of accommodation usually occurs in asthenopic persons who become ill with some unrelated condition, although it may also occur suddenly in otherwise healthy individuals, particularly children. As a general rule, accommodation recovers once the patient's illness is successfully treated. The transient loss of accommodation that can occur just before or after childbirth may be another example of this phenomenon, as may the accommodation paresis observed occasionally in chronic alcoholics.

The management of dynamic accommodation insufficiency is treatment of the underlying illness, after which the patient's symptoms often disappear. If accommodation insufficiency remains, the prescription of convex (plus) lenses is indicated, regardless of the patient's age. In patients with an associated convergence insufficiency, convergence exercises or base-out prisms added to the patient's near correction may be of benefit.

Accommodation Insufficiency Associated with Primary Ocular Disease

Iridocyclitis may cause profound dysfunction of the ciliary body. In the acute stage, there may be ciliary spasm and loss of accommodation. In the chronic stage, atrophy of the ciliary body results in accommodation insufficiency. The more severe the uveitis, the more commonly mydriasis and cycloplegia (internal ophthalmoplegia) are associated with it. In addition, viruses such as herpes zoster may produce a uveitis associated with a ciliary ganglionitis, resulting in a tonic pupil syndrome.

Glaucoma in children or young adults causes accommodation insufficiency from secondary atrophy of the ciliary body. The drugs used in the management of glaucoma affect the ciliary body as well as the iris. In patients who are still able to accommodate, miotic drugs frequently produce ciliary spasm with symptoms of blurred vision.

Choroidal metastases to the suprachoroidal space may produce cycloplegia and pupillary dilation from damage to the ciliary neural plexus.

Internal ophthalmoplegia associated with **contusion of the globe** is discussed in the section in this chapter related to the pupil. In most cases, when accommodation is paralyzed, the pupil is dilated and nonreactive. Recovery of accommodation is common, but full recovery of pupillary function is less likely. On rare occasions, the pupil is spared or recovers fully, but the ciliary muscle remains paralyzed. Following trauma to the globe, rupture of zonular fibers with partial subluxation of the lens may also produce loss of accommodation.

Iatrogenic trauma to the eye, such as that which occurs during retinal reattachment surgery, cryotherapy, or panretinal photocoagulation may injure the ciliary nerves, producing accommodation paresis and mydriasis. Laser applications at or anterior to the equator and long exposure times are important factors in the development of accommodation paresis following photocoagulation. Sector palsy of the iris sphincter can also occur after argon laser trabeculoplasty. In such cases, the palsy may be caused not by damage to the sphincter muscle but by damage to the parasympathetic nerves innervating it near the chamber angle.

Accommodation Insufficiency Associated with Neuromuscular Disorders

Some diseases produce myopathic changes in the smooth muscle fibers of the ciliary body. Isolated ocular involvement of this type is rare, however.

Myotonic dystrophy frequently produces degenerative changes in the lens, the region of the ora serrata, and the anterior chamber angle; it may also be associated with ocular hypotension.

Because other smooth muscle dysfunction occurs in such patients, the ciliary muscle also may be affected.

Myasthenia gravis may cause defective accommodation, and this may be the first symptom of the disorder. In almost all cases, the defect improves temporarily after an intravenous injection of edrophonium hydrochloride (Tensilon) or an intramuscular injection of neostigmine bromide (Prostigmin) and resolves with therapy.

Accommodation paralysis is a common and early sign of **botulism,** usually appearing suddenly about the fourth or fifth day of the illness. In some cases, it is the initial sign of nervous system involvement, usually heralding the onset of complete internal and external ophthalmoplegia and various bulbar palsies. It persists for as long as a year, if the patient survives.

Tetanus can produce accommodation paralysis. In most cases, the accommodation paralysis occurs in the setting of generalized ophthalmoparesis; however, some patients have normal eye movements and normally reactive pupils to light stimulation.

Accommodation Insufficiency Associated with Focal or Generalized Neurologic Didease

Accommodation paresis may be caused by both focal and generalized neurologic disorders that interrupt the innervation of the ciliary body. In some cases, focal lesions of the oculoparasympathetic pathway produce characteristic abnormalities of accommodation combined with disturbances of pupillary function, ocular motility, or both. In other instances, the parasympathetic innervation to the ciliary body is interrupted as part of the overall involvement of the nervous system.

Accommodation may become paretic in both eyes from lesions of the parasympathetic nuclei in the midbrain (e.g., following encephalitis). The pupils may or may not be affected. Vague visual complaints resulting from an abnormality of accommodation can be one of the earliest symptoms of pressure on the **dorsal mesencephalon,** either from hydrocephalus or from an extrinsic mass lesion such as a pineal tumor. These complaints may appear weeks before a deficiency of the pupillary light reaction becomes clinically evident. Some of these patients also develop accommodation spasm with blurring of distant vision as well as near vision. The patients thus become myopic as well as presbyopic (see below). Multiple sclerosis, Guillain-Barré syndrome, and ischemia can all cause accommodation paralysis through their effects on the mesencephalon, and some cases of bilateral internal ophthalmoplegia from syphilis may also occur from lesions in this location. In most patients, there are other signs of mesencephalic dysfunction.

Acute neurologic dysfunction of the hemispheres may cause accommodation insufficiency. The lesions that can produce this phenomenon include acute ischemic **stroke** and **hematoma**; thus far, reported cases are confined to the left cerebral hemisphere.

Wilson's disease is a hereditary disorder of copper metabolism that is characterized by a progressive degeneration of the CNS associated with hepatic cirrhosis. The neurologic syndrome frequently includes tremor and motor dysfunction. Ocular findings in patients with Wilson's disease include a peripheral corneal ring of copper deposition involving Descemet's membrane (Kayser-Fleischer ring), copper pigment under the lens capsule, and various ocular motor disturbances including jerky oscillations of the eyes, involuntary upgaze, paresis of upgaze, and slowed saccadic movements. Paresis of accommodation is common in such patients.

Most patients with **tonic pupil syndromes** initially have an accommodative paresis (see above). In rare cases, the ciliary muscle shows evidence of dysfunction even though the pupillary light and near reactions appear normal. In most cases of tonic pupil syndrome, particularly in Adie's syndrome, the accommodation insufficiency shows marked improvement over several months; however, because of denervation supersensitivity of the ciliary body, some patients have persistent tonic accommodation, and others have persistent fluctuations in accommodation.

Accommodation Insufficiency Associated with Systemic Disease

Children and adults may develop transient accommodation paresis following various systemic illnesses. In such cases, the accommodation paresis often appears to occur as an indirect complication of the systemic disorder rather than from direct damage to the ciliary body or its innervation. There are, however, certain systemic diseases that produce accommodation insufficiency through direct effects on the ciliary body and lens or on their innervation.

In patients who develop **diphtheria,** accommodative paralysis is usually bilateral and often occurs during or after the third week following the onset of infection. Patients typically have normal pupillary responses to light but almost no movement of the pupil during attempted near viewing. Recovery from this paralysis is common, but it may take several years.

Transient loss of accommodation may occur in patients with **diabetes mellitus,** particularly in the young. It develops in 14 to 19% of new diabetics in all age groups, but in 77% of patients under 30 years of age who also have refractive changes. Although the accommodation paresis may develop in patients with uncontrolled diabetes, it usually occurs after treatment has begun. Hyperopia and accommodation weakness develop concurrently within a few days after the patient's blood glucose has been lowered and then gradually return to normal over 2 to 6 weeks. Either metabolic or neurologic mechanisms can be responsible for accommodation paresis in a patient with this disease.

Severe accommodation and convergence insufficiency can occur after **decompression sickness.** The mechanism is unclear.

Accommodation Insufficiency Associated with Trauma to the Head and Neck

Symptoms of difficulty with focusing at near and at far, commonly associated with headache and pains about the eyes, are common complaints in patients who have experienced cerebral concussion or craniocervical extension injuries. These vague and ill-defined complaints are most prominent during the first weeks or months after injury. The persistence of such complaints for many months or even years is most common in patients who are seeking compensation for their injury through litigation.

An organic basis for these complaints is difficult, if not impossible, to establish. Objective signs are rarely present. Accommodation tests that depend upon volitional effort and subjective observations of the patient are obviously unreliable for the evaluation of these "accommodative" symptoms. Theoretically, any cerebral injury could impair the highly complex neurophysiologic system involved in the coordination of the near response. Similarly, abnormal input from the upper posterior cervical roots or contusion of the side of the cervical cord could theoretically disturb transmission in the ascending spinotegmental and spinomesencephalic pathways that influence parasympathetic outflow from the Edinger-Westphal nuclei. It seems likely that most patients who complain of difficulties with near vision after head trauma fall into three categories:

1. Those with a true postconcussive syndrome, with the symptoms being caused by disturbances in comprehension.
2. Those with reduced accommodation from asthenopia as an indirect complication of the injury.
3. Those who are attempting to gain material or psychologic compensation.

Accommodation Insufficiency and Paralysis from Pharmacologic Agents

Some pharmacologic agents that produce pupillary mydriasis after ocular instillation also produce cycloplegia, including atropine, scopolamine, homatropine, eucatropine, tropicamide, cyclopentolate, and oxyphenonium. None of these agents ever causes persistent paralysis of accommodation after discontinuation, although there may be some confusion when loss of accommodation occurs after treatment of a severe viral uveitis (e.g., herpes zoster, varicella) with a cycloplegic agent. In such cases, the accommodation paralysis occurs from the effects of the virus on the ciliary ganglion and not from the cycloplegic.

When cycloplegic agents or related substances are incorporated in medications that are taken internally or applied to the skin as ointments or plasters, there may be sufficient absorption to produce paresis of accommodation. In such cases, there is never complete paralysis of accommodation, and recovery begins shortly after the medication is discontinued.

Accommodation Paralysis for Distance: Sympathetic Paralysis

Lesions of the cervical sympathetic outflow may produce a defect that prevents the patient from accommodating fully from near to far, but most reports describe an *increase* in accommodative amplitude on the side of the Horner's syndrome. Accommodation paresis for distance may also occur periodically in patients with Raeder's paratrigeminal neuralgia.

ACCOMMODATION SPASM AND SPASM OF THE NEAR REFLEX

Accommodation Spasm Associated with Organic Disease

Accommodation crises or spasms produce an increase in myopia or pseudomyopia. Often, but not invariably, this increase is associated with convergence and miosis—that is, a **spasm of the near reflex.** In rare instances, these spasms are caused by or associated with a variety of diverse organic ocular motor and neurologic diseases, such as hepatic encephalopathy, neurosyphilis, ocular inflammation, Raeder's paratrigeminal syndrome, cyclic oculomotor palsy, coma, and myasthenia gravis.

Patients with both primary and secondary **aberrant reinnervation of the oculomotor nerve** have pupillary disturbances, and such patients may also have aberrant reinnervation of the ciliary body. Accommodation in these patients may thus be increased, compared with a normal age-matched population.

Accommodation Spasm Unassociated with Organic Disease

Many young persons, when undergoing a non-cycloplegic refraction, consistently accept overcorrecting concave (minus) lenses. When the same patients undergo a cycloplegic refraction, they are found to be emmetropic or at least significantly less myopic than they appeared to be when not cyclopleged. Such persons are exhibiting an increase or "spasm" of accommodation. In some patients, the accommodation spasm may be significant, as much as 10 diopters, and may persist for several years. Although accommodation spasm of such magnitude is often associated with excessive convergence that produces a variable esotropia with miosis, this is not invariably the case.

Spasm of accommodation occurs most often in patients who are malingering or who have conversion hysteria; in these patients, it usually occurs as intermittent attacks of accommodative spasm, convergence, and miosis—spasm of the near reflex. The degree of accommodation and convergence spasm in such patients is variable; however, miosis is always present and impressive (Fig. 15.35).

Spasm of the near reflex may be associated with headache, photophobia, defective vision for near and distance, inability to concentrate, and

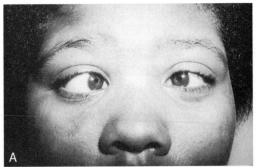

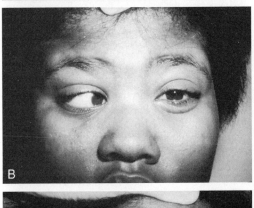

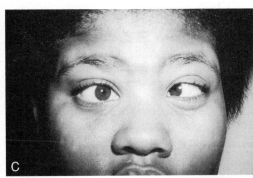

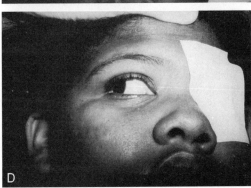

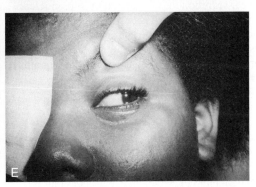

Figure 15.35. Spasm of the near reflex in an otherwise healthy 15-year-old woman. *A.* In primary position, the eyes are esotropic, and the pupils are constricted. *B.* On attempted left gaze, the left eye does not abduct, and both pupils become even smaller. *C.* On attempted right gaze, the right eye does not abduct, and both pupils become smaller. *D.* With the left eye patched, the right eye abducts fully on oculocephalic testing, and the pupil dilates. *E.* With the right eye patched, the left eye abducts fully on oculocephalic testing, and the pupil dilates.

diplopia with bilateral or unilateral limitation of horizontal eye movements. Because of these symptoms and signs, patients with this syndrome may initially be thought to have a unilateral or bilateral abducens nerve palsy or horizontal gaze palsy, and such patients may be subjected to extensive neurologic and neuroimaging investigations. The observation of **miosis** in a patient with apparent unilateral or bilateral limitation of abduction and severe myopia (8 to 10 diopters) is crucial in arriving at the correct diagnosis. This miosis generally resolves as soon as either eye is occluded with a hand-held occluder or patch. In addition, despite apparent

bilateral abduction weakness with both eyes open, such patients usually show full abduction in each eye when the opposite eye is patched and ductions are tested directly, or oculocephalic testing is performed. Refraction with and without cycloplegia will establish the presence of pseudomyopia. Of course, absence of these signs may indicate that the patient has organic spasm of the near reflex and requires a neurologic assessment.

The management of patients with spasm of the near reflex depends on the setting in which it occurs. Some patients require only simple reassurance that they have no irreversible visual or neurologic disorder. For others, psychiatric counseling or an amytal interview is appropriate. In some patients, symptomatic relief may be achieved with a cycloplegic agent and bifocal spectacles or reading glasses. Glasses with an opaque inner third of the lens can be used to treat some patients with spasm of the near reflex. These glasses are designed to occlude vision when the eyes are esotropic, thus interrupting the convergence spasm.

Accommodation Spasm from Pharmacologic Agents

Most of the cholinergic agents that are mentioned in the earlier section of this chapter concerning pharmacologically induced miosis also produce an increase in accommodation and, occasionally, accommodation spasm. Pilocarpine, physostigmine, and the organophosphate esters produce the most accommodation, whereas the effect of aceclidine on accommodation is minimal.

DISORDERS OF LACRIMATION

Tear secretion may be altered by supranuclear lesions as well as by lesions along the pathway from the brainstem to the lacrimal gland. In most cases, there are other neurologic abnormalities, particularly those that relate to facial or trigeminal nerve function.

TOPICAL DIAGNOSIS
Supranuclear Lesions

A few cerebral diseases produce distinct abnormalities of tear secretion. The most common abnormality is associated with signs of pseudobulbar palsy. The patient experiences inappropriate and unexpected spells of crying accompanied by profuse weeping. During the episodes, he or she shows all the outward expressions of grief without an inward emotional counterpart. These outbursts are extremely embarrassing to the patient and may be the principal reason that he or she seeks medical attention. These signs suggest hypothalamic involvement, usually in its posterior ventral region. This type of spontaneous crying can occur in patients with signs of pseudobulbar palsy from parkinsonism, various senile dementias, giant cell arteritis, hypothalamic tumors, encephalitis, meningitis, and even mass lesions such as recurrent craniopharyngioma with hypothalamic compression.

Brainstem Lesions

Abnormalities of tear secretion are seldom recognized in patients with lesions of the brainstem. Absence of tearing is not a consistent feature in patients with Möbius syndrome. The **congenital paradoxic gustolacrimal reflex** is a rare phenomenon that may be associated with congenital absence of ocular abduction or Duane's syndrome on the involved side (see below).

An acquired brainstem syndrome may produce unilateral involvement of the superior salivary nucleus when one of the small vessels supplying the area near the 4th ventricle at the level of the superior salivary nucleus becomes thrombosed. The vascular accident that develops when this vessel becomes occluded is characterized by a peripheral type of facial paralysis from inclusion of motor fibers in the lesion and an associated dry eye from involvement of the lacrimal nucleus. Salivary flow from the submaxillary gland is also decreased or absent. The rostral end of the vestibular nucleus lies in the immediate vicinity, and these patients usually have vertical or torsional nystagmus. The pathways and neurons concerned with lateral gaze may also be affected, causing an ipsilateral palsy of horizontal gaze.

It might be assumed that any lesion of the brainstem that involves the facial motor nucleus might automatically produce decreased tearing and loss of taste because of the proximity of the structures conveying these modalities. In fact, lesions in this area that produce facial weakness may spare both taste and tearing, because the motor fibers to the facial muscles are anatomically separate from the nerve's sensory-parasympathetic components.

Lesions Affecting the Nervus Intermedius, Facial Nerve Trunk, and Geniculate Ganglion

The secretory fibers to the lacrimal gland pass peripherally from the brainstem in the **nervus intermedius.** This nerve is adjacent to the facial nerve trunk and the vestibulocochlear nerve in the cerebellopontine angle and the internal auditory meatus, after which it joins the facial nerve before it reaches the geniculate ganglion (Figs. 15.36 and 15.37). Lesions in this area, usually tumors, can produce ipsilateral loss of hearing, vestibular palsy, facial palsy, loss of taste, hyperacusis, and a dry eye. Peripheral facial palsy

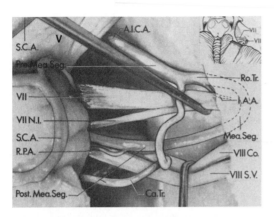

Figure 15.36. Relationships between nervus intermedius, facial nerve trunk, vestibulocochlear nerve trunk, and the superior cerebellar and anterior inferior cerebellar arteries. Nervus intermedius (*VII N.I.*) exits from the brainstem between the facial nerve trunk (*VII*) and the cochlear (*VIII Co.*) and superior vestibular (*VIII S.V.*) nerve trunks. Note relationships of the rostral (*Ro. Tr.*) and caudal (*Ca. Tr.*) trunks of the anterior inferior cerebellar artery (*A.I.C.A*) to the facial-vestibulocochlear nerve complex. *V,* trigeminal nerve; *S.C.A.,* superior cerebellar artery; *R.P.A.,* recurrent perforating artery; *I.A.A.,* internal auditory artery; *Mea, Seg.,* meatal segment. (Reprinted with permission from Martin RG, Grant JL, Peace D, et al. Microsurgical relationships of the anterior inferior cerebellar artery and the facial-vestibulocochlear nerve complex. Neurosurgery 1980;6:483–507.)

associated with ipsilateral reduction of reflex tearing usually suggests a lesion in the petrous bone, the cerebellopontine angle, or both. For example, many patients with vestibular schwannomas (acoustic neuromas) have a demonstrable but asymptomatic deficiency of tearing on the side of the lesion. This sign is often present *before* there is any gross clinical evidence of facial palsy or corneal hypesthesia. Thus, careful testing of reflex tearing in such patients may aid in initial diagnosis.

Occasional patients with small vestibular schwannomas report **excessive lacrimation** on the side of their deafness. This symptom may only be apparent during meals. The explanation for this rare gustolacrimal reflex is thought to be compression, demyelination, and short-circuiting of autonomic neural impulses in the nervus intermedius between the afferent fibers for taste and the secretomotor fibers for lacrimation (see below).

Lesions Affecting the Greater Superficial Petrosal Nerve

Any lesion that involves the floor of the middle fossa in the neighborhood of the gasserian ganglion may injure the lacrimal fibers in the greater superficial petrosal nerve (see Figs. 15.37 and 15.38). The resulting deficiency of tears on the affected side is rarely noted by the patient unless he or she has an associated palsy of the trigeminal or facial nerve and develops signs of keratitis from drying and exposure of the cornea. Acquired lesions that may damage the greater superficial petrosal nerve include nasopharyngeal tumors, meningeal sarcomas, schwannomas, inflammations of the gasserian ganglion (e.g., herpes zoster), petrositis, sphenoid sinus disease, aneurysms of the petrous portion of the carotid artery, fractures through the middle fossa, alcohol injections, and extradural operations for trigeminal neuralgia.

The finding of impaired tear secretion on the side of an acquired palsy of the abducens nerve is of great value because it indicates a lesion (usually extradural) in the middle fossa. Thus, patients with ''isolated'' abducens nerve palsies should also have careful testing of tear function in addition to other tests of facial and trigeminal nerve function. Most of the patients in whom we detect the combination of an abducens nerve palsy and ipsilateral decreased reflex tearing have nasopharyngeal tumors.

In the past, surgical section of the greater superficial petrosal nerve was advocated for the treatment of such disparate conditions as bullous keratopathy and atypical facial pain. This procedure has been supplanted by different techniques and is rarely performed.

Lesions Affecting the Sphenopalatine Ganglion

Lesions of the sphenopalatine ganglion produce unilateral diminution of reflex tearing, dryness of the nasal mucosa, and frequently paresthesia or hypesthesia in the area supplied by the maxillary division of the trigeminal nerve. The finding of diminished tearing in a patient with ipsilateral pain and hypesthesia in the cheek indicates a lesion, usually a malignant tumor, in the pterygopalatine fossa (Fig. 15.39). Unilateral reduction of tear secretion in a patient with a known tumor or infection of the maxillary (or

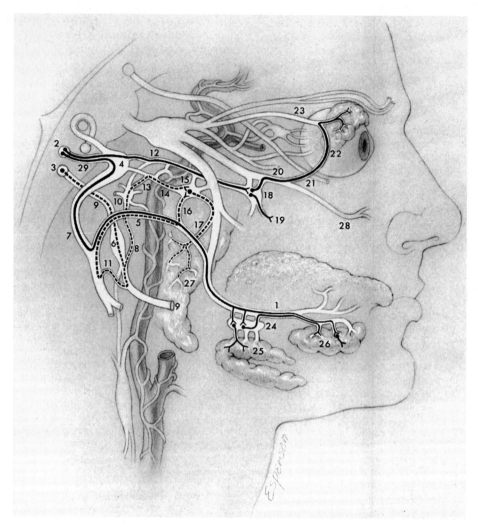

Figure 15.37. Secretomotor pathways for lacrimation and salivation: the efferent visceromotor (parasympathetic) outflow. *1*, lingual nerve; *2*, superior salivatory and lacrimal nucleus; *3*, inferior salivatory nucleus; *4*, geniculate ganglion of the seventh nerve; *5*, chorda tympani; *6*, petrosal ganglion; *7*, facial nerve; *8*, tympanic nerve; *9*, glossopharyngeal nerve; *10*, tympanic plexus; *11*, anastomotic branch (cranial nerves 9 to 7); *12*, greater superficial petrosal nerve; *13*, deep petrosal nerve; *14*, lesser superficial petrosal nerve; *15*, otic ganglion; *16*, anastomotic branch; *17*, auriculotemporal nerve; *18*, sphenopalatine ganglion; *19*, branches to nasal mucosa and palatine glands; *20*, maxillary division of trigeminal nerve; *21*, zygomatic nerve; *22*, zygomaticolacrimal anastomosis; *23*, lacrimal nerve; *24*, submaxillary ganglion; *25*, submaxillary gland; *26*, sublingual gland; *27*, parotid gland; *28*, infraorbital nerve; *29*, nervus intermedius.

sphenoid) sinus indicates extension of the disease beyond the confines of the sinus.

Some patients with an abducens nerve palsy have associated maxillary pain. Such patients usually have a lesion in the pterygopalatine fossa, most often a malignant nasopharyngeal tumor, and it is likely that the abducens nerve in some of these cases is affected in its extradural course posterior to the cavernous sinus. Transient abducens nerve palsy and decreased tearing may occur following a dental injection into the sphenopalatine area. This syndrome usually results from an inadvertent injection of anesthetic into the maxillary artery, a branch of which may supply the lateral rectus muscle via a meningeal-lacrimal anastomosis.

Lesions of the Zygomaticotemporal Nerve

Damage to the zygomaticotemporal nerve produces postganglionic denervation of the lacrimal gland. Such damage usually occurs from trauma involving the posterior lateral orbital wall. Occasionally, tumors in this area, particularly metastatic carcinoma, will damage these fibers, resulting in a reduction of reflex tearing.

DENERVATION SUPERSENSITIVITY

Postganglionic **parasympathetic** denervation of a salivary gland increases the excitability of cell membranes within the gland. The gland thus becomes supersensitive to its neurotransmitter substance, acetylcholine, and similar parasympathomimetic agents, such as pilocarpine and physostigmine. In addition, after degeneration of its postganglionic **sympathetic** nerve supply, the lacrimal gland becomes much more responsive to drugs such as pilocarpine, acetylcholine, and epinephrine. Finally, in patients with diminished tear secretion following trigeminal nerve root section for trigeminal neuralgia, subcutaneous administration of pilocarpine greatly increases the production of tears on the affected side compared with the normal side, whereas administration of neostigmine has no effect on the damaged side.

It appears from the above data that lacrimal denervation supersensitivity occurs following both pre- and postganglionic section of the parasympathetic fibers and from postganglionic section of the sympathetic fibers to the gland. Thus, testing for denervation supersensitivity has almost no value in the topical diagnosis of denervation and disease of the lacrimal gland.

PARADOXIC GUSTOLACRIMAL REFLEXES: CROCODILE TEARS

Unilateral profuse tearing in response to stimulation of taste receptors is a peculiar phenomenon that may be congenital but usually occurs after facial palsy. It can also be a rare but early sign of a vestibular schwannoma. Before discussing the congenital and acquired gustolacrimal reflexes, we review some of the afferent pathways responsible for transmission of gustatory stimuli and the adjacent efferent pathways to the salivary glands.

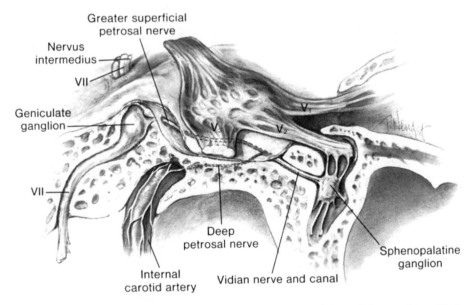

Figure 15.38.   Vertical section through the axis of the petrous pyramid of the temporal bone showing the location of the geniculate ganglion and the course of the greater superficial petrosal nerve from the geniculate ganglion to the sphenopalatine ganglion. Note that some sympathetic fibers leave the internal carotid artery at the foramen lacerum to form the deep petrosal nerve. This nerve joins with the greater superficial petrosal nerve to form the vidian nerve. Also note the connections between the sphenopalatine ganglion and the maxillary nerve trunk (V_2). V_1, ophthalmic nerve; V_3, mandibular nerve.

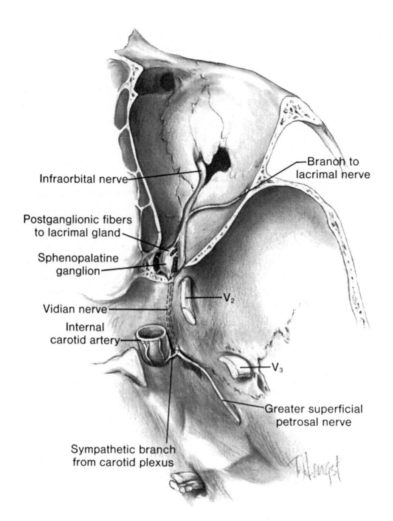

Branch to lacrimal nerve

Infraorbital nerve

Postganglionic fibers to lacrimal gland

Sphenopalatine ganglion

Vidian nerve

V_2

Internal carotid artery

V_3

Greater superficial petrosal nerve

Sympathetic branch from carotid plexus

Figure 15.39. Anatomic relations of the sphenopalatine ganglion, the vidian nerve, and the maxillary nerve behind the posterior wall of the orbit and maxillary antrum, viewed from above.

Anatomy of the Gustolacrimal Reflex

Anatomy of the Gustatory Pathways

Sensory fibers from the taste buds in the anterior two-thirds of the tongue pass centripetally with the lingual branch of the mandibular nerve, split off under the base of the skull in the chorda tympani, and in this nerve pass through the petrotympanic fissure, the middle ear, and a special canal in the posterior wall of the tympanic cavity to the facial canal, then upward with the trunk of the facial nerve to the geniculate ganglion, where the cell bodies of these bipolar sensory neurons are located (Fig. 15.40). In the geniculate ganglion, the gustatory fibers pass centrally as the nervus intermedius. Upon entering the pons, they turn caudally as the tractus solitarius and finally synapse in the rostral end of the nucleus solitarius. Gustatory fibers from the posterior third of the tongue reach the nucleus solitarius via the glossopharyngeal nerve.

Anatomy of the Secretomotor (Parasympathetic) Nerves to the Salivary Glands

Preganglionic salivary neurons arise in two sets of nuclei in the brainstem and follow two separate pathways to their parasympathetic ganglia (see Fig. 15.40). Salivary neurons of the

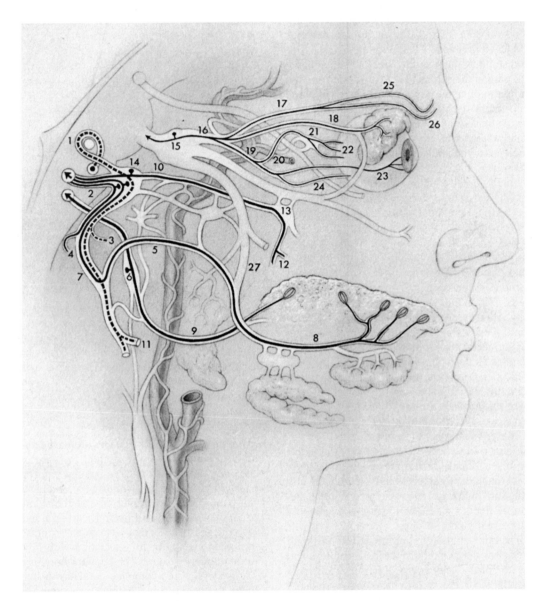

Figure 15.40. Sensory pathways for lacrimal and salivary reflexes. Afferent components of the trigeminal, facial, and glossopharyngeal nerves (*solid lines*). The motor outflow to the facial muscles is indicated as a dashed line. *1*, motor root of facial nerve; *2*, nervus intermedius; *3*, motor nerve to stapedius muscle; *4*, sensory fibers from eardrum and external auditory canal; *5*, chorda tympani; *6*, petrosal ganglion; *7*, facial nerve; *8*, lingual nerve; *9*, glossopharyngeal nerve; *10*, greater superficial petrosal nerve; *11*, motor branches to face; *12*, sensory fibers from soft palate and tonsillar region; *13*, sphenopalatine ganglion; *14*, geniculate ganglion; *15*, gasserian ganglion; *16*, ophthalmic division of the trigeminal nerve; *17*, frontal nerve; *18*, lacrimal nerve; *19*, nasociliary nerve; *20*, sensory root of ciliary ganglion; *21*, ciliary ganglion; *22*, short ciliary nerves; *23*, long ciliary nerve; *24*, infratrochlear nerve; *25*, supraorbital nerve; *26*, supratrochlear nerve; *27*, mandibular nerve.

superior salivary nucleus leave the lower pons with the lacrimal fibers and the nervus intermedius, pass through the geniculate ganglion without synapsing, proceed down the facial nerve, and leave the facial canal with the chorda tympani. With this nerve, they join the lingual nerve and pass to the submandibular ganglion and the diffuse sublingual ganglia where they synapse with the postganglionic neurons that innervate the submandibular and sublingual salivary glands. Salivary neurons of the **inferior salivary nucleus** leave the medulla with the fibers of the glossopharyngeal nerve and pass through the jugular foramen with the vagus and spinal accessory nerves. These salivary fibers pass through the petrous ganglion of the glossopharyngeal nerve without synapsing, branch off at the base of the skull, and ascend as the tympanic nerve (of Jacobson) to the tympanic cavity through a small canal in the undersurface of the petrous portion of the temporal bone on the jugular fossa. Within the tympanic cavity, the tympanic nerve divides into branches that form the tympanic plexus and are contained in grooves on the surface of the promontory. It is in this location that an anastomosing branch from the tympanic plexus joins the greater superficial petrosal nerve through a foramen in the roof of the tympanic cavity. The secretory fibers leave the tympanic cavity, course through the anterior surface of the petrous bone, enter the middle fossa as the lesser superficial petrosal nerve, and leave through a foramen in the base of the middle fossa (or through the foramen ovale) to end in the otic ganglion. In this ganglion, the preganglionic secretory fibers synapse with neurons that supply the parotid gland.

The otic ganglion lies at the base of the skull medial to the mandibular nerve and inferior to the foramen ovale. It has a sensory root from the fibers of the glossopharyngeal and facial nerves via the lesser superficial petrosal nerve, a motor root from the nerve to the internal pterygoid muscle, and a sympathetic root from the carotid sympathetic plexus. The otic ganglion gives origin to three communicating nerves: (1) the nerve to the pterygoid canal; (2) a twig to the chorda tympani; and (3) the auriculotemporal nerve supplying the postganglionic secretory fibers to the parotid gland. Two motor branches supply the tensor tympani and the tensor veli palatini.

General Considerations Concerning the Gustolacrimal Reflex

The syndrome of unilateral lacrimation associated with eating and drinking is often called "the syndrome of crocodile tears." The term appears to derive from the notion that "the crocodile, a harmful reptile, will weep over a man's head after he has devoured the body and then eat up the head too." A more appropriate designation is the "gustolacrimal reflex." Although this phenomenon is rare compared with the frequency of facial palsy (which usually precedes the appearance of the gustolacrimal reflex), it is not uncommon.

In most patients, the symptom of unilateral tearing during meals is little more than an inconvenience. In some patients, however, the tearing is so profuse that they must hold a handkerchief to their cheek to absorb the flow of tears.

Types of Gustolacrimal Reflexes

It is possible to distinguish at least three separate types of gustolacrimal reflexes. A congenital variety is often associated with congenital paralysis of abduction. One acquired variety has onset either in the initial stage of a facial palsy or without evidence of facial palsy. A second acquired variety develops after a facial palsy.

Congenital Gustolacrimal Reflex

Unilateral tearing associated with mastication can be a congenital phenomenon. In some patients, it is associated with congenital paralysis of ipsilateral abduction; in others, it is associated with paralysis of horizontal gaze to the side of the tearing. Congenital bilateral tearing associated with mastication may also occur as an isolated phenomenon or in association with bilateral abduction weakness or bilateral horizontal gaze paralysis (i.e., complete paralysis of horizontal gaze). In some patients, chewing and sucking motions seem to provide more powerful stimuli for unilateral lacrimation than do gustatory stimuli alone. The designation "salivary-lacrimal" reflex seems more appropriate in such cases, which presumably result from abnormal differentiation of the lacrimal and the salivary nuclei in the pons associated with a supranuclear or nuclear abnormality of the abducens nerve.

During the development of a brainstem nucleus, there is a dispersion and differentiation of the elements of the nucleus related to the growth of the gray reticular substance. It is likely that in the congenital gustolacrimal syndrome, this differentiation fails to occur, leaving instead a more ''atavistic state.'' In addition, traumatic facial and abducens nerve palsies can occur at the time of birth, and the former might also result in the gustolacrimal syndrome. In support of a central developmental origin of the congenital gustolacrimal reflex is the occurrence of the reflex in some patients with Duane's retraction syndrome, a disorder known to result from defective development of the abducens nucleus and anomalous reinnervation of the lateral rectus muscle. In addition, similar synkinesias may occur with developmental abnormalities of the midbrain.

Acquired Gustolacrimal Reflex with Onset in the Early Stage of Facial Palsy

The gustolacrimal reflex may develop within days to weeks after the appearance of a facial palsy. This phenomenon cannot be explained by misdirection of regenerating autonomic fibers. Rather, one must postulate that there is short-circuiting of nerve impulses between compressed demyelinated elements in the afferent and efferent autonomic portions of the nervus intermedius. The theory may be particularly attractive for those cases in which the gustolacrimal reflex disappears when the proximal portion of the facial nerve is decompressed. However, the first connections made by sprouting collateral branches are not necessarily permanent connections, and an inappropriate connection can be replaced some months later by a connection that will restore function toward the pre-injury state.

Acquired Gustolacrimal Reflex Following Facial Palsy or Section of the Greater Superficial Petrosal Nerve

The most common type of gustolacrimal reflex develops weeks or months after a total facial palsy from a lesion in the proximal portion of the nerve. The syndrome may follow skull fracture, herpes zoster oticus, or idiopathic facial palsy (Bell's palsy) with reduction in reflex tearing and unilateral loss of taste in the anterior two-thirds of the tongue.

The syndrome of crocodile tears may occur following surgical section of the greater superficial petrosal nerve where it exits from the petrous bone. It was once thought that the syndrome occurred from misdirected fibers from regenerating salivary axons that grow into the greater superficial petrosal nerve; however, many of these patients have little or no lacrimal secretion on the affected side until they begin to eat, at which time their tear secretion becomes copious. It is therefore more likely that the post-surgical gustolacrimal reflex results from collateral axon sprouting from glossopharyngeal preganglionic salivary nerves where the tympanic branch joins the greater superficial petrosal nerve. The salivary axons that reinnervate the sphenopalatine ganglion (and the lacrimal gland) are sprouts of intact fibers going to the otic ganglion and the parotid gland. This mechanism explains how salivary axons could circumvent a sectioned greater superficial petrosal nerve. In support of this mechanism is the finding that anesthetic block of the glossopharyngeal nerve at the jugular foramen stops the reflex lacrimation, as does sectioning of the glossopharyngeal nerve in the posterior fossa.

Many patients with an acquired gustolacrimal reflex require no intervention because they are accustomed to the problem. When relief of the disorder is required, various modes of therapy can be tried, including anticholinergic drugs, subtotal resection of the palpebral lobe of the lacrimal gland, and resection of the tympanic branch of the glossopharyngeal nerve just proximal to the lesser superficial petrosal nerve. This transtympanic operation is easily performed with modern otologic techniques and appears to be the most definitive and rational approach to the problem of crocodile tears in the patient with an acquired gustolacrimal reflex following facial palsy.

DRUG EFFECTS

Lacrimation may be altered by the effects of topical and systemic agents on the main lacrimal gland, its nerve supply, or the accessory lacrimal glands. In many cases, tearing is produced through irritation of the corneal epithelium, as an allergic reaction, or from the effects of an agent on other components of tears; however, some drugs, including methacholine and pilocarpine, appear to induce tearing by their direct parasympathomimetic action on the secretory cells of the lacrimal gland. The number of agents that reduce tear secretion is small and includes psychotropic drugs and practolol.

GENERALIZED DISTURBANCES OF AUTONOMIC FUNCTION

Pupillary and accommodation abnormalities may occur as part of generalized dysfunction of various portions of the autonomic nervous system. These disorders include, but are not restricted to, familial dysautonomia (Riley-Day syndrome); congenital familial sensory neuropathy with anhidrosis; hereditary anhidrotic ectodermal dysplasia; neural crest syndrome; congenital cholinergic nervous system dysfunction; tonic pupils, areflexia, and progressive segmental hypohidrosis (Ross syndrome); primary acquired autonomic dysfunction (Shy-Drager syndrome); acute pandysautonomia; autonomic hyperreflexia; and the Miller Fisher variant of Guillain-Barré syndrome (ophthalmoplegia, ataxia, and areflexia).

FOR MORE INFORMATION:

See Walsh & Hoyt's *Clinical Neuro-Ophthalmology,* 5th edition, Volume 1, Chapter 20, pp. 847–897, Chapter 21, pp. 899–915, Chapter 22, pp. 917–931, and Chapter 24, pp. 933–1040.

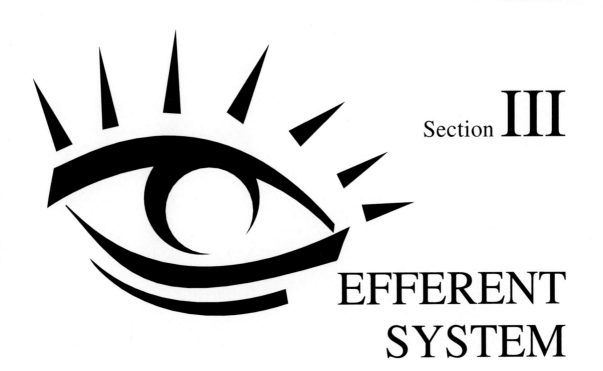

Section **III**

EFFERENT
SYSTEM

CHAPTER 16

Examination of Ocular Motility and Alignment

HISTORY

A careful history should always precede a complete examination of the ocular motor system. Patients with ocular motor disorders may complain of a number of visual difficulties, including diplopia, visual confusion, blurred vision, and the vestibular symptoms of vertigo, oscillopsia, or tilt.

DIPLOPIA

Because misalignment of the visual axes causes the image of an object of interest to fall on noncorresponding parts of the two retinas, usually the fovea of one eye and extrafoveal retina of the other eye, a sensory phenomenon occurs that is usually interpreted as **diplopia,** the visualization of an object in two different spatial locations. Depending on the nature of the misalignment, the diplopia may be horizontal, vertical, torsional, or a combination of these.

Diplopia that results from ocular misalignment disappears with either eye closed—it is a **binocular** phenomenon. Binocular diplopia is almost never caused by intraocular disease, although it may occur in rare patients in the setting of a monocular macular lesion, such as a subretinal neovascular membrane. The pathophysiology of binocular diplopia with uniocular disease is unclear, but it may represent the establishment of rivalry between central and peripheral fusion mechanisms.

Diplopia that persists with one eye closed,

monocular diplopia, is rarely caused by neurologic disease. In almost all cases, it is produced by local ocular phenomena, including uncorrected astigmatism or other refractive errors, corneal and iris abnormalities, cataract, and macular disease. Most patients with this type of monocular diplopia recognize a difference in the intensity of the two images that they see. One image is fairly clear, but the second image is perceived as "fuzzy" and may be described as a "ghost image" that overlaps the clear image.

Cases of monocular diplopia and polyopia are occasionally reported in patients with central nervous system (CNS) disease. Patients with "cerebral polyopia" usually do not complain of overlapping images and generally see each image with equal clarity (see Chapter 13). In addition, the monocular diplopia in these patients is always seen with *both* eyes (i.e., with either eye covered). Such patients usually have lesions in the parieto-occipital region. The mechanism of cerebral diplopia-polyopia is unknown.

Monocular diplopia is occasionally described by patients after surgery to correct congenital strabismus. In such patients, it is believed that a portion of the extrafoveal retina in the previously deviated eye has been used as a "fovea" for many years. Once the true foveas of the two eyes are aligned, there is apparently a sensory conflict in the previously deviated eye between the true fovea and that portion of the retina that previously corresponded to the fovea of the opposite eye. Such patients may complain of monocular diplopia and binocular triplopia. These symptoms usually disappear with time.

Monocular diplopia may be a complaint of persons with no evidence of ocular or cerebral disease. Such patients should not undergo extensive neurologic or neuroimaging evaluations.

It should be evident from the above discussion that in any patient complaining of "double vision," one must first determine if the double vision is binocular or monocular. If it is monocular, and the patient is otherwise healthy, the examiner may concentrate on ocular disorders, rather than on neurologic or myopathic disorders that affect ocular alignment. In patients with binocular diplopia, the eyes are presumably misaligned, and the examiner should ascertain if the diplopia is

- horizontal, vertical, or oblique
- better or worse in any particular direction of gaze
- different when viewing at distance or near
- affected by head posture

VISUAL CONFUSION

In patients with misalignment of the visual axes, the maculae of the two eyes are simultaneously viewing two different objects or areas. Thus, both macular images may be interpreted as existing at the same point in space. This sensory phenomenon is called **visual confusion.** Patients with visual confusion complain that the images of objects of interest are superimposed on inappropriate backgrounds.

BLURRED VISION

Misalignment of the visual axes does not always produce diplopia or visual confusion. In some patients, the images of an object seen by noncorresponding parts of the retina are so close together that the patient does not recognize diplopia but instead complains that the vision is blurred when both eyes are open. Similarly, some patients interpret visual confusion not as image superimposition but as simple "blurred vision." Blurred vision that exists only with both eyes viewing is quite common in the early stages of an ocular motor nerve paresis. In such patients, the blurred vision clears completely if **either eye** is closed.

Blurred vision that resolves with one but not either eye closed usually suggests a primary visual sensory disturbance. Blurred vision that does not resolve with either eye closed also usually occurs from visual sensory disease but may also occur in some patients with disorders of saccades (e.g., saccadic oscillations such as ocular flutter) and in patients with impaired pursuit leading to disordered tracking.

VESTIBULAR SYMPTOMS: VERTIGO, OSCILLOPSIA, AND TILT

Patients with disorders that affect the vestibular system may complain of disequilibrium or unsteadiness, symptoms that reflect imbalance of vestibular tone. A common complaint of patients with vestibular imbalance is **vertigo,** the illusory sensation of motion of self or of the environment. Vertigo usually reflects a mismatch among vestibular, visual, and somatosensory inputs concerning the position or motion of one's body in space. Although it is helpful to question patients with vertigo as to the direction of their vertiginous illusions, they are often uncertain because their vestibular sense indicates head rotation in one direction, whereas their eye movements (the slow phases of vestibular nystagmus) are producing visual image movements that connote rotation of the head in the opposite direction. It is best to evaluate the vestibular sense alone by asking the patient about the perceived direction of self-rotation with the **eyes closed,** thus eliminating conflicting visual stimuli.

Oscillopsia is an illusory to-and-fro movement of the environment that may be horizontal, vertical, torsional, or a combination of these directions. It is usually caused by an instability of fixation from mechanical or neurologic disorders. When oscillopsia is produced or accentuated by head movement, it is usually of vestibular origin. Oscillopsia is rarely present when ocular motor dysfunction is congenital.

A third group of vestibular symptoms include the perception of **tilts,** static rotations of the perceived world or the body. These complaints usually reflect a disturbance of the otolith organs from either peripheral or central causes. When dealing with such patients, as with patients who complain of vertigo, the examiner should ask about the perception of the positions of the body with the eyes closed, to eliminate conflicting visual stimuli.

EXAMINATION

The examination of the ocular motor system generally consists of the assessment of (1) fixation and gaze-holding ability, (2) range of monocular and binocular eye movements, (3) ocular alignment, and (4) performance of versions (saccades, pursuit). In addition, depending on the findings of the basic examination, it may be appropriate to test the vestibulo-ocular and optokinetic reflexes and to attempt to mechanically move the eyes using forced duction testing.

FIXATION AND GAZE-HOLDING ABILITY

Principles

In a normal, awake person, the eyes are never absolutely still. Fixation is interrupted by three distinctive types of miniature eye movements:

1. Microsaccades, with an average amplitude of about 6 minutes of arc and a mean frequency of about 2 per second.
2. Continuous microdrift at rates of less than 20 minutes of arc/second.
3. Microtremor, consisting of high-frequency (40 to 60 Hz) oscillations of 5 to 30 seconds of arc.

Square-wave jerks—spontaneous, horizontal saccades of about 0.5°, followed about 200 msec later by a corrective saccade and occurring at a rate of less than 9 per minute—can also be observed during fixation in most normal individuals.

When no efforts are being made toward ocular fixation or accommodation, the eyes are said to be in a "physiologic" position of rest. With total ophthalmoplegia, there is usually a slight divergence of the visual axes, and this position usually also occurs during sleep, deep anesthesia, and death.

Technique

In patients complaining of intermittent diplopia, visual confusion, or strabismus, tests of sensory fusion (e.g., stereoacuity) and fixation should be performed before the eyes are dissociated by tests of monocular visual function (e.g., visual acuity, color vision, visual fields).

The initial part of the ocular motor examination should consist of a careful study of fixation. The patient should be instructed to focus on a distant target, and the eyes should be observed carefully. Attention can be controlled by asking the patient to describe the target. If strabismus is present, any preference for fixation with one eye should be noted. Constant or intermittent monocular and binocular eye movements, whether conjugate or dissociated, should be noted. Subtle degrees of abnormal fixation can often be easily detected during the ophthalmoscopic examination. The types of fixation abnormalities that may be observed are described in Chapters 18 and 19 of this text.

RANGE OF EYE MOVEMENTS

Principles

To discuss eye movements, it is necessary to have a frame of reference against which any movement may be quantified. Accordingly, the **primary** position of the eyes is arbitrarily designated as that position from which all other ocular movements are initiated or measured. For practical purposes, the globe can be considered to rotate around a fixed point that lies 13.5 mm posterior to the corneal apex and 1.6 mm nasal to the geometric center of the globe.

All movements of the globe around the hypothetical center of rotation can be analyzed in terms of a coordinate system with three axes perpendicular to each other and intersecting at the center of rotation (Fig. 16.1). These three axes are called the X, Y, and Z axes of Fick. The Y axis is equivalent to the visual axis; the Z axis is vertical (around which the eye rotates

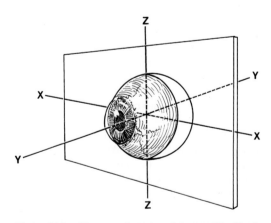

Figure 16.1. The axes of rotation of the eye. The Y axis corresponds to the line of sight when the eye is in the primary position, looking straight ahead.

horizontally); and the X axis is horizontal (around which the eye rotates vertically). These axes are stable with respect to a frontal plane, fixed in the skull, that corresponds roughly with the equatorial plane of the eye when it is directed straight ahead (Listing's plane).

Rotations of either eye alone without attention to the movements of the other eye are called **ductions.** Horizontal rotation (rotation around the Z axis of Fick) is termed **adduction** if the anterior pole of the eye is rotated nasally (i.e., inward or medially) and **abduction** if the anterior pole of the eye is rotated temporally (i.e., outward or laterally). Vertical rotation (around the X axis) is called **elevation** (or sursumduction) if the anterior pole of the eye rotates upward and **depression** (or deorsumduction) if it rotates downward.

Rotation around either the horizontal or vertical axis places the eye in a **secondary** position of gaze. In achieving this position, there is no rotation of the globe around the Y axis (i.e., there is no torsion).

The oblique positions of gaze are called **tertiary** positions. They are achieved by a simultaneous rotation around the horizontal and vertical axes, a movement that can be considered to occur around an oblique axis lying in Listing's plane. When an eye moves obliquely out of primary position, the vertical axis of the globe tilts with respect to the X and Z axes of Fick; however, this tilt is considered ''false torsion,'' because it is not a true rotation around the Y axis but rather an apparent movement with respect to the planar coordinate system. The amount of false torsion associated with any particular oblique position of gaze is constant, regardless of how the eye reaches that position (Donders' law). Tertiary positions of gaze are thus positions of gaze associated with false torsion.

True ocular torsion is defined by the direction of the rotation around the Y axis of Fick (i.e., the visual axis) relative to the nose. If the 12 o'clock region of the limbus rotates toward the nose, the movement is called **intorsion** (incycloduction; incyclotorsion). If the same area rotates away from the nose, the movement is called **extorsion** (excycloduction; excyclotorsion).

True ocular torsion occurs only minimally during voluntary eye movements. Torsion occurs mainly as part of the involuntary compensatory eye movements that take place during head tilt. In this setting, the torsion movements are called **countertorsion** or **counter rolling.** Countertorsion has two components, dynamic and static. **Dynamic countertorsion** occurs during head tilt and reflects the semicircular canal-induced torsional vestibulo-ocular reflex (VOR). **Static countertorsion** persists at a given angle of any head tilt, but the amount of rotation is minor compared with that which occurs from dynamic countertorsion. Static countertorsion reflects a tonic otolith-ocular reflex. Each utricle influences both eyes in both directions but primarily controls tilt to the contralateral side.

Most investigators find that static countertorsion represents only about 10% of the total amount of torsion associated with any large head tilt. Dynamic and static torsion apparently work within a small range to attempt to keep the sensory vertical raphes of each retina perpendicular to the horizon and may represent a partial compensatory mechanism for retinal tilt with further adaptation occurring within the CNS.

To discuss the independent action of any individual extraocular muscle or any pair of extraocular muscles is strictly a hypothetical convenience. In any actual rotation of the globe, all six muscles are involved and act as a single muscle unit with a single axis of rotation at any given moment. The complete muscle unit can produce an infinite variety of rotations consistent with Listing's and Donders' laws that together state that when the line of fixation passes from the primary to any other position, the angle of false torsion is the same as if the eye had arrived at this position by turning around a fixed axis perpendicular to the initial and final positions of the line of fixation. Nevertheless, some studies show that Listing's and Donders' laws are not precisely followed in that some true torsion does develop during eccentric gaze.

Within the concept of a single muscle unit, it nevertheless seems acceptable to discuss the actions of the extraocular muscles in the setting of individual antagonist pairs. The two horizontal rectus muscles have only the primary action of either adduction (for the medial rectus) or abduction (for the lateral rectus). The primary action of the two vertical rectus muscles is vertical eye movement (elevation for the superior rectus; depression for the inferior rectus), with both muscles additionally having secondary actions of adduction and torsion (intorsion for the superior rectus; extorsion for the inferior rectus).

Torsion is the primary action of the two oblique muscles, with the superior oblique producing intorsion and the inferior oblique producing extorsion. The secondary actions of these muscles are abduction and vertical movement (depression for the superior oblique; elevation for the inferior oblique).

Normal eye movements are binocular. Such movements are called **versions** if the movements of the two eyes are in the same direction and **vergence** movements if they are in opposite directions (i.e., divergence or convergence). For practical purposes, the extraocular muscles of each eye work in pairs during both versions and vergence movements, with one muscle of each eye contracting (the **agonist**) while its opposing muscle relaxes (the **antagonist**). The three agonist-antagonist muscle pairs for each eye are the medial and lateral rectus muscles, the superior and inferior rectus muscles, and the superior and inferior oblique muscles. Whenever an agonist muscle receives a neural impulse to contract, an equivalent inhibitory impulse is sent to the motor neurons supplying the antagonist muscle so that it will relax. This is called **Sherrington's law of reciprocal innervation.**

For the eyes to move together to produce a horizontal version, the lateral rectus of one eye and the medial rectus of the opposite eye must contract together. These muscles constitute a **yoke pair.** The other two yoke pairs are the superior rectus muscle of one eye and the inferior oblique muscle of the other eye, and the superior oblique muscle of one eye and the inferior rectus muscle of the other eye. Implicit in the concept of a yoke pair is that such muscles receive equal innervation so that the eyes move together. This is the simplest statement of **Hering's law of motor correspondence.**

Techniques

When testing the range of ocular movement, the examiner should ask the patient to follow a target through the full range of movement, including the cardinal (or diagnostic) positions of gaze. The eyes are tested individually with one eye covered and together with both eyes open. The normal range of movements is fairly stable throughout life for all directions except upgaze. Normal abduction is usually 50°; adduction, 50°; and depression, 45°. Upward gaze decreases somewhat with advancing age. There is a progressive decrease in upward rotation of the eyes from 40° in patients 5 to 14 years of age to only 16° in patients 85 to 94 years of age. Thus, limitation of upward gaze in an older individual may simply be age-related and not necessarily a new, pathologic process.

When the range of motion is limited, it is necessary to determine if the limitation is mechanical, and if not, whether the disturbance is supranuclear or peripheral.

Several tests may be used to determine if a mechanical restriction of ocular motion is present. Mechanical limitation of motion (such as that seen in patients with thyroid ophthalmopathy or orbital floor fracture with entrapment) can be inferred if intraocular pressure increases substantially when the patient attempts to look in the direction of gaze limitation. The intraocular pressure measurements are most easily performed using a Tono-Pen or a pneumatic tonometer, although any instrument may be used.

Mechanical limitation of motion can more reliably be detected with **forced duction** (or traction) testing. In such tests, an attempt is made to move the eye forcibly in the direction(s) of gaze limitation while the patient is attempting to look in that direction (Fig. 16.2). The cornea is anesthetized using several drops of a topical anesthetic, such as proparacaine or tetracaine hydrochloride. The conjunctiva is further anesthetized by holding a cotton swab or cotton-tipped applicator soaked with 5 to 10% cocaine against it for about 30 seconds. The conjunctiva is then grasped with a fine-toothed forceps near the limbus on the side opposite the direction in which the eye is to be moved. The patient is instructed to try to look in the direction of limitation, and an attempt is made to move the eye in that direction (i.e., opposite that in which mechanical restriction is suspected). If no resistance is encountered, the motility defect is not restrictive; however, if resistance is encountered, then mechanical restriction exists. In some patients, particularly those who are cooperative and have substantial limitation of movement, the forced duction test can be performed simply by asking the patient to look in the direction of limitation and then attempting to move the eye by placing a cotton-tipped applicator stick against the eye on the opposite side just posterior to the limbus. Other investigators recommend using a suction device to perform and quantify forced duction testing.

Forced ductions can also be used to test re-

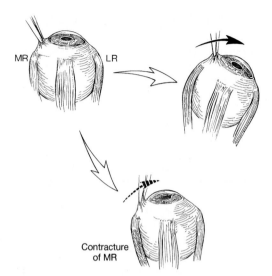

Contracture
of MR

Figure 16.2. Forced duction testing. After the eye has been anesthetized with topical proparacaine and cocaine, the conjunctiva just posterior to the limbus is grasped with a fine-toothed forceps at a point opposite the direction of limitation. An attempt is then made to rotate the eye in the direction of limitation. If no mechanical limitation is present, the eye can be moved fully into the direction of limitation (*solid black arrow*). If mechanical limitation is present, the eye will resist attempts to rotate it into the field of limitation (*dashed black arrow*).

striction of the oblique muscles. For this test, the conjunctiva is grasped near the limbus at the 3 o'clock and 9 o'clock position with toothed forceps. Retropulsion of the globe is then applied, putting the oblique muscles on stretch. The eye is then moved from medially to laterally in an arc that follows the orbital rim while depressed (to test the inferior oblique muscle) or elevated (to test the superior oblique muscle). During this process, a distinct bump is encountered as the globe passes over the stretched oblique tendon or muscle. The resistance of this bump to passage of the globe is an indication of the tightness of the muscle.

Often, particularly on children or when testing restriction of the oblique muscles, the forced duction test can be performed only under general anesthesia (Fig. 16.3). It should be remembered, however, that succinylcholine, which is often given to patients under general anesthesia, produces tonic contraction of the extraocular muscles, thereby altering the results of the forced duction test.

In addition to the forced duction test, mechanical determination of muscle force can be used to assess the function of apparently paretic muscles with contracture of their antagonists. An estimate of active muscle force present in patients with limitation of ocular motility can be made by stabilizing the anesthetized eye with a toothed forceps in a position near the limbus on the side of the limitation while the patient attempts to move the eye into the field of the limitation (Fig. 16.4). A tug on the forceps indicates that a contraction of the suspected paralytic muscle has occurred, and the results of this test can even be quantified.

Nonrestrictive limitation of eye movements may occur from disease of supranuclear or infranuclear structures. Because the workup and

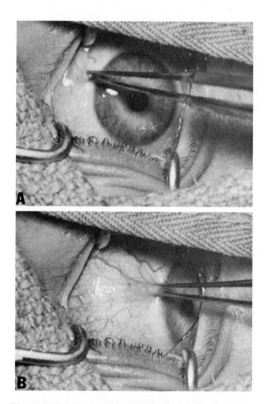

Figure 16.3. Forced duction testing in a patient under general anesthesia. *A.* The conjunctiva and episclera are grasped near the limbus with a fixation forceps. *B.* The eye is moved medially to test for mechanical restriction of adduction. Note that the eye can be moved medially without difficulty. (Reprinted with permission from von Noorden G, Maumenee AE. Atlas of Strabismus. 2nd ed. St. Louis: CV Mosby, 1973:113.)

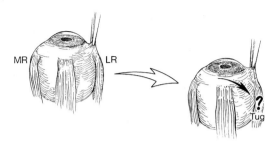

Figure 16.4.   Estimation of active, generated muscle force. After the eye has been anesthetized with topical proparacaine and cocaine, the conjunctiva just posterior to the limbus is grasped with a fine-toothed forceps on the side of the limitation. The examiner then holds the eye while the patient attempts to look in the direction of limitation. If there is an intact nerve supply to the muscle that could move the eye into the field of limitation, the examiner will feel a tug on the forceps.

management of the patient will vary considerably depending on the location of the lesion, it is imperative that supranuclear disorders be distinguished from infranuclear disorders. From a practical standpoint, supranuclear disorders that cause abnormalities in the range of eye movements usually result from lesions of the cerebral hemispheres or the brainstem premotor structures, whereas infranuclear disorders may be caused by lesions of the brainstem, ocular motor nerves, or the extraocular muscles themselves. In all cases, stimulation of the vestibular apparatus can be used to assess the integrity of the peripheral ocular motor pathways either by oculocephalic testing (the doll's head maneuver) or by caloric testing.

In the oculocephalic test, the awake patient is asked to fixate on a target straight ahead while the head (or the entire body) is rotated from side to side and up and down. A normal response consists of a conjugate eye deviation in the direction away from head or body rotation such that the eyes remain stable with respect to space despite the head movement. The remarkable integrity of this VOR can be tested by asking the patient to read a Snellen chart during head or body rotation. In patients with intact vestibular systems, there is no degradation of visual acuity, even with rotations of up to 40°/sec, whereas patients with vestibular disease have a rapid decline in this **dynamic visual acuity** with head rotation.

To perform the oculocephalic test in comatose patients, the eyelids are simply held open, and the rotational head movements are performed. The procedure can be modified for patients with severe neck rigidity or injuries that prevent neck flexion and extension. Such patients are placed on a stretcher with wheels. The stretcher is then sharply pushed in the direction of either the patient's head or feet. This maneuver does not produce a rotational stimulus but is simply a linear or translational movement that may stimulate otolith-ocular reflexes (which are minimal) and visual tracking. In fact, it probably functions as a full-field pursuit test, and similar results can be obtained using a slowly moving "optokinetic" tape or drum. Although these tests may not give exact information regarding the VOR, they nevertheless provide important information regarding ocular motility that may be otherwise impossible to obtain.

In unconscious patients, oculocephalic testing may be the most useful method of assessing eye movements. The VOR is often intact in such patients, whereas saccadic and pursuit eye movements are absent. Thus, rapid horizontal rotation of the head results in deviation of the eyes away from the direction of the head turn. The eyes then make an exponential drift back to primary position if the head rotation is maintained. Though not saccadic, this recentration of the eyes may be quite rapid, occurring with a time constant of less than 0.5 seconds in the most severe vegetative states. Normal responses during oculocephalic testing indicate that the nuclear and infranuclear ocular motor structures are intact and capable of being stimulated by an intact vestibular system. This test can also be used in patients with nonorganic limitation of gaze to show that a full range of eye movement can be elicited despite apparent gaze restriction during testing of voluntary eye movements.

Another way to stimulate the vestibular system is by caloric irrigation. In this test, performed in the light with the patient in a supine position, the external auditory canal is first inspected to make certain that the tympanic membrane is intact. The patient's head is flexed 30°. This places the lateral (horizontal) semicircular canals in a nearly vertical position allowing the thermal stimulus to induce maximal convection currents in the endolymph. Up to 200 mL of warm (44°C) or cold (30°C) water is infused into the external canal using a small tube fitted onto a syringe. In the awake patient, a normal response consists of conjugate nystagmus, with the slow phase toward the side of cold water irrigation (or away from the side of warm water irrigation) and the fast phase away from the side of cold water irrigation (or toward the side of warm water irrigation). The nystagmus occurs because an initial slow-phase movement of the eyes produced by stimulation of the vestibular system is followed by a refixation movement (quick phase or saccade). If the induced nystagmus is consistently less when one ear is irrigated, regardless of the stimulus temperature, a peripheral vestibular disturbance is present on that side. If the nystagmus is consistently greater in one direction, regardless of which ear is stimulated, the patient has a directional preponderance of the vestibular system that may occur with central or peripheral vestibular lesions and is otherwise nonlocalizing.

The eye movements that occur during caloric irrigation can best be observed by placing Frenzel's spectacles on the patient. These spectacles eliminate patient fixation and provide magnification for the examiner. Some models also provide illumination of the patient's eyes.

In practical terms, the caloric irrigation test is messy, uncomfortable for the awake patient, and usually useful only for detecting relatively gross asymmetry in vestibular function. Nevertheless, attempts have been made to quantify subtle vestibular dysfunction with this test. The duration of nystagmus after caloric irrigation seems to be a reproducible measure of vestibular function, and the slow-phase velocity of caloric stimulation nystagmus, as measured with electronystagmography, is a commonly used parameter for assessing vestibular function.

Vestibular function can also be tested with an air caloric apparatus that causes a continuous thermal change in the semicircular canals, thus avoiding the use of water. The test is thought by some to be more sensitive than water irrigation for detecting vestibular disorders.

In comatose patients with intact nuclear and infranuclear ocular motor structures and an intact vestibular system, a normal response is simply a tonic, conjugate ocular deviation toward the side of cold water irrigation and away from the side of warm water irrigation. There are no significant refixation movements, because all horizontal quick phases are generated by the paramedian pontine reticular formation (PPRF), which is not functioning in such patients. Absence of the VOR by either oculocephalic or caloric stimulation in comatose patients is consistently associated with poor outcome.

Caloric testing may be used to evaluate the integrity of vertical gaze by infusing warm or cold water simultaneously into both external auditory canals. A normal response in the awake individual is a conjugate jerk nystagmus with a slow phase that is upward when warm water is used and downward when cold water is used. A normal response in the comatose individual is a tonic, conjugate movement of the eyes upward (for warm water) or downward (for cold water). Although caloric testing is the best way to evaluate unilateral peripheral vestibular function, our experience with bilateral caloric irrigation suggests that it is of limited value in assessing the integrity of vertical gaze and that oculocephalic and rotation testing provide more accurate and reproducible results.

It is important to be aware that nystagmus can occasionally be induced by caloric testing in patients with abolished vestibular function. This **pseudocaloric nystagmus** always beats away from the affected ear, regardless of whether cold or warm water is used for irrigation. It can thus be distinguished from caloric nystagmus that beats away from the irrigated ear when cold irrigation is used and toward the irrigated ear when warm irrigation is used. Pseudocaloric nystagmus probably represents unmasking of a preexisting vestibular nystagmus through tactile (caloric) stimulation.

In some patients with paresis of upward gaze, **Bell's phenomenon** may be helpful in differentiating an infranuclear from a supranuclear lesion. Bell's phenomenon consists of outward and upward rolling of the eyes when forcible efforts are made to close the eyelids against resistance. It does not occur with blinks, and it is observed in only 50% of individuals during voluntary unrestrained lid closure. The presence of this movement in persons who cannot voluntarily elevate their eyes usually indicates that brainstem pathways between the facial nerve nucleus and that portion of the oculomotor nucleus responsible for ocular elevation are intact and, thus, that an upward gaze paresis is supranuclear in origin. Absence of a Bell's phenomenon has less diagnostic usefulness because about 10% of normal subjects do not have this facio-ocular movement. A downward Bell's response is present in up to 8% of normal individuals.

OCULAR ALIGNMENT

Principles

When the eyes are not aligned on the same object, **strabismus** is present. The strabismus may be congenital or acquired and may be caused by central or peripheral dysfunction. In some persons, particularly those with isolated congenital strabismus, the amount of ocular misalignment is unchanged regardless of the direction of gaze or of which eye is fixating the target. This type of strabismus is termed **comitant** or **concomitant.** On the other hand, when the amount of an ocular deviation changes in various directions of gaze, with either eye fixing or both, the strabismus is said to be **incomitant** or **noncomitant.** Congenital comitant strabismus is occasionally associated with other neurologic dysfunction, and acquired comitant strabismus may be a sign of intracranial disease. In addition, comitant strabismus may appear in otherwise normal children and adults, as well as in persons with neurologic or systemic disease, from **decompensation** of a preexisting phoria. Nevertheless, most instances of neuropathic or myopathic strabismus are of the incomitant variety.

Primary and Secondary Deviations

Any patient with a manifest deviation of one eye (heterotropia) will fixate a target with only one eye at a time. During viewing with that eye, the visual axis of the opposite (nonfixing) eye will be deviated a certain amount away from the target. Patients with a comitant strabismus have the same amount of deviation of the nonfixing eye regardless of the eye that is fixing or the field of gaze. Most patients with incomitant (and especially paralytic) strabismus tend to fix with the nonparetic eye if visual acuity is equal in the two eyes. In these patients, the deviation of the nonfixing eye is called the **primary** deviation. When such patients are forced to fix the same target with the paretic eye, the deviation that results, the **secondary** deviation, is always greater than the primary deviation (Fig. 16.5).

The explanation for this phenomenon is related to the position of the eyes within the orbits. When a single muscle is paretic, the deviation between the two eyes is proportional to the difference between the forces generated by the paretic muscle and its normal yoke muscle. Furthermore, the amount of force contributed by each muscle toward holding the eye in a specific

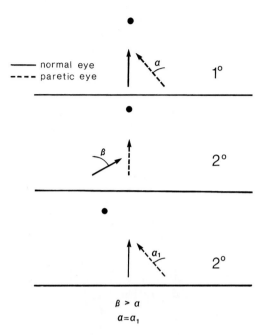

Figure 16.5. The principle of primary and secondary deviations. *Top:* When the normal eye fixes on a target directly ahead, the paretic eye deviates from the primary position by a certain amount (α). This is called the primary deviation. *Middle:* When the paretic eye fixes on a target in primary position, the normal eye also deviates from primary position by a certain amount (β), but this secondary deviation of the normal eye when the paretic eye is fixing is greater than the amount of deviation of the paretic eye when the normal eye is fixing ($\beta > \alpha$). *Bottom:* Although the common explanation of primary and secondary deviation is based on Hering's law of equal innervation to yoke muscles, some authors believe that the secondary deviation is greater than the primary deviation in paretic strabismus, because when the paretic eye is fixing in primary position it is forced farther into its field of limitation. If the paretic eye were fixing on an object in the opposite direction, the deviation of the eye from primary position (α_1) would be the same as if the normal eye were fixing on an object straight ahead ($\alpha = \alpha_1$). Thus, although Hering's law is maintained, the explanation for primary and secondary deviations is based upon the position of the eyes within the orbit and not upon which eye is fixing.

orbital position increases as the eye is moved into the direction of action of that muscle. Under normal circumstances, this force is equal for yoke pairs of muscles, obeying Hering's law. However, as the eyes move into the direction of action of the paretic muscle, the difference in forces generated by the normal and paretic yoke muscles increases, thus increasing the deviation between the two eyes. When this change in deviation is tested as a function of orbital position, it is actually found to be *independent* of which eye is fixing. Thus, when the paretic eye is fixating a target, it is held in an orbital position farther in the direction of action of the paretic muscle than when the nonparetic eye is fixating the same target. This results in a secondary deviation that is greater than the primary deviation simply because of the change in eye position toward the direction of action of the paretic muscle when the paretic eye is forced to take up fixation. The innervation to both muscles in the yoke pair is increased in that direction as predicted by Hering's law, and this increased innervation is more effective in the nonparetic mus-

cle. However, the innervation is not increased any more than if the nonparetic eye is forced to take up fixation in eccentric gaze to achieve the same final orbital position.

Past-Pointing and Disturbances of Egocentric Localization

Patients with paralytic strabismus often have anomalies of spatial localization called **past-pointing** or **false orientation.** If a patient is asked to point at an object in the field of action of a paretic muscle while the paretic eye is fixating, the patient's finger will point beyond the object *toward* the field of action of the paretic muscle (Fig. 16.6). During this test, it is impor-

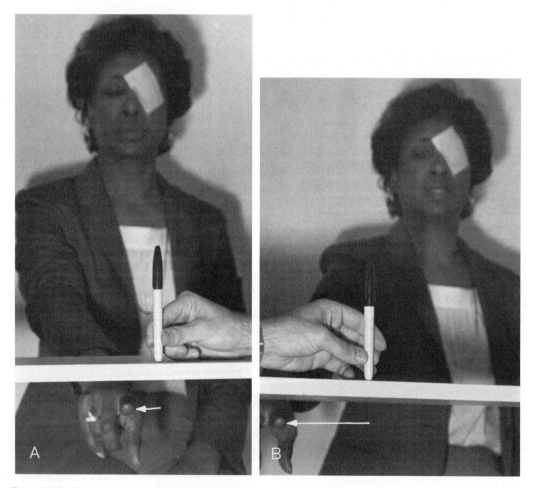

Figure 16.6. Past-pointing in a patient with a right sixth nerve paresis. *A.* In primary position, there is only a slight amount of past-pointing. *B.* In right gaze, however, the amount of past-pointing increases. The white arrows indicate the amount of past pointing (the difference between the actual target location and the area in space to which the patient points).

tant that the hand be covered or that the patient point rapidly toward the object so as to avoid visual correction of the error of localization while the hand is still moving toward the object.

Head Turns and Tilts

Patients with strabismus commonly turn or tilt the head to minimize diplopia. Head turns are frequently associated with paresis of the horizontal extraocular muscles, with the turn being toward the side of the weakness. Similarly, patients with vertical extraocular muscle paresis may carry their head flexed or extended. The majority of patients with such head turns adopt the particular posture to minimize or eliminate diplopia by moving the eyes away from the field of action of the paretic muscle; however, some patients adopt a head posture that actually increases the distance between the two images, allowing one of the images to be more easily ignored.

Head turns also occur in patients with congenital nystagmus. In such patients, keeping the eyes in an eccentric (null) position in the orbit by means of the head turn may result in reduction in the amplitude, frequency, or both of the nystagmus.

Head tilts are most commonly observed in patients with paresis of the oblique muscles, particularly the superior oblique. With an acquired superior oblique palsy, for example, the face is usually turned away from the paretic eye, the chin is down slightly, and the head is tilted toward the side opposite the paretic muscle. This permits fusion of images. Patients with congenital superior oblique palsy may adopt a similar head tilt or one in the opposite direction (i.e., toward the side of the paretic muscle) in order to more widely separate the images. Head tilts that occur from ocular causes often must be differentiated from nonocular torticollis.

Finally, we have observed patients whose head turns seem to be caused by central visual field defects and not by ocular misalignment. Such patients turn their heads toward the hemianopic field under both monocular and binocular conditions. The explanation for the head turn in these patients is unclear.

Techniques

Ocular alignment may be tested subjectively or objectively, depending on the circumstances

under which the examination is performed and the physical and mental state of the patient.

Subjective Testing

When a patient is cooperative, subjective testing of diplopia reliably indicates the disparity between retinal images. The simplest subjective tests of ocular alignment use colored filters to dissociate the deviation and to emphasize and differentiate the images so that the patient and the observer can interpret them. A fixation light is used to provide the image. A red filter held over one eye suffices in most cases; however, the addition of a green filter over the opposite eye gives better results in children, in patients with a tendency to suppress or ignore one of the images, and in patients with a slight paresis and good fusion ability who can overcome their deviation. The use of complementary colored filters, one over each eye, produces maximum dissociation of images because there is no part of the visible spectrum common to both eyes.

The red filter is always placed over the patient's right eye, and all questions posed to the patient relate to the relationship of the red image with respect to the white (or green) image. The patient is first asked if he or she sees one or two lights. If the patient sees two lights, he or she is then asked what color they are. After the appropriate answer, the patient is asked if the red light is to the right or left of the other light and if it is above or below the other light. The information thus received should be (1) that the patient sees two lights, one red and one white or green, and (2) that they are crossed (each image is perceived on the side opposite the eye that is seeing it) or uncrossed (each image is perceived on the same side as the eye that is seeing it), that the image relating to the right eye (red image) is higher or lower than the other image, or that the images are both horizontally and vertically separated.

It should be remembered that the image of an object is always displaced in the *opposite* direction to the position of the eye (Fig. 16.7). Thus, if an eye is exotropic, the patient will have **crossed** diplopia, and (with a red filter over the right eye) the patient will see the red image to the *left* of the other image. Similarly, if the patient has an esotropia, the red image will be seen to the *right* of the other image (**uncrossed** diplopia). If the patient has a vertical deviation of the eyes, the

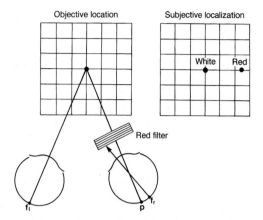

Figure 16.7. The principle of diplopia tests. A red filter is placed in front of the right eye, and the patient fixes a single light in the distance. If the eyes are misaligned, the light is imaged on the fovea of one eye (f_l) and the nonfoveal retina (p) of the opposite eye. The patient thus sees two images, white and red, in different locations in space.

eye that is higher will see the image of an object *below* that of the opposite eye.

Once a patient indicates that there is a clear separation of images when he or she is fixing on a light held straight ahead, the examiner can determine the area of maximum vertical separation, horizontal separation, or both, by having the patient look at a light held in the eight other cardinal positions of gaze (right, upper right, up, upper left, left, lower left, down, lower right).

In addition to the use of filters placed over one or both eyes, one can place a red Maddox rod over one eye and have the patient fixate on a white light. The ''rod'' is, in fact, a set of small half-cylinders aligned side by side in a frame in such a way that when the eye views a light through the cylinders, the image seen is that of a line perpendicular to the cylinder axis. Thus, if one views a white light with one eye covered by a red Maddox rod, the images will be those of a red line and a white light. The Maddox rod can be placed in such a manner as to produce a vertical, horizontal, or oblique line. Persons who are orthophoric see the line pass through the light. When the rod is oriented to produce the image of a vertical line, patients with a horizontal strabismus will see the line to the left or right of the light. When the rod is oriented so that a horizontal line image is produced, patients with a vertical strabismus will see the line above or below the light.

Torsional misalignment of the eyes (e.g., superior oblique palsy) can be tested with two Maddox rods, one over each eye. This is best performed using a trial lens frame. If both rods are oriented so as to produce a horizontal line image, an eye with torsional dysfunction will see the line as oblique, rather than horizontal. The patient is then asked to rotate the rod until the line is perceived as horizontal. By this method, the amount of torsion can be measured and followed. Traditionally, one clear (or white) and one red Maddox rod are used for this test. However, subjective torsion more reliably localizes to the paretic eye if two red Maddox rods are used and if the room is dark during testing.

Other subjective techniques to assess ocular misalignment may be used in which two test objects rather than one are presented to the patient in such a way that each object is viewed with only one eye (Fig. 16.8). The patient is then required to place the two objects in such a fashion that they appear to be superimposed. The objects only appear superimposed when their images fall on the fovea of each eye. Misalignment of the foveas results in the patient placing the objects in different locations in space. The eyes are differentiated and dissociated in various ways. Each eye may be presented with a different target, or complementary colors may be

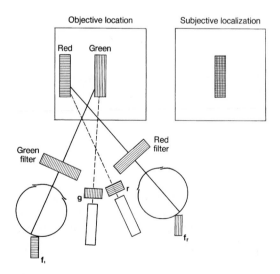

Figure 16.8. The principle of haploscopic tests. Red and green test objects are used, and the patient has a red filter placed in front of one eye and a green filter in front of the other eye.

placed into the visual field, either directly or by projection, with each eye being provided with a corresponding colored filter. These **haploscopic** tests include the use of a major amblyoscope, and the Hess screen and Lancaster red-green tests.

In general, the **Hess test** uses a gray or black screen marked with a tangent scale on which red targets are projected or positioned where the tangent lines cross. A green target or light is superimposed subjectively on the red fixation target. Complementary red and green filters are worn to permit (and stimulate) binocular dissociation, thus revealing the ocular deviation in each position of fixation. The test is performed with the patient 0.5 meter from the screen. The **Lancaster test** incorporates the same principles as the Hess screen but uses a two-dimensional grid rather than a tangent screen and is performed with the patient 1 or 2 meters from the grid.

Although the Hess and Lancaster tests use red and green colors to dissociate images as in the more simple ''red glass'' test described above, they differ from that test in principle. In the red glass test, one white fixation light is used that can be seen by each eye through the red and green (if used) filters. In the Hess or Lancaster tests, instead of a white light, two different color test objects are used. These are projected red and green lines that can only be perceived by the fovea of the eye that is viewing through the corresponding colored filter. Thus, the eye that is viewing through the red filter (usually the right eye) sees only the red line, whereas the eye that is viewing through the green filter (usually the left eye) sees only the green line. Each fovea perceives the image from its respective target as being located straight ahead. This is macular-macular projection (confusion). The binocular dissociation produced in this manner is sufficient to reveal even a minimal and well-controlled heterophoria. The patient, wearing the red filter over the right eye, is asked to superimpose the green line on the red line as each fixation position on the screen or grid is illuminated consecutively. The nonfixing left eye is deviated behind the green filter, but the patient merely guides the flashlight so that the green line is positioned where the deviated eye is pointing. At this point, the patient sees the red and green lights superimposed. The examiner, however, can see the deviation of the green line from the

red line and can plot the position of the green line onto a chart. The test is then repeated with the red and green filters reversed, so that the left eye now fixates the red line, and the field of the deviating right eye is plotted.

Not only is this test helpful in assessing the degree of deviation of both comitant and noncomitant strabismus at any given time, but it may be used in patients with paralytic strabismus to detect subtle changes in ocular alignment that occur over time. It thus may help in the planning and evaluation of therapy for such patients. In addition, subjective torsion of the eyes can be identified when the patient rotates one line at an oblique angle relative to the other line.

Objective Testing
CORNEAL LIGHT REFLEX

The simplest objective method of determining ocular alignment is the use of a hand light to cast a reflection on the corneal surfaces of both eyes in the cardinal positions of gaze. If the images from the two corneas appear centered, then the visual axes are usually correctly aligned. If the light reflexes are not centered, one can estimate the amount of misalignment based on the apparent amount of decentration of the light reflex (the **Hirschberg test**): with the fixation light held 33 cm from the patient, 1 mm of decentration equals 7° of ocular deviation.

Alternately, prisms can be placed over either of the eyes until the light reflexes appear centered (the **Krimsky test**). In general, prisms are always placed over the fixing eye; however, in circumstances where the nonfixing eye is so eccentric and limited in its excursion that centration of the light reflex is impossible or requires excessive prism over the fixing eye, holding the prism over the fixing eye results in a measurement of the deviation only in eccentric gaze. This is essentially the same as measuring the secondary, rather than the primary, deviation.

A number of conditions other than a heterotropia may cause decentration of the corneal light reflex and must be considered in order to interpret correctly tests based on centration of the light reflex. The **angle kappa** is defined as the angle between the visual line (the line connecting the point of fixation with the fovea) and the pupillary axis (the line through the center of the pupil perpendicular to the cornea). The angle is measured at the center of the pupil. It is considered positive when the light reflex is dis-

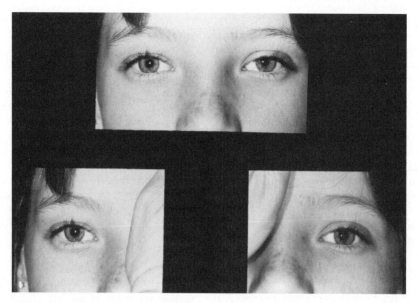

Figure 16.9. Positive angle kappa with the corneal light reflex test. With both eyes open (*top*) the eyes appear exotropic because the light reflection is decentered nasally in the left eye. The reflex remains centered in the right eye when the left eye is covered (*bottom left*). When the right eye is covered (*bottom right*), there is no shift of fixation, and the light reflection remains nasally displaced.

placed nasally, and negative when the light reflex is displaced temporally. A positive angle kappa may simulate an exodeviation (Fig. 16.9), and a negative angle kappa may simulate an esodeviation. Conversely, strabismus may be less apparent when a large angle kappa is associated with esotropia or a large negative angle is associated with exotropia.

Other ocular abnormalities that produce decentration of the corneal light reflex include eccentric fixation and ectopic macula (e.g., in patients with retinopathy of prematurity or other retinal disease with macular traction).

COVER TESTS

The most precise, objective methods of measuring ocular alignment are the **cover tests.** Although these tests require that the patient be able to fixate a target with either eye, they generally require less cooperation than do the subjective tests described above. The three types of cover tests used by most clinicians are the single-cover test, the cover-uncover test, and the alternate-cover (cross-cover) test.

In the **single-cover test,** the patient fixates an accommodative target at 33 cm (near target) or 6 meters (distant target). An opaque occluder is placed in front of one eye, and the examiner observes the opposite eye to see if it moves to take up fixation of the target (Fig. 16.10). If movement is observed, its direction and speed should be noted. The test is then repeated on the opposite eye. If the patient has a manifest ocular deviation (**heterotropia**), the previously nonfixing eye will be observed to change position in order to take up fixation when the fixing eye is covered. On the other hand, when the nonfixing eye is covered, no movement of the fixing eye will be observed (because it is already fixing on the target). This test is usually performed with the patient fixing in primary position and with the eyes in the other cardinal positions of gaze. Movements of as little as 1° can be easily observed.

In the **cover-uncover test**, the patient fixates on an accommodative target, and one eye is occluded. The behavior of that eye is then observed as the cover is removed (see Fig. 16.10). The direction of any deviation and the speed and rate of recovery to binocular fixation are noted.

If no movement of the uncovered eye is observed when the cover-uncover test is performed, an **alternate-cover test** may be used to detect a latent deviation of the eyes (**heteropho-**

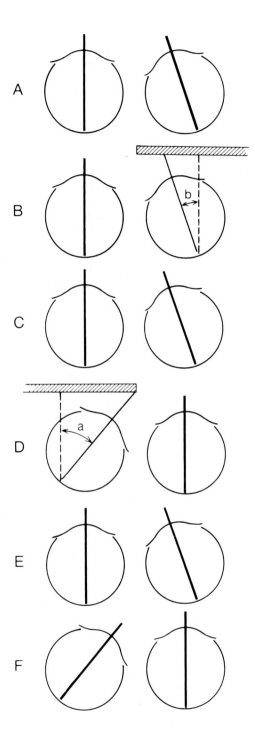

Figure 16.10. The single-cover and cover-uncover tests. In both tests, one eye is covered at a time; however, in the single-cover test, one eye is covered, and the opposite eye is observed. In the cover-uncover test, one eye is covered, and the behavior of that eye is observed when the cover is removed. *A.* Initially, with both eyes viewing, the left eye is fixating the target, and the right eye is esotropic. *B.* When the right eye is covered, no movement of the left (uncovered) eye is observed. *C.* Nor is any movement of the right eye observed when the cover is removed (*C*). *D.* When the left eye is covered, the right eye moves outward to take up fixation. Note that the deviation of the normal eye under cover (the secondary deviation, *a*) is greater than that of the paretic eye under cover (primary deviation, *b*). When the cover is removed, either (*E*) the left eye again takes up fixation, or (*F*) the paretic right eye continues to fixate.

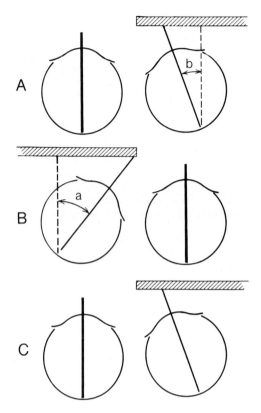

Figure 16.11. The alternate-cover test. This test prevents fusional vergence and thus tests both phorias and tropias but does not differentiate between them. In this test, the cover is quickly moved from one eye to the other, and any movement of either eye is noted. In this example, there is an esodeviation.

ria). Instead of occluding one eye and then taking the occluder away, first one eye and then the other is alternately occluded. The cover should remain in front of each eye long enough to allow the patient to take up fixation with the uncovered eye. This test prevents fusion and dissociates the visual axes. Any movement of either uncovered eye suggests that although the eyes are straight during binocular viewing, loss of fusion (i.e., by the alternate occlusion of the two eyes) results in a deviation of whichever eye is covered (Fig. 16.11).

The importance of distinguishing between heterophorias and heterotropias cannot be overemphasized, because patients with heterophorias have binocular central fusion, whereas patients with heterotropias do not.

If either the cover-uncover or alternate-cover

tests detect evidence of ocular misalignment, prisms can be used to neutralize the movement and thereby measure the deviation, whether it is a heterotropia or heterophoria. Prisms are placed in front of either eye such that the apex of the prism is oriented in the direction of the deviation, and the prism strength is altered until the deviation is no longer observed.

HEAD TILT TEST

When there is a vertical ocular deviation, it is often helpful to perform cover tests with the head tilted first toward one side and then toward the other. The patient is instructed to maintain fixation on a distant target, and the position of the eyes relative to each other is measured. The patient is then instructed to tilt his or her head to one side while maintaining fixation on the target, and the eyes are again examined to see if one eye has moved higher than the other. Measurements are made with the head tilted to each side.

This test is useful primarily in the diagnosis of superior oblique palsy, because patients with this disorder consistently show a hypertropia of the involved eye when the head is tilted toward the involved side. It has been suggested that the physiologic basis of this test lies in the fact that the vertical eye muscles are not driven in their usual yoked pairs when the head is tilted. Instead, the vestibular apparatus produces compensatory cyclorotation of the eyes by co-innervation of the ipsilateral (to the side of the tilt) superior oblique and superior rectus muscles, producing intorsion, and of the contralateral inferior oblique and inferior rectus muscles, producing extorsion.

When a patient with a trochlear nerve palsy tilts the head toward the affected side, intorsion of that eye should occur to keep the vertical meridian perpendicular to the horizon. As previously noted above, this intorsion is usually about 10° and is produced by the otolith-ocular reflex, resulting in synergistic contractions of the superior rectus and superior oblique muscles. If, however, the superior oblique muscle is paretic, its secondary actions, one of which is depression, is also impaired. The superior rectus muscle is therefore the only means by which the eye is intorted, and its main action, elevation of the eye, is unopposed.

THREE-STEP DIAGNOSTIC TEST

The head tilt test is best used as part of a "three-step" diagnostic test. This test is used to isolate the involved paretic muscle in concomitant or incomitant vertical deviations. It is only useful if the paresis is of a single cycloverted muscle. The steps are as follows:

1. The presence of a vertical heterotropia is determined in primary position. Depending on the eye that is hypertropic, one of four muscles may be paretic: the ipsilateral inferior rectus, the ipsilateral superior oblique, the contralateral superior rectus, or the contralateral inferior oblique. Thus, if the patient has a right hypertropia, the muscles that may be paretic are the right superior oblique, the right inferior rectus, the left superior rectus, or the left inferior oblique.

2. Whether the hypertropia increases in right or left horizontal gaze is determined. This reduces the potential paretic muscles to two. Thus, in a patient with a right hypertropia, if the deviation increases in right gaze, the affected muscles can only be the right inferior rectus (which has its maximum vertical action when the eye is in an abducted position) or the left inferior oblique (which has its maximum vertical action when the eye is in an adducted position). If the deviation increases in left gaze, the affected muscles could be either the right superior oblique or the left superior rectus.

3. The differential diagnosis between the two muscles, one in each eye, that are potentially responsible for the vertical heterotropia, is now made using the head tilt test as described above. Thus, if the patient has a right hypertropia that increases in left gaze, an increase in the hypertropia when the head is tilted to the right side indicates a paretic superior oblique muscle.

Although we believe the three-step test is extremely useful in patients with presumed trochlear nerve palsies, we find that its reliability in the diagnosis of pareses of other vertical muscles is questionable. Furthermore, restrictive ophthalmoplegia, myasthenia gravis, and skew deviation can mimic superior oblique palsy using the three-step test.

DIRECT OBSERVATION OF THE FUNDUS

A final objective method of determining ocular torsion is direct observation of the ocular fundus. The normal fovea is generally located about $7°$ below center of the optic disc (range, $0°$ to $16°$) or along a horizontal line originating from a point between the middle and lower thirds of the optic disc. When an eye is extorted, the foveal reflex rotates below this plane, whereas intorsion results in upward rotation of the reflex (Fig. 16.12). The amount of torsion can be determined using a variety of ophthalmoscopic and photographic methods.

PERFORMANCE OF VERSIONS

Versions may be tested by examining the saccadic, pursuit, vestibular, and optokinetic systems.

Clinical Examination of Saccades

Saccadic eye movements are examined clinically by instructing the patient to alternately fixate upon two targets—usually the examiner's finger and nose. Saccades in each direction can be examined in each field of gaze in both the horizontal and vertical planes. The examiner must determine if the saccades are (1) promptly initiated, (2) of normal velocity, and (3) accurate.

Saccadic latencies can be appreciated by noting the time it takes the patient to initiate the saccade. Abnormal voluntary saccadic velocities may be accentuated by using a hand-held drum or tape with repetitive patterns. Rotating the drum or passing the tape horizontally and vertically across the patient's visual field stimulates the optokinetic system to produce nystagmus. Abnormal saccadic velocities, particularly slowing, thus become more evident when the patient is forced to make multiple, repetitive saccades to refixate the passing targets. Altered saccadic velocities that occur in only one plane of movement can also be appreciated by using obliquely placed targets to stimulate oblique saccades. In such patients, the normal velocity component of the saccade (e.g., the horizontal) will be completed before the other component (e.g., the vertical), so that the trajectory appears L-shaped.

Disorders of saccadic accuracy—such as **saccadic dysmetria**—can be inferred from the direction and size of corrective saccades that the patient must make to ultimately acquire the fixation target. Because saccades as small as $0.5°$ can

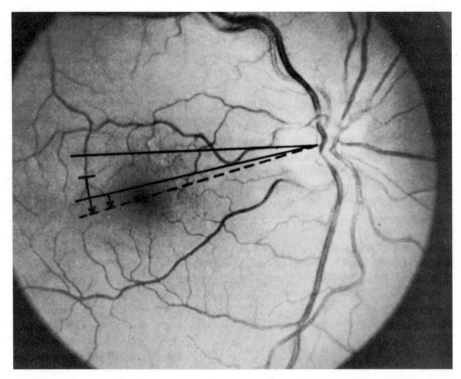

Figure 16.12. Torsion of the ocular fundus. Photograph of an extorted right fundus, direct view, with a dashed line drawn from the center of the optic disc through the fovea. The normal angular range of the fovea from the center of the disc is shown by the two solid lines. The amount of extorsion can be measured in degrees from the center of the normal range (*long arrow*) or from the limit of the normal range (*short arrow*). (Courtesy of Dr. David L Guyton.)

be easily identified during clinical observation, minimal degrees of saccadic dysmetria can be easily appreciated during the clinical examination. Normal persons may undershoot a target by a few degrees when refixations are large. Similarly, such individuals may overshoot a target during centripetal, and especially downward, saccades. This dysmetria is transient, however, gradually disappearing during repetitive refixations between the same targets.

When a saccadic abnormality is detected during the clinical examination, the examiner must attempt to localize the disturbance within the hierarchic organization of the saccadic eye-movement system. The first step in localization is to establish whether or not reflex types of saccades are affected by the disease process. Quick phases can be examined by spinning the patient in a swivel chair to elicit vestibular and optokinetic nystagmus. Next, an attempt should be made to determine if saccades can be performed without visual targets or in response to auditory

targets. This is achieved by asking the patient to refixate under closed lids. The eye movements thus generated can be observed, palpated, and even heard (with a stethoscope applied to the lids).

During the evaluation of saccadic eye movements, it is often helpful to observe gaze changes when the patient makes a combined eye-head movement to see if an accompanying head movement can facilitate the production of a saccade. This strategy is used by some patients with ocular motor apraxia. The effect of blinks should also be noted, because they may facilitate both the ability to initiate saccades and the subsequent saccadic velocity. Finally, fatigue of saccadic eye movements may be tested by asking the patient to repetitively refixate between two targets.

Clinical Examination of Pursuit

Patients with isolated deficiency of smooth pursuit do not usually complain of visual symptoms, because they can track moving objects with a series of saccades. Only very demanding tracking tasks (e.g., playing tennis, handball, or baseball) may cause patients with impaired pursuit to report difficulties. The vision of normal subjects deteriorates during tracking of targets moving at high frequencies, however, so that even complaints of inability to track fast-moving objects may not signify a disorder of smooth pursuit.

To test the pursuit system, the examiner should ask the patient to track a small target, such as a pencil tip held a meter or more from the eyes, with the head held still. The target should initially be moved at a low, uniform velocity. Pursuit movements that do not match the target velocity result in corrective saccades. If these are "catch-up" saccades, then the pursuit gain is low. If pursuit gain is too high, then "back-up" saccades are observed. Small children, uncooperative patients, or persons thought to have nonorganic blindness may be tested with a slowly rotating large mirror held before their eyes.

Although hand-held drums or tapes with repetitive targets do not truly test the optokinetic system, they do stimulate pursuit and may be useful in the detection of pursuit asymmetries and other abnormalities of the pursuit system.

The smooth-pursuit system can also be assessed using the VOR. The VOR normally generates eye movements that compensate for angular displacement of the head and maintain the visual axes "on target." If one observes a slowly moving target by moving the head, so that the target remains stationary relative to the head, the eye movements generated by the VOR are inappropriate and must be suppressed. The ability of a patient to suppress (or cancel) the VOR can be evaluated by using a central fixation target that moves in the same direction and at the same velocity as the head. Patients often do this best by fixating their thumbnail with their arm outstretched while being rotated in the examination chair. Persons with limb muscle weakness can be rotated in a wheelchair while fixating a target that rotates with the chair. When suppression of the VOR and pursuit are compared in normal human subjects, similar frequency response curves are obtained, leading to the hypothesis that suppression of the VOR depends directly on information derived from the smooth-pursuit system. This hypothesis is supported by the clinical observation that patients

with impaired smooth pursuit also have abnormal suppression of the VOR. The evaluation of VOR suppression is thus another way to test the integrity of the pursuit system. Deficits in VOR suppression, however, are nonlocalizing, because they may occur with either cerebral or cerebellar disease.

In some patients, it is difficult to test smooth pursuit because of spontaneous nystagmus; however, in some of these patients, the nystagmus is less prominent in a specific position of gaze (the null point). In these patients, cancellation of the VOR during head rotation can be tested with the eyes fixing on a target in this position. As with pursuit, the head rotation should be gentle at first. In patients with inadequate cancellation, the eyes are continually taken off target by the intact VOR, and corrective saccades therefore occur. An asymmetric deficit may imply a pursuit imbalance provided that the VOR is intact and symmetric: deficient cancellation of the VOR on rotation to one side corresponds to a low pursuit gain to that side. Furthermore, when there is a discrepancy between the performance of smooth pursuit and cancellation of the VOR (e.g., poor pursuit but good cancellation), one should suspect an inadequate or asymmetric VOR.

Clinical Examination of the Vestibular and Optokinetic Systems

The clinical methods used to test the vestibular system (oculocephalic and caloric testing) are described above. Although the optokinetic system can be tested in the laboratory (see below), the system cannot be tested as part of a routine clinical examination. As noted above, so-called "optokinetic" hand-held drums and tapes actually assess the smooth-pursuit system, not the optokinetic system.

QUANTITATIVE ANALYSIS OF EYE MOVEMENTS

Voluntary Eye Movements

Most disturbances of ocular motility and alignment can be detected during a standard clinical examination; however, some subtle abnormalities of the pursuit, saccadic, optokinetic, and vestibulo-ocular systems may be more easily and accurately assessed by performing a quantitative analysis of eye movements. The most common methods used to record eye movements are electro-oculography and infrared oculography. These techniques may be used to distinguish myopathic (restrictive) from neuropathic conditions that affect ocular motility and to determine the presence or absence of improvement of ocular motor function during therapy.

Although electro-oculography can yield reasonable recordings of horizontal eye movements, vertical measurements with this technique are affected by eyelid artifacts and nonlinearities. Changes in illumination and skin resistance also affect the readings with this method. Infrared oculography provides higher resolution measurements of both horizontal and vertical eye movements, but over a limited range, especially vertically. In addition, the signal is lost when the eyes are closed. Finally, neither electro-oculography nor infrared oculography measures ocular torsion.

The magnetic field-search coil method, which uses coils embedded in a silicone rubber ring that adheres to the sclera by suction, overcomes most of the problems that limit both electro-oculography and infrared oculography, and further advancements in this system using a digital microprocessor enable this technique to be used with great accuracy to measure almost all types of normal and abnormal eye movements.

The Vestibulo-Ocular Reflex

The oculocephalic and caloric tests that are performed in patients with apparent limitation of eye movement primarily test the function of the semicircular canals of the vestibular system. More extensive testing is usually directed toward determining gain, phase, and balance. Rotation tests give more accurate and reproducible results than do caloric tests, although the mental state of the patient while in darkness may influence the results. The gain of the VOR may be obtained by measuring the peak eye velocity in response to a velocity step (e.g., sudden sustained rotation at 60°/second) in darkness. This is usually done in vestibular laboratories equipped with servo-controlled chairs and eye-monitoring equipment, although portable systems for this purpose are available.

Although the otolith organs respond to linear acceleration, tests of their function are rarely performed. Several investigators have suggested that muscle responses that occur less than 100 msec after release into free-fall are part of a normal startle reflex that originates in the otoliths. Using this theory, otolith integrity can be measured by recording eye-blink reflexes that occur following sudden free-falls. Such testing may confirm the presence of otolith function in patients with impaired semicircular canal function or show impaired otolith function in patients with normal semicircular canal function.

The Optokinetic System

The hand-held "optokinetic" drums or tapes that are used to elicit smooth movements primarily test the pursuit system. True optokinetic testing requires a stimulus that fills the field of vision. A common technique is to have the patient sit inside a large, patterned optokinetic drum that is rotated around the patient. A true optokinetic stimulus induces a sensation of self-rotation. Another method of eliciting a true optokinetic response is rotation of an individual at a constant velocity in the light for over 1 minute. The sustained nystagmus that results is caused by purely visual stimuli (the vestibular response having died away); however, it is still difficult to separate its pursuit and optokinetic components.

FOR MORE INFORMATION:
See Walsh & Hoyt's *Clinical Neuro-Ophthalmology,* 5th edition, Volume 1, Chapter 27, pp. 1169–1188.

CHAPTER 17

Nuclear and Infranuclear Ocular Motility Disorders

The ocular motor system is separated anatomically and physiologically into infranuclear (peripheral), nuclear, internuclear, and supranuclear components. In this chapter, we consider ocular motor disturbances caused by congenital and acquired lesions of the nuclear and infranuclear neural structures—the lesions of the ocular motor nuclei and nerves.

Disorders that produce dysfunction of the oculomotor, trochlear, and abducens nerves may be located anywhere from the ocular motor nuclei to the termination of the nerves in the extraocular muscles within the orbit. Ocular motor nerve palsies may present in one of four ways:

1. As isolated partial or complete nerve palsies without any other neurologic signs and without symptoms except those related to the palsy itself.
2. In association with symptoms other than those related to the palsy (e.g., pain, dysesthesia, paresthesias) but without any signs of neurologic or systemic disease.
3. In association with other ocular motor

nerve palsies (e.g., the simultaneous onset of an oculomotor palsy and an abducens palsy) but without any other neurologic signs.
4. In association with neurologic signs other than the ocular motor nerve palsy.

Most large series that discuss the percentage of ocular motor nerve palsies caused by various etiologies do not take into account these various modes of presentation and thus are of limited value to the clinician. In the sections that follow, we discuss the features of ocular motor nerve palsies, the symptoms and signs that may accompany them relative to their known or presumed site of origin, the lesions that cause them, and their management.

OCULOMOTOR (THIRD) NERVE PALSIES

CONGENITAL

Congenital oculomotor nerve palsies are rare, compared with acquired palsies; however, they constitute nearly half of the oculomotor nerve pareses seen in children (Fig. 17.1). Most cases are unilateral, but bilateral cases also occur. As a general rule, patients with congenital oculomotor nerve palsies have no other neurologic or systemic abnormalities. Usually, these patients have some degree of amblyopia, and this may occur in either the paretic eye or nonparetic eye. Most cases of congenital oculomotor nerve palsy are sporadic; however, rare familial cases occur.

All patients with congenital oculomotor nerve palsy have some degree of ptosis and ophthalmoparesis, and nearly all have pupillary involvement. In most of these cases, the pupil is miotic rather than dilated, presumably because of misdirected oculomotor nerve regeneration (see below). Pupillary miosis as a result of aberrant regeneration appears to be much more frequent after congenital than acquired pupil-involving oculomotor palsy.

Abnormalities of the oculomotor nerve that are present at birth may be caused by absent or incomplete development of the nucleus, nerve, or both. Persons in whom this occurs may show varying degrees of oculomotor nerve dysfunction, depending on the severity of maldevelopment. It is likely that in most of these cases the oculomotor nuclear complex is intact, and the responsible lesion is in the nerve itself.

Injury to the oculomotor nerve during gestation, including amniocentesis, or at the time of delivery may produce a congenital oculomotor nerve palsy. Such patients may or may not have other physical signs of trauma or other neurologic signs. The mechanism of isolated oculomotor nerve palsy attributed to birth injury is not known, but it is probably damage to the sub-

arachnoid portion of the oculomotor nerve, either at its exit from the brainstem or just before it enters the cavernous sinus.

In addition to simple congenital oculomotor nerve palsy, several congenital syndromes implicate oculomotor maldevelopment with anomalous or paradoxic innervation of the extraocular muscles. These syndromes include (1) congenital adduction palsy with synergistic divergence, (2) atypical vertical retraction syndrome, and (3) cyclic oculomotor nerve paresis with cyclic spasm.

Congenital Adduction Palsy with Synergistic Divergence

Patients with this syndrome have congenital unilateral paralysis of adduction associated with simultaneous bilateral abduction on attempted gaze into the field of action of the paretic medial rectus muscle (Fig. 17.2). Most patients with congenital adduction palsy with synergistic divergence have no other neurologic abnormalities.

Electromyographic studies in patients with this condition suggest that it is caused by absent oculomotor nerve innervation of the affected medial rectus muscle, combined with absent or minimal innervation of the lateral rectus muscle by the abducens nerve but with a branch of the oculomotor nerve innervating the lateral rectus muscle (Fig. 17.3).

Vertical Retraction Syndrome

The main clinical feature of the vertical retraction syndrome is limitation of movement of the affected eye on elevation or depression, associated with a retraction of the globe and narrowing of the palpebral fissure (Fig. 17.4). There may be an associated esotropia or exotropia, more marked in the direction of the restricted vertical field of action. The superior rectus muscle is usually more affected than the inferior rectus muscle, so the retraction may be evident only during attempted depression of the eyes. The condition is usually unilateral, but bilateral cases have been reported. The results of both electrooculography and electromyography in patients with this condition are consistent with anomalous oculomotor innervation of the vertical rectus muscles of the affected eye.

Oculomotor Paresis with Cyclic Spasms (Cyclic Oculomotor Paresis)

Cyclic oculomotor paresis is usually unilateral and is, in the majority of cases, present from

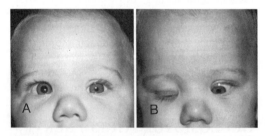

Figure 17.1. Congenital left oculomotor nerve palsy with aberrant regeneration in a child with a history of birth trauma. *A.* In primary position, there is a left hypotropia. Note the miotic left pupil. *B.* On attempted downward gaze, there is retraction of the left upper eyelid (pseudo-Graefe sign).

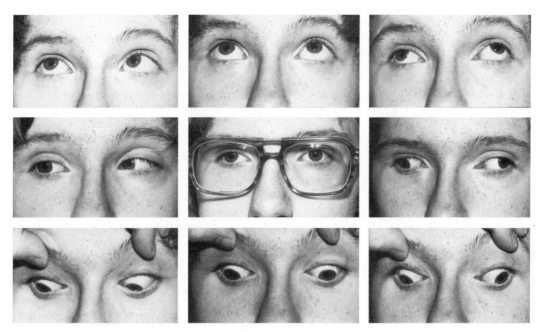

Figure 17.2.   Congenital right adduction palsy and synergistic divergence. Extraocular movements in nine fields of gaze. The right eye abducts somewhat on attempted right lateral gaze, but also abducts on right lateral gaze. (Reprinted with permission from Wilcox LM Jr, Gittinger JW Jr, Breinin GM. Congenital adduction palsy and synergistic divergence. Am J Ophthalmol 1981;91:1–7.)

birth. The typical patient with this condition has an oculomotor nerve paresis with ptosis, mydriasis, reduced accommodation, and ophthalmoparesis (Fig. 17.5 *Top* and 17.5 *Bottom left*). About every 2 minutes, the ptotic eyelid elevates, the globe begins to adduct, the pupil constricts, and accommodation increases (see Fig. 17.5 *Bottom right*). These spasms last 10 to 30 seconds and then give way to the paretic phase. Although most cases consist of alternating spasm and paresis of the entire oculomotor nerve, some patients show only the pupillary and accommodative signs of the syndrome. Such patients have no ptosis or diplopia at any time.

The cyclic movements seen in patients with cyclic oculomotor paresis are usually present when the oculomotor deficit is first discovered, but in some cases, the cyclic component develops several months to years after the onset of the paresis. Once present, the syndrome usually persists unchanged throughout life, although exceptions occur. The cycles continue even during sleep, although they do so at a reduced rate and amplitude; they subside only during deep sleep.

Most patients with unilateral cyclic oculomotor paresis have reduced visual acuity in the affected eye because of amblyopia. The syndrome is occasionally associated with other pathologic conditions, including birth trauma and congenital infections.

Associated movements of the eyes can influence the cycle of ocular motility in cyclic oculomotor paresis. In one series, 31 of 54 patients showed an increase in the extent and duration of the spastic phase with adduction or accommodation-convergence efforts. Attempted vertical gaze or forced eyelid closure had a similar effect in a few cases. Conversely, abduction efforts shortened and reduced the spasms and accentuated or prolonged the paretic phase. These influences of voluntary gaze efforts upon the cyclic movements did not appear immediately, but only after the effort was maintained for several seconds.

There are numerous theories regarding the pathogenesis of cyclic oculomotor paresis. The most likely explanation is that the original damage, caused at birth or in early childhood by trauma or infectious disease, affects the fibers of the intracranial portion of the oculomotor nerve,

Synergistic divergence

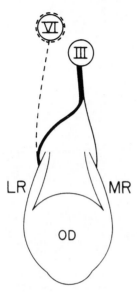

Figure 17.3. Anomaly of peripheral innervation that may explain synergistic divergence with congenital limitation of adduction. The oculomotor nerve provides major innervation of the lateral rectus muscle (which may or may not also be innervated by the abducens nerve). The thickness of the line representing the nerve represents quantitative innervation. Dashed lines indicate hypoplasia or aplasia of the abducens nucleus and/or nerve. *OD,* right eye; *LR,* lateral rectus muscle; *MR,* medial rectus muscle; *III,* oculomotor nucleus; *VI,* abducens nucleus. (Redrawn from Wilcox LM Jr, Gittinger JW Jr, Breinin GM. Congenital adduction palsy and synergistic divergence. Am J Ophthalmol 1981;91:1–7.)

followed by retrograde degeneration of the oculomotor neurons. When retrograde changes occur in the oculomotor neurons before the supranuclear connections of their cell bodies have matured, many of the supranuclear fibers fail to establish proper synaptic contacts with these cells. Instead, the fibers end diffusely in the neighborhood of the remaining motoneurons. Some of the injured nuclear cells recover, and regenerating nerve sprouts grow with their damaged axons haphazardly across the scar. Therefore, two cell populations exist in the oculomotor nucleus: normal neurons that escaped injury completely or recovered completely from slight damage, and neurons that have been severely damaged but remain alive. The cells of the first group transmit remnants of physiologic movements, whereas those of the second group are responsible for the abnormal cyclic spasms by a process of summation of subthreshold stimuli and rhythmic mass discharges.

Cyclic oculomotor paresis is usually a congenital condition. Rarely, cases occur after an acquired oculomotor nerve palsy, such as from a posterior fossa tumor. However, patients with true congenital oculomotor nerve paresis with cyclic spasms do not require any workup unless they have other evidence of neurologic disease, or they give a history of progressive neurologic dysfunction.

Cyclic oculomotor palsy usually continues throughout life. Nevertheless, in rare cases, the cycles disappear, and the patient is left with a persistent oculomotor nerve paresis.

ACQUIRED

Acquired dysfunction of the oculomotor nerve is far more common than its congenital counterpart, being caused by nearly every pathologic process.

Lesions of the Oculomotor Nucleus

Lesions that damage the oculomotor nucleus are not uncommon. When they occur, they often produce bilateral defects in ocular motility, eyelid position, or both. The bilaterality of involvement is explained by the anatomy of the nucleus and its fibers. Both levator palpebrae superioris muscles are innervated by a single, midline subnucleus located at the caudal end of the oculomotor nerve complex (Fig. 17.6). Thus, a lesion that damages this region produces a bilateral, symmetric ptosis. Symmetric ptosis that progresses rapidly to total ptosis, when neuropathic in origin, usually indicates a nuclear lesion with involvement of caudal midline structures. In some cases, the ptosis is isolated, whereas in others, there is associated ophthalmoplegia that may be significant or so minimal as to be overlooked.

Lesions of the oculomotor nuclear complex may spare the central caudal nucleus. Patients with such lesions have fixed, dilated pupils and ophthalmoparesis affecting one or more of the muscles innervated by the oculomotor nerve but no ptosis. Magnetic resonance imaging (MRI) can be used to confirm the rostral location of the lesion in these cases.

A second anatomic feature of the oculomotor nuclear complex that results in bilateral ocular damage is the nerve to the superior rectus mus-

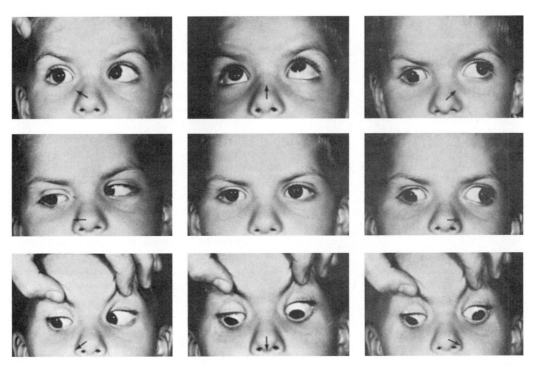

Figure 17.4. Synergistic vertical and horizontal divergence in a boy with congenital limitation of adduction and elevation of the right eye. On attempted left horizontal gaze (and to some extent on right horizontal gaze), the right eye abducts and shoots downward. Optokinetic stimuli and clockwise constant rotation in a Bárány chair caused divergent nystagmus. (Courtesy of Dr. Maurice Van Allen.)

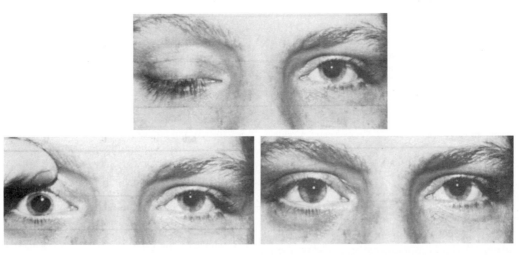

Figure 17.5. Right oculomotor paresis with cyclic spasm (cyclic oculomotor paresis) in a 21-year-old man. *Top:* Paretic phase with maximum ptosis. *Bottom left:* Paretic phase with eyelid held up to reveal markedly dilated right pupil. *Bottom right:* Spastic phase showing right eyelid in almost normal position and constricted right pupil. (Reprinted with permission from Fells P, Collin JRO. Cyclic oculomotor palsy. Trans Ophthalmol Soc UK 1979;99:192–196.)

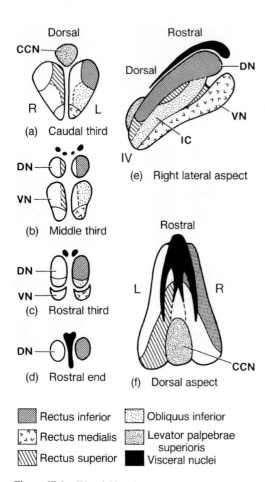

Dorsal

CCN

R   L

(a)   Caudal third

DN

VN

(b)   Middle third

DN

VN

(c)   Rostral third

DN

(d)   Rostral end

Rostral

Dorsal   **DN**

                                    VN

                                    IC

IV

(e)   Right lateral aspect

Rostral

L   R

                                    CCN

(f)   Dorsal aspect

▓ Rectus inferior   ░ Obliquus inferior

▚ Rectus medialis   ▒ Levator palpebrae
                              superioris
▨ Rectus superior   ■ Visceral nuclei

Figure 17.6. Warwick's schema of topographic organization within the oculomotor nucleus. Note the caudal dorsal midline position of caudal central nucleus (CCN), the motor pool for the levator palpebrae superioris. The motor pool of the superior rectus (*hashed area*) is **contralateral** to the extraocular muscle it innervates. The visceral (parasympathetic) nuclei are shown in black. *DN*, dorsal nucleus; *IC*, intermediate column; *IV*, tegion of the trochlear nucleus; *VN*, ventral nucleus. (Reprinted with permission from Warwick R. Representation of the extra-ocular muscles in the oculomotor nuclei of the monkey. J Comp Neurol 1953;98: 449–504.)

cle, which is crossed, its fibers passing through—but not originating from—the ipsilateral subnucleus for superior rectus function. Thus, the subnucleus for superior rectus function on either side of the brainstem gives rise to fibers that pass through the contralateral superior rectus subnucleus without synapse and innervate the **contralateral** superior rectus muscle. Lesions that affect this region thus cause not only

ipsilateral weakness of superior rectus, medial rectus, inferior rectus, inferior oblique, or a combination of these muscles, but also limitation of elevation in the contralateral eye from impairment of superior rectus function on that side. Such patients have bilateral limitation of upward gaze, occasionally worse on the contralateral side (Figs. 17.7 and 17.8).

Patients with damage to the oculomotor nuclear complex need not have ipsilateral pupillary dilation, but when the pupil is involved it indicates **dorsal, rostral** damage. Such damage is almost always bilateral and is frequently associated with infranuclear or supranuclear gaze palsies. Incomplete oculomotor nerve pareses, occasionally restricted to a nerve supplying a single extraocular muscle (e.g., isolated inferior rectus paresis), may be produced by focal lesions of the oculomotor nuclear complex.

Lesions of the oculomotor nucleus are most often caused by ischemia, usually from embolic or thrombotic occlusion of small, dorsal perforating branches of the mesencephalic portion of the basilar artery or, less often, from occlusion of the distal portion of the basilar artery itself ("top of the basilar syndrome"). Other etiologies include hemorrhage, infiltration by tumor, inflammation, brainstem compression, and, very rarely, cephalic tetanus, amyotrophic lateral sclerosis (ALS), and Kugelberg-Welander disease.

Involvement of the immediate premotor mesencephalic structures located adjacent to the oculomotor nuclei complex may produce difficulties with ocular motility that may initially appear indistinguishable from direct damage to the nucleus itself. Such supranuclear defects can usually be distinguished from their nuclear and infranuclear counterparts by stimulation of the vestibular system using oculocephalic or caloric testing. When such tests reveal improvement in ocular motility, a supranuclear lesion is unquestionably present. On the other hand, if there is no improvement in ocular motility, either isolated infranuclear or (more commonly) a combination of infranuclear and supranuclear damage may be present.

Lesions of the Oculomotor Nerve Fascicle

Fascicular lesions of the oculomotor nerves produce both complete and incomplete palsies that cannot be differentiated clinically from palsies caused by lesions outside the brainstem

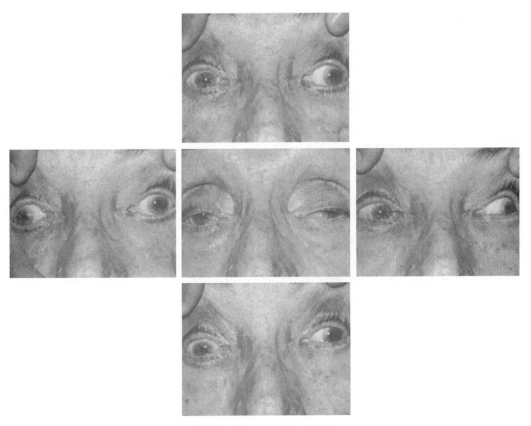

Figure 17.7.   Nuclear oculomotor nerve palsy. There is a complete left oculomotor nerve palsy. In addition, however, there is absence of elevation of the right eye. The right eye also has marked limitation of depression, suggesting that the lesion is not limited to the left oculomotor nerve nucleus but also involves the right nucleus as well. Neither oculocephalic nor caloric stimulation produced any improvement in vertical gaze.

(Fig. 17.9). Although most lesions that affect the fascicle produce an oculomotor nerve palsy with pupillary involvement, occasionally the pupil is spared. A fascicular oculomotor nerve palsy may occur as an isolated finding or in association with other brainstem signs. Thus, topical diagnosis of fascicular oculomotor nerve palsies depends either on the results of neuroimaging or on the coexistence of other neurologic signs (Fig. 17.10).

Fascicular oculomotor nerve palsies that are associated with other neurologic manifestations produce several characteristic syndromes. For example, lesions in the area of the brachium conjunctivum may produce ipsilateral oculomotor nerve palsy and cerebellar ataxia (**Nothnagel's syndrome**). The syndrome of ipsilateral oculomotor nerve palsy combined with contralateral involuntary movements is known as **Benedikt's syndrome** and reflects damage to the red nucleus, especially its dorsocaudal portion, through which the oculomotor fascicle passes (see Fig. 17.10). Mesencephalic lesions ventral to the red nucleus may damage fascicular oculomotor fibers and motor fibers in the cerebral peduncle, producing an oculomotor nerve palsy with contralateral hemiplegia or hemiparesis, including the lower face and tongue (**Weber's syndrome**) (Figs. 17.10 through 17.12). Simultaneous damage in the mesencephalon to the red nucleus *and* the brachium conjunctivum produces a syndrome with the features of both Benedikt's and Nothnagel's syndromes—oculomotor nerve paresis, contralateral asynergia, ataxia, dysmetria, and dysdiadochokinesia—called **Claude's syndrome** (see Fig. 17.10). The

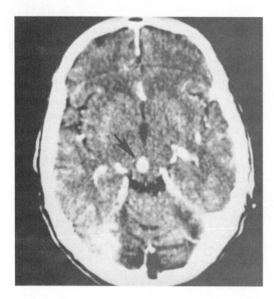

Figure 17.8. Computed tomographic scan in the patient whose appearance is seen in Figure 17.7. Note the enhancing lesion in the dorsal mesencephalon (*arrow*).

majority of mesencephalic syndromes are vascular in origin and are caused by occlusion or other injury to the vascular area of the basilar artery or perforating branches of the posterior cerebral artery; however, Claude's syndrome can result from thrombosis of the medial interpeduncular branch of the posterior cerebral artery.

Although divisional oculomotor nerve pareses are often caused by lesions in the cavernous sinus or posterior orbit (see below), anatomic separation into superior and inferior divisions begins in the brainstem. Thus, lesions of the oculomotor fascicles can cause isolated dysfunction of either the superior or inferior division of the oculomotor nerve. It is likely that fascicular lesions can also cause isolated weakness of only one of the muscles innervated by the oculomotor nerve.

As with nuclear oculomotor palsies, fascicular lesions may be ischemic, hemorrhagic, compressive, infiltrative, traumatic, or rarely, inflammatory. Because the fascicles are white matter tracts, demyelinating disease may also cause an oculomotor nerve paresis that may occur as an isolated phenomenon or associated with other neurologic manifestations. MRI is the optimum method of confirming the fascicular nature of an oculomotor nerve paresis.

Lesions of the Oculomotor Nerve in the Subarachnoid Space

Lesions that damage the oculomotor nerve in the interpeduncular fossa may be located anywhere from the emergence of the nerve at the ventral surface of the mesencephalon to the point at which the nerve penetrates the dura beside the posterior clinoid process to enter the cavernous sinus (Figs. 17.13 and 17.14). Interpeduncular damage to the oculomotor nerve may be partial or complete. In some cases, the palsy is initially incomplete but progresses over hours, days, weeks, or even months. In most cases, there is some degree of accommodative paresis, but pupillary involvement is variable and depends primarily on the nature of the lesion. Oculomotor nerve dysfunction that is produced by damage to its subarachnoid portion may occur as (1) isolated pupillary dilation with a reduced or absent light reaction, (2) ophthalmoplegia with pupillary involvement, or (3) ophthalmoplegia with normal pupillary size and reactivity.

Isolated Fixed, Dilated Pupil as the Sole Manifestation of Subarachnoid Oculomotor Nerve Palsy

Many different lesions that compress the oculomotor nerve from above and medially rarely may produce isolated pupillary dilation. Intracranial aneurysms, particularly those at the junction of the internal carotid artery and the posterior communication artery, are capable of producing a fixed dilated pupil in the early stages of oculomotor nerve involvement, but other signs of oculomotor nerve palsy usually develop within a few hours. Basilar artery aneurysms, however, can produce an isolated mid-dilated nonreactive or poorly reactive pupil that may be the only sign of an oculomotor nerve palsy for days or even weeks. Other extrinsic lesions in the interpeduncular cistern, such as cysts, can also produce this condition, as can intrinsic lesions of the oculomotor nerve, such as schwannomas or angiomas.

Basal meningitis, especially that caused by tuberculosis or syphilis, may damage the oculomotor nerve in the interpeduncular fossa and produce unilateral or bilateral internal ophthalmoplegia. Other infectious diseases associated with isolated internal ophthalmoplegia include leprosy, herpes zoster, chickenpox, smallpox, measles, diphtheria, scarlet fever, pertussis, and influenza; however, the lesion in such cases

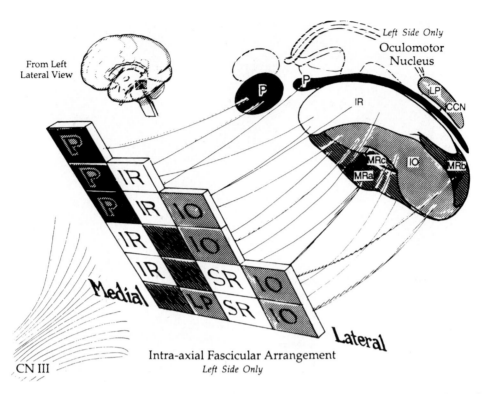

Figure 17.9. Proposed schematic arrangement of the fascicle of the oculomotor nerve (CN III) in a mediolateral and rostrocaudal plane. *IO,* inferior oblique; *IR,* inferior rectus; *LP,* levator palpebrae superioris; *MR,* medial rectus (subnuclei a, b, and c); *P,* pupillary sphincter; *SR,* superior rectus; *CCN,* central caudal nucleus. (Reprinted with permission from Ksiazek SM, Slamovits TL, Rosen CE, et al. Fascicular arrangement in partial oculomotor paresis. Am J Ophthalmol 1994;118:97–103.)

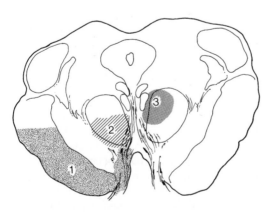

Figure 17.10. Diagram of a section through the mesencephalon showing regions in which the oculomotor nerve fascicle may be injured causing specific neurologic syndromes. *1.* Weber's syndrome. *2.* Benedikt's syndrome. *3.* Claude's syndrome.

more often involves the ciliary ganglion or the postganglionic fibers of the parasympathetic pathway to the eye and not the oculomotor nerve in the subarachnoid space.

Notwithstanding the case reports cited above, truly isolated pupillary dilation from involvement of the interpeduncular portion of the oculomotor nerve is *exceptionally rare.* The occurrence of a widely dilated, nonreactive pupil in an otherwise healthy patient, even a patient complaining of headache, is far more likely to be caused by either ciliary ganglion involvement (i.e., a tonic pupil) or direct pharmacologic blockade, both of which can be diagnosed easily by pharmacologic testing (see Chapter 15).

Subarachnoid Oculomotor Nerve Palsy with Pupillary Involvement

Lesions of the oculomotor nerve at its emergence from the brainstem may damage some of

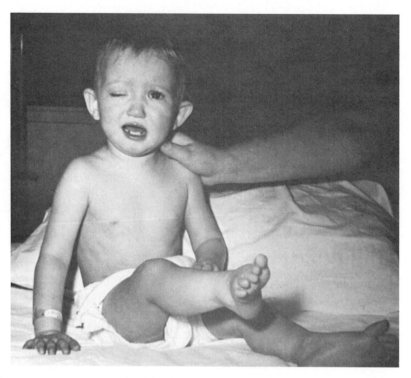

Figure 17.11. Weber's syndrome produced by a brainstem glioma infiltrating the mesencephalon. Note the oculomotor nerve palsy on the right, and the hemiplegia on the left.

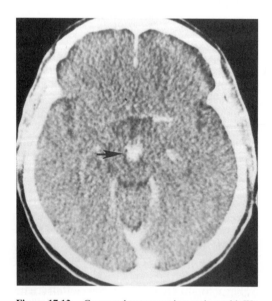

Figure 17.12. Computed tomogram in a patient with Weber's syndrome showing an enhancing lesion in the ventral mesencephalon (*arrow*). The lesion was thought to be a solitary metastasis from a breast carcinoma.

its rootlets, producing an isolated oculomotor nerve paresis. Most extrinsic lesions that damage the oculomotor nerve adjacent to the brainstem, however, produce a Weber's syndrome by compressing, infarcting, inflaming, or infiltrating the cerebral peduncle.

Intracranial aneurysms are the most common cause of isolated oculomotor nerve palsy with pupillary involvement, particularly (but not exclusively) when the patient has a history of sudden severe pain in or around the eye (Figs. 17.15 through 17.17). The aneurysms usually arise from the junction of the internal carotid and posterior communicating arteries; however, aneurysms located at the top of the basilar artery and aneurysms located at the junction of the basilar artery and superior cerebellar artery may produce a similar clinical picture. Such aneurysms may injure the oculomotor nerve by direct compression, from a small hemorrhage, or at the time of a major rupture.

One of the earliest signs of an oculomotor nerve palsy in a patient with a ruptured or expanding internal carotid-posterior communicat-

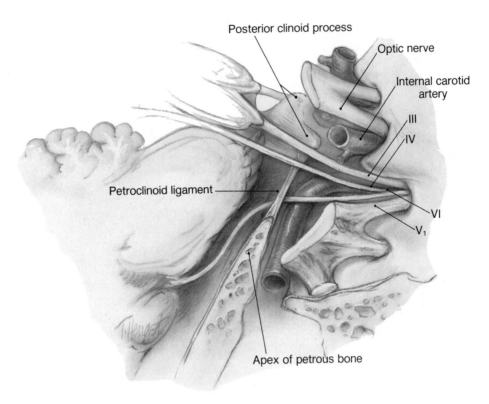

Figure 17.13.   Dissection to illustrate the subarachnoid and intracavernous courses of the ocular motor nerves. Note the long subarachnoid course of the trochlear nerve *(IV)* as it proceeds around the brainstem compared with the shorter courses of the oculomotor *(III)* and abducens *(VI)* nerves. Note also that the abducens nerve penetrates the dura at the base of the skull inferior to the points at which the oculomotor and trochlear nerves penetrate the dura. V_1, ophthalmic nerve.

ing artery aneurysm is a mild ptosis that may progress to a complete oculomotor nerve palsy within hours to a few days. However, ptosis may also be an early sign of an oculomotor nerve paresis caused by ischemia. The average interval from onset to development of maximum ophthalmoplegia can not be used to differentiate a microvascular etiology from a posterior communicating artery aneurysm.

Trauma to the oculomotor nerve during aneurysm surgery may produce a permanent or transient palsy. The trauma may be caused by direct manipulation of the nerve during surgery or by compression from the clip used to occlude the neck of the aneurysm.

A painful oculomotor nerve palsy with pupillary involvement may result from a posteriorly draining, low-flow carotid-cavernous sinus fistula. The fistula usually is of the spontaneous dural type, and the patient may be thought to have an aneurysm until angiography reveals the true etiology. The paresis may be complete or incomplete and may involve the pupil or be pupil-sparing. Some patients experience spontaneous resolution of the oculomotor nerve paresis weeks to months after onset of symptoms. Others may require treatment with hemostatic agents, embolization, or both.

Tumors and other compressive lesions, such as ectatic posterior cerebral or basilar artery vessels, can occasionally stretch or compress the oculomotor nerve in the interpeduncular fossa. In some instances, the patient has no complaint until minor trauma produces enough damage in an already compromised nerve to result in sudden dysfunction of the nerve with ophthalmoparesis, ptosis, and mydriasis. Intrinsic lesions of the oculomotor nerve, such as schwannomas or cavernous angiomas, can also produce an acute or progressive oculomotor nerve paresis (Fig. 17.18).

When paralysis of the oculomotor nerve oc-

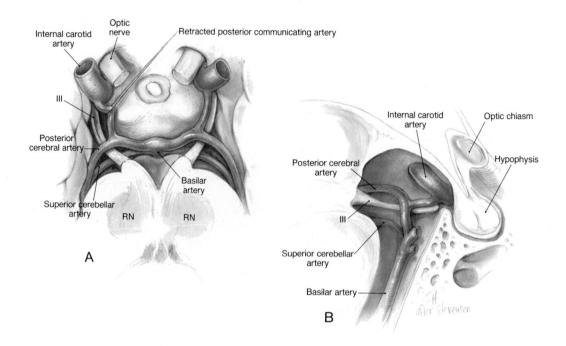

Figure 17.14.   The relationship of the oculomotor nerve to the intracranial arteries in the subarachnoid space. *A.* The oculomotor nerves (III) are viewed from above. On the left, the posterior communicating artery has been retracted to show the groove that it may produce through its contact with the oculomotor nerve. *RN,* red nucleus. *B.* Lateral view of the left oculomotor nerve (III) showing its arterial relationships.

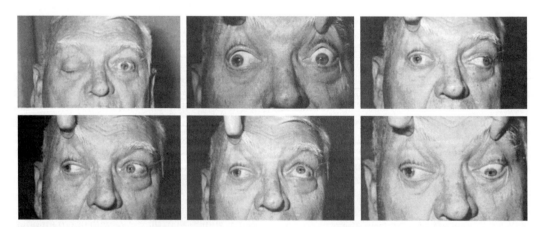

Figure 17.15.   Complete right oculomotor nerve palsy with involvement of the pupil. The patient also complained of severe right-sided retro-orbital pain.

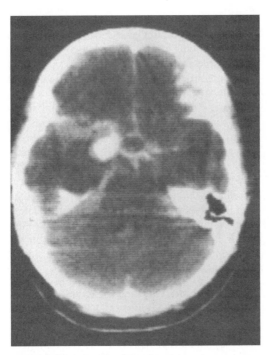

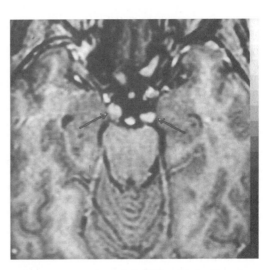

Figure 17.18.   T1-weighted magnetic resonance image (axial view) in a 31-year-old-woman with progressive bilateral pupillary-involved oculomotor pareses and neurofibromatosis. There are bilateral enhancing lesions in the interpeduncular cistern (*arrows*) consistent with schwannomas of the oculomotor nerves.

Figure 17.16.   Computed tomographic (CT) scan shows a large aneurysm at the junction of the right internal carotid and right posterior communicating arteries in the patient whose appearance is shown in Figure 17.15.

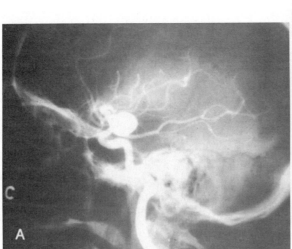

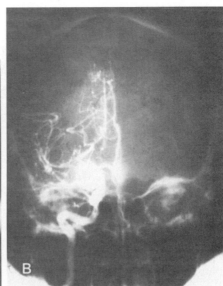

Figure 17.17.   Selective right internal carotid arteriogram showing large aneurysm at the junction of the right internal carotid and right posterior communicating arteries in the patient whose appearance is shown in Figure 17.15. *A.* Lateral view. *B.* Anteroposterior view.

curs in the setting of basilar meningitis, it is often bilateral and usually associated with other cranial nerve palsies. Nevertheless, meningitis, whether infectious, inflammatory, or neoplastic, occasionally produces isolated oculomotor nerve palsies, both with and without pupillary involvement. Various forms of the Guillain-Barré syndrome include oculomotor nerve involvement.

Vascular diseases, particularly diabetes mellitus, often produce an oculomotor nerve palsy that spares the pupil. Nevertheless, the pupil is involved in many cases. We believe that most cases of isolated, vasculopathic oculomotor nerve palsy with pupillary involvement are caused by lesions of the subarachnoid portion of the nerve.

Severe cranial trauma may produce oculomotor nerve palsy, both in isolation and in association with other cranial nerve palsies. Isolated involvement of the oculomotor nerve is usually caused by a frontal blow to a forward-moving head and, in most patients, is associated with skull fracture and concussion. Stretching, contusion, and avulsion are probably the major causes of the tissue damage.

An oculomotor nerve paresis can occur in rare patients with pseudotumor cerebri. The mechanism may be a direct effect of raised intracranial pressure (ICP) on the subarachnoid portion of the oculomotor nerve, the same mechanism that is believed to produce abducens nerve palsies in similar patients. A similar mechanism may be responsible for the development of an isolated oculomotor nerve palsy in patients with bilateral chronic subdural hematomas.

Because of the other important neural structures near the oculomotor nerve in the brainstem, cavernous sinus, and orbit, it is the subarachnoid space where a lesion of the oculomotor nerve is most likely to produce an oculomotor nerve palsy without other neurologic signs. Thus, it is possible that the oculomotor nerve palsies with pupillary involvement that occur in association with various viral syndromes, following immunization, and as part of a migraine syndrome are caused by lesions of the subarachnoid portion of the oculomotor nerve.

Subarachnoid Oculomotor Nerve Palsy with Pupillary Sparing

Ischemia is the most frequent cause of pupil-sparing oculomotor nerve palsies, particularly those that are unassociated with any other neurologic signs or symptoms (Fig. 17.19). In most instances, the patient has diabetes mellitus, but systemic hypertension, atherosclerosis, and migraine can all produce a similar clinical picture. Systemic lupus erythematosus may also produce a pupil-sparing oculomotor nerve paresis, and

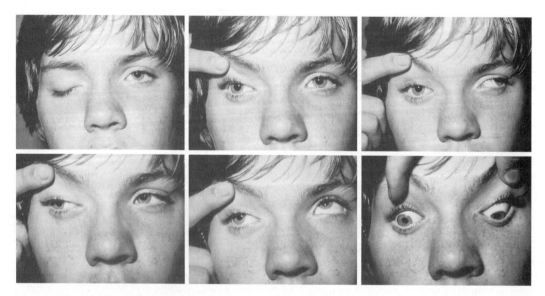

Figure 17.19.   Pupil-sparing oculomotor nerve palsy in a patient with diabetes mellitus.

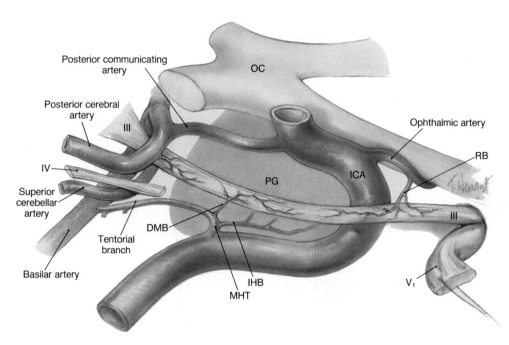

Figure 17.20. Vascular supply of the subarachnoid and intracavernous portions of the oculomotor nerve. In the subarachnoid space, the oculomotor nerve (III) receives vascular twigs from the posterior cerebral and superior cerebellar arteries, as well as from tentorial and dorsal meningeal branches (DMB) of the meningohypophyseal trunk (MHT) of the internal carotid artery (ICA). In the cavernous sinus, the nerve receives twigs from the tentorial, dorsal meningeal, and inferior hypophyseal branches (IHB) of the meningohypophyseal trunk and also from recurrent collateral branches (RB) of the ophthalmic artery. *IV*, trochlear nerve; V_1, ophthalmic division of the trigeminal nerve; *OC*, optic chiasm; *PG*, pituitary gland. (Redrawn from Nadeau SE, Trobe JD. Pupil sparing in oculomotor palsy: a brief review. Ann Neurol 1983;13:143–148.)

such a palsy may be the presenting sign of giant cell (temporal) arteritis. In cases of ischemic oculomotor nerve palsy, the lesion is most often located in the oculomotor nerve fascicle, where the pupillary efferent fibers are anatomically separate from the fibers to the extraocular muscles, or in the subarachnoid portion of the nerve, where the pupillary fibers occupy a peripheral location and receive more collateral blood supply than the main trunk of the nerve (Fig. 17.20). However, the intracavernous portion of the oculomotor nerve may be affected in some cases of diabetic and other ischemic oculomotor nerve pareses.

Patients with oculomotor nerve pareses caused by ischemia often have severe pain regardless of whether or not the pupil is involved. The pain may be so severe that it is difficult to distinguish from the pain caused by a ruptured or expanding aneurysm. Ischemic oculomotor nerve palsies characteristically resolve within 4 to 16 weeks without treatment. The resolution is almost always complete, and there is almost never evidence of aberrant regeneration (Fig. 17.21).

Although most pupil-sparing oculomotor nerve palsies (with or without associated pain) are caused by ischemia, such palsies may also be produced by subarachnoid compressive lesions, particularly aneurysms, but also ipsilateral temporal lobe astrocytomas and ipsilateral acute subdural hematomas. Such palsies are nearly always **incomplete** and are often accompanied by ocular or orbital pain. Patients with a painful, incomplete, pupil-sparing oculomotor nerve paresis should undergo MRI as well as either computed tomographic angiography (CTA) or MR angiography (MRA). Depending on the results of these studies, conventional angiography may be appropriate.

Both ischemic and compressive (especially aneurysmal) oculomotor nerve palsies may be associated with pain in and around the involved

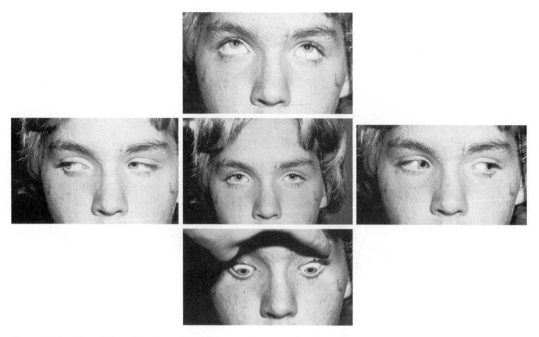

Figure 17.21. Resolution of pupil-sparing oculomotor nerve palsy in the patient seen in Figure 17.19. Improvement began to occur about 3 weeks following onset of the palsy.

eye. The explanation for this phenomenon is that sensory fibers from the ophthalmic division of the trigeminal nerve join the oculomotor nerve within the lateral wall of the cavernous sinus and run proximally along the nerve bundles to enter the brainstem. Although patients with aneurysms typically experience a more posterior, diffusely radiating headache than do patients with ischemia, it may be difficult to differentiate between ischemic and compressive involvement on the basis of the type of pain.

Other disorders that may be associated with isolated, pupil-sparing, oculomotor nerve palsies include viral inflammations, monoclonal gammopathy, various types of systemic lymphoma, and meningeal infiltration from chronic lymphocytic leukemia.

Subarachnoid Oculomotor Nerve Palsy from Involvement at or near Its Entrance to the Cavernous Sinus

The oculomotor nerve is particularly vulnerable to stretch and contusion injuries where it is firmly attached to the dura adjacent to the posterior clinoid process just posterior to the cavern-

ous sinus (Fig. 17.22). Frontal head trauma and aneurysms are common causes of injury at this site, as is surgery in the parasellar region.

Herniation of the hippocampal gyrus compresses the oculomotor nerve where it passes over the ridge of the dura associated with the attachment of the free edge of the tentorium to the clivus. As the herniating hippocampal gyrus descends into the tentorial incisura, it presses upon the upper surface of the ipsilateral oculomotor nerve that is running beneath it. As the supratentorial pressure increases and the uncal herniation pushes the mesencephalon laterally, the compressed oculomotor nerve is pulled more firmly into contact with the posterior clinoid process. Indeed, the oculomotor nerve may be deeply grooved where it is compressed upon the tentorial shelf between the free and the attached borders of the tentorium. The herniating cerebral mass ultimately reaches and impinges on the dorsal surface of the pons on the same side. Two factors that further embarrass conduction in the nerve are produced by this movement. First, each oculomotor nerve is stretched because its origin in the interpeduncular space is carried caudally by the herniating mesencephalon. Second, the basilar artery, which is tethered to the surface of the pons by numerous, short, pontine branches, moves downward with the herniating brainstem. The posterior cerebral arteries are therefore also drawn tightly down across the dorsal surface of the oculomotor nerves, producing even more compression (see Figs. 17.14 and 17.20).

Pupillary dilation is often the first sign of increasing cerebral edema or of an ipsilateral, expanding, supratentorial mass, such as an epidural, subdural, or intracerebral hematoma. This initial pupillary sign is caused by pressure on the peripheral portion of the nerve. The mydriasis is initially reversible but becomes irreversible with continued or repeated compression. In this setting, the direction of pressure is more significant than the degree of pressure. Mild compression

of the nerve against medial structures near its point of exit from the subarachnoid space almost always produces mydriasis, but the same amount of pressure applied directly to the nerve is much less likely to do so. In addition, neither direct compression of the cerebral hemisphere nor direct compression of the dorsal mesencephalon produces the unilateral pupillary dilation so characteristic of uncal herniation.

Initial evidence of transtentorial herniation with compression of the oculomotor nerve is pupillary dilation associated with a sluggish pupillary reaction to light. It is most likely that this effect is caused by pressure of the posterior cerebral artery on the superior surface of the oculomotor nerve where the pupillary fibers are concentrated. With increasing compression, additional signs of impaired oculomotor nerve function appear. The sequence of extraocular

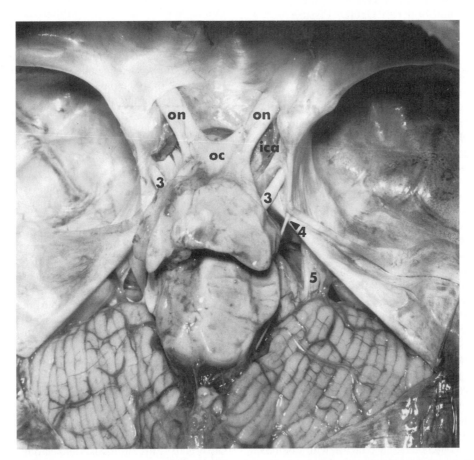

Figure 17.22. Base of the brain, showing position of the oculomotor (*3*) and trochlear (*4*) nerves as they penetrate the dura to enter the cavernous sinus. *5*, trigeminal nerve; *ica*, internal carotid artery; *oc*, optic chiasm; *on*, optic nerve.

muscle involvement is not consistent, but ptosis and medial rectus muscle weakness are usually the most apparent and easily demonstrable signs in the obtunded or semicomatose patient. Variations of this phenomena include subdural hematoma with contralateral pupillary dilation, ipsilateral complete oculomotor nerve palsy with pupillary involvement, and pupil-sparing oculomotor nerve palsy.

Recovery of oculomotor nerve function after herniation proceeds in the reverse order of the involvement. Thus, following improvement in eye movement and resolution of ptosis, the pupil may remain slightly dilated and sluggishly reactive to light for several days. Pupillary function is the least likely of all functions to return to normal.

Lesions of the Oculomotor Nerve within the Cavernous Sinus and Superior Orbital Fissure

Lesions within the cavernous sinus or superior orbital fissure may produce isolated oculomotor nerve dysfunction but more often cause a cranial polyneuropathy. When such a polyneuropathy is identified, the correct topical diagnosis can be made with relative ease.

Because the cavernous sinus contains structures that continue through the superior orbital fissure, it is often impossible to determine with certainty if the lesion is confined to the sinus, is in the fissure, or involves both structures. It is reasonable to consider damage in this region as a single entity, the **sphenocavernous syndrome.** This syndrome is characterized by paralysis or paresis of the oculomotor, trochlear, and abducens nerves, usually associated with involvement of the ophthalmic division (and in the cavernous sinus, the maxillary division) of the trigeminal nerve (Figs. 17.23 through 17.26). Involvement of the optic nerve either within the orbit or intracranially often causes visual loss. Because of the frequent involvement of the trigeminal nerve by lesions of the cavernous sinus and superior orbital fissure, patients with such lesions often complain of severe pain when they develop ophthalmoplegia. In many cases, there is oculosympathetic paresis, and there may be proptosis, edema of the eyelids, and chemosis of the conjunctiva. In patients with combined oculomotor paresis and sympathetic denervation, the pupil may be small or midposition and

poorly reactive. This appearance is almost pathognomonic of a cavernous sinus lesion.

The sphenocavernous syndrome may be produced by primary or secondary lesions within the cavernous sinus or superior orbital fissure or by lesions within the orbit or intracranial cavity that compress the cranial nerves that pass through these structures. Common lesions capable of producing the sphenocavernous syndrome include aneurysms, meningiomas, pituitary tumors, craniopharyngiomas, nasopharyngeal tumors, metastatic tumors, lymphoma, and infectious and inflammatory processes. Less common lesions include vascular malformations of the cavernous sinus, schwannomas, rhabdomyosarcoma, and multiple myeloma with and without deposition of amyloid.

Idiopathic granulomatous inflammation may produce a painful ophthalmoplegia from involvement of the cranial nerves within the cavernous sinus and superior orbital fissure: the **Tolosa-Hunt syndrome.** Patients with this syndrome typically improve rapidly and dramatically when treated with systemic corticosteroids; however, both spontaneous and steroid-induced remissions of symptoms and signs, sometimes of prolonged duration, occur in cases of painful ophthalmoplegia caused by tumors and aneurysms. Thus, because of the similarity of the symptoms, signs, and response to therapy of both inflammatory and noninflammatory lesions of the cavernous sinus (including ischemic lesions), patients with the syndrome of painful ophthalmoplegia require a complete assessment, including neuroimaging, a systemic evaluation for an underlying vascular or inflammatory disorder, and, in most cases, a lumbar puncture (Fig. 17.27). Although MRI is extremely useful in detecting a lesion of the cavernous sinus in a patient with painful ophthalmoplegia, the signal intensity within the cavernous sinus of patients with Tolosa-Hunt syndrome is similar to that of meningioma, lymphoma, metastatic tumor, and sarcoidosis. In addition, some cases of otherwise typical Tolosa-Hunt syndrome are characterized by sellar erosion, thus mimicking lesions with more destructive potential.

Vascular processes can produce a painful ophthalmoplegia from damage to structures in the cavernous sinus and superior orbital fissure. Cavernous sinus thrombosis and carotid-cavernous sinus fistulas can produce typical cavernous sinus syndromes, and painful ophthalmoplegia

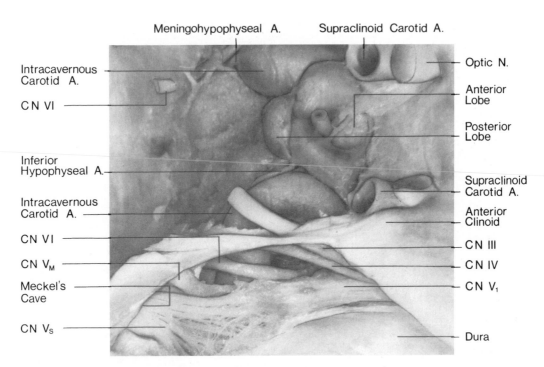

Figure 17.23. Superior lateral view of the right cavernous sinus, the anterior and posterior lobes of the pituitary gland, and the intracavernous structures including the internal carotid artery and the oculomotor (CN III), trochlear (CN IV), and abducens (CN VI) nerves. *CN Vm,* motor root of the trigeminal nerve; *CN Vs,* sensory root of the trigeminal nerve; *CN V₁,* ophthalmic division of the trigeminal nerve. (Reprinted with permission from Harris FS, Rhoton AL Jr. Anatomy of the cavernous sinus: a microsurgical study. J Neurosurg 1976;45:169–180.)

also occurs in patients with syphilis, giant cell (temporal) arteritis, diabetes mellitus, rheumatoid arthritis, and systemic lupus erythematosus.

The same lesions that produce the cavernous sinus syndrome may also cause **isolated oculomotor nerve dysfunction,** with and without pupillary involvement. In particular, extrinsic lesions, including pituitary adenomas, craniopharyngiomas, suprasellar aneurysms, and suprasellar meningiomas can cause isolated oculomotor nerve dysfunction. Lesions that infiltrate the cavernous sinus, such as multiple myeloma, metastatic carcinoma, and nasopharyngeal carcinoma may also produce an oculomotor nerve palsy, which may be the **initial sign** of the disease.

The ischemia that produces oculomotor nerve dysfunction in patients with diabetes mellitus is, at least in some instances, caused by a lesion in the intracavernous portion of the nerve. Similar lesions may be responsible for the isolated oculomotor nerve palsies that develop in patients with systemic hypertension, ophthalmoplegic migraine, herpes zoster ophthalmicus, and giant cell arteritis.

Trauma to the cavernous sinus and superior orbital fissure may produce an isolated oculomotor nerve palsy. Such palsies are usually associated with skull fracture and are caused by intraneural and perineural hemorrhage in the cavernous sinus or superior orbital fissure. Iatrogenic trauma to the cavernous sinus, such as that which may occur during endovascular treatment of an intracavernous aneurysm or a carotid-cavernous sinus fistula can also produce an isolated oculomotor nerve palsy.

In patients with compressive neuropathies caused by lesions within the cavernous sinus, neuroimaging studies usually establish the site of the lesion. In other instances, the development of an oculomotor nerve paresis that involves either the superior or inferior division of the oculomotor nerve may suggest a sphenocavernous (or an orbital) lesion. The importance of re-

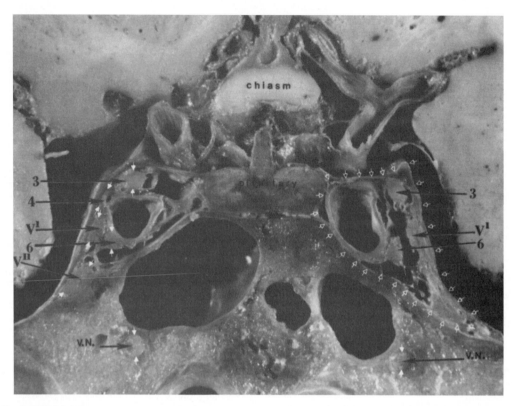

Figure 17.24. Transverse section through the optic chiasm, pituitary gland, and cavernous sinuses, showing the location of the ocular motor nerves. White hollow arrows (right side of photograph) indicate the boundaries of the cavernous sinus. White solid arrows (left side of photograph) outline boundaries of nerves. *3,* oculomotor nerve; *4,* trochlear nerve; *V^I,* ophthalmic division of the trigeminal nerve; *V^II,* mandibular division of the trigeminal nerve; *6,* abducens nerve; *VN,* vidian nerve. (Courtesy of Dr. William F. Hoyt.)

peated neuroimaging studies in patients presumed to have an intracavernous sinus oculomotor paresis that progresses despite normal initial neuroimaging cannot be overemphasized.

Lesions of the Oculomotor Nerve within the Orbit

The sphenocavernous syndrome is characterized by a painful ophthalmoplegia and is generally unassociated with visual loss from an optic neuropathy. Conversely, lesions in the apex of the orbit produce ophthalmoplegia that may or may not be painful but that are usually associated with loss of vision from optic neuropathy and variable proptosis. The distinction between these two entities—the sphenocavernous syndrome and the orbital apex syndrome—can thus often be made both on clinical grounds and by neuroimaging; however, it must be remembered

that many lesions extend from the cavernous sinus into the orbital apex and vice versa, so a clear separation of syndromes may be impossible. In addition, large intracranial mass lesions occasionally expand to such a degree that they compress the intracranial optic nerve and the subarachnoid or cavernous sinus portion of the oculomotor nerves and also prevent adequate venous drainage from the orbit, resulting in a ''pseudo-orbital apex syndrome.''

The oculomotor nerve enters the orbit as two separate divisions: the superior division, which innervates the levator palpebrae superioris and the superior rectus muscle; and the inferior division, which innervates the medial and inferior rectus muscle, the inferior oblique muscle, and the motor root of the ciliary ganglion. Thus, an incomplete oculomotor nerve paresis in the distribution of either division is often caused by a

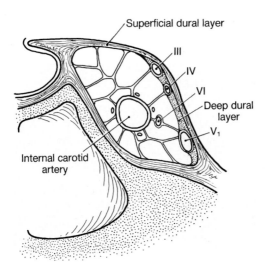

Figure 17.25.   Diagram of the cavernous sinus showing the location of the ocular motor nerves. Note that the lateral wall is composed of two layers: a superficial layer and a deep layer. The deep layer is formed by the sheaths of the oculomotor (III), trochlear (IV), and ophthalmic (V_1) nerves, with a reticular membrane between these sheaths. *VI*, abducens nerve. (Redrawn from Umansky F, Nathan H. The lateral wall of the cavernous sinus: with special reference to the nerves related to it. J Neurosurg 1982;56:228–234.)

lesion of either the sphenocavernous region or the orbital apex. However, as noted above, the oculomotor nerve has a divisional topographic arrangement beginning in the brainstem. Thus, divisional oculomotor nerve pareses may result from lesions not only in the cavernous sinus and orbital apex but also from lesions in the brainstem or subarachnoid space (Fig. 17.28). It is often impossible to determine if such a paresis is caused by a lesion within the orbit or the cavernous sinus unless there are other clinical signs of cavernous sinus or orbital disease, or unless neuroimaging studies are performed.

Processes within the orbit that can produce an oculomotor nerve palsy include inflammation, ischemia, infiltration, and compression. Trauma can also produce such a palsy. Oculomotor nerve palsies produced by orbital lesions may be complete or incomplete and usually involve the pupil. Other signs of orbital disease, including loss of vision, proptosis, and other ocular motor nerve pareses, are often but not invariably present.

Lesions of the Oculomotor Nerve of Uncertain or Variable Location

In many instances of isolated, oculomotor nerve palsy in both adults and children, the site of the lesion is unclear. In some cases, this is because the underlying condition can affect the nerve at many potential sites. For example, pa-

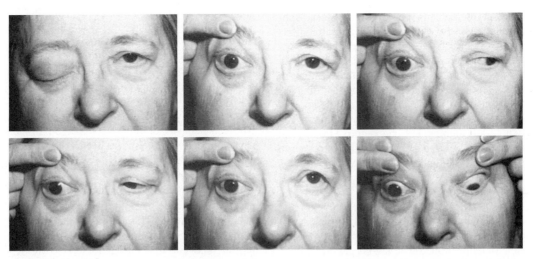

Figure 17.26.   Patient with cavernous sinus syndrome from basal meningioma. The patient has right proptosis associated with a complete right oculomotor nerve palsy, a right abducens nerve paresis, and a right Horner's syndrome. Note that the right pupil is slightly smaller than the left pupil.

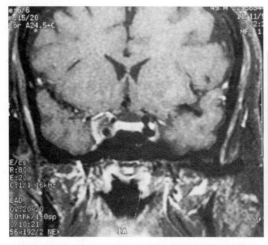

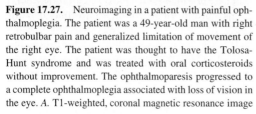

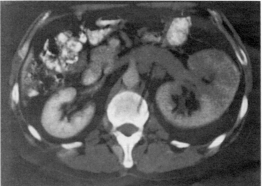

Figure 17.27. Neuroimaging in a patient with painful ophthalmoplegia. The patient was a 49-year-old man with right retrobulbar pain and generalized limitation of movement of the right eye. The patient was thought to have the Tolosa-Hunt syndrome and was treated with oral corticosteroids without improvement. The ophthalmoparesis progressed to a complete ophthalmoplegia associated with loss of vision in the eye. *A.* T1-weighted, coronal magnetic resonance image (MRI) after intravenous injection of paramagnetic contrast material reveals enlargement of the right cavernous sinus. *B.* CT scan of the abdomen reveals a left renal mass. The patient was found to have a metastatic renal cell carcinoma. (Reprinted with permission from Mehelas TJ, Kosmorsky GS. Painful ophthalmoplegia syndrome secondary to metastatic renal cell carcinoma. J Neuroophthalmol 1996;16: 289–290.)

tients with oculomotor nerve pareses in the setting of diabetes mellitus may have ischemic lesions involving the oculomotor nerve fascicle in the brainstem or the subarachnoid or cavernous sinus portions of the nerve. Similarly, the locations of the lesions in patients with systemic hypertension, carotid artery stenosis, systemic lupus erythematosus, periarteritis nodosa, ophthalmoplegic migraine, allergic granulomatous angiitis (Churg-Strauss syndrome), herpes zoster ophthalmicus, and giant cell arteritis may vary considerably. In other instances, there are no specific localizing signs, and no pathology is available. For example, transient, isolated oculomotor nerve palsies occasionally occur in patients with mumps and chickenpox. Finally, in some cases, the site of the oculomotor nerve palsy remains unknown despite extensive investigations. This is particularly true in cases of toxic ocular motor neuropathies.

The precise origin of isolated paresis of the inferior oblique muscle is unclear, but most cases are probably caused by lesions in the brainstem or in the orbit. Such patients generally have no other neurologic symptoms, and workups for other neurologic or myopathic disorders are invariably negative.

Recovery from Acquired Oculomotor Nerve Palsy

Oculomotor nerve paralysis, whether complete or incomplete, may have several outcomes. First, complete recovery may occur. In such cases, recovery may be complete within 1 to 2 weeks after the onset of symptoms. In other instances, notably those associated with diabetes mellitus, systemic hypertension, and ophthalmoplegic migraine, recovery does not begin for a month or more but is usually complete within 3 months. In still other cases, recovery can take much longer, sometimes as long as 3 years.

In some cases of oculomotor nerve palsy, the paralysis persists completely unchanged. In such cases, the nerve has usually been transected by trauma or chronic compression or has been infiltrated by tumor.

Finally, some patients with oculomotor nerve pareses experience partial recovery of oculomotor nerve function. This occurs especially after damage to the fascicular portion of the nerve. Partial recovery may be characterized by evidence of oculomotor nerve synkinesis (see below). In most cases, this synkinesis becomes apparent within 9 weeks after injury, but in other cases, there is no evidence of aberrant regeneration for as long as 3 to 6 months.

Acquired Oculomotor Synkinesis: Misdirection of Regenerating Fibers in the Oculomotor Nerve

Peripheral motor and sensory nerves, including the autonomic nerves, can regenerate. The regenerative process produces more axons than were present before the nerve was interrupted. Axons sprout from the proximal end of the severed nerve and from collateral nerves that have not been severely damaged. Cords of Schwann cells form in the peripheral segment of the nerve so that the new nerve fibers are conducted to the end organ. The newly formed neurons reach the empty tubes (Schwann's tubes) that contained functioning neurons before degeneration. Regenerating axons have the capacity to bridge long gaps in damaged nerves.

In peripheral nerves that innervate more than one muscle, misdirection of regenerating nerve fibers may occur. Thus, regenerating sprouts from axons that previously innervated one muscle group may ultimately innervate a different muscle group with a different function.

Following injury to the oculomotor nerve at any point along its pathway from the brainstem to the orbit, a syndrome of oculomotor nerve synkinesis may occur. In adults, evidence of synkinesis first appears about 9 weeks after injury, whereas in infants with oculomotor nerve palsy from birth trauma, such signs may be observed from 1 to 6 weeks following birth. Oculomotor nerve synkinesis is thought to occur from misdirection of regenerated axons in the nerve. Thus, the levator palpebrae superioris may receive fibers that were originally destined for the medial rectus muscle, or fibers originally intended for the superior rectus muscle may reach the inferior oblique, inferior rectus, or medial rectus muscles. The active elevation of the eyelid during

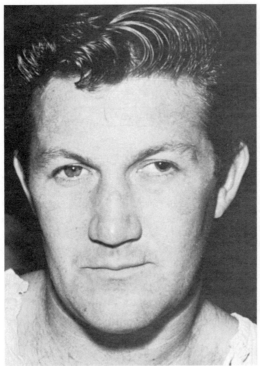

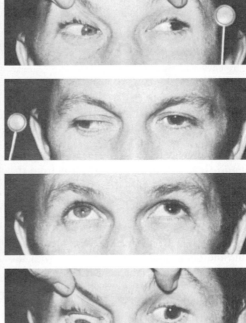

Figure 17.28. Paralysis of the inferior division of the left oculomotor nerve. Note that the left levator palpebrae superioris and the superior rectus muscle are not involved. This palsy occurred spontaneously and without pain. Neuroradio-logic investigations, including cerebral arteriography, were normal. The palsy cleared almost completely (the pupil remained slightly dilated) within 6 weeks. The etiology was never determined.

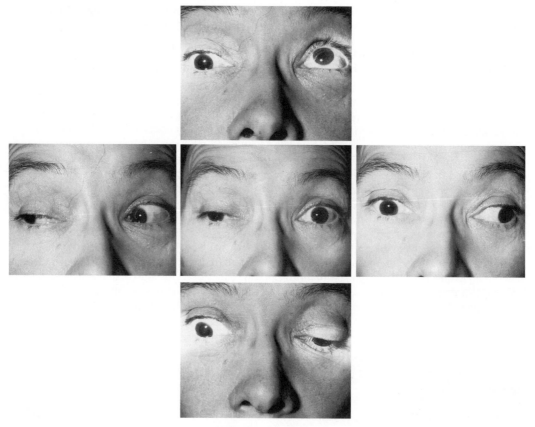

Figure 17.29.   Misdirected regeneration of the right oculomotor nerve following trauma (secondary aberrant regeneration). Note elevation of the right upper eyelid on attempted downward gaze and on attempted adduction of the right eye (pseudo-Graefe sign). Although the right pupil was markedly dilated and poorly reactive to light, it constricted slightly on attempted adduction of the eye.

attempted downward eye movement is called the **pseudo-Graefe sign** to distinguish it from the lid lag on downward gaze that occurs in patients with thyroid eye disease (Graefe's sign) (Fig. 17.29).

Fibers originally destined for any of the muscles innervated by the oculomotor nerve may reach the ciliary ganglion to synapse with the postganglionic parasympathetic fibers that innervate the iris sphincter muscle, the ciliary body muscle, or both. Often, this anomalous reinnervation of the pupil is easily observed because the pupil constricts only when the patient is asked to look in a direction requiring oculomotor nerve function (Fig. 17.30). In other cases, the pupil may appear to be permanently paralyzed in the mid-dilated position, but slit lamp biomicroscopy will enable the examiner to observe subtle abnormalities of pupillary movement that reflect misregeneration of the iris sphincter (Fig. 17.31). In still other cases, particularly in patients with congenital oculomotor palsy with aberrant regeneration, the pupil may be quite miotic. Segmental contraction of the iris sphincter to light may be observed in patients with aberrant regeneration of the oculomotor nerve, as may sector contractions of the iris sphincter during eye movements and abnormal pupillary unrest in eyes with pupils having no reaction to light. Because such pupils have a poor reaction to a light stimulus but do constrict during adduction, their reactions simulate the light-near dissociation of the Argyll Robertson pupil and have been called pseudo–Argyll Robertson pupils.

The ciliary body is innervated by postganglionic parasympathetic axons whose cell bodies

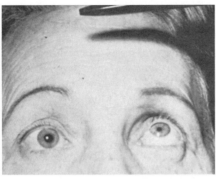

Figure 17.30.   Aberrant regeneration of the right oculomotor nerve with involvement of the pupil. *A.* During attempted elevation of the eyes, the right pupil remains mid-dilated. *B.* During depression of the eyes, the right pupil constricts.

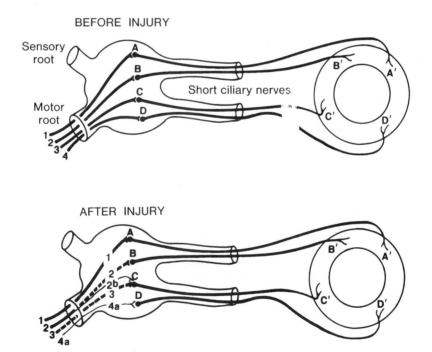

Figure 17.31.   Diagram of aberrant regeneration of the oculomotor nerve as it affects pupillary function. *Above:* Before injury, preganglionic fibers serving the pupillary light reaction synapse in the ciliary ganglion with axons that then proceed along short ciliary nerves to supply specific sectors of the iris sphincter. Thus preganglionic fiber *1* synapses with postganglionic fiber *A* to supply sector *A'* of the iris sphincter. *Below:* After injury to the preganglionic pathway, several phenomena may occur. A fiber may be undamaged (fiber *1*). A fiber may be completely destroyed and may never grow (fibers *3* and *4*), or it may be damaged, and regeneration may occur (fibers *2* and *2b*). In such a scenario, a collateral sprout could grow from a preganglionic fiber other than that originally intended for the iris sphincter. If fiber *4a* grew from a nerve originally destined for the inferior rectus muscle, then segment *D'* of the iris sphincter would constrict whenever the patient attempted to look downward. (Redrawn from Czarnecki JSC, Thompson HS. The iris sphincter in aberrant regeneration of the third nerve. Arch Ophthalmol 1978;96:1606–1610.)

are located in the ciliary body. Thus, patients with aberrant oculomotor regeneration develop aberrant reinnervation of the ciliary muscle. Such patients may become more myopic during attempted adduction and may develop increased intraocular pressure related to the direction of attempted gaze.

The signs of aberrant regeneration of the oculomotor nerve may be summarized as follows:

1. Horizontal gaze-eyelid synkinesis—elevation of the involved eyelid in attempted adduction of the eye.
2. Pseudo-Graefe sign—retraction and elevation of the eyelid on attempted downward gaze.
3. Limitation of elevation and depression of the eye with occasional retraction of the globe on attempted vertical movement.
4. Adduction of the involved eye on attempted elevation or depression.
5. Pseudo–Argyll Robertson pupil—the involved pupil does not react or reacts poorly and irregularly to light stimulation, but does constrict on adduction during conjugate gaze.
6. Monocular vertical optokinetic responses—the normal eye responds normally, but the involved eye has suppressed vertical responses.

The elevation of the eyelid that occurs in cases of oculomotor nerve misdirection may be more apparent during a combination of attempted downward gaze and adduction than on either movement alone.

The phenomenon of **secondary oculomotor nerve synkinesis** occurs in nearly all patients with congenital oculomotor nerve palsy; however, the majority of patients with this syndrome have experienced a primary, acute event that has produced a complete oculomotor nerve palsy. Secondary oculomotor nerve synkinesis occurs commonly following oculomotor nerve palsy from intracranial aneurysms, trauma (including surgical trauma), syphilis, and basal meningitis. As a general rule, synkinetic movements *do not occur* after ischemic insults to the nerve. Thus, in a patient suspected of having an ischemic oculomotor nerve palsy, particularly if there have been no previous episodes, the development of oculomotor synkinesis should suggest an alter-

native etiology, such as compression or inflammation.

Although the syndrome of acquired oculomotor nerve synkinesis occurs most frequently after acute oculomotor nerve palsy, it also occurs as a "primary" phenomenon; that is, without a preexisting acute oculomotor nerve paresis. Patients with **primary oculomotor nerve synkinesis** usually harbor slowly growing lesions of the cavernous sinus, usually meningiomas or aneurysms but also trigeminal schwannomas (Fig. 17.32). Slowly growing lesions in the subarachnoid space, including unruptured aneurysms, can also produce primary oculomotor nerve synkinesis. Lesions that cause primary aberrant regeneration grow so slowly that the mild oculomotor nerve damage that results does not produce major visual difficulties and, in addition, allows regeneration to occur.

EVALUATION AND MANAGEMENT OF PATIENTS WITH OCULOMOTOR NERVE PALSY

The evaluation of a patient with a congenital oculomotor nerve palsy is minimal. Generally, a careful systemic and neurologic assessment is all that is required. Such patients are at risk to develop amblyopia and must be managed with occlusion therapy. The decision to surgically correct ocular misalignment is based on the goals of the patient and the severity of the condition.

The evaluation of a patient with a congenital oculomotor nerve palsy depends on the associated symptoms and signs, the pattern of oculomotor nerve involvement, and the age of the patient. Acquired oculomotor nerve dysfunction may present in one of five ways:

1. *With a dilated, nonreactive or poorly reactive pupil without ophthalmoplegia or ptosis.* This presentation is **extremely rare** and usually occurs in the setting of a comatose or obtunded patient with an expanding supratentorial mass lesion. In the awake, alert patient with a widely dilated pupil, pharmacologic blockade or a tonic pupil are far more likely etiologies than compressive oculomotor nerve palsy. Nevertheless, it may be appropriate in some patients to obtain MRI, MRA, or CTA to determine if there is a basilar tip aneurysm or other mass lesion. Conven-

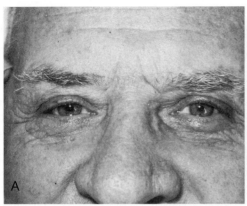
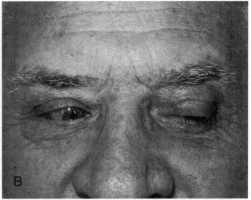

Figure 17.32.   Primary aberrant regeneration in a 63-year-old man. The patient had never had an acute oculomotor nerve palsy but had begun to notice intermittent diplopia. He was found to have a large right intracavernous trigeminal schwannoma. *A.* The patient has a small, intermittent exotropia caused by right medial rectus weakness. There is also slight anisocoria with a larger pupil on the right. *B.* On attempted gaze downward and to the left, the patient develops right upper eyelid retraction (pseudo-Graefe sign).

tional angiography is rarely indicated in such patients, unless noninvasive neuroimaging reveals abnormalities consistent with an aneurysm or other vascular lesion.

2. *With complete or incomplete ophthalmoparesis, ptosis, and a dilated, poorly reactive or nonreactive pupil.* This presentation may be produced by any pathologic process at any point along the pathway of the oculomotor nerve, but an intracranial aneurysm must be suspected and appropriate diagnostic studies immediately performed, particularly when this presentation is associated with orbital pain or headache. Tests include CT scanning without (looking for blood in the subarachnoid space) and with (looking for an intracranial aneurysm or other mass lesion) intravenous contrast, MRI, MRA, CTA, conventional angiography, or a combination of these techniques. None of these tests is 100% sensitive in detecting small intracranial aneurysms; however, both MRA and CTA, when performed correctly, can probably detect 95% of aneurysms 3 mm or greater in diameter. Nevertheless, conventional angiography remains the most sensitive test for detecting an intracranial aneurysm and should be performed in any patient in which this possibility is considered likely. Children

in the first decade of life are much less likely to harbor an intracranial aneurysm than are older children and adults. Nevertheless, oculomotor nerve palsies caused by aneurysms do occur in this age group. The decision to perform conventional angiography if noninvasive neuroimaging (e.g., MRI, MRA, CTA) reveals no abnormalities must be made on a case by case basis.

3. *With ophthalmoplegia and ptosis, but without any pupillary involvement.* Pupil-sparing oculomotor nerve palsies are most commonly caused by ischemia, but compression and inflammation may also produce them. Patients in this setting must be individualized; however, we believe that almost all cases of **complete but pupil-sparing** oculomotor nerve pareses are caused by ischemia and that patients with such pareses do not necessarily require neuroimaging. Conversely, patients with an **incomplete, pupil-sparing** oculomotor nerve paresis may require—in addition to measurement of systemic blood pressure, serum glucose, and sedimentation rate—noninvasive neuroimaging, such as standard MRI, MRA, CTA, or a combination of these studies, especially when pain accompanies the palsy. A lumbar puncture may also be appropriate in some of these patients. If these stud-

ies are negative, some patients may require arteriography to eliminate the possibility of an intracranial aneurysm. However, most older patients with incomplete, pupil-sparing oculomotor nerve pareses can be followed after a workup has been performed to determine if there is an underlying ischemic or inflammatory process (e.g., diabetes mellitus, giant cell arteritis, systemic hypertension). It must also be remembered that whenever the pupils are normal, an ophthalmoplegia may represent the effects of myopathic or neuromuscular disease (e.g., myasthenia gravis), rather than a neuropathy.

4. *With ophthalmoplegia, ptosis, and a small or midpositioned pupil.* Patients with this clinical picture usually have lesions in the cavernous sinus that have damaged not only the oculomotor nerve but also the oculosympathetic fibers.

5. *With misdirected (aberrant) regeneration.* Patients with **primary** aberrant regeneration have slowly growing mass lesions compressing or infiltrating the oculomotor nerve in the cavernous sinus or, less often, in the subarachnoid space.

Following diagnosis and treatment of the underlying disorder that has produced an oculomotor nerve palsy, one must wait to see if recovery will occur, and, if so, to what degree. Once it is clear that recovery of oculomotor nerve function will not be complete, the patient may have several choices.

In patients with partial recovery, various strabismus procedures may be of benefit in providing binocular single vision, at least in primary position, and ptosis surgery may also be used to improve the position of the affected eyelid. Botulinum toxin injections of the lateral rectus can realign the eyes for better fusion in patients with mild oculomotor nerve palsy who are awaiting improvement. Other patients seem content to simply patch the affected eye or are able to ignore the double image. An opaque contact lens provides a cosmetically acceptable means to alleviate subjective diplopia in these patients.

The management of patients with complete oculomotor nerve palsy is more difficult. Despite reports of cosmetic and functional success using surgical procedures that involve transposing or transplanting the superior oblique tendon, surgery rarely produces a satisfactory result from the standpoint of either the patient or the surgeon.

TROCHLEAR (FOURTH) NERVE PALSIES

Paralysis of the trochlear nerve is far less commonly recognized than paralysis of either the oculomotor or abducens nerves. However, trochlear nerve palsy is the most common cause of acquired vertical strabismus in the general population, other causes being ocular myopathies (e.g., dysthyroid eye disease), disorders of the neuromuscular junction (e.g., myasthenia gravis), incomplete oculomotor nerve paresis, and skew deviation. Trochlear nerve palsy causes partial or complete paralysis of the superior oblique muscle, usually associated over time with overaction of its antagonist, the ipsilateral inferior oblique muscle (Figs. 17.33 and 17.34). Patients with this disorder complain of vertical diplopia that is greatest in downgaze and to the opposite side. Such patients also have excyclotorsion when tested with double Maddox rods or Lancaster red-green glasses, particularly when the eye is in abduction, and this feature helps to distinguish trochlear nerve palsy from skew deviation, in which the higher eye is invariably intorted. The ability of the superior oblique muscle to intort the eye is particularly important when assessing superior oblique function in patients with an oculomotor nerve palsy. In such cases, the absence of intorsion when the patient attempts to depress the eye while it is abducted indicates lack of superior oblique function as well.

Most patients with trochlear nerve palsy have torticollis (Fig. 17.35). Such patients typically tilt the head to the side opposite the paralyzed superior oblique muscle. This spontaneous ocular torticollis is absent in patients with poor vision in either eye and in patients with large vertical fusional amplitudes that allow them to fuse in all positions of gaze. In addition, some patients with trochlear nerve palsy tilt their heads to the side of the palsy. This results in greater separation of images, thus allowing one of the images to be ignored.

CONGENITAL

Congenital trochlear nerve palsy is common. The etiology of congenital trochlear palsy is unknown; however, aplasia of the trochlear nerve

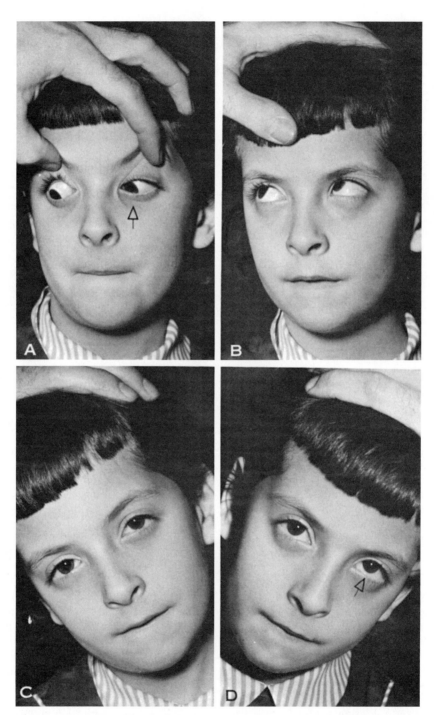

Figure 17.33. Left trochlear nerve palsy. *A.* Downward movement of the left eye (*arrow*) is limited in gaze down and right. *B.* Upward gaze to the right shows secondary overaction of the left inferior oblique muscle, the antagonist of the left superior oblique muscle. *C.* Head tilt to the right produces orthophoria and eliminates diplopia. *D.* Head tilt to the left results in upward deviation of the left eye (*arrow*). (Courtesy of Dr. R.D. Harley.)

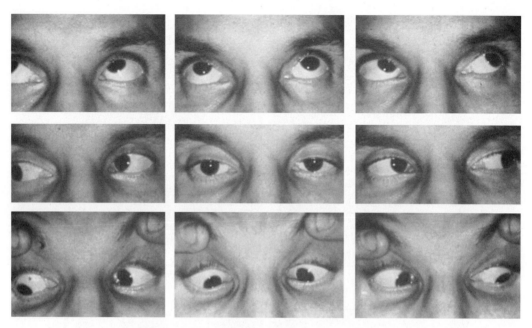

Figure 17.34. Bilateral trochlear nerve palsies in a 28-year-old man following a motorcycle accident. The patient suffered a severe blow to the vertex of his head. Note the patient's inability to depress either eye fully in adduction. There is bilateral overaction of both inferior oblique muscles. (Courtesy of Jacqueline Morris, C.O.)

nucleus appears to be responsible in some cases, and hypoplasia in others. Most congenital trochlear nerve palsies are sporadic; however, autosomal-dominant transmission occasionally occurs. Most patients with congenital trochlear nerve palsy are neurologically normal, but some patients have other neurologic deficits, including cerebral palsy, and many have some degree of facial asymmetry that may be obvious or subtle and easily overlooked.

Patients with congenital trochlear nerve palsy usually develop large vertical fusion amplitudes that, in association with a head tilt, allow them to compensate for their muscle weakness. Such patients may, however, develop diplopia from decompensation of the palsy after a minor head injury or without any antecedent event. When these patients are evaluated, a review of old photographs, such as a driver's license, often reveals a preexisting head tilt. In addition, direct measurement of vertical fusion amplitudes may also establish the diagnosis. Normal persons have a vertical fusion range of only 3 to 6 prism diopters, whereas patients with congenital superior oblique paresis may have 10 to 25 prism diopters of vertical fusion amplitude.

Congenital superior oblique palsy may be bilateral. In some instances, the patients appear to have a unilateral palsy until they undergo surgical correction, at which time the contralateral palsy becomes apparent. In most cases, however, careful measurements of both vertical and torsional deviation (including direct visualization of the ocular fundi to determine if torsion is present—see Chapter 16) permits differentiation between unilateral and bilateral palsies.

ACQUIRED

When an etiology can be determined, blunt head trauma, usually a direct orbital, frontal, basal, or oblique cranial blow, is the most common cause of isolated, acquired, unilateral and bilateral trochlear nerve palsy in both adults and children. As with other ocular motor nerve palsies, however, almost any pathologic process can damage the trochlear nerve at any point from its nucleus to its termination in the orbit where it innervates the superior oblique muscle.

Lesions of the Trochlear Nerve Nucleus

Lesions of the brainstem that damage the trochlear nerve nucleus cannot be localized with certainty on clinical grounds unless there are other neurologic signs suggesting intrinsic mesencephalic damage. Even when such signs are present, distinguishing nuclear from fascicular involvement is almost impossible. In addition, extrinsic lesions that compress the dorsal mesencephalon may damage the trochlear nerves as they emerge from the brainstem and at the same time produce damage to intrinsic brainstem structures. Cells of the trochlear nucleus are often damaged by lesions that involve the tegmentum at the junction of the pons and mesencephalon, particularly contusion and hemorrhage caused by impact against the tentorial margin. Other lesions that can produce intrinsic damage to the trochlear nerve nuclei include ischemia, primary and metastatic tumors, and vascular malformations (Figs. 17.35 and 17.36). Paresis of the superior oblique muscle with such lesions can, however, be obscured by associated conjugate or internuclear gaze defects. In such patients, the recognition of a trochlear nerve palsy becomes possible only after the supranuclear difficulties resolve.

Both unilateral and bilateral superior oblique paresis can be associated with Parinaud's dorsal midbrain syndrome from pineal tumors, aqueductal stenosis, and hydrocephalus; vertical diplopia in this setting is far more commonly caused by trochlear nerve dysfunction than previously recognized. Trochlear nerve palsy also can follow neurosurgical procedures in the posterior fossa. Although the oculomotor and trochlear motor nuclei can be slightly affected in ALS

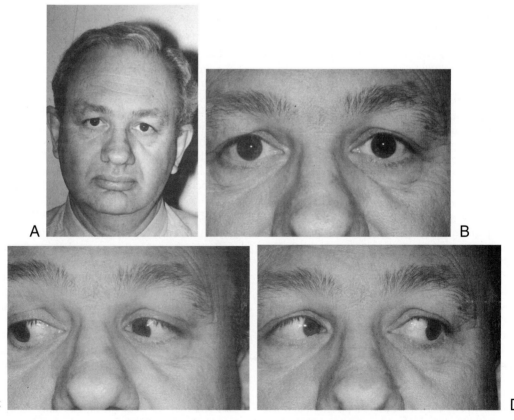

Figure 17.35.   Appearance of a 53-year-old man with an acute right trochlear nerve palsy. *A.* The patient has a moderate head tilt toward the left shoulder. *B.* In primary position, there is a small right hypertropia. *C.* On gaze right and down, both eyes move normally. *D.* On gaze left and down, there is underaction of the right superior oblique muscle, with an increased right hypertropia. (Courtesy of Dr. Steven R. Hamilton.)

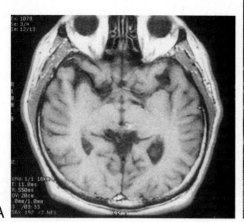
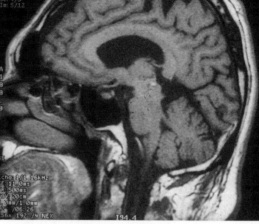

A   B

Figure 17.36. MRI performed on the patient whose appearance is shown in Figure 17.35. The study was performed when the patient did not recover in several months. T1-weighted axial (*A*) and sagittal (*B*) images show a small vascular malformation in the region of the left trochlear nucleus.

in a manner similar to that of the anterior horns, the degree of damage in most cases is less than that which would be expected to produce a significant ophthalmoplegia.

Lesions of the Trochlear Nerve Fascicle

Fascicular involvement of the trochlear nerves can be caused by the same processes that cause damage to the trochlear nuclei. These processes include compression, infiltration, ischemia, hemorrhage, trauma, and inflammation, particularly multiple sclerosis.

Because of the dorsal location of the trochlear fascicles, associated neurologic signs are of less help in the topographic diagnosis of such lesions than are neuroimaging studies. Nevertheless, two important associated signs that suggest that the site of a trochlear nerve paresis is the trochlear nucleus or fascicle are a central Horner's syndrome and a relative afferent pupillary defect (RAPD) unassociated with evidence of an optic neuropathy or optic tract syndrome.

The Horner's syndrome is caused by damage to descending sympathetic fibers in the dorsal brainstem, which are usually adjacent to the trochlear nerve nucleus. Thus, the Horner's syndrome is usually on the side opposite the trochlear nerve paresis (because the trochlear nerves are crossed). The only exception is if the lesion affects the postdecussation portion of the trochlear nerve fascicle, in which case both the trochlear nerve paresis and the Horner's syndrome are on the same side.

The RAPD is caused by damage to afferent pupillary fibers in the brachium of the superior colliculus (see Chapter 15). If the trochlear nerve paresis is caused by a lesion of the predecussation portion of the fascicle (or the trochlear nerve nucleus), the RAPD is on the same side as the trochlear nerve paresis, whereas if the paresis is caused by damage to the postdecussation portion of the fascicle, the RAPD is on the side opposite the trochlear nerve paresis (Fig. 17.37).

Lesions of the Trochlear Nerve in the Subarachnoid Space

The trochlear nerve is particularly susceptible to injury or compression as it emerges from the dorsal surface of the brainstem. Injuries in this location may avulse the rootlets of the emerging nerve, or there may be stretching or contusion injury from hemorrhage within the nerve.

When damage occurs to the trochlear nerves at their exit from the brainstem, both nerves are often involved, although in some cases the bilaterality of the condition may not be apparent unless the patient is carefully examined. Even then, the presence of bilateral palsies may first become apparent after the patient undergoes surgical correction of the apparent unilateral palsy.

As the trochlear nerve passes forward through the subarachnoid space, it may be damaged by trauma. In many cases, the site of damage is unclear. This is especially true when the palsy is accompanied by evidence of blunt trauma involving the ipsilateral or contralateral orbit. In such cases, patients may have both a trochlear nerve palsy and an orbital blowout fracture; in other cases, an orbital fracture is assumed because of the external appearance of the patient, when in fact the cause of the vertical diplopia is a trochlear nerve palsy. Nevertheless, in some patients, it is clear that the subarachnoid portion of the nerve has been damaged. This is particularly true when the trauma is iatrogenic. We have frequently encountered patients with unilateral trochlear nerve palsy after surgery for tentorial

meningiomas or large vestibular schwannomas (acoustic neuromas).

A trochlear nerve paresis may occur in patients immediately following an anterior temporal lobectomy for treatment of medically intractable epilepsy. The trochlear nerve palsy typically resolves completely within about 3 months and is thought to result from indirect traction on the subarachnoid portion of the trochlear nerve during surgery.

Trauma that is insufficient to produce a skull fracture or loss of consciousness may nevertheless cause a trochlear nerve palsy because of the extremely fragile nature of the nerve and its long subarachnoid course. Thus, a head injury that

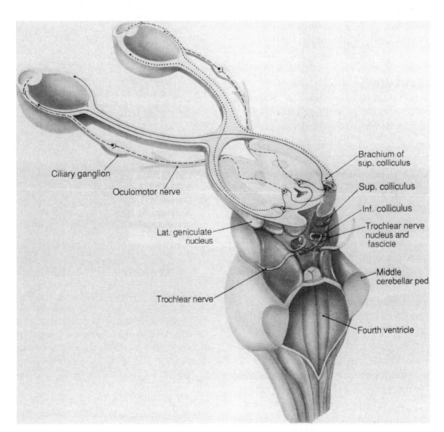

Figure 17.37.   Presumed site of damage in a young woman who developed a left trochlear nerve paresis and was found to have a left relative afferent pupillary defect unassociated with any visual sensory deficit. The shaded portion of the illustration indicates a lesion involving the brachium of the right superior colliculus and the right dorsal mesencephalon, including the right trochlear nucleus or the predecussation portion of the right trochlear nerve fascicle. The patient was found to have an anaplastic astrocytoma of the brainstem. (Reprinted with permission from Eliott D, Cunningham ET Jr, Miller NR. Fourth nerve paresis and ipsilateral relative afferent pupillary defect without visual sensory disturbance: a sign of contralateral dorsal midbrain disease. J Clin Neuro-ophthalmol 1991;11:169–171.)

would not be expected to cause either an oculo-motor or an abducens nerve paresis can produce a unilateral or bilateral trochlear nerve paresis. One must always be aware, however, that ocular motor nerve palsies that occur after apparently trivial head trauma, including trochlear nerve palsy, may be associated with asymptomatic basal intracranial tumors that have stretched, thinned, or infiltrated the nerve which, neverthe-less, has continued to function. Some of these patients have other neurologic signs. Thus, pa-tients who develop a trochlear nerve paresis after minor head trauma should be carefully checked for other ocular and neurologic defects and should undergo careful follow-up examinations or neuroimaging studies if there is any question as to an etiology for the trochlear nerve paresis other than trauma.

The subarachnoid portion of the trochlear nerve can occasionally be damaged by posterior fossa aneurysms. In most cases, the aneurysm arises from the junction of the basilar and supe-rior cerebellar arteries.

The subarachnoid portion of the trochlear nerve may also become affected in patients with basal meningitis. Syphilis, tuberculosis, sarcoid-osis, and Lyme disease are the most common causes.

Schwannomas of the trochlear nerve may pro-duce diplopia from trochlear nerve palsy by in-volvement of the nerve in the subarachnoid space (Fig. 17.38). In some cases, the schwannoma is located adjacent to the brainstem and may even compress it, producing neurologic deficits consistent with brainstem dysfunction. In other cases, diplopia is the only manifestation of the tumor. Other intrinsic lesions of the sub-arachnoid portion of the trochlear nerve include cavernous angiomas and arteriovenous malfor-mations.

Patients with posteriorly draining dural ca-rotid-cavernous sinus fistulas may develop an acute, painful trochlear nerve paresis. Because the fistula is draining posteriorly, such patients have none of the orbital congestive manifesta-tions usually associated with carotid-cavernous sinus fistulas, such as conjunctival chemosis, di-lation of conjunctival vessels, or proptosis.

The association of trochlear nerve palsy and elevated ICP is well documented. Some of these patients have pseudotumor cerebri, whereas oth-ers have hydrocephalus related to a variety of different processes, including blocked ventricu-

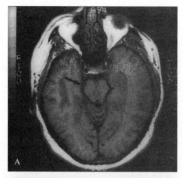
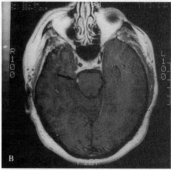
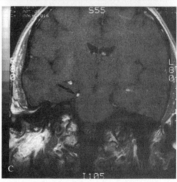

Figure 17.38. Neuroimaging in a 53-year-old man with vertical diplopia and a head tilt. An examination revealed a right trochlear nerve paresis. MRI was performed when the patient's diplopia did not improve within several months. *A.* T1-weighted axial MRI shows slight enlargement of the subarachnoid portion of the right trochlear nerve (*arrow*). *B.* T1-weighted axial MRI in same plane after intravenous injection of paramagnetic contrast material shows enhance-ment of the trochlear nerve in this region (*arrow*). *C.* En-hanced T1-weighted coronal MRI of same area shows loca-tion of the right trochlear nerve lesion just beneath the tentorium cerebelli (*arrow*). The signal characteristics of the lesion are most consistent with a schwannoma or meningi-oma of the trochlear nerve.

loperitoneal shunts. Indeed, bilateral trochlear nerve paresis may be a localizing sign of involvement of the superior medullary velum by a dilated sylvian aqueduct or downward pressure from an enlarged 3rd ventricle.

Lesions of the Trochlear Nerve within the Cavernous Sinus and Superior Orbital Fissure

Lesions that produce a cavernous sinus syndrome are discussed above. When such lesions produce combined ocular motor nerve palsies, the trochlear nerve is often involved. It is unusual, however, for isolated trochlear nerve palsy to occur from cavernous sinus disease, although ischemic conditions (e.g., diabetes mellitus) may conceivably affect the trochlear nerve in this location as they do the oculomotor nerve. In this respect, it is also possible that the isolated trochlear nerve palsy that occurs in some patients with herpes zoster may be produced by a local granulomatous angiitis that originates in the ophthalmic division of the trigeminal nerve and spreads to the sphenocavernous portion of the trochlear nerve. This cannot be the only mechanism, however, because trochlear nerve palsy also occurs in patients with geniculate herpes zoster (i.e., the Ramsay-Hunt syndrome).

Lesions of the Trochlear Nerve within the Orbit

Trauma (including surgical injury) may damage the trochlear nerve within the orbit; however, in many cases, it is impossible to ascertain if the damage has occurred to the nerve, the trochlea, the superior oblique muscle or tendon, or several of these structures. A similar problem arises in assessing patients with orbital inflammation, ischemia, or vascular malformations that are associated with superior oblique dysfunction. The superior oblique paralysis that occurs in patients with Paget's disease of the orbit and with hypertrophic arthritis may also be caused by mechanical disruption of the superior oblique tendon within the trochlea and not by damage to the trochlear nerve itself. The orbital portions of both the oculomotor and trochlear nerves may become ischemic after dental anesthesia.

Lesions of the Trochlear Nerve of Uncertain or Variable Location

Acquired, isolated paralysis of the superior oblique muscle without any systemic or neuro-logic signs or symptoms is not uncommon. In a substantial number of these patients, spontaneous recovery occurs within 1 to 4 months. When such palsies are truly acquired and not the result of decompensation of a preexisting congenital trochlear palsy, they are most likely inflammatory or ischemic in origin.

Recovery from Acquired Trochlear Nerve Palsy

Following the development of a trochlear nerve palsy, superior oblique function may:

- Recover completely, particularly in cases of ischemia or closed injury or after relief of compression from tumor or aneurysm.
- Recover incompletely, leaving the patient with mild but persistent vertical diplopia, torsional diplopia, or both.
- Show no recovery, as occurs primarily after mesencephalic injury or with transection of the trochlear nerve by trauma or compression.

EVALUATION AND MANAGEMENT OF TROCHLEAR NERVE PALSY

The diagnosis of a trochlear nerve palsy is made primarily by performing the "three-step test" (see Chapter 16). It must be emphasized that this test is only useful if the paresis is of a single cyclovertical muscle. Furthermore, although we believe the three-step test is extremely useful in patients with presumed trochlear nerve palsies, its reliability in the diagnosis of pareses of other vertical muscles is questionable. In addition, restrictive ophthalmoplegia, myasthenia gravis, and skew deviation can mimic a trochlear nerve palsy when they are evaluated using the three-step test.

The easiest method of treating the vertical or torsional diplopia experienced by patients awaiting resolution of an acquired or a decompensated congenital trochlear nerve palsy is occlusion of one eye with a patch or an opaque contact lens. In other cases, particularly those with mild vertical displacement, the use of a vertical press-on (Fresnel) prism may be of benefit, although some degree of diplopia in extremes of gaze is almost always present. In cases of acquired trochlear nerve palsy, no attempt at surgical correction should be considered until at least 8 to 12 months have elapsed without improvement in superior oblique function, unless the physician knows with certainty that the trochlear nerve has been severed (e.g., after intracranial surgery in which the nerve has been transected by accident or design and the cut ends not reapproximated with sutures).

When a trochlear nerve palsy has been stable over an appropriate period of time, one may attempt to correct persistent diplopia using any one of several operative procedures. These procedures are designed to (1) strengthen all or a portion of the superior oblique muscle, (2) weaken its antagonist, the ipsilateral inferior oblique muscle, or (3) weaken its yoke muscle, the contralateral inferior rectus muscle. The decision to use one or another of these procedures or to use several in combination depends on the results of a careful orthoptic examination. Similar considerations apply for the treatment of bilateral trochlear nerve palsies. The results of surgery for both congenital and acquired trochlear nerve palsies are usually excellent.

ABDUCENS (SIXTH) NERVE PALSIES AND NUCLEAR HORIZONTAL GAZE PARALYSIS

The abducens nerve is unique in that damage to its nucleus results not in ipsilateral abduction weakness but in horizontal gaze paralysis toward the side of the lesion. In addition, the precise anatomic location of the nerve produces syndromes that are different from those seen with damage to either the oculomotor or trochlear nerves.

CONGENITAL

Congenital absence of abduction as an isolated phenomenon is exceedingly rare but may occur from injury to the abducens nerve shortly before or during birth. That birth trauma is a significant factor indicated by an incidence of congenital abduction weakness in infants that increases progressively from 0% for deliveries by caesarean section, to 0.1% for spontaneous vaginal delivery, to 2.4% for forceps delivery, and to 3.2% for vacuum extraction. It is likely that the increased complexity of instrumentation during delivery is associated with this increased risk of abducens nerve palsy.

Congenital paralysis of conjugate horizontal eye movements occurs more frequently than does unilateral or bilateral abduction weakness. Congenital horizontal gaze palsy may occur as an isolated sporadic finding, or it may be familial. Histologic findings in patients with isolated bilateral horizontal gaze palsy include absent or hypoplastic abducens nuclei and absent abducens nerves.

Congenital absence of abduction, either alone or as part of a horizontal gaze palsy, is usually observed in association with other neurologic or systemic anomalies. For example, patients with cerebral palsy seem to have an increased prevalence of congenital abducens paresis. In addition, congenital paralysis of both abduction and horizontal gaze occurs in patients with a variety of skeletal abnormalities, including Klippel-Feil syndrome and progressive familial kyphoscoliosis. A syndrome of congenital horizontal gaze paralysis and ear dysplasia is also well described, and unilateral agenesis of the abducens nucleus and nerve (as well as the trochlear nucleus and nerve) can occur in patients with oculoauriculovertebral dysplasia-hemifacial microsomia (Goldenhar-Gorlin syndrome). The cervico-oculo-acoustic (Wildervanck syndrome) syndrome may be associated with a Klippel-Feil anomaly, congenital sensory neural deafness, and bilateral abducens nerve palsy.

Far more common are congenital disturbances of horizontal gaze associated with two conditions: Möbius syndrome and Duane's retraction syndrome (DRS).

Möbius Syndrome (Congenital Bulbar Paralysis)

Characteristically, this defect involves the face and horizontal gaze mechanisms bilaterally. Affected patients have a mask-like facies, with the mouth constantly held open. In some infants, this defect prevents adequate nursing. The eyelids often cannot be completely closed, and in some patients, they cannot be closed at all. There may be excess lacrimation and epiphora. Some patients have only an esotropia associated with unilateral or bilateral limitation of abduction, and some may even be able to converge. In most cases, however, the eyes are straight and do not move horizontally in either direction (Fig. 17.39). In rare cases, vertical eye movements are also abnormal.

Other congenital defects that are found in patients with this syndrome include deafness, webbed fingers or toes, supernumerary digits, atrophy of the muscles of the chest, neck, and particularly the tongue, and absence of the

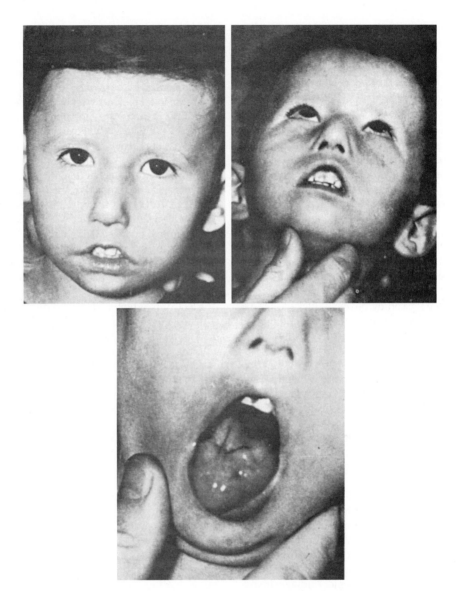

Figure 17.39.   Möbius syndrome in a 3-year-old boy. The boy had spontaneous vertical eye movements but no horizon- tal eye movements. Note bilateral facial palsy and atrophy of the tongue.

hands, feet, fingers, or toes. Occurring less fre- quently are low-set ears, a small mouth opening, micrognathia, epicanthal folds, abnormalities of lower cranial nerves causing speech and swal- lowing difficulties, congenital heart defects, tachypnea, or a combination of these abnormali- ties. There also appears to be an association of the Möbius syndrome with anosmia and hypogo- nadotrophic hypogonadism (Kallmann syn-

drome). Nearly all patients with Möbius syn- drome have some degree of mental retardation.

Most cases of Möbius syndrome are sporadic. Although autosomal-dominant pedigrees occur, we are aware of only two families with primary skeletal anomalies associated with a Möbius fa- cies and ocular motor dysfunction in more than one member. It is thought that the risk is no greater than 2% for another affected sibling in pedigrees in which the syndrome includes limb abnormalities.

Pathologic findings in patients with Möbius syndrome can be separated into four groups according to the neuropathologic findings in the brainstem nuclei. Group I consists of cases with hypoplasia or atrophy of cranial nerve nuclei. These cases are associated with an absence of, or decrease in, the number of neurons in the affected cranial nerve nuclei. Some of these cases have other associated anomalies, and there are no signs of necrosis or degenerations. It is likely that these central nervous system lesions are caused by maldevelopment rather than by acquired insults later in life.

Group II consists of cases in which, in addition to neuronal loss, there is evidence of active neuronal degeneration in the affected facial nerve nuclei. It is postulated that these neuronal changes are caused by physical injury to the facial nerve, arising from a malformed temporal bone or from application of forceps during delivery.

Group III consists of cases in which, in addition to a decrease in the number of neurons and reactive changes in the affected cranial nerve nuclei, there is frank necrosis of the tegmentum of the lower pons. These lesions are probably acquired later during fetal life rather than during early embryonic development, and both hypoxia and viral infections are implicated in their etiology.

Group IV consists of cases in which no lesions are found in the brainstem or cranial nerves. Some of these cases are associated with severe atrophy of the facial muscles and others with creatinuria. Thus, a primary myopathy may be responsible for these cases.

The diversity of pathologic findings in patients with Möbius syndrome suggests that the syndrome actually is a heterogeneous group of congenital disorders that in some cases are caused by developmental defects, and in others, by acquired hypoxic or other insults. This syndrome may be detected with prenatal ultrasonographic testing.

Duane's Retraction Syndrome (Stilling-Turk-Duane Syndrome)

Duane's retraction syndrome is a predominantly congenital eye movement disorder characterized by marked limitation or absence of abduction, variable limitation of adduction, and palpebral fissure narrowing and globe retraction on attempted adduction (Fig. 17.40). Vertical ocular movements are often noted on adduction, most frequently in an upward direction.

A disorder of horizontal eye movements is common to all patients with DRS. In most cases, the abnormalities are unilateral, but bilateral Duane's syndrome occurs in 15 to 20% of affected patients. The syndrome occurs more commonly in females than males, and the left eye is more frequently affected than the right. In most patients, gaze is directed toward the side of the unaffected eye, and in some instances, the face is turned toward the affected side to allow binocular single vision. Vision is almost always normal unless there is associated anisometropia. Thus, in the majority of cases, no treatment is necessary unless the patient has a marked head turn.

Electromyographic studies show that DRS is a neurogenic disorder in which branches of the oculomotor nerve innervate the lateral rectus muscle (Fig. 17.41). Retraction of the globe is produced by a co-contraction of horizontal rectus muscles. Autopsy studies have confirmed anomalous innervation of the extraocular muscles. Abducens nuclei and nerves are absent and the lateral rectus muscle is innervated by branches from the oculomotor nerve. Interestingly, in the region of the abducens nuclei, cell bodies representing internuclear neurons typically remain intact.

There are three types of DRS: Duane I type consists of limited or absent abduction with relatively normal adduction; Duane II consists of limited or absent adduction with relatively normal abduction; and Duane III is characterized by limited abduction and adduction. In all cases, an anomaly of ocular motor innervation involving the oculomotor and abducens nerves is thought to be responsible.

Although some cases may be caused by birth trauma, 30 to 50% of patients with DRS have associated congenital defects involving ocular, skeletal, and neural structures. The differentiation of these frequently affected structures occurs between the fourth and eighth weeks of gestation, coincident with the development of the ocular motor nerves. Thus, a teratogenic event during the second month of gestation may cause DRS. This theory is supported by the occurrence of DRS in children of mothers who have taken the drug thalidomide during pregnancy. In addi-

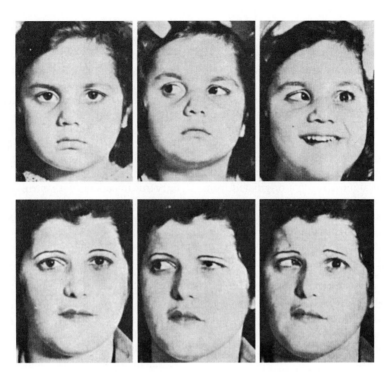

Figure 17.40.   Unilateral left Duane's retraction syndrome in a young girl (*above*) and her mother (*below*). The syndrome was present in five members of three generations. (Reprinted with permission from Laughlin RC. Hereditary paralysis of the abducens nerve. Report of a case. Am J Ophthalmol 1937;20:396–398.)

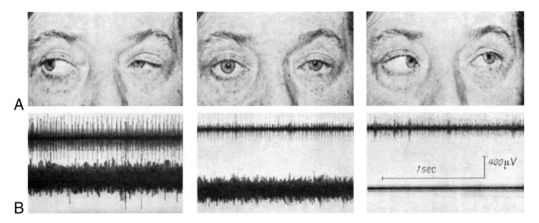

Figure 17.41.   Electromyogram in left Duane's retraction syndrome. Simultaneous recording from left lateral rectus (*a*) and medial rectus (*b*) muscles shows *paradoxic innervation* of the lateral rectus muscle during attempted adduction of the left eye. In fact, the lateral rectus muscle receives its maximal innervation during adduction and its minimal innervation during attempted abduction (upper right). The innervation pattern of the left medial rectus is normal. Note its inhibition during abduction of the eye. (Reprinted with permission from Huber A, Esslen E, Kloti R, et al. Zum problem des Duane syndromes. Albrecht von Graefes Arch Klin Exp Ophthalmol 1964;167:169–191.)

tion, genetic testing shows a defect in the long arm of chromosome 4 in some cases and a defect in chromosome 22 in others. Given the multitude of associated anomalies seen in DRS, multiple etiologies, including chromosomal disorders and trauma, may produce DRS. Most cases of DRS are sporadic, but familial unilateral and bilateral cases occur and constitute about 10% of observed cases.

An acquired form of DRS can occur in patients with brainstem tumors, presumably from anomalous neural impulses that originated from disruption of the oculomotor and abducens nerve nuclei and their connections. Acquired DRS can also occur after orbital trauma or damage to the ocular motor nerves during cavernous sinus or orbital surgery. In these cases, direct trauma to the oculomotor and abducens nerves, with interruption of their sheaths, presumably allows anomalous reinnervation to occur. Other acquired diseases of the extraocular muscles or of the orbit, including fibrosis or muscle inflammatory disease, may mimic DRS.

ACQUIRED

Lesions of the Abducens Nerve Nucleus

The abducens nucleus contains not only motoneurons that innervate the ipsilateral lateral rectus but also cell bodies of internuclear neurons that cross the midline and ascend in the contralateral medial longitudinal fasciculus (MLF) to synapse in the medial rectus subnucleus on that side (Fig. 17.42). Thus, lesions that damage the abducens nucleus produce a **conjugate gaze palsy** to the ipsilateral side, and lesions of both abducens nuclei completely eliminate conjugate horizontal gaze. **Neither unilateral nor bilateral isolated abduction weakness ever occurs from a lesion of the abducens nucleus.** In most but not all cases in which the abducens nucleus is damaged, an ipsilateral, peripheral, facial nerve palsy is also present. This palsy occurs because the facial nerve fascicle loops around the abducens nucleus before exiting from the brainstem (Fig. 17.43).

The horizontal gaze palsy that occurs from damage to the abducens nucleus is not always symmetric, perhaps because the cell bodies of the abducens motoneurons are more vulnerable than those of the internuclear neurons to certain insults, thus producing an asymmetric horizontal gaze paralysis that is worse in the abducting eye. Lesions of the abducens nucleus sometimes

damage the ipsilateral MLF, producing the **one-and-a-half syndrome.** This syndrome consists of a horizontal gaze palsy combined with an internuclear ophthalmoplegia (INO).

Lesions that produce intrinsic brainstem damage and cause acquired unilateral or bilateral paralysis of horizontal gaze from damage to the abducens nuclei include ischemia, infiltration, trauma, inflammation, and compression (Figs. 17.44 and 17.45). In many instances, however, several mechanisms play a role. This is particularly true in patients with intrinsic pontine hematomas. Horizontal gaze palsies may occur as part of the syndrome of familial pontine cavernous angiomas.

Patients with the Wernicke-Korsakoff syndrome often develop paralysis of conjugate gaze, presumably from a metabolic insult to the abducens nuclei. Patients with hepatic encephalopathy may develop a similar condition. Neuronal loss and gliosis can occur in the abducens nuclei of patients with ALS. In most of these cases, similar changes are observed in the other ocular motor nuclei. The relative susceptibility of some brainstem motor neuron groups to the neurodegenerative process that occurs in ALS is not completely understood.

Lesions of the Abducens Nerve Fascicle

When an abducens nerve palsy coexists with a gaze palsy to the same side from damage to both the abducens nucleus and the ipsilateral abducens nerve fascicle, identification of the peripheral nerve element in the gaze palsy cannot be assessed unless there is a marked asymmetry between the two eyes, with the abducting eye being more limited in movement than the adducting eye. In other instances, fascicular involvement of the abducens nerve produces an isolated abduction weakness that cannot be differentiated clinically from involvement outside the brainstem. However, most lesions that damage the abducens fascicle produce distinctive clinical syndromes from damage to the surrounding neurologic tissue.

A lesion in the pontine tegmentum may damage the abducens and facial nerve fascicles, the nucleus of the tractus solitarius, the central tegmental tract, the spinal tract of the trigeminal nerve (and its nucleus), the superior olivary nucleus, or a combination of these structures. Such a lesion may produce ipsilateral paralysis of abduction, ipsilateral facial palsy (flaccid), loss of

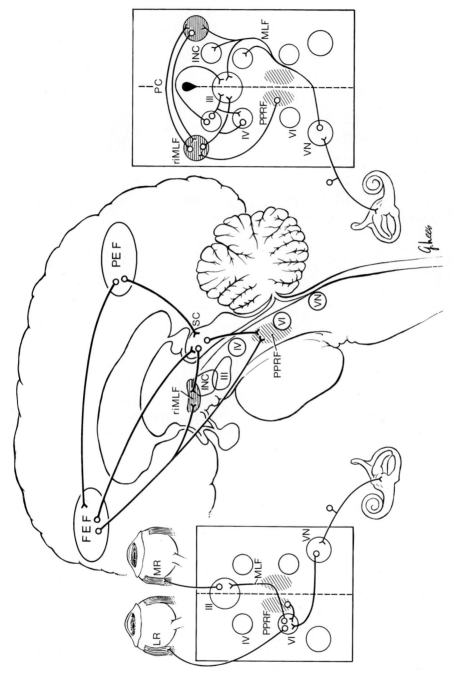

Figure 17.42.   Diagram on left shows that the abducens nucleus (VI) contains not only motoneurons that innervate the ipsilateral lateral rectus (LR) but also cell bodies of internuclear neurons that cross the midline and ascend in the contralateral medial longitudinal fasciculus (MLF) to synapse in the medial rectus subnucleus on that side (III). *MR*, medial rectus muscle; *PPRF*, paramedian pontine reticular formation; *VN*, vestibulbar nucleus; *IV*, trochlear nerve nucleus.

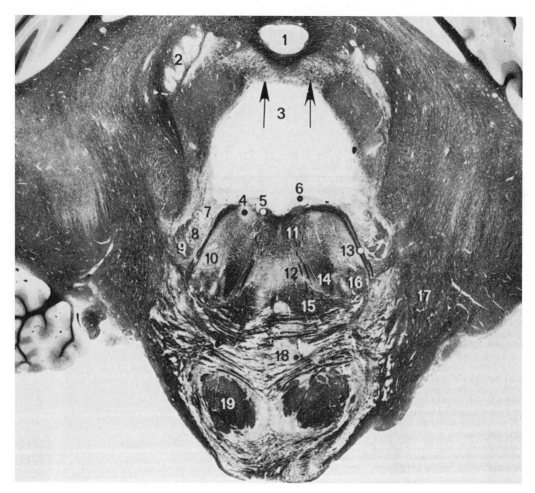

Figure 17.43. Transverse section through the caudal pons showing the abducens nuclei at the level of the facial genu. *1*, cerebellar vermis; *2*, dentate nucleus; *3*, 4th ventricle; *4*, abducens nucleus; *5*, genu of the facial nerve; *6*, facial colliculus; *7*, lateral vestibular nucleus; *8*, spinal nucleus of the trigeminal nerve; *9*, spinal tract of the trigeminal nerve; *10*, facial nucleus; *11*, medial longitudinal fasciculus; *12*, reticular formation; *13*, fasciculus of facial nerve; *14*, central tegmental tract; *15*, medial lemniscus and trapezoid body; *16*, spinal and trigeminal nuclei; *17*, middle cerebellar peduncle; *18*, pontine nuclei and transverse pontine fibers; *19*, pyramidal tract. The arrows show the position of the cerebellar fastigial nuclei. (Reprinted with permission from Ghuhbegovic N, Williams TH. The Human Brain: A Photographic Guide. Hagerstown, MD: Harper & Row, 1980.)

taste from the anterior two-thirds of the tongue, ipsilateral central Horner's syndrome, ipsilateral analgesia of the face, and ipsilateral peripheral deafness. Together, these signs comprise the syndrome of the anterior inferior cerebellar artery—**Foville's syndrome.** The clinical expression of this syndrome is rarely complete, and many of its features may occur in association with ipsilateral paralysis of horizontal gaze rather than ipsilateral paralysis of abduction, indicating nuclear, rather than fascicular, involvement.

A lesion in the ventral paramedian pons may damage, in addition to the ventral portion of the abducens fascicle, the corticospinal tract, the ventral portion of the facial nerve fascicle, or both. Such a lesion produces an ipsilateral abducens palsy and a contralateral hemiplegia, with (**Millard-Gubler syndrome**) or without (**Raymond-Cestan syndrome**) ipsilateral peripheral facial paralysis (Fig. 17.46).

Fascicular lesions of the abducens nerve may be produced by ischemia, tumor compression or infiltration, infection, demyelination, and other

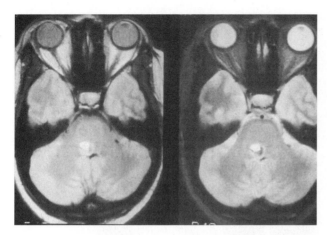

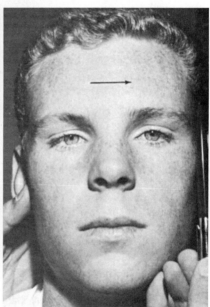

Figure 17.44. MRI in a 62-year-old woman with a slowly progressive right horizontal gaze paresis and ipsilateral facial weakness. Axial proton-density (*left*) and T2-weighted (*right*) images demonstrate a lesion in the region of the right abducens nerve nucleus. An evaluation revealed breast carcinoma with evidence of systemic metastases, and the lesion was thought to be a metastasis.

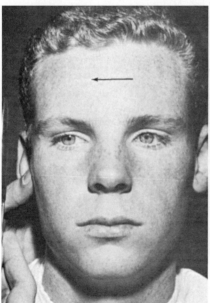

Figure 17.45. Acute bilateral paralysis of horizontal gaze in a 16-year-old boy with multiple sclerosis. Two weeks after this photograph was obtained, all neurologic signs had resolved.

inflammation. For example, although the abducens nerve palsies that occur in association with diabetes mellitus are usually assumed to occur from involvement of the subarachnoid or cavernous sinus portion of the nerve, some patients with isolated abducens nerve pareses in the setting of diabetes mellitus have MRI evidence of small hemorrhagic or ischemic brainstem lesions. The most common inflammation causing a fascicular abducens nerve paresis is demyelination.

Lesions of the Abducens Nerve in the Subarachnoid Space

Causes of abducens nerve damage in the subarachnoid space are many and varied. The long course of the nerve is usually cited as an explanation for its frequent involvement; however, the course of the trochlear nerve is longer and yet trochlear nerve pareses occur less frequently than do abducens nerve pareses. In fact, the location and course of the abducens nerve, rather than its length, are the major factors that lead to

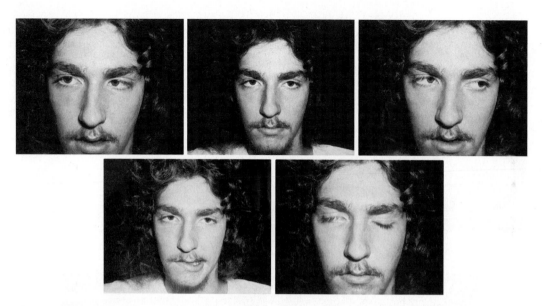

Figure 17.46. Millard-Gubler syndrome in a 23-year-old man with an intrapontine hemorrhage. The patient has a right abducens nerve paresis, a right peripheral facial nerve paresis, and a left (contralateral) hemiparesis.

an abducens nerve paresis. The abducens nerve lies along the ventral surface of the pons and is bound to that structure by the anterior inferior cerebellar artery. The nerve may therefore be compressed by this vessel, the posterior inferior cerebellar artery, or the basilar artery, particularly when the vessel is atherosclerotic or dolichoectatic. Aneurysms of these vessels may also cause abducens paralysis. In most of these cases, there are no other cranial nerve findings, but there may be severe headache.

After its exit from the pons, the abducens nerve passes almost vertically through the subarachnoid space to pierce the dura overlying the clivus. During its course, it is vulnerable to damage from a variety of processes in the posterior fossa, including descent of the brainstem associated with vertex blows, space-occupying masses above the tentorium (transtentorial herniation), posterior fossa masses, and structural abnormalities (e.g., Chiari malformations). In these settings, the abducens nerve may be stretched and injured at its attachment at either the pons or the clivus. Trauma may be direct, including neurosurgical, or indirect from blunt, closed head injury. Both unilateral and bilateral abducens paralysis, usually associated with other neurologic signs and symptoms, have been reported in patients placed in halo-pelvic traction.

Meningitis—whether bacterial, neoplastic, spirochetal, or viral—may produce abducens nerve paralysis (Fig. 17.47). As with other ocular motor nerve palsies produced by meningitis, abducens nerve palsies are often bilateral. Patients with the acquired immune deficiency syndrome (AIDS) are particularly prone to develop meningitis caused by a variety of opportunistic organisms, including various mycobacteria, *Cryptococcus neoformans, Toxoplasma gondii,* cytomegalovirus, and herpes simplex virus. In such patients, unilateral as well as bilateral abducens nerve palsies frequently occur, often in combination with other cranial and ocular motor nerve palsies. Both unilateral and bilateral abducens nerve paresis can also occur in patients with idiopathic hypertrophic cranial pachymeningitis, a condition characterized by chronic, nongranulomatous inflammation of the meninges (Fig. 17.48).

Basal tumors may directly damage the subarachnoid portion of the abducens nerve. Meningioma and chordoma may produce both unilateral and bilateral abducens palsies without any other neurologic signs and symptoms. A chronic, isolated painless abducens paresis can be the only sign of a trigeminal schwannoma. Vestibular schwannomas (acoustic neuromas) may cause abducens palsy but almost never as

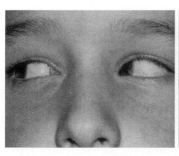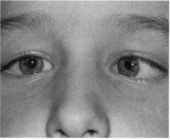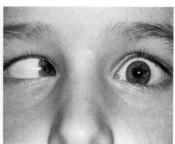

Figure 17.47. Left abducens nerve palsy in a 7-year-old boy with aseptic meningitis. It was assumed that the palsy was caused by damage to the abducens nerve in the subarachnoid space. The palsy cleared without treatment.

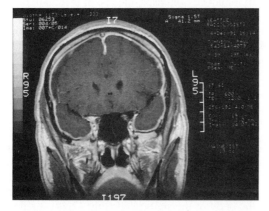

Figure 17.48. Neuroimaging in a 39-year-old man with a slowly progressive right abduction deficit associated with headache. Axial T1-weighted MRI shows diffuse meningeal enhancement as well as inflammatory changes in the right cavernous sinus. Biopsy of the meninges established a diagnosis of idiopathic hypertrophic cranial pachymeningitis. The disease was arrested with cranial irradiation and immunotherapy.

their sole manifestation. Similarly, although the abducens nerve may be damaged by exophytic spread of intrinsic posterior fossa tumors such as glioma, medulloblastoma, or ependymoma, patients with these tumors almost always have other neurologic symptoms and signs. As with the oculomotor and trochlear nerves, schwannomas of the subarachnoid portion of the abducens nerve may produce an isolated abducens paralysis. Cavernous angiomas of the nerve may produce a similar clinical picture.

Changes in ICP may produce abducens palsy. Patients with increased ICP commonly develop both unilateral and bilateral abducens palsies. In such instances, the palsies may represent false localizing signs of intracranial tumors.

A unilateral (and occasionally bilateral) abducens palsy may develop after a lumbar puncture, whether or not there is increased ICP. The incidence of this complication is 0.25%. Significant features of this syndrome are the delayed appearance of the paresis (5 to 14 days after the lumbar puncture) and the invariable recovery, usually within 4 to 6 weeks. Similar cases occur after shunting for hydrocephalus, after spinal anesthesia, and after myelography performed with water-soluble contrast material.

Spontaneous intracranial hypotension may cause severe headaches and unilateral or bilateral abducens nerve paresis. MRI in such cases usually reveals diffuse enhancement and thickening of the meninges, and attempted lumbar puncture is usually unsuccessful in obtaining cerebrospinal fluid because of the low ICP. The abducens pareses generally resolve and the MR abnormalities disappear when the hypotension is treated or resolves spontaneously.

Abducens nerve paresis that results from increased ICP probably occurs because the abducens nerve becomes compressed between the pons and the basilar artery or clivus or is stretched along the sharp edge of the petrous temporal bone. Similar mechanisms may be responsible for the abducens nerve palsies that develop following the sudden production of a low-pressure state such as that which occurs after lumbar puncture, after cerebrospinal fluid shunting, or spontaneously.

Although anteriorly draining dural carotid-cavernous sinus fistulas frequently cause an abducens nerve paresis from compression or ischemia of the abducens nerve in the cavernous sinus (see below), dural carotid-cavernous sinus fistulas that drain posteriorly into the inferior petrosal sinus may also produce an acute abducens nerve paresis that is unassociated with the chemosis, proptosis, and redness normally associated with an anteriorly draining fistula. The palsy usually is unilateral, and it may be isolated or associated with other ocular motor nerve pareses.

Lesions of the Extradural Portion of the Abducens Nerve at the Petrous Apex

After the abducens nerve penetrates the dura overlying the clivus, it passes beneath the petroclinoid (Gruber's) ligament. In this region, it is adjacent to the mastoid air cells. In patients with severe mastoiditis, the inflammatory process may extend to the tip of the petrous bone, producing localized inflammation of the meninges in the epidural space and a classic condition called **Gradenigo's syndrome.** The adjacent abducens nerve becomes inflamed and paretic. In addition, because the gasserian ganglion and facial nerve are also nearby, such patients have severe pain on the ipsilateral side of the face and around the eye and may also develop facial paralysis. Abducens paresis may not occur until 2 to 3 days following the onset of pain. Photophobia and lacrimation are often present, and corneal sensation may be diminished. In some patients, meningitis develops, whereas in others, only a localized inflammation occurs. Because of the prompt and almost universal use of antibiotics in children with known or presumed acute otitis media, the incidence of Gradenigo's syndrome is extremely low.

Lesions other than inflammation can involve the petrous apex and produce symptoms suggesting Gradenigo's syndrome. These lesions include tumors and aneurysms of the intrapetrosal segment of the internal carotid artery. Thus, patients presenting with the petrous apex syndrome should be carefully evaluated with appropriate neuroimaging studies before it is concluded that the involvement is inflammatory.

When lateral sinus thrombosis or phlebitis extends into the inferior petrosal sinus, the abducens nerve may become paretic. A similar situation may occur when one jugular vein (particularly the right jugular) is ligated during radical neck dissection. Thrombosis of the inferior petrosal sinus may explain the abducens nerve palsy that sometimes occurs in patients with mastoiditis. In other cases, however, a

pseudotumor cerebri syndrome develops, and the abducens palsy is secondary to increased ICP.

The abducens nerve may be injured in its petrous segment when the skull is fractured. In some of these cases, longitudinal fractures of the temporal bone are responsible.

Abducens nerve pareses caused by lesions in the superior aspect of the sphenopalatine (pterygopalatine) fossa often present with a typical clinical picture that includes loss of tearing, irritation of the eye on the side of the paresis, and trigeminal sensory neuropathy in the distribution of the maxillary division of the trigeminal nerve. In a majority of cases, the lesion is a malignant tumor (e.g., nasopharyngeal carcinoma) that has extended through foramina at the base of the skull and has spread beneath the dura to damage the extradural portions of the abducens and trigeminal nerves.

Lesions of the Abducens Nerve in the Cavernous Sinus and Superior Orbital Fissure

Abducens nerve paralysis, either isolated or in combination with other cranial neuropathies, may occur from lesions within the cavernous sinus. The location of the abducens nerve within the body of the sinus itself (Fig. 17.49)—rather than in the deep layer of the lateral sinus wall where the oculomotor, trochlear, and ophthalmic nerves are located—predisposes it to damage from intracavernous vascular lesions, including aneurysms, direct and dural carotid-cavernous fistulas, and rarely internal carotid artery dissection.

Tumors that infiltrate the cavernous sinus as well as those that compress the structures within it may produce isolated abducens palsy. These include meningioma, metastatic carcinoma, nasopharyngeal carcinoma, Burkitt's lymphoma, pituitary adenoma with and without apoplexy, craniopharyngioma, and a variety of other rare lesions in the region of the optic chiasm and cavernous sinus, including suprasellar germinomas, osteogenic sarcomas, teratomas, and multiple myeloma or plasmacytoma. When such lesions are sufficiently large, they may involve both cavernous sinuses and produce bilateral abducens nerve palsies.

Ischemic conditions, such as hypertension, diabetes mellitus, giant cell arteritis, systemic lupus erythematosus, and migraine, may damage

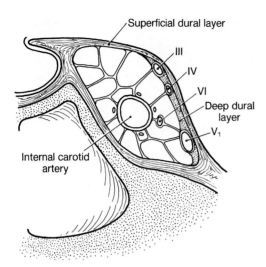

Figure 17.49.   Diagram of the cavernous sinus showing that the lateral wall is composed of two layers: a superficial layer and a deep layer. The deep layer is formed by the sheaths of the oculomotor (III), trochlear (IV), and ophthalmic (V₁) nerves, with a reticular membrane between these sheaths. Note that the abducens nerve, *VI*, is located within the body of the cavernous sinus, not within the lateral wall as are the other ocular motor nerves. (Redrawn from Umansky F, Nathan H. The lateral wall of the cavernous sinus. With special reference to the nerves related to it. J Neurosurg 1982;56:228–234.)

the abducens nerve within the cavernous sinus, as may both granulomatous (e.g., tuberculosis, sarcoidosis, or the Tolosa-Hunt syndrome) and nongranulomatous (e.g., sphenoid sinus abscess or idiopathic hypertrophic pachymeningitis) inflammation. Herpes zoster may also produce abducens palsy from involvement of the abducens nerve in the cavernous sinus.

Although isolated involvement of the abducens nerve by cavernous sinus pathology is not rare, it is far more common for such involvement to be associated with other neurologic signs and symptoms, even if there are no other ocular motor nerve palsies. One of the more important of these cavernous sinus syndromes consists of the combination of isolated abducens paralysis and ipsilateral postganglionic Horner's syndrome (Fig. 17.50). This syndrome can occur in association with primary and traumatic intracavernous aneurysms and with both benign and malignant tumors that arise in or invade the cavernous sinus. The occurrence of this syndrome is explained by the anatomic course of the oculo-

sympathetic fibers within the cavernous sinus which leave the internal carotid artery and join briefly with the abducens nerve before separating and fusing with the ophthalmic division of the trigeminal nerve (Fig. 17.51).

Lesions of the Abducens Nerve within the Orbit

The abducens nerve has a very short course in the orbit, piercing the lateral rectus muscle only a few millimeters from the superior orbital fissure. For this reason, isolated involvement of this nerve within the orbit is rare, although it may occur in patients with a primary orbital schwannoma that originates from the sheath of the orbital portion of the abducens nerve. Abducens nerve paresis can also occur following injection of an anesthetic solution in preparation for mandibular surgery. In many cases, the neural etiology of the orbital process is obvious. In other cases, however, differentiation between neural and muscular involvement producing abduction weakness may not be possible.

Lesions of the Abducens Nerve of Uncertain or Variable Location

Transient isolated abducens nerve palsy occurs rarely, but especially in children. Such palsies are probably caused most often by an underlying vascular or inflammatory lesion. Indeed, many (but certainly but not all) of these patients have associated systemic vascular disease, particularly hypertension, diabetes mellitus, or cardiac disease, or they have a history of a recent vaccination or an illness compatible with a viral syndrome. Some patients, particularly but not exclusively children, have recurrences of such "benign" transient palsies. The location of the lesion in such cases is unknown. Similarly, the location of the lesion that produces abducens palsy as a part of the ophthalmoplegic migraine syndrome or as part of drug intoxications is unclear.

Chronic, Isolated Abducens Nerve Paralysis

Most patients who develop abducens nerve pareses either experience spontaneous improvement of the paresis or are found to have an underlying lesion that has caused the paresis. Some patients, however, do not recover and have no obvious lesion despite an extensive evaluation (see below). We follow such patients at regular intervals, obtaining an interval history and per-

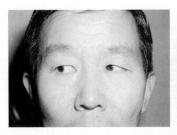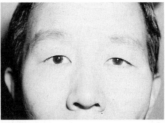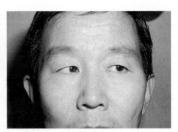

Figure 17.50. Left abducens nerve paresis associated with left postganglionic Horner's syndrome in a patient with a nasopharyngeal carcinoma. Note the mild left ptosis and miosis.

forming a complete examination each time the patient is seen. If, during this time, the patient develops other neurologic signs or the paresis worsens, a complete workup, including neuroimaging and an otolaryngologic evaluation, is performed. If no changes occur over a 3-month period, we perform or repeat a complete assessment of the patient. Although many patients with isolated, chronic abducens nerve palsies that last more than 6 months follow a completely benign course, a substantial number of such patients harbor basal tumors that may be amenable to treatment if identified at an early stage.

Spontaneous recovery of an abducens nerve palsy does not eliminate the presence of a neoplastic process. The possible mechanisms for recovery in such cases include remyelination, axon regeneration, relief of transient compression (e.g., resorption of hemorrhage), restoration of impaired blood flow, slippage of a nerve previously stretched over the tumor, or immune responses to the tumor.

EVALUATION AND MANAGEMENT OF ABDUCENS NERVE PALSY

There is a tendency to assume that all patients with an esotropia associated with unilateral or bilateral abduction weakness have an abducens nerve paresis. In fact, the physician encountering such a patient should first consider the possibility that the condition is myopathic (e.g., thyroid eye disease) or neuromuscular (e.g., myasthenia gravis). A careful history and examination directed at these possibilities may be sufficient to eliminate them as etiologies. Alternatively, the physician may need to perform further studies, including orbital ultrasonography, orbital imaging, thyroid function studies, serum assay for antireceptor antibodies, and single-fiber electromyography.

Once the physician is satisfied that an abducens nerve paresis is likely, he or she should initiate an evaluation that, like the evaluation performed in patients with an oculomotor nerve palsy, depends on the associated symptoms and signs and the age of the patient. All patients with a presumed abducens nerve palsy *must* undergo a thorough neurologic assessment, particularly with respect to the first eight cranial nerves and the integrity of the oculosympathetic pathway. If other neurologic signs (e.g., trigeminal sensory neuropathy, facial paresis, hearing loss, Horner's syndrome) are present, such patients should undergo neuroimaging. If patients have mild redness, swelling, or proptosis of the affected eye, an evaluation for a spontaneous dural carotid-cavernous sinus fistula or even cavernous sinus thrombosis should be performed. Patients with septic cavernous sinus thrombosis nearly always have prominent systemic manifestations of sepsis.

If a patient with an apparent abducens nerve paresis has no other findings and has underlying systemic vascular disease or is in the vasculopathic age group (i.e., over age 60), and if the onset of the palsy is sudden, the patient should be followed at regular intervals, with an interval history obtained and a complete examination performed each time the patient is seen. If, during this time, the patient develops other neurologic signs or the paresis worsens, a complete workup, including neuroimaging and an otolaryngologic evaluation, is performed. If no changes occur over a 3-month period, a complete reassessment of the patient should be performed. On the other hand, if the patient is under age 60 and has no risk factors for ischemic or inflammatory disease, we perform MRI with careful attention to the pathway of the abducens nerve from the brainstem to the orbit. A lumbar

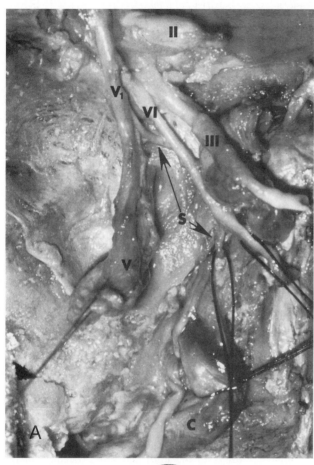

Figure 17.51. Oculosympathetic connections with the abducens nerve in the cavernous sinus. *A.* The sympathetic nerve (*S*) enters the cavernous sinus with the internal carotid artery (*C*). Within the sinus, it joins briefly (*short arrow*) with the abducens nerve (*VI*). It then separates from the nerve (*long arrow*) and joins with the ophthalmic branch (*V₁*) of the trigeminal nerve (*V*). *III*, oculomotor nerve; *II*, optic nerve. (Reprinted with permission from Parkinson D, Johnston J, Chaudhur A. Sympathetic connections to the fifth and sixth cranial nerves. Anat Rec 1978;191:221–226.) *B.* Drawing of relationship of oculosympathetic fibers, abducens nerve, and trigeminal nerve. *III*, oculomotor nerve; *IV*, troclear nerve; *V*, trigeminal neve; *V₁*, ophthalmic trunk; *V₂*, maxillary trunk; *V₃*, mandibular trunk; *VI*, abducens nerve.

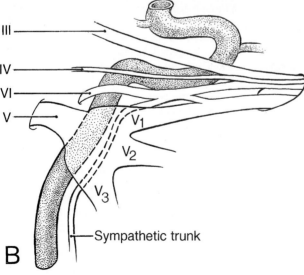

puncture may be indicated in some patients, as may MRA or CTA and an otolaryngologic assessment.

Abducens nerve paralysis may or may not resolve, and the resolution may be complete or incomplete. Ischemic pareses patients almost always recover completely, usually within 2 to 4 months, whereas some degree of spontaneous recovery of traumatic abducens pareses occurs in 30 to 54% of patients and may take more than 1 year. Among patients who do not recover, serious pathology (e.g., tumor, stroke, aneurysm) is often present, emphasizing the importance of performing an evaluation in patients whose abducens nerve palsy does not recover within 3 to 6 months.

As is the case with trochlear nerve function, patients whose abducens nerve is transected during a neurosurgical procedure may recover abducens nerve function if the cut ends of the nerve are rejoined with sutures at the time of surgery.

Strabismus surgery should not be considered to correct an abducens nerve palsy until at least 8 to 10 months have passed without improvement, unless it is known that the abducens nerve is no longer intact. During this period, some patients prefer to occlude one eye, whereas others are able to ignore their diplopia or visual confusion. Although a patch is the simplest manner in which to occlude one eye, an opaque contact lens can also be used. Patients under 8 years old should undergo alternate patching of the eyes to prevent amblyopia. In most patients with unilateral abducens paresis, prisms are not of great benefit, although they are occasionally useful in achieving binocular single vision in primary position.

Chemodenervation of the antagonist medial rectus muscle with botulinum toxin can be used to treat patients with both acute and chronic abducens nerve palsy. We believe that early use of botulinum toxin in patients with acute abducens nerve palsy does not affect the eventual outcome of the condition and that chemodenervation therapy is generally less beneficial than surgery in the treatment of chronic abducens nerve palsy.

Surgery, when required, usually consists of either weakening of the ipsilateral medial rectus muscle combined with strengthening of the ipsilateral lateral rectus muscle or some type of vertical muscle transposition procedure, often combined with chemodenervation of the ipsilateral medial rectus muscle with botulinum toxin.

DIVERGENCE WEAKNESS AND ITS RELATIONSHIP TO ABDUCENS NERVE PALSY

Weakness of divergence appears to be a well-defined entity. It is diagnosed by five criteria:

1. There is sudden uncrossed, horizontal diplopia at distance.
2. The angle of strabismus remains unchanged or may decrease on horizontal gaze to either side.
3. When an object is brought near to the patient, the two images approach each other and become fused when the object is at a distance of 25 to 40 cm from the patient.
4. Ductions are full.
5. Fusion divergence is reduced or absent.

Divergence weakness should not be confused with convergence spasm because patients with the latter condition maintain an esotropia at near, have miotic pupils, have reduced distance visual acuity from induced myopia, and show normal fusional divergence.

One should distinguish between the syndromes of **divergence insufficiency,** in which an otherwise perfectly healthy patient develops the sudden onset of esotropia at distance, and **divergence paralysis,** in which the patient has associated neurologic disease. Divergence insufficiency is most frequently observed in young adults in the third and fourth decades of life, although it may occur at any age. In most instances, divergence insufficiency is a self-limited condition that can be treated with base-out prisms if needed. In other cases, however, extraocular muscle surgery is necessary.

Divergence paralysis appears to be produced by the same types of neurologic disorders that cause abducens paralysis, including intracranial masses, increased ICP, multiple sclerosis, epidemic encephalitis, syphilis, intracranial hemorrhage, head trauma, acute lymphoblastic leukemia, brainstem ischemia, medication effect, and as the initial sign in the Miller Fisher syndrome. We see divergence paralysis most often in patients with multiple sclerosis and in patients with increased ICP from brain tumor or pseudotumor cerebri.

The explanation for the occurrence of divergence paralysis is controversial. Some physicians believe that divergence paralysis does not exist and that all such cases are really bilateral abducens nerve pareses. Other investigators postulate the existence of a divergence center in the brainstem.

Whatever the pathogenesis of divergence weakness, patients with this disorder should be assumed to have neurologic disease until proven otherwise and should undergo an evaluation that includes neuroimaging. If no abnormalities are found, the patients may be followed or treated with prisms or surgery as noted above.

CYCLIC ESOTROPIA AND ITS RELATIONSHIP TO ABDUCENS NERVE PALSY

Cyclic, or alternate-day, esotropia is a rare condition characterized by a regularly recurring esotropia that may, at first, be mistaken for an unusual form of abducens paralysis. It usually appears in children 3 to 4 years old, but it also occurs in adults. It may ultimately become constant. The condition is unrelated to visual activity, accommodation, or the interruption of fusion. On esotropic days, a constant deviation of 30 to 40 prism diopters is typical. Cyclic esotropia occurs without any abnormalities of eyelid or pupillary activity, suggesting that it is not caused by oculomotor nerve hyperactivity. Most cases occur with regular 48-hour cycles. Although cyclic esotropia usually begins spontaneously, it may develop after strabismus surgery for an intermittent exotropia, after cataract extraction, in association with retinal detachment, in patients with optic atrophy, after traumatic aphakia, and after removal of 3rd ventricular tumors.

The etiology of cyclic esotropia is unknown. Circadian rhythmicity occurs in a variety of physiologic processes, including intraocular pressure, temperature, headache, and psychologic states. Among the suggested causes are an abnormal hypothalamic "biologic clock," incomplete or unusual cerebral dominance, prior encephalitis, and trauma. Cyclic esotropia may be a strabismus interrupted by periodic intervals of fusion, rather than normal function intermixed with periods of disturbance. Thus, central adaptation to a peripheral defect may be partly responsible for some forms of this phenomenon.

The appropriate treatment for cyclic esotropia is surgery aimed at correcting the maximum ocular deviation. Patients usually obtain good results with straight eyes and central fusion. Once corrected, the cyclic pattern does not recur, and there is no overcorrection on previously straight days.

DIAGNOSIS OF INFRANUCLEAR OPHTHALMOPLEGIA

In patients with monocular ophthalmoplegia that appears to involve more than one ocular motor nerve, or in patients with bilateral ophthalmoplegia, several possibilities must be considered. First, the etiologies may not, in fact, be neurologic. Myopathies or disorders of the neuromuscular junction may be responsible (see Chapters 20 and 21). Second, when the etiology is neurologic, the lesion may reside anywhere from the brainstem to the orbit. Intrinsic brainstem lesions may produce mixtures of ocular motor nerve pareses on one or both sides combined with supranuclear disorders of gaze. Extrinsic masses adjacent to the brainstem (especially those that grow along the clivus) and lesions within or adjacent to the cavernous sinus, such as meningiomas and pituitary adenomas, are particularly prone to produce both unilateral and bilateral ocular motor polyneuropathies. Pathologic processes including ischemia, hemorrhage, inflammation, compression, infiltration, metabolic dysfunction, toxic reactions, trauma, and degeneration may all be responsible. In most cases, the clinical history and a careful examination, when combined with appropriate neuroimaging, systemic, and otolaryngologic studies, are sufficient to identify the site and nature of the disease process.

Recurrent cranial nerve palsies may occur in patients with or without a family history of such phenomena. Some of these patients have an underlying systemic vasculopathy, most often diabetes mellitus. Others have no evidence of a systemic illness but may be found to have an asymptomatic meningeal process. Still other patients have no clinical or laboratory evidence of systemic or neurologic disease. In most cases, there is involvement of the ocular motor nerves followed or preceded by facial nerve paralysis. The relationship of such palsies to the Tolosa-Hunt syndrome, particularly when they are associated with pain, is unclear.

The effects of exogenous agents on the ocular motor system may be separated into peripheral ocular motor neuropathies, abnormal supranuclear responses (including abnormalities of the vestibulo-ocular reflex), extrapyramidal reactions, neuromuscular blockade of extraocular muscles, and myotoxic reactions. Drugs that produce damage to the ocular motor system by mechanisms involving the ocular motor nerves rarely occur compared with toxic optic neuropathies. They occur sporadically from systemic ingestion of a heterogenous group of compounds. These palsies may be confined to a single ocular motor nerve, or they may be associated with signs of other cranial or spinal nerve involvement. Toxic cranial nerve palsies, particularly ocular motor palsies, display no characteristic features by which they can be identified as toxic. Thus, presumptive diagnosis depends on history or laboratory data indicating exposure to a neurotoxic compound. The diagnosis may be further supported by other physical findings suggesting neurotoxicity and by improvement or clearing of signs following cessation of exposure to the drug in question.

Some of the substances that have been said to produce toxic ocular motor nerve pareses include antirabies vaccine, arsenic, arsphenamine, aspirin, carbon tetrachloride, chloroquine, colchicine, cytosine arabinoside, dichloroacetylene, diphenylhydantoin, ethylene glycol, gelse-

mium sempervirens, isoniazid, lead, nitrofurans, pamaquine, phenylbutazone, piperazine, thalidomide, thallium, trichloroethylene, Orthoclone OKT3, vincristine, and interferon α-2a. In none of these cases is the precise mechanism of damage clearly understood.

HYPERACTIVITY OF THE OCULAR MOTOR NERVES

Several ocular motor syndromes are characterized by hyperactivity, rather than hypoactivity, of one or more of the ocular motor nerves. The most common of these are ocular neuromyotonia and superior oblique myokymia (SOM).

OCULAR NEUROMYOTONIA

Ocular neuromyotonia is characterized by brief, episodic contractions of muscles supplied by the oculomotor, trochlear, or abducens nerves. The condition is usually unilateral, but bilateral cases occur. In most cases, the extraocular muscles corresponding to only one of the ocular motor nerves are affected; however, some patients have involvement of muscles innervated by more than one of the ocular motor nerves on one side (Fig. 17.52). In most patients, ocular

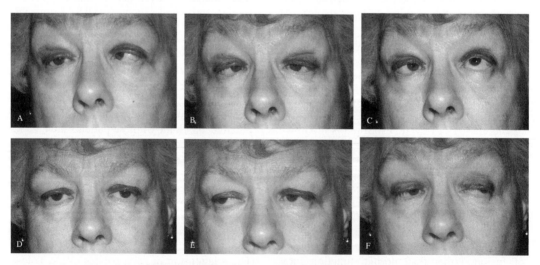

Figure 17.52. Ocular neuromyotonia. Appearance of a 62-year-old woman who had been treated with whole brain radiation for a pituitary tumor 15 years prior to her presentation. The patient had paroxysmal spasms of adduction of the right eye, left eye (A), or both eyes (B), lasting several seconds. The pupils remained normal during the spasms, and there was no evidence of accommodation spasm as might be expected if the patient was experiencing spasm of the near response. In addition, there was occasional spasm of elevation of the left eye (C). Between episodes of spasm, the eyes were straight (D) and horizontal gaze to the right (E) and left (F) was normal. The spasms initially responded to quinine (tonic water) but later required carbamazepine.

neuromyotonia is permanent; however, it resolves spontaneously in some patients and disappears with treatment in others.

Most patients who develop ocular neuromyotonia have previously received radiation therapy to the base of the skull. This is not always the case, however. For example, some patients have received radiation indirectly, as occurred in a patient who develop ocular neuromyotonia many years after he underwent myelography with iophendylate (Pantopaque, Thorotrast), a substance that is weakly radioactive. Other patients have developed the condition in the setting of dysthyroid orbitopathy.

The pathogenesis of ocular neuromyotonia is unclear. It is postulated that unstable membranes of injured ocular motor axons generate spontaneous impulses, which produce involuntary sustained and inappropriate ocular muscle contraction.

The evaluation of patients with ocular neuromyotonia, particularly those without a history of prior radiation therapy, should include MRI of the brain, with particular attention to the suprasellar region and posterior fossa. Carbamazepine is often effective in treating this condition.

SUPERIOR OBLIQUE MYOKYMIA (SUPERIOR OBLIQUE MICROTREMOR)

Superior oblique myokymia is characterized by typical symptoms of monocular blurring of vision or tremulous sensations in the eye. Patients typically experience brief episodes of vertical or torsional diplopia, vertical or torsional oscillopsia, or both. Attacks usually last less than 10 seconds but may occur many times per day. The attacks may be brought on by looking downward, by tilting the head toward the side of the affected eye, or by blinking. The eye movements of SOM are often difficult to appreciate on gross examination, although they are usually apparent during examination with the ophthalmoscope or slit lamp biomicroscope. They consist of spasms of cyclotorsional and vertical movements.

The majority of patients with SOM have no underlying disease, although cases have been reported following trochlear nerve palsy, after mild head trauma, in the setting of multiple sclerosis, after brainstem stroke, in a patient with a dural arteriovenous fistula, and in patients with cerebellar tumor. The etiology of SOM may be neuronal damage and subsequent regeneration, leading to desynchronized contraction of muscle fibers.

Superior oblique myokymia spontaneously resolves in some patients. Other patients are not bothered by their symptoms and thus do not need treatment. For patients whose symptoms are particularly distressing, both medical and surgical therapy are available. Individual patients may respond to a number of drugs, including carbamazepine, baclofen, and topically or systemically administered β-adrenergic blocking agents. Patients who do not respond to drug therapy, who develop side effects from the drugs, or who do not wish to take drugs for their condition may experience complete relief of symptoms after extraocular muscle surgery, the most successful of which is tenectomy of the affected superior oblique muscle combined with ipsilateral inferior oblique myectomy.

SYNKINESES INVOLVING THE OCULAR MOTOR AND OTHER CRANIAL NERVES

A *synkinesis* is a simultaneous movement or a coordinated set of movements of muscles supplied by different nerves or different branches of the same nerve. Normally occurring cranial synkineses are exemplified by sucking, chewing, conjugate eye movements, and Bell's phenomenon.

Abnormal cranial nerve synkineses occur most commonly in DRS (see above) and in the Marcus Gunn jaw-winking phenomenon (trigemino-ocular motor synkinesis). Similar synkineses involving various facial and neck muscles and the extraocular muscles occur in rare patients. A synkinesis between the superior oblique muscle (innervated by the trochlear nerve) and one of the muscles elevating the tongue and hyoid (innervated by the trigeminal, facial, or hypoglossal nerve) can cause double vision produced by swallowing. Similarly, bobbing movements of the eyes may be associated with jaw movements, suggesting a complex form of trigemino-ocular motor synkinesis similar to the classic Marcus Gunn jaw-winking phenomenon but involving more than just the levator muscle.

FOR MORE INFORMATION:

See Walsh & Hoyt's *Clinical Neuro-Ophthalmology,* 5th edition, Volume 1, Chapter 25, pp. 1043–1099; and Chapter 28, pp. 1189–1281.

CHAPTER 18

Supranuclear and Internuclear Ocular Motor Disorders

Supranuclear ocular motor disorders can be caused by lesions in the brainstem, cerebellum, or cerebral hemispheres. Internuclear ocular motor disorders, by definition, are caused by damage to brainstem pathways that coordinate the movements of the two eyes. In this chapter, we discuss the features and causes of supranuclear and internuclear ocular motor disorders.

OCULAR MOTOR SYNDROMES CAUSED BY LESIONS OF THE MEDULLA

The medulla contains a number of structures that are important in the control of eye movements: vestibular nuclei, perihypoglossal nuclei, medullary reticular formation, inferior olive, and restiform body (Fig. 18.1). The perihypoglossal nuclei consist of the nucleus prepositus hypoglossi (NPH), which lies in the floor of the 4th ventricle, the intercalatus nucleus, and ventrally the nucleus of Roller. These nuclei have rich connections with other ocular motor structures (Figs. 18.2 and 18.3). The NPH and the adjacent medial vestibular nucleus (MVN) are of critical importance for holding horizontal positions of gaze (the neural integrator). These structures also participate in vertical gaze-holding, although more rostral structures, especially the interstitial nucleus of Cajal (INC), also contribute. When lesions are present in the paramedian structures of the medulla, nystagmus—commonly upbeat, but sometimes horizontal with a gaze-evoked component—is the most common finding.

Lesions of the **inferior olivary nucleus** or its connections may produce the **oculopalatal myoclonus syndrome** (see Fig. 18.1). This condition usually develops weeks to months after a brainstem or cerebellar infarction, although it may also occur with degenerative conditions. The term *myoclonus* is misleading, because the movements of affected muscles are to-and-fro and are approximately synchronized, typically at a rate of 2 to 4 cycles/second.

The ocular movements present in a majority of cases consist of pendular oscillations that are often vertical but may have a horizontal or torsional component. Predominantly vertical oscillations are usually associated with symmetric bilateral palatal myoclonus. Mixed vertical-torsional movements, sometimes disconjugate and with a seesaw quality, are associated with unilateral or asymmetric palatal myoclonus. Occasionally, patients develop the eye oscillations without movements of the palate (ocular myoclonus). Eyelid closure may bring out the vertical ocular oscillations. The nystagmus sometimes disappears with sleep, but the palatal movements usually persist. Occasionally, the oscillations resolve spontaneously. Gabapentin and ceruletide may partially ameliorate the eye oscillations. The main pathologic finding with palatal myoclonus is hypertrophy of the inferior olivary nucleus; this may be identified during life by magnetic resonance imaging (MRI).

Occasionally, acute disease processes are restricted to the **vestibular nuclei.** For example, vertigo may be the sole symptom of an exacerbation of multiple sclerosis (MS) and of brainstem ischemia. Nystagmus caused by disease of the vestibular nuclei may be purely horizontal, vertical, or torsional. Mixed patterns also may occur. Moreover, nystagmus from a central vestibular lesion can mimic that caused by peripheral vestibular disease. Dolichoectasia of the basilar artery may produce a variety of combinations of central and peripheral vestibular syndromes. Microvascular compression of the vestibulocochlear nerve may also give rise to paroxysmal vertigo.

WALLENBERG'S SYNDROME (LATERAL MEDULLARY INFARCTION)

Typically, lesions of the vestibular nuclei also affect neighboring structures, especially the cer-

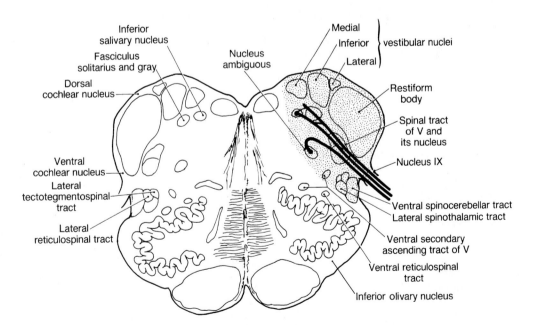

Figure 18.1. Schematic drawing of the medulla oblongata. The specific neural structures that are commonly damaged in Wallenberg's syndrome are shaded.

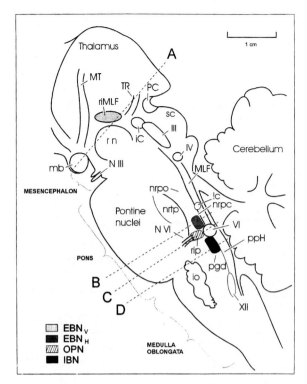

Figure 18.2. Sagittal view of a human brainstem showing the location of saccadic premotor neurons. Shaded areas mark the location of premotor saccadic neurons: excitatory medium-lead burst neurons of the horizontal *(EBN_H)* system in the nucleus reticularis pontis caudalis (nrpc) and of the vertical *(EBN_V)* system in the rostral interstitial nucleus of the medial longitudinal fasciculus *(riMLF)*. Inhibitory medium-lead burst neurons *(IBN)* are present in the nucleus paragigantocellularis dorsalis *(pgd)* and omnipause neurons *(OPN)* are present in the nucleus raphe interpositus (rip). The dashed lines *A, B, C,* and *D* indicate the planes of the corresponding sections shown in Figure 18.3. *III*, oculomotor nucleus; *IV*, trochlear nucleus; *VI*, abducens nucleus; *XII*, hypoglossal nucleus; *iC*, interstitial nucleus of Cajal; *io*, inferior olive; *mb*, mammillary body; *MLF*, medial longitudinal fasciculus; *MT*, mammillothalamic tract; *N III*, oculomotor nerve; *NVI*, abducens nerve; *lc*, locus ceruleus; *nrtp*, nucleus reticularis glossi; *rn*, red nucleus; *sc*, superior colliculus; *TR*, tractus retroflexus. (Reprinted with permission from Horn AKE, Buttner-Ennever JA, Buttner U. Saccadic premotor neurons in the brainstem: functional neuroanatomy and clinical implications. Neuro-ophthalmology 1996;16:229–240.)

Figure 18.3. Transverse sections through the human brainstem at levels indicated in Figure 18.2 to show the localization of saccadic premotor neuron groups (*shaded areas*) from rostral to caudal (*A–D*). A. The rostral interstitial nucleus of the medial longitudinal fasciculus *(riMLF)*. B. The nucleus reticularis pontis caudalis *(nrpc)*. C. The nucleus raphe interpositus *(nrp)*. D. The nucleus paragigantocellularis dorsalis *(pgd)*. E–H. Magnified views of the areas containing premotor saccadic neurons in *A–D*. Immunoreactive human neurons (only within the relevant areas) are indicated by dots. E. The riMLF contains vertical medium-lead burst neurons *(EBN_V)* *(arrow)*. F. The area containing horizontal excitatory medium-lead burst neurons *(EBN_H)* is confined to the medial part of the nrpc *(arrow)*. G. The saccadic omnipause neurons *(OPN)* are located within the rip, scattered at the midline *(arrow)*. H. The horizontal inhibitory medium-lead burst neurons *(IBN)* lie within the medial part of the pgd. *cm*, centromedian nucleus; *CTT*, central tegmental tract; *dmpn*, dorsomedial pontine nuclei; *gc*, gigantocellular nucleus; *H*, field of Forel; *hb*, habenular nuclei; *LL*, lateral lemniscus; *lv*, lateral vestibular nucleus; *mb*, mammillary body; *ML*, medial lemniscus; *MLF*, medial longitudinal fasciculus; *mv*, medial vestibular nucleus; *nd*, dorsal thalamic nucleus; *nrtp*, nucleus reticularis tegmenti pontis; *NV*, trigeminal nerve; *NVI*, abducens nerve; *NVII*, facial nerve; *ov*, nucleus ovalis; *pc*, parvocellular nucleus; *ppH*, nucleus prepositus hypoglossi; *rn*, red nucleus; *sn*, substantia nigra; *so*, superior olive; *sv*, superior vestibular nucleus; *TR*, tractus retroflexus; *Vm*, motor trigeminal nucleus; *Vs*, sensory trigeminal nucleus; *VI*, abducens nucleus; *VII*, facial nucleus. (Reprinted with permission from Horn AKE, Buttner-Ennever JA, Buttner U. Saccadic premotor neurons in the brainstem: functional neuroanatomy and clinical implications. Neuro-ophthalmology 1996;16:229–240.)

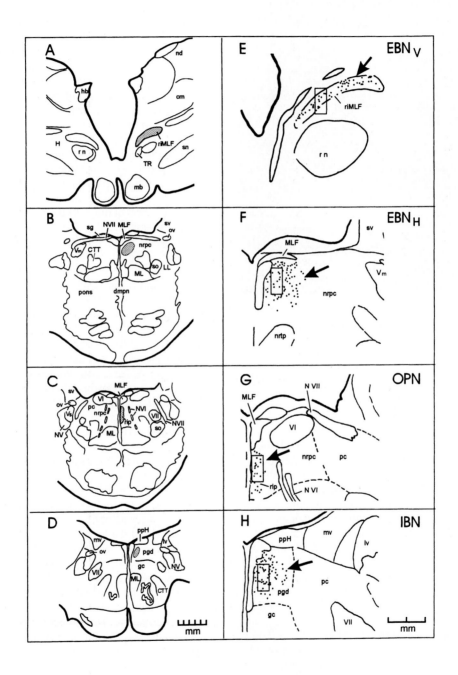

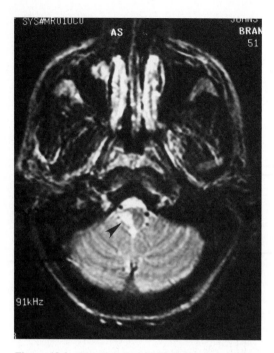

Figure 18.4. Neuroimaging of Wallenberg's syndrome. The T2-weighted magnetic resonance image (MRI), axial view, in a 51-year-old man with Wallenberg's syndrome—characterized in part by lateropulsion of saccades toward the right side, a skew deviation with the right eye being hypotropic, and the ocular tilt reaction—shows a hyperintense area (*arrowhead*) consistent with an infarct on the right side of the medulla.

ebellar peduncles and perihypoglossal nuclei. The best recognized syndrome involving the vestibular nuclei is caused by a lateral medullary infarction (Wallenberg's syndrome) (see Fig. 18.1). The typical findings of Wallenberg's syndrome are **ipsilateral** impairment of pain and temperature sensation over the face, central Horner's syndrome, limb ataxia, and a bulbar disturbance causing dysarthria and dysphagia. **Contralaterally,** pain and temperature sensation are impaired over the trunk and limbs. The facial nerve may also be affected if the infarct extends more rostrally. The disorder is most commonly caused by occlusion of the ipsilateral vertebral artery; occasionally, the posterior inferior cerebellar artery (PICA) is selectively involved (Fig. 18.4). Dissection of the vertebral artery (either spontaneous or traumatic, such as following chiropractic manipulation) is occasionally the cause. Rarely, demyelinating disease produces this syndrome.

The symptoms of Wallenberg's syndrome include vertigo and a variety of unusual sensations of body and environmental tilt, often so bizarre as to suggest a psychogenic origin. Patients may report the whole room tilted on its side or even upside down; with their eyes closed, they may feel themselves to be tilted. Similar symptoms are occasionally reported in patients without signs of lateral medullary infarction and may be caused by transient brainstem or cerebellar ischemia. Such symptoms may also occur with lesions in the cerebral hemispheres.

Lateropulsion, a compelling sensation of being pulled toward the side of the lesion, is often a prominent complaint of patients with Wallenberg's syndrome and is also evident in the ocular motor findings. If the patient is asked to fixate straight ahead and then gently close the lids, the eyes deviate conjugately toward the side of the lesion. This is reflected by the corrective saccades that the patient must make on eye opening to reacquire the target. Lateropulsion may even appear with a blink.

Saccadic eye movements are also affected by lateropulsion (Fig. 18.5). Horizontally, saccades directed toward the side of the lesion usually overshoot the target, and saccades directed away from the side of the lesion undershoot the target; this is referred to as **ipsipulsion** of saccades and should be differentiated from the **contrapulsion** of saccades that occurs with infarcts from occlusion of the superior cerebellar artery (SCA; see below). Quick phases of nystagmus are similarly affected in Wallenberg's syndrome, so saccades directed away from the side of the lesion are smaller than those directed toward the lesion. On attempting a purely vertical refixation, the patient produces an oblique saccade directed toward the side of the lesion. Corrective saccades then bring the eyes back to the target. With time, vertical saccades may become more perverse; S-shaped saccadic trajectories can appear a week or more after the onset of the illness and may reflect an adaptive strategy to correct the saccadic abnormality. **Torsipulsion**—inappropriate torsional saccades during attempted horizontal or vertical saccades—also may occur, often in association with torsional nystagmus.

When present, spontaneous **nystagmus** in Wallenberg's syndrome is usually horizontal or mixed horizontal-torsional with a small vertical component. In primary position, the slow phase is directed toward the side of the lesion, although

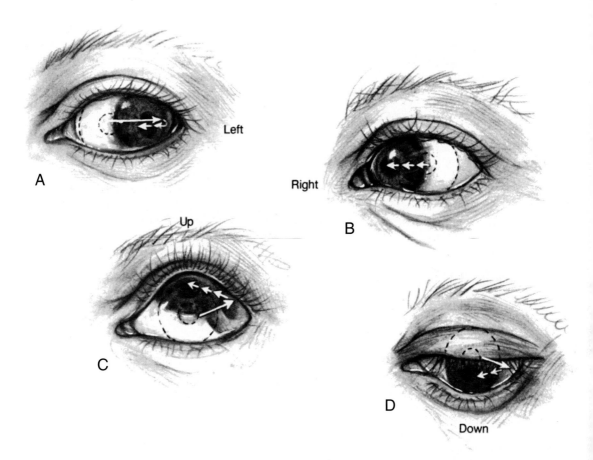

Figure 18.5. Lateropulsion of saccades in a patient with a left Wallenberg's syndrome. *A.* On attempted leftward gaze, the patient overshoots the target and must make a corrective saccade. *B.* On attempted rightward gaze, the patient makes a series of hypometric saccades. *C–D.* On attempted upward and downward gaze, the eyes move obliquely to the left and must make several refixation movements back to center. (Redrawn from Kommerell G, Hoyt WF. Lateropulsion of saccadic eye movements: electro-oculographic studies in a patient with Wallenberg's syndrome. Arch Neurol 1973;28:313–318.)

it may reverse direction in eccentric positions, suggesting coexistent abnormalities of the gaze-holding mechanism. Lid nystagmus (synkinetic lid twitches with horizontal quick phases) can also occur. The **ocular tilt reaction** (OTR; see below) commonly occurs in Wallenberg's syndrome, as does a **skew deviation,** with an ipsilateral hypotropia. The eyes counter-roll toward the side of the lesion, but unequally, so that there is a cyclodeviation. The lower eye is usually more extorted. Some patients show ipsilateral head tilt. The skew deviation and head tilt arise from imbalance in pathways mediating otolith responses (Fig. 18.6). The subjective sensations of tilt or inversion of the world probably also reflect involvement of central projections from the gravireceptors, the utricle and saccule.

Smooth pursuit is usually impaired in Wallenberg's syndrome, particularly for tracking targets moving away from the side of the lesion. Caloric testing usually shows intact horizontal canal function. During both rotational and caloric testing, there is a **directional preponderance** of slow phases, usually toward the side of the lesion. Head nystagmus also occurs in some patients.

Many of the findings in Wallenberg's syndrome, including the bizarre visual disturbances and the skew deviation, may reflect imbalance of otolith influences caused by direct damage

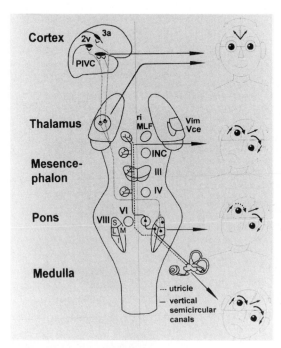

Figure 18.6. Graviceptive pathways from the otoliths and vertical semicircular canals mediating the vestibular reactions in the roll plane. The projections from the otoliths and the vertical semicircular canals to the ocular motor nuclei (trochlear nucleus *IV*, oculomotor nucleus *III*, abducens nucleus *VI*) and the supranuclear centers of the interstitial nucleus of Cajal *(INC)*, and the rostral interstitial nucleus of the medial longitudinal fasciculus *(riMLF)* are shown. They subserve vestibuloocular reflex (VOR) in three planes. The VOR is part of a more complex vestibular reaction that also involves vestibulospinal connections via the medial and lateral vestibulospinal tracts for head and body posture control. Furthermore, connections to the assumed vestibular cortex (areas *2v* and *3a* and the parietoinsular vestibular cortex, *PIVC*) via the vestibular nuclei of the thalamus (*Vim*, *Vce*) are depicted. Graviceptive vestibular pathways for the roll plane cross at the pontine level. Ocular tilt reaction (OTR) is depicted schematically on the right in relation to the level of the lesion—ipsiversive OTR with peripheral and pontomedullary lesions, contraversive OTR with pontomesencephalic lesions. In vestibular thalamus lesions, the tilts of the subjective visual vertical may be contraversive or ipsiversive; in vestibular cortex lesions, they are preferably contraversive. OTR is not induced by supratentorial lesions above the level of INC. (Reprinted with permission from Brandt T, Dieterich M. Vestibular syndromes in the roll plane: topographic diagnosis from brainstem to cortex. Ann Neurol 1994;36:337–347.)

to the caudal aspects of the vestibular nuclei. Damage to the restiform body, which carries olivocerebellar projections, may also account for some of the ocular motor findings, especially the steady-state deviation of the eyes toward the side of the lesion and the ipsipulsion of saccades. Ipsipulsion of saccades, with deviation of the eyes to the side of the lesion, can be produced experimentally by lesions of the fastigial nucleus. This finding supports the hypothesis that in Wallenberg's syndrome, the interruption of climbing fiber input to the dorsal cerebellar vermis releases Purkinje cell inhibition upon the underlying fastigial nucleus, thus leading to the equivalent of a lesion in the fastigial nucleus. An analogous increase in Purkinje cell inhibition from the flocculus to the vestibular nucleus may also play a role in the ipsilateral steady-state deviation of the eyes and the nystagmus (slow phase toward the side of the lesion) seen in these patients.

SYNDROME OF THE ANTERIOR INFERIOR CEREBELLAR ARTERY

The anterior inferior cerebellar artery (AICA) supplies portions of the vestibular nuclei, adjacent dorsolateral brainstem, and inferior lateral cerebellum. In addition, the AICA is the origin of the labyrinthine artery in most persons and also sends a twig to the cerebellar flocculus in the cerebellopontine angle. Consequently, ischemia in the distribution of the AICA may cause vertigo, vomiting, hearing loss, facial palsy, and ipsilateral limb ataxia, along with gaze-holding and pursuit deficits as well as vestibular nystagmus (Fig. 18.7). The ocular motor signs reflect a combination of involvement of the labyrinth, vestibular nuclei, and the flocculus (see below).

SKEW DEVIATION AND THE OCULAR TILT REACTION

Skew deviation is a vertical misalignment of the visual axes caused by a disturbance of prenuclear inputs. Torsional and horizontal deviations may be associated findings. The hypertropia may be the same in all positions of gaze (comitant), or it may vary and may even alternate (e.g., right hypertropia on right gaze, left hypertropia on left gaze) (incomitant or noncomitant). When skew deviation is incomitant—and especially in the pattern of an individual muscle palsy—it can only be differentiated from a vertical extraocular

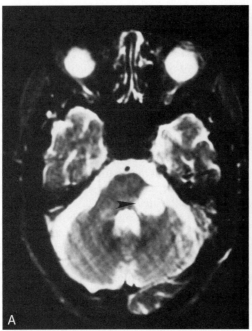
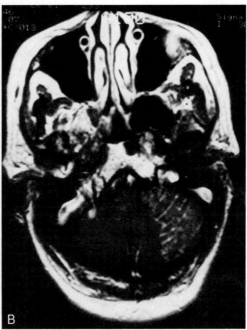

Figure 18.7. Neuroimaging of an infarct in the territory of the left anterior inferior cerebellar artery (AICA). *A.* T2-weighted axial MRI scan shows hyperintense area in the region of the left middle cerebellar peduncle (*arrowhead*). *B.* T1-weighted axial MRI scan after intravenous injection of paramagnetic contrast material shows diffuse enhancement in the distal distribution of the AICA involving the left cerebellar hemisphere. The 69-year-old patient had, among other manifestations, left-beating gaze-evoked nystagmus.

muscle palsy by the coexistence of signs of central neurologic dysfunction. Rarely, patients show a slowly **alternating skew deviation,** with each eye being hypertropic for about 30 seconds to a minute.

In some patients, skew deviation is associated with ocular torsion and head tilt, the **ocular tilt reaction,** which may be tonic (sustained) or paroxysmal (see Fig. 18.6). Such patients also show a deviation of the subjective vertical. The ocular torsion may be dissociated, producing a cyclodeviation. The OTR is usually attributed to an imbalance in otolith-ocular and otolith-collic reflexes that are part of a phylogenetically old righting response to a lateral tilt of the head. In patients with more rostral lesions, interruption of descending pathways involved with controlling head posture may also contribute to the head tilt of the OTR.

Skew deviation occurs with a variety of abnormalities in the vestibular periphery, brainstem, or cerebellum and as a reversible finding with raised intracranial pressure (ICP) from supra-

tentorial tumors or pseudotumor cerebri. In infants, a skew deviation may be the harbinger of a subsequent horizontal strabismus.

Why does skew deviation occur with lesions at a variety of sites throughout the posterior fossa? Current evidence suggests that skew deviation occurs whenever peripheral or central lesions cause an **imbalance of otolithic inputs** (see Fig. 18.6). An imbalance of posterior semicircular canal inputs may also play a role, although in this setting, nystagmus should also be present.

A knowledge of the anatomic pathways involved in the otolith-ocular reflexes is helpful in the topologic diagnosis of skew deviation, because lesions at various sites along these pathways can cause this condition. In lateral-eyed animals, tilting the head laterally around the longitudinal (anterior-posterior) axis causes a disjunctive, vertical (skew) deviation (i.e., one eye goes up, the other goes down) that acts to hold the visual axis of each eye close to the horizontal. In human subjects, who are frontal eyed, a static head tilt (ear to shoulder) causes sustained conjugate counter-rolling of the eyes (ocular torsion) that is about 10% of the head roll; thus, the static ocular response does not compensate for the head tilt and is thought to be vestigial. In contrast, peripheral or central lesions that disrupt otolithic inputs often cause large amounts of skew deviation (e.g., 7°) and ocular torsion (e.g., 25°). Usually, any pathologic head tilt (ear to shoulder) is contralateral to the hypertropic eye, and the ocular torsion is such that the upper poles of the eyes rotate toward the lower ear. It is postulated that the contralateral head tilt is a compensatory response to the perceived tilt of the subjective visual vertical, although it may also reflect direct involvement of descending projections from the vestibular nuclei or the INC to cervical motoneurons.

Lesions of the **vestibular organ or its nerve** can cause both skew deviation and the OTR by producing an imbalance in utricle inputs. The OTR may also occur as a component of **Tullio's phenomenon,** which is characterized by sound-induced vestibular symptoms. It occurs in patients with perilymph fistula either at the oval or round window, with other abnormal communications between the membranous labyrinth (particularly the anterior semicircular canal) and the perilymph space, or with abnormalities of the ossicular chain and its connection with the membranous labyrinth.

The utricle projects predominantly to the ipsilateral lateral vestibular nucleus, whereas the saccule projects to the y-group of vestibular nuclei. Thus, disease of the **vestibular nuclei** (e.g., as part of Wallenberg's lateral medullary syndrome) may also cause skew deviation with hypotropia on the side of the lesion. In addition, some patients show an ipsilateral head tilt and disconjugate ocular torsion. The latter is an excyclotropia, with excyclodeviation of the ipsilateral, lower eye, but small or absent incyclodeviation of the contralateral, higher eye. It is the absence of excyclotorsion in the hypertropic eye that allows a skew deviation to be differentiated from a trochlear nerve palsy (see Chapters 16 and 17).

Skew deviation is encountered in some patients with **cerebellar lesions.** Some of these patients show an alternating skew deviation that is characterized by a hyperdeviation of the abducting eye. This abnormality also may be analogous to a phylogenetically old, otolith-mediated, righting reflex present in lateral-eyed animals, which in this case is related to the ocular motor response that compensates for fore and aft pitch of the head. Although coexistent involvement of the brainstem is likely in some of these patients, skew deviation also occurs in some patients who appear to have pure cerebellar disease. This suggests that just as the cerebellum governs the semicircular canal-ocular reflex, it also influences the otolith-ocular reflexes. Indeed, downbeat nystagmus, which is sometimes attributable to disease of the flocculus (see below and Chapter 19), commonly coexists with skew deviation.

Utricular projections from the vestibular nuclei probably cross the midline and ascend in the medial longitudinal fasciculus (MLF). Therefore, unilateral **internuclear ophthalmoplegia** (INO) is often associated with a skew deviation. The INO usually is on the side of the hypertropic eye, possibly because lesions of one MLF cause an imbalance of ascending otolithic inputs.

In the **midbrain,** otolith projections contact the oculomotor and trochlear nerve nuclei, as well as the INC. Mesencephalic lesions in or around the INC thus may cause skew deviation and the OTR (see Fig. 18.6). When the head tilt is sustained (tonic), it is contralateral to the side of the lesion; in addition, there is usually a hypertropia that is ipsilateral to the lesion and a conjugate cyclotorsion that is characterized by intorsion of the ipsilateral eye. Associated defects of vertical eye movements and oculomotor or trochlear nerve function are common, including seesaw nystagmus. Combined prenuclear and fascicular or nuclear lesions in the midbrain may create torsion of one eye and the OTR. In some patients, the skew deviation (with or without a head tilt) is not sustained but paroxysmal. An irritative mechanism has been proposed and, indeed, stimulation in the region of the INC causes an ipsilateral OTR. Microvascular compression may also cause a paroxysmal skew deviation with torsional nystagmus.

Rarely, skew deviation slowly alternates or varies in magnitude over the course of a few minutes. The periodicity of the phenomenon is reminiscent of periodic alternating nystagmus, and the two phenomena can, in fact, coexist. Patients with this condition usually have midbrain lesions.

OCULAR MOTOR SYNDROMES CAUSED BY LESIONS OF THE CEREBELLUM

Clinicians are appropriately cautious in attributing eye movement abnormalities specifically to cerebellar dysfunction, because the brainstem is so frequently damaged in patients with lesions of the cerebellum. Nevertheless, most clinical and experimental studies provide convincing evidence that cerebellar lesions alone can cause specific ocular motor abnormalities (Figs. 18.8 and 18.9). In essence, three principal syndromes can be identified: the syndrome of the dorsal vermis and underlying posterior fastigial nuclei; the syndrome of the flocculus and paraflocculus; and the syndrome of the nodulus and ventral uvula. The main features of each of these syndromes are summarized in Table 18.1.

LOCATION OF LESIONS AND THEIR MANIFESTATIONS

Experimental lesions of the **dorsal vermis** (lobules VI and VII) and of the underlying fastigial nuclei (called the fastigial oculomotor region or FOR) cause saccadic dysmetria, typically hypometria, when the vermis alone is involved, and hypermetria when the deep nuclei are affected (see Fig. 18.9). Lesions of the deep nuclei may sometimes lead to macrosaccadic oscillations, an extreme degree of hypermetria.

The pattern of saccadic dysmetria that occurs in cerebellar disease, as well as whether corrective saccades occur, may also vary with the type of visual stimulus. Saccades to remembered targets may be more dysmetric in some patients, whereas in other patients, only corrective saccades are dysmetric. Saccadic dysmetria may be present for externally triggered movements to a visual target but not for internally triggered saccades during scanning of a visual scene. Mild deficits of pursuit may also be produced by lesions of the dorsal vermis, as may defects in motion perception. Bilateral symmetric lesions of the deep nuclei do not lead to pursuit deficits, although unilateral lesions lead to a contralateral deficit, probably because of an imbalance in eye acceleration signals.

Experimental lesions of the **flocculus and paraflocculus** cause gaze-evoked nystagmus, rebound nystagmus, and downbeat nystagmus (see Fig. 18.8). Such lesions also cause impaired smooth tracking, either with eyes alone (smooth pursuit) or with eyes and head; postsaccadic drift; and loss of some adaptive capabilities, such as the ability to adjust the gain and direction of the vestibulo-ocular reflex (VOR) or the pulse-step match for saccades. Unilateral lesions produce ipsilateral deficits in pursuit and gaze holding. In patients with cerebellar disease, pursuit defects with the head still, defects in combined eye-head tracking, and gaze-holding deficits frequently occur together, reflecting their common substrate in the flocculus and vestibular nuclei. Quantitatively, however, pursuit with the head still is sometimes relatively more impaired. Patients with cerebellar disease may show phase errors during tracking, but there is some preservation of predictive capability. The ability to generate anticipatory smooth eye movements of high speed at the onset of tracking is also impaired in some patients with cerebellar lesions.

Experimental lesions of the **nodulus** lead to an increase in the duration of vestibular responses that predisposes the animal to the development of periodic alternating nystagmus. Such lesions also produce other abnormalities of the "velocity-storage mechanism," including a failure of tilt suppression of postrotatory nystagmus and loss of habituation. Positional nystagmus usually occurs with lesions of the nodulus.

Another ocular motor sign attributable to a focal cerebellar lesion is torsional nystagmus during vertical pursuit. Patients with lesions in the middle cerebellar peduncle show this phenomenon. The direction of the torsional nystagmus changes with the direction of the pursuit, with the eye velocity of the slow phase of the torsional nystagmus being directly proportional to the eye velocity of the slow phase of pursuit. This finding probably relates to the fact that smooth pursuit is organized in, and superimposed on, a phylogenetically old vertical "labyrinthine-optokinetic" coordinate system. Thus, for a pure vertical pursuit movement to occur, opposite torsional components must cancel (as is the case for pure vertical vestibular nystagmus). The middle cerebellar peduncle probably carries information to and from the cerebellum (perhaps between the flocculus and the nucleus reticularis tegmenti pontis in the pons) that contains vertical pursuit signals encoded with a torsional component.

Other signs occur in patients with lesions restricted to the cerebellum that cannot yet be attributed to dysfunction of a particular part of

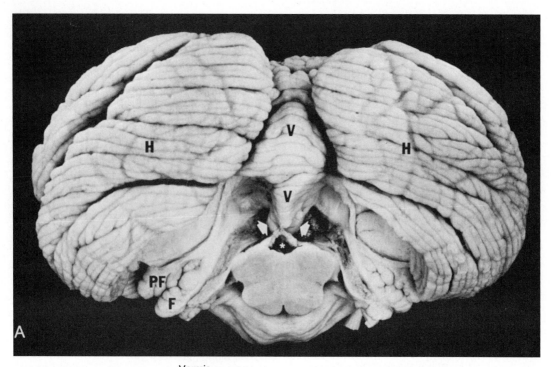

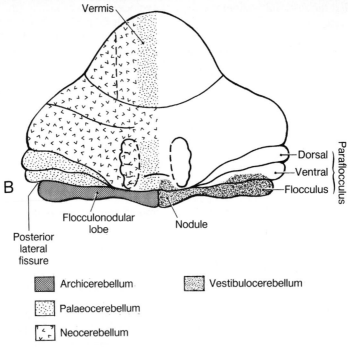

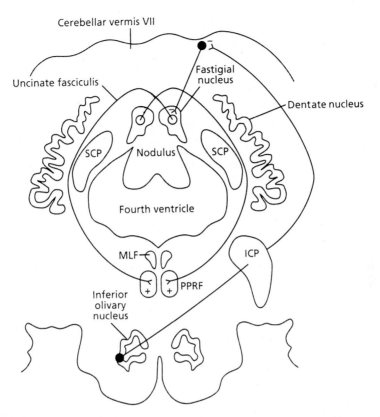

Figure 18.9. Schema of projections from the inferior olivary nuclei through the inferior cerebellar peduncle *(ICP)* to lobule VII of cerebellar cortex, where Purkinje cells inhibit the fastigial nucleus *(FN)*. The caudal part of the fastigial nucleus probably excites the contralateral paramedian pontine reticular formation *(PPRF)* via its projections in the uncinate fasciculus. A lesion in the left inferior cerebellar peduncle increases Purkinje cell activity, leading to decreased firing of the ipsilateral fastigial nucleus and decreased activation of the contralateral (right) paramedian pontine reticular formation. This causes ipsipulsion of saccades. A lesion of the left uncinate fasciculus (from the right fastigial nucleus) decreases activity in the ipsilateral paramedian pontine reticular formation, causing contrapulsion of saccades. *MLF*, medial longitudinal fasciculus; *SCP*, superior cerebellar peduncle. (Reprinted with permission from Sharpe JA, Morrow MJ, Newman NJ, et al. Continuum, Neuro-ophthalmology. American Academy of Neurology, 1995.)

Figure 18.8. The human cerebellum. *A.* Anterior inferior view shows the cerebellar hemispheres *(H)*, vermis *(V)*, flocculus *(F)*, and paraflocculus *(PF)*. *White arrowheads*, nodulus; *asterisk*, 4th ventricle. (Reprinted with permission from Ghuhbegovic N, Williams TH. The Human Brain: A Photographic Guide. Hagerstown, MD: Harper & Row, 1980.) *B.* Schematic drawing of the subdivisions of the human cerebellum. The left half of the drawing shows the three main subdivisions: the archicerebellum—the flocculonodular lobe; the paleocerebellum—the anterior vermis, the pyramis, the uvula, and the paraflocculus; and the neocerebellum. The right half of the diagram shows the structures of the vestibulocerebellum—the flocculonodular lobe and the dorsal and ventral parafloccculi. (After Brodal A. Neurological Anatomy in Relation to Clinical Medicine. 3rd ed. New York: Oxford University Press, 1981.)

Table 18.1
Localization of Cerebellar Eye Movement Abnormalities

STRUCTURE	FUNCTION	DISORDER
Dorsal vermis and posterior fastigial nucleus	Saccade accuracy, smooth pursuit	Saccadic dysmetria, impaired pursuit
Flocculus and paraflocculus	Retinal-image stabilization (smooth tracking with head still or free suppression of inappropriate vestibular nystagmus, holding positions of gaze, adaptive control of the VOR and pulse-step match)	Impaired smooth pursuit, VOR cancellation and fixation suppression of caloric nystagmus; gaze-evoked, rebound, centripetal and downbeat nystagmus; postsaccadic drift; inappropriate amplitude or direction of the VOR
Nodulus and ventral uvula	Control of low-frequency response of the VOR	Periodic alternating nystagmus, impaired tilt suppression of post-rotatory nystagmus, positional nystagmus, impaired habituation of the VOR, increased duration of vestibular responses.

the cerebellum. They include square-wave jerks, esotropia ("divergence paralysis") with alternating skew deviation, disconjugate (poorly yoked) saccades with disconjugate gaze-evoked nystagmus, divergent nystagmus, centripetal nystagmus, primary-position upbeating nystagmus, increased responsiveness of the cervicoocular reflex, and impaired responses to linear translation (L-VOR).

The cerebellum is also important in long-term **adaptive functions** that keep eye movements appropriate to the visual stimulus. For example, adaptation of the gain of the VOR is impaired in patients with cerebellar lesions. This adaptive or "repair shop" function of the cerebellum probably accounts for both the enduring nature of the ocular motor deficits that accompany diffuse cerebellar lesions and, perhaps, the somewhat variable effects of cerebellar lesions. Thus, inherent, idiosyncratic abnormalities in brainstem or peripheral ocular motor mechanisms that are normally "repaired" by the cerebellum may reappear after cerebellar lesions.

ETIOLOGIES

Developmental Anomalies

The **Arnold-Chiari malformation** is an anomaly of the hindbrain involving the caudal cerebellum (including the vestibulocerebellum, flocculus, paraflocculus [tonsils], uvula, and nodulus) and the caudal medulla. In the type 1 malformation, the cerebellar tonsils are displaced caudally into the foramen magnum, and

the medulla is elongated. A meningomyelocele usually is not present. Such patients often present with symptoms in adult life. In the type 2 malformation, both the 4th ventricle and the inferior vermis extend below the foramen magnum, the brainstem and spinal cord are thin, and a lumbar meningomyelocele is usually present. Patients with a type 2 malformation usually present in childhood, but in milder cases, the onset of symptoms is delayed until adulthood. Presenting symptoms include oscillopsia that is brought on or exacerbated by head movements, and Valsalva-induced dizziness, vertigo, cervical pain, and headaches. A variety of ocular motor abnormalities, especially downbeat nystagmus (both spontaneous and positional), occur in patients with the Chiari malformation (Table 18.2). Diagnosis is by MRI, with sagittal views of the craniocervical junction being most useful (Fig. 18.10). Patients often improve after suboccipital decompression, although it may take months for the eye movement abnormalities to diminish. A similar ocular motor syndrome may be observed in patients with other lesions located at the craniocervical junction.

The **Dandy-Walker syndrome** consists of a malformation of the cerebellar vermis, a membranous cyst of the 4th ventricle, and malformations of the cerebellar cortex and deep cerebellar nuclei. Patients with this condition often show a mild saccadic dysmetria, although some patients have normal eye movements. Ocular motor abnormalities, including nystagmus and strabis-

Table 18.2
Eye Signs in the Chiari Malformation

1. Downbeat nystagmus (occasionally with a torsional component), worse on lateral gaze
2. Sidebeat nystagmus (primary position, unidirectional, horizontal nystagmus)
3. Periodic alternating nystagmus
4. Divergent nystagmus
5. Esotropia
6. Gaze-evoked nystagmus
7. Rebound nystagmus including torsional rebound
8. Impaired pursuit (and VOR cancellation)
9. Impaired OKN with slow build-up of eye velocity in response to a constant-velocity stimulus
10. Convergence nystagmus
11. Divergence paralysis
12. Skew deviation accentuated or alternating on lateral gaze
13. Saccadic dysmetria
14. Internuclear ophthalmoplegia
15. Increased VOR gain
16. Shortened VOR time constant
17. Positional nystagmus

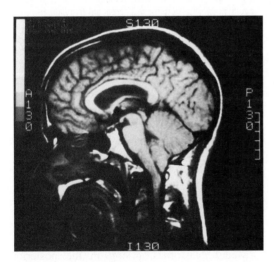

Figure 18.10. Neuroimaging of an Arnold-Chiari malformation. T1-weighted sagittal MRI shows herniation of cerebellar tonsils below the foramen magnum (*arrowhead*). Note flattening of the brainstem in this region.

mus, also occur in patients with agenesis of the vermis or hypoplasia of the entire cerebellum. Other rare syndromes associated with anomalous cerebellar development include Coffin-Siris syndrome (developmental delay, hypoto-

nia, cutaneous changes, and abnormalities of the roof of the 4th ventricle) and Joubert's syndrome (a variable combination of episodic tachypnea, psychomotor retardation, retinal dystrophy, torsional nystagmus, skew deviation, ocular motor apraxia, agenesis of the cerebellar vermis, and fibrosis of the extraocular muscles).

Degenerative Diseases

Many degenerative processes can affect the cerebellum or its connections and produce cerebellar eye signs. These disorders include the cerebellar cortical degenerations, ataxia telangiectasia, and various spinocerebellar and olivopontocerebellar degenerations (OPCDs), such as Machado-Joseph disease (a variant of autosomal-dominant spinocerebellar disease type 3) and Friedreich's ataxia. Moreover, many of these conditions also affect brainstem structures. Thus, other, presumably noncerebellar, ocular motor signs may be present (e.g., slow saccades, prolonged saccadic latencies, decreased or absent vestibulo-ocular responses, and ophthalmoplegia). It remains to be proved whether eye movement abnormalities can be used to reliably detect extracerebellar involvement or early signs of disease in persons at risk for developing hereditary ataxias. In general, patients with Friedreich's ataxia show a decrease of vestibulo-ocular responses and prominent square-wave jerks. Slow saccades point to brainstem involvement, as occurs with the spinocerebellar degenerations.

Paraneoplastic cerebellar degeneration is a rare remote effect of cancer, usually occurring with breast, ovarian, or small-cell lung cancer, and typically associated with serum and cerebrospinal fluid anti-Yo antibodies. The onset of symptoms is usually acute or subacute, with the development of severe midline and appendicular ataxia, dysarthria, and downbeat nystagmus. Pathologic studies indicate total loss of Purkinje cells in patients with this condition. Such patients have lost all output from the cerebellar cortex, and the common finding of primary-position downbeat nystagmus thus tends to confirm that asymmetric, inhibitory projections of the cerebellum to the central connections of the semicircular canals can be the cause of this nystagmus. A cerebellar syndrome may also complicate treatment of cancer or leukemia with cytosine arabinoside.

Periodic vertigo and ataxia syndromes, often responsive to acetazolamide, may be associated with prominent cerebellar eye signs, especially downbeat nystagmus. Such syndromes may be associated with migraine, essential tremor, or myokymia. Some are mapped to chromosome 19 and are best considered as channelopathies.

Vascular Diseases

The cerebellum is supplied by three branches of the vertebrobasilar circulation: the PICA, the AICA, and the SCA. Occlusion of one or more of these vessels often produces concurrent brainstem infarction, making precise clinicopathologic correlation difficult. Infarction in the distribution of the distal PICA may cause a syndrome of acute vertigo and nystagmus that often simulates an acute peripheral vestibular lesion. These symptoms probably reflect a central vestibular imbalance created by asymmetric infarction of the vestibulocerebellum. The vestibulocerebellum normally has a tonic inhibitory effect upon the vestibular nuclei, and patients with lesions in this region may have prominent gaze-evoked nystagmus that helps differentiate this cerebellar lesion from an acute peripheral vestibulopathy.

Infarction in the territory of the AICA, the branches of which often supply the flocculus, may cause vertigo, vomiting, hearing loss, facial palsy, and ipsilateral limb ataxia, along with gaze-holding and pursuit deficits as well as vestibular nystagmus (see Fig. 18.7). The ocular motor signs reflect a combination of involvement of the labyrinth, vestibular nuclei, and the flocculus.

Infarction in the territory of the SCA causes ataxia of gait and limbs and vertigo (Fig. 18.11). A characteristic abnormality is **saccadic contrapulsion.** This consists of an overshooting of contralateral saccades and an undershooting of ipsilateral saccades. Attempted vertical saccades are oblique, with a horizontal component away from the side of the lesion. Thus, this saccadic disorder is the opposite of the saccadic ipsilpulsion seen in Wallenberg's syndrome (see above) and probably reflects interruption of outputs from the fastigial nucleus running in the uncinate fasciculus next to the superior cerebellar peduncle. Infarction restricted to the posterior-inferior vermis can selectively impair pursuit and optokinetic eye movements.

Mass Lesions

Cerebellar hemorrhage, tumors, infarcts, abscesses, cysts, and extra-axial hematomas may

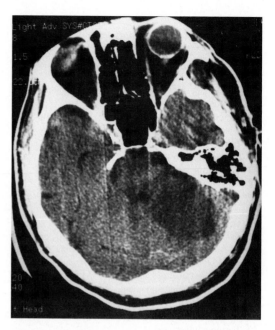

Figure 18.11. Neuroimaging of infarct in the territory of the superior cerebellar artery (SCA) in a 69-year-old man with hypertension. Computed tomographic scan shows a large hypodense area in the left cerebellar hemisphere corresponding to the distribution of the left SCA. The patient had a left horizontal gaze palsy from compression of the left side of the brainstem.

all cause cerebellar eye signs by direct damage to the cerebellar parenchyma. Cerebellar lesions, however, may also compress the brainstem and produce additional signs. Vertical or horizontal gaze disorders can occur, depending on whether the direction of compression is rostral or forward, respectively. The oculomotor, trochlear, and abducens nerves may also be affected. Ocular motor dysfunction may also be caused by secondary obstructive hydrocephalus and increased ICP.

Medulloblastomas arising in the posterior medullary velum frequently produce or are associated with positional nystagmus. Involvement of the nodulus and uvula are presumably responsible for this finding and may also account for the inability to suppress postrotational nystagmus by tilting the head. Tumors within the 4th ventricle may affect the cerebellar nuclei, vestibulocerebellum, and dorsal medulla. Upbeating nystagmus may occur in such cases.

Vestibular schwannomas (acoustic neuromas) may compress the cerebellar flocculus (which lies in the cerebellopontine angle) and produce eye signs of vestibulocerebellar lesions, including Brun's nystagmus in which there is a coarse nystagmus beating to the side of the lesion (reflecting a gaze-holding deficit) and a fine nystagmus beating away from the side of the lesion (reflecting a vestibular imbalance). Asymmetry of the caloric responses correlates with tumor size, and rotational testing may reveal abnormalities in some of these patients. MRI is the most sensitive and specific method used to detect small lesions in this region. Acute cerebellar hemorrhage frequently causes nystagmus, gaze palsy (usually toward the side of the lesion), abducens nerve palsy, and skew deviation. These signs are, caused, in part, by compression of the brainstem.

OCULAR MOTOR SYNDROMES CAUSED BY LESIONS OF THE PONS

LESIONS OF THE INTERNUCLEAR SYSTEM: INTERNUCLEAR OPHTHALMOPLEGIA

Among the fibers that comprise the MLF, many carry a conjugate horizontal eye movement command from abducens internuclear neurons in the pons to the medial rectus subdivision of the **contralateral** oculomotor nuclear complex in the midbrain (Fig. 18.12). Other fibers in the MLF carry signals for holding vertical eye position, for vertical smooth pursuit, and for the vertical VOR.

Manifestations

Lesions of the MLF produce **internuclear ophthalmoplegia** (Fig. 18.13). When the lesion is unilateral, the INO is characterized by weakness of adduction ipsilateral to the side of the lesion (Fig. 18.14). This weakness can vary from a complete loss of adduction beyond the midline to a mild decrease in the velocity of adduction without any limitation in range of motion. The fibers subserving horizontal gaze in the MLF each carry commands for all types of conjugate eye movements. Thus, vestibular slow phases, pursuit and optokinetic following movements, and saccades and quick phases of nystagmus are all affected by the MLF lesion. The weakness of adduction, however, may be more obvious for saccades because damaged axons, especially those that are demyelinated, show a greater de-

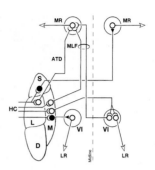

Figure 18.12. The direct horizontal VOR pathway from horizontal semicircular canal *(HC)* to medial rectus *(MR)* subnucleus of the oculomotor nucleus and to the abducens nucleus *(VI)*. Excitatory second-order vestibular neurons project to the medial rectus subnuclei through the medial longitudinal fasciculus *(MLF)* and the ascending tract of Deiters *(ATD)*. Axons of the ascending tract of Deiters actually course through the abducens nucleus without synapse (not shown). The abducens nucleus contains motoneurons of the lateral rectus muscle *(LR)* and internuclear neurons that project through the opposite medial longitudinal fasciculus to the medial rectus subnucleus on that side. *Hollow symbols:* excitatory neurons. *Solid symbols:* inhibitory neurons. Inhibition of internuclear neurons in the ipsilateral abducens nucleus is not illustrated. *S,* superior vestibular nucleus; *L,* lateral vestibular nucleus; *M,* medial vestibular nucleus; *S,* descending vestibular nucleus. (Reprinted with permission from Sharpe JA, Johnston JL. The vestibulo-ocular reflex: clinical, anatomic and physiologic correlates. In: Sharpe JA, Barber HO, eds. The Vestibulo-Ocular Reflex and Vertigo. New York: Raven Press, 1993:15–39.)

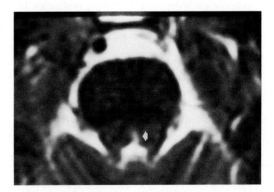

Figure 18.13. Neuroimaging in a patient with a left internuclear ophthalmoplegia. T2-weighted MRI, axial view, shows a tiny area of hyperintensity consistent with an infarct in the region corresponding to the location of the left medial longitudinal fasciculus *(arrowhead)*. The patient also had a skew deviation.

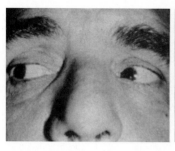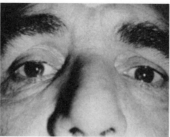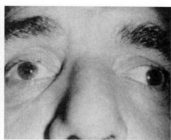

Figure 18.14. Unilateral, right internuclear ophthal-moplegia in a 32-year-old man with multiple sclerosis. Note complete lack of adduction in the right eye on attempted left horizontal gaze.

fect when carrying high-frequency as opposed to low-frequency impulses. This dissociation is reflected in a "pulse-step mismatch" that occurs because saccade speed (determined by the high-frequency "pulse" of innervation) is diminished out of proportion to the limitation in range of adduction (determined by the low-frequency "step" of innervation). This **adduction lag** is brought out clinically by asking the patient to make large-amplitude (which require the highest speeds) horizontal saccades back and forth across the midline or by using an "optokinetic" tape or drum with repetitive symbols to produce nystagmus that allows easy comparison of the movements of the two eyes.

When patients with INO are able to converge, despite absence of voluntary adduction, a caudal lesion with preservation of the medial rectus subdivision of the oculomotor nuclear complex can be assumed. Patients with INO and intact convergence were said to have a **posterior internuclear ophthalmoplegia** by Cogan. Although the presence of intact convergence is important in such cases, the absence of convergence in the setting of an INO (the "anterior" internuclear ophthalmoplegia of Cogan) does not necessarily imply a rostral lesion involving the medial rectus nuclear subdivision. Some patients simply are not able to produce a strong convergence effort, and the vertical disparity that occurs when a unilateral INO is associated with a skew deviation (see below) also may interfere with convergence effort.

In some patients with an INO, abducting saccades in the affected eye may also be slow or "fractionated." This phenomenon may reflect impaired inhibition of the affected medial rectus. Slowing of abducting saccades tends to be more prominent in bilateral INO, probably because of damage to extra-MLF pathways running through the pontine tegmentum.

The second cardinal sign of an INO is **nystagmus on abduction in the contralateral eye.** This nystagmus consists of a centripetal (inward) drift, followed by a corrective saccade that may be hypermetric, hypometric, or orthometric. It is present in nearly all patients with INO. A number of mechanisms could account for the abduction nystagmus of INO, and they may not be mutually exclusive:

1. An increase in convergence tone.
2. Impaired inhibition of the medial rectus contralateral to the lesion.
3. Interruption of descending internuclear fibers that project to the abducens nucleus.
4. A gaze-evoked nystagmus.
5. Adaptation to the contralateral medial rectus weakness.

The cause of abduction nystagmus must relate either to lesions outside the MLF or to an adaptive response to the initial adduction weakness.

Skew deviation (see Fig. 18.15) commonly occurs with unilateral INO but is rarely seen with bilateral INO. When skew deviation is associated with an INO, the higher eye is usually on the side of the lesion. In this setting, it is usually easy to differentiate the skew deviation from a trochlear nerve palsy, particularly when the higher eye shows intorsion rather than extorsion using double Maddox rods, the Lancaster red-green test, or fundus observation.

Dissociated vertical nystagmus (downbeat in the ipsilateral eye, torsional in the contralateral eye) may occur with an INO. This pattern of dissociated nystagmus reflects the finding that posterior semicircular canal pathways mediating

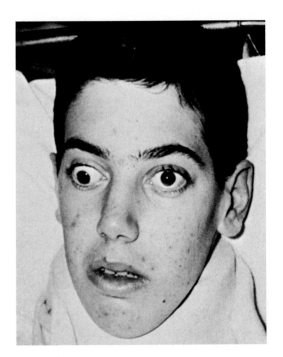

Figure 18.15. Skew deviation in a patient following an operation on the posterior fossa for a superiorly placed vermis tumor. The deviation persisted for 3 weeks. The patient also had a left internuclear ophthalmoplepia.

excitation pass through the MLF, but some anterior semicircular canal pathways do not. Patients with a unilateral INO may also have an ipsiversive torsional nystagmus (top poles of the eyes cyclorotate so as to beat toward the side of the lesion). The torsional nystagmus is sometimes dissociated and is usually but not always associated with a skew deviation. It may relate to interruption of pathways between the vestibular nuclei and the INC. Some patients with bilateral

INO have impaired fixation. In such patients, sporadic bursts of monocular abducting saccades may occur in each eye.

Patients with bilateral INO have bilateral adduction weakness and abducting nystagmus (Fig. 18.16). Such patients also have impaired vertical vestibular and pursuit eye movements and impaired vertical gaze holding with gaze-evoked nystagmus on looking up or down.

Many patients with an INO have no visual symptoms, particularly when there is no limitation of adduction. In other cases, either limitation of adduction or skew deviation may cause diplopia that is horizontal, vertical, or oblique. Patients with INO occasionally complain of oscillopsia. Horizontal oscillopsia usually occurs from either the adduction lag or the abduction nystagmus, whereas vertical oscillopsia occurs during head movements and is caused by a deficient vertical VOR. In many patients, visual symptoms become less bothersome or resolve completely, either because of recovery of function of MLF axons or because of central adaptive mechanisms.

Lesions that damage the MLF may also damage the abducens nucleus, fascicle, or both on either side of the brainstem. Lesions that damage the MLF on one side and the ipsilateral abducens nucleus produce the one-and-a-half syndrome (see below), whereas lesions that damage the ipsilateral abducens fascicle produce horizontal ophthalmoplegia in the ipsilateral eye from the combination of an INO and an abducens nerve palsy. Lesions that damage the MLF on one side and the paramedian pontine reticular formation (PPRF) or abducens nucleus on the opposite side produce a horizontal gaze palsy toward the side of the damaged PPRF or abducens nucleus. In such cases, the INO cannot be diagnosed because of

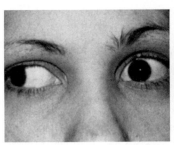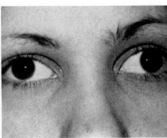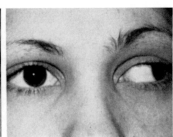

Figure 18.16. Bilateral internuclear ophthalmoplegia in a young woman with multiple sclerosis. The pupils have been dilated with mydriatics.

Table 18.3
Etiology of Internuclear Ophthalmoplegia

1. Multiple sclerosis (commonly bilateral); post-irradiation demyelination
2. Brainstem infarction (commonly unilateral), including complication of arteriography; hemorrhage
3. Brainstem and 4th ventricular tumors and mesencephalic clefts
4. Chiari malformation, and associated hydrocephalus and syringobulbia
5. Infection: bacterial, viral and other forms of meningoencephalitis; in association with AIDS
6. Hydrocephalus; subdural hematoma; supratentorial arteriovenous malformation
7. Nutritional disorders: Wernicke's encephalopathy and pernicious anemia
8. Metabolic disorders: hepatic encephalopathy, maple syrup urine disease, abetalipoproteinemia, Fabry's disease
9. Drug intoxications: phenothiazines, tricyclic antidepressants, narcotics, propranolol, lithium, barbiturates, D-penicillamine, toluene
10. Cancer: either due to carcinomatous infiltration or remote effect
11. Head trauma, including cervical hyperextension or manipulation
12. Degenerative conditions: progressive supranuclear palsy
13. Syphilis
14. Pseudo-internuclear ophthalmoplegia of myasthenia gravis and Fisher's syndrome

the overriding horizontal gaze palsy. Damage to the MLF on one side and to the contralateral abducens nerve fascicle will produce abduction weakness of the contralateral eye combined with adduction weakness of the ipsilateral eye. In this setting, there will be a "pseudo-horizontal gaze palsy" on attempted horizontal gaze away from the side of the MLF lesion. The diagnosis may be suspected in a patient who appears to have a horizontal gaze palsy that is asymmetric, with one eye (usually the adducting eye) being much more limited than the other.

Etiologies

Table 18.3 summarizes some etiologies of INO. In general, a unilateral INO is most commonly caused by ischemia, although even in these cases there is often subtle involvement of the other side. Bilateral INO is commonly caused by demyelination. Although MRI frequently shows a lesion in the MLF in patients with INO (see Fig. 18.13), there are many exceptions.

LESIONS OF THE ABDUCENS NUCLEUS

Lesions of the abducens nucleus cause an ipsilateral palsy of horizontal conjugate gaze because

the abducens nucleus contains two groups of neurons: abducens motoneurons that innervate the ipsilateral lateral rectus muscle and abducens internuclear neurons that innervate the contralateral medial rectus motor neurons via the MLF (Fig. 18.17). Vergence movements of the eyes are spared however, so adduction is possible with a near stimulus. Most often, the abducens nucleus is affected in association with adjacent tegmental structures, particularly the genu of the facial nerve, the MLF, and the PPRF (Fig. 18.18). Lesions restricted to the abducens nucleus can often be distinguished from those in the adjacent caudal PPRF, because only in the latter may pursuit and vestibular movements be spared, and only in the former may ipsilateral saccades in the contralateral field be spared by virtue of intact inhibition upon the contralateral abducens nucleus. Gaze-evoked nystagmus on contralateral gaze also occurs in patients with presumed abducens nucleus lesions. Possible mechanisms for the gaze-evoked nystagmus include damage to adjacent vestibular or NPH pathways that are involved in neural integration for gaze holding, or damage to the paramedian cells and tracts that lie in part in the rostral abducens nucleus and have reciprocal connections with the cerebellar flocculus, a structure also involved in gaze holding.

LESIONS OF THE PARAMEDIAN PONTINE RETICULAR FORMATION

The PPRF, which corresponds principally to medial portions of the nucleus pontis centralis caudalis, contains burst neurons that are important in the generation of saccades, and the paramedian nucleus raphe interpositus contains pause neurons that inhibit burst neurons at all times except during saccades.

Destructive lesions of the PPRF, such as infarction and hemorrhage, tend to affect all cell groups, along with fibers of passage that convey pursuit and vestibular signals to the ipsilateral abducens nucleus. **Unilateral** destructive lesions cause an ipsilateral, conjugate, horizontal gaze palsy. With acute lesions, the eyes may be deviated contralaterally. Nystagmus occurs when gaze is directed into the intact contralateral field of movement with quick phases directed away from the lesioned side; this is usually accentuated in darkness. Ipsilaterally directed saccades and quick phases are small and slow and do not carry the eye past the midline. Vertical saccades may be slightly slow, and an inappropriate horizontal component, directed away from

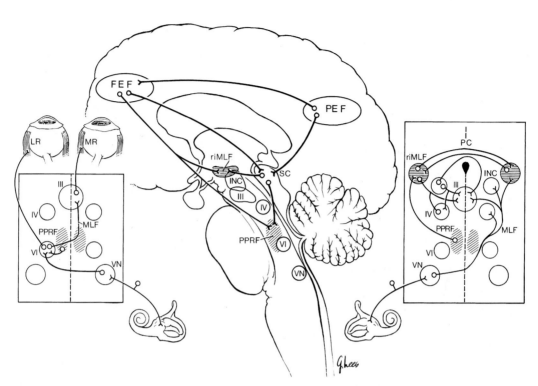

Figure 18.17. Summary of saccadic and vestibular eye movement control. The center figure shows the supranuclear connections from the frontal eye fields *(FEF)* and the parietal eye field *(PEF)* to the superior colliculus *(SC)*, rostral interstitial nucleus of the medial longitudinal fasciculus *(riMLF)*, and the paramedian pontine reticular formation *(PPRF)*. The FEF, PEF, and SC are involved in the production of saccades. The schematic drawing on the left shows the brainstem pathways for horizontal gaze. Axons from the cell bodies located in the PPRF travel to the ipsilateral abducens nucleus *(VI)*, where they synapse with abducens motoneurons whose axons travel to the ipsilateral lateral rectus muscle *(LR)* and with abducens internuclear neurons whose axons cross the midline and travel in the medial longitudinal fasciculus *(MLF)* to the portions of the oculomotor nucleus *(III)* concerned with medial rectus *(MR)* function (in the contralateral eye). The schematic drawing on the right shows the brainstem pathways for vertical gaze. Important structures include the riMLF, PPRF, the interstitial nucleus of Cajal *(INC)*, and the posterior commissure *(PC)*. Note that axons from cell bodies located in the vestibular nuclei *(VN)* travel directly to the abducens nuclei and, most via the MLF, to the oculomotor nuclei. *IV*, trochlear nucleus.

the side of the lesion, may occur during attempted vertical saccades.

Smooth-pursuit movements and slow phases of optokinetic nystagmus may be preserved in both directions within the intact field of movement of a patient with a lesion of the PPRF, but they usually cannot bring the eyes across the midline. Sometimes horizontal pursuit is asymmetrically impaired, more so for contralateral target motion. In some patients with PPRF lesions, vestibular stimuli drive the eyes past the midline. Presumably, in such individuals either the ipsilateral abducens nucleus and its direct vestibular input are intact, or the PPRF lesion is more rostral. With more restricted lesions, usually hemorrhages, both smooth pursuit and the VOR are preserved, but saccades are absent or slow. Occasionally in such patients, vestibular stimuli can drive only the contralateral adducting eye and not the ipsilateral abducting eye into the ipsilateral field. This finding implies a lesion of one PPRF and the ipsilateral abducens nerve but sparing the abducens nucleus.

Bilateral lesions restricted to the PPRF are uncommon. Discrete infarction or tumor can cause a selective loss of saccades, leaving smooth pursuit and the VOR relatively preserved. Such a selective deficit implies loss or dysfunction of saccadic burst neurons but sparing of fibers of passage conveying smooth pursuit and the VOR. Patients with horizontal gaze palsies may substitute convergence for impaired conjugate adduction and then cross-fixate to extend their range of view. Furthermore, during the recovery phase

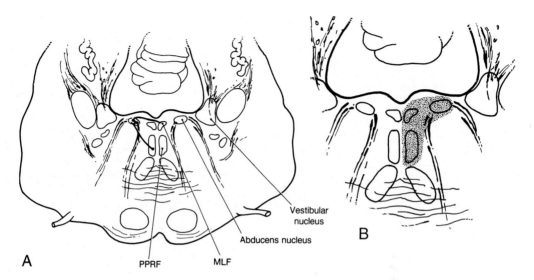

Figure 18.18.   Drawing of the pons at the level of the abducens nuclei. *A*. Drawing illustrates the important structures involved in the production of horizontal gaze. *MLF*, medial longitudinal fasciculus; *PPRF*, paramedian pontine reticular formation. Note that neurons project from the PPRF to the abducens nucleus and that neurons in the abducens nucleus are both motoneurons whose axons represent the abducens nerve and internuclear neurons whose axons ascend in the *contralateral* MLF. *B*. The areas that may be involved when a one-and-a-half syndrome is present. Note that involvement of either the abducens nucleus or the PPRF can cause the horizontal gaze palsy. Damage to the ipsilateral medial longitudinal fasciculus produces the internuclear ophthalmoplegia. (Modified from Sharpe JA, Rosenberg MA, Hoyt WF, et al. Paralytic pontine exotropia: a sign of acute unilateral pontine gaze palsy and internuclear ophthalmoplegia. Neurology 1974;24:1076–1081.)

from bilateral gaze palsies from vascular lesions, involuntary synkinetic divergence and convergence movements may appear with horizontal or vertical gaze. Bilateral pontine lesions may abolish all horizontal eye movements, but reflexive eye movements may be spared, particularly with chronic lesions such as tumors.

Bilateral pontine lesions may impair vertical eye movements. It is well established that signals for vertical vestibular and smooth-pursuit eye movements ascend in the MLF and other pathways through the pons, and it also seems likely that pontine lesions can cause impairment of vertical saccades. This view is supported by reports of abnormal (usually slow) vertical saccades in patients with discrete, bilateral pontine lesions and by similar findings in monkeys with bilateral neurotoxic lesions of the PPRF. Pause cells project rostrally to vertical burst neurons located in the midbrain. Pontine lesions, therefore, may lead to desynchronization of vertical (and horizontal) burst neuron discharge and, consequently, to slow vertical (and horizontal) saccades.

COMBINED UNILATERAL CONJUGATE GAZE PALSY AND INTERNUCLEAR OPHTHALMOPLEGIA (ONE-AND-A-HALF SYNDROME)

Combined lesions of the abducens nucleus or PPRF and adjacent MLF on one side of the brainstem cause an ipsilateral horizontal gaze palsy and an INO. The only preserved horizontal eye movement is abduction of the contralateral eye, hence the name **one-and-a-half syndrome** (Figs. 18.18 and 18.19). Patients with this condition may have an exotropia when attempting to look straight ahead; the eye opposite the side of the lesion deviates outward. This strabismus is thought to be caused by the unopposed drives of the intact pontine gaze center. Thus, the condition is often called **paralytic pontine exotropia.**

Many patients, however, have an esotropia or no deviation in primary position (as with many cases of INO). The spared abduction saccades of the contralateral eye are followed by centripetal drift, so a nystagmus similar to that of the abducting eye in INO is present.

Occasionally, the ipsilateral horizontal vestib-

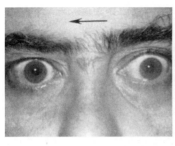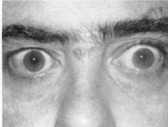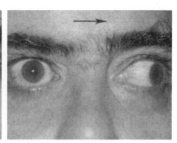

Figure 18.19.   One-and-a-half syndrome in a 23-year-old man with multiple sclerosis. Arrows indicate direction of attempted gaze. All ocular motor signs cleared within 3 months after onset.

ular responses are preserved when voluntary gaze is abolished, suggesting that the pontine lesion is more rostral in the PPRF or more discrete in the caudal PPRF, thus sparing the vestibular projections to the abducens nucleus. Although attempts at conjugate (version) movements elicit no adduction, vergence movements may be preserved in such cases. Ocular bobbing may accompany the one-and-a-half syndrome.

The one-and-a-half syndrome may result from brainstem ischemia, hemorrhage, tumor infiltration, trauma, or demyelination.

SLOW SACCADES FROM PONTINE LESIONS

Certain metabolic, toxic, and degenerative conditions can cause selective deficits of ocular motility suggestive of predominant loss of one population of brainstem neurons concerned with eye movements. Such a process may explain both slow saccades and saccadic oscillations (see Chapter 19) in patients with lesions in the pons.

Slow saccades are characteristic of many degenerative and metabolic diseases (Table 18.4). Horizontal saccades may be slowed in patients with spinocerebellar or olivopontocerebellar degenerations; vertical saccades are often relatively less affected in such patients. In diseases that principally affect the midbrain, such as progressive supranuclear palsy (PSP), vertical saccades are the first to become slow. In some patients with slow saccades, blinks of the eyelids may actually speed up the movements. Patients with spinocerebellar degenerations usually make saccades that have normal amplitudes despite their low velocity. PSP, however, causes both slow and small horizontal saccades. Patients with slow saccades may use a variety of strategies of eye-head coordination to move their eyes more quickly to the target.

Table 18.4
Etiology of Slow Saccades

1. Olivopontocerebellar atrophy and related spinocerebellar degenerations
2. Huntington's disease
3. Progressive supranuclear palsy
4. Parkinson's disease (advanced cases) and related diseases; Lytico-Bodig
5. Whipple's disease
6. Lipid storage diseases
7. Wilson's disease
8. Drug intoxications: anticonvulsants, benzodiazepines
9. Tetanus
10. Dementia: Alzheimer's disease (stimulus-dependent) and AIDS-associated
11. Lesions of the paramedian pontine reticular formation
12. Internuclear ophthalmoplegia
13. Peripheral nerve palsy; diseases affecting the neuromuscular junction and extraocular muscle; restrictive ophthalmopathy
14. Paraneoplastic syndromes

OCULAR MOTOR SYNDROMES CAUSED BY LESIONS OF THE MESENCEPHALON

SITES AND MANIFESTATIONS OF LESIONS

Disturbances of vertical eye movements from midbrain lesions usually are caused by damage to one or more of three main structures: the posterior commissure, the rostral interstitial nucleus of the medial longitudinal fasciculus (riMLF), and the interstitial nucleus of Cajal (see Figs. 18.2, 18.3, and 18.17).

Posterior Commissure

Lesions of the **posterior commissure** cause a syndrome characterized by loss of upward gaze and a number of other associated findings (Table 18.5 and Figs. 18.20 through 18.22). The condition is known by a variety of names: Parinaud's

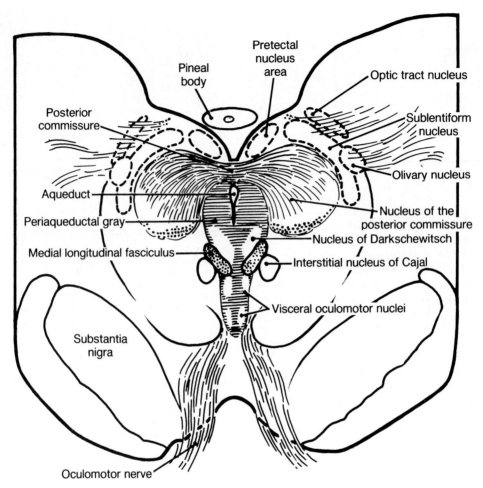

Figure 18.20. Drawing of the major pretectal nuclei. Note relationship of the posterior commissure to other structures. (Reprinted with permission from Carpenter MB, Pierson RJ. Pretectal region and the pupillary light reflex: an anatomical analysis in the monkey. J Comp Neurol 1973;149:271–300.)

syndrome, Koerber-Salus-Elschnig syndrome, pretectal syndrome, dorsal midbrain syndrome, and the sylvian aqueduct syndrome. Unilateral midbrain lesions can also create the same ocular motor syndrome, but probably by interrupting the afferent and efferent connections of the posterior commissure.

Although paralysis of upward gaze has, in the past, been ascribed to destruction of the superior colliculi, this is not the case. Experimental lesions restricted to the superior colliculus in nonhuman primates produce no limitation of upward gaze but rather defects in latency and accuracy for saccades and increased numbers of inappropriate saccades.

The vertical gaze deficit (Fig. 18.23) caused by

lesions of the posterior commissure usually affects all types of eye movements, although the VOR and Bell's phenomenon may sometimes be spared. Below the horizontal meridian, vertical saccades can be made but are usually slow. Acutely, the eyes may be tonically deviated downward (**setting-sun sign**); this finding is prominent in premature infants who have suffered intraventricular hemorrhage. Transient downward deviation of the eyes occasionally occurs in healthy neonates, but in such cases, the eyes can be easily driven above the horizontal meridian by the vertical doll's head maneuver. Tonic upward deviation of the eyes occurs in some patients with midbrain lesions. Oculogyric crises may also occur in patients with midbrain

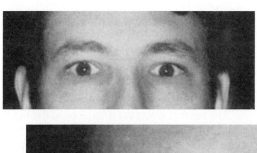
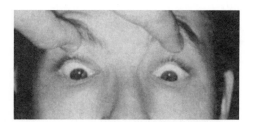
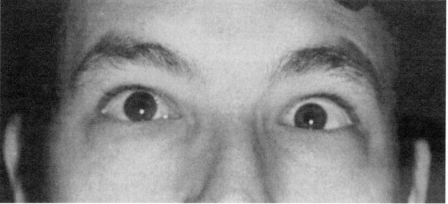

Figure 18.21. Appearance of a patient with Parinaud's dorsal midbrain syndrome. *Above left:* The eyes are straight in primary position. Note bilateral upper eyelid retraction. *Above right:* Downward gaze is normal. *Below:* There is marked limitation of upward gaze bilaterally, worse on the left, producing a right hypertropia. (Reprinted with permission from Bajandas FJ, Aptman M, Stevens S. The sylvian aqueduct syndrome as a sign of thalamic vascular malformation. In: Smith JL, ed. Neuro-Ophthalmology Focus 1980. New York: Masson, 1979:401–406.)

lesions. Episodic tonic upgaze may occur in otherwise normal infants and in patients with cerebellar ataxia.

The dorsal midbrain syndrome is also characterized by disturbances of horizontal eye movements, especially vergence. In some patients, convergence is paralyzed, whereas in others it is excessive, resulting in **convergence spasm.** During horizontal saccades, the abducting eye may move more slowly than its adducting fellow eye. This finding is called **pseudo-abducens palsy** and may reflect an excess of convergence tone. It may lead to an early symptom of posterior commissure lesions—reading difficulty caused by a transient inability to find, and to focus both eyes on, the beginning of the next line when a horizontal saccade is made.

Convergence-retraction nystagmus may occur in patients with disease of the midbrain (Fig. 18.24). This disorder presumably results from damage to the posterior commissure, because it can be produced by experimental lesions restricted to this structure. Convergence-retrac-

tion nystagmus is best regarded as a saccadic disorder because it consists of asynchronous, opposed saccades.

Eyelid abnormalities occur in patients with dorsal midbrain lesions. The most common is eyelid retraction (Collier's tucked lid sign), but ptosis may occasionally occur (see Fig. 18.21). In some cases, the eyelid abnormalities are more significant than the eye movement abnormalities.

Pupillary size and reactivity are commonly abnormal in patients with lesions of the midbrain in the region of the posterior commissure (see Chapter 15). The pupils are usually large and react better to an accommodative stimulus than to light (i.e., light-near dissociation).

A variety of disease processes can affect the region of the posterior commissure (Table 18.6). Pineal tumors produce the dorsal midbrain syndrome either by direct pressure on the posterior commissure or by causing obstructive hydrocephalus. Hydrocephalus may produce this syndrome by enlarging the aqueduct and 3rd ventricle or the suprapineal recess, thus stretching or

Table 18.5
Features of the Dorsal Midbrain Syndrome

1. Limitation of upward eye movements (Parinaud's syndrome):
   Saccades
   Smooth pursuit
   Vestibulo-ocular reflex
   Bell's phenomenon
2. Lid retraction (Collier's sign); occasionally ptosis
3. Disturbances of downward eye movements:
   Downward gaze preference ("setting sun" sign)
   Downbeating nystagmus
   Downward saccades and smooth pursuit may be impaired, but vestibular movements are relatively preserved
4. Disturbances of vergence eye movements:
   Convergence-retraction nystagmus (Koerber-Salus-Elschnig syndrome)
   Paralysis of convergence
   Spasm of convergence
   Paralysis of divergence
   "A" or "V"-pattern exotropia
   Pseudo-abducens palsy
5. Fixation instability (square-wave jerks)
6. Skew deviation
7. Pupillary abnormalities (light-near dissociation)

compressing the posterior commissure. Shunt dysfunction may produce Parinaud's syndrome before dilation of the ventricles is apparent on neuroimaging or measures of ICP are consistently high.

Rostral Interstitial Nucleus of the Medial Longitudinal Fasciculus

The **rostral interstitial nucleus of the medial longitudinal fasciculus,** which lies in the prerubral fields of the mesencephalon, contains the burst neurons that generate vertical and torsional saccades (see Figs. 18.2, 18.3, and 18.17). The riMLF lies dorsomedial to the rostral half of the red nucleus, medial to the fields of Forel, lateral to the periventricular gray and the nucleus of Darkschewitsch, and immediately rostral to the INC. The right and left riMLF are connected, probably via the posterior commissure dorsally and perhaps also by a commissure that lies ventral to the aqueduct. Bilateral experimental lesions of the riMLF abolish all vertical and torsional saccadic movements.

Lesions of the riMLF are usually infarcts in the distribution of a small perforating vessel (the posterior thalamosubthalamic paramedian artery) that arises between the bifurcation of the basilar artery and the origin of the posterior communicating artery (Figs. 18.23, and 18.25 through 18.28). This vessel may be paired or single. It supplies structures that include the riMLF, rostromedial

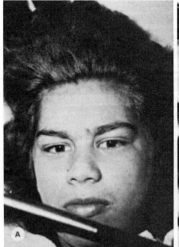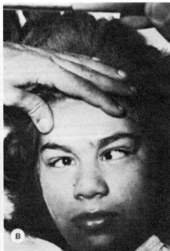

Figure 18.22. Dorsal midbrain syndrome. *A.* Gaze straight ahead. *B.* On attempted upward gaze, the patient develops convergence-retraction nystagmus.

red nucleus, adjacent subthalamus, the posterior inferior portion of the dorsomedial nucleus, and the parafascicular nucleus of the thalamus. Lesions of the riMLF usually produce a downgaze palsy, mainly affecting saccades. Rarely, they cause a complete vertical gaze palsy.

Unilateral lesions of the riMLF produce slowed or abolished saccades in the vertical plane. Unilateral lesions also cause a contralaterally beating torsional nystagmus, a tonic torsional deviation to the contralateral side, and a deficit in generating ipsilateral directed torsional quick phases (top pole rolling to the side of the lesion).

Bilateral lesions of the riMLF are more common than unilateral lesions. They cause either loss of downward saccades or loss of all vertical

saccades (Fig. 18.29). Although vertical smooth pursuit and the VOR may be affected with lesions in this area, this probably reflects damage to nearby structures, such as the MLF and INC.

The vertical one-and-a-half syndrome consists of loss of all downward movements and selective loss of upward movements in one eye or impairment of all upward eye movements and a selective deficit of downward saccades in the eye on the side of the lesion. Unilateral lesions of the midbrain can produce combined upgaze and downgaze palsies, isolated upgaze palsies, or a monocular elevator palsy, as well as the vertical one-and-a-half syndrome. Lesions of the adjacent **periaqueductal gray matter** of the midbrain may cause an imbalance of the vertical gaze-holding mechanism.

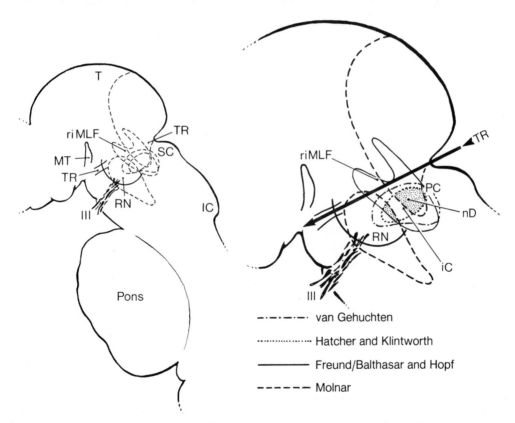

Figure 18.23.   Locations of lesions producing isolated paralysis of upward gaze. *Left:* The schematic drawing of four lesions giving rise to upward gaze paralysis have been superimposed on a sagittal section of the human brainstem. *Right:* The enlargement of the lesions shows that the common areas involved *(stippled regions)* include the interstitial nucleus of Cajal *(iC)*, the nucleus of Darkschewitsch *(nD)*, and fibers of the posterior commissure *(PC)*. *IC,* inferior colliculus;

MT, mammillothalamic tract; *riMLF,* rostral interstitial nucleus of the medial longitudinal fasciculus; *RN,* red nucleus; *SC,* superior colliculus; *T,* thalamus; *TR,* tractus retroflexus; *III,* oculomotor nerve. (Redrawn from Büttner-Ennever JA, Büttner U, Cohen B, et al. Vertical gaze paralysis and the rostral interstitial nucleus of the medial longitudinal fasciculus. Brain 1982;105:125–149.)

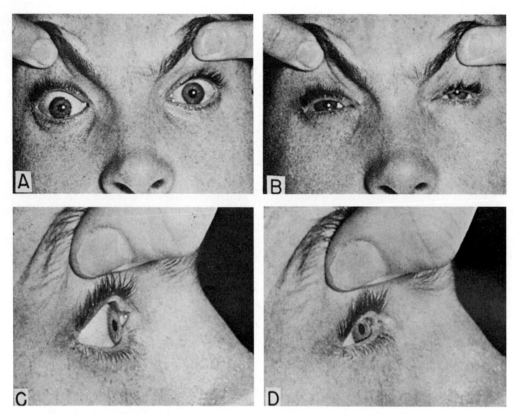

Figure 18.24. Dorsal midbrain syndrome. *A*. Position of eyes in primary position. *B*. Retraction on attempted upward gaze. *C*. Lateral view of right eye when the patient is looking straight ahead. *D*. On attempted upward gaze, obvious retrac-

tion of the globe occurs. (Reprinted with permission from Lyle DJ, Mayfield FH. Retraction nystagmus: a case report. Am J Ophthalmol 1954;37:177–182.)

Interstitial Nucleus of Cajal

Lesions restricted to the **interstitial nucleus of Cajal** may produce two distinct deficits: an ocular tilt reaction (see above) and a defect in vertical pursuit and vertical gaze holding. In the OTR, there is a contralesional tonic torsional deviation and a contralesional beating torsional nystagmus. A jerk seesaw nystagmus may occur in patients with lesions that damage the INC, and the INC may also contribute to dynamic properties of the VOR, so-called velocity storage. Lesions in the midbrain produce a change in the phase of the VOR, and electric stimulation of the INC in humans produces torsional nystagmus and the OTR.

Other Sites and Manifestations

Unilateral, paramedian midbrain lesions sometimes cause impairment of ipsilateral, horizontal smooth pursuit by affecting the descend-

ing smooth-pursuit pathway. Contralateral saccades may also be affected, but the horizontal VOR tends to be spared (Roth-Bielschowsky phenomenon). Paramedian midbrain lesions also often damage the oculomotor nerve nucleus, thereby producing a combination of nuclear and prenuclear deficits. Lesions that damage the oculomotor nucleus are characterized by bilateral elevator and eyelid weakness, because the superior rectus subnucleus is located contralaterally, and the levator subnucleus is located in the midline (see Chapter 17). Pupillary abnormalities are common in patients with such lesions. Occasionally, large midbrain lesions also cause complete loss of horizontal eye movements.

Rarely, midbrain lesions selectively impair the function of both elevator muscles (the superior rectus and inferior oblique muscles) of one eye. This **double elevator palsy** is thought to be supranuclear in origin, because in the primary

Table 18.6
Etiology of Disorders of Vertical Gaze

1. **Tumor.** Classically, pineal germinoma or teratoma in an adolescent male; also pineocytoma, pineoblastoma, glioma, metastasis
2. **Hydrocephalus.** Usually aqueductal stenosis leading to dilation of the 3rd ventricle and aqueduct or enlargement of the suprapineal recess with pressure on the posterior commissure
3. **Vascular.** Midbrain or thalamic hemorrhage or infarction; subdural hematoma
4. **Metabolic.** Lipid storage disease: Niemann-Pick variants, Gaucher's disease, Tay-Sachs disease; maple syrup urine disease; Wilson's disease; kernicterus
5. **Drug-induced.** Barbiturates, carbamazepine, neuroleptic agents
6. **Degenerative.** Progressive supranuclear palsy, Huntington's disease, cortical basal degeneration, Lytico-Bodig syndrome, diffuse Lewy body disease; miscellaneous degenerations
7. **Miscellaneous.** Multiple sclerosis, Whipple's disease, hypoxia, encephalitis, syphilis, aneurysm, neurosurgical procedure, mesencephalic clefts, tuberculoma, trauma, benign transient form of childhood

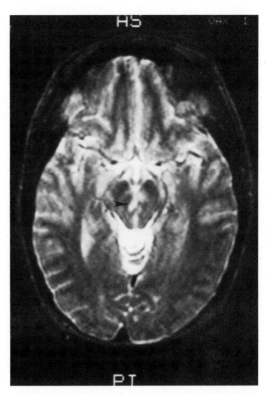

Figure 18.25. Neuroimaging of a lesion in a patient with bilateral conjugate vertical saccadic gaze palsy and cognitive dysfunction. T2-weighted axial MRI shows a hyperintense midline lesion (*arrowhead*) affecting the region of the rostral interstitial nucleus of the medial longitudinal fasciculus.

position the eyes are nearly straight, and only when the patient looks upward does a vertical disconjugacy become evident. This condition may be acquired, occurring most often in patients with midbrain infarction or tumor, but it also may be congenital.

When the condition is acquired, the lesion may be ipsilateral or contralateral to the eye with the palsy. Because the superior rectus is a stronger elevator than the inferior oblique, certainty of weakness of the latter muscle is sometimes lacking. If, however, both the inferior oblique and the superior rectus muscles are clearly weak, a nuclear lesion is unlikely, because these two muscles are supplied by the ipsilateral and contralateral oculomotor subnuclei, respectively. More likely, prenuclear inputs to the oculomotor nuclei are impaired in such patients, in whom the VOR is variably affected.

A monocular elevator palsy may be associated with a contralateral downgaze palsy. Occasionally, a "monocular elevator palsy" may be caused by a lesion selectively involving the inferior oblique and superior rectus muscle fascicles of the oculomotor nerve as it exits the brainstem. In most instances, however, a monocular paresis of elevation results from causes other than midbrain disease, such as thyroid ophthalmopathy, blowout fracture of the orbit, or myasthenia gravis.

NEUROLOGIC DISORDERS THAT PRIMARILY AFFECT THE MESENCEPHALON

Progressive Supranuclear Palsy

Progressive supranuclear palsy is a degenerative disease of later life characterized by disturbances of tone and posture leading to falls, difficulties with swallowing and speech, and mental slowing. The disturbance of eye movements is usually present early in the course of the disease, but it occasionally is noted late or not at all. The condition is usually fatal within 6 years of onset, death commonly being caused by aspiration pneumonia. Although familial cases of PSP occur and appear to be inherited in an autosomal-dominant fashion, the disease is usually sporadic.

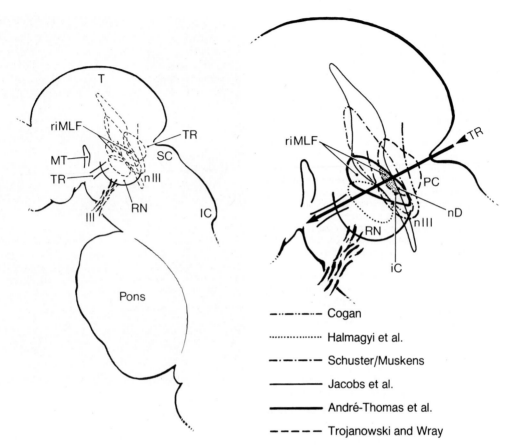

Figure 18.26. Locations of lesions producing isolated paralysis of downward gaze. *Left:* Sagittal section through the human brainstem on which the bilaterally destroyed areas in the six autopsied cases of isolated downward gaze paralysis are superimposed. *Right:* The enlargement of the lesions shows that the common area destroyed in these cases (*stippled region*) lies dorsal to the red nucleus at the level of the tractus retroflexus *(TR)*—that is, around the rostral interstitial nucleus of the medial longitudinal fasciculus *(riMLF)* and the nucleus of Darkschewitsch *(nD). iC,* interstitial nucleus of Cajal; *IC,* inferior colliculus; *MT,* mammillothalamic tract; *PC,* posterior commissure; *RN,* red nucleus; *SC,* superior colliculus; *T,* thalamus; *III,* oculomotor nerve; *n III,* oculomotor nucleus. (Redrawn from Büttner-Ennever JA, Büttner U, Cohen B, et al. Vertical gaze paralysis and the rostral interstitial nucleus of the medial longitudinal fasciculus. Brain 1982;105:125–149.)

A variety of eyelid abnormalities occur in patients with PSP. These include typical blepharospasm, apraxia of eyelid closing or opening, lid retraction, and lid lag. More than one of these abnormalities may coexist in a single patient.

The initial ocular motor deficit of PSP consists of **impairment of vertical saccades and quick phases.** Downward saccades are usually affected first and are usually more severely impaired than upward saccades, at least in the early stages of the disease. Impaired saccades are at first slow and later also small, with eventual complete loss of voluntary vertical refixations. Vertical smooth pursuit is usually relatively preserved,

and the VOR is intact until later in the disease, although a characteristic nuchal rigidity may make the vertical doll's head maneuver difficult.

Many patients with PSP first complain of visual difficulties related to the disturbance of vertical, and particularly downward, saccades. These complaints include problems with near tasks, particularly reading and eating. Such patients can be helped by providing them with a separate set of reading glasses so that they don't have to use bifocal or progressive-lens glasses, which require them to look downward through a small lower area of the spectacle lens for near viewing.

Horizontal eye movements also show characteristic disturbances in patients with PSP. Typical abnormalities include impaired fixation with square-wave jerks, impaired pursuit, impaired vestibular cancellation, and saccades and quick phases that are small and eventually slow. In some patients, the abnormality of voluntary horizontal eye movements resembles an INO; however, vestibular stimulation may overcome the limitation of adduction in such cases. Convergence eye movements are also commonly impaired in patients with PSP. Late in the disease, the ocular motor deficit may progress to a complete ophthalmoplegia.

PSP is a diffuse brainstem disorder, although cortical involvement may also be important. Both computed tomographic (CT) scanning and MRI show atrophy of the midbrain and dilation of the quadrigeminal cisterns, cerebral aqueduct, and 3rd and 4th ventricles. Histologically, neuronal loss, neurofibrillary tangles, and gliosis principally affect the brainstem reticular formation and

the ocular motor nuclei. The midbrain may bear the brunt of the early pathology, accounting for the relative vulnerability of vertical saccades. Thus, the slow, vertical saccades probably result from dysfunction of burst neurons in the riMLF, whereas the neck stiffness, often with dorsiflexion, may be caused by damage to the INC, which contributes to the control of eye-head movements. Abnormalities are also present in the nucleus raphe interpositus in the pons in which omnipause neurons, important for control of velocity and amplitude of both horizontal and vertical saccades, are located. Pursuit abnormalities may reflect damage to the deep pontine nuclei.

The differential diagnosis of PSP includes a similar syndrome caused by multiple infarcts affecting the basal ganglia, internal capsule, and midbrain. Hydrocephalus may also mimic PSP, and PSP should be differentiated from the pathologically distinct cortical-basal ganglion degeneration, which may affect vertical and horizontal

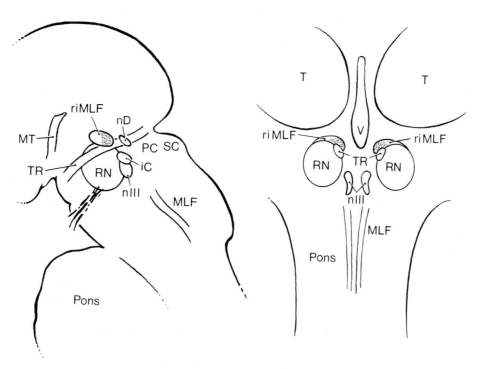

Figure 18.27.   Smallest area critical for the selective mediation of downgaze (*stippled area*). *Left:* Sagittal view of the brainstem as seen from the midline. *Right:* Coronal view of the critical region as seen from a rostral approach. Note that the involved region is rostral to the posterior commissure *(PC)* in a region that has been designated as the rostral interstitial nucleus of the medial longitudinal fasciculus *(riMLF)*. *iC*, interstitial nucleus of Cajal; *MLF*, medial longitudinal

fasciculus; *MT*, mammillothalamic tract; *nD*, nucleus of Darkschewitsch; *n III*, oculomotor nucleus; *RN*, red nucleus; *SC*, superior colliculus; *T*, thalamus; *TR*, tractus retroflexus; *V*, 3rd ventricle. (Redrawn from Pierrot-Deseilligny C, Chain F, Gray F, et al. Parinaud's syndrome: electro-oculographic analysis of six cases with deductions about vertical gaze organization in the premotor structures. Brain 1982; 105:667–696.)

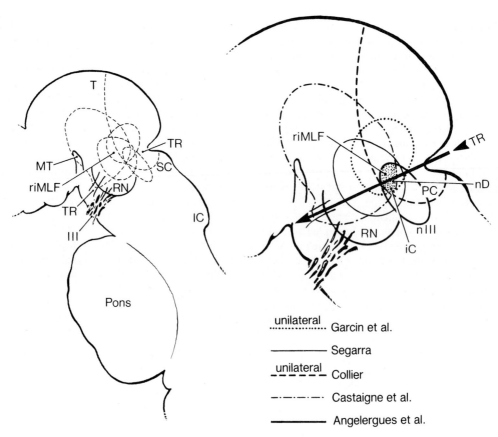

unilateral
·················· Garcin et al.

——————— Segarra

unilateral
– – – – – Collier

–·–·–·– Castaigne et al.

——————— Angelergues et al.

Figure 18.28. Locations of brainstem lesions that produce paralysis of both upward and downward gaze. *Left:* Five *unilateral* or *bilateral* lesions producing upward and downward gaze paralysis are superimposed on a sagittal section of the human brain. *Right:* The enlargement shows the common area involved (*stippled region*). This area includes parts of the rostral interstitial nucleus of the medial longitudinal fasciculus (*riMLF*), the interstitial nucleus of Cajal (*iC*), and the nucleus of Darkschewitsch (*nD*). *IC*, inferior colliculus; *MT*, mammillothalamic tract; *PC*, posterior commissure; *RN*, red nucleus; *SC*, superior colliculus; *T*, thalamus; *TR*, tractus retroflexus; *III*, oculomotor nerve; *n III*, oculomotor nucleus. (Redrawn from Büttner-Ennever JA, Büttner U, Cohen B, et al. Vertical gaze paralysis and the rostral interstitial nucleus of the medial longitudinal fasciculus. Brain 1982;105:125–149.)

gaze but which also causes focal dystonia, ideomotor apraxia, alien hand syndrome, myoclonus, and an asymmetric akinetic-rigid syndrome with late onset of gait or balance disturbances. PSP must also be differentiated from Parkinson's disease. Although upward gaze may be limited in both PSP and Parkinson's disease, impaired downward gaze, slow vertical saccades, abnormal horizontal saccades, and square-wave jerks are much more characteristic of PSP. Diffuse Lewy body disease may present a problem in differential diagnosis and mimic PSP or Parkinson's disease. Other basal ganglia disorders that may mimic PSP include idiopathic striatopallidodentate calcification, autosomal-dominant parkin-

sonism and dementia with pallidopontonigral degeneration, multisystem atrophy (MSA), and OPCD.

Whipple's Disease

Whipple's disease is a rare, multisystem infectious disorder characterized by weight loss, diarrhea, arthritis, lymphadenopathy, and fever that may involve and even be confined to the central nervous system (CNS). This disease can cause a defect of ocular motility that may mimic PSP. Initially, vertical saccades and quick phases are abnormal; eventually, however, all eye movements may be lost. A highly characteristic finding is pendular vergence oscillations and concurrent contractions of the masticatory muscles, **oculo-**

masticatory myorhythmia. The pendular vergence oscillations are always associated with a vertical saccade palsy. Ophthalmoplegia may occur in association with myorhythmia of the leg, but not of the eyes or jaw. Whipple's disease can be diagnosed using molecular analysis and can be treated with antibiotics.

OCULAR MOTOR SYNDROMES CAUSED BY LESIONS OF THE THALAMUS

Thalamic lesions are characterized by disturbances of both horizontal and vertical gaze. Conjugate deviation of the eyes **contralateral** to the

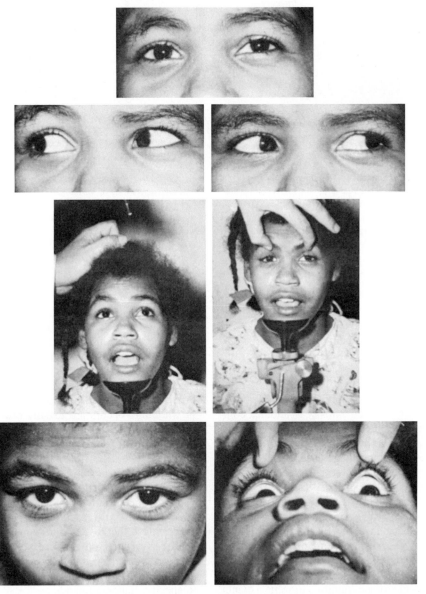

Figure 18.29. Supranuclear vertical ophthalmoplegia in a patient with a metabolic storage disease (DAF syndrome). *Top:* In primary position, the patient's eyes are straight. She is also able to make normal voluntary horizontal eye movements. *Middle:* The patient cannot make voluntary upward or downward vertical eye movements. *Bottom:* On oculocephalic testing, full vertical ocular excursions are elicited. (Reprinted with permission from von Noorden GK, Maumenee AE. Atlas of Strabismus. 2nd ed. St Louis: CV Mosby, 1973:161.)

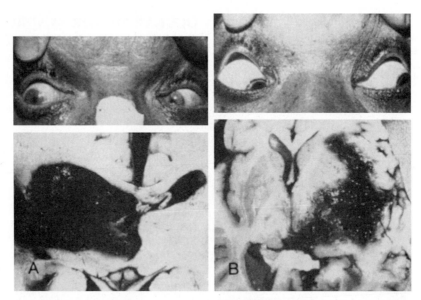

Figure 18.30. Contralateral ("wrong-side") gaze deviation with supratentorial, thalamic-basal ganglia hemorrhage. *A, top:* The patient's eyes are deviated to the right. *A, bottom:* Coronal section immediately posterior to the mammillary bodies shows a left intracerebral hemorrhage involving the thalamus, internal capsule, and basal ganglia. *B, top:* In another patient, the eyes are deviated down and left. *B, bottom:* Horizontal section through the mid-diencephalon reveals a right intracerebral hemorrhage involving the pretectum, thalamus, posterior limb of the internal capsule, globus pallidus, and putamen. In both patients, the hemorrhage also involved the lateral midbrain tegmentum. (Reprinted with permission from Keane JR. Contralateral gaze deviation with supratentorial hemorrhage: three pathologically verified cases. Arch Neurol 1975;32:119–122.)

side of the lesion (also called wrong-way deviation) may occur with hemorrhage affecting the medial thalamus (Fig. 18.30). The cause of this contraversive deviation is unclear, but it may be an irritative phenomenon.

Forced downward deviation of the eyes, with convergence and miosis, is another common feature of thalamic hemorrhage; affected patients appear to peer at their noses. In autopsied cases, the hemorrhage usually extends into or compresses the midbrain. Hence, forced downward deviation of the eyes may represent either an irritant effect of the hemorrhage on structures responsible for downward gaze or an imbalance created by an acute upgaze palsy. Resolution of the downward deviation occurs after treatment of raised ICP; thus, traction on mesencephalic structures or hydrocephalus may be responsible for the condition in some patients.

Esotropia occurs in patients with caudal thalamic lesions and may be quite marked. Although it is usually associated with downward gaze de-

viation, it may occur as an isolated finding. The esotropia that occurs with thalamic lesions may reflect a disturbance of vergence inputs to the oculomotor nuclei.

Combined lesions of the thalamus and midbrain may cause paresis of convergence. Patients in whomthis occurs are usually orthophoric in primary position during distance viewing but develop a significant exotropia during attempted near viewing.

Patients with posterolateral thalamic infarctions may have disturbances of the subjective visual vertical (either ipsilateral or contralateral). The ocular tilt reaction is not present, however, unless the rostral midbrain is also damaged. Associated disturbances of arousal and short-term memory occur in some patients with thalamic lesions and may be caused by damage to specific thalamic nuclei.

Patients with central thalamic lesions show defects in double-step saccade paradigms, suggesting that information for saccades programmed using extraretinal information about eye position must pass through the thalamus and possibly the internal medullary lamina.

Patients with lesions of the pulvinar develop difficulties in shifting attention and gaze into the contralateral hemifield, manifested by a paucity and prolonged latency of visually guided saccades. These results indicate the importance of this thalamic nucleus in directing visual attention.

OCULAR MOTOR ABNORMALITIES AND DISEASE OF THE BASAL GANGLIA

A number of diseases characterized by damage to the basal ganglia are associated with specific disturbances of ocular motility and alignment.

PARKINSON'S DISEASE

Patients with Parkinson's disease may show a number of ocular findings. Steady fixation is often disrupted by square-wave jerks, and upward gaze is often moderately restricted, although this abnormality frequently is observed in normal, elderly persons. Convergence insufficiency is a particularly common and often symptomatic disturbance.

Saccades in Parkinson's disease are characteristically hypometric, particularly when patients are asked to perform rapid, self-paced refixations between two stationary targets. Saccades made in anticipation of the appearance of a target light or to a remembered target location are also hypometric, and patients with Parkinson's disease have difficulty in generating sequences of memory-guided saccades to all types of stimuli. In contrast, saccades made **reflexively** to novel visual stimuli are of normal amplitude and usually promptly initiated. Patients with mild Parkinson's disease perform normally on the antisaccade task, but with advanced disease, errors increase, especially when patients are also taking anticholinergic drugs.

Clinically, the saccadic initiation defect to command or to continuously visible targets appears to be more marked in the vertical plane. Upward saccades especially may be hypometric. In contrast, vertical saccades to randomly appearing visual targets are normal. If downward saccades are abnormal, or the velocity of vertical saccades in either direction is decreased, PSP is a more likely diagnosis than Parkinson's disease.

Eye-head movements may be abnormal in Parkinson's disease. Affected patients tend not to move their heads unless instructed to do so. During rapid eye-head gaze shifts in response to either predictable or nonpredictable step displacements of the target, patients show increased latency and slowing of head or eye movements.

Smooth-pursuit movements are usually impaired in Parkinson's disease, although the defect is minimal in mildly affected patients. During tracking of a target moving in a predictable, sinusoidal pattern, pursuit gain (eye velocity/target velocity) is decreased, leading to catch-up saccades. Because the catch-up saccades are hypometric, however, the cumulative tracking eye movement is less than that of the target, and this may be the main mechanism for defective smooth tracking. Visual cancellation of the VOR is abnormal so that during combined active eye-head tracking, gain (gaze velocity/target velocity) is reduced.

Patients with the syndrome of amyotrophic lateral sclerosis + parkinsonism + dementia (Lytico-Bodig syndrome)—which is encountered in the inhabitants of the islands of the South Pacific Ocean, including Guam—may show more severe deficits than patients with idiopathic Parkinson's disease, including limitation of vertical gaze. Patients with diffuse Lewy body disease, Creutzfeldt-Jakob disease, multisystem atrophy, cortical-basal ganglion degeneration, and PSP must also be distinguished from idiopathic Parkinson's disease. Antisaccade testing is abnormal in cortical-basal ganglion degeneration and in PSP (see above).

Oculogyric crises, once encountered mainly in patients with postencephalitic parkinsonism, now occurs primarily as a side effect of drugs, especially neuroleptic agents. A typical attack begins with feelings of fear or depression, which give rise to an obsessive fixation of a thought. The eyes typically deviate upward and sometimes laterally (Fig. 18.31); they rarely deviate downward. During the period of upward deviation, the movements of the eyes in the upper field of gaze appear nearly normal. Affected patients have great difficulty looking down, except when they combine a blink and downward saccade. Thus, the ocular disorder may reflect an imbalance of the vertical gaze-holding mechanism. Anticholinergic drugs promptly terminate both the thought disorder and the ocular devia-

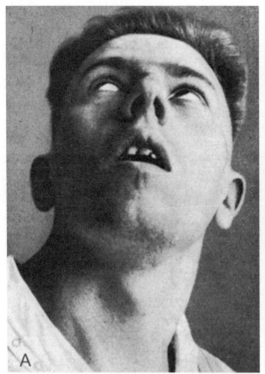
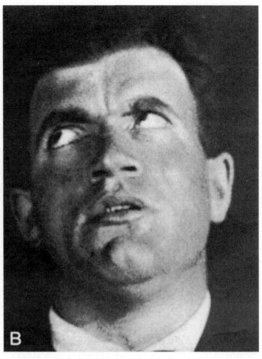

Figure 18.31. Oculogyric crisis in patients with postencephalitic parkinsonism. *A.* In a young man. Note hyperextension of neck, opening of the mouth, and conjugate deviation of the eyes up and to the right. *B.* In a middle-aged man. Again, the eyes are conjugately deviated up and to the right. (Reprinted with permission from Kyrieleis W. Die Augenv-

eränderungen bei entzündlichen Erkrankungen des Zentralnervensystems. III. Die nichteitrigen entzündlichen Erkrankungen des Zentralnervensystems. A. Die nichteitrige epidemische Encephalitis (Encephalitis epidemica, lethargica). In: Schieck F, Brückner A, eds. Kurzes Handbuch der Ophthalmologie. Vol 6. Berlin: Julius Springer, 1931:712–738.)

tion, a finding that suggests that the disorders of thought and eye movements are linked by a pharmacologic imbalance common to both.

Oculogyric crises are distinct from the brief upward ocular deviations that occur in Tourette's syndrome, Rett's syndrome, and in most patients with tardive dyskinesia. In some patients with tardive dyskinesias, however, the upward eye deviations are longer lasting and also have the characteristic neuropsychologic features of oculogyric crises, thus making the differentiation between the two entities difficult, if not impossible.

In general, treatment of Parkinson's disease with dopaminergic drugs such as L-dopa does not seem to improve the ocular motor deficits, except for saccadic accuracy (i.e., saccades become larger). Occasionally, reversal of saccadic slowing occurs with treatment, and newly diag-

nosed patients with idiopathic Parkinson's disease may experience improved smooth pursuit after institution of dopaminergic therapy.

HUNTINGTON'S DISEASE

Huntington's disease produces disturbances of voluntary gaze, particularly **saccades.** The disease is caused by a genetic defect of the IT15 gene (the "Huntington" gene) on chromosome 4, producing a CAG triplet repeat. Initiation of saccades in patients with Huntington's disease may be difficult. Such patients show prolonged latencies, especially when the saccade is to be made on command or in anticipation of a target moving in a predictable fashion. An obligatory blink or head turn may be used to start the eye moving. Saccades may be slow in the horizontal or vertical plane. This deficit can often be detected early in the disease if eye movements are measured, but it may not be evident clinically until late in the course. Saccades may be slower in patients who become symptomatic at an earlier age, and such persons are more likely to have inherited the disease from their father. Longitudinal studies of saccades can be used to quantify the progression of the disease.

Smooth pursuit may be impaired with decreased gain in patients with Huntington's disease, but it often is relatively spared compared with saccades. By contrast, gaze holding and the VOR are preserved. Late in the disease, rotational stimulation causes the eyes to deviate tonically with few or no quick phases.

Fixation is abnormal in some patients with Huntington's disease because of saccadic intrusions. Thus, these patients have difficulty initiating voluntary saccades but show an excess of extraneous saccades during attempted fixation. Studies reveal an excessive distractibility in, for example, an antisaccade task. A second finding is that saccades to visual stimuli are made at normal latency, whereas those made to command are delayed. These findings may be related to the parallel pathways that control the various types of saccadic responses. On the one hand, disease affecting either the frontal lobes or the caudate nucleus, which inhibits the pars reticulata of the substantia nigra (SNpr), may lead to difficulties in initiating voluntary saccades in tasks that require learned or predictive behavior. On the other hand, Huntington's disease also affects the SNpr. Because the SNpr inhibits the superior colliculus and therefore suppresses reflexive saccades to visual stimuli, one might expect excessive distractibility during attempted fixation. The slowing of saccades may reflect damage to saccadic burst neurons, but at least some pathologic evidence suggests that disturbance of prenuclear inputs, such as the superior colliculus or frontal eye fields (FEF), is responsible.

Despite the nearly ubiquitous finding of abnormal eye movements in patients with Huntington's disease, some persons with the disease who are evaluated before they become symptomatic show normal eye movements. Thus, routine testing of eye movements cannot be regarded as a reliable method for determining which offspring of affected patients will go on to develop the disease. The abnormal eye movements that occur in patients with Huntington's disease may improve in patients treated with sulpiride.

OTHER DISEASES OF BASAL GANGLIA

A number of conditions other than Parkinson's and Huntington's diseases that affect the basal ganglia cause abnormal eye movements. Hepatolenticular degeneration (Wilson's disease) and juvenile dystonic lipidosis (Niemann-Pick type 2s) are discussed below. Other conditions include caudate hemorrhage, which is sometimes associated with ipsilateral gaze preference, and, rarely, Sydenham's chorea. Patients with bilateral lesions in the lentiform nucleus show prominent abnormalities in saccades that require an internal representation of the target (remembered saccades, saccades to sequences, predictive saccades) but have normal responses for visually guided saccades, including antisaccades (which are nonetheless triggered by a visual target). Defects in control of predictive pursuit eye movements may also be a feature of striatal damage.

Patients with Tourette syndrome may show a variety of ocular abnormalities, including blepharospasm and eye tics that are sometimes associated with involuntary gaze deviations; however, saccades, fixation, and pursuit are normal when tested using conventional laboratory paradigms. The gaze deviations that occur in patients with Tourette syndrome must be distinguished from benign eye movement tics, which children often outgrow.

Routine ocular motor functions are normal in most patients with essential blepharospasm. In some studies, however, abnormal saccade latencies are seen for both visually guided and memory-guided saccades, suggesting a possible basal ganglia localization. Patients with spasmodic torticollis may show abnormalities in vestibular function, including the torsional VOR. Patients with tardive dyskinesia may show increased saccade distractibility.

OCULAR MOTOR SYNDROMES CAUSED BY LESIONS IN THE CEREBRAL HEMISPHERES

ACUTE UNILATERAL LESIONS

Following an acute destructive lesion of one cerebral hemisphere, the eyes usually deviate conjugately toward the side of the lesion (Prevost's or Vulpian's sign) (Fig. 18.32). Gaze deviations are more common after large strokes involving predominantly the right post-Rolandic cortex (Fig. 18.33). Visual hemineglect often ac-

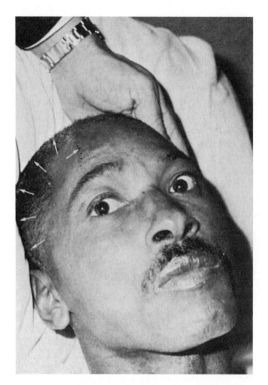

Figure 18.32. Persistent hemispheral (supranuclear) horizontal gaze palsy following severe frontal head trauma. Five weeks before this photograph was taken, the patient sustained a severe blow to the head, causing a depressed right frontal skull fracture. Operation disclosed extensive contusion and necrosis of the right frontal lobe (*arrows* indicate the site of the surgical incision). The patient had akinetic mutism and was hemiplegic on the right side. His eyes remained in right conjugate gaze at all times, but he could follow a very slowly moving target to the left.

gaze palsies associated with pontine lesions (see above). When quick phases of caloric nystagmus directed away from the side of the lesion are absent, consciousness is usually impaired (consequent to shift of intracranial contents), but exceptions occur. Sometimes, in addition to ipsiversive deviation of the eyes, there is a small-amplitude nystagmus with ipsilateral quick phases. The slow phases of this nystagmus may reflect unopposed pursuit drives directed away from the side of the lesion. Vertical saccades may be abnormal; they are dysmetric with an inappropriate horizontal component toward the side of the lesion. Because both hemispheres usually must be activated to elicit a purely vertical saccade, the loss of one hemisphere may be the cause of such oblique saccades.

When acute right cerebral hemisphere lesions cause conjugate deviation of the eyes, the lesions are located predominantly in the subcortical frontoparietal region and the internal capsule. In the left hemisphere, the lesions are usually larger, covering the entire frontotemporoparietal area. The larger the lesion, the more persistent the conjugate deviation. Both the pursuit and the saccade deficits associated with conjugate deviation of the eyes are predominantly contralateral, but as the conjugate deviation resolves, an ipsilateral pursuit defect becomes more apparent. Craniotopic defects in saccades and especially pursuit may outlast the conjugate deviation, being greater in the field contralateral to the lesion. The initial conjugate deviation may reflect the effect on eye movements of cerebral hemisphere asymmetries in attention mechanisms, whereas the more enduring eye movement defects after the conjugate deviation resolves may reflect more specific defects in motor control mechanisms mediated by the hemispheres.

Conjugate eye deviation is occasionally "wrong way"—contralateral to the side of the lesion. The lesions are almost always hemorrhagic, most commonly in the thalamus (see above). Affected patients usually have signs of rostral brainstem dysfunction and a shift of midline structures. Epileptic phenomena, impairment of ipsilateral pursuit pathways, and more caudal damage to descending pathways near the brainstem are evoked as explanations. In most cases, the last cause seems most plausible. Acute hemisphere lesions may cause epileptic seizures with contralateral deviation of the eyes or nys-

companies such gaze deviations. Gaze deviation that occurs after a stroke usually resolves within a few days to a week. Persistence of gaze deviation in this setting occurs only if there is a previous lesion in the contralateral frontal lobe. In general, for comparably sized lesions, ocular motor defects—both pursuit and saccades—are more profound when the lesion is in the nondominant hemisphere.

In the acute phase, patients may not voluntarily direct their eyes toward the side of the intact hemisphere, in part because of neglect. Shortly thereafter, however, vestibular stimulation usually produces a full range of horizontal movement (with the slow phase), in contrast to most

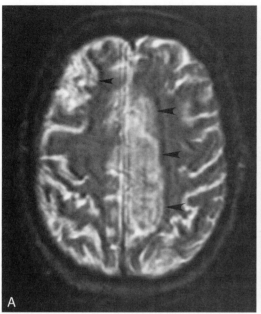 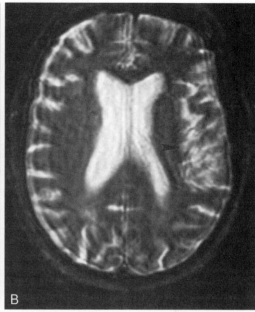

Figure 18.33. Neuroimaging of an acute infarct in the territory of the left anterior cerebral and middle cerebral arteries. *A.* T2-weighted axial MRI shows diffuse hyperintensity in the distribution of the left anterior cerebral artery (*large arrowheads*). Note also small area of hyperintensity in the right frontal region, consistent with an old infarct (*small arrowhead*). *B.* T2-weighted MRI at a lower plane reveals an area of hyperintensity in the region of the left middle cerebral artery (*arrowhead*). The patient had a supranuclear conjugate gaze paresis to the left side and right hemineglect. He also had difficulty generating rightward saccades. The ocular motor signs were transient as expected from a left-sided cerebral lesion.

tagmus, often with an associated head turn (see below).

PERSISTENT DEFICITS CAUSED BY LARGE UNILATERAL LESIONS

Persistent ocular motor deficits caused by lesions such as hemidecortication for intractable seizures are summarized in Table 18.7. Although there may be no resting deviation of the eyes, forced eyelid closure may cause a contralateral **spastic** conjugate eye movement, the mechanism of which is not understood (Fig. 18.34). This tonic deviation (Cogan's sign) differs from the tonic deviation associated with Wallenberg's syndrome; in the former, active or attempted eyelid closure is necessary to cause the eyes to deviate, whereas in the latter, the deviation occurs even with eyes open in darkness. Cogan's sign occurs most frequently in patients with parietotemporal lesions.

In primary position, a small-amplitude nystag-

mus may be present that is best seen during ophthalmoscopy. It is characterized by slow phases directed toward the side of the intact hemisphere and may represent an imbalance in smooth pursuit tone. Horizontal pursuit gain (eye velocity/target velocity) is low for tracking of targets moving toward the side of the lesion for all stimulus velocities. For targets moving slowly toward the intact hemisphere, the eye movements may be too fast (pursuit gain > 1); for higher target velocities, pursuit gain toward the intact side is normal. This disturbance of smooth pursuit probably reflects loss of both posterior (occipital-parietal-temporal) and frontal influences (Fig. 18.35).

A convenient way to demonstrate the asymmetry of smooth pursuit that occurs with large hemisphere lesions is with a hand-held "optokinetic" tape or drum. The response is decreased when the stripes are moved or the drum is rotated toward the side of the lesion. At the bedside, this response

Table 18.7
Persistent Effects of Large Unilateral Lesions of the Cerebral Hemispheres upon Ocular Motor Function

Fixation	In darkness, eyes usually drift away from the side of the lesion. This may also be evident during fixation (on ophthalmoscopic examination[a]) as nystagmus with quick phases toward the side of the lesion; square-wave jerks.
Saccades	Slower saccades to both sides, especially contralaterally; latency longer for small saccades directed contralateral to the side of the lesion; inaccurate (hypometric and hypermetric) saccades into the "blind" hemifield.
Smooth pursuit	Reduced pursuit gain toward the side of the lesion; smooth pursuit gain away from the side of the lesion may be increased for low-velocity targets.
Optokinetic	Reduced gain for stimuli directed toward the side of the lesion; impaired optokinetic afternystagmus; may be relatively preserved compared with pursuit, with prolonged build-up of slow-phase velocity.[b]
Vestibular	During sinusoidal rotation, VOR gain in darkness may be slightly asymmetric (greater for eye movements away from the side of the lesion); with attempted fixation of an imagined or real stationary target, the asymmetry is increased.
Forced eyelid closure	Eyes usually deviate conjugately away from the side of the lesion ("spasticity of conjugate gaze").

[a] Remember that the direction of eye movements appears inverted during ophthalmoscopy.
[b] Recorded in patients with parietal lobe lesions.

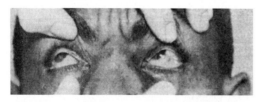

Figure 18.34. Conjugate lateral deviation of the eyes on forced closure of the eyelids in a patient with a tuberculoma of the left occipitoparietal region. (Reprinted with permission from Cogan DG. Neurologic significance of lateral conjugate deviation of the eyes on forced closure of the lids. Arch Ophthalmol 1948;39:37–42.)

is usually judged by the frequency and amplitude of quick phases; but because these quick-phase variables also depend on slow-phase velocity, a decreased response may reflect impaired slow-phase generation, impaired quick-phase generation, or a combination of the two.

Hemidecortication causes abnormalities of both contralateral and ipsilateral horizontal saccades. Saccades are usually slower than normal for refixations into and sometimes out of the hemianopic field. Saccadic latency is also prolonged in both directions. For small refixations, contralaterally directed saccades have greater latencies than ipsilateral saccades. Prolonged saccadic reaction time may reflect: (1) defects in visual detection because of the hemianopia, (2) defects in directing visual attention, and (3) abnormal motor programming. Saccadic accuracy is impaired asymmetrically: most contralaterally directed saccades do not put the eye on target.

The horizontal VOR may be mildly asymmetric in hemidecorticate patients, with the gain (eye velocity/head velocity) being greater for compensatory eye movements directed away from the side of the lesion. More asymmetry appears when visual fixation and vestibular stimulation are combined (during rotation while fixating a stationary object), probably reflecting the ipsilateral smooth-pursuit deficit. The asymmetry is still present during head rotation if the patient imagines a stationary object.

FOCAL LESIONS

Ocular motor disturbances that occur from focal lesions of the cerebral hemispheres depend on a variety of factors, including the location and size of the lesion and whether the lesion is unilateral or bilateral.

Occipital Lobe Lesions

A small, unilateral lesion of either occipital lobe causes a contralateral homonymous visual field defect without any significant disturbance of ocular motor function; however, a large, unilateral lesion of either occipital lobe usually causes a contralateral homonymous hemianopia and an ocular motor deficit (saccadic dysmetria) that is related primarily to the field defect. Saccades into the hemianopic visual field are dysmetric, usually hypometric, and similar patterns of saccades are seen with acoustic targets, implying some degree of common motor programming, perhaps influenced by associated defects in directing spatial attention. Characteristic patterns also occur in patients who have hemianopic

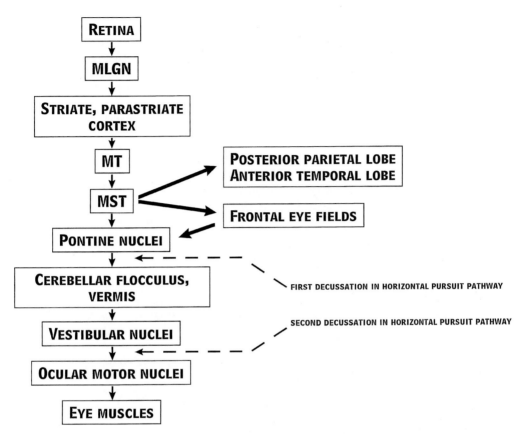

Figure 18.35.   Schematic flow of visual motion and motor signals that generate smooth pursuit. Dashed lines indicate double decussation of pathway for horizontal pursuit. *MLGN,* magnocellular lateral geniculate nucleus; *MT,* middle temporal visual area; *MST,* medial superior temporal area. (Reprinted with permission from Morrow MJ, Sharpe JA. Smooth pursuit eye movements. In: Sharpe JA, Barber HO, eds. The Vestibulo-Ocular Relfex and Vertigo. New York: Raven Press, 1993:141–162.)

dyslexia. Patients with hemianopia usually show a variety of compensatory strategies to increase saccadic accuracy, unless hemineglect is also present. These strategies include a staircase of search saccades with backward, glissadic drifts; a deliberate overshooting saccade to bring the target into the intact hemifield of vision; and with predictable targets, saccades using memory of previous attempts. Rapid gaze shifts achieved by combined movements of eye and head also show increased latency of head movements and development of compensatory strategies when looking to the side of the hemianopia. Smooth pursuit remains intact with unilateral lesions of the striate cortex, as long as the moving stimulus is presented to the intact hemifield. Optokinetic nystagmus elicited at the bedside is usually symmetric, unless subcortical pathways involved in smooth tracking are also affected.

Parietal Lobe Lesions

Unilateral lesions of the parietal lobes, especially those involving the inferior parietal lobule and underlying deep white matter, cause abnormalities of ocular tracking of moving targets, including an asymmetry of smooth pursuit and of optokinetic nystagmus as tested at the bedside with hand-held drums or tapes. Lesions at the temporoparietooccipital junction probably affect secondary visual areas that are important for motion processing and for programming of smooth-pursuit eye movements (see Fig. 18.35). One such area is likely to be the human homologue of what in monkeys is called the middle temporal (MT) visual area.

Lesions of MT in monkeys impair the ability to estimate the speed of a moving target that is within the affected visual field, although stationary objects can be seen and accurately localized. The ocular motor consequences of this **scotoma for motion** are that saccades made to targets moving in the affected, contralateral hemifield

are inaccurate and that the initiation of smooth pursuit is impaired. Such a behavior deficit occurs in patients with lesions affecting the temporoparietooccipital cortex.

Lesions of adjacent cortex (including Brodmann areas 19 and 39) (Fig. 18.36), which probably correspond to the medial superior temporal

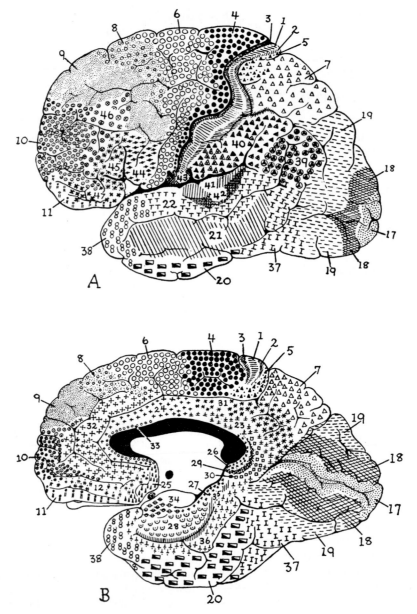

Figure 18.36. Cytoarchitectural map of the human cortex. *A*. Convex surface. *B*. Medial surface. The cortical areas of greatest importance with respect to visual sensory and ocular motor activity are areas 8, 17, 18, and 19. (Reprinted with permission from Strong OS, Elwyn A. Human Neuroanatomy. 3rd ed. Baltimore: Williams & Wilkins, 1953.)

(MST) visual area and underlying white matter lead to a **directional defect** in smooth pursuit that is characterized by impaired tracking (reduced gain) for targets moving toward the side of the lesion, irrespective of the visual hemifield in which the target lies.

In some patients, pursuit gain away from the side of the parietal lobe lesion is also somewhat reduced, especially when the eyes move into the contralateral field of gaze. This phenomenon probably results from contralateral neglect. In other patients, contralateral pursuit gain is increased. Subcortical, thalamic, and brainstem lesions may cause an ipsilateral defect from damage to the descending pathway for smooth pursuit. In human patients with parietal lesions, optokinetic nystagmus is often impaired in response to stimuli moving toward the side of the lesion, although it may be relatively spared compared with foveal tracking. Optokinetic afternystagmus and circularvection (the sensation of self-rotation) may also be impaired.

Unilateral lesions of the parietal lobe may affect saccadic initiation, causing an increase in saccadic latencies, either bilaterally or only for saccades to contralateral targets. These changes are independent of any visual field defect. The latency defects are enhanced when the fixation target remains on and a new target appears in the periphery (the ''overlap'' task) and are diminished when the fixation target is extinguished before the presentation of the new target in the periphery (the ''gap'' task). Other deficits reported with unilateral parietal lesions include inaccuracy and hypometria of contralaterally directed visually guided saccades, saccadic slowing, and disturbances of predictive saccadic tracking. Memory-guided saccades are especially impaired, being both delayed and inaccurate. These changes in saccades are more prominent with right hemisphere lesions. The saccade defects associated with parietal lesions may be caused, in part, by difficulties in shifting attention from one position to another in extrapersonal space, but there are no strict correlations between attention and the ocular motor deficits.

Bilateral parietal lobe lesions may cause acquired ocular motor apraxia, particularly if the lesions are large (see below). When smooth pursuit is possible, it is particularly limited with higher acceleration target motion.

Temporal Lobe Lesions

In patients with posterior temporal lesions, fixation-suppression of caloric-induced nystagmus is impaired when slow phases are directed away from the side of the lesion. This abnormality may reflect impairment of visual-motion or smooth-pursuit pathways rather than any effect on vestibular nystagmus per se. Patients with homonymous hemianopia and lesions affecting the temporal lobes may lack the sensation of self-rotation (circularvection) that normally occurs during full-field optokinetic stimulation, compared with patients who have an homonymous hemianopia from occipital lesions and who do experience circularvection. These findings support the localization of the vestibular cortex to the superior temporal gyrus and, perhaps, the adjacent parietal cortex. Patients with parieto-insular lesions may have tilts of the subjective visual vertical, usually contraversive. This is not associated with a skew deviation, although occasionally there is some monocular torsion. Patients with lesions in the same area may also have a defect in generating memory-guided saccades after a vestibular (rotational) stimulus. Finally, patients with lesions in the medial temporal lobe—the hippocampus—show marked impairment of generating sequences of saccades, whereas their spatial memory is intact. Seizures emanating in the temporal lobes may cause a variety of vestibular sensations. Although a mild feeling of dizziness is common with a variety of seizure types, a true sensation of rotation, called ''tornado epilepsy,'' is a rare but well-described epileptic phenomenon.

Frontal Lobe Lesions

Lesions of the frontal lobe may produce an ipsilateral conjugate deviation of the eyes that resolves with time. Rarely, contralateral deviation occurs with acute frontal lesions or fronto-parietal lesions. Enduring deficits after frontal lobe lesions include abnormalities of saccades and smooth pursuit. Three areas within the frontal lobes that play an important role in the control of eye movements are: (1) the frontal eye fields, (2) the supplementary eye fields (SEF) in the supplementary motor area, and (3) the prefrontal cortex (PFC) (see Figs. 18.17 and 18.36).

Unilateral FEF lesions lead to a slight increase in saccade latency to reflexively triggered saccades with a predominantly contralateral hypometria. Latencies are greatest in the overlap task (when the initial fixation target remains on, even after the peripheral target appears), suggesting a role for the FEF in disengagement from central fixation. Saccades may show a prolonged latency to predictable target jumps, particularly in patients with right-sided frontal lesions. Patients with this condition show a bilateral deficit in latency and accuracy for saccades to a remembered visual target but not for remembered saccades after a vestibular (rotation) input. With attempted vertical saccades, a horizontal component directed toward the side of the lesion often causes an oblique movement. Mild slowing of contralateral saccades occurs in some patients. Deep, unilateral frontal lobe lesions cause increased latency for contralateral saccades. This deficit is probably caused by damage of efferent and afferent connections of the FEF.

Patients with unilateral frontal lesions show defects in the antisaccade task. This requires the subject to suppress a reflexive glance toward a peripheral visual target and, instead, look toward its mirror location in the contralateral visual field. Patients with unilateral frontal lobe lesions that involve the PFC have difficulty in suppressing the reflexive glance, especially if the visual stimulus appears in the visual hemifield contralateral to the side of the lesion. Patients with lesions in the FEF alone do not have this problem. On the other hand, patients with either PFC or FEF lesions show difficulty in generating the antisaccade when the target lies in the visual hemifield ipsilateral to the lesion. After PFC lesions, there is also a deficit in *both* vestibular (rotation) and visually guided memory saccades. Lesions affecting the SEF, especially in the left hemisphere, impair the ability of patients to make a remembered sequence of saccades. Likewise, patients with such lesions cannot make a memory-guided saccade to a visual target, but they can do so after a body rotation. In a double-step paradigm in which subjects had to be able to use nonretinal, corollary discharge information about the saccade to the first target to compute the size and direction of the second saccade, patients with frontal lesions were able to make the appropriate computation about the size and direction of the saccade; that is, their spatial computation was intact, although they had defects in latency.

Patients with unilateral frontal lobe lesions also show pursuit deficits (see Fig. 18.35). The FEF, SEF, and perhaps the PFC play a role in this abnormality. The defects are in both initiation and maintenance (more so at higher target speeds and frequencies). If lesions are in the SEF, defects are ipsilateral; if lesions are in the FEF, defects are bilateral but usually are greater for ipsilateral tracking. Patients with SEF lesions may have delayed reversal with periodic constant-velocity stimuli, implying impaired anticipation of the target trajectory. Saccades to moving targets are also inaccurate in some of these patients. Patients with lesions affecting the FEF may also show craniotopic as well as directional (ipsilateral) defects in pursuit. Tracking in the field contralateral to the lesion is worse than in the ipsilateral field. Visual exploration deficits may also play a role in some of the eye movement deficits seen with frontal lesions.

Acute bilateral frontal or frontoparietal lesions may produce a striking disturbance of ocular motility that is called **acquired ocular motor apraxia.** It is characterized by loss of voluntary control of eye movements, both saccades and pursuit, with preservation of reflex movements, including the VOR and quick phases of nystagmus. There is also relative preservation of saccades made to visual targets compared with internally guided saccades made on command and with blinking or head movements. Voluntary movements of the eyes are limited in the horizontal and usually also in the vertical plane. The defect of voluntary eye movements probably reflects disruption of descending pathways both from the FEF and the parietal cortex so that the superior colliculus and brainstem reticular formation are bereft of their supranuclear inputs.

OCULAR MOTOR APRAXIA

Ocular motor apraxia is characterized by an impaired ability to generate saccades on command (Fig. 18.37). In congenital ocular motor apraxia (COMA), an abnormality in eye movements may be recognized shortly after birth, when the child does not appear to fixate upon objects normally and may be thought to be blind. Between ages 4 to 6 months, characteristic thrusting horizontal head movements develop, sometimes with prominent blinking or even rubbing the eyelids, when the child attempts to change fixation. In children with poor head control, development of head thrusting may be delayed or absent. Almost all patients also show a defect in generating quick phases of nystagmus, which can usually be appreciated at the bedside

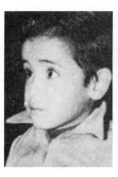 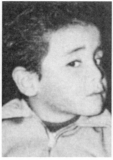 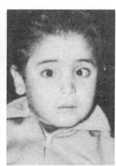

Figure 18.37.   Congenital ocular motor apraxia. The patient was looking to the right (*left*) when he was told to glance at the camera. His head rapidly moved to the left, while the eyes remained deviated toward the right. As a result, the patient's head had to turn farther to the left in order to permit fixation ahead (*center*). Once the patient was able to fixate on the camera, his head turned slowly back to the right until it was straight (*right*). (Reprinted with permission from Urrets-Zavalia A, Remonda C. Congenital ocular motor apraxia. Ophthalmologica 1957;134:157–167.)

by manual spinning of the patient, either when holding the child out at arm's length or by rotating the child on a swivel chair (if necessary sitting in an adult's lap). Despite difficulties in shifting horizontal gaze, vertical voluntary eye movements are normal, an important differential diagnostic point because **most acquired cases of ocular motor apraxia cause defects in both the horizontal and vertical planes.**

The head thrusts made by patients with COMA probably reflect one of several adaptive strategies to facilitate changes in gaze. Younger patients appear to use their intact VOR, which drives their eyes into an extreme contraversive position in the orbit. As the head continues to move past the target, the eyes are dragged along in space until they become aligned with the target. The head then rotates backward, and the eyes maintain fixation as they are brought back to the primary position in the orbit by the VOR. In contrast, older patients appear to use the head movement alone to trigger the generation of a saccadic eye movement that cannot normally be made with the head still. This strategy may reflect the use of a phylogenetically old linkage between head and saccadic eye movements that occurs reflexively in afoveate animals when they desire to redirect their center of visual attention.

The cause of COMA is unknown. One theory is that it may reflect a delay in the normal development of the mechanisms by which humans assume voluntary control over eye movements. Delayed psychomotor development (especially in learning to read and in speech), infantile hypo-

tonia, strabismus, incoordination, torsional nystagmus, and clumsiness occur in some patients. Associated anomalies, especially agenesis of the corpus callosum and cerebellar dysplasia and hypoplasia (for example, as part of Joubert's syndrome), are found in a number of patients with COMA. Most likely, however, such anomalies are markers of abnormal development rather than being directly responsible for the eye movement disorder. COMA is occasionally familial, and it has been reported in monozygotic twins. Patients with COMA usually improve with age, with the head movements becoming less prominent as the patients are better able to direct their eyes voluntarily.

A variety of disorders that directly damage the brainstem mechanisms for generating saccades—including structural or degenerative processes within the pontine and mesencephalic reticular formations—are characterized by the development of a strategy of head thrusting or blinking to shift the gaze that superficially resembles COMA. These disorders usually can be differentiated from COMA because all types of saccades and quick phases (both horizontal and vertical) are typically affected, and because saccades may be slow. In the early stages of these diseases, however, the ocular motor apraxia may be indistinguishable from COMA. Thus, patients with ataxia telangiectasia (Louis-Bar syndrome, 11q22-23) and its variants (ataxia-oculomotor apraxia syndrome of Aicardi), Gaucher's disease (types 2 and 3, 1q21-31), Niemann-Pick disease type 2s, Pelizaeus-Merzbacher disease,

Cockayne's syndrome, Huntington's disease, hepatolenticular degeneration, vitamin E deficiency, some of the peroxisome disorders, Whipple's disease, and many other storage diseases and aminoacidurias may appear to have COMA or at least COMA-like eye movements (see Fig. 18.29).

ABNORMAL EYE MOVEMENTS AND DEMENTIA

Patients with various dementing processes have abnormal eye movements, reflecting either disturbances in cerebral cortical structures or in other subcortical structures that may also be affected by that particular disease. Excessive errors on the antisaccade test, particularly when associated with a "visual grasp reflex," are a useful indicator of an organic process when pseudodementia is a diagnostic consideration in a patient with a possible cognitive decline.

Patients with Alzheimer's disease have excessive numbers of square-wave jerks and defects in saccade latency and, occasionally, accuracy and velocity. Alzheimer's disease patients show longer mean fixation durations and a reduced number of exploring saccades when viewing simple but not complex scenes, perhaps reflecting a motivation deficit. Impairment of spatially directed attention may also be reflected in eye-movement abnormalities, and a Balint-like syndrome may develop. Pursuit abnormalities also occur in patients with Alzheimer's disease.

Patients with Creutzfeldt-Jakob disease may show limitation of vertical gaze and slow vertical saccades as well as two rare forms of nystagmus, periodic alternating nystagmus and centripetal nystagmus. Cerebellar eye signs are typically found in another prion disorder, Gerstmann-Sträussler-Scheinker disease.

Patients with infection by the human immunodeficiency virus (HIV) show a number of ocular motor abnormalities that usually reflect the effects of an opportunistic infection or coexistent neoplasia. In addition, HIV encephalopathy itself can cause disturbed ocular motility, including errors on the antisaccade task; increased fixation instability; increased latencies of horizontal and, especially, vertical saccades; acquired ocular motor apraxia; cerebellar and brainstem signs, including gaze-evoked and dissociated nystagmus; slow saccades; and decreased, but especially asymmetric, pursuit gain.

OCULAR MOTOR MANIFESTATIONS OF SEIZURES

Abnormal eye and head movements are common manifestations of epileptic seizures. A variety of eye movements can occur in this setting, including horizontal or vertical gaze deviation and conjugate, retractory, or monocular nystagmus. Epileptic convergence nystagmus also occurs with periodic lateralizing epileptiform discharges and with burst-suppression patterns. The seizure focus may arise from any lobe, although the lesions usually are more posterior. Epileptic nystagmus occurs with typical absence seizures and with infantile spasms.

Patients with epileptic foci affecting the temporoparietooccipital cortex may show either ipsiversive or contraversive eye deviation and nystagmus. Overall, contraversive deviation of the eyes is more common than ipsiversive deviation during seizures. In cases with posterior foci (temporal, parietal, or occipital lobes), experimental studies suggest that eye movements may be mediated by projections via either the superior colliculus or the FEF. Thus, saccades may be generated by more than one of the descending parallel pathways. Frontal lobe foci are also reported to cause contraversive deviations unless they are bilateral, in which case vertical deviations also may occur.

Head turning is a common accompaniment of epileptic gaze deviation. In patients who are conscious during the seizure, a frontal focus is likely, and the initial direction of head turning is usually, but not invariably, contralateral to the seizure focus. A contralateral focus is also likely in a patient who shows marked, sustained, and unnatural lateral positioning of his or her head and eyes. In patients who are unconscious during the seizure, the focus may arise from any lobe, and head turning may be toward or away from the side of the lesion. Seizures that originate in the superior temporal lobes may cause a variety of vestibular sensations, and occipital lobe seizures may produce oscillopsia. Rarely, seizures are precipitated by movements of the eyes, such as convergence or sustained lateral deviation.

EYE MOVEMENTS IN STUPOR AND COMA

The ocular motor examination is especially useful for evaluating the unconscious patient, because both arousal and eye movements are controlled by neurons in the brainstem reticular formation. Comatose patients do not make eye movements that depend upon cortical visual processing. Voluntary saccades and smooth pursuit are in abeyance, and quick phases of nystagmus also may be absent. The ocular motor examination of the unconscious patient, therefore, consists of observing the resting position of the eyes, looking for any spontaneous movements, and reflexively inducing eye movements.

Gaze Deviations

Conjugate, horizontal deviation of the eyes is common in coma. When the coma is caused by a lesion above the brainstem ocular motor decussation between the midbrain and pons, the eyes are usually directed toward the side of the lesion and away from the hemiparesis that typically is present. A vestibular stimulus, however, can usually drive the eyes across the midline. If the conjugate deviation is caused by a lesion below the ocular motor decussation, the eyes will be directed away from the side of the lesion and toward the hemiparesis. The latter is typically seen with pontine lesions, but also in some patients with thalamic and, rarely, hemispheric disease above the thalamus (so-called wrong-way deviations).

Intermittent deviation of the eyes and head is usually caused by seizure activity. At the onset of each attack, gaze is usually deviated contralateral to the side of the seizure focus and may be followed by nystagmus with contralaterally directed quick phases. Toward the end of the seizure, gaze drifts to an ipsilateral (paretic) position.

Tonic downward deviation of the eyes, often accompanied by convergence, occurs in patients with thalamic hemorrhage and with lesions affecting the dorsal midbrain. It may be induced by unilateral caloric stimulation, after the initial horizontal deviation subsides, in patients with coma induced by sedative drugs. Forced downward deviation of the eyes can also be seen in patients with nonorganic (feigned) coma or seizures.

Tonic upward deviation of the eyes is uncommon in coma, but it may occur following an hypoxic-ischemic insult, even when no pathologic lesions are found in the midbrain. Patients who survive after manifesting this ocular motor disturbance typically develop downbeating nystagmus, the upward drift of which is thought to be caused by loss of inhibition on the upward vertical VOR. Upward deviation of the eyes also occurs as a component of oculogyric crisis, which usually occurs as a side effect of certain drugs, especially neuroleptic agents. Tonic uninhibited elevation of the lids (**eyes-open coma**) may also occur in unconscious patients and may be related to pontomesencephalic dysfunction.

Deviations of the visual axes in coma may be caused by skew deviation, a decompensated phoria, or paralysis of one or more of the ocular motor nerves. Restrictive ophthalmopathy, particularly blow-out fracture of the orbit, may be an additional mechanism in patients who have had facial trauma. Diagnosis of the cause of the deviation depends upon determining if the range of movement of the eyes induced by head rotation or caloric stimulation (see below) is reduced in a pattern corresponding to specific extraocular muscle weakness. In addition, assessment of the pupils and other brainstem reflexes may help. Pupillary involvement is an early sign of uncal herniation, and disturbances of eye movements usually follow (see Chapter 15). Vertical tropias are usually caused by skew deviation or trochlear nerve palsy, the latter being particularly common following head trauma (see Chapter 17). Bilateral abducens palsy occurs when increased ICP compromises the nerves as they bend over the petroclinoid ligament. Occasionally, skew deviation and INO occur in patients with metabolic encephalopathy or drug intoxication.

Spontaneous Eye Movements

Spontaneous eye movements that occur in unconscious patients may help establish the etiology of the coma (Table 18.8). **Slow conjugate or disconjugate roving eye movements** are similar to the eye movements of light sleep but slower than the rapid eye movements (REM) of paradoxic or REM sleep. Their presence indicates that brainstem gaze mechanisms are intact.

Other types of spontaneous eye movements consist of various forms of vertical to-and-fro movements, often called ''bobbing.'' Typical **ocular bobbing** consists of intermittent, usually conjugate, rapid downward movement of the eyes followed by a slower return to the primary position. Reflex horizontal eye movements are usually absent. Ocular bobbing is a classic sign of intrinsic pontine lesions, usually hemorrhage, but it also occurs in patients with cerebellar lesions that compress the pons and in some cases of metabolic or toxic encephalopathy. **Inverse bobbing** also occurs in this setting. This eye

Table 18.8
Spontaneous Eye Movements Occurring in Unconscious Patients

TERM	DESCRIPTION	CAUSES
Ocular bobbing	Rapid, conjugate, downward movement; slow return to primary position	Pontine strokes; other structural, metabolic or toxic disorders
Ocular dipping or inverse ocular bobbing	Slow downward movement; rapid return to primary position	Unreliable for localization; follows hypoxic-ischemic insult or metabolic disorder
Reverse ocular bobbing	Rapid upward movement; slow return to primary position	Unreliable for localization; may occur with metabolic disorders
Reverse ocular dipping or converse bobbing	Slow upward movement; rapid return to primary position	Unreliable for localization; pontine infarction and with AIDS
Ping-pong gaze	Horizontal conjugate deviation of the eyes, alternating every few seconds	Bilateral cerebral hemispheric dysfunction
Periodic alternating gaze deviation	Horizontal conjugate deviation of the eyes, alternating every 2 minutes	Hepatic encephalopathy; disorders causing periodic alternating nystagmus and unconsciousness
Vertical myoclonus	Vertical pendular oscillations (2–3 Hz)	Pontine strokes
Monocular movements	Small, intermittent, rapid monocular horizontal, vertical, or torsional movements	Pontine or midbrain destructive lesions, perhaps with coexistent seizures

movement abnormality, which is also called **ocular dipping**, is characterized by a slow downward movement, followed by a rapid return to midposition. **Reverse bobbing** consists of rapid deviation of the eyes upward and a slow return to the horizontal, whereas **converse bobbing** (also called **reverse dipping**) is characterized by a slow upward drift of the eyes that is followed by a rapid return to primary position. These variants of ocular bobbing are less reliable for localization than is straightforward ocular bobbing. Nevertheless, the occurrence in some patients of several different types of ocular bobbing during the course of their illness suggests a common underlying pathophysiology. Because the pathways that mediate upward and downward eye movements differ anatomically, and probably pharmacologically, it seems likely that these movements represent a varying imbalance of mechanisms for vertical gaze in the setting of bilateral horizontal gaze paralysis.

Rarely, large-amplitude pendular vertical oscillations occur in the acute phase of a brainstem stroke. This **vertical myoclonus** may have a pathogenesis similar to that of acquired pendular nystagmus.

Repetitive vertical eye movements, including variants of ocular bobbing, may contain **conver-gent-divergent** components. Such movements are usually caused by disease affecting the dorsal midbrain.

Monocular bobbing movements may occur as a synkinesis with jaw movement. Such movements are similar to those seen in the congenital condition called the Marcus Gunn jaw-winking phenomenon and primarily involve the neural pathways to the inferior rectus muscle.

Ping-pong gaze consists of slow, horizontal, conjugate deviations of the eyes that alternate every few seconds. Although ping-pong gaze can occur in patients with posterior fossa hemorrhage, it is usually a sign of bilateral infarction of the cerebral hemispheres. Sometimes, oscillations with a periodicity similar to that of ping-pong gaze can be induced transiently by a rapid head rotation in patients with bilateral hemisphere disease.

Rapid, small-amplitude, vertical eye movements may be the only manifestation of epileptic seizures in patients with coexistent brainstem injury. Rapid, monocular eye movements with horizontal, vertical, or torsional components, which occur in coma, may also indicate brainstem dysfunction.

Identification of patients who are conscious but quadriplegic—the **locked-in syndrome** or de-efferented state—depends on identifying preserved voluntary vertical eye movements. The syndrome is typically caused by pontine infarction and is characterized in part by a variable loss of voluntary and reflex horizontal movements, such that eyelid or vertical eye movements may be the only means of communication during the acute illness. The locked-in syndrome also occurs with midbrain lesions, in which case ptosis and ophthalmoplegia may be present.

Reflex Eye Movements

Reflex eye movements may be elicited in unconscious patients either by head rotation (the oculocephalic or doll's head maneuver) or by caloric stimulation (see Chapter 16). Head rotation, with the patient supine, stimulates the labyrinthine semicircular canals, the otoliths, and neck muscle proprioceptors. However, eye rotations induced by head rotation in unconscious individuals principally result from the effects of the semicircular canals and their central connections, that is, the VOR (Figs. 18.12 and 18.38). Head rotations should not be used in unconscious patients unless it is certain that no neck injury or abnormality is present. Conventionally, high-frequency (1 to 2 Hz) quasi-sinusoidal rotations or position-step stimuli are applied; the latter consists of a sudden head turn to a new position. Both horizontal and vertical rotations should be performed. If small-amplitude head rotations are performed, the adequacy of the VOR can be estimated by observing the optic disc of one eye with an ophthalmoscope.

Caloric irrigation of the external auditory meatus causes convection currents of the vestibular endolymph that displace the cupula of a semicircular canal; thus, this procedure also tests the VOR. The canal stimulated depends on the orientation of the head; for example, with the head elevated 30° from the supine position, the horizontal canals are principally stimulated. Before caloric stimulation, the physician should always check that the tympanic membrane is intact. Usually only about 5 mL of ice water need be introduced into the external auditory meatus, but large quantities (100 mL or more) may be necessary to induce a response in some comatose patients.

Caloric stimulation with ice water may sometimes be a more effective stimulus than head rotation, in part because of the sustained nature of the stimulus and in part because of the arous-

ing effect of the cold water. Combined cold caloric stimulation and head rotation may be the most effective stimulus in the deeply unconscious patient. This usually produces tonic deviation of the eyes toward the irrigated ear in patients with intact vestibular function.

In testing reflex eye movements in unresponsive patients, it is important to note: (1) the magnitude of the response, (2) whether the ocular deviation is conjugate, (3) the dynamic response to position-step head rotations, and (4) the occurrence of any quick phases of nystagmus, particularly during caloric stimulation. Impaired abduction suggests an abducens nerve palsy. Impaired adduction usually indicates either an INO or an oculomotor nerve palsy, although occasionally impaired adduction to vestibular stimulation may be observed in patients with metabolic coma or drug intoxication. Vertical responses may be impaired with disease of the midbrain or bilateral lesions of the MLF. Pontine lesions may abolish the reflex eye movements in the horizontal plane but spare the vertical responses. When reflex eye movements are present in an unresponsive patient, the brainstem is likely to be structurally intact. When reflex eye movements are abnormal or absent, the cause may be structural disease, profound metabolic coma, or drug intoxication.

If reflex eye movements are intact in an unconscious patient, the eyes are carried into a corner of the orbit when the head is rapidly rotated horizontally to a new position (velocity step stimulus). If the head is held stationary in its new position, the eyes may slowly drift back to the midline. This implies that the gaze-holding mechanism (neural integrator) is not functioning normally. Patients with more rapid centripetal drift may have more severe brain injury.

Quick phases of nystagmus are usually absent in acutely unconscious patients. Their presence, without a tonic deviation of the eyes, should raise the possibility of nonorganic (i.e., feigned) coma. In patients who are stuporous but uncooperative, caloric nystagmus may be a useful way of inducing eye movements that cannot be initiated voluntarily. Patients who survive coma but who are left in a persistent vegetative state, with severe damage of the cerebral hemispheres but preservation of the brainstem, regain nystagmus with caloric or rotational stimulation.

During syncope, normal subjects develop downbeat nystagmus and tonic upward devia-

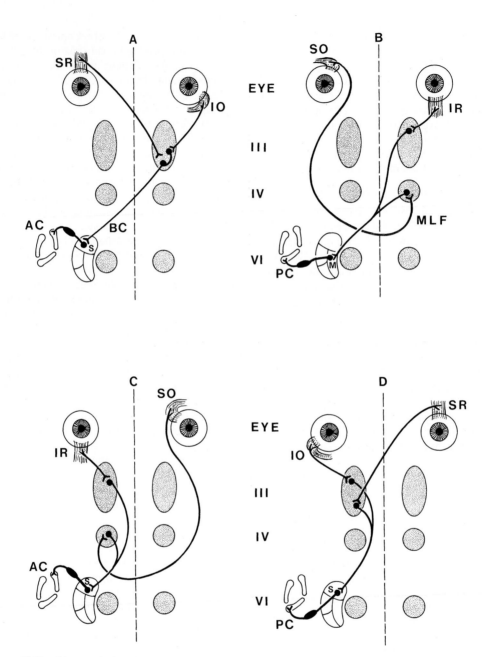

Figure 18.38. Direct vertical vestibulo-ocular projections from the vertical semicircular canals. *A–B.* Excitatory connections. *C–D.* Inhibitory connections. *A.* Excitatory afferents from the anterior semicircular canals *(AC)* synapse in the superior vestibular nucleus *(S)*, and their signals are relayed via the brachium conjunctivum *(BC)* to ocular motor subnuclei that drive the ipsilateral superior rectus *(SR)* and contralateral inferior oblique *(IO)* muscles. *B.* Excitatory afferents from the posterior semicircular canals *(PC)* synapse in the medial vestibular nucleus *(M)*, and their signals are relayed via the contralateral medial longitudinal fasciculus *(MLF)* to the ocular motor subnuclei that drive the ipsilateral superior oblique *(SO)* and contralateral inferior rectus *(IR)* muscles. *C.* Inhibitory afferents from the anterior semicircular canals. *D.* Inhibitory afferents from the posterior semicircular canals. (Redrawn from Ghelarducci B, Highstein SM, Ito M. In: Baker R, Berthoz A, eds. Control of Gaze by Brain Stem Neurons. New York: Elsevier/North-Holland Biomedical Press, 1977:167–175.)

tion of the eyes. Most also exhibit an increased amplitude of the VOR. These findings are most compatible with cerebellar hypoperfusion.

OCULAR MOTOR MANIFESTATIONS OF SOME METABOLIC DISORDERS

Some babies who ultimately develop normally show transient ocular motor disturbances, including upward or downward deviation of the eyes (but with a full range of reflex vertical movement), intermittent opsoclonus, and skew deviation. However, abnormal eye movements also occur in many metabolic diseases that affect the nervous system, particularly inborn errors of metabolism, in infants, children, and adults.

The **lipid storage diseases** are often characterized by gaze palsies. Tay-Sachs disease impairs vertical and, subsequently, horizontal eye movements. Adult-onset hexosaminidase deficiency also preferentially affects vertical gaze. Variants of Niemann-Pick disease that begin after the first year of life (e.g., the sea-blue histiocyte syndrome or juvenile dystonic lipidosis) are characterized by deficits of voluntary vertical eye movements, particularly saccades and smooth pursuit; vertical vestibular and horizontal eye movements are relatively preserved (see Fig. 18.29). Gaucher's disease is associated with a prominent deficit of horizontal gaze, and slow saccades may be a prominent finding in adults with this condition.

Pelizaeus-Merzbacher disease is an X-linked recessive leukodystrophy with severe cerebellar signs, including saccadic dysmetria. Some patients with this condition also show difficulty initiating saccades and pendular nystagmus.

Wernicke's encephalopathy is characterized by the triad of ophthalmoplegia, mental confusion, and gait ataxia. It is caused by thiamine deficiency and is most commonly encountered in alcoholics. The ocular motor findings include weakness of abduction, gaze-evoked nystagmus, primary-position vertical nystagmus, impaired vestibular responses to caloric and rotational stimulation, INO, the one-and-a-half syndrome, and horizontal and vertical gaze palsies that may progress to total ophthalmoplegia. The ophthalmoplegia is almost always bilateral but may be asymmetric. Lesions are found in the ocular motor and vestibular nuclei, as well as in the paraventricular regions of the thalamus, the hypothalamus, periaqueductal gray matter, superior vermis of the cerebellum, and dorsal motor nucleus of the vagus.

Most likely, affected areas of the brain contain neurons that use high amounts of glucose and, therefore, are particularly dependent upon thiamine, an important coenzyme in glucose metabolism. Administration of thiamine usually causes rapid improvement of the ocular motor signs, although complete recovery may take several weeks. Coexistent magnesium deficiency should also be treated. In patients with Wernicke's disease who go on to develop Korsakoff's syndrome, which is primarily characterized by a severe and enduring memory loss, ocular motor abnormalities may persist. The ocular motor abnormalities include slow and inaccurate saccades, impaired smooth pursuit, and gaze-evoked nystagmus.

Leigh's syndrome is a subacute necrotizing encephalopathy of infancy or childhood characterized by psychomotor retardation, seizures, and brainstem abnormalities, including eye movements. It is invariably fatal. It is an inherited disorder of mitochondrial function and can be caused either by abnormalities of mitochondrial DNA or by chromosomal disease. Both the disturbances of ocular motility and the pathologic findings resemble those caused by experimental thiamine deficiency or Wernicke's encephalopathy.

Deficiency of vitamin E may cause a progressive neurologic condition characterized by areflexia, cerebellar ataxia, and loss of joint position sense. Ocular motor involvement includes progressive gaze restriction, sometimes with strabismus. There usually is a dissociated ophthalmoplegia and nystagmus in which adduction is fast but with a limited range and abduction is slow but with a full range (the posterior INO of Lutz). The combination of ocular motor findings in patients with vitamin E deficiency probably reflects a mixture of central and peripheral pathology. Vitamin E deficiency is more common in children, in whom it may be caused by abetalipoproteinemia (Bassen-Kornzweig disease). It is also reported in adults who have bowel or liver diseases that interfere with fat absorption or as part of an inherited ataxia caused by a defect of chromosome 8q13, the site of the α-tocopherol transfer protein gene.

Hepatolenticular degeneration, also called

Wilson's disease, is an inherited disorder of copper metabolism that is transmitted in an autosomal-recessive fashion. The defect is in a copper-transporting ATPase gene at q14.3 on chromosome 14. The classic clinical picture is a movement disorder with psychiatric symptoms and associated liver disease. Ocular motor disorders in hepatolenticular degeneration include a distractibility of gaze, with inability to voluntarily fix upon an object unless other competing visual stimuli are removed. Slow saccades and apraxia of eyelid opening can also occur.

Amyotrophic lateral sclerosis is associated with various eye movement disorders, including nystagmus, saccade disturbances that suggest a frontal lobe disturbance, and pursuit impairment. However, the existence of multisystem diseases in which motor neuron degeneration is just one neurologic feature makes specific clinical diagnoses difficult.

EFFECTS OF DRUGS ON EYE MOVEMENTS

Many substances affect eye movements (Table 18.9). In some cases, the drug induces abnormalities of eye movements at therapeutic concentrations (e.g., anticonvulsants). In other cases, abnormalities of eye movements develop only when concentrations of the drug in the CNS are inappropriately elevated. In still other cases, the eye movement abnormalities are caused by substances not meant for internal use.

Patients with drug-induced abnormalities of eye movements most often complain of diplopia, caused by ocular misalignment, or oscillopsia, caused by spontaneous nystagmus or an inappropriate VOR. Many drugs have their effect on central vestibular and cerebellar connections, and they cause ataxia and gaze-evoked nystagmus.

Although all classes of eye movements may be affected by **therapeutic doses** of various drugs, smooth pursuit, eccentric gaze holding, and convergence are particularly susceptible. For example, diazepam, methadone, phenytoin, barbiturates, chloral hydrate, and alcohol all impair smooth-pursuit tracking.

At **toxic levels,** neuroactive drugs can impair all eye movements, particularly when consciousness is also impaired. Phenytoin may cause a complete ophthalmoplegia in an awake patient, and therapeutic levels may cause ophthalmoplegia in patients in stupor. Phenytoin and diazepam can lead to opsoclonus. The tricyclic antidepressants may cause complete ophthalmoplegia or an INO in stuporous patients. Lithium causes a variety of abnormalities, including fixation instability and downbeat nystagmus.

In addition to drugs, certain **toxins** can cause abnormal eye movements. Some, such as chlordecone and thallium, cause saccadic oscillations. Intoxication with hydrocarbons can cause a vestibulopathy, and exposure to trichloroethylene and other solvents may affect pursuit, suppression of the VOR, and saccades. Prolonged exposure to toluene, especially in glue-sniffing addiction, may lead to a variety of ocular motor disturbances, including pendular and downbeat nystagmus, saccadic oscillations, and INO. Tobacco has a number of ocular motor effects. It causes upbeat nystagmus, impaired pursuit, decreased saccade latency, and increased square-wave jerks during pursuit, although performance is normal on the antisaccade test. Cocaine can affect eye movements, with opsoclonus being the most dramatic abnormality.

Ototoxicity, especially that associated with administration of aminogylcosides, is an important cause of loss of the VOR. Intravenous gentamycin is most often responsible. Its toxicity may be insidious, occurring without hearing symptoms and even with normal blood levels and relatively short periods of administration. Some patients who develop ototoxicity may be genetically predisposed to its toxic side effects. Topical (intratympanic) gentamicin is used to purposefully ablate labyrinthine function as part of the treatment of intractable Ménière's syndrome or Tullio's phenomenon, but it may occasionally lead to unwanted labyrinthine loss when used to treat external ear infections. Cisplatin is probably not as vestibulotoxic as originally thought.

FOR MORE INFORMATION:

See Walsh & Hoyt's *Clinical Neuro-Ophthalmology,* 5th edition, Volume 1, Chapter 25, pp. 1043–1099, Chapter 26, pp. 1101–1167; and Chapter 29, pp. 1283–1349.

Table 18.9
Effects of Drugs on Eye Movements

DRUG	REPORTED EFFECTS
Amphetamines	Reduced saccadic latency
	Increased AC/A ratio
Baclofen	Reduced VOR time constant
	Complete paralysis of gaze
Benzodiazepines	Reduced velocity and increased duration of saccades
	Impaired smooth pursuit
	Decreased gain and increased time constant of VOR
	Divergence paralysis
Beta-adrenergic blocking agents	Internuclear ophthalmoplegia
Carbamazepine	Decreased velocity of saccades
	Impaired smooth pursuit
	Gaze-evoked nystagmus
	Oculogyric crisis
	Downbeat nystagmus
	Complete paralysis of gaze
Chloral hydrate	Impaired smooth pursuit
Ethyl alcohol	Reduced peak velocity of saccades
	Increased latency of saccades
	Hypometric saccades
	Impaired smooth pursuit and VOR suppression
	Gaze-evoked nystagmus
	Position-induced nystagmus
	Reversed compensation of cerebellar lesions
Lithium carbonate	Saccadic dysmetria
	Impaired smooth pursuit
	Gaze-evoked nystagmus
	Downbeat nystagmus
	Oculogyric crises
	Internuclear ophthalmoplegia
	Complete paralysis of gaze
	Opsoclonus
Methadone	Hypometric saccades
	Impaired smooth pursuit
Nitrous oxide	Reduced peak velocity of saccades
	Impaired smooth pursuit
Phenobarbital and other barbiturates	Reduced peak saccadic velocity
	Gaze-evoked nystagmus
	Impaired vergence
	Decreased VOR gain
	Perverted caloric responses
	Vertical nystagmus
	Partial or complete paralysis of gaze
Phenothiazines	Oculogyric crises
	Internuclear ophthalmoplegia
Phenytoin	Impaired smooth pursuit and VOR suppression
	Gaze-evoked nystagmus
	Downbeat nystagmus
	Periodic alternating nystagmus
	Complete paralysis of gaze
	Convergence spasm
Tobacco	Upbeat nystagmus in darkness (cigarettes)
	Square-wave jerks (nicotine)
	Impaired pursuit (nicotine)
Toluene	Pendular nystagmus
	Internuclear ophthalmoplegia
Tricyclic antidepressants	Internuclear ophthalmoplegia
	Complete paralysis of gaze
	Opsoclonus

CHAPTER 19

Nystagmus and Related Ocular Motility Disorders

This chapter concerns abnormal eye movements that disrupt steady fixation and thus degrade vision. In order for humans to see an object optimally, the image of the object must be held steady over the foveal region of the retina. Although the visual system can tolerate some motion of images on the retina, if this motion becomes excessive (more than about 5°/second for Snellen optotypes), vision declines and patients may experience illusory motion of the seen world, oscillopsia. Furthermore, if the image of the object is moved from the fovea to peripheral retina, it will be seen less clearly.

In healthy persons, three separate mechanisms interact to prevent deviation of the line of sight from the object of regard. The first is **fixation,** which has two distinct components: (1) the visual system's ability to detect retinal image drift and program corrective eye movements, and (2) the suppression of unwanted saccades that would take the eye off target. The second mechanism is the **vestibulo-ocular reflex** (VOR), by which eye movements compensate for head perturbations at short latency and thus maintain clear vision during locomotion. The third mechanism is **eccentric gaze-holding,** the ability of the brain to hold the eye at an eccentric position in the orbit against the elastic pull of the suspensory ligaments and extraocular muscles, which tend to return it toward primary position. For all three gaze-holding mechanisms to work effectively, their performance must be precise. This requires continuous recalibration by adaptive mechanisms that monitor the visual consequences of eye movements.

The two types of eye movements that disrupt steady fixation are **nystagmus** and **saccadic intrusions.** The essential difference between the two lies in the **initial** eye movement that takes the line of sight off the object of regard. For nystagmus, it is a **slow** drift (or "slow phase"). After this initial slow eye movement, corrective or other abnormal eye movements may follow. Thus, nystagmus may be defined as a repetitive, to-and-fro movement of the eyes that is initiated by a slow phase (drift). Saccadic intrusions, on the other hand, are inappropriate rapid eye movements that take the eye off target and thus prevent steady fixation. They include a spectrum of abnormal movements, ranging from single saccades to sustained saccadic oscillations.

It is important to realize that not all nystagmus is pathologic. Normally, **physiologic nystagmus** preserves clear vision during self-rotation. Under most circumstances, such as during locomotion, head movements are small and the VOR is able to generate eye movements that compensate for them. Consequently, the line of sight remains pointed at the object of regard. In response to large head or body rotations, however, the VOR alone carries the eyes to the limits of their range, where they can no longer preserve clear vision. Thus, during sustained rotations, quick phases occur that reset the eyes into their working range. This is **vestibular nystagmus.** If rotation is sustained for several seconds, the vestibular afferents no longer accurately signal head rotation, and visually driven or **optokinetic nystagmus** takes over to stop excessive slip of images of stationary objects on the retina. Additional examples of physiologic nystagmus are **arthrokinetic** and **audiokinetic nystagmus** (see below). Both vestibular and optokinetic nystagmus act to hold retinal images steadily. Pathologic nystagmus, on the other hand, causes excessive drift of images of stationary objects on the retina and thus degrades vision. Pathologic nystagmus may also produce oscillopsia. An exception is congenital nystagmus, which may be associated with normal visual acuity and which seldom causes oscillopsia.

Nystagmus, both physiologic and pathologic, may consist of alternating slow drifts (slow phases) in one direction and corrective, resetting

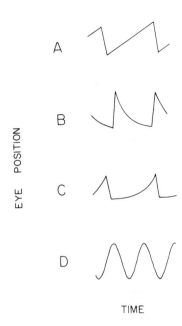

Figure 19.1.   Four common slow-phase waveforms of nystagmus. *A.* Constant velocity drift of the eyes. This occurs in nystagmus caused by peripheral or central vestibular disease and also with lesions of the cerebral hemisphere. The added quick-phases give a "saw-tooth" appearance. *B.* Drift of the eyes back from an eccentric orbital position toward the midline (gaze-evoked nystagmus). The drift shows a negative exponential time course, with decreasing velocity. This waveform reflects an unsustained eye position signal caused by a "leaky" neural integrator. *C.* Drift of the eyes away from the primary position with a positive exponential time course (increasing velocity). This waveform suggests an unstable neural integrator and is usually encountered in congenital nystagmus. *D.* Pendular nystagmus, which is encountered as a type of congenital nystagmus and with acquired brainstem disease. (Reprinted with permission from Leigh RJ, Zee DS. The Neurology of Eye Movements. 2nd ed. Philadelphia: FA Davis, 1991.)

saccades (quick phases) in the other. This form of nystagmus is called **jerk nystagmus** (Fig. 19.1*A*). Pathologic nystagmus may, however, also consist of smooth oscillations of approximately equal velocity and amplitude: **pendular nystagmus** (Fig. 19.1*D*). Conventionally, clinicians describe jerk nystagmus according to the direction of the quick phase. Thus, if the slow movement is upward, the nystagmus is described as "downbeating"; if the slow movement is to the right, the nystagmus is "left-beating." Although it is convenient to describe the frequency, amplitude, and direction of the quick phases of the nystagmus, it should be remembered that **it is the slow phase that reflects the underlying abnormality.**

Nystagmus may occur in any plane, but it is usually predominantly horizontal, vertical, or torsional. Physiologic nystagmus is almost always conjugate; that is, both eyes move in the same direction, usually with the same amplitude and frequency. Pathologic nystagmus, on the other hand, may have different amplitudes in the two eyes, may go in different directions leading to different trajectories of nystagmus in the two eyes, or may have different temporal properties—that is, phase shift between the two eyes—leading to movements that are sometimes in opposite directions. The first case is often called dissociated nystagmus; the latter is often called disconjugate nystagmus.

It is often possible to diagnose the cause of nystagmus by taking a careful history and systematically examining the patient. The physician should ask about the duration of the nystagmus, if it is accompanied by other neurologic symptoms, and if it interferes with vision and causes oscillopsia. The physician should also determine if nystagmus or attendant visual symptoms are worse when the patient is viewing far or near objects or when the patient is in motion, or if the visual symptoms are affected by different gaze angles (e.g., worse on right gaze). If the patient habitually tilts or turns the head, the physician should determine whether or not these features are evident on old photographs.

Before assessing eye movements, the physician must examine the afferent visual pathway, looking for signs of retinal or optic nerve dysfunction. The stability of fixation should be assessed with the eyes close to primary position, viewing near or far targets, and at eccentric gaze angles. It is often useful to record the direction and amplitude of nystagmus for each of the cardinal positions of gaze. If the patient has a head turn or tilt, the eyes should be observed in various directions of gaze when the head is in that position as well as when the head is held straight. During fixation, each eye should be occluded in turn to check for latent nystagmus (see below).

Subtle forms of nystagmus, such as those that are intermittent and those with low amplitude or variable velocity, require careful prolonged observation over 2 to 3 minutes. In some cases, low-amplitude nystagmus may be detected only

by viewing the patient's retina with an ophthalmoscope; the direction of horizontal or vertical jerk nystagmus is inverted when viewed through the ophthalmoscope.

The effect of removal of fixation on nystagmus should always be noted. Removal of fixation is often achieved by eyelid closure; nystagmus is then evaluated by recording eye movements, by palpating the globes, or by auscultation with a stethoscope. Lid closure itself may affect nystagmus, however, and it is better to evaluate the effects of removing fixation with the eyelids open.

One method is to observe the nystagmus when the patient wears Frenzel goggles. These goggles consist of 10- to 20-diopter spherical convex lenses placed in a frame that has its own light source. The goggles defocus the patient's vision, thus preventing fixation of objects, and they also provide the examiner with a magnified, illuminated view of the patient's eyes. Lacking these goggles, the examiner can simply use two high-plus spherical lenses from a trial case. He or she can also note the effect of transiently covering the viewing eye during ophthalmoscopy in an otherwise dark room.

Evaluation of nystagmus is incomplete without a systematic examination of each functional class of eye movements (vestibular, smooth-pursuit, saccades, vergence), because different forms of nystagmus can be directly attributed to abnormalities of some of these movements. It is often helpful to measure the nystagmus waveform because the shape of the slow phase often provides a pathophysiologic signature of the underlying disorder. To properly characterize nystagmus, it is important to measure eye position and velocity, as well as target position, during attempted fixation at different gaze angles, in darkness, and during vestibular, optokinetic, saccadic, pursuit, and vergence movements. Common slow-phase waveforms of nystagmus are shown in Figure 19.1.

Conventionally, nystagmus is measured in terms of its amplitude, its frequency, and their product, intensity. However, visual symptoms caused by nystagmus usually correlate best with the speed of the slow phase and the extent of displacement of the image of the object of regard from the fovea.

There are many different methods available for recording eye movements, but many patients with nystagmus cannot accurately point their

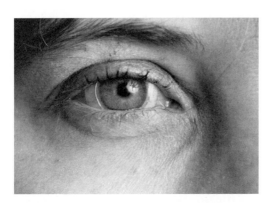

Figure 19.2.   A method for precise measurement of horizontal, vertical, and torsional eye rotations. The subject is wearing a silastic annulus embedded in which are two coils of wire, one wound in the frontal plane (to sense horizontal and vertical movements) and the other effectively in the sagittal plane (to sense torsional eye movements). When the subject sits in a magnetic field, voltages are induced in these search coils that can be used to measure eye position. (Reprinted with permission from Leigh RJ, Zee DS. The Neurology of Eye Movements. 2nd ed. Philadelphia: FA Davis, 1991.)

eyes at visual targets. In such cases, precise measurement is best achieved with the magnetic search coil technique (Fig. 19.2), because the contact lens that the patient wears can be precalibrated on a protractor-gimbal device. In addition, this is the only technique that permits precise measurement of horizontal, vertical, and torsional oscillations over an extended range of amplitudes and frequencies.

Our classification of nystagmus starts by relating the various forms of nystagmus to disorders of visual fixation, the VOR, or eccentric gaze-holding. In addition, the adaptive processes that optimize these eye movements may be affected by disease, and we discuss these recalibration mechanisms as we deal with each class of nystagmus.

NYSTAGMUS ASSOCIATED WITH DISEASE OF THE VISUAL SYSTEM AND ITS PROJECTIONS TO BRAINSTEM AND CEREBELLUM

ORIGIN AND NATURE OF NYSTAGMUS ASSOCIATED WITH DISEASE OF THE VISUAL PATHWAYS

Disorders of the visual pathways are often associated with nystagmus. The most obvious

example is the nystagmus that invariably accompanies blindness. At least two separate mechanisms can be identified: the visual fixation mechanism itself and the visually mediated calibration mechanism that optimizes its action.

The smooth visual fixation mechanism stops the eyes from drifting away from a stationary object of regard. The fixation mechanism that generates smooth eye movements to correct for drifts of the eyes depends upon the motion detection (magnocellular) portion of the visual system. This motion-vision system is inherently slow, with a response time of about 100 msec that encumbers all visually mediated eye movements, including fixation, smooth pursuit, and optokinetic responses. If the response time is delayed further—by disease of the visual system—attempts by the brain to correct eye drifts may actually increase retinal error rather than reduce it and may lead to ocular oscillations.

Vision is also needed for recalibrating and optimizing all types of eye movements. These functions depend on visual projections to the cerebellum, the structure some authors call "the ocular motor repair shop." Thus, signals from secondary visual areas concerned with motion-vision project to the cerebellum via the pontine nuclei and middle cerebellar peduncle. For example, neurons in the dorsolateral pontine nuclei and Purkinje cells in the cerebellar flocculus both encode visual-motion signals. Visual signals for recalibration may also pass via the inferior olive, which sends climbing fibers to the cerebellum. If the ocular motor system is to be recalibrated, visual signals need to be compared with eye movement commands. It is not certain how or where this function is performed. Candidate regions include the paramedian tracts (PMT) in the lower pons, where cells receive inputs from almost all ocular motor structures and project to the cerebellar flocculus, and the pathways that coordinate conjugate and vergence movements via connections between nucleus reticularis tegmenti pontis and cerebellar nucleus interpositus. Lesions at any part of this visual-motor recalibration pathway can deprive the brain of signals that hold each of the eyes on the object of regard, the result being drifts of the eyes off target, leading to nystagmus.

Disease affecting various parts of the visual system from retina to cortical visual areas and interrupting visual projections to pons and cerebellum may be associated with nystagmus.

CLINICAL FEATURES OF NYSTAGMUS
ASSOCIATED WITH LESIONS
AFFECTING THE VISUAL PATHWAYS

Retinal disorders causing blindness, such as
Leber's congenital amaurosis, lead to continuous jerk nystagmus. This nystagmus has components in all three planes and changes direction
over the course of seconds or minutes (Fig.
19.3A). The drifting "null point"—the eye position at which nystagmus changes direction—probably reflects inability to "calibrate"
the ocular motor system. Nystagmus occurs in
patients with a variety of hereditary retinal disorders. Some, but not all, show the increasing-velocity waveform (see Fig. 19.1C) that was once
thought to be specific for congenital nystagmus

(see below). Loss of vision later in life also
causes nystagmus, however. Seesaw nystagmus,
for example, developed in a patient who progressively lost vision from retinitis pigmentosa.

Optic nerve disease is commonly associated
with pendular forms of nystagmus. With unilateral disease of the optic nerve, such as tumors
or compression, nystagmus largely affects the
abnormal eye (monocular nystagmus), with low-
frequency, bidirectional drifts that are more
prominent vertically and unidirectional drifts
with quick phases that occur horizontally (see
Fig. 19.3B). When disease such as demyelination affects both optic nerves, the amplitude of
nystagmus is often greater in the eye with poorer
vision.

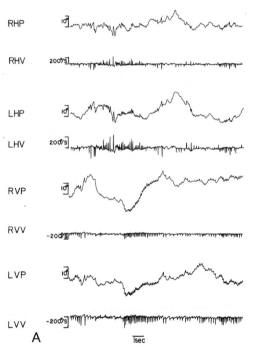

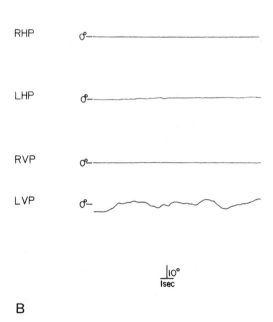

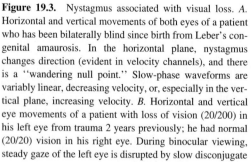

Figure 19.3. Nystagmus associated with visual loss. *A.*
Horizontal and vertical movements of both eyes of a patient
who has been bilaterally blind since birth from Leber's congenital amaurosis. In the horizontal plane, nystagmus
changes direction (evident in velocity channels), and there
is a "wandering null point." Slow-phase waveforms are
variably linear, decreasing velocity, or, especially in the vertical plane, increasing velocity. *B.* Horizontal and vertical
eye movements of a patient with loss of vision (20/200) in
his left eye from trauma 2 years previously; he had normal
(20/20) vision in his right eye. During binocular viewing,
steady gaze of the left eye is disrupted by slow disconjugate

drifts that are more prominent vertically. *RHP,* horizontal
gaze position of right eye; *RHV,* horizontal gaze velocity of
right eye; *LHP,* horizontal gaze position of left eye; *LHV,*
horizontal gaze velocity of left eye; *RVP,* vertical gaze position of right eye; *RVV,* vertical gaze velocity of right eye;
LVP, vertical gaze position of left eye; *LVV,* vertical gaze
velocity of left eye. Upward deflections indicate rightward
or upward gaze movements. Measurements were made using
the magnetic search coil technique. (Reprinted with permission from Leigh RJ, Thurston SE, Tomsak RL, et al. Effect
of monocular visual loss upon stability of gaze. Invest Ophthalmol Vis Sci 1989;30:288–292.)

The phenomenon of nystagmus predominantly affecting the eye with poorer vision is not confined to primary optic nerve disease, however, and occurs in patients with profound amblyopia. Oscillations may also occur after development of a dense cataract or in high myopia in childhood. They may disappear when vision is restored, or they may persist, leading to oscillopsia. The former findings support the contention that these ocular oscillations are primarily caused by loss of vision rather than by any primary disorder of the ocular motor system. The origin of vertical drifts that occur in a blind eye is unknown but has been attributed to disturbance of either the vertical vergence mechanism or a monocular visual stabilization system.

In infants, the appearance of monocular, vertical, pendular nystagmus raises the possibility of an anterior visual pathway tumor, and neuroimaging studies are indicated. However, monocular oscillations in children are sometimes due to spasmus nutans. Monocular visual impairment, such as amblyopia, also leads to horizontal nystagmus. If it is present from birth, the features of this nystagmus are those of latent nystagmus. These conditions are discussed below.

Parasellar and suprasellar lesions, such as pituitary tumors, may be associated with seesaw nystagmus, a form of pendular nystagmus in which one half-cycle consists of elevation and intorsion of one eye and synchronous depression and extorsion of the other eye; during the next half-cycle, the vertical and torsional movements reverse (Fig. 19.4). Such lesions probably produce this unique type of nystagmus by compressing the midbrain and causing damage to the interstitial nucleus of Cajal (INC) or its connections (see below). However, seesaw nystagmus also occurs in a mutant strain of dogs that lack an optic chiasm and in patients in whom neuroimaging and visual-evoked responses suggest a similar developmental defect. Seesaw nystagmus also developed in a patient with progressive visual loss from retinitis pigmentosa. Thus, it remains possible that visual inputs, especially crossed visual inputs, are important for optimizing vertical-torsional eye movements.

Horizontal nystagmus is a documented finding in patients with unilateral disease of the **cerebral hemispheres,** especially when the lesion is large and posterior. Such patients show a constant-velocity drift of the eyes toward the intact hemisphere (i.e., quick phases directed toward the side of the lesion). The nystagmus is often low-amplitude and is sometimes appreciated only by viewing the ocular fundus with a direct ophthalmoscope. Such patients usually also show asymmetry of horizontal smooth pursuit (impaired toward the side of the lesion). This asymmetry of visual tracking suggests that the cause of the nystagmus in such patients is an imbalance of pursuit tone. Whether this asymmetry occurs primarily from impairment of parietal cortex concerned with directing visual attention or from disruption of cortical areas important for processing motion-vision remains unclear.

ACQUIRED PENDULAR NYSTAGMUS AND ITS RELATIONSHIP TO DISEASE OF THE VISUAL PATHWAYS

Acquired pendular nystagmus (Fig. 19.5) is one of the more common types of nystagmus and is the oscillation associated with most distressing visual symptoms. Its pathogenesis remains unclear, and more than one mechanism may be responsible. It is encountered in a variety of conditions (Table 19.1), including several disorders of myelin, cerebellar degenerations, oculopalatal myoclonus, and Whipple's disease.

Acquired pendular nystagmus usually has horizontal, vertical, and torsional components, although one component may predominate. (In congenital pendular nystagmus, however, the oscillation usually is predominantly horizontal, with a small torsional and a negligible vertical component.) The horizontal, vertical, and tor-

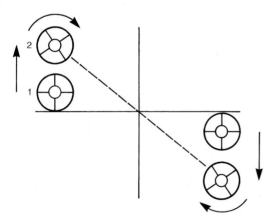

Figure 19.4. Seesaw nystagmus. As the right eye elevates, it also intorts. At the same time, the left eye depresses and extorts. The right eye then depresses and extorts, while the left eye elevates and intorts.

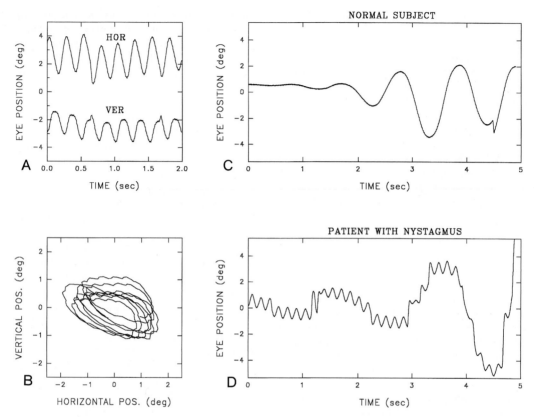

Figure 19.5. Acquired pendular nystagmus. *A.* Time plots of nystagmus of the patient's right eye while fixating a central visual target. The horizontal *(HOR)* and vertical *(VER)* records have been offset from zero eye position for convenience of display. Upward deflections correspond to rightward or upward eye rotations. *B.* Nystagmus trajectory seen as a scan path of eye movements in the horizontal and vertical planes corresponding to the time plot in *A.* The scan path corresponded to the direction of oscillopsia that the patient reported. *C–D:* Examples of ocular oscillations induced by imposing an effective delay in visual feedback. *C.* Normal subject. An effective delay in visual feedback of 480 msec was imposed at time zero. The subject developed ocular oscillations at about 1.0 Hz. *D.* Patient with multiple sclerosis and acquired pendular nystagmus. The effects of imposing an electronic delay of 480 msec. The oscillations of her nystagmus (unchanged at 6.5 Hz) were superimposed upon growing 0.67 Hz oscillations induced by the electronic manipulation. (Panels *C* and *D,* reprinted with permission from Averbuch-Heller L, Zivotofsky AZ, Das VE, et al. Investigations of the pathogenesis of acquired pendular nystagmus. Brain 1995;188:369–378.)

sional components of each eye's oscillations usually have the same frequency. If the horizontal and vertical oscillatory components are in phase, the trajectory of the nystagmus is oblique. If the horizontal and vertical oscillatory components are out of phase, the trajectory is elliptical (see Fig. 19.5*B*). A special case is a phase difference of 90° and equal amplitude of the horizontal and vertical components, in which case the trajectory is circular. When the oscillations of each eye are compared, the nystagmus may be conjugate, but often the trajectories are dissimilar, in which case the size of oscillations is different (sometimes appearing monocular), and there may be an asynchrony of timing (phase shift). The latter may reach 180°, in which case the oscillations are convergent-divergent.

The temporal waveform of acquired pendular nystagmus usually approximates a sine wave, but more complex oscillations sometimes occur. The frequency of oscillations of acquired pendular nystagmus ranges from 1 to 8 Hz, with a typical value of 3.5 Hz. For any particular patient, the frequency tends to remain fairly constant; only rarely is the frequency of oscillations different in the two eyes. In some patients, the

Table 19.1
Etiology of Pendular Nystagmus

Visual loss (including unilateral disease of the optic nerve)
Disorders of central myelin
• Multiple sclerosis
• Pelizaeus-Merzbacher disease
• Cockayne's syndrome
• Toluene abuse
Oculopalatal myoclonus
Acute brainstem stroke
Whipple's disease
Spinocerebellar degenerations
Congenital nystagmus

nystagmus stops momentarily after a saccade—so-called postsaccadic suppression. Acquired pendular nystagmus may be suppressed or brought out by eyelid closure. In some patients with this condition, smooth pursuit may be intact, so tracking eye movements occur with nystagmus superimposed.

Acquired Pendular Nystagmus with Demyelinating Disease

Acquired pendular nystagmus is a common feature of a variety of disorders of central myelin, including acquired disorders such as multiple sclerosis (MS), congenital disorders such as Pelizaeus-Merzbacher disease, and toluene abuse. Because concurrent optic neuritis often coexists in patients with MS who have pendular nystagmus, prolonged response time of the visual processing might be responsible for the ocular oscillations. Evidence to support this notion comes from the observation that oscillations are larger in the eye with evidence of more severe optic nerve demyelination. However, the nystagmus often remains unchanged in darkness, when visual inputs should have no influence on eye movements. In normal subjects, it is possible to induce spontaneous ocular oscillations by experimentally delaying the latency of visual feedback during fixation (see Fig. 19.5C); however, the frequency of these induced oscillations is less than 2.5 Hz, which is lower than in most patients with pendular nystagmus. When this experimental technique is applied to patients with acquired pendular nystagmus, it does not change the characteristics of the nystagmus but instead superimposes lower-frequency oscillations similar to those induced in normal subjects (see Fig.

19.5D). Thus, disturbance of visual fixation from visual delays cannot be held accountable for the high-frequency oscillations that often characterize acquired pendular nystagmus. A more likely possibility is that visual projections to the cerebellum are impaired, leading to instability in the reciprocal connections between brainstem nuclei and cerebellum that are important for recalibration. Thus, it may be relevant that internuclear ophthalmoplegia (INO) is common in these patients, suggesting involvement of brainstem regions close to the cell groups of the PMT. In patients in whom the oscillations are predominantly convergent-divergent, it is possible that instability arises in connections between nucleus reticularis tegmenti pontis and cerebellar nucleus interpositus, both of which are important for vergence control. Processes other than demyelination may also affect these pathways.

Oculopalatal Myoclonus

Acquired pendular nystagmus may be one component of the syndrome of **oculopalatal** (pharyngo-laryngo-diaphragmatic) **myoclonus.** This condition usually develops several months after brainstem or cerebellar infarction, although it may not be recognized until years after the stroke. Oculopalatal myoclonus also occurs with degenerative conditions. The term ''myoclonus'' is misleading, because the movements of affected muscles are to-and-fro and are approximately synchronized, typically at a rate of about 2 cycles per second. The palatal movements should really be termed ''tremor,'' rather than myoclonus, and the eye movements should be called ''pendular nystagmus.'' Although the palate is most often affected, movements of the eyes may be associated with movements of the facial muscles, pharynx, tongue, larynx, diaphragm, mouth of the Eustachian tube, neck, trunk, and extremities.

The ocular movements of oculopalatal myoclonus typically consist of pendular oscillations that are often vertical, although they may have a small horizontal or torsional component. If the palatal myoclonus is unilateral, the pendular oscillations consist of a mixed vertical-torsional movement, with the eye on the side of the palatal myoclonus intorting as it rises and extorting as it falls. The opposite eye, however, extorts as it rises and intorts as it falls, similar to what is observed in seesaw nystagmus. The movements may be somewhat disconjugate with some or-

Figure 19.6. Pathology of oculo-palatal myoclonus. A section through the cerebellum and medulla shows marked demyelination of the right dentate nucleus and restiform body (*double arrows*). The left inferior olive is hypertrophic and shows mild demyelination (*arrow*). (Reprinted with permission from Nathanson M. Palatal myoclonus: Further clinical and pathophysiological observations. Arch Neurol Psychiatr 1956;75: 285–296.)

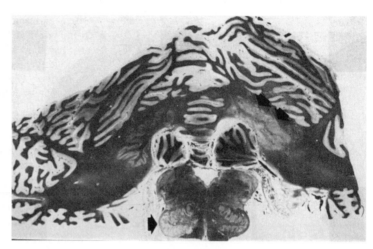

bital position dependency, and some patients show cyclovergence (torsional vergence) oscillations. The eye oscillations may be disconjugate, both horizontally and vertically. Eyelid closure may bring out the vertical ocular oscillations. The nystagmus sometimes disappears with sleep, but the palatal movements usually persist. Once established, the condition is usually intractable, and spontaneous remission is uncommon. Occasionally, patients develop the eye oscillations without movements of the palate, especially following brainstem infarction.

The main pathologic finding with palatal myoclonus is hypertrophy of the inferior olivary nucleus (Fig. 19.6). This change may be diagnosed during life using magnetic resonance imaging (MRI). There may also be destruction of the contralateral dentate nucleus. It is postulated that the nystagmus of oculopalatal myoclonus results from an instability in the projection from the inferior olive to the cerebellar flocculus, a structure thought to be important in the adaptive control of the VOR. It is also possible that projections from the cell groups of the PMT to the cerebellum are impaired in this condition.

Convergent-Divergent (Vergence) Pendular Oscillations

Vergence pendular oscillations are often small in amplitude and thus often overlooked by clinicians. They occur in patients with MS, brainstem stroke, and cerebral Whipple's disease.

In Whipple's disease, the oscillations typically have a frequency of about 1.0 Hz and are accompanied by concurrent contractions of the masticatory muscles, a phenomenon called "oculomasticatory myorhythmia." Supranuclear paralysis of vertical gaze also occurs in this setting and is similar to that encountered in progressive supranuclear palsy (see Chapter 18).

There are two possible explanations for the convergent-divergent nature of vergence pendular oscillations: a phase shift between the eyes, produced by dysfunction in the normal yoking mechanisms, or an oscillation affecting the vergence system itself. The latter explanation is more likely, because patients who have been studied show no phase shift (i.e., the oscillations are conjugate) vertically, and because the relationship between the horizontal and torsional components is similar to that occurring during normal vergence movements (excyclovergence with horizontal convergence).

NYSTAGMUS CAUSED BY VESTIBULAR IMBALANCE

Nystagmus related to imbalance in the vestibular pathway can be caused by damage to peripheral or central structures. The characteristics of the nystagmus vary greatly, depending on which portion of the pathway is damaged. Thus, it usually is possible to distinguish nystagmus caused by peripheral vestibular imbalance from nystagmus caused by central vestibular imbalance.

NYSTAGMUS CAUSED BY PERIPHERAL VESTIBULAR IMBALANCE

Clinical Features

Disease affecting the peripheral part of the vestibular pathway (i.e., the labyrinth and the vestibular nerve) causes nystagmus with linear slow phases (see Fig. 19.1*A*). Such unidirectional slow-phase drifts reflect an imbalance in the level of tonic neural activity in the vestibular nuclei. If peripheral disease leads to reduced activity in, for example, the vestibular nuclei on the left side, the vestibular nuclei on the right side will drive the eyes, in a slow phase, to the left. In this example, quick phases will be directed to the right, away from the side of the lesion. Paradoxically, some patients show nystagmus with a horizontal component that beats *toward* the side of the lesion. In such cases, the nystagmus may be a ''recovery nystagmus,'' which represents the effects of a central adaptation process. An imbalance of vestibular tone usually also causes vertigo and a tendency to fall toward the side of the lesion. Apart from these attendant symptoms, two features of the nystagmus itself are useful in identifying the vestibular periphery as the culprit: its trajectory (direction) and whether or not it is suppressed by visual fixation.

The trajectory of peripheral vestibular nystagmus is related to the geometric relationships of the semicircular canals. For example, complete unilateral labyrinthine destruction leads to a mixed horizontal-torsional nystagmus (the sum of canal directions from one ear); in benign paroxysmal positional vertigo (BPPV), a mixed upbeat-torsional nystagmus reflects posterior semicircular canal stimulation. Pure vertical or pure torsional nystagmus almost never occurs with peripheral vestibular disease, because this would require selective lesions of individual canals from one or both ears, an unlikely event.

Nystagmus caused by disease of the vestibular periphery often is more prominent, or may only become apparent, when visual fixation is prevented. The reason for this is that when visually generated eye movements are working normally, as they usually are in patients with peripheral vestibular disease, they will slow or stop the eyes from drifting due to vestibular imbalance.

Another common, but not specific, feature of nystagmus caused by peripheral vestibular disease is that its intensity increases when the eyes are turned in the direction of the quick phase: **Alexander's law.** This phenomenon probably reflects an adaptive strategy developed to counteract the drift of the vestibular nystagmus and so establish an orbital position (i.e., in the direction of the slow phases) in which the eyes are

quiet and vision is clear. This phenomenon forms the basis for a common classification of unidirectional nystagmus. Nystagmus is called ''first degree'' if it is present only on looking in the direction of the quick phases; ''second degree'' if it is also present in the primary position; and ''third degree'' if it is present on looking in all directions of gaze. Some patients with peripheral vestibular disease develop a horizontal nystagmus in upgaze, with convergence, or during vertical smooth-pursuit movements.

Nystagmus Induced by Change of Head Position

Peripheral vestibular nystagmus is often influenced by head movements or a change in head position. This feature can be used to aid in the diagnosis. If the patient can tolerate it, he or she can be placed in one of several head-hanging positions (head straight back or turned to the right or left) and immediately observed for changes in the nystagmus after a change from one head position to another. This technique is especially helpful in the diagnosis of patients with BPPV, who transiently develop mixed upbeat and torsional nystagmus when the affected posterior semicircular canal is placed in a dependent position. Such patients usually complain of brief episodes of vertigo precipitated by change of head position, such as when they turn over in bed or look up to a high shelf. The condition may follow head injury or viral neurolabyrinthitis.

To test for nystagmus and vertigo in a patient with possible BPPV, the examiner should turn the patient's head toward one shoulder and then quickly move the head and neck together into a head-hanging (down 30° to 45°) position. About 2 to 5 seconds after the affected ear is moved to this dependent position, a patient with BPPV will report the onset of vertigo, and a mixed upbeat-torsional nystagmus, best viewed with the patient wearing Frenzel goggles, will develop. The direction of the nystagmus changes with the direction of gaze. When the patient looks toward the dependent ear, the nystagmus becomes more torsional; when the patient looks toward the higher ear, the nystagmus becomes more vertical. This pattern of nystagmus corresponds closely to stimulation of the posterior semicircular canal of the dependent ear (which causes slow phases mainly by activating the ipsilateral superior oblique and contralateral inferior rectus muscles). The nystagmus increases for up to 10 seconds, but it then fatigues and is usually gone by 40 seconds. When the patient sits back up, a similar but milder recurrence of these symptoms occurs, with the nystagmus being directed opposite to the initial nystagmus. Repeating this procedure several times will decrease the symptoms and make the signs more difficult to elicit. This **habituation** of the response is of diagnostic value, because a clinical picture similar to that of BPPV can be caused by cerebellar tumors, MS, or posterior circulation infarction. With such central processes, however, there is no latency to onset of nystagmus and no habituation of the response with repetitive testing. In some patients, a paroxysm of horizontal nystagmus beating toward the ground and accompanied by vertigo is induced by sudden horizontal head turns performed as the patient lies supine. This may be a lateral canal variant of BPPV.

Studies show that otolithic debris in the respective canals (canalolithiasis) interferes with the flow of endolymph or movement of the cupula and is probably responsible for BPPV and its variants. Several useful bedside procedures can be used to treat the syndrome (see below).

Nystagmus that persists after a horizontal change in head position (e.g., with the subject supine and the head turned to the right or left) is less specific than transient nystagmus induced by changes in head position. Indeed, some otherwise normal subjects develop nystagmus that is horizontal with respect to the head and that is evident behind Frenzel goggles during static, horizontal positional testing. Such positional nystagmus may remain beating in the same direction whether the head is turned to the right or left, or it may change direction with lateral head turn such that it is either always beating toward the earth (geotropic) or away from the earth (ageotropic or apogeotropic). Sustained geotropic and ageotropic nystagmus probably reflect the effects of changing otolithic influences and may be encountered with either peripheral or central vestibular lesions. Only if such nystagmus is present during visual fixation does it suggest the possibility of central disease, however (see below). Occasionally, disease affecting central vestibular connections, such as a cerebellar tumor, brainstem infarction, or MS, may produce nystagmus associated with postural vertigo and severe nausea with vomiting. These manifestations may suggest a peripheral lesion; however, the charac-

teristics of the nystagmus are usually central, rather than peripheral.

In patients who have symptomatically recovered from a unilateral, peripheral vestibulopathy, nystagmus can often be induced following vigorous head shaking in the horizontal or the vertical plane for 10 to 15 seconds. After horizontal head shaking, patients may show horizontal nystagmus with quick phases directed away from the side of the lesion. After vertical head shaking, patients with unilateral peripheral vestibular lesions may show less prominent nystagmus with horizontal quick phases directed toward the side of the lesion.

Rarely, hyperventilation-induced nystagmus occurs in patients with vestibular schwannomas (acoustic neuromas) and after vestibular neuritis. This nystagmus has slow phases directed away from the side of the lesion, and there is often a prominent torsional component.

Nystagmus Induced by Proprioceptive and Auditory Stimuli

It is uncertain whether or not an imbalance of cervical inputs can produce a nystagmus similar to that caused by peripheral vestibular disease. In normal human subjects, eye movements generated from cervical proprioception—the cervico-ocular reflex (COR)—play little role in the stabilization of gaze, although the COR does increase in responsiveness in persons who have lost vestibular function and in certain patients with cerebellar disease. However, the entity of cervical nystagmus is not well established.

The perception of passive body motion relies primarily on vestibular and visual information. However, an illusion of body rotation accompanied by a conjugate, horizontal, jerk nystagmus—**arthrokinetic nystagmus**—can be induced when the horizontally extended arm of a normal, stationary subject is passively rotated about a vertical axis in the shoulder joint. The slow phase of the nystagmus is in a direction opposite to that of the arm movement. The mean slow-phase velocity increases with increasing arm velocity, and the nystagmus continues for a short time following cessation of arm movement (arthrokinetic after-nystagmus). The existence of arthrokinetic circularvection and nystagmus suggests that there exists in normal humans a functionally significant somatosensory-vestibular interaction within the central vestibular system, at least for afferent pathways, carrying position and kinesthetic information from the joints.

Normal stationary subjects in darkness may experience illusory self-rotation when exposed to a rotating sound field. This illusion is generally accompanied by **audiokinetic nystagmus,** which is conjugate and horizontal, with the slow phase in the direction opposite to that of the experienced self-rotation. Neither the illusory self-rotation nor the nystagmus occurs when the subject is exposed to a rotating sound field in the light—that is, when a stable visual environment is present. The occurrence of nystagmus during illusory self-rotation indicates that apparent as well as actual body orientation can influence ocular motor control. However, because auditory stimulation does not elicit illusory self-rotation or nystagmus when a stable visual environment is present, visual information must dominate auditory information in determining apparent body orientation and sensory localization.

Taken together, these findings indicate that although vestibular and visual inputs play the major role in generating eye movements that compensate for head movements, normal mechanisms of body orientation and localization can also use perceptions of body movements and somatosensory and auditory afferents. Thus, these are examples of physiologic nystagmus. On the other hand, patients who develop vestibular symptoms and nystagmus when exposed to certain sounds—**Tullio's phenomenon**—have either pathologic stimulation of otolithic organs or a congenital or acquired fistula in the bony labyrinth.

Peripheral Vestibular Nystagmus Induced by Caloric or Galvanic Stimulation

Nystagmus induced by caloric stimulation of one ear has all the features of that caused by unilateral or asymmetric peripheral vestibular disease. During caloric stimulation, a temperature gradient across the temporal bone induces a convection current in the endolymph of a semicircular canal if it is orientated earth-vertically. Before attempting to induce caloric nystagmus, the physician must first check that the tympanic membrane is visible and intact. The subject is then placed supine and the neck is flexed 30°. A cold stimulus (30°C) induces horizontal slow-phase components directed toward the stimulated ear (quick phases in the opposite direction).

With a warm stimulus (44°C) and the same head orientation, quick phases are toward the stimulated ear (hence the mnemonic **COWS**: cold–opposite, warm–same).

Caloric stimulation is an important way to test each peripheral labyrinth. Bedside testing with ice-cold water is especially useful in the evaluation of the unconscious patient. In this setting, tonic eye deviation indicates preservation of pontine function. Induction of caloric nystagmus is also a useful way to confirm preservation of consciousness in patients feigning coma. Suppression of caloric nystagmus by visual fixation depends on pathways important for visually mediated eye movements.

NYSTAGMUS CAUSED BY CENTRAL VESTIBULAR IMBALANCE
Clinical Features

Three common forms of nystagmus are thought to be caused by imbalance of central vestibular connections. These are downbeat, upbeat, and torsional nystagmus.

Downbeat nystagmus occurs in a variety of disorders (Table 19.2), but it is most commonly associated with disease affecting the cerebellum, the craniocervical junction, or the blood vessels in these regions. It may also be a manifestation

Table 19.2
Etiology of Downbeat Nystagmus

Cerebellar degeneration, including familial periodic ataxia, paraneoplastic degeneration
Craniocervical anomalies, including Arnold-Chiari malformation, Paget's disease, basilar invagination
Infarction of brainstem or cerebellum
Dolichoectasia of the vertebrobasilar artery
Multiple sclerosis
Cerebellar tumor, including Hemangioblastoma
Syringobulbia
Encephalitis
Head trauma
Toxic-metabolic
• Anticonvulsant medication
• Lithium intoxication
• Alcohol
• Wernicke's encephalopathy
• Magnesium depletion
• Vitamin B_{12} deficiency
• Toluene abuse
Congenital
Transient finding in otherwise normal infants

of drug intoxication. Downbeat nystagmus is usually present with the eyes in primary position, but its amplitude may be so small that it can only be detected by viewing the ocular fundus with an ophthalmoscope. In addition, it may occur intermittently. Generally, Alexander's law is obeyed. Thus, nystagmus intensity is greatest in downgaze and least in upgaze. Usually the waveform is linear, but it may be increasing in velocity (see Fig. 19.1C). The latter is usually the case if Alexander's law is violated (i.e., when the nystagmus increases in upgaze). This phenomenon may reflect an unstable gaze-holding mechanism (see below). Most often, it is brought out best by having the patient look down and to one side. Downbeat nystagmus may also be evoked by placing the patient in a head-hanging position. Convergence may influence the amplitude and frequency of the nystagmus or convert it to upbeat nystagmus. Some patients show combined divergent and downbeat nystagmus. In most patients, removal of fixation (e.g., with Frenzel goggles) does not substantially influence slow-phase velocity, although the frequency of quick phases may diminish.

A variety of ocular motor abnormalities often accompany downbeat nystagmus and reflect coincident cerebellar dysfunction. Vertical smooth pursuit and the vertical VOR are abnormal because of impaired ability to generate smooth downward eye movements; such asymmetries cannot simply be attributed to superimposed nystagmus. Sometimes, the VOR for upward eye movements is hyperactive, with a gain exceeding 1.0. Impairment of horizontal gaze-holding, smooth pursuit, and combined eye-head tracking also commonly coexist. Vertical diplopia usually reflects associated skew deviation. The visual consequences of downbeat nystagmus are oscillopsia and postural instability.

Upbeat nystagmus that is present with the eyes close to primary position occurs in many clinical conditions (Table 19.3). Nystagmus intensity is usually greatest in upgaze, and it usually does not increase on right or left gaze. As with downbeat nystagmus, slow phases are often increasing in velocity if Alexander's law is violated (see Fig. 19.1C). Removal of visual fixation has little influence on slow-phase velocity. Convergence may enhance or suppress upbeat nystagmus or convert it to downbeat nystagmus. Placing the patient in a head-hanging position

increases the nystagmus in some persons. It should be noted that the nystagmus in many patients with BPPV is upbeating. However, this is a transient phenomenon brought on by quickly placing the patient with the affected side down. Furthermore, the nystagmus of BPPV has a torsional component, and its direction depends upon the direction of gaze. As is the case with downbeat nystagmus, patients with upbeat nystagmus often show asymmetries of vertical vestibular and smooth-pursuit eye movements as well as associated cerebellar eye movement findings.

Torsional nystagmus is a less commonly recognized form of central vestibular nystagmus than downbeat or upbeat nystagmus. It is often difficult to detect except by careful observation of conjunctival vessels or by noting the direction

Table 19.3
Etiology of Upbeat Nystagmus

Cerebellar degenerations
Multiple sclerosis
Infarction of medulla, midbrain, or cerebellum
Tumors of the medulla, midbrain, or cerebellum
Wernicke's encephalopathy
Brainstem encephalitis
Behçet's syndrome
Meningitis
Leber's congenital amaurosis or other congenital disorder
   of the anterior visual pathways
Thalamic arteriovenous malformation
Organophosphate poisoning
Tobacco
Associated with middle ear disease
Congenital
Transient finding in otherwise normal infants

Table 19.4
Etiology of Torsional Nystagmus

Syringobulbia, with or without syringomyelia and Chiari
   malformation
Brainstem stroke (Wallenberg's syndrome) or arteriovenous
   malformation
Brainstem tumor
Multiple sclerosis
Oculopalatal myoclonus
Head trauma
Congenital
Associated with the ocular tilt reaction

of retinal movement on either side of the fovea, using an ophthalmoscope or contact lens. Although both peripheral vestibular and congenital nystagmus may have torsional components, purely torsional nystagmus, like purely vertical nystagmus, indicates disease affecting central vestibular connections, including demyelination, infarction (e.g., Wallenberg's syndrome), arteriovenous malformation, tumor, and syringobulbia (Table 19.4). Torsional nystagmus shares many of the features of downbeat and upbeat nystagmus, including modulation by head rotations, variable slow-phase waveforms, and suppression by convergence. It is also probably a common finding in patients with the ocular tilt reaction (see Chapter 18). Nonrhythmic but continuous torsional eye movements may be a feature of paraneoplastic encephalopathy.

Horizontal nystagmus in primary position from central vestibular imbalance is an uncommon but well-documented phenomenon. The underlying disorder usually is a Chiari (Arnold-Chiari) malformation. The slow-phase waveform in this form of nystagmus may be of the increasing-velocity type, making distinction from congenital nystagmus potentially difficult. However, patients with acquired central vestibular horizontal nystagmus typically report recent onset of visual symptoms such as oscillopsia,

and measurements usually demonstrate an associated vertical component that is absent in congenital nystagmus. Patients with horizontal nystagmus that is present in the primary position should always be observed continuously for 2 to 3 minutes to exclude the possibility that the nystagmus is actually periodic alternating nystagmus (PAN, see below).

Pathogenesis of Central Vestibular Nystagmus

Downbeat nystagmus is usually associated with lesions of the vestibulocerebellum (see Figs. 18.8 and 18.9)—the flocculus, paraflocculus, nodulus, and uvula—and the underlying medulla. Upbeat nystagmus is most commonly reported in patients with medullary lesions (Fig. 19.7; also see Figs. 18.1 through 18.3). These lesions affect the perihypoglossal nuclei and adjacent medial vestibular nucleus (MVN)—structures important for gaze holding—and the ventral tegmentum, which contains projections from the vestibular nuclei that receive inputs from the anterior semicircular canals. Upbeat nystagmus also occurs in patients with lesions affecting the anterior vermis of the cerebellum or the adjacent brachium conjunctivum and midbrain. Thus, it would seem that lesions at several distinct sites can cause both upbeat and downbeat nystagmus.

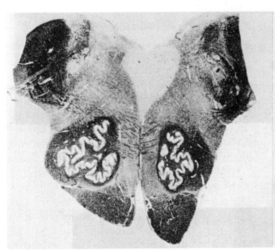
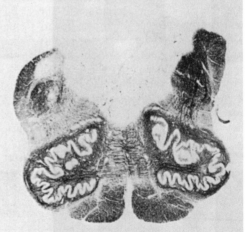
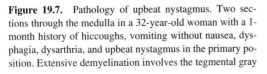

Figure 19.7. Pathology of upbeat nystagmus. Two sections through the medulla in a 32-year-old woman with a 1-month history of hiccoughs, vomiting without nausea, dysphagia, dysarthria, and upbeat nystagmus in the primary position. Extensive demyelination involves the tegmental gray matter in the region of the pontomedullary junction. (Reprinted with permission from Fisher A, Gresty M, Chambers B, et al. Primary position upbeating nystagmus. A variety of central positional nystagmus. Brain 1983;106:949–964.)

However, it is possible to account for these findings by considering the fundamental anatomic fact that, unlike the horizontal vestibular system which is right-left symmetric, the connections for vertical vestibular responses are dissimilar for upward or downward eye movements, both anatomically and pharmacologically. These up-down asymmetries involve connections subserving: (1) the vertical VOR, (2) the otolith-ocular reflexes, (3) the vestibulocerebellum, (4) the network for eccentric gaze holding (neural integrator), and (5) the smooth-pursuit system.

Excitatory projections for the vertical VOR from the posterior semicircular canals, which mediate downward eye movements, synapse in the MVN and then cross dorsally in the medulla beneath the nucleus prepositus hypoglossi (NPH) to reach the contralateral medial longitudinal fasciculus (MLF) (see Fig. 18.38). Experimental lesions that damage this pathway cause upward eye drifts and downbeat nystagmus. On the other hand, it appears that excitatory connections from the anterior semicircular canals, which mediate upward eye movements, take different routes. Indeed, more than one pathway may contribute. Central imbalance of otolithic inputs may also contribute to vertical nystagmus. The case for the cerebellar flocculus being an important structure in the production of downbeat nystagmus rests on the finding that Purkinje cells send inhibitory projections to the central connections of the anterior semicircular canal but not to the posterior canal. This asymmetry of inhibitory projections accounts for the finding that experimental flocculectomy causes downbeat nystagmus. This lesion disinhibits the projections to the anterior canal but not to the posterior canal, causing the eyes to drift up and producing downbeat nystagmus. A neural network that includes the vestibulocerebellum and the NPH and adjacent MVN is also thought to be important for the eccentric gaze-holding mechanism (see below). Lesions of the vestibulocerebellum may cause instability of this network, making the eyes drift at increasing velocity away from primary position in the vertical or horizontal planes. Finally, it has been suggested that the characteristics of downbeat nystagmus could be explained by a central imbalance in smooth pursuit with cerebellar lesions. Resolution of upbeat or downbeat nystagmus after the first few months of life in otherwise normal infants may reflect calibration of pursuit

or gaze-holding mechanisms as the visual system becomes fully myelinated.

PERIODIC ALTERNATING NYSTAGMUS

PAN is a spontaneous horizontal nystagmus, present in primary gaze, that reverses direction approximately every 2 minutes (Fig. 19.8). Because the period of oscillation is about 4 minutes, the disorder may be missed unless the examiner observes the nystagmus for several minutes. As the nystagmus finishes one half-cycle (e.g., of right-beating nystagmus), a brief transition period occurs during which the eyes may be stable, or there may be upbeating or downbeating nystagmus or small to-and-fro saccadic movements before the next half-cycle (e.g., of left-beating nystagmus) starts. A congenital form of PAN also exists (see below), but this is usually much less regular in the timing of reversal of direction and shows slow-phase waveforms typical of congenital nystagmus. PAN must be differentiated from "ping-pong gaze," an ocular deviation that reverses direction not over several minutes but every few seconds and that is usually encountered in unconscious patients with large bihemispheric lesions.

In most patients with acquired PAN, the nystagmus has the same characteristics in light or in darkness. Smooth pursuit and optokinetic nystagmus are usually impaired. Vestibular stimuli are able to reset the oscillations, and critically timed rotational stimuli can stop PAN for several minutes.

Acquired PAN occurs in association with a number of conditions (Table 19.5), many of which affect the cerebellum. If the neurologic disorder also damages the brainstem mechanism for generating quick phases, patients may develop a more severe disorder of eye movements, called "periodic alternating gaze deviation." PAN may also develop in patients who develop progressive loss of vision from ocular causes, including vitreous hemorrhage and cataract. In such cases, the nystagmus resolves when vision is restored.

The pathogenesis of PAN is becoming increasingly clear. Experimental ablation of the nodulus and uvula of the cerebellum in monkeys causes PAN when the animals are placed in a dark room. One function of the nodulus and uvula is to control the time course of rotationally induced nystagmus—so-called "velocity storage." Thus, following ablation of the nodulus

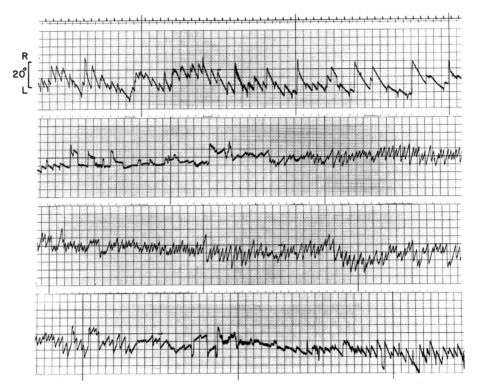

Figure 19.8.   Periodic alternating nystagmus in a patient who had undergone a biopsy of a posterior fossa mass (cryptococcal abscess), which required the cerebellar vermis to be split. The four parts of this horizontal electro-oculographic record are continuous; the time scale at the top is in seconds. The period of the oscillations was about 4 minutes. (Reprinted with permission from Leigh RJ, Robinson DA, Zee DS. A hypothetical explanation for periodic alternating nystagmus: Instability in the optokinetic-vestibular system. Ann NY Acad Sci 1981;374:619–635.)

Table 19.5
Etiology of Periodic Alternating Nystagmus

Chiari malformations and other hindbrain anomalies
Multiple sclerosis
Cerebellar degenerations
Cerebellar tumor, abscess, cyst, and other mass lesion
Creutzfeldt-Jakob disease
Ataxia-telangiectasia
Brainstem infarction
Anticonvulsant medications
Infections affecting cerebellum, including syphilis
Hepatic encephalopathy
Trauma
Following visual loss (from vitreous hemorrhage or cataract)
Congenital nystagmus

and uvula, the duration (velocity storage) of rotationally induced nystagmus is excessively prolonged. It is postulated that normal vestibular repair mechanisms reverse the direction of this nystagmus, thus producing the oscillations of PAN. These oscillations would ordinarily be blocked by visual stabilization mechanisms that tend to suppress nystagmus, but disease of the cerebellum that causes PAN usually also impairs these mechanisms. There is evidence that control of the velocity-storage mechanism by the nodulus and uvula is achieved by inhibitory pathways that use gamma-amino-butyric acid type B ($GABA_B$). This is consistent with the observation that the $GABA_B$ agonist baclofen is able to abolish PAN caused by both experimental and clinical lesions of the nodulus and uvula.

Two other unusual disorders may be related to PAN. One, which was observed in a blind person, is **periodic alternating windmill nystagmus,** in which oscillations occur in both the horizontal and vertical planes, 90° out of phase. The other consists of paroxysms of mixed torsional-horizontal-vertical nystagmus that occur every 2 minutes in association with nausea. In the latter patient, the initial mechanism was probably paroxysmal hyperactivity in one vestibular nucleus complex, unlike PAN, in which prolongation of the vestibular response is the initial mechanism. However, in both entities, an adaptive mechanism appears to influence the nystagmus every 2 minutes. This is perhaps the most direct evidence that **dysfunction of an ocular motor recalibration mechanism can lead to nystagmus.**

SEESAW AND HEMI-SEESAW NYSTAGMUS

In seesaw and hemi-seesaw nystagmus, one half-cycle consists of elevation and intorsion of one eye and synchronous depression and extorsion of the other eye; during the next half-cycle, the vertical and torsional movements reverse (see Fig. 19.4). The waveform may be pendular or jerk. In the latter case, the slow phase corresponds to one half-cycle. A seesaw component is present in many central forms of nystagmus, and seesaw nystagmus may be congenital, or it may occur in association with a variety of acquired disorders (Table 19.6).

Jerk seesaw nystagmus (hemi-seesaw nystagmus) occurs in patients with lesions in the region of the INC. Such patients often have a contralateral ocular tilt reaction (see Chapter 18). With a right INC lesion, the reaction consists of a left head tilt, a skew deviation with a right hypertropia, tonic intorsion of the right eye and extor-

Table 19.6
Etiology of Seesaw Nystagmus

Mesodiencephalic disease*
Parasellar masses
Brainstem stroke
Septo-optic dysplasia
Chiari malformation
Syringobulbia
Retinitis pigmentosa
Head trauma
Congenital form, including transient finding in albinism

* Includes hemi-seesaw nystagmus

sion of the left eye, and misperception that earth-vertical is tilted to the left. Rarely, the ocular tilt reaction is paroxysmal in form, in which case it is ipsilateral to the INC lesion. Some patients with this condition also show corresponding paroxysms of jerk seesaw nystagmus. Corrective, ipsilesional quick phases may occur if the adjacent rostral interstitial nucleus of the MLF (riMLF) is intact. If the riMLF is also damaged, however, either no quick phases or contralesional quick phases may be observed.

Pendular seesaw nystagmus occurs most often in patients with large tumors in the region of the optic chiasm and diencephalon, and, thus, these oscillations have been attributed to either compression of the diencephalon or to the effects of chiasmal visual field defects. Pendular seesaw nystagmus also occurs in patients with visual loss caused by primary ocular disease, including retinitis pigmentosa. Thus, as discussed above, it is possible that visual loss inactivates the recalibration mechanism for eye movements. One aspect of the vestibular responses concerns movements to compensate for head roll motion if the subject looks at an object located off the midsagittal plane; in this case, a seesaw rotation of the eyes is the geometrically appropriate compensation. Normal calibration of this response, which would require that motion-visual information be sent to the cerebellum, could be impaired with large suprasellar lesions, leading to the pendular variant of seesaw nystagmus. Thus, both the jerk and pendular variants of seesaw nystagmus probably arise from imbalance or miscalibration of vestibular responses that normally function to optimize gaze during head rotations in roll.

NYSTAGMUS DUE TO ABNORMALITY OF THE MECHANISM FOR HOLDING ECCENTRIC GAZE

GAZE-EVOKED NYSTAGMUS

Nystagmus that is induced by turning the eye to an eccentric position in the orbit is called **gaze-evoked nystagmus.** It is the most common form of nystagmus encountered in clinical practice. Although the terms ''gaze-evoked nystagmus,'' ''end-point nystagmus,'' and ''gaze-paretic nystagmus'' are often used synonymously, ''gaze-evoked nystagmus'' is a general term that includes both physiologic and pathologic nystagmus. When the nystagmus is physiologic, the

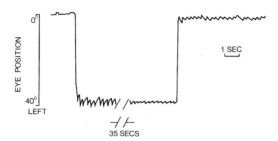

Figure 19.9. Gaze-evoked and rebound nystagmus from a patient with familial cerebellar degeneration. On looking to the far left, the patient develops gaze-evoked nystagmus that, after about 35 seconds, shows reduction of slow-phase velocity. When the eyes are then returned to primary position, the nystagmus reverses direction (rebound nystagmus). (Reprinted with permission from Zee, DS, Yee, RD, Cogan, DG, et al. Ocular motor abnormalities in hereditary cerebellar ataxia. Brain 1976;99:207–234.)

term "end-point nystagmus" is appropriate (see below). When the nystagmus is associated with a paresis of gaze, as in patients with ocular motor nerve palsies or weakness of the extraocular muscles, the term "gaze-paretic nystagmus" should be used.

Gaze-evoked nystagmus usually occurs on lateral or upward gaze, seldom on looking down. If fixation is impaired or prevented (e.g., in darkness), the slow phases consist of centripetal drifts that may have an exponentially decaying waveform (see Figs. 19.1B and 19.9). If visual fixation is possible, however, the slow phases have a more linear profile.

To understand how gaze-evoked nystagmus arises, one must consider the neural command required to hold the eye steadily at an eccentric position in the orbit. When the eye is turned toward a corner of the orbit, the fascia and ligaments that suspend the eye exert an elastic force to return toward primary position. Overcoming this elastic restoring force requires a tonic contraction of the extraocular muscles. This is achieved by an eye-position signal to the ocular motoneurons, called a "step," that is generated by the gaze-holding network, also called the neural integrator. This network includes the vestibulocerebellum, the NPH and MVN in the medulla, and the INC in the midbrain. Gaze-evoked nystagmus is caused by a deficient step, such that the eyes cannot be maintained at an eccentric orbital position and are pulled back toward primary position by the elastic forces of the or-

bital fascia. Corrective quick phases then move the eyes back toward the desired position in the orbit. Frequently, lesions that produce gaze-evoked nystagmus also impair visual fixation and smooth pursuit.

Gaze-evoked nystagmus may be caused by a variety of medications, including alcohol, anticonvulsants, and sedatives. Gaze-evoked nystagmus may also be caused by structural lesions that damage the gaze-holding neural network. Experimental lesions of the NPH/MVN region effectively abolish horizontal gaze-holding function and also partially impair vertical gaze holding. Inactivation of the INC abolishes vertical gaze-holding function. Experimental flocculectomy greatly, but not completely, impairs horizontal gaze holding, besides causing downbeat nystagmus.

Rarely, cerebellar lesions cause the gaze-holding mechanism to become unstable, so that the eyes drift with increasing velocity away from primary position in either the vertical or the horizontal plane. This "gaze-instability nystagmus" often violates Alexander's law.

Differences between Physiologic "End-Point" Nystagmus and Pathologic Gaze-Evoked Nystagmus

Gaze-evoked nystagmus is commonly encountered in normal persons, in which cases it is called "end-point nystagmus." It typically occurs on looking far laterally and is poorly sustained. The nystagmus is primarily horizontal. It is usually symmetric, but it may be asymmetric, being more prominent on looking to one side than to the other. In some persons, the nystagmus is sustained, occurs with less than full deviations of the eye, and may be slightly dissociated or have a torsional component. This physiologic form of gaze-evoked nystagmus can be differentiated from that caused by disease, because the former has lower intensity (i.e., slower drift) and, most importantly, is not accompanied by other ocular motor abnormalities. Pathologic gaze-evoked nystagmus, on the other hand, is accompanied by other defects of eye movements, such as impaired smooth pursuit.

Dissociated Nystagmus

A special type of pathologic gaze-evoked nystagmus is dissociated or "ataxic" nystagmus. This type of nystagmus is most commonly encountered with an INO. Dissociated nystagmus

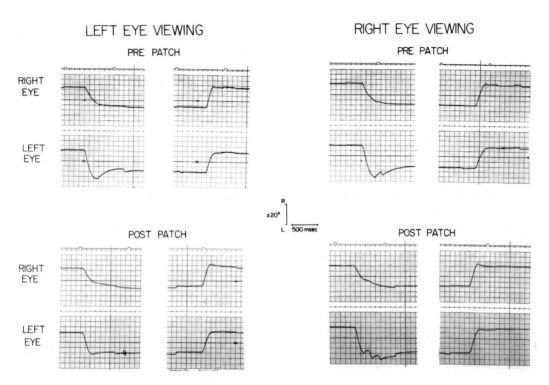

Figure 19.10. Effects of habitual monocular viewing on the eye movements of a patient with unilateral, right internuclear ophthalmoplegia. Pre-patch data were obtained after habitual binocular viewing, but the patient preferred to fixate with the right eye. Post-patch data were obtained after 5 days of patching of the right eye to ensure habitual left eye viewing. Left and right eye viewing refer to the viewing conditions at the time the eye movements were recorded. After patching, note the decrease in the abduction nystagmus of the left eye (decrease in the size of the abduction saccadic pulse and of the backward post-saccadic drift), with a commensurate decrease in the size of the saccadic pulse and increase of the onward post-saccadic drift for the adduction saccades made by the right eye. These changes were independent of which eye was viewing during the recording session. Patching led to little change in the adducting saccades made by the left eye or abducting saccades made by the right eye (vertical bar indicates +20°; horizontal bar, 500 msec). (From Zee DS, Hain TC, Carl JR. Abduction nystagmus in internuclear ophthalmoplegia. Ann Neurol 1987;21: 383–388.)

is, in fact, a series of saccades followed by post-saccadic drift that occurs when the patient attempts to look laterally away from the side of the lesion. Because the saccades initiate the oscillations, this ocular motor abnormality is not a true nystagmus, but rather a series of saccadic pulses. Consider, for example, a patient with a right-sided INO (Fig. 19.10, top panels). When the patient attempts to look to the left, the adducting saccades of the right eye are slow and hypometric. Each consists of a hypometric pulse, followed by a glissadic drift of the eye toward the target. Abducting saccades in the left eye are hypermetric, overshooting the target, and are followed by a glissadic backward drift of the

eye. A series of such small saccades and drifts gives the appearance of dissociated nystagmus. Because of the difference in the velocity of the adducting saccades in the eye on the side of the lesion and the abducting saccades in the contralateral eye, comparison of horizontal saccades made by each eye is most useful in making the diagnosis of an INO. When the INO is subtle, moving an optokinetic tape or rotating an optokinetic drum toward the side of the affected medial rectus muscle induces asymmetric quick phases, with smaller-sized movements in the affected eye.

Several explanations have been offered to account for dissociated nystagmus in INO, but the most plausible suggestion is that it is an attempt by the brain to adaptively "correct" hypometric saccades caused by the weak medial rectus muscle. To compensate for the weakness of the medial rectus, there is an adaptive increase in innervation to the adducting eye and, because of Hering's law of equal innervation, there is a commensurate change in the innervation to the normal, abducting eye. Although this adaptive change may help get the paretic eye on target, it leads to overshooting saccades and postsaccadic drift of the abducting eye if the patient attempts to fixate with the ipsilesional eye. Support for this interpretation comes from the observation that patching the eye with the adduction weakness for several days almost abolishes the overshoot and pulse-step mismatch of the abducting eye, when the latter eye fixates (Fig. 19.10, bottom left panel). Indeed, surgically induced medial rectus weakness leads to a similar nystagmus, and this nystagmus also resolves if the eye with the weak medial rectus is patched for several days. Both myasthenia gravis and the Miller Fisher syndrome may also produce a dissociated nystagmus similar to that seen in an INO.

Dissociated nystagmus characterized by larger movements in the **adducting** eye occurs when some patients with abducens nerve palsy look into the paretic field. Indeed, whenever a patient habitually prefers to fixate with a paretic eye, the normal eye will show a dissociated nystagmus while looking in the direction of action of the paretic muscle, regardless of the pathogenesis of the weakness.

Gaze-Evoked Nystagmus in Familial Paroxysmal Ataxia

Familial paroxysmal ataxia is a dominantly inherited, genetically heterogeneous disorder that is characterized by attacks of generalized ataxia, dysarthria, and gaze-evoked rebound and downbeat nystagmus. One form with onset in early childhood is characterized by very brief attacks and myokymia. It is caused by a mutation in a potassium channel gene on chromosome 12. Another form has a later onset, longer attacks, and interictal gaze-evoked nystagmus. The mutation in this form is on chromosome 19, close to the locus for familial hemiplegic migraine. Both types of familial paroxysmal ataxia usually respond to treatment with acetazolamide (Diamox).

Bruns' Nystagmus

Tumors in the cerebellopontine angle, such as meningiomas or schwannomas of the vestibulocochlear nerve (i.e., acoustic neuromas), may produce a low-frequency, large-amplitude nystagmus when the patient looks toward the side of the lesion and a high-frequency, small-amplitude nystagmus when the patient looks toward the side opposite the lesion. The nystagmus that occurs on gaze toward the side of the lesion is gaze-evoked nystagmus caused by defective gaze holding, whereas the nystagmus that occurs during gaze toward the side opposite the lesion is caused by vestibular imbalance. This special nystagmus is called **Bruns' nystagmus.**

CONVERGENCE-RETRACTION NYSTAGMUS

So-called **convergence-retraction nystagmus** is characterized by quick phases that converge or retract the eyes on attempts to look up. It is elicited either by asking the patient to make an upward saccade or by using a hand-held "optokinetic" drum or tape and moving the stripes or figures down. This maneuver produces normal slow, downward, following eye movements, but upward quick phases are replaced by rapid convergent movements, retractory movements, or both. Affected patients usually have impaired or absent upward gaze. The deficit in upgaze may be observed for both pursuit and saccadic eye movements; however, in some cases, upward pursuit appears normal, whereas upward saccades are obviously abnormal (pursuit-saccadic dissociation).

Convergence-retraction nystagmus is commonly produced by lesions of the mesencephalon that damage the posterior commissure, such as pineal tumors, and is usually part of the more extensive disorder of eye movements, pupillary reactivity, and eyelid position called Parinaud's syndrome (see Chapter 18). Convergence-retraction nystagmus is, in fact, a saccadic disorder rather than a true nystagmus because the primary, adductive movements are asynchronous adducting saccades. Electromyography in such cases demonstrates simultaneous contraction of all four rectus muscles during each quick phase. During horizontal saccades, the abnormal pattern of convergent innervation manifests itself as slowing of the abducting eye: "pseudo-abducens palsy." Convergence-retraction nystagmus may also be a manifestation of epileptic seizures, and it may occur in association with a Chiari malformation. Convergence-retraction nystagmus is usually intermittent, being determined by saccadic activity, and it thus can be differentiated from other, more continuous, forms of disjunctive nystagmus, such as convergent-divergent pendular nystagmus and the oculomasticatory myorhythmia that is characteristic of Whipple's disease (see above).

Jerk-waveform **divergence nystagmus** is diagnosed infrequently, but it may occur in patients with cerebellar disease, such as the Chiari malformation. In such cases, a combined divergent and downbeat nystagmus produces slow phases that are directed upward and inward.

CENTRIPETAL AND REBOUND NYSTAGMUS

If a patient with gaze-evoked nystagmus attempts to look eccentrically for a sustained period, the nystagmus may begin to decrease in amplitude and may even reverse direction so that the eye begins to drift centrifugally ("centripetal nystagmus"). If the eyes are then returned to the primary position, a short-lived nystagmus with slow drifts in the direction of the prior eccentric gaze occurs. This is called **rebound nystagmus** (see Fig. 19.9). Both centripetal and rebound nystagmus may reflect an attempt by brainstem or cerebellar mechanisms to correct for the centripetal drift of gaze-evoked nystagmus. Rebound nystagmus typically occurs in patients with cerebellar disease, but it has been reported following experimental lesions in the region of the NPH and MVN and in normal subjects with typical gaze-evoked nystagmus. Other lesions reported to cause this type of paroxysmal nystagmus include lateral medullary infarction and tumors confined to the flocculus. Rebound nystagmus may be explained by a sustained eye-position signal causing an imbalance of central vestibular mechanisms.

CONGENITAL FORMS OF NYSTAGMUS

Here we review those forms of nystagmus that develop during infancy. Although some patients with congenital nystagmus show visual abnormalities, others with similar ocular oscillations do not. Furthermore, the presence of any type of waveform, such as pendular (see Fig. 19.1D) or jerk (see Fig. 19.1A), does not suggest pathogenesis or indicate if the nystagmus is associated with visual system anomalies. Thus, the underlying mechanisms are not fully understood. Three distinct syndromes are currently recognized: congenital nystagmus, latent nystagmus, and spasmus nutans.

CONGENITAL NYSTAGMUS
Clinical Features

Congenital nystagmus is usually diagnosed during infancy, but it occasionally presents during adult life, when it may create a diagnostic problem, especially if the patient has other neurologic symptoms, such as headaches or dizziness. Certain clinical features usually differentiate congenital nystagmus from other ocular oscillations. It is almost always conjugate and horizontal, even on up or down gaze. A small torsional component to the nystagmus is probably common but is difficult to identify clinically. Only rarely is congenital nystagmus purely vertical or torsional. Congenital nystagmus is usually accentuated by the attempt to visually fixate a distant object and also by attention or anxiety. Eyelid closure and convergence usually suppress it, but occasionally congenital nystagmus is evoked by viewing a near target. Its intensity may also be influenced by viewing the vertical lines of an optokinetic tape. Congenital nystagmus often decreases when the eyes are moved into a particular position in the orbit, called the "null" region. In some patients, the direction of the nystagmus periodically reverses direction, but seldom in the regular manner encountered in the acquired form of PAN (see above). In some patients, the direction of the nystagmus is influenced by which eye is viewing, with the nystagmus beating away from the covered eye. This is similar to latent nystagmus (see below).

The most distinctive feature of congenital nystagmus is its waveforms, the most common of which are increasing-velocity (see Fig. 19.1C) and pendular (see Fig. 19.1D). Frequently superimposed on these waveforms, which may be combined, are **foveation periods,** the hallmark of congenital nystagmus. During each cycle, usually after a quick phase, there is a brief period when the eyes are still and pointed at the object of regard. With jerk waveforms, the quick phases (saccades) may brake the oscillation or bring the eyes to the target. With pendular waveforms, the oscillation is flattened by a foveation period when the eyes are closest to the target (Fig. 19.11). The particular waveform that is seen in a patient with congenital nystagmus de-

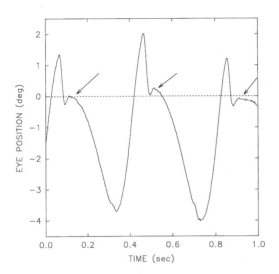

Figure 19.11.   A pendular type of congenital nystagmus waveform with superimposed quick phases. Note that following each quick phase, "foveation periods" occur (indicated by arrows), at which time the eye is close to desired fixation point (0° indicated by the dashed line) and eye velocity is low (i.e., the image is on the fovea and image slip is low).

pends in part upon the patient's age. Most infants show large-amplitude "triangular" waveforms. Shortly thereafter, the waveform becomes pendular, but it changes again to a jerk type as the patient reaches about 1 year of age. These waveforms are so characteristic of congenital nystagmus that reliable records of eye position and velocity will often establish the diagnosis.

Foveation periods are only rarely reported in acquired forms of nystagmus. They are probably one reason why most patients with congenital nystagmus do not complain of oscillopsia, despite otherwise nearly continuous movement of their eyes, and why many have normal visual acuity, as opposed to most patients with acquired nystagmus who complain of oscillopsia, blurred vision, or both. Foveation periods are not invariably present in congenital nystagmus. When they are absent or poorly developed, visual acuity is usually impaired.

Up to 30% of patients with congenital nystagmus also have strabismus. Another commonly described associated finding in such patients is "inverted pursuit" or "inverted optokinetic nystagmus." With a hand-held optokinetic drum or tape, quick phases are directed in the same direction as the drum rotates or the tape moves,

a response that is the reverse of normal. In fact, based on measurements made of tracking during the foveation period, it has been shown that both smooth-pursuit and optokinetic eye movements are preserved in at least some persons with congenital nystagmus. Similarly, vestibular responses are generally normal in patients with congenital nystagmus and, if judged by retinal image stability during foveation periods, performance is also normal and allows a similar view of the world whether the patient is stationary or in motion. However, in patients with associated visual disorders such as albinism, vestibular responses to lower frequencies of head rotations and optokinetic responses may be impaired. Occasional patients exhibit congenital nystagmus only during attempted smooth tracking, and others can voluntarily release or inhibit their congenital nystagmus, suggesting that fixation plays some role in the oscillations.

Head turns are common in patients with congenital nystagmus and are used to bring the eyes close to the "null" position in the orbit, where nystagmus is minimal. The observation of such a head turn in childhood photographs is often helpful in diagnosing congenital nystagmus. Another strategy used by patients with either congenital or latent nystagmus (see below) is to purposely induce an esotropia to suppress the nystagmus. Such an esotropia requires a head turn to direct the viewing eye at the object of interest. This phenomenon is called the "nystagmus blockage syndrome."

Some patients with congenital nystagmus also show head oscillations. Such head movements cannot act as an adaptive strategy to improve vision unless the VOR is negated. In fact, head movements are *not* compensatory in most patients with congenital nystagmus and tend to increase when the individual attends to an object, an effort that also increases the nystagmus. It seems probable, therefore, that both the head tremor and the ocular oscillations are the consequence of a common disordered neural mechanism.

Pathogenesis

Nystagmus developing early in life and showing some of the waveform characteristics of congenital nystagmus in humans, occurs in mutant dogs who lack the normal hemidecussation of fibers in the optic chiasm and in normal monkeys who are subjected to monocular visual deprivation in infancy. It is also associated with a variety of visual system disorders in humans, including ocular and oculocutaneous albinism, achromatopsia, retinal cone dystrophy, optic nerve hypoplasia, Leber's congenital amaurosis, retinal coloboma, aniridia, corectopia, congenital stationary night-blindness, Chédiak-Higashi syndrome, Joubert syndrome, and peroxisomal disorders. In addition, failure to develop a normal optic chiasm may predispose the patient to congenital seesaw nystagmus. Because of the many diagnostic possibilities, a complete ophthalmologic evaluation must be performed in patients with congenital nystagmus associated with decreased visual acuity or visual dysfunction, and an electroretinogram should be considered.

Congenital nystagmus, both with and without associated visual system abnormalities, may be familial. Several modes of inheritance have been reported and, in X-linked forms, the mothers may show subtle ocular motor abnormalities. However, there may be considerable differences in waveforms among members of a single family with hereditary congenital nystagmus. Although some cases of congenital nystagmus have been ascribed to pre-, peri-, or postnatal insults, this requires confirmation.

The known anatomic variations of the anterior visual system in persons with congenital nystagmus—such as excessive crossing at the chiasm in association with albinism or absent crossing of nasal fibers in achiasmatic subjects with congenital seesaw nystagmus—have led to the development of models for congenital nystagmus based on "miswiring" of visual pathways. A model that proposes that maladaptation to early visual deprivation leads to instability of the gaze-holding mechanisms has also been proposed. Further work is required to validate these models.

LATENT (OCCLUSION) NYSTAGMUS
Clinical Features

True **latent nystagmus** is a jerk nystagmus that is absent when both eyes are viewing but appears when one eye is covered. This conjugate nystagmus is characterized by quick phases that beat toward the side of the fixating eye. In most patients, a nystagmus is also present when both eyes are uncovered. This nystagmus, which is called "manifest latent nystagmus," is usually of low amplitude. It apparently occurs because only one eye is fixating, and vision from the other deviated eye is suppressed. Latent nystagmus usually reverses direction upon covering the other eye. In some patients, however, it is present when one eye is covered but is absent when

the other is covered. Occasional patients can control their latent nystagmus at will. Latent nystagmus is usually associated with strabismus, typically esotropia. Amblyopia is frequent; binocular vision with normal stereopsis is rare.

The slow phase of latent nystagmus usually shows a decaying velocity waveform when the eyes are close to primary position (see Fig. 19.1B), in contrast to the increasing velocity waveform of congenital nystagmus. A number of studies suggest that foveation may occur during the slowest part of the drift if the amplitude of the nystagmus is large, and immediately after the quick phase if the amplitude is small. Latent nystagmus usually follows Alexander's law, with the nystagmus being greatest on looking in the direction of the quick phases, away from the covered eye. Some patients turn the head to keep the viewing eye in an adducted position, where nystagmus is minimal. This strategy and other mechanisms used by patients to reduce latent or congenital nystagmus are part of a phenomenon called "the nystagmus blockage syndrome." Occasionally, congenital and latent nystagmus coexist, in which case the waveforms may be quite complex. Rarely in such patients, if vision is clearer with the latent nystagmus waveforms than with the congenital nystagmus waveforms, the patients switch from congenital to latent nystagmus as one eye becomes esotropic and the other takes up fixation. In addition to strabismus, patients with latent nystagmus frequently show an upward deviation of the covered eye (alternating sursumduction or dissociated vertical deviation). In such patients, the nystagmus often has a torsional component. Latent nystagmus is quite common, and accurate diagnosis is important to avoid inappropriate investigations. It should be differentiated from gaze-evoked nystagmus in association with strabismus, especially abducting nystagmus occurring with INO, in which an exotropia may be present.

Pathogenesis

Latent nystagmus is thought to be caused by a defect in cortical motion processing that results from lack of development of binocular vision. This view is supported by the finding that persons with latent nystagmus show impaired initiation of smooth pursuit in a specific pattern: nasal target motion evokes more vigorous pursuit than temporal motion, and upward motion evokes more pursuit than downward motion.

A second, related theory is that latent nystagmus is caused by an imbalance in the subcortical optokinetic system, perhaps secondary to a loss of cortical motion detectors. This would account for the temporal-nasal directional predominance of monocular optokinetic responses shown by some patients with latent nystagmus and by normal infants prior to maturation of cortical vision.

A third proposal is that latent nystagmus is caused by a defect in the influence of the internal representation of egocentric coordinates upon the direction of gaze. Support for this hypothesis comes from the observation that a patient with lifelong monocular blindness was able to reverse the direction of his latent nystagmus by attempting to view from his blind eye.

It is also possible that an abnormality of extraocular proprioception predisposes to latent nystagmus, because extraocular proprioception is important for the normal development of binocularity. These proposed mechanisms may not be mutually exclusive.

SPASMUS NUTANS

Spasmus nutans is characterized by the triad of nystagmus, head nodding, and an anomalous head position, such as torticollis. It usually begins in the first year of life, although it may not be detected until the child is 3 or 4 years old. Neurologic abnormalities are absent, although strabismus or amblyopia may coexist. The syndrome is sometimes familial. Spasmus nutans spontaneously remits, usually within 1 to 2 years after onset, although it may last for over 8 years.

The most consistent feature of spasmus nutans is the nystagmus, although head nodding may be the first abnormality to be noticed. Because the nystagmus is usually intermittent and has a small-amplitude, high-frequency (3 to 11 Hz) pendular waveform, it can easily be overlooked. When recognized, however, it has a shimmering quality. The nystagmus of spasmus nutans almost always differs in the two eyes, and it may even be uniocular (Fig. 19.12). Other distinguishing features are the variability of the ampli-

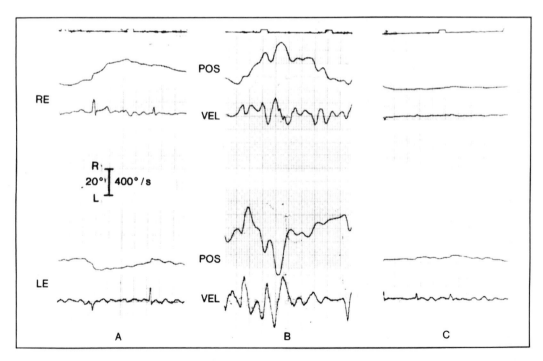

Figure 19.12. Examples of nystagmus of spasmus nutans from one child during a single recording session. *A.* There are binocular oscillations with no phase difference between the eyes. *B.* There are binocular oscillations with approximately 180° phase difference between the eyes. *C.* There are uniocular oscillations of the left eye. *LE,* left eye; *RE,* right eye; *POS,* position; *VEL,* velocity. Timing marks, at top of records, indicate 1-second intervals. (From Weissman BM, Dell'Osso LF, Abel LA, et al. Spasmus nutans: a quantitative prospective study. Arch Ophthalmol 1987;105:525–528.)

tude of nystagmus in each eye and the difference in the phase relationship between the two eyes. Even over the course of a few seconds or minutes, the oscillations may variably be conjugate, disconjugate, dissociated, or purely monocular (see Fig. 19.12). The plane of the nystagmus is predominantly horizontal, but it may have vertical or torsional components. It may sometimes be brought out by evoking the near response.

The head nodding of spasmus nutans is irregular, with horizontal or vertical components. It is usually more prominent when the child attempts to inspect something of interest. About two-thirds of the patients have an additional head tilt or turn. In some patients, the head nodding appears to turn off the nystagmus; however, it is unclear if head nodding, turning, or tilting are always adaptive strategies adopted to reduce the nystagmus or if they are simply another manifestation of the underlying abnormality in the central nervous system.

Two main clinical decisions must be made by the physician who sees a child with eye and head oscillations. The first is to determine if the nystagmus is associated with a tumor of the anterior visual sensory pathway, particularly an optic chiasmal glioma. A careful ophthalmologic evaluation must be performed in all children, with particular emphasis on the anterior visual system. If there is any suggestion that the child has optic nerve or chiasmal dysfunction, neuroimaging studies should be performed. The second clinical decision is to determine if the ocular motor disturbance is actually spasmus nutans, which will resolve over time, or congenital nystagmus, which probably will not. Spasmus nutans usually can be differentiated from congenital and latent nystagmus by its intermittency, high frequency, and dissociated characteristics. If the child will cooperate, eye movement recordings often help differentiate between these two entities.

EYE MOVEMENTS DURING EPILEPTIC SEIZURES

Patients with epileptic foci affecting portions of the cortex concerned with the programming of smooth pursuit and saccades may show either ipsiversive or contraversive eye deviation and nystagmus. With activation of cortical saccade regions, initial contraversive eye deviation is followed by contralaterally beating quick phases. This can be distinguished clinically from activation of pursuit regions that results in ipsiversive gaze deviation followed by contralaterally beating quick phases, with the slow phases moving the eyes across the midline. In patients with epileptic saccadic activity, the underlying focus usually affects the occipitotemporoparietal junction.

Contraversive quick phases in epileptic patients may result from two different mechanisms. First, they may be primary contraversive saccades that are caused by epileptic activity in the saccadic regions, and that are followed by centripetal drift from impaired gaze-holding. Such drifts are often seen in patients taking antiepileptic medications. Second, they may be secondary, reflexive contraversive saccades that are correcting a slow ipsiversive deviation across the midline that is caused by epileptic activation of either the smooth-pursuit or optokinetic regions. The second mechanism produces true nystagmus, whereas the first is actually a saccadic disorder.

To induce epileptic nystagmus in awake patients, the frequency of discharge must be high (above 10 spikes per second) and must affect the temporoparietooccipital junction area. In patients with coexistent brainstem lesions, the only manifestation of such activity may be rapid, small-amplitude, vertical eye movement. The absence of horizontal movements in such patients reflects dysfunction of the paramedian pontine reticular formation (PPRF).

EYELID NYSTAGMUS

Upward movements of the eyelids frequently accompany upward movements of vertical nystagmus. In fact, the absence of lid nystagmus in a patient with upbeat nystagmus may suggest disconnection between the premotor signals for the superior rectus and levator palpebrae superioris, implicating the region between the riMLF and the oculomotor nerve nucleus. For the same reasons, lid nystagmus unaccompanied by vertical eye nystagmus may reflect midbrain lesions. In patients with long-standing compression of the central caudal nucleus, "midbrain ptosis" may occur and may lead to lid nystagmus.

Twitches of the eyelid occasionally accompany horizontal nystagmus. In some patients, eyelid nystagmus may be dampened by convergence, whereas in other patients, eyelid nystagmus may be induced by convergence. The latter is called **Pick's sign.** In both types of cases, lesions are often present in the medulla, cerebellum, or both structures. The curious association of eyelid nystagmus with convergence may occur because the eyelid normally retracts with near effort. Therefore, any compromise of lid function will become more evident on attempts to converge. The eyelid nystagmus has been likened to the pathologic form of gaze-evoked nystagmus that occurs in patients with cerebellar disease and that is often associated with downward drifts of the eyelids, followed by corrective rapid upward movements.

SACCADIC INTRUSIONS

Several types of inappropriate saccadic eye movements may intrude upon steady fixation. These are schematized in Figure 19.13, and actual recorded examples are shown in Figure 19.14. Saccadic intrusions must be differentiated from nystagmus, in which, as noted above, a drift of the eyes from the desired position of gaze is the primary abnormality, and from saccadic dysmetria (see Fig. 19.13A), in which the eye overshoots or undershoots a target, sometimes several times, before achieving stable fixation. Because all of these movements are often rapid and brief, it may be necessary to measure eye and target position as well as eye velocity to identify accurately the saccadic abnormality.

SQUARE-WAVE JERKS

Square-wave jerks, also called *Gegenrucke,* are a common finding in healthy persons, particularly the elderly. They are small, conjugate saccades, ranging from 0.5° to 5.0° in size, that take the eye away from and—after about 200 msec—return it to the fixation position (see Figs. 19.13C and 19.14A). They are often more prominent during smooth pursuit and are most easily detected during ophthalmoscopy. They are also present in darkness.

Square-wave jerks with an increased frequency (up to 2 Hz) occur in certain cerebellar syndromes, in progressive supranuclear palsy, and in cerebral hemispheric disease. In such cases, they are called ''square-wave oscillations.'' These movements are commonly mistaken for nystagmus. Cigarette smoking increases the frequency of square-wave jerks.

MACROSQUARE-WAVE JERKS
(SQUARE-WAVE PULSES)

Macrosquare-wave jerks are large eye movements, typically greater than 5°, that occur

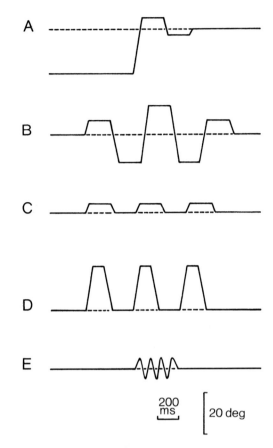

Figure 19.13. Schematic drawings of various saccadic oscillations. *A.* Saccadic dysmetria: saccades with inappropriate amplitudes that occur in response to target jumps. *B.* Macrosaccadic oscillations: hypermetric saccades about the position of the target. *C.* Square-wave jerks: small, inappropriately occurring saccades away from and back to the position of the target. *D.* Macrosquare-wave jerks: large, uncalled-for saccades away from and back to the position of the target. *E.* Ocular flutter: to-and-fro, back-to-back saccades without an intersaccadic interval. (From Leigh, RJ, Zee, DS. The Neurology of Eye Movements. 2nd ed. Philadelphia: FA Davis, 1991.)

at a frequency of about 2 to 3 Hz. After taking the eye off the target, they return it after a latency of about 80 msec (see Fig. 19.13D). These eye movements occur in light or darkness, but they occasionally are suppressed during monocular fixation. Macrosquare-wave jerks occur in bursts and vary in amplitude. They are encountered in disease states that disrupt cerebellar outflow, such as MS.

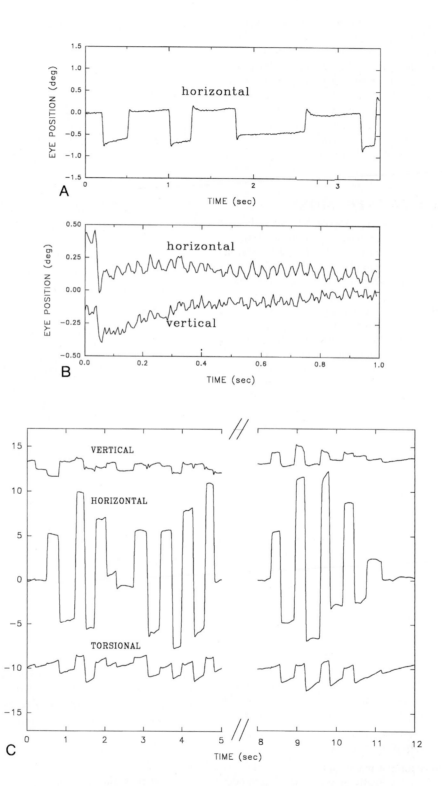

MACROSACCADIC OSCILLATIONS

Macrosaccadic oscillations usually consist of horizontal saccades that occur in bursts, initially building up and then decreasing in amplitude, with intersaccadic intervals of about 200 msec (see Figs. 19.13*B* and 19.14*C*). Originally described in cerebellar patients, macrosaccadic oscillations are thought to be an extreme form of saccadic dysmetria, in which the patient's saccades are so hypermetric that they overshoot the target continuously in both directions and, thus, oscillate around the fixation point. They are usually induced by a gaze shift, but they may also occur during attempted fixation or even in darkness. They may have vertical or torsional components and, occasionally, the former may be quite prominent clinically.

SACCADIC PULSES, OCULAR FLUTTER, AND OPSOCLONUS

Saccadic pulses are brief intrusions upon steady fixation. They are produced when a saccadic pulse is unaccompanied by a step command. The eye movement thus consists of a saccade away from the fixation position, with a rapid drift back. Saccadic pulses may occur in series or as doublets. They are encountered in some normal persons and in patients with MS.

There is a continuum between saccadic pulses and saccadic oscillations without an intersaccadic interval. The latter may occur in one direction, usually the horizontal plane, in which case they are called **ocular flutter** (see Fig. 19.13*E*), or they may be multivectorial, in which case they are termed **opsoclonus** or **saccadomania.** The frequency of oscillations is usually high, typically 10 to 15 cycles per second, being higher with smaller size movements. Ocular flutter may be intermittent and mainly associated with voluntary saccades (flutter dysmetria) and intermittent flutter-type head movements. Occasionally, the amplitude of the oscillations is very small (microflutter). In such cases, the movements may be detected only with a slit lamp or an ophthalmoscope or by using eye movement recordings. Such "microflutters" sometimes have components in all three planes (see Fig. 19.14*B*).

Sustained opsoclonus is a striking finding, in which multidirectional conjugate saccades, usually of large amplitude, interfere with steady fixation, smooth pursuit, or convergence. These movements usually persist during sleep. Opsoclonus is often accompanied by myoclonus—brief jerky involuntary limb movements. In such cases, the condition is called the "opsoclonus-myoclonus syndrome." In children, this syndrome is also called "dancing eyes and dancing feet." Ataxia and encephalopathy may also accompany opsoclonus.

The reported causes of ocular flutter and opsoclonus are summarized in Table 19.7. Drugs are a common cause, but the opsoclonus-myoclonus syndrome can also be a manifestation of remote cancer (i.e., a paraneoplastic condition), infection, autoimmune disturbance, metabolic insult, and vascular disease. In about 50% of cases, the etiology remains obscure.

In children, about half of the cases of opsoclonus and ocular flutter are paraneoplastic and associated with tumors of neural crest origin, such as neuroblastoma. In adults, opsoclonus occurs most often in association with lung, breast, and ovarian cancer. Various autoantibodies can be detected in sera of some patients with opsoclo-

◀———————————————————————

Figure 19.14. Actual recordings of saccadic oscillations. *A.* Horizontal saccadic intrusions (square-wave jerks) that repeatedly move the image of regard off the fovea. The patient had progressive supranuclear palsy. *B.* Diagonal microsaccadic flutter that was detectable only with an ophthalmoscope but, because of its high frequency, caused oscillopsia and impaired vision in this patient, who was otherwise well. *C.* Two segments of macrosaccadic oscillations from the right eye of a patient with a pontine infarction. Fixation is interrupted by bursts of saccadic intrusions that are time-locked in the horizontal, vertical, and torsional planes. The return saccade usually overshoots the central fixation point. Torsional and vertical tracings have been off- set for convenience of display. Upward deflections correspond to rightward, upward, or clockwise eye rotations, with respect to the patient. (Panels *A* and *B* reprinted with permission from Leigh RJ, Averbuch-Heller L, Tomsak RL, et al. Treatment of abnormal eye movements that impair vision: strategies based on current concepts of physiology and pharmacology. Ann Neurol 1994;36:129–141, 1994. Panel *C* reprinted with permission from Averbuch-Heller L, Kori AA, Rottach KG, et al. Dysfunction of pontine omnipause neurons causes impaired fixation: macrosaccadic oscillations with a unilateral pontine lesion. Neuro-ophthalmology 1996; 16:99–106.)

Table 19.7
Etiology of Ocular Flutter and Opsoclonus*

Viral encephalitis
Component of the syndrome of myoclonic encephalopathy
  of infants ("dancing eyes and dancing feet")
Paraneoplastic
• Neuroblastoma
• Other tumors
Trauma (in association with hypoxia and sepsis)
Meningitis
Intracranial tumors
Hydrocephalus
Thalamic hemorrhage
Multiple sclerosis
Hyperosmolar coma
Associated with systemic disease
• Viral hepatitis
• Sarcoid
• AIDS
• Other
Side effects of drugs
• Lithium
• Amitriptyline
• Phenytoin
• Diazepam
Toxins
• Chlordane
• Thallium
• Strychnine
• Toluene
• Organophosphates
Transient phenomenon of healthy neonates

* Not all case reports have documented the abnormality with eye
movement recordings.

nus. Of these, anti-Ri antibody is the most common. It is reported in association with cancer of the breast or pelvic organs and, less commonly, in patients with small-cell carcinoma of the lung or bladder cancer. A second antibody, anti-Hu, was reported with opsoclonus in two children with neuroblastoma and in an adult with small-cell lung cancer. This is an antineuronal antibody that is usually associated with paraneoplastic sensory neuronopathy, cerebellar degeneration, and limbic encephalitis.

When opsoclonus occurs as a manifestation of brainstem encephalitis, it is often a benign and self-limited condition. Paraneoplastic opsoclonus-myoclonus differs from other paraneoplastic syndromes in that spontaneous remissions may occur irrespective of the underlying tumor. Children with paraneoplastic opsoclonus

generally have a better oncologic prognosis than those without the neurologic syndrome, irrespective of disease stage. Regardless of the tumor, neurologic outcome is unpredictable, and cure from cancer may still be associated with severe neurologic sequela, or vice versa, in both children and adults.

VOLUNTARY SACCADIC OSCILLATIONS OR "VOLUNTARY NYSTAGMUS"

Some normal persons possess or develop the ability to voluntarily induce saccadic oscillations. These movements are called "psychogenic flutter" or **voluntary nystagmus.** Voluntary nystagmus is found in about 5 to 8% of the population and may occur as a familial trait. The oscillations are conjugate, with frequency and amplitude similar to those encountered in ocular flutter and opsoclonus. Although usually confined to the horizontal plane, voluntary nystagmus can occasionally be vertical or torsional. It may even be accompanied by a head tremor. Voluntary nystagmus can be produced in the light or dark and with the eyes open or closed. It causes oscillopsia and reduced visual acuity and is often accompanied by eyelid flutter, a strained facial expression, and convergence. Some patients who are able to produce voluntary nystagmus are also able to superimpose voluntary saccades on smooth movements during tracking of a target moving with constant acceleration.

It is important to distinguish voluntary nystagmus, which has no pathologic significance, from pathologic forms of nystagmus or saccadic oscillations, such as ocular flutter, that require a complete evaluation.

PATHOGENESIS OF SACCADIC INTRUSIONS

The saccadic command is generated by burst neurons of the brainstem reticular formation that project monosynaptically to ocular motoneurons. The burst neurons for horizontal saccades are located in the PPRF, whereas the burst neurons for vertical and torsional saccades are located in the riMLF. Burst neurons discharge only during saccadic eye movements. The activity of all saccadic burst neurons is gated by omnipause neurons, which are crucial for suppressing unwanted saccades during fixation and slow eye movements. The omnipause neurons are located in the caudal pons within the raphe interpositus nucleus (RIP), adjacent to the abducens nucleus. Inputs into omnipause neurons arise in the superior colliculus, frontal eye fields, and mesencephalic reticular formation (MRF).

During steady fixation, the threshold for electrical stimulation of saccades in either the frontal eye fields or the superior colliculus is elevated. Presumably, this elevation in threshold is mediated through the projections of these cells to the omnipause neurons. In the rostral superior colliculus, a distinct population of "fixation neurons" has been identified, whereas in the frontal eye fields, neurons active during suppression of saccades have been identified. Pharmacologic inactivation at both sites leads to disruption of fixation by saccadic intrusions, but not by flutter or opsoclonus. Furthermore, inactivation of the MRF may cause saccadic intrusions. Thus, impairment of any of these projections to the omnipause neurons can lead to saccadic intrusions, explaining the increased incidence of square-wave jerks with cerebral hemispheric disease and in progressive supranuclear palsy, in which the MRF and superior colliculus are both damaged.

The pathogenesis of saccadic oscillations without an intersaccadic interval (e.g., ocular flutter and opsoclonus) seems closely related to the properties of the burst neurons themselves. Burst neurons have very high discharge rates (up to 1000 spikes/second), and they discharge vigorously even for small saccades. Burst neurons are controlled by local feedback circuits in the brainstem, and any delays in this feedback could produce saccadic oscillations under certain conditions.

Theoretically, disease affecting omnipause neurons or their afferents from the superior colliculus might be expected to lead to saccadic oscillations such as ocular flutter and opsoclonus. For example, a complete absence of cells in the omnipause region was demonstrated in a patient with paraneoplastic saccadic oscillations, presumably from autoimmune destruction of normal tissue. Some experimental data are in conflict with this hypothesis, however, because chemical lesions of the omnipause neurons are reported to cause slowing of both horizontal and vertical saccades. There also is some evidence that impaired glycinergic transmission may play a role in the pathogenesis of both ocular flutter and opsoclonus.

Cerebellar dysfunction has traditionally been blamed for ocular flutter and opsoclonus. Experimental lesions of the cerebellum do not produce these oscillations, however, even though striking saccadic dysmetria can be produced when the dorsal vermis, and especially the caudal fastigial nucleus of the cerebellum, are inactivated. It remains possible that the fastigial nucleus, which projects to burst neurons, increases the excitability of these cells, thus leading to flutter.

TREATMENTS FOR NYSTAGMUS AND SACCADIC INTRUSIONS

Ideally, knowledge of the pathogenesis of a form of nystagmus should suggest the treatment. However, such knowledge is still lacking for many forms of nystagmus and saccadic intrusions. Although a number of drugs are reported to improve nystagmus in individual patients, few have been subjected to controlled clinical trials. When drug treatments fail or effective drugs cannot be tolerated by the patient, certain optical devices or surgery on the extraocular muscles can be tried (Table 19.8).

PHARMACOLOGIC TREATMENTS

Most nystagmus caused by **peripheral vestibular imbalance** spontaneously resolves over the course of a few days. Present approaches use vestibular suppressants for 24 to 48 hours, primarily for severe vertigo and nausea. If the nystagmus persists after this time, exercises are used to accelerate the brain's ability to redress the imbalance. In the case of BPPV, maneuvers to displace otolithic debris from the affected semicircular canal and exercises to sustain recovery are usually effective.

Basic pharmacologic studies have provided insights concerning the treatment of central forms of vestibular nystagmus. Of special interest is GABA, which has been shown to play a role in both vestibular eye movements and eccentric gaze holding. **Acquired PAN,** which is thought to be partly caused by abnormal prolongation of velocity storage, is abolished by baclofen, a $GABA_B$ agonist, and this response occurs with both experimental and clinical lesions of the nodulus and uvula. Furthermore, **downbeat nystagmus,** which may be caused by a central vestibular imbalance, also improves in some patients who are treated with baclofen. Baclofen is less effective in treating congenital nystagmus, including congenital PAN.

There is also evidence that nicotinic acetyl-

Table 19.8
Treatments for Nystagmus and Its Visual Consequences*

DRUGS
Baclofen
Gabapentin
Clonazepam
Valproate
Trihexyphenidyl
Benztropine
Scopolamine
Isoniazid
Carbamazepine
Barbiturates
Alcohol
Cannabis
Acetazolamide

OPTICAL DEVICES
Prisms (base-in or base-out)
Retinal image stabilization

SPECIAL PROCEDURES
Botulinum toxin
Anderson-Kestenbaum
Cüppers

OTHER MEASURES
Biofeedback
Acupuncture
Cutaneous head and neck stimulation

* For further details, see Leigh RJ, Averbuch-Heller L, Tomsak RL, et al. Treatment of abnormal eye movements that impair vision: strategies based on current concepts of physiology and pharmacology. Ann Neurol 1994;36:129–141.

cholinergic mechanisms play a role in vestibular-mediated vertical eye movements. Nicotine can produce upbeat nystagmus in normal subjects in darkness, intravenous physostigmine may increase the intensity of downbeat nystagmus, and scopolamine suppresses downbeat nystagmus in some patients.

The $GABA_A$ agonist clonazepam is effective in reducing **downbeat nystagmus** in a variety of patients with different lesions. Patients with downbeat nystagmus should be given a single 1–2 mg dose of clonazepam to determine whether long-term therapy is likely to be effective. Baclofen can also be used to reduce the velocity of both upbeat and downbeat nystagmus and thus eliminate or reduce associated oscillopsia in selected patients. Intravenous scopolamine may reduce downbeat nystagmus and improve oscillopsia, as may trihexyphenidyl.

Increased acetylcholine esterase activity and cholinergic denervation supersensitivity has been reported in the hypertrophied inferior olivary nucleus of patients with oculopalatal myoclonus, which, as noted above, is actually a form of **acquired pendular nystagmus.** This finding prompted trials of anticholinergic agents for other forms of acquired pendular nystagmus. The neuropharmacology of acquired pendular nystagmus is unknown, and more than one mechanism may be involved. This type of nystagmus used to be treated with barbiturates, but sedative side effects limit the use of this class of drugs. Although initial studies showed that individual patients were helped by trihexyphenidyl, only a few patients have subsequently responded to tridihexethyl chloride, and anticholinergic side effects are not tolerated. Intravenous scopolamine can effectively reduce nystagmus and improve vision, but it is not practical to prescribe scopolamine by intravenous injection for patients with acquired nystagmus.

Prompted by the reports that GABAergic agents are important for normal function of the gaze-holding mechanism, investigators tested the effect of a single oral 600 mg dose of the anticonvulsant gabapentin in patients with acquired pendular nystagmus. The drug was well tolerated, and visual acuity improved in several patients, associated with reduction or abolition of the nystagmus and the development of foveation periods. In another study, gabapentin that was given daily in divided doses totalling 900–1500 mg produced long-term benefit in patients with acquired pendular nystagmus, and the drug is currently being evaluated in multicentered controlled clinical trials.

Valproate, which also has GABAergic properties, may help some patients with acquired pendular nystagmus. Isoniazid has also been proposed as treatment for acquired pendular nystagmus. Palatal myoclonus may respond to carbamazepine in some patients.

Improvement in **seesaw nystagmus** has been reported in some patients treated with alcohol, baclofen, and clonazepam, given separately or in combination. All symptoms of **familial episodic ataxia with nystagmus,** including the nystagmus, usually respond to treatment with acetazolamide.

Experimental evidence suggests that treatment with GABA agonists might prevent inappropriate **saccadic intrusions.** In fact, several benzodiazepines (e.g., diazepam, clonazepam) and the barbiturate phenobarbital may be effective in abolishing high-amplitude square-wave jerks and macrosaccadic oscillations. There is also evidence that amphetamines can suppress square-wave jerks in some patients.

Propranolol, verapamil, clonazepam, and thiamine have all been reported to diminish microsaccadic **ocular flutter** in individual patients. In patients with **paraneoplastic opsoclonus,** treatment of the tumor is not necessarily associated with resolution of the ocular movement disorder. Opsoclonus associated with neural crest tumors in children usually responds to corticosteroid treatment; however, up to 50% of such children have persistent neurologic disabilities, including ataxia, poor speech, and cognitive problems. Similar responses to steroids may occur in children with parainfectious or idiopathic opsoclonus. Although preferential responses to adrenocorticotrophic hormone (ACTH) rather than to steroids have been reported, there are no controlled studies comparing both substances.

In adults with paraneoplastic opsoclonus, the course of the opsoclonus is also largely independent of the underlying tumor. It may not improve following tumor therapy, although it tends to wax and wane, and it may spontaneously resolve in some patients with untreated tumor. Treatment with ACTH or steroids has not been uniformly successful in such cases, although both plasmapheresis and intravenous immunoglobulin therapy have occasionally proved effective. Biotin-responsive opsoclonus was described in a patient with multiple carboxylase deficiency.

In patients with opsoclonus-myoclonus syndrome, immunoadsorption therapy (plasma exchange through a protein A column that binds immune complexes and the Fc portion of IgG molecules) was effective in abolishing both opsoclonus and myoclonus.

OPTICAL TREATMENTS

Convergence prisms provide one optical approach that often benefits patients whose nystagmus dampens when they view a near target. Typically recommended are 7.00 prism diopter base-out prisms combined with −1.00 diopter spheres to compensate for accommodation, although the spherical correction may not be needed in presbyopic individuals. In some patients with congenital nystagmus, the improvement of vision that results from nystagmus suppression when they wear base-out prisms is sufficient for them to qualify for a driver's license. Some patients with acquired nystagmus also benefit from the use of convergence prisms, whereas patients whose nystagmus is worse during near viewing may benefit from wearing base-in (divergence) prisms.

Theoretically, it should be possible to use prisms to help patients whose nystagmus is reduced or absent when the eyes are moved into a particular position in the orbit: the "null region." For patients with congenital nystagmus, there is usually some horizontal eye position in which the nystagmus is minimized, whereas downbeat nystagmus may decrease or disappear in upgaze. In practice, patients use head turns to bring their eyes to the optimum position, and only rarely are prisms that produce a conjugate shift helpful.

A different approach to the treatment of nystagmus is the use of an optical system that stabilizes images on the retina. This system consists of a high-plus spectacle lens worn in combination with a high-minus contact lens. The system is designed on the principle that stabilization of images on the retina could be achieved if the power of the spectacle lens focused the primary image close to the center of rotation of the eye. However, such images are then defocused, and a contact lens is required to extend the clear image back onto the retina. Because the contact lens moves with the eye, it does not negate the effect of retinal image stabilization produced by the spectacle lens. With such a system, it is possible to achieve up to about 90% stabilization of images upon the retina.

There are several limitations to the system, however. One is that it disables all eye movements (including the VOR and vergence movements) and thus is useful only when the patient is stationary and is viewing monocularly. Another limitation is that with the highest power components (contact lens of −58.00 diopters and spectacle lens of +32 diopters) the field of view is limited. Some patients with ataxia or tremor (such as those with MS) have difficulty inserting the contact lens. However, initial problems posed by rigid polymethyl methacrylate contact lenses can be overcome by using gas-permeable or even soft contact lenses. Most patients do not need the highest power components for oscillopsia to be abolished and vision to be improved.

In selected patients, the device may prove useful for limited periods of time, such as when the patient wishes to watch a television program.

Contact lenses alone sometimes suppress congenital nystagmus. This effect is not from the mass of the lenses but is probably mediated via trigeminal afferents.

The main therapy for latent nystagmus consists of measures to improve vision, particularly patching for amblyopia in children.

BOTULINUM TOXIN AS TREATMENT OF NYSTAGMUS

An approach to treatment of nystagmus that has gained popularity is injection of botulinum toxin into either the extraocular muscles or the retrobulbar space. The major side effect is ptosis. The main reservation expressed by most investigators is the temporary nature of the treatment and the necessity for repeated injections, with their attendant risk. Furthermore, patients tend not to be pleased with the results, because of ptosis, diplopia, increase of nystagmus in the noninjected eye, or keratitis. Thus, botulinum toxin may abolish nystagmus and improve vision in some patients, but its limited period of action and side effects may limit its therapeutic value.

SURGICAL PROCEDURES FOR NYSTAGMUS

Two surgical procedures may be effective for certain patients with congenital nystagmus: the Anderson-Kestenbaum operation and artificial divergence operation.

The Anderson-Kestenbaum procedure is designed to move the attachments of the extraocular muscles so that the new primary position of the eyes is at the null position. It is performed after first making careful eye movement measurements of nystagmus intensity with the eyes in various positions of gaze and determining the approximate null position. The appropriate extraocular muscles are then weakened or strengthened as necessary to achieve the required shift in the position of the null. The Anderson-Kestenbaum procedure not only shifts and broadens the null region but also results in decreased nystagmus outside the region. It is of uncertain value in the treatment of acquired forms of nystagmus.

The artificial divergence operation of Cüppers is a second procedure designed to reduce nystagmus. It may be helpful in patients whose congenital nystagmus dampens or is suppressed during near viewing and who have stereopsis.

Studies comparing these two methods indicate that the artificial divergence operation generally results in a better visual outcome than the Anderson-Kestenbaum procedure alone.

Several authors recommend performing large recessions of all of the horizontal rectus muscles for treatment of patients with congenital nystagmus. Although modest improvements in visual acuity are reported, some of the patients develop postoperative diplopia. Other authors report improvement with tenectomies of the horizontal rectus muscles in patients with no null position or a null position at 0°.

The role of surgery in the treatment of acquired nystagmus is not well established, although it is clear that suboccipital decompression improves downbeat nystagmus in Chiari syndromes and also prevents progression of other neurologic deficits.

OTHER FORMS OF TREATMENT

A variety of methods other than those described above have been used to treat nystagmus, principally the congenital variety. Electrical stimulation or vibration over the forehead may suppress congenital nystagmus. It is postulated that this effect, like wearing contact lenses, is exerted via the trigeminal system, which receives extraocular proprioception. Acupuncture administered to the neck muscles may suppress congenital nystagmus in some patients via a similar mechanism. Biofeedback has also been reported to help some patients with congenital nystagmus. The role of any of these treatments in clinical practice has yet to be demonstrated.

FOR MORE INFORMATION:
See Walsh & Hoyt's *Clinical Neuro-Ophthalmology,* 5th edition, Volume 1, Chapter 31, pp. 1461–1505.

CHAPTER 20

Myopathies Affecting the Extraocular Muscles

DEVELOPMENTAL DISORDERS OF EXTRAOCULAR MUSCLE

Anomalous development of extraocular muscles is probably more common than the literature would indicate. Many of these anomalies are recognized only during surgical procedures or at autopsy. The most common congenital anomalies of the extraocular muscles are agenesis, anomalous insertions or origins, and the adherence and fibrosis syndromes.

AGENESIS OF THE EXTRAOCULAR MUSCLES

Most cases of **agenesis** of the extraocular muscles involve only a single muscle. Isolated agenesis of the lateral rectus muscle, medial rectus muscle, inferior rectus muscle, superior rectus muscle, and superior oblique muscle are all well described, particularly in children with craniostenoses. Indeed, vertical strabismus in patients with craniostenosis is usually not of

neuropathic origin but is myopathic, caused either by maldevelopment of extraocular muscles or by the mechanical effects of orbital asymmetry on muscle action.

ANOMALIES OF EXTRAOCULAR MUSCLE LOCATION

An abnormal **insertion** of an extraocular muscle is occasionally responsible for ocular motor dysfunction. In its mildest form, this may simply occur as a bifid insertion of the medial, lateral, or superior rectus muscles. The insertions of the superior and inferior oblique muscles vary widely, so it is often difficult to state when they are truly abnormal. Nevertheless, in some patients, the insertions of one or the other of these muscles is clearly abnormal. For example, the superior oblique tendon may insert on the undersurface of the superior rectus muscle, or the inferior oblique tendon may be attached to the lateral rectus muscle. The insertions of the four rectus muscles are much less variable, and thus abnormal insertions are more easily recognized (Fig. 20.1). Abnormal insertions of extraocular muscles, like agenesis of the muscles, often occur in children with craniostenosis.

Abnormal **origins** of extraocular muscles are quite rare. They appear to affect the inferior oblique muscle more than any of the other extraocular muscles.

Occasionally, an extraocular muscle shows underaction because of an abnormally increased length. In other instances, an anomalous muscle slip or fibrous band is present (Fig. 20.2). This

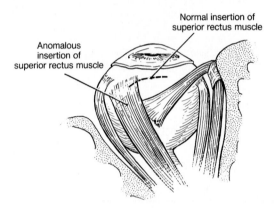

Figure 20.1. Anomalous insertion of the superior rectus muscle in a patient with strabismus. Note that the superior rectus muscle inserts just superior to the lateral rectus muscle. (Redrawn from Rosenbaum AL, Jampolsky A. Pseudoparalysis caused by anomalous insertion of superior rectus muscle. Arch Ophthalmol 1975;93:535–537.)

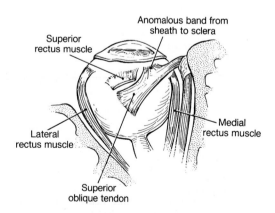

Figure 20.2. Anomalous tendon sheath resulting in tethering of the superior rectus and preventing normal vertical gaze. (Redrawn from Raab EL. Superior oblique tendon sheath syndrome: an unusual case. Ann Ophthalmol 1976; 8:345–347.)

phenomenon may be responsible for some cases of the superior oblique tendon sheath syndrome **(Brown's syndrome)**. Patients with this syndrome show absence of elevation in adduction, improvement of elevation in the primary position, and normal or near-normal elevation in abduction (Fig. 20.3). Forced-duction testing shows mechanical limitation of motion upward and inward of the affected eye, but upward saccadic velocities are normal. The cause of the congenital form of the superior oblique tendon sheath syndrome is unknown, but a restrictive band posterior and inferior to the globe may be responsible in the majority of patients.

CONGENITAL ADHERENCE AND FIBROSIS SYNDROMES

There are two main types of adherence syndromes associated with defective eye movements. In one type, there are adhesions between the sheaths of the lateral rectus and inferior oblique muscles that make it impossible to abduct the eye. The disorder is usually bilateral. The second type is characterized by adherence between the sheaths of the superior rectus and superior oblique muscles, preventing elevation of the affected eye.

Congenital fibrosis of all the extraocular muscles is quite rare. It is an autosomal-dominant disorder mapped to the centromeric region of chromosome 12. The syndrome is characterized by:

- Fibrosis of all the extraocular muscles
- Fibrosis of Tenon's capsule
- Adhesions between muscles, Tenon's capsule, and globe
- Inelasticity and fragility of the conjunctiva
- Absence of elevation or depression of the eyes
- Little or no horizontal movement
- Eyes fixed 20° to 30° below the horizontal
- Blepharoptosis
- Chin elevation (Fig. 20.4)

In nearly all patients, the condition is unassociated with systemic, neuropathic, or generalized myopathic abnormalities, but some patients have facial diparesis, and individual patients have inguinal hernias and cryptorchidism or a cleft palate. The syndrome is usually bilateral, but unilateral cases occur.

Histopathologic findings in some patients

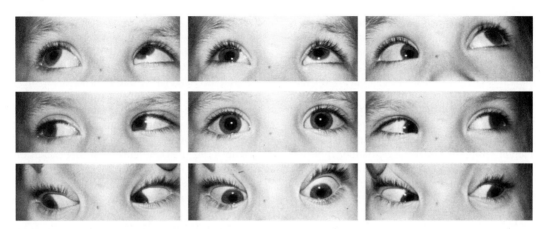

Figure 20.3. Four-year-old child with congenital Brown's superior oblique tendon sheath syndrome. Note marked limitation of upward movement of the right eye when the eye is adducted, compared to mild limitation of upward movement of the eye when it is abducted. The patient was able to fuse in the primary position. (Courtesy of Jacqueline E. Morris, C.O.)

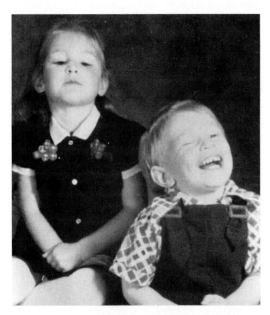

Figure 20.4. Congenital fibrosis syndrome in a brother and sister. Because of the bilateral ptosis and ophthalmoplegia, both children have adopted a head posture with the chin elevated. (Courtesy of Dr. Stewart M. Wolff.)

with these syndromes include replacement of muscle tissue with fibrous tissue and degenerative changes in the muscles. In other patients, however, the muscles are normal or show minimal pathologic changes. Electron microscopic evaluation in some cases reveals active fibrocyte proliferation and absence of striated muscle tissue. Extensive neuropathologic analysis of a single case showed absence of the superior division of the oculomotor nerve and its corresponding motor neurons; atrophy and fibrotic replacement of the levator palpebrae superioris and superior rectus; and abnormalities in all of the extraocular muscles, not just those innervated by the superior division of the oculomotor nerve. These findings suggest that dominantly inherited congenital fibrosis of the extraocular muscles is actually caused by an abnormality of development of their innervation, similar to Duane's retraction syndrome (see Chapter 17).

CONGENITAL MYOPATHIES

Some congenital, primarily nonprogressive myopathies affect the extraocular muscles. Although the disorders in this group are similar to one another clinically and are called collectively **structurally defined congenital myopathies,** they have distinctive morphologic features. The primary congenital myopathies are

1. Central core myopathy
2. Nemaline myopathy
3. Centronuclear (or myotubular) myopathy
4. Multicore disease
5. Congenital fiber type disproportion.

A second group of congenital myopathies is yet to be characterized fully. These disorders generally present with congenital hypotonia or with early-onset generalized weakness that does not progress. Some have ocular features, but others do not. Skeletal deformities, such as high-arched palate, scoliosis, and a slender body habitus often mark these myopathies as beginning in utero; however, disparate phenotypes, in which symptoms appear and even progress in adult life, without dysmorphic features to mark a developmental onset, also occur in nemaline, centronuclear, and multicore myopathies.

Most congenital myopathies are mild and nonprogressive or slowly progressive. Some cases, however, are severe, relentlessly progressive, or both, resulting in substantial debilitation.

Congenital myopathies must be differentiated from other causes of congenital hypotonic weakness. For example, Werdnig-Hoffman disease (acute or type 1 spinal muscular atrophy) is neurogenic, uniformly fatal, and rarely if ever affects extraocular muscles. In fact, ptosis or external ophthalmoplegia probably indicates that a congenital hypotonic disorder is a myopathy. More chronic forms of spinal muscular atrophy also spare extraocular muscles. Congenital myotonic dystrophy, neonatal myasthenia gravis, and infant botulism commonly cause hypotonia, weakness, facial paresis, and ophthalmoparesis (see below and Chapter 21).

In **central core disease,** muscle fibers exhibit a well-defined, round, central core that lacks mitochondria. Inheritance is autosomal dominant.

The muscular weakness appears in early childhood. Marked hypotonia is rarely noted, but motor milestones are usually slightly delayed. The lower extremities are most severely affected, particularly proximally. The facial, sternocleidomastoid, and trapezius muscles may be slightly affected. Extraocular muscles are occasionally involved. Central core disease is caused by a mutation in the ryanodine receptor calcium channel (19q13.1). Patients with this condition are also at risk for malignant hyperthermia, with which central core disease is allelic.

In **nemaline myopathy** (also called ''rod myopathy''), myriad minute rod-shaped granules are present in most of the muscle fibers (Fig. 20.5). Patients with this condition typically have a dysmorphic, elongated, weak face and a high-arched palate. Ptosis and ophthalmoparesis occasionally occur and may be severe (Fig. 20.6).

In **centronuclear myopathy,** most muscle fibers show centrally located nuclei around which there is a small area devoid of enzymatic activity (Fig. 20.7). Because there are wide differences among patients with this disease with respect to mode of inheritance, age of onset, clinical severity, presence or absence of ocular signs, and histochemical abnormalities, this morphologic syndrome must subsume several different disorders.

Early-onset centronuclear myopathy, the most common variety, is characterized clinically by severe neonatal hypotonia, relatively slight delay in motor development, diffuse muscle

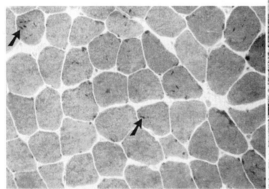 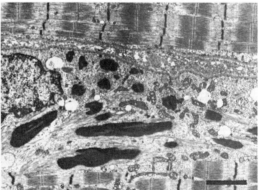

A   B

Figure 20.5. Histopathology of nemaline myopathy. *A.* Muscle biopsy shows small collections of rod-like structures (*arrows*). Modified Gomori trichrome stain (scale = 100 microns). *B.* Electron micrograph of the biopsy specimen shows a cluster of rod bodies adjacent to a nucleus at the periphery of a fiber in longitudinal section (scale = 2 microns). (Reprinted with permission from Wright RA, Plant GT, Landon DN, et al. Nemaline myopathy: an unusual cause of ophthalmoparesis. J Neuroophthalmol 1997;17: 39–43.)

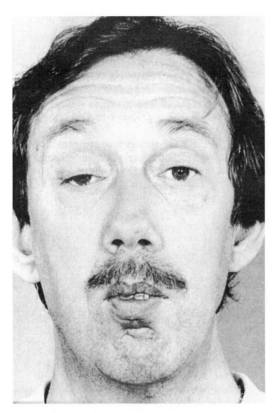

Figure 20.6. Appearance of a 45-year-old man with nemaline myopathy. Note bilateral asymmetric ptosis. The patient must use the frontalis muscle to help raise the eyelids. (Reprinted with permission from Wright RA, Plant GT, Landon DN, et al. Nemaline myopathy: an unusual cause of ophthalmoparesis. J Neuroophthalmol 1997;17:39–43.)

weakness with easy fatigability, scapular winging, and waddling gait, and severe dysfunction of the flexors of the feet. In addition, patients with this disorder have bilateral facial and masticatory weakness as well as ptosis and external ophthalmoplegia (Fig. 20.8). There is generalized areflexia without myotonia or fasciculation. A few patients have cataracts. The course of the disease is generally slowly progressive, with some patients becoming severely disabled by the fourth decade of life. The disorder causes death in some persons; however, other patients who are severely affected in early childhood may nevertheless remain stable or progress slowly. An autosomal-recessive transmission pattern is thought to be operative in the majority of cases, but an autosomal-dominant gene with variable expression is also possible.

In some cases of centronuclear myopathy, muscle weakness does not appear until adulthood. Most patients with this **late-onset** form of centronuclear myopathy have muscle wasting and weakness, mainly of trunk and limb-girdle muscles. Unlike the early-onset form of centronuclear myopathy, extraocular muscle involvement and ptosis are rare in this form of the disease.

A severe **neonatal form** of centronuclear myopathy occurs only in males and is linked to chromosome Xq28. Death from respiratory failure usually occurs in the first few hours or days of life. The few affected children who are able to overcome these neonatal difficulties show a slow improvement in their motor condition but manifest ptosis and external ophthalmoplegia.

Multicore disease is a congenital, nonprogressive myopathy in which the primary histopathologic change is multiple, focal loss of normal sarcomeric cross-striations. These foci of myofibrillar disruption are devoid of mitochondria (Fig. 20.9), giving affected muscle fibers a punched-out appearance like central core disease, but the lesions are smaller and multiple. The disorder is not linked to central core disease or to malignant hyperthermia. Most cases of multicore disease are sporadic, but inheritance in some families seems to be autosomal dominant or autosomal recessive.

Clinically, most cases of multicore disease share the usual pattern of a benign congenital myopathy: floppiness at birth, delayed motor development, and a generalized reduction in muscle bulk. Facial weakness may be present. Ocular involvement includes isolated, bilateral ptosis, mild limitation of ocular movement, and complete external ophthalmoplegia (Fig. 20.10). Cardiac abnormalities are sometimes present and include congenital defects and hypertrophy of cardiac muscle. Most patients have a nonprogressive course, but mild worsening of signs may occur both in early-onset and late-onset cases.

In patients with **congenital fiber type disproportion** (CFTD), type 1 fibers are significantly smaller than type 2 fibers (Fig. 20.11). Children with this disorder are hypotonic at birth. Other features include a long thin face, open mouth, and a high-arched palate. Muscle weakness is diffuse. Affected persons are generally of short stature and low body weight, and they frequently have skeletal abnormalities, particularly congen-

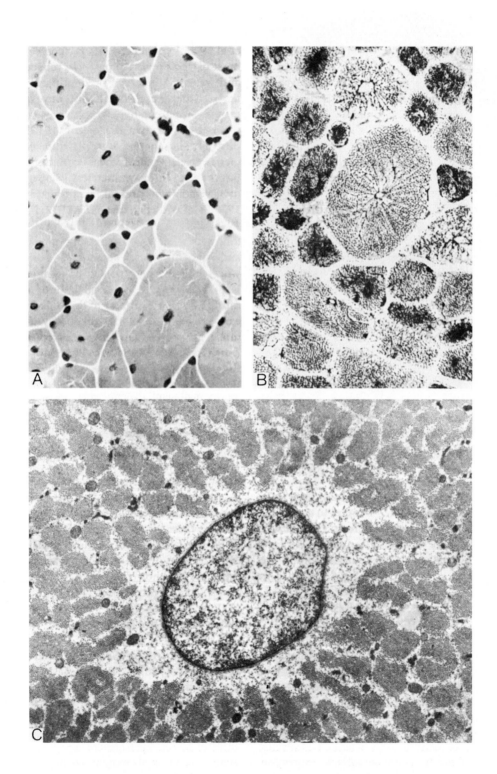

It is clear that individual patients may show structural alterations of muscle fibers that are "characteristic" of more than one type of congenital myopathy. The frequency with which such associations are encountered suggests some relationship among the different structural congenital myopathies. It is therefore likely that either the structural alterations are, in fact, insufficient to permit an exact classification of these disorders or that the production of structural abnormalities occurs as a continuum during muscle development and thus allows multiple patterns to emerge.

MUSCULAR DYSTROPHIES

The term **muscular dystrophy** is used to describe a group of genetically determined disorders that cause **progressive** weakness and wasting of the skeletal muscles and that are assumed to affect the muscle cell directly. Some forms cause death after 15 to 20 years, whereas others are compatible with a normal life expectancy. The distinction between the terms myopathy and dystrophy breaks down, however, when it is realized that some glycogenolytic myopathies, like acid maltase deficiency, can progress inexorably like dystrophies, and some dystrophies, like Becker dystrophy, may hardly progress at all. Although the diagnosis of this group of disorders cannot be established by morphology alone, histologic examination of an affected muscle can exclude other myopathies (e.g., the congenital myopathies and the mitochondrial myopathies). In others, molecular genetic testing can provide the correct diagnosis.

Muscular dystrophies are historically subdivided on the basis of age of onset, mode of inheritance, and clinical features:

1. The dystrophin-deficient dystrophies, including the severe X-linked pseudohypertrophic muscular dystrophy of Duchenne, with its more benign "Becker" variant.
2. The dystrophin-associated glycoprotein

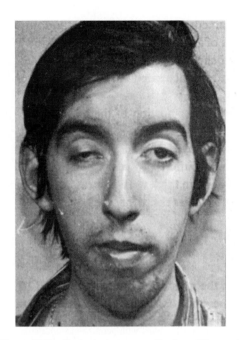

Figure 20.8. Centronuclear myopathy in a 20-year-old man with generalized muscular weakness, a high-arched palate, moderate scoliosis, and winged scapulae. (Reprinted with permission from Jadros-Santel D, Grcevic N, Dogan S, et al. Centronuclear myopathy with type 1 fiber hypotrophy and "fingerprint" inclusions associated with Marfan's syndrome. J Neurol Sci 1980;45:43–56.)

ital hip dislocation. Deep-tendon reflexes are weak or absent. Respiratory problems may occur within the first 2 years of life, after which patients generally slowly improve. Bilateral ptosis and ophthalmoplegia rarely occur (Fig. 20.12).

Some congenital myopathies are characterized histologically primarily by **intracytoplasmic inclusion bodies** within affected muscle fibers. These myopathies include **fingerprint body myopathy, reducing body myopathy,** and **congenital (neuro)myopathy with cytoplasmic bodies.** One patient with reducing body myopathy had a mild bilateral ptosis and diffuse muscle weakness.

Figure 20.7. Histopathology of centronuclear myopathy. *A.* Note centrally located nuclei in most of the fibers (hematoxylin and eosin stain, ×160). *B.* Radial disposition of the intermyofibrillary network in the large fibers can be seen with NADH-tetrazolium reductase stain (×160). *C.* Electron micrograph of a single fiber shows a small area devoid of organelles surrounding the centrally located nucleus (×14,000). (Reprinted with permission from Fardeau M. Congenital myopathies. In: Mastaglia FL, Walton JN, eds. Skeletal Muscle Pathology. Edinburgh: Churchill Livingstone, 1982:161–203.)

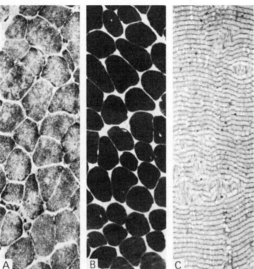

Figure 20.9. Histopathology of multicore disease. *A.* Small defects and irregularities are present in the intermyofibrillar network of involved skeletal muscle fibers; NADH-tetrazolium reaction (×135). *B.* Myofibrillar ATPase reaction after preincubation at pH 4.35 showing type 1 fiber uniformity (×135). *C.* A thick section of epoxy-embedded skeletal muscle shows several foci of disrupted myofibrillar striations (×340). *D.* Electron micrograph of an involved skeletal muscle fiber shows a small focus of sarcomeric disorganization. (Reprinted with permission from Fardeau M. Congenital myopathies. In: Mastaglia FL, Walton JN, eds. Skeletal Muscle Pathology. Edinburgh: Churchill Livingstone, 1982:161–203.)

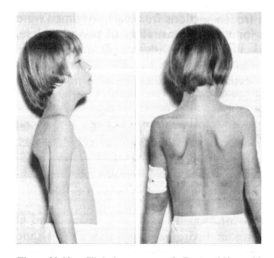

Figure 20.10. Clinical appearance of a 7-year-old boy with multicore disease. He has bilateral ptosis, lordosis, and slight elbow contractures. The truncal and extremity muscles are slightly decreased in bulk. (Reprinted with permission from Engel AG, Gomez MR, Groover RV. Multicore disease: a recently recognized congenital myopathy associated with multifocal degeneration of muscle fibers. Mayo Clin Proc 1971;46:666–681.)

disorders that may resemble Duchenne or Becker dystrophy, including mutations of merosin and the α-, β-, γ-, or δ-sarcoglycans.

3. Various limb-girdle dystrophies, including severe childhood-onset autosomal-recessive (chromosome 13) muscular dystrophy, juvenile scapulohumeral dystrophy of Erb, pelvifemoral dystrophy of Leyden and Möbius, and adult-onset autosomal-dominant limb-girdle dystrophy.

4. The fascioscapulohumeral dystrophy of Landouzy and Déjérine.

5. Distal dystrophies (myopathies) of Welander, Miyoshi, and others.

6. Various congenital muscular dystrophies; including Fukuyama dystrophy, muscle-eye-brain disease, and Walker-Warburg syndrome.

7. Myotonic muscular dystrophy.

8. Proximal myotonic myopathy.

9. Oculopharyngeal dystrophy.

Only the last four of these disorders are of neuro-ophthalmologic importance.

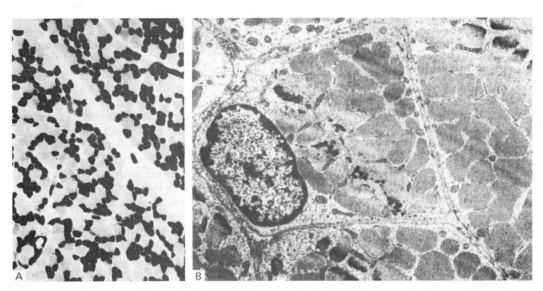

Figure 20.11. Histopathology of congenital fiber type disproportion. *A.* Myofibrillar ATPase reaction after preincubation at pH 4.65 shows that all type 1 fibers are small (× 135). *B.* Electron micrograph shows normal appearance of small, type 1 fibers (× 5850). (Reprinted with permission from Fardeau M. Congenital myopathies. In: Mastaglia FL, Walton JN, eds. Skeletal Muscle Pathology. Edinburgh: Churchill Livingstone, 1982:161–203.)

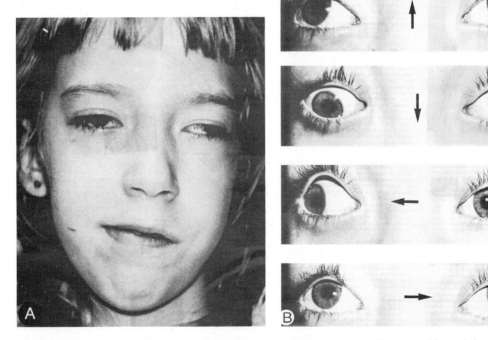

Figure 20.12. Clinical appearance of an 8-year-old girl with congenital fiber type disproportion. *A.* The patient has myopathic facies, bilateral ptosis and exotropia. *B.* The patient has profound ophthalmoparesis. Only abduction of the right eye is normal. (Reprinted with permission from Owen JS, Kline LB, Oh SJ, et al. Ophthalmoplegia and ptosis in congenital fiber type disproportion. J Pediatr Ophthalmol Strabismus 1981;18:55–60.)

CONGENITAL MUSCULAR DYSTROPHIES

A number of patients have dystrophic muscle pathology associated with symptoms that are present at birth and a variable clinical course. These patients are said to have congenital muscular dystrophy (CMD). CMD is by no means rare; it is believed to represent 16% of childhood muscular dystrophies and 9% of all neuromuscular disorders in children.

Patients with CMD show generalized muscle involvement at birth. Muscle atrophy and weakness are symmetric and predominate in proximal muscles. Neither ptosis nor ophthalmoplegia are present in patients with the most common forms of simple CMD confined to skeletal muscle, such as merosin-deficient congenital muscular dystrophy, the sarcoglycanopathies, and the mutations in other dystrophin-associated glycoproteins. However, nonmuscular ocular involvement is frequent in three congenital dystrophy syndromes that are really multisystemic disorders of eye, brain, and skeletal muscle: the Fukuyama type of CMD, so-called "muscle-eye-brain disease," and the Walker-Warburg syndrome.

Fukuyama Congenital Muscular Dystrophy

Patients with Fukuyama dystrophy have CMD associated with central nervous system (CNS) involvement, including mental retardation and convulsions. Children are severely weak from birth, and only a few children are able to walk without assistance. Most survive beyond infancy to remain relatively stable, but the average life span is only 8 to 10 years. Serum creatinine kinase (CK) is elevated and the muscle biopsy shows myopathic and fibrotic changes. Neuroimaging reveals ventricular enlargement and hypoplasia of the cerebellar vermis as well as severe magnetic resonance imaging (MRI) signal abnormalities in white matter. It is transmitted as an autosomal-recessive trait with no sex predilection, a high incidence of consanguinity, and a high frequency of affected siblings. The gene localization is 9q31–33.

Ocular involvement in Fukuyama congenital muscular dystrophy is inconsistent, but it is milder than that in muscle-eye-brain disease and Walker-Warburg syndrome (see below). Ocular findings include occasional optic nerve hypoplasia and optic atrophy, pathologic high myopia, cataracts, retinal abnormalities, and weakness of the orbicularis oculi muscles.

Muscle-Eye-Brain Disease

Muscle-eye-brain disease is also characterized by severe congenital hypotonic weakness from both progressive CNS disease and congenital muscular dystrophy. Although the cerebral and visual abnormalities are severe, most patients reach adult age (average age of death is 18). As in Fukuyama dystrophy, the serum CK is elevated, and muscle biopsy shows mild myopathy with fibrosis.

Ocular abnormalities are more consistent and severe in muscle-eye-brain disease than in Fukuyama dystrophy, but they are less uniform than in Walker-Warburg syndrome. High myopia is common. Ocular findings in postmortem cases include severe generalized loss of retinal ganglion cells, retinochoroidal scars, a pronounced preretinal membrane and gliosis, mottled retinal pigment epithelium, and mild optic nerve and chiasm atrophy with reactive gliosis.

Walker-Warburg Syndrome

The Walker-Warburg syndrome has more severe findings than either Fukuyama dystrophy or muscle-eye-brain disease. Although the neuropathologic features are the same as those of muscle-eye-brain disease, they are more extensive. The ocular malformations are also more severe. Typical ocular features include retinal dysplasia and nonattachment, persistent hyperplastic primary vitreous, optic nerve atrophy, microphthalmia, corneal opacities, congenital cataract, and congenital glaucoma. The serum CK is elevated.

MYOTONIC MUSCULAR DYSTROPHY

The most prevalent inherited neuromuscular disease in adults is **myotonic dystrophy,** a multisystem disorder characterized by myotonia and progressive wasting and weakness of distal muscles. Many patients are recognized instantly by their characteristic frontal balding, long face, ptosis, hollowing of the masseter and temporalis muscles, slackened mouth, facial weakness, and thin neck and limbs. Other features include intellectual impairment, testicular atrophy, excessive daytime somnolence, insulin resistance, and cardiac conduction defects. The most important finding on physical examination is **myotonia**—involuntary delayed relaxation following a contraction, such as after sustained handgrip. However, most patients with myotonic dystrophy complain of weakness, not the myotonia.

Genetics

Myotonic dystrophy is an autosomal-dominant disease that is highly variable in severity and age of onset. It exhibits "anticipation," the phenomenon of increasing severity of inherited disease in successive generations of an affected family. The prevalence is approximately 5 per 100,000.

The genetic defect is amplification of an unstable trinucleotide CTG repeat located in an untranslated region of the gene that encodes myotonin-protein kinase on chromosome 19. The number of CTG repeats ranges from about 50 in patients who are mildly affected to thousands in severely affected patients. Amplification of the CTG repeat is the molecular basis for genetic anticipation.

Men and women are equally at risk, with one exception. When myotonic dystrophy presents at birth (i.e., congenital myotonic dystrophy), weakness is severe, and mental retardation is the rule. Paternal inheritance of very large CTG repeats is genetically inhibited, accounting for maternal inheritance of the congenital form.

Clinical Manifestations

Myotonia of the skeletal muscles is distinctive diagnostically but is often inconstant. It is almost always present electromyographically after the age of 5 years, but it may vary clinically from inapparent to severe. Severity may vary during the day, usually being most severe early in the morning or during rest after exercise. It may be increased by excitement and by cold. It can often be brought out by asking the patient to shake hands. In affected persons, the handclasp is continued after an attempt is made to release the grasp. In some instances, it may be impossible to open the eyelids after they are forcibly closed. Tapping the muscles with a hammer or finger is often sufficient to induce a prolonged contraction. Repetition of a movement eventually abolishes the myotonia.

From the patient's perspective, myotonia is eclipsed in importance by **weakness.** Weakness and wasting of the muscles of the jaw and face cause the temples to appear sunken and the face to become narrowed, appear lengthened, and

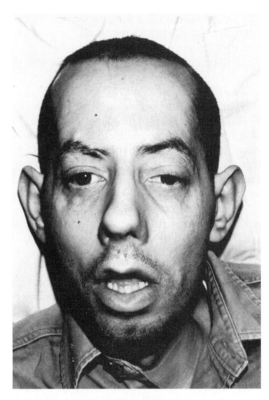

Figure 20.13.   Clinical appearance of a 56-year-old man with myotonic dystrophy. Note bilateral ptosis, exotropia, myopathic facies, and frontal baldness typical of this disorder.

lose its expression (Fig. 20.13). The voice becomes monotonous and frequently has a nasal twang, either through atrophy or myotonia of the palatal muscles. It may be impossible for the patient to hold the head up for any length of time because of weakness of the paraspinal muscles, and the sternocleidomastoid muscles and other neck flexors are often wasted until they become mere cords.

Muscle wasting is often most apparent distally in the forearms and hands, ankle dorsiflexors, and quadriceps, leading to the erroneous diagnosis of neuropathy. In congenital or early-onset severe disease, weakness and hypotonia may be more proximal or universal.

Cardiac conduction defects occur in 90% of patients with myotonic dystrophy and include first-degree heart block, left anterior hemiblock, right bundle-branch block, and complete heart block. These defects can cause syncope or sudden death. Mitral valve prolapse occurs with a higher prevalence than in the normal population, but it is seldom clinically significant and does not require antibiotic prophylaxis. Fatal cases of congestive failure occur but are rare except for cor pulmonale.

Weakness of the respiratory muscles of the chest and diaphragm produces hypoventilation, especially nocturnally, leading to disordered sleep and daytime hypersomnolence. Central respiratory drive may also be decreased in patients with myotonic dystrophy. Aspiration and pneumonia frequently complicate the lives of affected patients and may cause death.

Prominent **structural changes in the brain** are infrequent in patients with myotonic dystrophy. Enlargement of the 3rd ventricle and basal cisterns may be present, particularly in patients with severe mental retardation. MRI reveals nonspecific abnormalities in a significant percentage of patients with myotonic dystrophy. These abnormalities include changes consistent with cerebral atrophy and high-signal areas on T2-weighted images in the subcortical white matter.

Many but not all patients with myotonic dystrophy have **mild mental retardation,** although it may require as many as three or four generations before mental retardation becomes evident in the pedigree of a family with this disorder. Even patients without overt mental retardation may have altered cognitive and personality function.

Patients with myotonic dystrophy may have a variety of **skeletal abnormalities,** particularly frontal bossing, hyperostosis interna, or diffuse thickening of the calvaria that, with cranial muscle wasting, contribute to the V-shaped or "hatchet-faced" appearance. Other common deformities include high-arched palate, prognathism or micrognathism, small sella turcica, scoliosis, kyphosis, and pectus excavatum.

Gastrointestinal symptoms occur in three of every four patients with myotonic dystrophy and may be caused by striated or smooth muscle involvement. Evaluation of dysphagia by cine-esophagography can demonstrate aspiration from impaired cricopharyngeal coordination or relaxation, diminished esophageal motility, cardiospasm, or esophageal dilation. Other gastrointestinal symptoms include constipation, fecal incontinence, intermittent diarrhea, urinary retention, and epigastric pain. Uterine inertia produces prolonged labor, and there is a high rate of fetal loss. Impaired colonic motility is associated with fecal impaction and megacolon. Prolonged relaxation of the anal sphincters is caused by reflex-induced myotonia.

As myotonic dystrophy progresses, diminished 17-ketosteroid levels and **infertility** occur in both men and women. This is associated with testicular atrophy in men and fetal wastage in women. Insulin resistance is common, but overt diabetes mellitus is not.

Ocular Involvement

A variety of ocular disturbances occur in patients with myotonic dystrophy. **Ptosis** is frequently present and may be mild or profound (Figs. 20.13 and 20.14). In addition, there may be **weakness of the orbicularis oculi muscles,** producing infrequent blinking and difficulty closing the eyes. When the orbicularis is affected, there may be bilateral lower lid retraction or delayed opening of the eyes after forceful closure. The combination of ptosis and orbicularis weakness, particularly when combined with ophthalmoparesis, may suggest a diagnosis of myasthenia gravis or chronic progressive external ophthalmoplegia (CPEO) (see below).

Abnormal eye movements are present in many patients with myotonic dystrophy. In its mildest form, the ocular motor involvement consists of slowed saccades in patients who have a full range of eye movements and no visual complaints. In other patients, however, there are varying degrees of ophthalmoparesis. Rare patients even have an eye movement disorder simulating a bilateral internuclear ophthalmoplegia (see Fig. 20.14). Pathologic examination of extraocular muscles from affected patients suggests that the ophthalmoplegia is caused by primary muscle involvement similar to that found in other voluntary muscles in the body.

Cataract is the most common ocular abnormality in patients with myotonic dystrophy, occurring in nearly 100% of patients with the disease. Even if lens changes are not visible by ophthalmoscope, slit lamp biomicroscopy will usually reveal some lens opacification, although some patients with severe myotonic dystrophy nevertheless have clear lenses. The severity of the cataract is not related to the severity of the disease.

Myotonic cataracts have two major features. The first has been described as "iridescent dust"

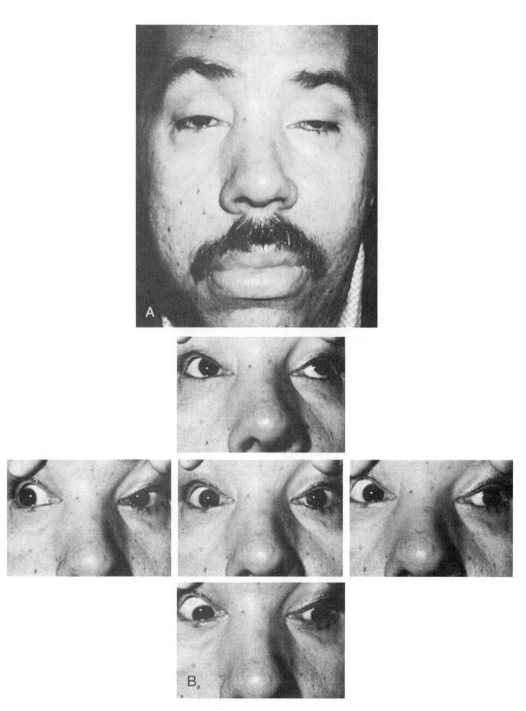

Figure 20.14.   Severe ptosis (*A*) and ophthalmoplegia (*B*) in a 49-year-old man with myotonic dystrophy. (Courtesy of Dr. Thomas L. Slamovits.)

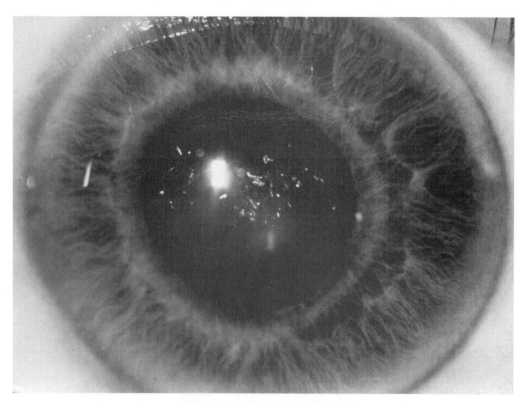

Figure 20.15.   Cataract in a patient with myotonic dystrophy consists of numerous dot opacities, each having a different
color. The opacities were located primarily in the posterior subcortical region of the lens.

or ''fine points mixed with colored crystals.''
These abnormal areas are located in a thin band
of anterior and posterior cortex just beneath the
lens capsule (Fig. 20.15). The crystals may be
opaque and white, but they are more often red,
green, or blue. They are often globular in shape,
but they may be quite irregular. The second characteristic feature of myotonic cataracts is a stellate grouping of opacities at the posterior pole
along the posterior suture lines (Fig. 20.16). The
stellate configuration is thought to be a later
stage than that of the colored crystals.

Nonspecific corneal changes occur in some
patients with myotonic dystrophy. Such changes
often take the form of a corneal epithelial dystrophy that can reduce visual acuity in one or both
eyes and that may worsen after cataract extraction.

Sluggish pupillary responses may occur in
patients with myotonic dystrophy, particularly
those who have slow and limited eye movements. The pupils in such patients also (1) tend

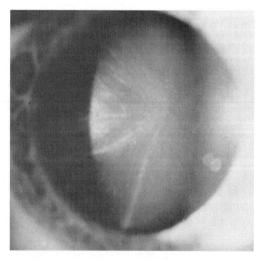

Figure 20.16.   Cataract in a patient with myotonic dystrophy consists of spoke-like opacities of the posterior subcortical region of the lens.

to be miotic, (2) react sluggishly and incompletely to both light and near stimuli, (3) react normally to psychosensory stimuli, and (4) do not tend to fatigue on repeated stimuli any more than normal pupils. Although changes in pupillary reaction may be detected with pupillographic techniques, most patients with myotonic dystrophy appear clinically to have normally reactive pupils.

Vascular abnormalities of the iris occur in many patients with myotonic dystrophy. These iris neovascular tufts can usually be identified by slit lamp biomicroscopy. They show leakage of dye after intravenous injection of fluorescein. In most cases, they are of no consequence, but they can bleed spontaneously or after mild ocular trauma, resulting in a hyphema.

The **ciliary processes may be short and depigmented** in patients with myotonic dystrophy. These abnormalities may explain the finding of **ocular hypotony** in many patients with this disorder.

Retinal abnormalities occur in patients with myotonic dystrophy. The involvement ranges from abnormalities of dark adaptation and electroretinography in patients with no visual complaints and normal-appearing fundi to decreased vision with pigmentary retinopathy involving the macula, peripheral retina, or both (Fig. 20.17). Regardless of the degree of retinopathy, it is not as severe as retinitis pigmentosa and does not cause blindness.

Abnormal visual-evoked potentials may be found in patients with myotonic dystrophy who have no visible retinal abnormalities and a normal electroretinogram (ERG). The abnormalities include reduced amplitude and prolonged latency, and they occur even in patients with apparently normal visual acuity and no evidence of any retinal abnormality by either clinical examination or electrophysiologic testing. Thus, at least some patients with myotonic dystrophy have dysfunction in the visual sensory conducting system other than at the retinal level.

Pathology

The pathologic findings in patients with myotonic dystrophy, like the clinical manifestations, are extensive and variable. In the earliest stages of the disease, a muscle biopsy may appear completely normal or show only a slight excess of central nuclei. As the disease progresses, nuclei appear increased in number, located centrally, and arranged in long rows (Fig. 20.18).

Other pathologic abnormalities include variation in the caliber of the fibers, myofiber degen-

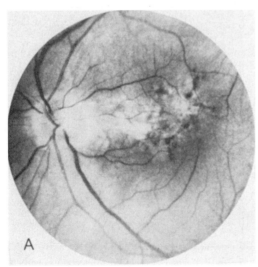
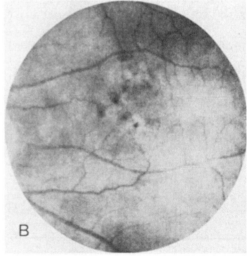

Figure 20.17. Chorioretinopathy in myotonic dystrophy. *A.* Posterior pole of the left eye in a 50-year-old man. Note the streaklike arrangement of the pigment clumps radiating from the fovea as well as the white streak extending between the disc and the macula. *B.* Posterior pole of left eye in a 36-year-old woman. Note pigment clumps and surrounding white streaks in the macula. (Reprinted with permission from Burian HM, Burns CA. Ocular changes in myotonic dystrophy. Am J Ophthalmol 1967;63:22–34.)

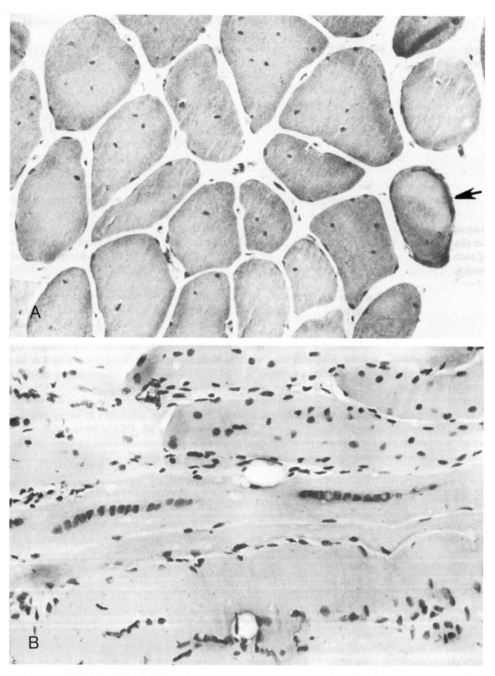

Figure 20.18. Histopathology of skeletal muscle fibers in myotonic dystrophy. *A.* Cross-section of involved muscle shows variation in both diameter and shape of fibers. Sarcolemmal nuclei are increased in number, and many have a central location. The arrow shows "ringbinden" (×340). *B.* One fiber in longitudinal section contains rows of central sarcolemmal nuclei (×340). (Reprinted with permission from Aström KE, Adams RD. Myotonic disorders. In: Mastaglia FL, Walton JN, eds. Skeletal Muscle Pathology. Edinburgh: Churchill Livingstone, 1982:266–286.)

eration and regeneration, ringed fibers (''ring-binden''), myofibrils with an aberrant course, sarcoplasmic masses of tightly packed disordered myofilaments, focal areas of myofibrillar disruption and Z-band streaming, and associated secondary changes in mitochondria or the sarco-tubular system.

In the advanced stages of the disease, a large proportion of the total fiber population is lost and is replaced by connective tissue and fat cells. The extraocular muscles may undergo similar changes.

Diagnosis and Treatment

The patient's presentation for cataract extraction may be the family's initial presentation, and it is therefore incumbent on the neuro-ophthalmologist to recognize the syndrome. The diagnosis is supported by findings of myotonia on an electromyogram (EMG) and multihued speckled cataracts on slit lamp examination. Testing of deoxyribonucleic acid (DNA) for the CTG repeat can be performed when the diagnosis is not clinically obvious, thus eliminating the need for a muscle biopsy.

When troublesome, myotonia can be treated with phenytoin or other drugs, but few patients request this therapy. Distal weakness causing footdrop is treated with ankle-foot orthoses. Cardiac conduction defects may require pacemakers.

Treatment of ophthalmoparesis is usually unnecessary because the limitation of eye movement in patients with myotonic dystrophy is usually symmetric. Thus, such patients do not commonly complain of diplopia. Prisms can be used to treat patients with diplopia in primary position.

Treatment of ptosis is somewhat problematic in patients with myotonic dystrophy because of the commonly associated orbicularis weakness. If the eyelids are raised to a ''normal'' level, such patients may develop severe tearing and irritation from exposure keratopathy, and some may even develop corneal ulceration leading to blindness. Thus, the eyelids should be raised only when ptosis is interfering with function and only as high as needed to improve vision.

PROXIMAL MYOTONIC MYOPATHY

Proximal myotonic myopathy (PROMM) is an autosomal-dominant disorder that has certain features in common with myotonic dystrophy but that has a different clinical presentation and no abnormal enlargement of the CTG repeat in the myotonic dystrophy gene. The chromosome localization and the gene responsible for this disorder are unknown, but there is no linkage to the gene loci for myotonic dystrophy, muscle sodium channel disorders, or muscle chloride disorders.

The clinical features of PROMM are muscle stiffness, myotonia, weakness, muscle pain, and cataracts. These problems can occur singly or in various combinations. Initial symptoms usually develop between 20 and 60 years of age. Many patients first complain of intermittent stiffness in the thigh muscles of one or both legs and of intermittent grip myotonia. In other patients, cataracts are the first manifestation of the disorder. These may appear in late childhood or early adolescence and are indistinguishable from those in myotonic dystrophy, being posterior subcapsular, iridescent, multicolored opacities. Cardiac arrhythmias occur in some patients.

EMG usually reveals myotonic discharges in affected patients, including those without obvious clinical myotonia. However, these discharges are scarce and difficult to detect. Muscle biopsy usually reveals a nonspecific myopathy. In contrast to myotonic dystrophy, there are no ringbinden or subsarcolemmal masses, and there is no evidence of selective type 1 fiber atrophy.

The prognosis of PROMM is more favorable than that of myotonic dystrophy. Most patients do not show any deterioration of mental status, dysarthria, dysphagia, or respiratory failure. Nonsteroidal anti-inflammatory drugs and muscle relaxants can be used to treat the muscle pain experienced by these patients, and antimyotonia therapy, including mexiletine, phenytoin, and acetazolamide, can be used to treat patients with severe myotonic stiffness and grip myotonia. Cataract surgery may be warranted in some patients.

OCULOPHARYNGEAL DYSTROPHY

Oculopharyngeal dystrophy is inherited as an autosomal-dominant trait mapped to chromosome 14q11.2–13 in the region of the gene for myosin heavy chains. Many affected families with this disorder are of French-Canadian heritage.

The two essential clinical characteristics of oculopharyngeal muscular dystrophy are ptosis and dysphagia (Fig. 20.19). Although neither

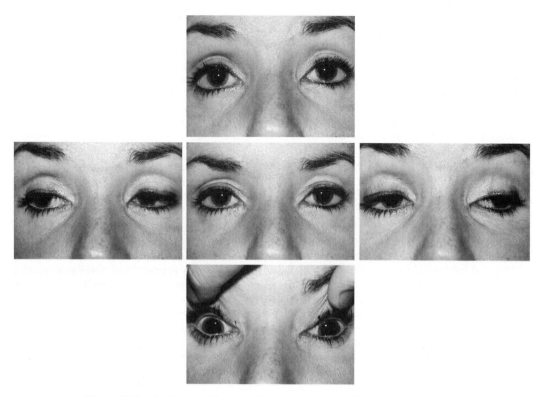

Figure 20.19. Ptosis and ophthalmoplegia in a patient with oculopharyngeal dystrophy.

symptom usually presents until late in life, mild ptosis usually precedes any significant dysphagia, often by several years.

The best way to assess the onset and familial occurrence is by examining old family photographs for ptosis. The ptosis in patients with oculopharyngeal muscular dystrophy is eventually always bilateral, rarely complete, and usually symmetric, although one eyelid may become ptotic weeks or months before the other. External ophthalmoplegia is present in most patients. By comparison, limb-muscle weakness is mild and proximal, if it is present at all. This is not a rare condition. Patients with oculopharyngeal muscular dystrophy comprised 33% of patients with acquired ptosis in one series.

Dysphagia may be disabling. At first there is difficulty only in swallowing solid foods, but eventually swallowing liquids also becomes difficult, and several attempts at swallowing may be necessary to empty the upper pharynx. Examination of the swallowing mechanisms in affected patients usually reveals weak movements in the pharynx and larynx. Ingested material may

thus be aspirated, resulting in recurrent pneumonitis. Some patients with severe dysphagia are treated successfully with cricopharyngeal myotomy, but a percutaneous feeding gastrostomy is a more practical treatment and is more commonly used.

Oculopharyngeal dystrophy is a primary myopathy with degenerative changes, fibrosis, abundant central nuclei, altered myofibrils, Z-bands, and other nonspecific changes. The characteristic lesions, however, are an extensive accumulation of autophagic vacuoles in non-necrotic myofibers (Fig. 20.20) and nuclear inclusions in striated muscle (Fig. 20.21).

ION CHANNEL DISORDERS (MYOTONIA)

Myotonia, as noted above, is a phenomenon in which muscle fibers have a pathologically persistent activity after a strong contraction or are continuously active when they should be relaxed. Myotonia is identified physiologically as a delay in muscle relaxation after percussion or electric stimulation of a muscle, or after a voluntary contraction. The phenomenon is caused by mutations affecting chloride, sodium, and calcium ion channels in surface membranes. It persists after blockage of either the peripheral nerve or the neuromuscular junction. In patients with myotonia, the spontaneous action potentials as recorded in the EMG are high-frequency discharges of single muscle fibers that wax and wane in both amplitude and frequency. When translated into sound, these discharges produce a noise resembling that of a dive-bomber or a motorcycle engine.

Clinical myotonia is a common feature of a number of different genetically determined, primary muscle diseases, including autosomal-dominant myotonia congenita, autosomal-recessive myotonia, paramyotonia congenita, the familial periodic paralyses, myotonic muscular dystrophy (see above), and chondrodystrophic myotonia.

MYOTONIA CONGENITA

Autosomal-dominant and autosomal-recessive **myotonia congenita** result from allelic mu-

tations of the chloride channel gene encoded on chromosome 7q35. Myotonic symptoms, noted in the first years of life and often worse in males than females, frequently lessen by the second or third decade of life. Myotonia of limb muscles is more likely to occur when strenuous exertion is initiated after a period of rest; it is then followed by transient weakness. Unlike paramyotonia, the myotonia is not aggravated by cooling, and long-lasting paralysis does not occur. This is one of only a few neuromuscular disorders in which prominent hypertrophy can occur, particularly in the masseter, proximal arms, thighs, calves, and extensor digitorum brevis.

Patients with myotonia congenita often have eyelid myotonia. At the very least, lid lag is usually present, and frank blepharospasm may occur in some patients after forced closure of the eyelids. Strabismus is said to occur in some patients, but not ptosis or generalized ophthalmoplegia. Swallowing and voice are spared, but chewing is sometimes affected.

The pathophysiology of the myotonia is

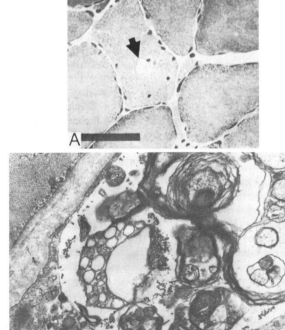

Figure 20.20. Vacuoles within an affected muscle in a patient with oculopharyngeal dystrophy. The rimmed vacuole (*arrow*) in *A* corresponds to an autophagic vacuole within a muscle fiber (*B*). *A.* Gomori trichrome stain (bar = 50 microns). *B.* Electron micrograph (bar = 1 micron). (Reprinted with permission from Schmalbruch H. The muscular dystrophies. In: Mastaglia FL, Walton J, eds. Skeletal Muscle Pathology. Edinburgh: Churchill Livingstone, 1982:235–265.)

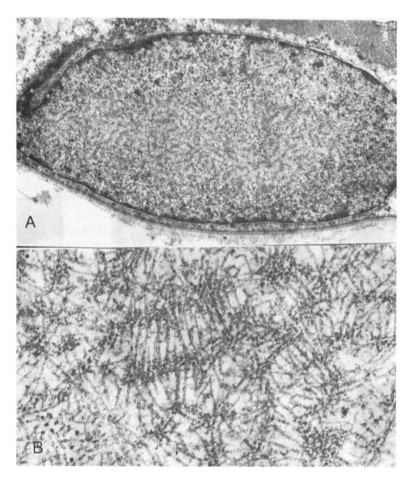

Figure 20.21. Nuclear inclusions in skeletal muscle of patients with oculopharyngeal dystrophy. *A.* Transverse section of a muscle fiber shows a subsarcolemmal nucleus that contains abundant filamentary inclusions arranged in palisades ($\times 13,000$). *B.* At higher magnification, the intranuclear inclusions can be seen to consist of tubular filaments that do not have any specific orientation. (Reprinted with permission from Tomé FMS, Fardeau M. Nuclear inclusions in oculopharyngeal dystrophy. Acta Neuropathol 1980;49:85–87.)

thought to be caused by both low chloride channel conductance and abnormal reopening of sodium channels. Specific genetic diagnosis is possible. Treatment, which is most often successful with Mexiletene or quinine, and less so with procainamide or phenytoin, is best undertaken several days before vigorous activity, rather than on a regular basis.

PARAMYOTONIA CONGENITA

Paramyotonia congenita is a condition characterized by autosomal-dominant inheritance, paradoxic myotonia (i.e., myotonia that worsens with exercise), exacerbation of myotonia by cold, and periodic attacks of weakness. The disorder is caused by mutations in the sodium channel gene and is allelic to hyperkalemic periodic paralysis, accounting for the great overlap between the two syndromes. Neither ptosis nor ophthalmoplegia occur in patients with this disease; however, some patients show myotonic lid lag similar to that observed in other myotonic disorders, including myotonia congenita. Paramyotonia may be induced by placing ice cubes over the eyelids. Specific genetic diagnosis is available. Paramyotonia often responds to Mexiletene and acetazolamide, but not usually to drugs like quinine or phenytoin.

PERIODIC PARALYSIS

Familial periodic paralysis is a rare syndrome characterized by abnormal flux of potassium across muscle membranes and by spells of severe flaccid weakness in the limb muscles. The spells last minutes to hours and are provoked by rest following exercise. Bulbar and ocular muscles are rarely affected, and respiratory muscles are almost never affected. The syndrome is subdivided into hyper-, hypo-, and normokalemic types, but all three types share onset by the third decade of life, greater severity in males, autosomal-dominant inheritance, and oliguria preceding attacks.

Examination shows normal strength between attacks, but if the attacks are frequent and not treated, mild fixed proximal weakness may develop. Myotonia, especially eyelid myotonia, may be seen. In rare patients, hypo- or hyperkalemia causes a complicating cardiac arrhythmia.

During paralytic attacks, muscles are inexcitable, and deep-tendon reflexes are hypoactive or absent. The histologic hallmark is a vacuolar myopathy most consistently associated with the permanent myopathy that develops after repeated attacks.

Hypokalemic periodic paralysis is caused by mutations in the dihydropyridine receptor calcium channel encoded at chromosome 1q31–32, but the pathophysiologic mechanism by which these mutations alter potassium flux across muscle membrane is incompletely understood. The age of onset is from about 5 years to the fourth decade of life. Attack frequency is highly variable, but attacks are often more severe and longer lasting (up to 24 hours) than the spells in hyperkalemic periodic paralysis (see below). Attacks can be precipitated by carbohydrate loading and rest before exercise (e.g., the classic Sunday morning athlete after a night of pizza and beer). Weakness of extraocular muscles or ptosis rarely occurs, but eyelid myotonia is common, causing lid lag (Fig. 20.22). The myotonia in hypokalemic periodic paralysis is confined to lid muscles. Thus, EMG evidence of myotonia in limb muscles makes other forms of periodic paralysis more likely.

The diagnosis of hypokalemic periodic paralysis is made by serial electrolyte determinations, electrocardiogram (ECG), exclusion of thyrotoxicosis (an important acquired cause of hypokalemic periodic paralysis in young Hispanic and Asian men), electromyography, the McManis exercise test, and insulin/glucose provocative testing if necessary.

Acute treatment is with oral intake of potassium chloride and gentle exercise. Acetazolamide can help prevent further attacks. Thyrotoxic periodic paralysis requires specific antithyroid therapy.

Hyperkalemic periodic paralysis is caused by mutations in the sodium channel α-subunit gene at 17q13.1–13.3, causing defective sodium channel inactivation. Attacks of paralysis usually present before 10 years of age and are often milder and shorter than those in patients with hypokalemic periodic paralysis. They occur after fasting or during rest following exercise. Cranial muscles are affected in about half the cases. Myotonia may be prominent by both examination and EMG studies. Muscle hypertrophy may be present. Sensory symptoms occur but without sensory signs.

Eyelid abnormalities may be significant in patients with hyperkalemic periodic paralysis. Such patients, particularly young children, may have transient attacks of "staring." In adults, the sclera above the cornea is visible when the patient looks down after looking upward (Fig. 20.23). Lid lag is commonly present during attacks but may disappear after repeated up and down movements of the eyes. It may be brought

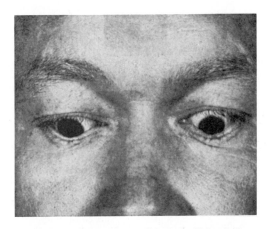

Figure 20.22. Lid lag in hypokalemic familial periodic paralysis. The upper lids floated down about 20 seconds after the photograph was taken. (Reprinted with permission from Resnick JS, Engel WK. Myotonic lid lag in hypokalemic periodic paralysis. J Neurol Neurosurg Psychiatry 1967;30: 47–51.)

on by placing an ice cube against the eyelids for several minutes.

Diagnosis is made by serial electrolyte determinations, ECG, EMG studies, and exercise testing. Provocative testing with potassium loading is rarely indicated. Specific molecular diagnosis is possible.

Acute attacks are not often severe enough to require treatment other than ingestion of simple carbohydrates. Prophylaxis against further at-

tacks, to forestall any permanent weakness, requires thiazide diuretics.

Normokalemic periodic paralysis is rare. Its nosologic distinction from hyperkalemic periodic paralysis is unclear because serum potassium may be normal in some patients with hyperkalemic periodic paralysis, normokalemic patients may have potassium-sensitive periodic paralysis, and at least one family with normokalemic periodic paralysis displayed the common

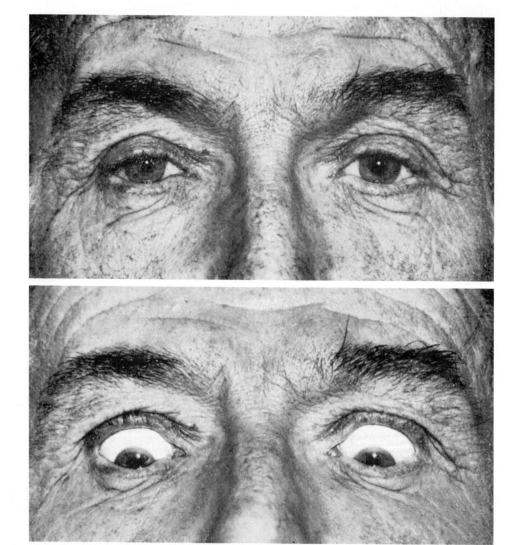

Figure 20.23. Lid retraction and lag in hyperkalemic familial periodic paralysis. *Top:* The eyelids are in normal position when the patient is looking straight ahead. *Bottom:* When the patient looks down, there is marked lid retraction and lid lag that disappear within 1 minute. (Reprinted with permission from McArdle B. Adynamia episodica hereditaria and its treatment. Brain 1962;85:121–148.)

sodium channel mutation associated with hyper-kalemic periodic paralysis.

SCHWARTZ-JAMPEL SYNDROME (CHONDRODYSTROPHIC MYOTONIA)

Schwartz-Jampel syndrome is a rare syndrome of dwarfism, abnormalities of long bones and the face, blepharospasm, and myotonic symptoms. The facial appearance of blepharospasm, puckered lips, myokymic twitching of the chin, low-set ears, receding chin, a high-pitched forced voice, and high-arched palate is distinctive. Frequent ophthalmologic features include myopia, cataract, strabismus, and nystagmus. Most early case series suggested that the typical EMG discharges are true myotonic potentials generated in muscle. This condition is not a true myotonia, because EMG discharges from affected muscles are abolished by *d*-tubocurarine. This finding suggests that the abnormal activity of affected muscles may be generated from the presynaptic region of the neuromuscular junction. The continuous muscle fiber activity may be considered a form of neuromyotonia. The pertinent gene is localized to chromosome 1p34–36.1.

MITOCHONDRIAL MYOPATHIES (MITOCHONDRIAL ENCEPHALOMYOPATHIES)

The mitochondrial encephalomyopathies are a genetically and biochemically diverse set of disorders that are defined by structural abnormalities of mitochondria on muscle biopsy. The histologic hallmark of these disorders is the abnormal accumulation of increased numbers of enlarged mitochondria beneath the sarcolemma of affected muscle fibers. Because of their irregular appearance and their strikingly dark red color when stained with the modified Gomori trichrome stain, these abnormal muscle fibers are called **ragged-red fibers** (RRF) (Fig. 20.24). In patients with ophthalmoplegia, RRF are usually present in skeletal muscles. They are also found in the orbicularis oculi muscle and in the extraocular muscles of affected patients.

When viewed with the electron microscope, the mitochondria in affected muscle fibers appear more numerous and more variable in size than in normal muscle fibers. The mitochondria are often enlarged, with distorted or disorganized cristae that are sometimes arranged concen-

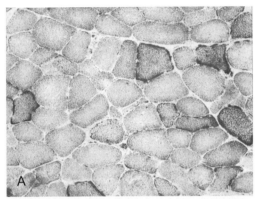

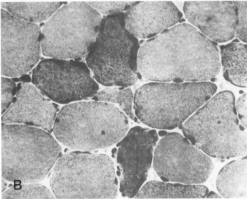

Figure 20.24. "Ragged-red" fibers in chronic progressive external ophthalmoplegia (CPEO). *A.* Succinate dehydrogenase reaction shows increased activity at the periphery of some muscle fibers in a patient with CPEO. Although mitochondrial protein synthesis is reduced in affected fibers, the activity of this enzyme is preserved because the protein subunits of Complex II (succinate dehydrogenase-ubiquinone reductase) are encoded exclusively by the nuclear genome. *B.* A group of three ragged-red fibers surround an atrophic, angulated muscle fiber. Modified Gomori trichrome stain. (Reprinted with permission from Morgan-Hughes JA. Mitochondrial myopathies. In: Mastaglia FL, Walton J, eds. Skeletal Muscle Pathology. Edinburgh: Churchill Livingstone, 1982:309–339.)

trically. Paracrystalline inclusions are invariably present within the cristae, and similar inclusions may also be observed outside cristae (Fig. 20.25). In most cases, RRF reflect the presence of mutations in mitochondrial DNA (mtDNA).

MITOCHONDRIAL DISORDERS ASSOCIATED WITH EXTERNAL OPHTHALMOPLEGIA

Chronic progressive external ophthalmoplegia is the most frequent manifestation of mitochondrial myopathies. Indeed, among patients with mitochondrial myopathies, 90% have ocular or ocular motor abnormalities, and CPEO is the presenting feature in about two-thirds of the patients. Of course, a chronic progressive external ophthalmoplegia may occur in association with a variety of myopathic and other disorders (e.g., Graves' disease, myasthenia gravis, and brainstem glioma). It should be clear, therefore, that this is simply a clinical sign and not a nosologic entity.

Generalized skeletal muscle weakness is present in most patients with CPEO. Nevertheless, ptosis and ophthalmoplegia can occur in the absence of weakness in other muscles. In patients who are not born with obvious external ophthalmoplegia, **ptosis** is usually the first evidence of involvement and may precede ophthalmoparesis

by months to years (Fig. 20.26). The ptosis is slowly progressive and tends to become complete in most cases. Characteristically, it is bilateral, but unilateral ptosis can be present for years before the opposite side becomes involved or ophthalmoparesis is observed. As the ptosis progresses, it eventually interferes with vision, and the patient must tilt the head backward and use the frontalis muscles to elevate the eyelids (see Fig. 20.26). The ptosis is fixed, unlike the variable, fatigable ptosis in myasthenia gravis. Rare patients have complete ophthalmoplegia and no significant ptosis.

Because **limitation of ocular movements** is generally symmetric, most patients with CPEO do not complain of diplopia and are not aware of a problem with ocular motility until it is of such severity that it limits peripheral vision or

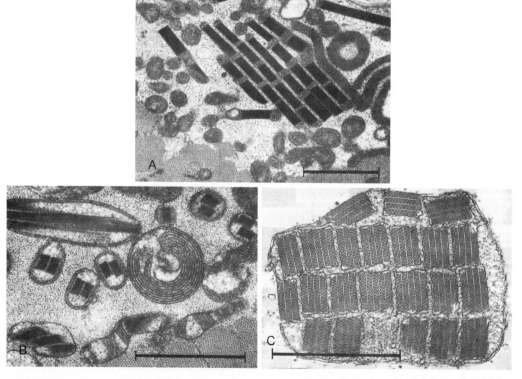

Figure 20.25. Mitochondrial inclusions in chronic progressive external ophthalmoplegia. *A.* Intramembrane crystals arranged in chains separated by transverse mitochondrial cristae. *B.* Mitochondria contain ''parking lot'' inclusions or multiple concentric cristae embedded in glycogen (bar = 2 microns). *C.* An enlarged mitochondrion contains 22 intracrystal paracrystalline inclusions (bar = 1 micron). (Reprinted with permissions from Morgan-Hughes JA. Mitochondrial myopathies. In: Mastaglia FL, Walton JN, eds. Skeletal Muscle Pathology. Edinburgh: Churchill Livingstone, 1982:309–339.)

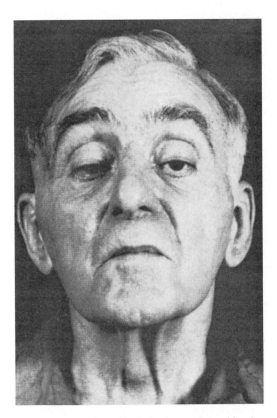

Figure 20.26. Myopathic facies in a patient with mitochondrial cytopathy and chronic progressive external ophthalmoplegia. Note flat, expressionless facial features associated with continuous wrinkling of the frontalis muscles and a posterior head tilt in order to compensate for bilateral ptosis. (Courtesy of Dr. I. Lewis and the Canadian Medical Association Journal.)

until someone points it out to them. For this reason, immobility of the eyes is usually severe when such patients are first examined (Fig. 20.27). In many cases, downward movements are relatively intact compared with upward and horizontal movements.

In the rare patients who have asymmetric limitation of movement and complain of double vision, prism therapy or surgery may be used to improve ocular alignment, at least temporarily. Surgery to raise the eyelids can be performed in patients with severe ptosis that prevents them from functioning normally, but because such patients may also have weakness of the orbicularis oculi muscles, care must be taken to avoid raising the eyelids so much that the patient develops

exposure keratopathy from inability to close the eyes.

Both ultrasonography and computed tomographic (CT) scanning in patients with CPEO show thin, presumably atrophic, extraocular muscles (Fig. 20.28). The thinning is usually symmetric.

Kearns-Sayre syndrome (KSS) represents a severe form of CPEO associated with multisystem involvement. KSS is characterized by the combination of CPEO and pigmentary retinopathy before the age of 20 years, together with one or more of the following: complete heart block, cerebrospinal fluid (CSF) protein >1 mg/mL, cerebellar ataxia, short stature, deafness, dementia, and endocrine abnormalities. The occurrence of similar mutations of mtDNA in CPEO and KSS supports the view that these disorders are part of a continuous spectrum of the same disease.

In most instances, the retinopathy that occurs in patients with KSS is different from that seen in patients with the group of hereditary retinal disorders collectively known as retinitis pigmentosa, hence the use of the term **pigmentary retinopathy** to emphasize the distinction. Although cases of CPEO associated with what appears to be typical retinitis pigmentosa probably occur, the pigmentary retinopathy of KSS generally can be differentiated from retinitis pigmentosa by both clinical and electrophysiologic criteria.

The pattern of retinal involvement in KSS is particularly important. In contrast to retinitis pigmentosa, which usually affects the peripheral and midperipheral retina, at least initially, the retinopathy of KSS usually occurs initially in the posterior fundus (Fig. 20.29). Severe involvement of the peripapillary zone is typical. In this region, retinal epithelial atrophy frequently results in increased visibility of the choroidal vessels and the appearance of ''choroidal sclerosis,'' although rare cases occur in which a pattern of choroideremia is present. In advanced cases, a metallic sheen or mottled fluorescent appearance surrounds the optic nerve. ''Bonespicule'' pigment formation, a common feature of retinitis pigmentosa, rarely occurs.

Examination of affected fundi usually shows diffuse depigmentation of the retinal pigment epithelium with a characteristic mottled ''salt and pepper'' pattern of pigment clumping similar to that seen in patients with congenital ru-

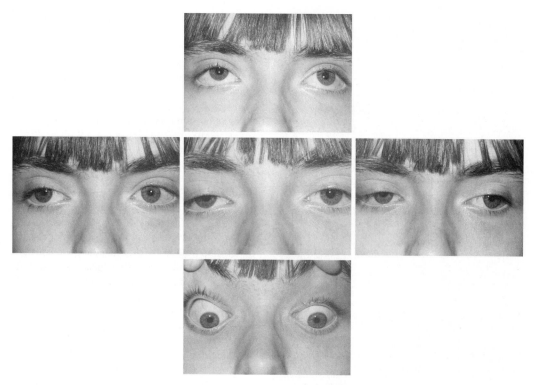

Figure 20.27.   Moderate ptosis and severe external ophthalmoplegia in a patient with mitochondrial cytopathy. The patient had no evidence of retinopathy or cardiac disease.

bella. This appearance may be most marked around the macula. Visual symptoms such as night blindness or diminished visual acuity are generally mild and occur in only about 40 to 50% of patients. However, there are rare cases of KSS with CNS involvement in which bone-spicule formation and pigment clumping in the macula are associated with profound loss of visual acuity.

Although exceptions exist, dark adaptometry and electroretinography are usually normal or only mildly abnormal in patients with KSS. In most cases in which there are abnormal electrophysiologic studies, observable retinal abnormalities are present. The primary defect on pathologic studies of KSS is in the retinal pigment epithelium.

Patients with KSS typically have **cardiac conduction disturbances.** The actual time of onset and the frequency of cardiac involvement in patients with KSS is variable. In some cases, the onset of heart block occurs simultaneous with the onset of ocular disturbances. In others, the

cardiac disturbances develop several years after the onset of ptosis and ocular motor dysfunction. Any patient with CPEO and a pigmentary retinopathy or neurologic dysfunction but with a normal ECG should be warned of the possibility of future cardiac disease, and the symptoms of such disease should be explained. In addition, such patients should undergo cardiac examinations at regular intervals, regardless of their age.

Although the cardiac dysfunction that occurs in patients with KSS can often be managed effectively with an artificial pacemaker, patients may die suddenly, even after insertion of a pacemaker. Such patients die not because of a cardiac arrhythmia but because of a decreased ventilatory response to hypoxia and hypercarbia caused by deficient brainstem respiratory control mechanisms. Cardiac failure in patients with KSS can be successfully treated with cardiac transplantation.

Up to 25% of patients with CPEO have **weakness of nonocular muscle groups.** Facial muscles, particularly the orbicularis oculi muscles, may be affected. Such patients may thus be unable not only to open the eyelids but also to close them tightly (Fig. 20.30). With involvement of the frontalis muscle, there is an increasing inability to wrinkle the forehead and use the frontalis to help open the eyelids. This results in an apparent worsening of ptosis. All muscles of the face may eventually become affected, and the face thus becomes thin and expressionless. In some patients, the muscles of mastication become involved. With progression of the disease, there is often weakness and wasting of the neck and shoulder muscles. Although the muscles of

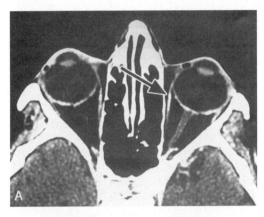
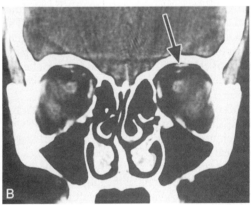

Figure 20.28. Computed tomographic scanning of extraocular muscles in a patient with chronic progressive external ophthalmoplegia. *A.* Axial view shows marked thinning of left medial rectus muscle (*arrow*). *B.* Coronal view shows similar thinning of left superior rectus muscle (*arrow*). (Reprinted with permission from Wallace DK, Sprunger DT, Helveston EM, et al. Surgical management of strabismus associated with chronic progressive external ophthalmoplegia. Ophthalmology 1997;104:695–700.)

the extremities may be involved, the weakness is often so mild that some patients are unaware that they have any weakness, and others deny weakness even though they can be observed to alter their behavior to compensate for mild extremity weakness (e.g., lifting a coffee cup with two hands to avoid spilling).

Patients with KSS usually have evidence of **neurologic dysfunction.** Abnormalities include cerebellar ataxia, pendular nystagmus, vestibular dysfunction, hearing loss, impaired intellectual function, and peripheral neuropathy. In addition, in many patients there is elevation of CSF protein content. Spongiform changes in the brain are present in almost every patient in whom an autopsy is performed. CNS involvement in KSS is reflected in MRI abnormalities in the brainstem, globus pallidus, thalamus, and the white matter of the cerebrum and cerebellum. In addition, regional abnormalities of brain metabolism are demonstrated in patients with KSS using MR spectroscopy (MRS).

Endocrine dysfunction is common in patients with KSS. In addition to short stature, hypoparathyroidism with low or absent parathyroid hormone levels is well documented, and tetany may be a presenting symptom. Short stature is present in 38% of cases; gonadal dysfunction after puberty affecting both sexes occurs in 20% of cases; and diabetes mellitus is found in 13% of patients, half of whom require insulin. Dysthyroidism, hyperaldosteronism, and hypomagnesemia are uncommon. Bone or tooth abnormalities and calcification of the basal ganglia are found both in patients with and without hypoparathyroidism.

MITOCHONDRIAL GENETICS

Mitochondria are the only cellular organelles, aside from the nucleus, containing DNA. The mtDNA is a 16,569 base pair circle of double-stranded DNA. The majority of the 67 or so mitochondrial proteins are encoded by the nuclear genome, translated on cytoplasmic ribosomes, and transported into mitochondria. Mitochondrial DNA encodes 13 mitochondrial proteins as well as the two ribosomal ribonucleic acids (rRNAs) and 22 transfer RNAs (tRNAs) required to translate these proteins. Oxidative phosphorylation is carried out by the four multiprotein complexes of the respiratory chain and adenosine triphosphate (ATP) synthetase (Complex V). The mtDNA encodes seven subunits of

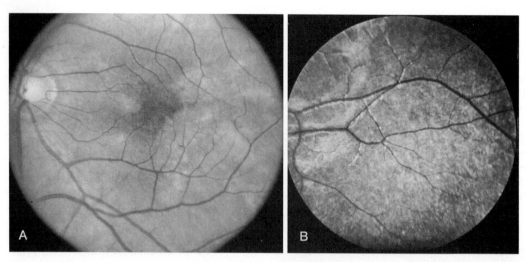

Figure 20.29. Pigmentary retinopathy in Kearns-Sayre syndrome. *A.* Posterior pole of a 17-year-old man shows mild pigmentary disturbance with pigment clumping overlying white streaks. Note resemblance to retinopathy of myotonic dystrophy (see Fig. 20.17). *B.* Stippled retinal pigmentary disturbance in a 35-year-old woman with Kearns-Sayre syndrome.

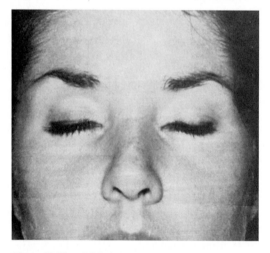

Figure 20.30. Orbicularis oculi weakness in a patient with Kearns-Sayre syndrome. The patient is attempting to close her eyelids as tightly as possible.

Complex I (NADH-ubiquinone reductase), one subunit of Complex III (ubiquinol-cytochrome c reductase), three subunits of Complex IV (cytochrome c oxidase), and two subunits of ATP synthetase. Because the protein subunits of Complex II (succinate dehydrogenase-ubiquinone reductase) are encoded exclusively by the nuclear genome, Complex II activity is not impaired by mutations of the mitochondrial genome.

Mitochondria lack efficient mechanisms for DNA repair, and mutations of mtDNA (i.e., point mutations and deletions) increase with age. Because individual mitochondria typically contain 10 to 100 copies of mtDNA, such mutations produce a mixture of mutant and normal mtDNA, a condition called **heteroplasmy.** The random segregation of these molecules as cells divide during development can produce populations of cells highly enriched in either mutant or normal mtDNA, depending when in the course of development these mutations occur.

Mitochondrial protein synthesis depends exclusively on mitochondrial-encoded tRNAs, which use a genetic code different from that of nuclear-encoded tRNAs. Because the genes encoding mitochondrial tRNAs are distributed along the entire length of the mtDNA, large deletions of mtDNA invariably result in the loss of several tRNAs. Deletions of mtDNA are associated with an overall reduction in the translation of mitochondrial mRNAs, including those located outside of the deleted region.

The severity of dysfunction within an affected cell appears to correlate with the proportion of deleted mtDNA. RRF are the morphologic correlates of impaired mitochondrial protein synthesis in muscle fibers. The morphologic changes associated with RRF are segmental and related to local variations in the proportion of deleted mtDNA along individual muscle fibers.

The function of mitochondrial tRNAs can also be impaired by point mutations in highly conserved regions of tRNA genes. Mitochondrial protein synthesis cannot be maintained in the presence of homoplasmic mutations that result in the inactivation of essential tRNAs. In contrast, heteroplasmic mutations can be complemented by tRNAs encoded by normal mtDNA within the same mitochondrion.

Although most cases of CPEO are sporadic, some are hereditary. Because mtDNA is maternally transmitted, **point mutations in mtDNA** show a maternal pattern of inheritance. Mothers pass these mutations to offsprings of both sexes, but the mutations are only passed to subsequent generations through the female line. Maternal inheritance of CPEO is associated with point mutations in highly conserved regions of mitochondrial tRNAs. The best characterized of these mutations is the A→G transition of nucleotide-3243 of tRNA$^{Leu(UUR)}$ (i.e., the A3243G transition). This mutation is most often associated with the clinical phenotype called **MELAS syndrome** (*m*itochondrial *e*ncephalomyopathy, *la*ctic *a*cidosis, and *s*troke-like episodes). MELAS syndrome is characterized by: (1) stroke before the age of 40 years; (2) encephalopathy characterized by seizures, dementia, or both; and (3) evidence of mitochondrial dysfunction characterized by lactic acidosis, RRF in skeletal muscle, or both. This illustrates a recurring theme in mitochondrial diseases—a given mutation of mtDNA can be associated with more than one disease phenotype, in this case CPEO and MELAS.

Most cases of CPEO and KSS are sporadic and associated with **single deletions of mtDNA.** Deleted mtDNAs appear to be distributed to a wider variety of tissues in KSS than CPEO. Duplications of mtDNA are also found in patients with either diabetes mellitus or Pearson's syndrome, a mitochondrial disease characterized by infantile sideroblastic pancytopenia, insufficiency of the pancreas, and hepatic dysfunction.

In sporadic cases of KSS and CPEO, all the mutant mtDNAs within an individual have the same deletion. These deletions differ among patients in both size and location, except for one, 4,977-bp long, that is found in more than one-third of all patients with deletions (i.e., the so-called common deletion). The common deletion is flanked by a perfect 13–base pair direct repeat in the normal mitochondrial genome, suggesting that homologous recombination may play a role in this deletion.

Deletions of mtDNA impair mitochondrial protein synthesis; the severity of dysfunction within an affected cell correlates with the proportion of deleted mtDNA. The close association between deletions of mtDNA and dysfunction of the extraocular muscles may be related to the relatively high metabolic activity of these muscles, which are tonically active while the eyes are maintained in primary position.

Autosomal-dominant and autosomal-recessive ophthalmoplegia are associated with **multiple deletions of mtDNA.** These deletions occur at multiple sites, involving a large portion of mtDNA, and most of them seem to be flanked by direct sequence repeats, shown to be "hot spots" in the case of single large deletions. The dominant mutation maps to nuclear chromosome 10q23.3–24.3, demonstrating that the nuclear genome plays an important, but as yet undefined, role in regulating the replication of mtDNA. The recessive mutation, which presumably is also associated with the nuclear genome, has not been mapped.

A number of different clinical phenotypes are associated with autosomal-dominant ophthalmoplegia, including various combinations of muscle weakness and atrophy, exercise intolerance, lactic acidosis, cataract formation, hearing loss, ataxia, tremor, mental retardation, and peripheral neuropathy.

Autosomal-recessive ophthalmoplegia is associated with the **MNGIE syndrome** (*mi*tochondrial *n*euro*g*astro*i*ntestinal *e*ncephalomyopathy). Patients with the MNGIE syndrome also have mild peripheral neuropathy, leukoencephalopathy, and gastrointestinal symptoms (recurrent nausea, vomiting, or diarrhea) with intestinal dysmotility. By contrast, a disablingly severe *s*ensory *a*taxic *n*europathy with *d*ysarthria and *o*phthalmoplegia (**SANDO**) occurs as a sporadic disorder in association with multiple mitochondrial DNA deletions.

It is important to distinguish the mitochondrial myopathies from autosomal-dominant oculopharyngeal muscular dystrophy (see above) and myasthenia gravis (see Chapter 21), because these disorders have distinct therapeutic and genetic implications. Muscle biopsy is the single

most useful diagnostic tool for evaluating patients with suspected mitochondrial disease. The
presence of RRF on muscle biopsy, in excess of
what can be accounted for by age, establishes
the diagnosis of mitochondrial myopathy.

Mutations of mtDNA (both deletions and
point mutations) can be detected in muscle,
blood, and other biopsied tissue using the polymerase chain reaction. It is clear, however, that
a single mutation of mtDNA may be associated
with more than one phenotype.

All patients with known or presumed CPEO
should undergo a careful ophthalmologic assessment, including a dilated ophthalmoscopic examination to determine if a pigmentary retinopathy is present. In addition, patients with CPEO
that is associated with pigmentary retinopathy,
neurologic dysfunction, or both should undergo
an immediate assessment of cardiac function.
Patients in whom no disturbances are found
should nevertheless be monitored with periodic
ECGs.

ENCEPHALOMYOPATHY WITH OPHTHALMOPLEGIA FROM VITAMIN E DEFICIENCY

A condition called **abetalipoproteinemia** or
the **Bassen-Kornzweig syndrome** is characterized by acanthocytosis, pigmentary retinopathy,
progressive ataxia, and neuropathy. It results
from the lack of apolipoprotein B, which is essential to the transport of fat-soluble vitamins.
The syndrome is caused by lack of vitamin E
because of impaired intestinal absorption of lipids and lipid-soluble vitamins. In fact, the neurologic disorder of abetalipoproteinemia is identical with that observed in other forms of human
vitamin E deficiency, whether caused by malabsorption, cholestatic liver disease with impaired
secretion of bile salts, bowel resection, or cystic
fibrosis. The neurologic signs in patients with
vitamin E deficiency include ataxia, areflexia,
and loss of vibratory sensation due both to demyelinating neuropathy and neuronal degeneration of the cerebellum. The ocular motor abnormalities in patients with this disorder include
abnormally slow voluntary saccades, slow or absent fast components of vestibular and optokinetic nystagmus, strabismus, pseudointernuclear
ophthalmoplegia with dissociated nystagmus in
the **adducting eye** on attempted horizontal gaze,

and moderate to severe progressive external
ophthalmoplegia.

Some patients with abetalipoproteinemia develop unilateral ptosis when they look to the
right or left. The ptosis is always on the side of
the abducting eye. The etiology of this "alternating ptosis" is unclear, but it may represent development of, or unmasking of, a preexisting,
ocular motor-levator synkinesis. Many patients
with vitamin E deficiency syndromes develop
pigmentary retinopathy in addition to ocular
motor abnormalities. This retinopathy is similar
in appearance and visual outcome to the retinopathies observed in patients with mitochondrial
cytopathies.

In patients with the vitamin E deficiency syndrome, the neurologic defects, including the
ocular motor disturbances, can be improved if
the serum vitamin E level is restored to normal
with supplemental vitamin E therapy, administered via either an oral or parenteral route. Other
fat-soluble vitamins should also be administered.

INFLAMMATORY MYOPATHIES

The term "myositis" can be used for any disorder in which inflammation affects muscle. The
inflammation may be confined to a single muscle or may be diffuse. Inflammatory myopathies
may be separated into two major categories: myopathies caused by an identified infective agent
and idiopathic inflammatory myopathies.

INFECTIVE MYOSITIS

Infective myositis may be caused by bacteria,
viruses, parasites, or fungi. **Bacteria** that produce pyomyositis are commonly *Staphylococ-
cus aureus, Streptococcus pyogenes,* and *Clostridium welchii.* These and other bacteria usually
produce ophthalmoparesis indirectly when there
is a generalized, suppurative orbital inflammation with swelling of soft tissues. On rare occasions, however, true extraocular myositis occurs
from direct muscle invasion by bacteria. The
bacteria usually gain entrance to the orbit from
infected paranasal sinuses, often after trauma.
Recognition is important because of the immediate need for antibiotics.

Viruses associated with an infective myopathy include the influenza virus and the Coxsackie A and B viruses. The extraocular muscles
are not affected in the majority of cases.

Although many **parasites** can theoretically involve the extraocular muscles, the most frequent and best-known form of parasitic infestation of muscle in general and extraocular muscle in particular is **trichinosis.** The causative agent, *Trichinella spiralis,* is a nematode that is usually acquired in humans as the result of ingesting raw or incompletely cooked pork, bear meat, or horse meat. After penetration of the small intestine, the larvae enter the lymphatic system and the bloodstream and are disseminated widely throughout the body. Involvement of the extraocular muscles is common (Fig. 20.31), occurring second in frequency after involvement of the diaphragm.

Patients with trichinosis often develop ocular signs early in the course of the disease. Chemosis of the conjunctiva is characteristic and primarily occurs over the extraocular muscles. There is a varying degree of ophthalmoparesis from muscle involvement, and movement of the eyes is painful. Other ocular signs include proptosis, optic neuritis, and retinal ischemia.

Parasites other than *Trichinella spiralis* that produce infective myopathies include *Cysticercus, Echinococcus, Toxoplasma gondii, Sarcocystis,* and *Trypanosoma.* These parasites produce ophthalmoparesis by direct invasion of the extraocular muscles.

A variety of **fungi** can produce orbital inflammation with limitation of ocular motility. As with other infective agents, the inflammatory response may be granulomatous or nongranulomatous and may produce ophthalmoplegia through inflammation of ocular motor nerves, extraocular muscles, or soft tissue. The fungi most commonly responsible for orbital inflammation include organisms from the class Phycomycetes (mucormycosis) and *Aspergillus.*

IDIOPATHIC MYOSITIS
Myositis Limited to the Orbit

Local inflammatory conditions may produce limitation of ocular motility. Such conditions may be focal, as in the acquired form of **Brown's superior oblique tendon sheath syndrome.** The acquired form of this syndrome differs from its congenital counterpart (see above) in that it is often intermittent and is associated with inflammation and scarring, either within the superior oblique tendon or next to the anterior sheath. It may occur following superior oblique surgery, retinal detachment surgery, or trauma; in association with paranasal sinus disease; or with either the adult or juvenile forms of rheumatoid arthri-

tis. Most cases of acquired Brown's syndrome are intermittent. Although persistent cases imply predominant scarring and contracture rather than inflammation, some respond to local injections of corticosteroids.

More diffuse involvement of one or more extraocular muscles occurs in the condition that is called **orbital myositis** or the myositic form of idiopathic inflammatory orbital pseudotumor. Patients with this condition usually experience sudden diplopia associated with orbital pain that ranges from mild to excruciating, conjunctival chemosis and injection, and, occasionally, proptosis (Figs. 20.32 and 20.33). Ultrasonography, CT scanning, and MRI show enlargement of one or more extraocular muscles, and biopsies of involved muscles show infiltration with chronic inflammatory cells. Orbital myositis may occur not only as an isolated phenomenon but also in association with systemic disorders characterized by vasculitis or granulomatous inflammation, including systemic lupus erythematosus, rheumatoid arthritis, sarcoidosis, and Wegener's granulomatosis.

Systemic Myositis

Dermatomyositis should not be considered polymyositis with a rash. Rather, it is a systemic vasculopathic autoimmune disorder with histopathologic abnormalities and disease mechanisms distinct from polymyositis. Fever, skin lesions, arthritis, Raynaud's phenomenon, gastrointestinal manifestations, and even cardiac dysfunction may occur in this disease, but weakness of proximal limb-girdle muscles is most often the dominant feature. The skin signs are distinctive: heliotrope orbital/malar rash, Gottron's nodules and periungual erythema, and extensor surface rash. When skin manifestations are transient or slight, the diagnosis may be missed. The distinctive skeletal muscle pathology indicates the diagnosis: perifascicular myofiber necrosis or atrophy; deposition of complement-mediated immune complexes on capillary endothelium, resulting in capillary destruction; primary inflammation surrounding non-necrotic myofibers; and sometimes perivascular inflammation. Ophthalmoplegia is extremely rare in patients with dermatomyositis.

In **polymyositis,** signs are limited to skeletal muscle, and proximal weakness predominates in legs over arms. Less than 25% of patients have either muscle pain or dysphagia. Although the

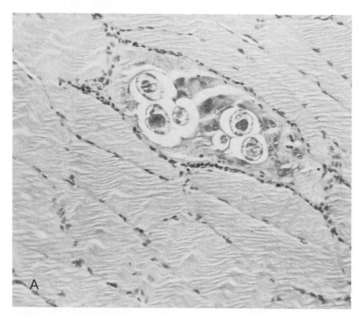

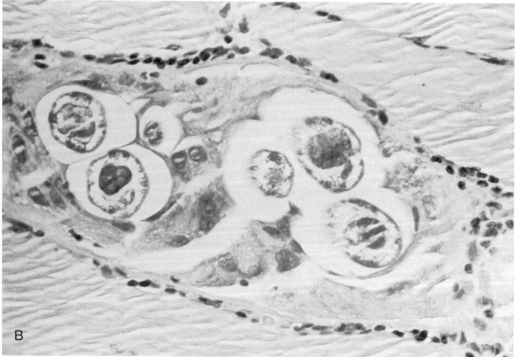

Figure 20.31. Trichinosis involving the extraocular muscles. *A.* Several cysts are present within a single extraocular muscle fiber, surrounded by chronic inflammatory mononuclear cells. *B.* Higher power view of cysts. (Courtesy of Dr. W. Richard Green.)

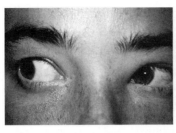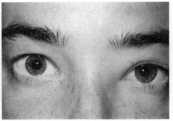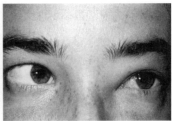

Figure 20.32. Orbital myositis affecting only the left medial rectus muscle in a 20-year-old woman. The nasal conjunctiva of the left eye is chemotic, and the patient cannot abduct the left eye fully.

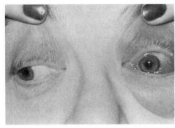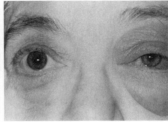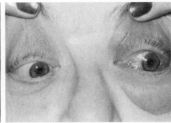

Figure 20.33. Orbital myositis affecting several extraocular muscles of the left eye in a 54-year-old woman. The patient shows proptosis, diffuse eyelid edema, conjunctival chemosis, and ophthalmoparesis.

face and jaw may be weak, ptosis and ophthalmoplegia are uncommon. If they occur, one should consider myasthenia gravis as an overlapping second autoimmune disease. The muscle biopsy in polymyositis shows myofiber necrosis, regeneration, and primary inflammation, but none of the perifascicular or vascular changes of dermatomyositis.

ENDOCRINE MYOPATHIES

GRAVES' DISEASE

Perhaps the most common systemic disorder associated with diplopia, ophthalmoparesis, and infiltration of extraocular muscles is Graves' disease (Fig. 20.34). Graves' orbitopathy often occurs in the context of mild hyperthyroid myopathy, producing mild proximal limb muscle weakness. The serum CK activity is normal in hyperthyroid myopathy. Myasthenia gravis is also increased in frequency in patients with Graves' disease, potentially producing diagnostic confusion about the pathophysiology of the ophthalmoparesis. Graves' orbitopathy may occur months or even years before there is any clinical or laboratory evidence of thyroid dysfunction. Such persons are said to have "euthyroid Graves' disease."

The extraocular muscles are the primary focus of thyroid disease within the orbit, and motility disturbances are found in more than 80% of patients with Graves' disease. Both imaging studies (i.e., ultrasonography, CT scanning, MRI) and pathologic examination of affected muscles demonstrate involvement of the muscle tissue itself with sparing of the muscle tendons (Fig. 20.35). This finding is in contrast to involvement of the muscles by idiopathic inflammatory pseudotumor or orbital myositis that tend to involve the tendon as well as the muscle.

Pathologic examination of extraocular muscles in patients with Graves' disease reveals lymphocyte and plasma cell infiltration along with edema within the endomysium of the extraocular muscles. Although there is some controversy, the primary autoimmune target in Graves' ophthalmopathy appears to be orbital fibroblasts, rather than muscle cells.

In the early stages of extraocular muscle involvement, the muscles become enlarged, resulting in limitation of ocular motility. If this limitation is symmetric among the muscles of both eyes, patients will not complain of diplopia even though they may have severe limitation of ocular motility. In most cases, however, asymmetric in-

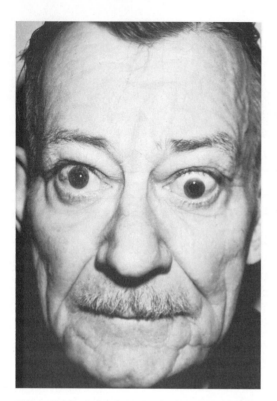

Figure 20.34. Clinical appearance of a 65-year-old man with Grave's ophthalmopathy. Note marked upper and lower eyelid retraction, bilateral proptosis, and marked left hypotropia.

filtration, orbital venous congestion, and trichinosis may all produce large extraocular muscles.

Patients with clinical and imaging evidence of thyroid eye disease should undergo appropriate tests of thyroid function to determine the state of the thyroid and pituitary glands and the need for therapy. Patients with systemic and laboratory evidence of dysthyroidism who have evidence of orbitopathy should have an aggressive approach to normalization of their systemic disease. Patients who are hypothyroid should be treated with replacement therapy. Although there is evidence that radioablation of the thyroid gland can produce or exacerbate the ocular manifestations in patients with hyperthyroidism, this therapy is effective in rendering patients permanently euthyroid. Such patients may benefit from treatment with low-dose (0.5 mg/kg/day) prednisone, beginning just before radioablation

volvement of the two eyes or of the extraocular muscles in one eye causes diplopia that may be vertical, horizontal, or oblique, caused by mechanical restriction of the affected muscles (Fig. 20.36).

As thyroid eye disease progresses, the infiltration and edema of the extraocular muscles produces loss of muscle tissue, and the muscles become fibrotic. In such cases, proptosis may be minimal despite severe diplopia. In addition to diplopia, involvement of extraocular muscles may produce proptosis, swelling of the conjunctiva and eyelid, and optic neuropathy from compression of the optic nerve by swollen muscles in the orbital apex.

In patients suspected of having Graves' disease as the cause of their diplopia, ultrasonography, CT scanning, and MRI are the most important tests to obtain. Diseases such as inflammatory orbital pseudotumor, tumor in-

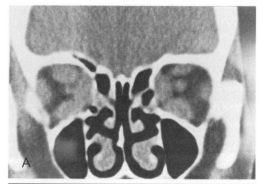

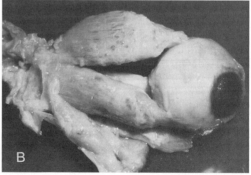

Figure 20.35. Appearance of the extraocular muscles in Graves' ophthalmopathy. *A.* Computed tomographic scan, coronal view, shows generalized enlargement of all extraocular muscles, worse on the right side. *B.* Pathologic specimen from a patient with Graves' ophthalmopathy shows marked enlargement of all extraocular muscles. (*B:* Courtesy of Drs. Ralph C. Eagle, Jr., and W. Richard Green.)

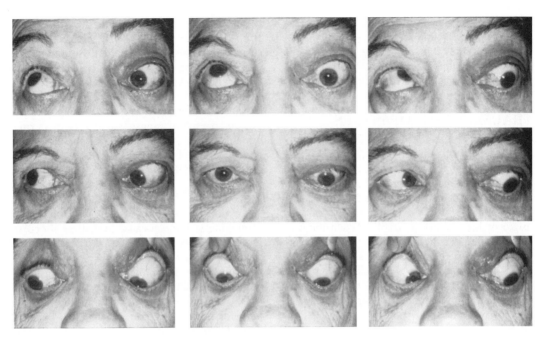

Figure 20.36.   Marked vertical strabismus in a 63-year-old woman with Graves' ophthalmopathy. Note inability of the left eye to elevate above the midline. Despite the marked extraocular muscle involvement, the patient showed almost no proptosis. (Courtesy of Jacqueline E. Morris, C.O.)

and continuing for about 1 month following radioablation before beginning a 2-month taper of the medication. This treatment may prevent Graves' ophthalmopathy from developing or, if it is already present at the time of the radioablation, from exacerbating.

Treatment of the orbitopathy associated with Graves' disease is extremely successful. Irritation and swelling can be treated with a short (1 to 2 month) course of systemic corticosteroids or with low-dose (2000 cGy) orbital radiation therapy. Proptosis can be treated with orbital decompression using a variety of techniques. Strabismus can be treated with prisms, surgery, or both.

The optic neuropathy of Graves' disease can be treated with systemic corticosteroids, low-dose radiation therapy, or orbital decompression. The decision as to which technique to use is based on several factors, including the general health of the patient, the severity of visual loss, and the presence or absence of other orbital manifestations of the disease, particularly proptosis. Patients who do not respond to one form of therapy almost always respond to another, and eventually more than 90% of patients experience resolution of the optic neuropathy.

OTHER ENDOCRINE MYOPATHIES

Proximal muscle weakness is a common finding in patients with **Cushing's syndrome** and can be caused both by hypokalemia and by a direct effect of cortisol on muscle-cell protein turnover, producing atrophy. The diagnosis rests on the typical cushingoid habitus, normal serum CK, and elevated urinary 24-hour free cortisols. It remits with successful treatment of the underlying condition. Some patients with Cushing's syndrome develop ophthalmoparesis and mild exophthalmos, probably from direct involvement of the extraocular muscles. Ultrasonography and other imaging studies in such patients often show enlargement of the extraocular muscles.

Patients on long-term **systemic corticosteroid therapy** may develop bilateral proptosis and limitation of ocular motility. It is possible that the orbital tissue changes in these patients represent a local toxic myopathy similar to that observed in Cushing's syndrome.

Endocrine myopathies occur with hyperpara-thyroidism, hypoparathyroidism, acquired hypo-thyroidism, adrenal insufficiency, and acromeg-aly. The myopathic features tend to be mild and similar in all cases. Extraocular muscle involve-ment is rare.

TRAUMATIC MYOPATHIES

Trauma is probably the most common cause of isolated extraocular muscle damage. When the injury is not associated with orbital fracture, ocular motor dysfunction may be caused by intramuscular edema and hemorrhage, by mus-cle laceration, or by avulsion of the muscle origin or insertion (Fig. 20.37). When there is an associated orbital fracture, the same mecha-nisms of injury may occur. In addition, how-ever, the extraocular muscles and surrounding tissue may be injured by bone fragments or become entrapped within the fracture site, pro-ducing restriction of ocular motility (Fig. 20.38).

Iatrogenic trauma to the orbit may also pro-duce ocular motor dysfunction by direct muscle injury. Extraocular muscle imbalance occurs occasionally after retinal detachment surgery, usually related to the size and location of the silicone material used during a scleral buckling procedure. Inadvertent injury to the extraocular muscles may occur during both cataract and glaucoma surgery. The superior rectus muscle may be injured by a bridle suture placed to stabilize the eye during surgery; however, the most common injury is damage to the inferior rectus muscle, inferior oblique muscle, or both from the toxic effects of the local anesthetic (usually lidocaine or Marcaine). Both transient and permanent extraocular muscle imbalance occur after blepharoplasty, usually from injury to the superior oblique tendon. Injury to the extraocular muscles may occur during surgery on the paranasal sinuses, particularly during ethmoidectomy, because both the medial rectus and superior oblique muscles are adjacent to the medial orbital wall.

OTHER MYOPATHIES

Any local orbital process that acts as a space-occupying lesion can cause limitation of ocular motility simply by its mass effect. **Tumors** within the muscle cone typically produce limita-tion of motion in this manner. In addition, rhab-domyosarcoma may occasionally arise in one or more of the extraocular muscles, producing limi-tation of motion; however, because such patients typically present in childhood or adolescence with rapidly progressive proptosis, the diagnosis is rarely in question.

Discrete and diffuse metastases of carcinomas and lymphomas to the extraocular muscles are common (Fig. 20.39). In such cases, CT scan-ning and MRI may show focal or generalized enlargement of the infiltrated extraocular muscle or muscles.

Infiltration of extraocular muscles can occur in patients with **amyloidosis.** Amyloid is a homogeneous, eosinophilic, extracellular pro-tein that may be demonstrated with light mi-

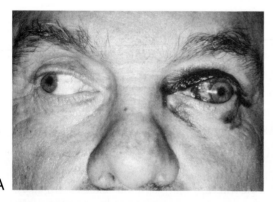

A

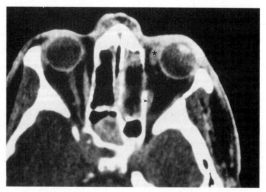

B

Figure 20.37. Iatrogenic traumatic myopathy. The patient had horizontal diplopia following a transnasal endoscopic sinus procedure. *A.* The patient is looking to the right. He has a marked exotropia and cannot adduct the left eye at all.

B. Axial CT scan shows that the left medial rectus muscle has been lacerated. One can clearly see a proximal (*asterisk*) and a distal (*arrowhead*) segment of the muscle.

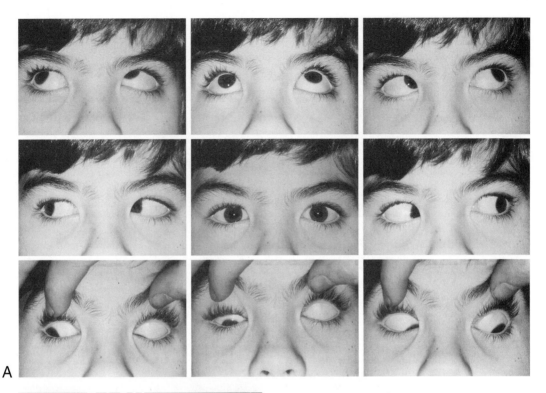

A

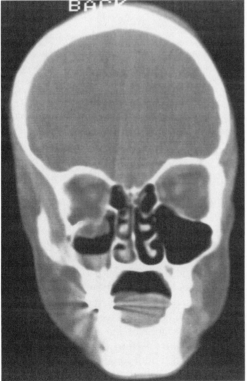

B

Figure 20.38. Entrapment of the inferior rectus muscle caused by a blowout fracture of the orbit. *A.* Clinical appearance of a 10-year-old boy with a right orbital floor fracture. Note inability of the right eye to fully elevate or depress. *B.* Coronal CT scan of the patient shows a dehiscence in the floor of the right orbit with prolapse of tissue into the maxillary sinus. Note that there is a soft tissue density in the floor of the sinus, indicating either swollen mucosa or blood. (Courtesy of Dr. Nicholas T. Iliff.)

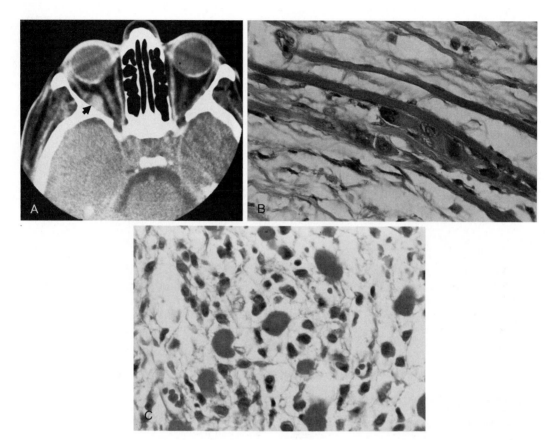

Figure 20.39. Metastatic carcinoma involving the extraocular muscles. *A.* CT scan from a patient with metastatic breast carcinoma shows a focal enlargement of the right lateral rectus muscle (*arrow*) in a woman complaining of painless diplopia. She had no proptosis. Although a needle biopsy of the muscle was nondiagnostic, the patient had resolution of diplopia and improvement in the appearance of the muscle following orbital irradiation. (Courtesy of Drs. C. Citrin and B. Brown.) *B.* Longitudinal section of an extraocular muscle in a patient with metastatic carcinoma shows malignant cells between muscle fibers. *C.* Cross-section of an extraocular muscle in a patient with metastatic carcinoma and proptosis shows that individual muscle fibers are separated by tumor cells and interstitial edema. (Courtesy of Dr. W. Richard Green.)

croscopy by its characteristic staining properties with metachromatic dyes and Congo red, and with electron microscopy by its composition of fine, rigid, nonbranching fibrils. Amyloidosis is classified on the basis of its clinical features into three general categories: (1) primary (systemic or localized; familial or sporadic), (2) secondary, and (3) amyloidosis associated with multiple myeloma. Although only small, clinically insignificant deposits of amyloid in the eye occur in secondary amyloidosis, extraocular muscle infiltration is common in primary amyloidosis and also occurs in patients with amyloidosis associated with multiple my-

eloma. In some patients, the involvement is subclinical, producing no ocular motor dysfunction, whereas in other cases, varying degrees of proptosis and ophthalmoparesis are present, depending upon the extent of extraocular muscle load (Fig. 20.40).

Patients with high-flow carotid-cavernous sinus fistulas or arteriovenous malformations often develop enlargement of the extraocular muscles because of the greatly **increased venous pressure within the orbit.** Similarly, in rare patients, tumors or aneurysms in the anterior temporal fossa may compress draining orbital veins and produce a similar picture. Patients with such lesions may thus have diplopia from both ocular motor nerve palsies and from swelling of the extraocular muscles themselves (Figs. 20.41 and 20.42).

Localized ischemia of extraocular muscles can produce clinical limitation of ocular motility. At least some patients with giant cell arteritis who develop diplopia and ophthalmoplegia do so from ischemic extraocular myopathy rather than from ischemia of the ocular motor nerves or brainstem. Ischemia of the extraocular muscles also is probably responsible for at least some cases of ophthalmoparesis that occur in association with other systemic vascular diseases, particularly those characterized by vasculitis (e.g., periarteritis nodosa, systemic lupus erythematosus).

Skeletal myopathy is occasionally a presenting feature of adult **celiac disease.**

Patients with **skeletal muscle storage diseases** usually present in one of two ways. First, there may be pain, weakness, and rhabdomyolysis that are induced by exercise or fasting. This presentation occurs in patients with impaired metabolism of glycogen (symptoms after brief exercise) or of fatty acids (symptoms after extended exercise or fasting) that reduces the rate at which skeletal muscle can generate high-energy phosphate bonds. Plasma membrane integrity is thus compromised, and rhabdomyolysis occurs. Patients with myophosphorylase deficiency (McArdle's disease), muscle phosphofructokinase deficiency (Tarui's disease), and carnitine palmityl acyltransferase deficiency present with exercise-induced weakness. Most patients with these disorders have no disturbances of ocular motility or alignment.

A second presentation in patients with skeletal muscle storage diseases is fixed muscle weakness. In these patients, excess glycogen or triglyceride causes disruption of myofibrillar architecture. Deposits in extraocular muscle could be responsible for strabismus in occasional patients. Patients with acid maltase deficiency

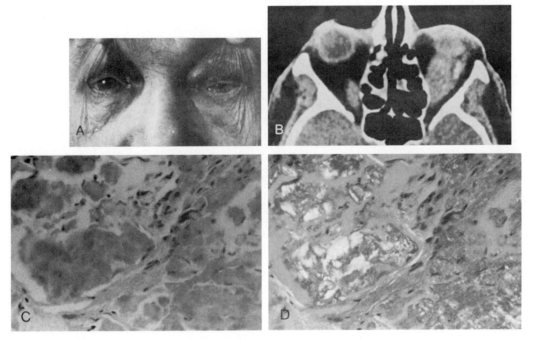

Figure 20.40.   Orbital amyloidosis. *A.* A patient with multiple myeloma has complete ptosis and ophthalmoplegia. (Reprinted with permission from Raflo GT, Farrell TA, Sioussat RS. Complete ophthalmoplegia secondary to amyloidosis associated with multiple myeloma. Am J Ophthalmol 1981; 92:221–224.) *B.* In another patient with proptosis and ophthalmoparesis, the left inferior rectus muscle is markedly enlarged. *C.* Biopsy of this muscle shows large amounts of amorphous material that stain positively for amyloid. *D.* A phase-contrast photomicrograph of the field shown in *C* reveals that the amorphous material is birefringent, a characteristic of amyloid. (Courtesy of Dr. Thomas C. Spoor.)

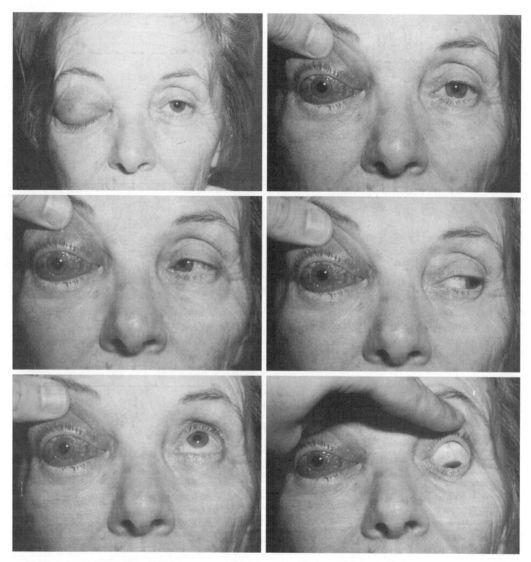

Figure 20.41. Clinical appearance of a 54-year-old woman with a traumatic fistula between the right internal carotid artery and the cavernous sinus. Note right proptosis, conjunctival hyperemia and chemosis, and almost complete ophthalmoplegia. Moderate dilation and poor reactivity of the right pupil to light indicate that the patient's ophthalmoplegia is caused by a combination of mechanical and neuropathic involvement.

(Pompe's disease), brancher enzyme deficiency (Andersen's disease), debrancher enzyme deficiency, and carnitine deficiency have fixed muscle weakness.

Drug-induced toxic myopathies are rare without the superimposition of another risk factor, such as renal insufficiency, hepatic insufficiency, malnutrition, or a concomitant drug interaction, that elevates levels of the offending drug. Biologic toxins affect muscles through direct, cell-specific interactions. Drugs and toxins can cause muscle weakness by affecting muscle fibers or their neuromuscular junctions. Direct effects on muscle include: (1) myonecrosis with or without myoglobinuria (e.g., ethanol in the malnourished; lovastatin or its

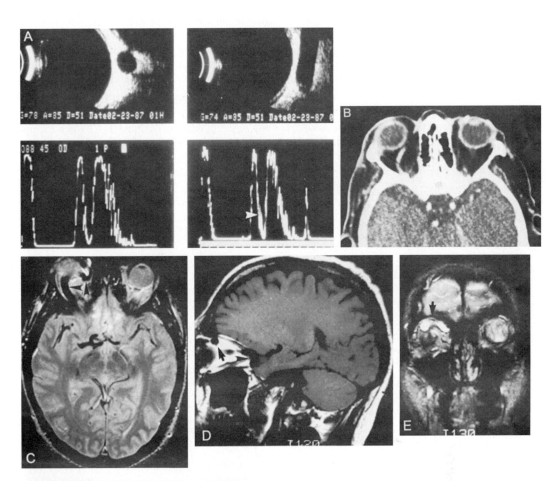

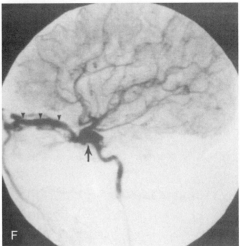

Figure 20.42. Diagnostic tests in patients with enlarged extraocular muscles and other clinical evidence of a direct carotid-cavernous sinus fistula. *A.* Orbital ultrasonography (A and B modes) shows enlargement ''of the superior ophthalmic vein.'' The lower right A-scan shows blurring of the spikes within the vein (*arrowhead*). This appearance is caused by rapid blood flow within the vessel. *B.* CT scan, axial view, shows an enlarged superior ophthalmic vein in a patient with a direct carotid-cavernous sinus fistula on that side. *C–E.* Magnetic resonance images in a patient with a carotid-cavernous sinus fistula. *C.* T2-weighted axial image, shows an enlarged superior ophthalmic vein on the side of the fistula. The vein appears as a black curvilinear structure beginning at the apex of the orbit and continuing forward in the superolateral orbit as a curvilinear tubular structure (*arrowhead*). A small portion of the nasal component of the vein is also seen (*arrowhead*). *D.* T1-weighted sagittal image shows the most posterior and anterior components of the enlarged vein (*arrowheads*). *E.* Short TR and TE image, coronal view, shows the enlarged superior ophthalmic vein as a white curvilinear structure that curves from lateral to medial in the anterosuperior orbit (*arrowhead*). *F.* Selective left internal carotid arteriogram shows a direct carotid-cavernous sinus fistula (*arrow*) draining anteriorly into the superior ophthalmic vein (*arrowheads*).

analogues taken concomitantly with cyclosporine) and (2) excessive autophagy (e.g., chloroquine, colchicine, amphiphilic drugs). Undoubtedly, myotoxic reactions also occur in extraocular muscles, but there are few well-documented cases.

The venom of the beaked sea snake, *Enhydrina schistosa,* produces an unusual myotoxic reaction that apparently can involve the extra-ocular muscles. The primary clinical manifestations of this type of poisoning are trismus, flaccid paresis of the extremities, and myoglobinuria. In severe poisoning, there may be ptosis and limitation of ocular motility.

FOR MORE INFORMATION:

See Walsh & Hoyt's *Clinical Neuro-Ophthalmology,* 5th edition, Volume 1, Chapter 25, pp. 1043–1052 and Chapter 30, pp. 1351–1406.

Disorders of Neuromuscular Transmission

Acetylcholine (ACh), the substance that mediates neuromuscular transmission in striated and cardiac muscle, is synthesized chiefly in the motor nerve terminals and is stored in vesicles for subsequent release (Fig. 21.1). It is estimated that each vesicle, or "quantum," contains about 10,000 ACh molecules. Neuromuscular transmission begins with the release of the contents of the vesicles by a process of exocytosis that occurs at specialized release sites. The probability of vesicular binding and release at these sites depends directly on calcium concentrations in nerve terminals. The vesicle release sites are located directly opposite the areas of highest concentration of ACh nicotinic receptors on the postsynaptic membranes (see Fig. 21.1), thus minimizing the distance that the transmitter must travel to reach the receptor site. When ACh combines with its receptor, a transient increase of permeability to sodium and potassium ions occurs, resulting in membrane depolarization.

The entire process of neuromuscular transmission is rapid, on the order of a millisecond. It is terminated by the removal of ACh, in part by its diffusion away from the neuromuscular junction, but mostly by the action of acetylcholinesterase, which rapidly hydrolyzes ACh. The amplitude of the muscle endplate potential depends on the number of ACh molecules that interact with receptor molecules. Any change that reduces the probability of interaction—and thus the safety margin—may result in failure of neuromuscular transmission.

The ACh receptor of skeletal muscle is opened when binding sites are occupied by the agonist, ACh. Blocking agents such as α-bungarotoxin or curare bind at or near the same site, preventing access to ACh. ACh receptors in muscle cells undergo active turnover by endocytosis and subsequent lysosomal degradation.

MYASTHENIA GRAVIS

Myasthenia gravis is a disease characterized clinically by muscle weakness and fatigability, attributable to too few available ACh receptors at neuromuscular junctions. Receptor depletion is mediated by one or more antibodies directed against ACh receptors, resulting in impaired neuromuscular transmission. Myasthenia gravis is the most common disorder that affects the neuromuscular junction.

Autoimmune myasthenia gravis affects all races and ages, with an incidence of 4 to 5 per 100,000. The incidence is both age and gender dependent, peaking in young women and older men. Patients with thymomas are more likely to

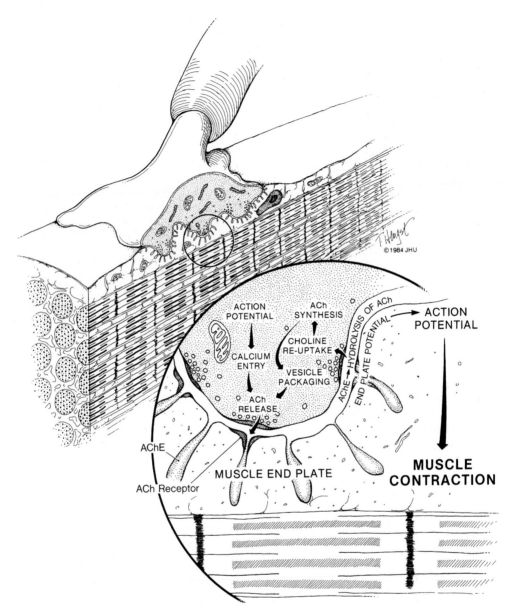

Figure 21.1. Drawing of the normal neuromuscular junction. Note the sites of acetylcholine *(ACh)* release, the location of acetylcholine receptors, and the location of acetylcholinesterase *(AChE)*.

be over 30 years old and male. Neonatal myasthenia gravis affects about one in seven babies born to myasthenic mothers.

ETIOLOGY AND PATHOGENESIS

Myasthenic patients have less than one-third of the ACh receptors present in normal persons.

This reduction in number of available ACh receptors is caused by the actions of antibodies to those receptors (see Fig. 21.1). Such antibodies are found in the serum of 80 to 90% of patients with generalized myasthenia gravis. Anti-ACh receptor antibodies reduce the number of available receptors via three mechanisms: (1) receptor blockade, (2) complement-mediated membrane damage, and (3) accelerated degradation of the receptor.

Across patients, the serum anti-ACh receptor antibody concentration does not correlate well with disease severity. However, for an individual patient, a significant relative reduction in antibody titer (50% or more) is often associated with marked clinical improvement. Some "antibody-negative" patients have mild or localized disease (e.g., ocular myasthenia), whereas others have generalized, even severe disease. Acquired antibody-negative myasthenia gravis is nonetheless autoimmune, because it responds to immunotherapy and pheresis and can be passively transferred. Therefore, anti-ACh receptor antibodies must be present in such patients, even though they are not detectable by conventional radioimmunoassay techniques.

In myasthenia gravis, the amount of ACh released from the presynaptic terminal both at rest and after sustained activity is normal; however, because of the reduced number of available ACh receptors, the amplitude of endplate potentials at some neuromuscular junctions may be too low to trigger an action potential. If transmission is sufficiently impaired at enough neuromuscular junctions, the muscle becomes weak. Normally, with sustained muscle activity, the amount of ACh released from the presynaptic nerve terminal is reduced with each successive impulse, but because of the large safety factor, transmission is not affected and strength is maintained. In myasthenia gravis, however, the reduced ACh results in further impaired impulse transmission at even more neuromuscular junctions. This is the basis of muscle fatigability and electrophysiologic decrement in myasthenia gravis.

The anti-ACh receptor antibody is the result of a T-cell-dependent B-cell response. The thymus contains the strategic mix to mount an immune attack on the ACh receptor. The central role of the thymus is underscored by the observations that two-thirds of myasthenic patients have thymic hyperplasia with germinal center formation, and about 10% have thymomas. In addition, most patients with myasthenia gravis improve after thymectomy (see below).

SYMPTOMS AND SIGNS

The hallmark clinical feature of myasthenia gravis is variability in the strength of the affected muscles. Weakness varies from day to day and from hour to hour, typically increasing toward evening. Transient weakness is often associated with physical exertion. Affected muscles fatigue if contraction is maintained or repeated. This must be differentiated from the neurasthenic "fatigue" of tiredness or depression. The most commonly affected muscles, in descending frequency, are:

- The levator palpebrae superioris, the extraocular muscles, and orbicularis oculi.
- The proximal limb muscles, especially triceps brachii, deltoids, and iliopsoas.
- The muscles of facial expression, mastication, and speech.
- The neck extensors.

The levator palpebrae superioris and extraocular muscles are initially affected in about 70% of cases, and these muscles are eventually affected in over 90% of patients. When weakness of these muscles is combined with weakness of the orbicularis oculi, the combination is highly suggestive of myasthenia gravis.

Ptosis and Other Signs of Levator Palpebrae Superioris Dysfunction

Ptosis may occur as an isolated sign or in association with extraocular muscle involvement. It is characterized by its fluctuating nature and frequently shifts from one eye to the other. It is often initially unilateral but eventually almost always becomes bilateral (Fig. 21.2). When signs are limited to one eye, despite seeming myasthenic features, it is essential to image the orbit and brain for a mass lesion. When ptosis is bilateral, it is usually asymmetric, but severe symmetric ptosis may occur, particularly in patients with severe ophthalmoplegia. The ptosis is frequently absent when the patient awakens, but it appears later in the day, becoming most pronounced in the evening. Repeated closures of the eyelids may make ptosis appear or may worsen it when it is initially minimal. Similarly, prolonged upward gaze will often result in gradual lowering of the eyelids (Fig. 21.3).

Enhancement of ptosis often occurs in patients with myasthenia gravis. Such patients, who appear to have either unilateral or symmetric bilateral ptosis, will have worsening of ptosis on one side when the opposite eyelid is elevated and held in a fixed position (Fig. 21.4). The explanation of this "seesaw" phenomenon is Hering's law of equal innervation, which relates to the levator muscles as it does to the extraocular muscles. Manual eyelid elevation decreases the effort required for eyelid elevation ipsilaterally and thus results in relaxation of the contralateral levator palpebrae superioris and consequent worsening ptosis on that side. This is a corollary to the contralateral eyelid retrac-

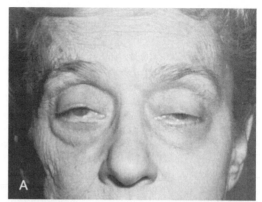

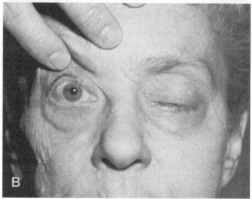

Figure 21.4. Enhanced ptosis in a 78-year-old woman with myasthenia gravis. *A.* The patient has bilateral ptosis. *B.* When the right eyelid is elevated, the patient develops increased (enhanced) ptosis on the opposite side.

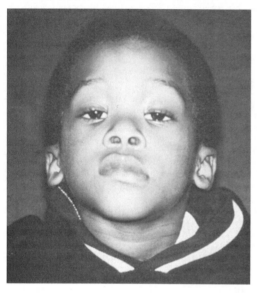

Figure 21.2. Bilateral ptosis in a 5-year-old boy with myasthenia gravis.

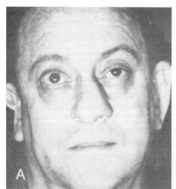
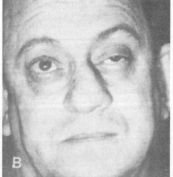
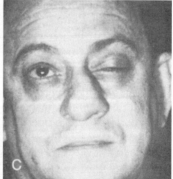

Figure 21.3. Increasing ptosis on maintained upward gaze in a patient with myasthenia gravis. *A–C.* Three frames from a movie showing progressive ptosis over a 3-minute period as the patient maintained fixation above the horizontal meridian. (Reprinted with permission from Cogan DG. Myasthenia gravis: a review of the disease and a description of lid twitch as a characteristic sign. Arch Ophthalmol 1965; 74:217–221.)

tion that is often seen in patients with unilateral ptosis.

Enhancement of ptosis is not pathognomonic for myasthenia gravis. It can be seen in patients with congenital ptosis and in patients with acquired ptosis from causes other than myasthenia. Nevertheless, in a patient with an appropriate history, the observation of enhancement of ptosis is highly suggestive of myasthenia gravis.

The presence of an eyelid twitch response, the so-called **Cogan's lid twitch,** is characteristic of myasthenia gravis. When the patient's eyes are directed downward for 10 to 20 seconds and the patient is then instructed to make a vertical saccade back to primary position, the upper eyelid elevates and either slowly begins to droop or twitches several times before settling into a stable position (Fig. 21.5). This eyelid twitch phenomenon is caused by the rapid recovery and easy fatigability of myasthenic muscle.

Transient, **spontaneous eyelid retraction** occurs in some patients with myasthenia gravis without evidence of thyroid dysfunction (Fig. 21.6). This phenomenon, which usually occurs on return of the eyes from upward gaze to primary position, may be caused by post-tetanic facilitation of the levator palpebrae superioris. It should be noted, however, that there is an increased prevalence of thyroid eye disease among patients with myasthenia gravis (see below), and persistent bilateral eyelid retraction or unilateral eyelid retraction without contralateral ptosis in a patient with myasthenia should suggest a diagnosis of coincident thyroid ophthalmopathy.

Ophthalmoparesis and Other Abnormalities of Eye Movement

Involvement of the extraocular muscles, like ptosis, is extremely common in patients with myasthenia gravis, although the reason for this is unknown. Possible explanations include:

1. Minimal weakness of the extraocular muscles is likely to be symptomatic, in contrast to that in limb muscles.
2. Extraocular muscles show anatomic and physiologic differences from limb muscles; 80% are single-innervated twitch fibers, and such fibers, which have high nerve firing frequencies, may be more sensitive to fatigue.
3. The morphologic and physiologic properties of extraocular muscles may make

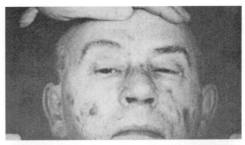
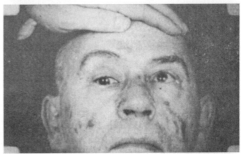
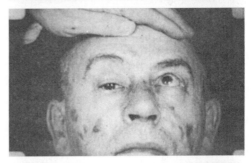
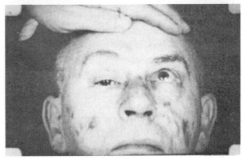

Figure 21.5.   Cogan's eyelid twitch phenomenon in a patient with myasthenia gravis. The photograph is made from successive frames of a movie. As the patient looks upward, the left eyelid elevates fully while the right eyelid elevates only partially. The right eyelid then immediately becomes successively more ptotic. The entire process takes only a few seconds. In motion, this transient eyelid elevation gives the appearance of a twitch. (Reprinted with permission from Cogan DG. Myasthenia gravis: a review of the disease and a description of lid twitch as a characteristic sign. Arch Ophthalmol 1965;74:217–221.)

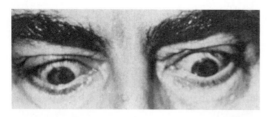

Figure 21.6. Transient, bilateral, asymmetric upper eyelid retraction in a patient with myasthenia gravis. The retraction occurred following prolonged upgaze. It persisted for several seconds and then resolved. (Reprinted with permission from Puklin JE, Sacks JG, Boshes B. Transient eyelid retraction in myasthenia gravis. J Neurol Neurosurg Psychiatry 1976; 39:44–47.)

them especially sensitive to a loss of functional ACH receptors. They may be more accessible to circulating antibodies and have a low safety factor.

4. The antigenic properties of extraocular muscles may differ from those of limb muscles.

In most cases, disturbances of ocular motility and alignment are associated with ptosis; however, cases without clinical involvement of the levator muscles occur. There is no set pattern to extraocular muscle involvement. All degrees of ocular motor dysfunction, from apparent involvement of a single isolated muscle to complete external ophthalmoplegia, occur. Thus, the abnormalities may mimic ocular motor nerve palsies, internuclear ophthalmoplegia, or gaze palsies.

The medial rectus muscle seems to be more frequently affected than the other extraocular muscles. This involvement may produce either a variable, incomitant strabismus or a clinical picture simulating unilateral or bilateral internuclear ophthalmoplegia with weakness of adduction of one eye and abducting nystagmus in the opposite eye (Fig. 21.7).

Some patients develop blurred distant vision from pseudomyopia. This phenomenon apparently results from "substitute convergence" that is used by the patient to compensate for bilateral weakness of the medial rectus muscles. Such patients usually have normal accommodation (see below).

Individual muscles other than the medial rectus may also be selectively involved in patients with myasthenia gravis. Some patients develop

an acute and isolated inferior rectus paresis as the initial sign of myasthenia gravis, whereas others develop sudden weakness of the superior oblique muscle that mimics a trochlear nerve paresis. The involvement of multiple muscles innervated by the oculomotor nerve may mimic a pupil-sparing oculomotor nerve palsy. A "double elevator palsy" (unilateral limitation of upward gaze) may also be observed in patients with myasthenia gravis.

Many patients with myasthenia gravis present either with dysfunction of extraocular muscles in one eye that are innervated by more than one cranial nerve or with dysfunction of muscles in both eyes. Bilateral paralysis of upward gaze can mimic a dorsal midbrain syndrome, and horizontal gaze limitation may erroneously suggest a lesion of the pons (see Chapter 18).

As myasthenia gravis progresses, weakness of the extraocular muscles may simulate the progressive external ophthalmoplegia encountered in patients with mitochondrial myopathies (see Chapter 20). In severely affected patients, there may be complete external ophthalmoplegia. This is almost always associated with complete or almost complete ptosis.

The tendency for affected muscles, including the extraocular muscles, to fatigue may cause patients with a full range of eye movements to show fatigue on sustained eccentric gaze. Such patients show a "muscle-paretic" fatigue that may be mistaken for a brainstem or cerebellar process.

Even in patients in whom the clinical examination does not reveal evidence of fatigue of eye muscles, recordings of eye movements may demonstrate a variety of ocular motor abnormalities. Saccades are typically abnormal, with four main types of abnormalities being present:

1. hypermetric saccades
2. hypometric saccades that begin with normal velocity but ultimately show a decrease in velocity (intrasaccadic fatigue) and undershoot the target
3. small, jerking ("quiver") eye movements
4. gaze-evoked nystagmus

In addition, the velocity and amplitude of saccades decrease after repetitive refixations in many patients.

Not all features of myasthenic eye movements can be ascribed solely to changes in peripheral mechanisms. The brain monitors the accuracy

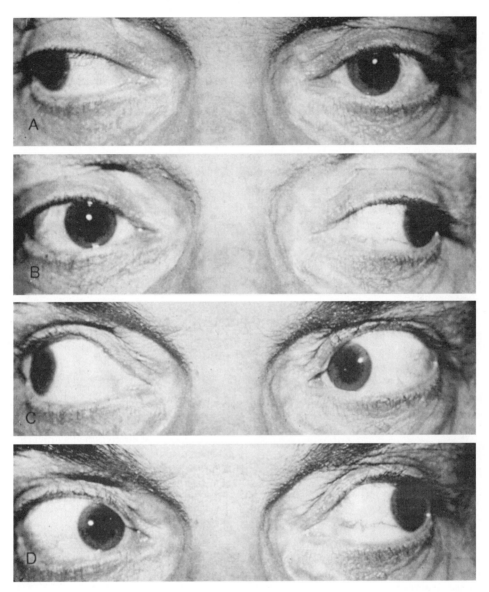

Figure 21.7.   Pseudo-internuclear ophthalmoplegia in a patient with myasthenia gravis. *A.* On attempted rightward gaze, there is adduction lag of the left eye. Note bilateral ptosis. *B.* On attempted leftward gaze, there is adduction lag of the right eye. *C–D.* Following intravenous administration of edrophonium chloride (Tensilon), there is marked improvement of adduction of both the left eye (*C*) and the right eye (*D*). (Reprinted with permission from Glaser JS. Myasthenic pseudo-internuclear ophthalmoplegia. Arch Ophthalmol 1966;75:363–366.)

of saccades and makes appropriate innervation changes to optimize ocular motor performance; thus, when myasthenia causes paretic saccades, central adaptation is stimulated. Patients with myasthenia gravis often show hypometric large saccades but **hypermetric** small saccades. Saccadic hypermetria occurs because the central nervous system has adaptively increased the size of the saccadic pulse in an attempt to overcome the myasthenic weakness.

Nystagmus

As noted above, some patients with myasthenia gravis have involvement of one or both medial rectus muscles, producing a syndrome that mimics a unilateral or bilateral internuclear ophthalmoplegia with abduction nystagmus. Others develop upgaze paresis and convergence-retraction nystagmus that mimics a dorsal midbrain syndrome.

Although they are rare, isolated abduction nystagmus and delayed nystagmus (following a change in gaze) may occur as presenting signs of myasthenia gravis. The nystagmus occurs because myasthenic fatigue limits the ability to hold the eye steady after a saccade. Depending on whether the pulse or the step is more affected, the resulting pulse-step mismatch causes a forward or backward postsaccadic drift. This type of nystagmus is called muscle-paretic nystagmus and probably occurs when the tonic fibers are fatigued. In this setting, the fast-twitch fibers are relatively spared, because they only discharge vigorously during saccades or quick phases.

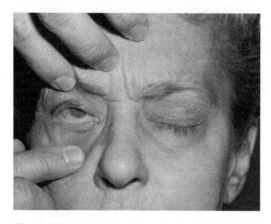

Figure 21.8. Weakness of the orbicularis oculi in a 76-year-old woman with severe myasthenia gravis. The patient is attempting to forcefully close her eyelids while the examiner attempts to open them. Note the relative ease with which the examiner is able to open the eyelids on the right and the lack of tight eyelid closure on the left.

Orbicularis Oculi Involvement

Patients with myasthenia gravis often have involvement of the orbicularis oculi muscles that may not be apparent when ptosis or ophthalmoplegia predominate. The combination of ptosis, ophthalmoplegia, and weakness of the orbicularis oculi is found in only a few disorders, myasthenia gravis being the most common. Patients suspected of having myasthenia gravis should therefore have testing of orbicularis oculi strength by having the patient forcefully shut the eyes while the examiner manually attempts to open the eyelids against the forced lid closure (Fig. 21.8).

A sign of weakness of the orbicularis oculi muscle that may be observed in patients with myasthenia gravis is the "peek sign." Upon gentle eyelid closure, the orbicularis oculi muscle contracts, initially achieving eyelid apposition; however, the muscle rapidly fatigues, and the palpebral fissure widens, thereby exposing the sclera. The patient thus appears to "peek" at the examiner (Fig. 21.9). A similar phenomenon in some patients with myasthenia gravis is probably responsible for ectropion of the lower eyelid that develops as the day progresses.

Pupillary Function and Accommodation

Most patients with myasthenia gravis have no obvious disturbances of pupillary size or function. Nevertheless, rare patients have anisocoria, others have sluggishly reactive pupils that improve after intravenous injection of edrophonium chloride (Tensilon), and still others show pupillary fatigue during constant light stimulation in the eyes. In addition, in many patients with myasthenia gravis who have no pupillary abnormalities on clinical examination, pupillography shows reduced velocity and acceleration of pupillary constriction to both light and near stimuli, suggesting that the iris sphincter can be

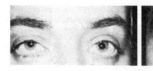 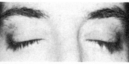 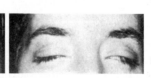

Figure 21.9. The orbicularis oculi "peek" phenomenon in myasthenia gravis. *Left:* The patient is fixing straight ahead. Note mild bilateral ptosis. *Middle:* On voluntary eyelid closure, there is initial apposition of the lid margins bilaterally. *Right:* Within 2 seconds, the eyelids slip apart, exposing the sclera. (Reprinted with permission from Osher RH, Griggs RC. Orbicularis fatigue: the "peek" sign of myasthenia gravis. Arch Ophthalmol 1979;97:677–679.)

involved in myasthenia gravis. It should be emphasized that in most patients with myasthenia, pupillary dysfunction is **not clinically significant** and should not confuse the diagnosis. Thus, in patients with nonspecific ocular motility disturbances and clinically normal pupillary responses, myasthenia gravis should be strongly considered in the differential diagnosis. Conversely, when ocular motor disturbances occur in the setting of a dilated, poorly reactive pupil, myasthenia gravis should not be considered as a cause.

Diminished accommodation may occur in patients with myasthenia gravis, and some patients with myasthenia demonstrate progressive weakening of accommodation during prolonged convergence. These abnormalities typically improve after an intravenous injection of Tensilon or an intramuscular injection of neostigmine methylsulfate (Prostigmin), and they tend to resolve or improve when the patient is treated with an anticholinesterase agent.

Nonocular Features

In patients with generalized involvement of skeletal muscles, the facies may be characteristic, showing a generalized weakness of expression (Fig. 21.10). Weakness frequently affects the neck extensors (head "ptosis") and proximal limb muscles. When the muscles of expression, phonation, articulation, swallowing, and chewing are affected, there may be a characteristic facial "snarl," dysarthric speech, nasal regurgitation of liquids, and the need to prop the jaw closed. When the muscles of respiration or swallowing are involved, the term "myasthenic

crisis" indicates the gravity of the disease. Rarely, myasthenia gravis can present with respiratory insufficiency alone. In some patients, the stapedius muscle is involved, resulting in hyperacusis or a decrease in the intensity of sound required to elicit an acoustic reflex.

There is usually a history of fluctuation and fatigability (worse with repeated activity; improved by rest). In women, weakness may worsen in relation to the menstrual cycle. If the weakness occurs in a vague and variable pattern, it may be misinterpreted as having a psychogenic origin. Patients may complain of pain in weak muscles, especially in the neck, back, and around the eyes, but this complaint may be attributable to the extra effort required to maintain posture and fusion.

On physical examination, the findings are limited entirely to the lower motor unit, without loss of reflexes or altered sensation or coordination. The differential diagnosis of blepharoptosis and facial weakness is fairly limited to myasthenia gravis, myotonic dystrophy, oculopharyngeal dystrophy, and mitochondrial myopathy.

DIAGNOSTIC TESTING

The tests devised to diagnose myasthenia gravis include clinical tests, pharmacologic tests, repetitive nerve stimulation, an assay for anti-ACh receptor antibody, and single-fiber electromyography (EMG).

Clinical Tests

Two clinical tests may be helpful in supporting the diagnosis of myasthenia gravis: the sleep test and the ice test. They are particularly useful

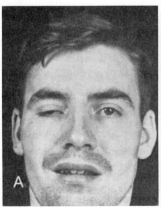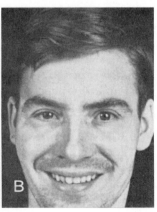

Figure 21.10. Clinical appearance of a patient with myasthenia gravis before and after intramuscular injection of neostigmine methylsulfate (Prostigmin). *A.* Prior to injection there is bilateral ptosis, more marked on the right side, as well as generalized weakness of the facial muscles. The patient had been asked to smile as widely as possible. *B.* At 15 minutes after intramuscular injection of Prostigmin, the patient's ptosis has disappeared, and his facial musculature now appears to function normally. (Reprinted with permission from Mattis RD. Ocular manifestations of myasthenia gravis. Arch Ophthalmol 1941;26:969–982.)

in very young, elderly, or ill patients for whom pharmacologic testing may be difficult or considered potentially dangerous.

Sleep Test

The majority of patients with myasthenia gravis show marked improvement in ptosis, ocular motor dysfunction, or both immediately upon awakening from sleep. This improvement lasts 2 to 5 minutes, following which the ptosis and ophthalmoparesis recur. Patients with ptosis and ophthalmoparesis caused by disorders other than myasthenia show no such improvement after sleep. This phenomenon can be used as a test of myasthenia gravis: the **sleep test.**

The sleep test is performed as follows. The external appearance of the patient is observed and photographed, and the patient is then taken to a room where he or she can lie down and go to sleep. The patient is awakened 30 to 45 minutes later, immediately observed, and photographed to determine if there has been any improvement in eyelid position, ocular motility and alignment, or both (Fig. 21.11).

The sleep test is a safe, moderately sensitive, and specific way to confirm a presumptive diagnosis of myasthenia gravis.

Ice Test

The use of local cooling to eliminate ptosis in patients with possible myasthenia gravis is a rapid, simple, and inexpensive test with a high degree of specificity and sensitivity. The **ice test** is particularly useful in patients in whom the use of anticholinesterase agents is contraindicated by either cardiac status or age. Local cooling from 35°C to 28°C reduces decrement, neuromuscular jitter, and weakness, and all of these effects are reversed on rewarming. Cooling the eyelids with an ice pack improves ptosis in almost all patients with myasthenia, but not in patients with congenital ptosis or ptosis attributable to oculomotor nerve palsy or various myopathies.

The ice test is performed as follows. The size of the palpebral fissure is measured, photographed, or both. A surgical glove containing crushed ice or ice cubes is then applied to the

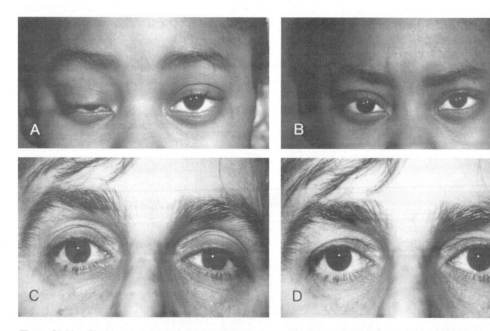

Figure 21.11. The sleep test for myasthenia gravis. *A.* A 10-year-old girl has right ptosis. Note use of the frontalis to help elevate the eyelid. *B.* After 30 minutes of sleep, the ptosis has resolved. The frontalis is no longer contracted. *C.* A 48-year-old man has bilateral symmetric ptosis. *D.* After 30 minutes of sleep, the ptosis has resolved. (Reprinted with permission from Odel JG, Winterkorn JMS, Behrens MM. The sleep test for myasthenia gravis: a safe alternative to Tensilon. J Clin Neuroophthalmol 1991;11:288–292.)

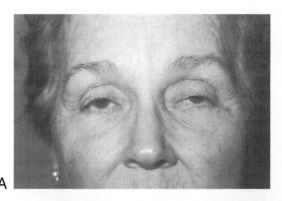

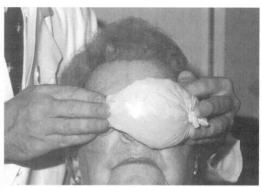

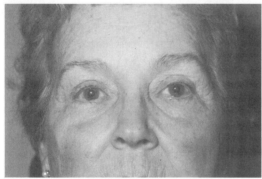

Figure 21.12.   The ice test for myasthenia gravis. The patient was a 73-year-old woman with a history of cardiac disease and bilateral ptosis of 3-months' duration. *A.* Appearance of the patient before the ice test. *B.* Placement of a surgical glove containing ice over the closed eyelids. *C.* Immediately upon removing the glove, it can be seen that the ptosis has resolved.

more involved eyelid for 2 minutes, with the opposite lid serving as a control. After 2 minutes, the glove is removed, and the size of the palpebral fissure is immediately measured or photographed (Fig. 21.12).

The test is considered positive if the size of the palpebral fissure is greater after cooling. This difference is usually greater than 2 mm in patients with myasthenia gravis. The improvement in ptosis typically lasts less than 1 minute.

Pharmacologic Tests

The abnormal fatigability of skeletal muscles may be evaluated by observing or quantifying their strength before and after the injection of an anticholinesterase agent. Nearly any objectively quantifiable motor endpoint can be used, such as millimeters of ptosis at rest, timed fatigue of the lids on upgaze, vital capacity, timed swallow of 4 oz of water by straw (the ''slurp test,'' especially useful in children), forward arm abduction time, or the cine-esophagram. Anticholinesterase pharmacologic testing has a sensitivity of about 50 to 75% in myasthenia gravis. Thus, when myasthenia gravis is strongly suspected,

and pharmacologic testing is negative or cannot be performed, patients should undergo more extensive electrophysiologic and serologic tests.

Edrophonium Chloride (Tensilon) Test

Edrophonium chloride (**Tensilon**) is a rapidly acting and quickly hydrolyzed anticholinesterase. It competes with ACh for acetylcholinesterase and thus allows prolonged and repetitive action of ACh at the synapse. It is commonly chosen because of the rapid onset (30 seconds) and short duration (about 5 minutes) of its effect.

In patients with ptosis, Tensilon has particular value. An intravenous dose of 10 mg is usually used. Once the position of the eyelids is verified, a test dose of 2 mg of Tensilon is injected, and the patient is observed carefully for any idiosyncratic reaction (see below) or for improvement in ptosis. If definite improvement occurs, the test is considered positive and is terminated. If no improvement occurs within about 2 minutes and the patient has no adverse reaction to the medication, the remaining 8 mg of the dose is injected either as a single bolus or in 2–4 mg increments given 2 minutes apart as the patient is observed.

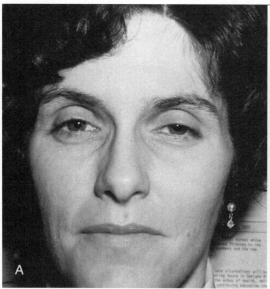 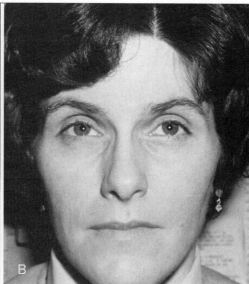

Figure 21.13. The Tensilon test for myasthenia gravis. The patient was a 27-year-old woman with ptosis and intermittent diplopia. *A.* Before injection of Tensilon, the patient has bilateral ptosis and weakness of facial musculature. *B.* One minute following an intravenous injection of 2 mg of Tensilon, the patient's ptosis has disappeared, and her facial muscles appear to function more normally.

A positive response is elevation of one or both eyelids, sometimes accompanied by an improvement in facial expression, which lasts not just a few seconds but 2 to 5 minutes (Fig. 21.13). If no improvement in eyelid position occurs within about 3 minutes, the test is negative. Occasionally, a paradoxic reaction—worsening of ptosis—may occur following administration of Tensilon. Similarly, nearly all patients experience transient quivering of the eyelids, lacrimation, and salivation. These responses do not constitute a positive test.

Tensilon may also be used in patients without ptosis but with diplopia. Such patients are best tested by having them hold a red glass over one eye (or use red-green glasses), fixate a distant white light, and describe the relative positions of the two lights seen (red and white or green). Tensilon is then injected, and the patient is asked to describe any change in the position of the two lights. Another option is to use the Lancaster red-green test and the Hess screen to plot the position of the two eyes before and after the injection of Tensilon. This technique provides an extremely accurate determination of eye position.

It is not sufficient simply to ask a patient if his or her diplopia resolves after injection of Tensilon, because patients with diplopia may have a change in ocular alignment without recognizing a corresponding change in diplopia. Thus, a patient with an objectively positive Tensilon test may have no subjective awareness that his or her strabismus has improved unless the improvement is substantial.

When ocular motility is minimally affected, a careful study of eye movements before and after intravenous injection of Tensilon may be particularly helpful in diagnosis. Small changes in saccadic accuracy, particularly the development of saccadic hypermetria, suggest myasthenia gravis. Saccadic fatigability during repetitive refixations or optokinetic nystagmus, which is reversed by Tensilon, is also a useful sign.

Because Tensilon is a peripheral anticholinesterase agent, it allows ACh to accumulate briefly in ganglia, at parasympathetic nerve endings, and at neuromuscular junctions in all types of muscle—cardiac, smooth, and striated. It is the transient excess of ACh at **nicotinic** synapses that produces a positive test in patients with myasthenia gravis, but this same excess may also produce **muscarinic** cholinergic side effects from a brief overstimulation of the parasympathetic nervous system. Minor side effects of Tensilon testing include fainting, dizziness, and involuntary defecation. Severe side effects are uncommon, but rare patients experience severe bradycardia, apnea, and even cardiac arrest.

Although most side effects associated with the Tensilon test can probably be prevented by pretreating patients with an intramuscular injection of atropine sulfate, such reactions are exceedingly rare. Accordingly, we do not pretreat our patients with atropine, but we always have the drug available during the test. In addition, we do not perform Tensilon (or Prostigmin) tests in older patients, particularly those with known cardiac disease. Instead, we rely on the results of a sleep test or an ice test (see above) to direct a further diagnostic evaluation. Should it be necessary to perform a Tensilon test in a patient with cardiac disease, we always have an intravenous line in place and have the patient hooked up to an electrocardiograph machine.

A positive Tensilon test is almost, but not always, indicative of myasthenia gravis. However, a negative Tensilon test in no way rules out myasthenia gravis. We have seen patients in whom several Tensilon tests were unequivocally negative but who had other evidence of myasthenia gravis. We have also seen patients who had several negative Tensilon tests before a positive Tensilon or Prostigmin test was observed. In patients suspected of having myasthenia gravis, a negative Tensilon test should be followed either by a Prostigmin test or by other nonocular diagnostic tests (see below).

Neostigmine Methylsulfate (Prostigmin) Test

Because of the transient nature of both ocular and systemic changes in muscle strength that occur following administration of Tensilon, the neostigmine methylsulfate (**Prostigmin**) test remains an exceptionally valuable method of diagnosing myasthenia gravis, particularly in patients with diplopia but without ptosis. The longer duration of the effects of this drug is sufficient to permit repeated testing of muscle strength and evaluation of ocular motility. In adults with obvious ptosis and ophthalmoparesis, we generally combine 0.6 mg of atropine sulfate with 1.5 mg of Prostigmin in a 3 mL syringe and inject the mixture into one of the deltoid or gluteal muscles. A change in ocular motility or alignment and an improvement in

ptosis is usually apparent within 15 minutes and is most obvious 30 to 45 minutes following the injection (see Fig. 21.10).

When there is only minor ophthalmoparesis, we perform quantitative measurements of ocular motility and alignment before and after Prostigmin injection. In such cases, we perform prism-cover testing in primary position at distance and near and in the cardinal positions of gaze. We also measure the extent of ductions for the cardinal positions of gaze. These measurements are repeated 30 to 45 minutes following intramuscular injection of Prostigmin. The extent of the difference between preinjection and postinjection measurements determines if the test is positive or negative.

We find the Prostigmin test to be particularly helpful in the diagnosis of myasthenia gravis in children in whom intravenous injection of Tensilon may be accompanied by crying and lack of cooperation, precluding any meaningful assessment of its effect. In such patients, Prostigmin is injected and by the time the Prostigmin takes effect, the child has stopped crying and can be observed and the eye movements measured if necessary. In children, the amount of Prostigmin given is related to body weight and is usually 0.04 mg/kg, not exceeding a total dose of 1.5 mg (the adult dose).

As with Tensilon, a positive Prostigmin test usually, but not always, indicates myasthenia gravis. A positive response to Prostigmin may occur in patients with such diverse entities as multiple sclerosis, brainstem tumors, and congenital ptosis.

A negative Tensilon test does not preclude a positive Prostigmin test. Furthermore, a negative Prostigmin test, like a negative Tensilon test, does not rule out myasthenia gravis.

Electrophysiologic Tests

The primary electrophysiologic technique used in the diagnosis of myasthenia gravis consists of eliciting a decremental response to **repetitive supramaximal motor nerve stimulation** (Fig. 21.14). Supramaximal electric stimuli are delivered at a rate of 2 to 3 Hz to the appropriate nerves, and compound muscle action potentials (CMAPs) are recorded from muscles. A rapid decrement in amplitude of ≥ 10 to 15% is considered abnormal. The diagnosis of myasthenia gravis can be confirmed in about 95% of patients with this technique, provided that sev-

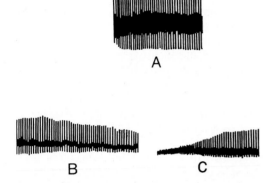

Figure 21.14. Drawing of the results of an electromyogram during repetitive nerve stimulation in (*A*) a normal person, in (*B*) a patient with myasthenia gravis, and in (*C*) a patient with the Lambert-Eaton myasthenic syndrome. Note the decremental response in myasthenia gravis and the facilitation response in the myasthenic syndrome.

eral clinically weak muscles, including a proximal one such as the deltoid, are studied.

The diagnostic application of repetitive nerve stimulation may be falsely negative when temperature is uncontrolled. Decremental responses are not pathognomonic of myasthenia gravis, because low-level decrement may be seen in Lambert-Eaton myasthenic syndrome, amyotrophic lateral sclerosis, and even polymyositis. A normal test does not exclude myasthenia gravis. Nevertheless, the diagnosis is highly probable if a reduced safety factor is demonstrable, and if it is promptly corrected by Tensilon or Prostigmin.

Endplate potentials reach the threshold for triggering an action potential of the muscle fiber with random variability, and this results in a variable latency between a nerve stimulus and the action potential of the responding muscle fiber. The latencies of responses of fibers belonging to the same motor unit are therefore not quite synchronous. The variability between any fiber and a reference fiber from the same unit is called "jitter." When the safety factor for transmission is low, these latency variabilities (jitters) are increased. There are also more response failures ("blocking"). Both blocking and jitter are increased by exercising or heating the muscle. Jitter can be detected in human muscles using suitably selective electrodes, and the latencies can be studied statistically during either voluntary contraction or indirect stimulation—**single-fiber electromyography.**

An experienced electrophysiologist is required to perform single-fiber EMG. Increased jitter may have causes other than defective neuromuscular transmission (such as denervation), and the results are considered positive only in the context of normal fiber density and a routine electromyogram. Single-fiber EMG is a highly sensitive test. It is positive in 88 to 99% of patients with myasthenia gravis. Like the Tensilon and Prostigmin tests, however, the single-fiber EMG may be negative initially, only to be positive several months later.

If a clinically weak muscle has normal jitter at all endplates, the diagnosis of myasthenia gravis can be excluded. In ocular myasthenia, the sensitivity of repetitive nerve stimulation is low, even in facial muscles, whereas the sensitivity of single-fiber EMG is high, especially in the frontalis muscle. In generalized myasthenia, the sensitivity of repetitive nerve stimulation is high, about that of anti-ACh receptor antibody, and the sensitivity of single-fiber EMG is highest (>95%).

Anti-Acetylcholine Receptor Antibody Assay

A radioimmunoassay using human ACh receptor labeled with $^{125}I\alpha$-bungarotoxin to detect antireceptor antibodies is one of the standard diagnostic tests for myasthenia gravis. Although the presence of anti-ACh receptor antibodies is specific for myasthenia gravis, antibodies are not detectable in about 15% of all patients subsequently proven to have myasthenia and in no more than 50% of patients with weakness confined to eyelid or extraocular muscles. Some assays measure all antireceptor antibodies; others specifically measure antibodies that produce blocking of the ACh-binding site on the receptor or antibodies that accelerate degradation (modulation) of the ACh receptor. False-positive results are extremely rare but sometimes occur in patients with amyotrophic lateral sclerosis.

Additional Tests

Because a thymic tumor is found in about 10% of patients with myasthenia gravis, part of the evaluation of a patient with suspected or proven myasthenia gravis should be imaging of the mediastinum. Computed tomographic (CT) scanning and magnetic resonance imaging (MRI) are probably equally sensitive.

In addition, a complete blood count, erythrocyte sedimentation rate, antinuclear antibody test, and thyroid function tests should be performed because of the increased prevalence of other autoimmune diseases in myasthenic patients (see below).

Systemic corticosteroids are often used to treat patients with myasthenia gravis (see below). Thus, any patient suspected of having this disorder should be tested for diabetes mellitus and should undergo a skin test for tuberculosis, because both diseases could be worsened by the administration of systemic corticosteroids.

DISORDERS ASSOCIATED WITH MYASTHENIA GRAVIS

Patients with myasthenia gravis have a much higher prevalence of other autoimmune disorders than do otherwise normal persons. Disorders of the thyroid gland, including subclinical disease indicated by serum antibody studies, are more frequent in a myasthenic population than in a normal population. Such patients are as commonly hypothyroid as hyperthyroid. The incidence of hyperthyroidism before, during, and after detectable myasthenia gravis is about 5%. If all thyroid disorders are considered, the prevalence may be as high as 9% in males and 18% in females.

Many of these patients have dysthyroid symptoms that precede myasthenic symptoms by months or years. In other cases, dysthyroid symptoms may be subsiding when symptoms and signs of myasthenia gravis first appear and vice versa. The linkage between them must be the genetic and other factors predisposing to autoimmunity. All diseases of the thyroid gland are over-represented, including nontoxic goiter, spontaneous myxedema, Hashimoto's disease, Graves' disease, and thyroid carcinoma.

Other autoimmune disorders also occur more commonly in patients with myasthenia than in the normal population. Rheumatoid arthritis and ankylosing spondylitis are common in myasthenics and their relatives. Aplastic anemia associated with a thymic tumor can occur in patients with myasthenia, as can pernicious anemia. Other immune-mediated disorders occasionally associated (individually and familially) with myasthenia gravis are systemic lupus erythematosus, pemphigus vulgaris, ulcerative colitis, sarcoidosis, Sjögren's syndrome, diabetes mellitus, and autoimmune hepatitis. Primary adrenal insufficiency of the autoimmune type is rare.

Associated disorders that probably have an immunologic basis or cause immunodeficiency in patients with myasthenia gravis are acrocyanosis, hemolytic anemia, nephritis, the reticuloses, Satoyoshi's syndrome, herpes zoster, Kaposi's sarcoma, and lymphoid tumor of the orbit.

FOCAL OR OCULAR MYASTHENIA

Although about 75% of patients with myasthenia gravis initially present with ptosis, diplopia, or both, about 60% of these patients eventually develop other signs and symptoms, including proximal muscle weakness, difficulty with speech, and difficulty swallowing. The remainder of patients whose manifestations remain localized to the eyelids and extraocular muscles are said to have "ocular myasthenia gravis." In general, patients with only ocular manifestations at onset who go on to develop systemic manifestations do so within 2 years; however, there are too many exceptions to this rule to adequately reassure patients or clinicians. Because limb muscles are depleted of ACh receptors even in apparently ocular myasthenia, all myasthenia gravis should be considered generalized.

TREATMENT

Most patients with myasthenia gravis can lead full and productive lives with proper therapy. Treatment includes cholinesterase inhibitors, thymectomy, immunosuppressive drugs, and, for patients with ocular manifestations, local therapy.

Cholinesterase Inhibitors

Anticholinesterase agents are the first-line therapy for patients with myasthenia gravis. These drugs prolong the action of ACh by slowing its degradation at the neuromuscular junction, thereby enhancing neuromuscular transmission. Although most patients experience some benefit from anticholinesterase agents, the response is often incomplete, particularly in patients with ocular manifestations, necessitating additional therapy.

Pyridostigmine bromide (**Mestinon**) is the most widely used anticholinesterase. Its onset of action occurs within 30 minutes and peaks at 1 to 2 hours. Anticholinesterases are safe, well-tolerated drugs, although they should be used with caution in patients with asthma or cardiac conduction defects. The most common side effect is diarrhea, which is dose-related. Other symptoms of cholinergic excess are tearing, sialorrhea, and fasciculations. These usually do not interfere with treatment. Excessive amounts of anticholinesterases may cause increased weakness that is reversible after decreasing or discontinuing the drug.

Thymectomy

Thymectomy is recommended for patients with myasthenia gravis in two settings.

First, patients between puberty and 50 years of age who are inadequately controlled on Mestinon alone may benefit from thymectomy. Thymectomy results in clinical improvement in about 85% of such patients, with drug-free remission in up to 35% and reduced medication requirements in up to 50%. The benefit from thymectomy is delayed, however, rarely occurring within 6 months and usually requiring 2 to 5 years for demonstrated efficacy. The surgery is more difficult in older patients because of involution of thymic tissue beyond middle age, and such patients are less likely to improve after thymectomy.

Second, thymectomy should be performed in any patient with a thymoma, regardless of the patient's age, because these tumors may spread locally and become invasive, even though they rarely metastasize.

Thymectomy is an elective procedure and should be performed when the control of myasthenia is optimal. Patients with significant weakness often benefit from a course of plasmapheresis weeks to days before planned surgery. Plasmapheresis may also be necessary after surgery if patients have significant postoperative weakness, a common occurrence. When both thymectomy and immunosuppressive medications are to be used to treat a patient with myasthenia gravis, thymectomy is usually performed before placing the patient on medication. This avoids poor wound healing and reduces the potential risk of postoperative infection related to immunosuppression. If immunosuppressive therapy after thymectomy is indicated, it is generally begun 2 to 6 weeks postoperatively for prednisone or 1 to 2 weeks postoperatively in the case of azathioprine (Imuran).

A number of different approaches can be used to perform a thymectomy, including a median sternotomy and limited transcervical or endoscopic transcervical approaches. If thymomatous tissue cannot be completely excised, nonferro-

magnetic clips should be placed at the site of remaining tumor, and postoperative radiotherapy administered.

Immunosuppressive Drugs

When anticholinesterase agents are ineffective, and thymectomy is unwarranted or cannot be performed, three drugs can provide chronic immunosuppression: prednisone, azathioprine, and cyclosporine. The choice among them is made by considering two factors: how the toxicity profile fits the patient, and how fast the patient must improve. Factors by which to compare the use of these drugs are outlined in Table 21.1.

Corticosteroids (Prednisone)

Corticosteroids are indicated when myasthenia gravis symptoms are insufficiently controlled by anticholinesterase agents and are sufficiently disabling to the patient that the frequent side effects of these drugs are worth the risk. "Sufficient control" is best defined functionally for each individual patient. For example, some patients are willing to live with moderate generalized weakness or to patch one eye to eliminate diplopia, whereas for others even mild ptosis or diplopia is intolerable. Corticosteroids can produce improvement in patients with all degrees of weakness, from diplopia to severe respiratory involvement. Diplopia, which is rarely corrected by anticholinesterase agents alone, usually responds extremely well to steroid treatment. Older men with myasthenia gravis seem to respond particularly well to steroid therapy.

More than 80% of myasthenic patients can be expected to improve with steroid treatment alone. Improvement usually begins within 2 to 3 weeks after beginning treatment, although maximum benefit may not occur for up to 6 months or more.

There are no absolute contraindications to the use of corticosteroids, but relative contraindications include severe obesity, diabetes mellitus, uncontrolled hypertension, ulcer disease, osteoporosis, or ongoing infections. Long-term treatment with steroids requires medical attention by an experienced physician. Patients who are unable or unwilling to be followed closely should *never* be treated with steroids.

Patients with moderate to severe generalized weakness or significant respiratory insufficiency or bulbar weakness are at risk of a transient steroid-induced exacerbation and should be admitted to the hospital for initiation of steroid therapy

Table 21.1.
Standard Immunotherapy in Myasthenia Gravis

DRUG	USUAL ADULT DOSE	TIME TO ONSET OF IMPROVEMENT	TIME TO MAXIMAL IMPROVEMENT	TOXICITY/EFFICACY MONITORING
Prednisone	Gradually increasing to 60 mg q.d. orally followed by q.o.d. regimen	2–3 weeks	3–6 months	Weight Blood pressure Fasting blood glucose Electrolytes Ophthalmic examination Bone density, 24 h urine calcium, 25-OH vitamin D (especially in postmenopausal women)
Cyclosporine (Sandimmune)	5 mg/kg/day orally, divided b.i.d. (125–200 mg b.i.d.)	2–12 weeks	3–6 months	Blood pressure Serum creatinine Blood urea nitrogen Cyclosporine level, 12 h trough by RIA Amylase Cholesterol
Azathioprine (Imuran)	2–3 mg/kg/day orally (100–250 mg daily)	3–12 months	1–2 years	WBC (maintain >3500) Differential (goal, <1000 lymphocytes) MCV (goal, >100 fl) Platelets Liver function tests Amylase

and observation. Nearly 50% of such patients have an exacerbation, which lasts days and occurs most commonly during the second 5 days of induction. The cause of this initial steroid-induced deterioration is not clear.

If a patient has mild myasthenia gravis or purely ocular involvement and can be reliably monitored at about weekly intervals, outpatient initiation of prednisone may be performed. Therapy is usually begun at a dose of 5–10 mg of prednisone per day. The dose is then increased every week by 5 mg until a response occurs. This usually happens at a dose of 35–60 mg/day.

Once a patient receiving daily prednisone experiences a clinical response to the medication, the dosage is kept constant until the improvement levels off or 3 months, whichever comes first. When the patient reaches a plateau of improvement, the total dose is changed to alternate-day therapy and tapered gradually to seek the smallest effective dose. It often takes *more than 1 year* to determine the minimum requirement for a given patient. It is extremely important to taper the drug very gradually.

Physicians must make their patents familiar with the unfortunately long list of side effects of chronic steroid therapy. Almost every patient will gain weight and develop part of the cushingoid habitus. Other side effects include hypertension, hyperglycemia, osteoporosis, ulcers, dyspepsia, adrenal insufficiency, and infections caused by opportunistic organisms.

Azathioprine

Azathioprine can be used effectively as initial therapy in myasthenia gravis. The manner in which azathioprine is most often used derives from its chief disadvantage—beneficial effects may take 6 months or more to appear. It therefore tends to be used as additional therapy in patients whose myasthenia is not adequately controlled after thymectomy and corticosteroid therapy. The combination affords the relatively rapid onset of immunosuppression produced by the steroids and allows tapering of corticosteroids once the azathioprine has had time to take effect. The addition of azathioprine also allows a reduction of steroid dosage in otherwise well-controlled patients who experience unacceptable side effects of prednisone and in patients who require a chronic maintenance dose of prednisone of more than about 50 mg on alternate days.

Patients who are unable or unwilling to be followed medically should *never* be treated with azathioprine. Approximately 10% of patients are unable to tolerate or continue azathioprine because of abnormal liver function, bone marrow depression, or an idiosyncratic reaction consisting of flu-like symptoms of fever and myalgia.

Cyclosporine

Cyclosporine is an immunosuppressive agent with efficacy similar to azathioprine. It has the advantage of a more prompt effect, usually occurring within weeks. However, worrisome side effects include nephrotoxicity and hypertension, in addition to facial hirsutism, gastrointestinal disturbance, headache, tremor, convulsions, and rarely hepatotoxicity. Visual complications of cyclosporine include reversible cerebral blindness, complex visual hallucinations, and rarely optic disc swelling.

Although occasionally used as a first-line immunosuppressive drug in patients with myasthenia gravis, cyclosporine is more commonly used in patients in whom corticosteroids or azathioprine treatment has either failed or has resulted in excessive toxicity.

Short-Term Immunotherapies

Plasmapheresis, also called plasma exchange, depletes circulating anti-ACh receptor antibodies and can therefore produce short-term improvement in patients with myasthenia gravis. Plasmapheresis is used primarily to stabilize patients in myasthenic crisis and for short-term management of patients undergoing thymectomy, in order to avoid corticosteroids and immunosuppressants. Less commonly, it is used as adjuvant therapy in severely ill patients who are slow to respond to immunosuppressants. Repeated plasmapheresis as a chronic form of therapy, either because the patient is intolerant or unresponsive to conventional immunosuppressant treatment, is rarely indicated.

Plasmapheresis works rapidly in patients with myasthenia gravis, with objective improvement measurable within days of treatment. Improvement in the individual patient correlates roughly with reduction in anti-ACh receptor antibody titers. The beneficial effects of plasmapheresis are temporary, lasting only days to weeks, unless concomitant immunosuppressive agents are used. Even "antibody-negative" patients may improve after plasmapheresis. The major risks are related to problems of vascular access and include infection, thrombosis, perforation, sepsis,

arrhythmia, anaphylactic shock, pulmonary embolism, and systemic hemorrhage from disseminated intravascular coagulopathy.

The indications for use of **intravenous human immune globulin** (HIG) are the same as those for plasmapheresis—to produce rapid improvement so as to get the patient through a difficult period of myasthenic weakness. When patients respond, the onset is within 4 to 5 days, and the maximum response occurs within 1 to 2 weeks of initiation of therapy. The effect is transient but may be sustained for weeks to months, allowing intermittent chronic therapy. The mechanism of action of HIG in myasthenia gravis is unknown, but it has no consistent effect on the measurable amount of anti-ACh receptor antibody. Adverse reactions occur in less than 10% of patients and are generally mild. They include allergy, headache, fluid overload, and various gastrointestinal symptoms. HIG is very expensive.

Comparison of Immunotherapeutic Options

Each of the available immunotherapeutic options for myasthenia gravis has its advantages and disadvantages. Prednisone generally acts rapidly and is effective, but it has substantial side effects. Azathioprine is safe and moderately effective but slow. Cyclosporine is about equal to azathioprine in effectiveness and much more rapid in its effects, but it is expensive, with more serious side effects. Cyclophosphamide is a potent but highly toxic immunosuppressive drug and is therefore reserved for special cases.

Both plasmapheresis and intravenous HIG are often useful for the short-term management of acute problems, or as pre- or post-operative therapy. However, the effects of both are transient, and their costs are extremely high.

Local Treatment

Patients with ocular symptoms alone may not require systemic therapy. Ptosis, the single most frequent finding and complaint, may be reduced in many patients by placing a wire attachment on the top of one or both sides of a spectacle frame to keep the eyelids elevated. Almost invariably, patients develop irritation of the eyes from exposure because these "ptosis crutches" prevent normal blinking, but many patients nevertheless prefer this method of treatment. This is particularly true when the amount or type of medication required to relieve the ptosis has intolerable side effects.

Ptosis surgery can be performed in some patients with myasthenia gravis, particularly in patients who are refractory to appropriate medical therapy, thymectomy, or both, or in whom ptosis is the only (or predominant) finding. Success is sometimes short-lived, however, because myasthenic ptosis is variable and can recur.

Some patients with intermittent diplopia may require no therapy, but most are sufficiently bothered that some type of treatment is usually necessary. In patients with diplopia along a relatively fixed plane, prisms can be used, particularly when there is a relatively comitant deviation. Some patients may be content to wear prisms that correct their diplopia only in primary position. Other patients may prefer to wear a patch over one eye.

Rare patients improve with small doses of botulinum toxin A. Such treatment may be preferable to anticholinesterases, because those medications often do not improve ocular symptoms.

Extraocular muscle surgery is rarely warranted in patients with myasthenia gravis and diplopia unless the strabismus has been stable for at least a year, and no other treatment options are available.

PROGNOSIS

In considering the prognosis of patients with myasthenia gravis, there are two areas of concern: the tendency for patients with ''ocular myasthenia'' to develop systemic symptoms and signs, and the treatment response of ocular as compared with systemic symptoms and signs.

It is important to emphasize that myasthenia gravis is never truly focal. Patients with symptoms apparently restricted to the eyes still have a systemic disease, as one would expect with an antibody-mediated process. From 50 to 80% of patients who present with purely ocular symptoms and signs eventually develop generalized myasthenia, usually—but not invariably—within 2 years of onset of the disorder. Increasing duration of pure ocular myasthenia is associated with a decreasing risk of late generalized symptoms. Patients older than 50 years of age at onset are at substantially greater risk to develop generalized myasthenia complicated by ventilatory insufficiency, whereas younger age at onset is associated with a more benign outcome.

About 10 to 20% of patients with ocular myasthenia gravis undergo a spontaneous remission.

Remissions may be permanent, but relapses may occur up to 14 years after remission and may cause recurrent and progressive worsening of symptoms.

Of all ocular signs, ptosis appears to be the most responsive to therapy. Ptosis usually improves with anticholinesterase therapy, corticosteroid therapy, or after thymectomy. Diplopia is more refractory to treatment than is ptosis. Many patients show no improvement in diplopia with anticholinesterase agents and require patching of one eye, immunosuppressive therapy, thymectomy, or a combination of these modalities to achieve improvement or remission.

MYASTHENIC CRISIS

A patient with myasthenia gravis is said to be in ''myasthenic crisis'' when he or she experiences significant acute respiratory insufficiency or dysphagia. Any patient with myasthenia gravis who reports dyspnea or dysphagia should be evaluated promptly. The two most helpful measurements of respiratory function in myasthenic patients are forced vital capacity and negative inspiratory force. Arterial blood gas measurements are not a good determinant because they may be normal despite imminent respiratory failure.

Physicians should have a high suspicion of infection as a potential precipitating cause of myasthenic crisis. Patients with myasthenia gravis are frequently immunosuppressed; furthermore, reduced respiratory function increases their vulnerability to pneumonia. Myasthenic patients with respiratory insufficiency (or post-thymectomy) can benefit from periodic inflation of the lungs with intermittent positive pressure therapy to reduce atelectasis and the risk of pneumonia.

NEONATAL MYASTHENIA GRAVIS

Preparations for the contingency of neonatal myasthenia should be made in the delivery room for all myasthenic mothers, because it is not possible to predict from the severity or laboratory features of the mother's myasthenia (even antibody positivity) whether or not an infant will be affected. Affected infants have weak suck and cry and may have generalized weakness or impaired swallowing and breathing. The disorder may be recognized any time in the first 72 hours and abates spontaneously after 2 to 3 weeks as passively transferred myasthenic antibody from the mother is cleared. Treatment requires only anticholinesterase agents and support of vital functions.

PEDIATRIC MYASTHENIA

Autoimmune myasthenia gravis can occur at any age. Thus, the challenge in "juvenile-onset" myasthenia is to distinguish antibody-mediated disease from gene mutations affecting ion channels (see below). Juvenile-onset autoimmune myasthenia gravis differs little from adult-onset disease, except that it frequently improves with age. It responds to anticholinesterase agents and immunotherapy. The optimum age for thymectomy and immunosuppressive agents in such patients is controversial.

CONGENITAL MYASTHENIC SYNDROMES

Congenital myasthenia gravis is actually a group of genetic neuromuscular transmission disorders. These conditions can be differentiated from acquired autoimmune myasthenia gravis on the basis of clinical, electromyographic, electrophysiologic, cytochemical, structural, and molecular genetic grounds.

Many, but not all cases present neonatally or in infancy with ptosis, fluctuating ophthalmoparesis, poor feeding, and respiratory difficulty. Symptoms may be episodic or may demonstrate fatigability that is worsened by crying, activity, or fever. Persistence of symptoms, rather than a transient monophasic course, distinguishes a congenital myasthenic syndrome from neonatal myasthenia gravis. Some syndromes may not even present until adolescence or adulthood. Serum anti-ACh receptor antibodies are absent. In many cases, siblings or parents are affected, but a negative family history does not exclude autosomal-recessive inheritance. The Tensilon test, which relies on intact acetylcholinesterase and normal channel open times for its effect, is negative in many congenital myasthenic syndromes.

Congenital myasthenic syndromes may be separated into those in which the defect is primarily presynaptic and those in which the defect is primarily postsynaptic. The major syndromes in which the defect is presynaptic are related to defects in ACh synthesis, mobilization, or release. Postsynaptic syndromes are mainly those caused by endplate acetylcholinesterase deficiency and ACh receptor deficiency, as well as the slow-channel syndrome.

PRESYNAPTIC CONGENITAL MYASTHENIC SYNDROMES

Presynaptic congenital myasthenic disorders were previously called "familial infantile myasthenia." They are transmitted in an autosomal-recessive fashion and are characterized by fluctuating ptosis, feeding difficulties during infancy, easy fatigability on exertion, and episodic apnea following crying, vomiting, or febrile illnesses. Symptoms respond to neostigmine but not to prednisone, and they improve with age.

No circulating anti-ACh receptor antibodies are found. The number of motor endplates is normal, but the endplates themselves have abnormally small synaptic vesicles. The postsynaptic regions are normal. Electrophysiologic studies suggest a presynaptic defect in ACh resynthesis or mobilization. The defective step or steps in ACh synthesis are unknown but could involve choline re-uptake, ACh assembly via choline acetyltransferase, or vesicle packaging. A related autosomal-recessive presynaptic syndrome marked by less episodic symptoms is associated with a paucity of synaptic vesicles and reduced quantal release.

POSTSYNAPTIC CONGENITAL MYASTHENIC SYNDROMES

Congenital Acetylcholinesterase Deficiency

In patients with **congenital acetylcholinesterase deficiency,** weakness, atrophy, fatigability, and ophthalmoparesis are usually recognized in the first 2 years of life (Fig. 21.15). Autosomal-recessive inheritance is the rule. In most pa-

Figure 21.15. Congenital myasthenic syndrome caused by acetylcholinesterase deficiency. *A.* A 16-year-old boy with bilateral ptosis, facial and skeletal muscle weakness, reduced muscle bulk, and scoliosis. *B–C.* Electron cytochemical localization of acetylcholinesterase activity. *B.* Patient's endplate shows no reaction after incubation with α-bungarotoxin. *C.* Control endplate from a normal subject shows marked reaction after only 30 minutes of incubation. (Reprinted with permission from Engel AG, Lambert EH, Gomez MR. A new myasthenic syndrome with end-plate acetylcholinesterase deficiency, small nerve terminals, and reduced acetylcholine release. Ann Neurol 1977;1: 315–330.)

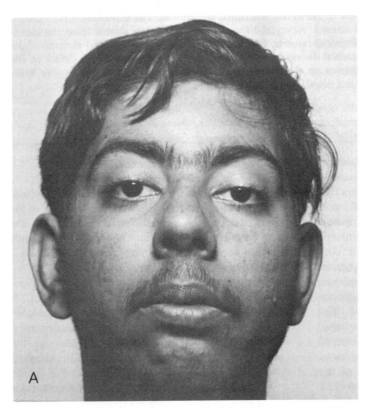

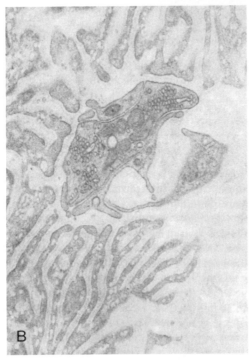

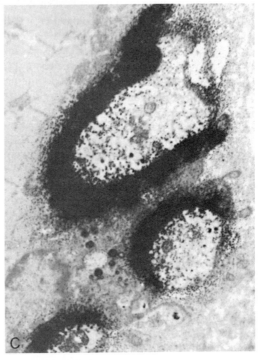

tients, pupillary light responses are abnormally slow. These patients typically show no response to treatment with either Mestinon or corticosteroids. There are no circulating antibodies to ACh receptors, there are normal numbers of ACh receptors on muscle biopsy, and acetylcholinesterase is absent from the motor endplates by cytochemistry.

Electromyographic studies in patients with congenital acetylcholinesterase deficiency show decremental responses at 2-Hz stimulation, postactivation facilitation, and postactivation exhaustion. Microelectrode studies reveal a prolonged delay of miniature endplate potentials (mepps), potentials that are generated by the resting tonus of the muscle, not by specific muscle stimulation. However, the most distinguishing electrophysiologic finding is a reduplicated CMAP response to single stimuli. This is caused by absent acetylcholinesterase, the action of which is normally the rate-limiting step for termination of the action of ACh. The physiology is similar to that of organophosphate poisoning.

Primary Acetylcholine Receptor Deficiency

Patients with autosomal-recessive **primary acetylcholine receptor deficiency** present with poor feeding and ptosis in the neonatal period. They eventually develop generalized fatigue and complete external ophthalmoplegia by 13 years of age. Slight limb and facial weakness are present. There is a severe reduction in mepp amplitude, and ACh receptors are quantitatively reduced. This syndrome may be caused by a molecular mutation in the ACh receptor itself, possibly at or near the ACh binding site, or in a part of the molecule that affects receptor insertion or turnover. Unlike patients with congenital acetylcholinesterase deficiency, patients with a congenital deficiency of ACh receptors improve when treated with anticholinesterase agents, such as Mestinon.

Slow-Channel Syndrome

In **slow-channel syndrome,** the age of onset, rate of progression, severity, and pattern of weakness are highly variable. Atrophy is common. Some patients have predominant involvement of cervical, scapular, and finger extensor muscles. Ophthalmoparesis and ptosis are often prominent (Fig. 21.16). The diseases confused with this disorder include mitochondrial myopathy, myotonic dystrophy, congenital myopathy, spinal muscular atrophy, limb-girdle dystrophy, Möbius syndrome, and peripheral neuropathies.

Like congenital acetylcholinesterase deficiency, slow-channel syndrome is characterized by reduplicated CMAP responses to single stimuli. Mepps and endplate potentials are low in amplitude and prolonged in duration because of greatly prolonged ion channel open times. Acetylcholinesterase staining of endplates is normal. This physiology predicts that such patients should be unresponsive to, or even worsened by, anticholinesterase agents, and that is precisely the case.

Slow-channel syndrome is an example of cellular excitotoxicity. The result of this open-channel cationic toxicity is not only a myasthenic syndrome but a fixed, vacuolar myopathy.

ACQUIRED DISORDERS OF NEUROMUSCULAR TRANSMISSION OTHER THAN MYASTHENIA GRAVIS

As with congenital ''myasthenic'' syndromes, acquired disorders of neuromuscular transmission may be caused by presynaptic or postsynaptic abnormalities. In addition, some syndromes are characterized by *both* pre- and postsynaptic abnormalities. Most of the acquired disorders of neuromuscular transmission are caused by the effects of exogenous agents on the neuromuscular junction.

LAMBERT-EATON MYASTHENIC SYNDROME

Clinical Features

Lambert-Eaton myasthenic syndrome is characterized primarily by weakness but also by fatigability, hyporeflexia, and autonomic dysfunction. Weakness is proximal and more prominent in legs and truncal muscles than in arms. Ocular and bulbar muscles are sometimes affected, but mildly so, in contrast to their prominent involvement in myasthenia gravis. Weakness is more disabling than life threatening, because the disorder rarely produces respiratory failure. Therefore, Lambert-Eaton myasthenic syndrome is really part of the differential diagnosis of acquired myopathy in adults. It is not often confused with myasthenia gravis, although the two

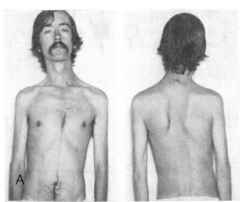

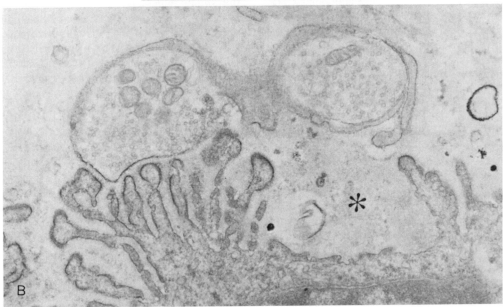

Figure 21.16. Congenital myasthenic syndrome caused by an abnormality of the acetylcholine-induced calcium ion channel. *A.* The 29-year-old patient has moderate bilateral ptosis, scoliosis, and moderate atrophy of cervical, shoulder, arm, forearm, and torso muscles. *B.* Localization of acetylcholine receptors with horseradish peroxidase-labeled α-bungarotoxin. There is no activity observed in areas where junctional folds have degenerated (asterisk). Electron dense deposits in the synaptic space probably contain calcium. (From Engel AG, Lambert EH, Mulder DM, et al. Investigations of 3 cases of a newly recognized familial, congenital myasthenic syndrome. Trans Am Neurol Assoc 1979;104: 8–11.)

autoimmune disorders may coexist. Reflexes are reduced or absent, but muscle wasting is infrequent. Autonomic symptoms and signs include dry mouth, decreased sweating, erectile impotence, and loss of the pupillary light reflex.

Lambert-Eaton myasthenic syndrome is autoimmune and is associated commonly with carcinoma (especially small-cell lung cancer) or other autoimmune disorders. Paraneoplastic Lambert-Eaton myasthenic syndrome often presents before (sometimes 2 to 3 years before) the discovery of the neoplasm.

As in myasthenia gravis, sex and age affect case incidence. Two-thirds of all cases are paraneoplastic. These are mostly in men. One-third are primarily autoimmune and are mostly in women. This accounts for the overall male predominance of about 4 to 1 in the disorder. Although most affected patients are adults, the disorder can also occur in children. The myasthenic syndrome may develop in patients with pernicious anemia, thyroid disease, or Sjögren's syndrome.

Pathophysiology

The neuromuscular transmission defect in Lambert-Eaton myasthenic syndrome is presynaptic. It is caused by impaired release of ACh at motor nerve terminals because of antibodies directed against voltage-gated calcium channels in the motor nerve terminal and cholinergic autonomic nerve terminals. These antibodies reduce the number of calcium channels and thus the probability of synaptosomal release of ACh at active zones. Small-cell carcinomas enriched in voltage-gated calcium channels provide the shared antigenic stimulus in paraneoplastic Lambert-Eaton myasthenic syndrome. Synthesis and mobilization of ACh are unimpaired, and the amount of depolarization produced by single quanta is normal. The impaired release results in endplate potentials that are too small to trigger muscle action potentials. As a result, muscles fatigue and evoked CMAPs are low in amplitude.

The normal increased mobilization of calcium that occurs in the nerve terminal immediately following exercise or electric activation of motor nerves at rates above 10 Hz transiently increases the release of ACh, the resultant endplate potential amplitude, and therefore muscle strength. This **facilitation** is the basis for the electrophysiologic diagnosis, but it is only occasionally evident on physical examination. Repetitive nerve stimulation reveals decrement at 2 Hz but marked (40 to 1000%) facilitation of the compound muscle action potential after brief exercise or 50-Hz stimulation (see Fig. 21.14C). Single-fiber EMG reveals increased jitter and blocking that improve as units fire at higher rates. As in myasthenia gravis, failure of neuromuscular transmission and weakness worsen when the temperature is raised.

Ocular Manifestations

In contrast to myasthenia gravis, ocular symptoms are rare in Lambert-Eaton syndrome, but ptosis and both clinical and subclinical ocular motor involvement do occur in some patients. Just as fatigable ptosis after sustained upgaze is a clinically useful sign in myasthenia gravis,

paradoxic lid elevation after sustained upgaze may be a clinically useful sign in Lambert-Eaton syndrome.

Therapy

In general, the Lambert-Eaton myasthenic syndrome responds to therapy less well than does myasthenia gravis. A combined approach to therapy includes treatment of any underlying cancer, pharmacotherapy of the neuromuscular transmission defect, and immunosuppression.

Because the syndrome may precede the discovery of a tumor by several years, the evaluation should include not only an initial extensive search for underlying malignancy, including chest CT scanning or MRI, but also frequent surveillance if the initial evaluation is negative. Partial, rarely complete remission may be achieved by removal or control of the underlying cancer with surgery, radiation therapy, or chemotherapy.

Because the main defect in Lambert-Eaton myasthenic syndrome is impaired release of ACh from the nerve terminal, neuromuscular transmission is best treated by drugs that enhance release. Aminopyridine drugs are potassium channel blockers that, by prolonging the duration of an action potential, increase nerve terminal calcium uptake by enhancing the activation of voltage-gated calcium channels. As a result, ACh release (and release of other neurotransmitters at other synapses) is greatly increased. The aminopyridine of choice is **3,4-diaminopyridine,** which repairs the neuromuscular transmission defect, improves muscle strength quantitatively, ameliorates autonomic symptoms, and significantly improves functional measures of strength and well being. The risk of seizures from drug toxicity increases with doses over 80–100 mg per day. Other toxicity includes paresthesias, gastric upset, and insomnia.

As in myasthenia gravis, **anticholinesterase agents** can partially repair the neuromuscular transmission defect in Lambert-Eaton myasthenic syndrome by preventing breakdown of ACh in the synaptic cleft and prolonging the effect of ACh at receptors, even though the primary defect is presynaptic. The effect in Lambert-Eaton myasthenic syndrome is modest. Thus, anticholinesterases are usually used to supplement other forms of therapy.

Immunotherapy is indicated when treatment of the underlying malignancy or treatment with

3,4-diaminopyridine or pyridostigmine provides insufficient or no benefit and when the potential benefits of immunosuppressants are believed to outweigh the potential risks. Because Lambert-Eaton myasthenic syndrome rarely remits spontaneously, treatment needs to be continued indefinitely. Immunosuppressants by themselves do not often produce complete symptomatic remission.

NEUROMUSCULAR DISORDERS CAUSED BY TOXINS

Toxins that disturb neuromuscular transmission may be acquired from many sources, including bacteria, arthropods, and snakes. Treatment depends on the recognition of the specific toxin, the availability of antitoxin, and supportive therapy.

Toxins That Damage Presynaptic Neuromuscular Transmission

Arthropod Envenomation

SPIDERS

Envenomation by the female black widow spider, *Latrodectus mactans,* causes diffuse central and peripheral nervous system stimulation with vasoconstriction, hypertension, and autonomic hyperactivity. The effects on muscle and neuromuscular transmission begin 15 to 60 minutes after envenomation, with muscle cramps involving the trunk and extremities. Black widow spider venom increases the release of ACh quanta at vertebrate neuromuscular junctions until the vesicles in the nerve terminal become depleted.

The venom of the brown widow spider, *Latrodectus geometricus*, has similar properties but causes intermittent release of ACh.

TICKS

Paralysis may occur in humans as a result of a salivary toxin elaborated by female **ticks.** In most cases, irritability precedes paralysis by 12 to 24 hours. Paralysis of the legs usually occurs first, often associated with pain, paresthesias, and numbness. In severe cases, paralysis of the upper extremities begins within 24 hours. Bulbar paralysis quickly follows, and death may occur from respiratory paralysis. Cerebellar ataxia is frequently present. Myoclonic twitching and choreiform movements may occur.

Ocular signs occur late in the course of tick paralysis. The pupils dilate and do not react to either light or near stimulation. The extraocular muscles may become paralyzed, usually in association with the onset of facial paralysis. Photophobia may occur and is often severe.

Electrophysiologic studies of patients with tick paralysis reveal slowing of motor and sensory nerve conduction. Endplate potentials at neuromuscular junctions from patients poisoned with toxin from North American ticks (*Dermacentor andersoni, Dermacentor variabilis*) are normal, but toxin from the Australian tick (*Ixodes holocyclus*) produces a temperature-dependent reduction in evoked release of transmitter, suggesting that presynaptic inhibition of ACh release may contribute to paralysis.

Patients with tick paralysis do not respond to anticholinesterase agents because the pathology is presynaptic. The treatment is to remove the offending tick immediately and to provide supportive measures, including assisted ventilation, until the intoxication phase subsides. The neurologic symptoms and signs usually resolve after the tick is removed, and the ultimate prognosis is therefore favorable. If the tick is not removed before bulbar signs appear, however, death may occur despite supportive measures.

SCORPIONS

Scorpion toxin increases ACh release at the neuromuscular junction secondarily by inducing repetitive potentials in nerve terminal membrane. The scorpion sting results in serious visceral effects, but neuromuscular transmission is little affected. Nevertheless, some patients develop abnormal eye movements after being stung. The abnormal movements are generally involuntary, conjugate, slow, and roving, but occasionally they are dysconjugate. A primary-position unsustained nystagmus may occur. Neurologic and systemic manifestations of the envenomation, including the abnormal eye movements, generally resolve within 1 hour after treatment with species-specific antivenom and within 24 hours when only symptomatic treatment is given.

Snake Envenomation

The venom of the Papuan taipan snake, *Oxyuranus scutellatus canni,* contains a variety of toxins, including neurotoxins, a procoagulant, and a calcium channel blocking toxin. Envenomed patients usually develop local tender lymphadenopathy, abdominal pain, and a systemic consumption coagulopathy within 1 to 2 hours of the bite. Signs of neurotoxicity become evident over the next few hours, with progressive ptosis, external ophthalmoplegia, paralysis of bulbar muscles, and weakness of respiratory and peripheral musculature. Many envenomed patients require intubation and assisted ventilation for several days until the effects of the venom begin to dissipate.

Botulism

Botulism occurs in three forms: food-borne, wound, and infantile. The disease is produced by a polypeptide toxin elaborated by the organism *Clostridium botulinum*. It is the most potent poison known. A cholinergic synapse may be blocked by as few as 10 molecules of toxin.

- In **food-borne botulism,** symptoms begin about 8 to 36 hours after food containing the toxin is eaten. The toxin is intact because proper cooking that normally would denature the toxin has not been performed.
- In **wound botulism,** organisms contaminating wounds produce toxin that is absorbed systemically. Nearly all cases develop from extremity wounds that occur outside the home. Symptoms begin 4 to 17 days after the injury, with an average incubation time of 7 days. Wounds that cause botulism may appear clinically uninfected; however, when the wound is carefully explored and cultured, the organism is usually found.
- In **infantile botulism,** organisms in the gastrointestinal tract produce toxin that is systemically absorbed.

At least eight types of botulinum toxin are characterized (A, B, Cα, Cβ, D, E, F, and G). Types A and B are the most common causes of botulism in the United States, although type E should be suspected when seafood is thought to be the source of the infection.

The diagnosis of botulism depends on clinical, epidemiologic, and electrophysiologic findings and may be confirmed by the discovery of the toxin, the organism, or both in food, stool, or a wound. Signs of infantile botulism are constipation, listlessness, poor suck, regurgitation, and generalized weakness. In children and adults, the symptoms of botulism include nausea, vomiting, blurred vision, dysphagia, and pooling of secretions in the mouth and pharynx, followed by diplopia and generalized weakness that mainly affects proximal muscles.

Examination of affected patients reveals facial, pharyngeal, and generalized proximal weakness, but normal sensation. Urinary retention and hypoactive bowel sounds are frequently present.

Ophthalmologic findings include dilated, nonreactive or poorly reactive pupils, ptosis, and ophthalmoparesis or ophthalmoplegia (Fig. 21.17). Rapid quivering eye motions are present in some patients with botulism. These eye movements are observed during attempts to refixate laterally placed objects and occur only in association with severe ophthalmoparesis. The quivering motions are composed of multiple hypometric saccades, many of which have subnormal, variable velocities. It is likely that, by blocking ACh release at the neuromuscular junction, botulinum toxin limits the duration of saccadic burst innervation reaching extraocular muscle.

EMG establishes the diagnosis of botulism. The findings suggest a presynaptic disorder analogous to Lambert-Eaton myasthenic syndrome. Motor and sensory nerve conduction velocities are normal. The amplitude of the evoked muscle action potential is usually reduced. There may be no decrement at low rates of stimulation. Following exercise or at high stimulus frequencies, significant facilitation is present. Single-fiber EMG shows increased jitter and blocking. These abnormalities are less prominent at higher frequencies of innervation. Fibrillations in affected muscles may appear about 2 weeks after the disorder begins.

Botulism is treated with bivalent (A and B) or trivalent (A, B, and E) antitoxin, 20,000 to 40,000 units, 2 to 3 times per day, in addition to removal of stomach and intestinal contents. In patients with wound botulism, the most important treatment is to open and extensively débride the wound. Penicillin or another antibiotic should be given, with the choice of the antibiotic being based on sensitivities from wound culture. Full respiratory and nutritional support may be required. Patients with botulism do not respond to treatment with anticholinesterase agents.

Botulinum toxins impair neuromuscular transmission presynaptically by interfering with the exocytotic release of ACh vesicles after the stimulus-induced influx of calcium into the nerve terminal. Both spontaneous and stimulus-in-

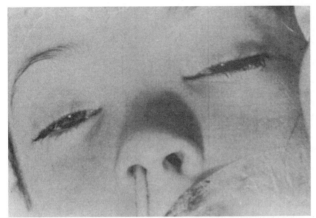

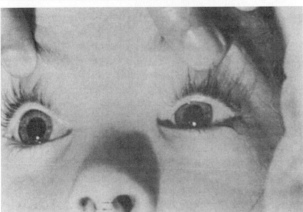

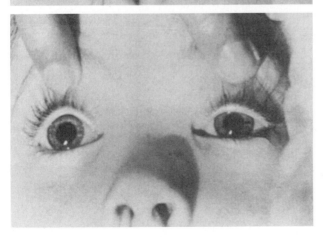

Figure 21.17.   Clinical appearance of an 8-year-old girl who developed wound botulism after she fell from a horse and sustained a compound fracture of the humerus. Although the wound appeared clean, *Clostridium botulinum* was cultured from it. *Top:* The patient has severe bilateral ptosis. *Middle:* On attempted rightward gaze, there is marked limitation of movement of both eyes. Note dilated pupils. *Bottom:* On attempted leftward gaze, there is almost no movement of the eyes. The patient was quadriparetic but was awake and alert. She recovered completely within several months.

duced release of ACh quanta are affected. Recovery eventually occurs when nerve fibers sprout, and new neuromuscular junctions are established, but the process may take months to years.

Like *Clostridium botulinum, Clostridium tetani* produces a neurotoxin that blocks the calcium-dependent release of ACh at neuromuscular junctions, but this effect is overshadowed by its effects on the central nervous system.

Toxins That Damage Both Pre- and Postsynaptic Neuromuscular Transmission

Envenomation by poisonous snakes is an important problem around the world. Of the four largest families of poisonous snakes—*Elapidae:* cobras, coral snakes, mambas, kraits; *Hydrophiidae:* sea snakes; *Viperidae:* old world vipers; and *Crotalidae:* rattlesnakes and related species—only the first two have venom with potent neuromuscular blocking properties. (The South American rattlesnake, *Crotalus durissus terrificus*, is an exception.)

In most cases of *Elapidae* envenomation, neuromuscular blocking activity of the venoms is a major cause of death and disability. Envenomation is followed in minutes to hours by signs of neuromuscular blockade resembling that caused by competitive neuromuscular blocking drugs. Patients initially develop bilateral ptosis, ophthalmoparesis, and dysphagia, followed later by tongue, laryngeal, and pharyngeal weakness. Respiratory paralysis eventually occurs, leading to death if patients are not treated. Many of the symptoms show improvement with anticholinesterase agents, although antivenom administration and ventilatory and cardiocirculatory support are the mainstays of treatment.

Sea snake venoms not only produce primary myopathic damage but also show nondepolarizing postjunction neuromuscular blocking activity similar to that produced by *Elapidae* toxins. It is likely, therefore, that at least some of their toxicity is caused by neuromuscular transmission failure in addition to direct muscle damage.

Persons bitten by the South American rattlesnake show symptoms similar to those with *Elapidae* envenomation. One of the toxins in the venom of this snake is crotoxin, which produces neuromuscular blockade. This toxin reduces the evoked release of ACh, possibly by interfering with calcium entry or subsequent release mechanisms.

NEUROMUSCULAR DISORDERS CAUSED BY DRUGS

The common settings in which the effects of drugs appear are: (1) in a patient at increased risk because of abnormally increased drug concentration; (2) as part of a drug-induced generalized immunologic disorder; (3) with delayed re-

Table 21.2.
Drugs That Cause Neuromuscular Disorders

DRUGS THAT AFFECT POSTSYNAPTIC
NEUROMUSCULAR TRANSMISSION
- Neuromuscular Blockers
  Alcuronium
  Curare
  Pancuronium
  Succinylcholine
  Vecuronium
- Anticholinesterase Agents
  Ambenonium
  Echothiophate
  Neostigmine
  Organophosphate and carbamate insecticides
  Physostigmine
  Pyridostigmine
- D-Penicillamine
- Phenothiazines
  Chlorpromazine
  Promazine
- Trimethaphan

DRUGS THAT AFFECT BOTH PRE- AND POSTSYNAPTIC
NEUROMUSCULAR TRANSMISSION
- Corticosteroids
- Antiarrhythmic Drugs
  Procainamide
  Quinidine
- Antibiotics
  Aminoglycosides
  Monobasic amino acid antibiotics (lincomycin, clindamycin)
  Tetracyclines
  Polymyxin drugs
- Anticonvulsants
  Mephenytoin
  Phenytoin
  Trimethadione
- β-Adrenergic Blocking Drugs
  Oxyprenolol
  Practolol
  Propranolol
  Timolol
- Chloroquine
- Cisplatin (*cis*-diamminedichloroplatinum)
- Lithium
- Magnesium

covery of strength following general anesthesia during which neuromuscular blocking agents may have been used; and (4) unmasking or worsening of myasthenia gravis or the myasthenic syndrome (Table 21.2). Drug-induced disturbances of neuromuscular transmission usually resemble naturally occurring myasthenia gravis, causing prominent ptosis and ophthalmoparesis as well as variable degrees of facial, bulbar, and extremity muscle weakness. Respiratory difficulties may occur early and are often severe. Treatment consists of discontinuing the offending agent and reversing the block with various agents, including calcium gluconate, potassium, and anticholinesterases.

Certain commonly used drugs produce neuromuscular transmission disturbances in patients through actions that are restricted to postsynaptic mechanisms (see Table 21.2). Such drugs can "unmask" subclinical myasthenia gravis. It is rare for such drug effects to be important clinically in patients with normal neuromuscular transmission. Antibiotics, antihypertensives, and neuromuscular blockers in particular are cited based on experimental electrophysiologic data; at times, such drugs are listed as "contraindicated" in myasthenia gravis. This made more

sense in an era before widespread availability of sophisticated respiratory monitoring and intensive care units. Several common drugs implicated as peripherally acting neuromuscular blockers, such as phenytoin, calcium channel blockers, and propranolol, can be used perfectly safely in vivo.

In antibiotic usage, a nonblocking agent should always be chosen if possible, but an effective aminoglycoside should never be routinely avoided in favor of a cephalosporin, for example, if the antibiotic sensitivities do not support that decision. In a severe infection, or when a myasthenic patient is already on a ventilator, the indicated antibiotic should be used despite its potential effects on neuromuscular transmission.

A variety of drugs act at both pre- and postsynaptic sites of the neuromuscular junction to disturb transmission in humans (see Table 21.2). These drugs fall into several classes, including steroids, antiarrhythmic drugs, antibiotics, anticonvulsants, and β-adrenergic blockers.

FOR MORE INFORMATION:
See Walsh & Hoyt's *Clinical Neuro-Ophthalmology,* 5th edition, Volume 1, Chapter 30, pp. 1406–1444.

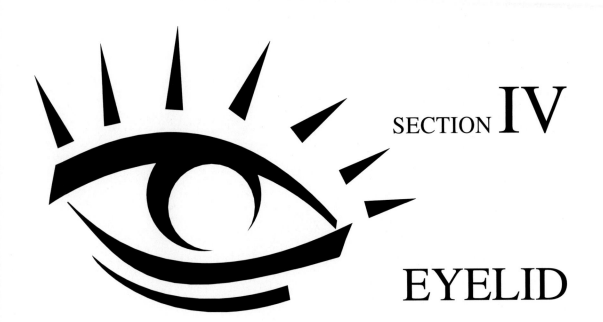

SECTION IV

EYELID

CHAPTER 22

Abnormal Eyelid Position and Movement

ABNORMALITIES OF EYELID OPENING	ABNORMALITIES OF EYELID CLOSURE
Insufficient Opening of the Eyelid: Ptosis	Insufficiency of Eyelid Closure
Inappropriate Elevation of the Upper Eyelid: Eyelid Retraction	Excessive or Anomalous Eyelid Closure: Hyperactivity of the Orbicularis Oculi Muscle

Detailed observation of eyelid position and movement is an important, but often neglected part of the neuro-ophthalmologic examination. In evaluating the eyelids, one should note the resting position of the upper and lower eyelids, evaluate the ability of the upper eyelid to open, and evaluate the various aspects of eyelid opening and closing, including voluntary, reflex, and spontaneous blinking, as well as the lid movements accompanying eye movements (Figs. 22.1 and 22.2).

All lid movements result from the interaction of four simple forces (Fig. 22.3):

1. An active closing force produced by the orbicularis oculi.
2. An active opening force generated by the levator palpebrae superioris.
3. An active opening force generated by a smooth muscle, Müller's muscle (also called the superior tarsal muscle).
4. Passive lid-closing forces produced by stretching of ligaments and tendons of the eyelid.

With an understanding of these forces, it is possible to determine which element(s) of the lid system any disorder affects. For example, blinks result from a cessation of the tonically active levator palpebrae followed by a transient burst of the normally quiescent orbicularis oculi. The active orbicularis oculi force combined with passive lid closing forces rapidly lower the lid. When the orbicularis oculi activity terminates, the tonic levator palpebrae activity resumes. This action slowly raises the eyelid until the passive closing forces match the active opening forces generated by the levator palpebrae. Moving the lid in conjunction with vertical eye movements only involves changes in the activity of the levator palpebrae muscle. The levator palpebrae receives an eye movement input qualitatively identical with that of its developmental progenitor, the superior rectus. As the eye elevates, the tonic activity on the levator palpebrae increases and raises the eyelid. With decreases in levator palpebrae activity, the passive downward forces pull the lid down until the passive closing and active opening forces again match.

ABNORMALITIES OF EYELID OPENING

INSUFFICIENT OPENING OF THE EYELID: PTOSIS

A deficiency of levator tonus produces the clinical sign called blepharoptosis or **ptosis.** Ptosis may be produced by damage to the motor system controlling eyelid elevation and position at any level of the pathway, from the cerebral cortex to the levator muscle itself. Topical diagnosis of ptosis depends upon the character of the deficiency and upon evidence of neuropathic, neuromuscular, aponeurotic, developmental, mechanical, or myopathic disease.

The degree of ptosis can be quantified clinically by measuring the vertical length of the

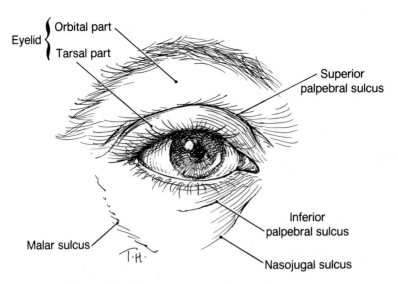

Figure 22.1. Superficial anatomy of the orbit and eyelids.

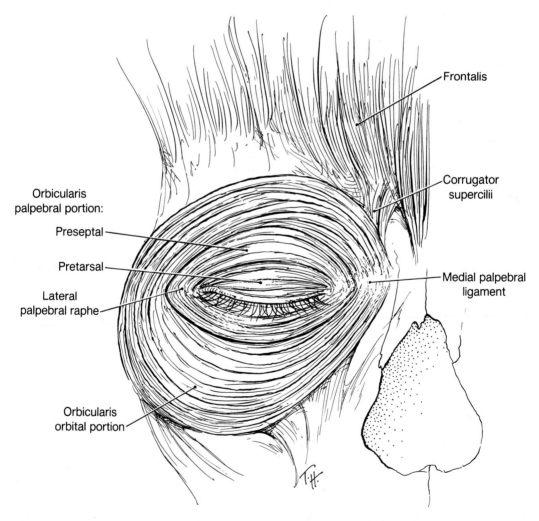

Figure 22.2. Anatomy of the orbicularis oculi muscle and associated muscles.

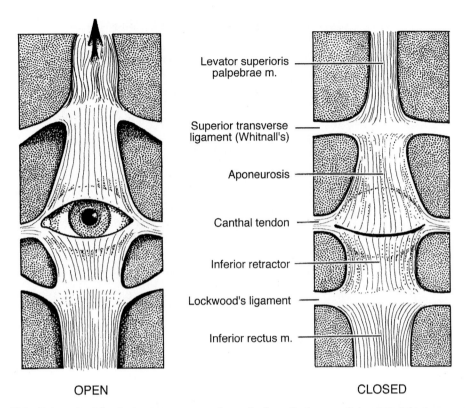

Levator superioris
palpebrae m.

Superior transverse
ligament (Whitnall's)

Aponeurosis

Canthal tendon

Inferior retractor

Lockwood's ligament

Inferior rectus m.

OPEN   CLOSED

Figure 22.3. Schematic of the elastic structures responsible for the passive forces acting on the upper and lower eyelid. Elevating the lid to the open position or in upward gaze, increases the tension along the orbicularis oculi (not shown), Whitnall's ligament, the canthal-tarsal complex, and Lockwood's ligament. Relaxation of the levator palpebrae releases this stored elastic energy causing the eyelid to close or descend on downgaze. (Reprinted with permission from Sibony PA, Manning KA, Evinger C. Eyelid movements in facial paralysis. Arch Ophthalmol 1991;109:1555–1561.)

palpebral fissure (about 9 mm in normal subjects) assuming the lower eyelid is normally positioned. A more useful measure is the distance between the upper lid margin and the midcorneal reflex when the globe is in primary position. This is called the **uMRD.** Ptosis can be defined as an uMRD less than 2 mm or an asymmetry of more than 2 mm between eyes. Using this definition, most patients with ptosis exhibit a contraction of the superior visual field to 30° or less.

Equally important is an assessment of levator function measured by determining the excursion of the upper eyelid from extreme downgaze to extreme upgaze while immobilizing the frontalis muscle. From 12 to 17 mm of upper lid movement is considered a normal levator excursion. Levator function is reduced in patients with neurogenic, developmental, and myopathic processes, whereas patients with acquired aponeurotic defects usually have relatively normal levator excursions.

Neurogenic Ptosis
Ptosis from Supranuclear Deficiency of Levator Innervation

Most cases of neuropathic ptosis are caused by lesions of the oculomotor nucleus or nerve or of the oculosympathetic pathway; however, both unilateral or bilateral **cortical ptosis** can be caused by damage to various disparate regions of the cerebral hemisphere, including the temporal lobe, the temporo-occipital region, the angular gyrus, and the frontal lobe. The precise anatomic pathways responsible for this type of ptosis are uncertain.

Unilateral cortical ptosis is a rare manifestation of hemisphere dysfunction. It is usually, al-

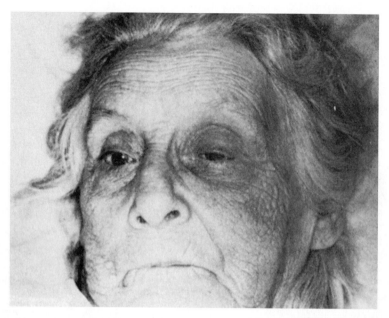

Figure 22.4. Unilateral supranuclear ptosis. This patient developed a left hemiparesis after a hemispheral cerebrovascular accident. Note the acquired left ptosis that occurred at the same time. (Reprinted with permission from Caplan LR. Ptosis. J Neurol Neurosurg Psychiatry 1974;37:1–7.)

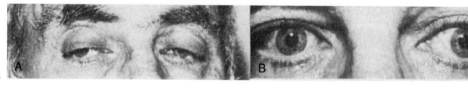

A   B

Figure 22.5. Bilateral supranuclear ptosis with recovery. *A.* The patient has bilateral severe ptosis. Computed axial tomography revealed evidence of bilateral frontal lobe infarctions. *B.* Two months later, the patient's ptosis has completely resolved. (Reprinted with permission from Krohel GB, Griffin JF. Cortical blepharoptosis. Am J Ophthalmol 1978;85:632–634.)

though not invariably, contralateral to the lesion. Unilateral ptosis can occur contralateral to lesions of the angular gyrus, contralateral to temporal lobe seizure foci, contralateral to a frontal lobe arteriovenous malformation (AVM), and contralateral more often than ipsilateral to ischemic damage to hemispheric structures (Fig. 22.4).

Bilateral cortical ptosis is associated most frequently with extensive nondominant hemisphere lesions. In most instances, the ptosis is accompanied by midline shift, gaze deviation to the right, and other signs of right hemisphere dysfunction. The ptosis is often asymmetric, perhaps because of an associated ipsilateral facial weakness or possibly asymmetric supranuclear input. In the setting of cerebral infarction, the ptosis is transient, lasting from several days to 5 months or more (Fig. 22.5). On rare occasions, it is accompanied by other supranuclear eyelid disturbances, such as blepharospasm or involuntary levator inhibition. The association of cerebral ptosis and reflex blepharospasm with nondominant hemisphere lesions suggests a cortical asymmetry in the control of eyelid position.

The extrapyramidal system primarily affects the eyelids by modifying the excitability of the blink reflex, although it may modulate eyelid position to a limited extent. In one series, for example, 10 of 70 patients with Parkinson's disease had ptosis. A more common extrapyramidal insufficiency of eyelid opening is **apraxia of eyelid opening** (AEO). Because most patients with AEO have motor system dysfunction involving the extrapyramidal or pyramidal systems, this finding is not, by definition, an apraxia. Consequently, alternative terms are often used for this condition, including "akinesia of lid function," "blepharocolysis," "eyelid freezing," "focal eyelid dystonia," and "supranuclear involuntary levator palpebrae inhibition." The main clinical features of AEO are: (1) a transient inability to initiate lid opening; (2) the absence of any significant evidence of orbicularis oculi contraction, such as lowering of the brow beneath the orbital rim (Charcot's sign); (3) frontalis contraction during attempts to open the eyelids; and (4) the absence of any other signs of neural or myopathic dysfunction. AEO most commonly occurs in patients with progressive supranuclear palsy, Parkinson's disease, atypical parkinsonism including that induced by methyl-phenyl-tetrahydropyridine (MPTP) and, less commonly, in patients with essential blepharospasm, Shy-Drager syndrome, adult-onset Hallervorden-Spatz disease, Huntington's chorea, cerebral diplegia with parkinsonism, frontotemporal gunshot injury, right hemisphere stroke, Wilson's disease, and amyotrophic lateral sclerosis/parkinsonism-dementia complex. In rare instances, AEO occurs as an isolated finding.

Electromyographic (EMG) studies show that patients with AEO can be separated into several groups related to the activity of their levator and orbicularis oculi muscles. The first group consists of patients who exhibit intermittent variable periods of levator inhibition without any orbicularis oculi activity. Such patients may occasionally experience typical episodes of blepharospasm. The second group consists of patients with a variant of blepharospasm in which involuntary contractions are limited to the pretarsal segment of the orbicularis oculi. The third group have "motor persistence" of the pretarsal orbicularis oculi—an inability to inhibit pretarsal orbicularis contractions after voluntary eyelid closure. Because it may be impossible to distinguish "involuntary levator inhibition" from pretarsal blepharospasm without an EMG, it is more accurate to describe such patients using a less specific term, such as "involuntary eyelid closure."

Treatment of involuntary eyelid closure caused by supranuclear inhibition of levator activity is not particularly successful. Individual case reports suggest that several drugs may be useful, including desipramine and L-dopa. Injection of the orbicularis oculi and frontalis muscles with botulinum toxin type A produces variable results, depending on the degree of orbicularis contraction that accompanies the levator inhibition.

Ptosis from Paradoxic Supranuclear Inhibition of Levator Tonus

Ptosis may be a component of a variety of oculopalpebral synkinesias, although lid position in primary gaze may be normal in some of these cases. The causes of paradoxic levator inhibition (and excitation) are obscure and may involve a variety of mechanisms, including misdirection of regenerating peripheral nerve fibers, ephaptic transmission, and disturbances in the supranuclear pathways responsible for levator tonus, excitation, and inhibition.

In cases of **paradoxic levator inhibition,** eyelid posture may be normal or slightly ptotic when the patient is staring straight ahead. As the patient adducts the eye on the affected side, the eyelid drops abruptly because of a loss of levator muscle tone. On abduction, the levator contracts, and the eyelid returns to a normal posture. The synkinesia may be unilateral (Fig. 22.6) or bilat-

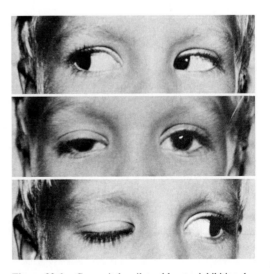

Figure 22.6.   Congenital, unilateral levator inhibition during left horizontal gaze. (Courtesy of Dr. C. Hedges.)

eral (Fig. 22.7). It may occur as an isolated inner-vational anomaly or in association with other congenital anomalies of the extraocular muscles, such as Duane's retraction syndrome, esotropia, or underaction of the superior rectus. The inverse of this pattern—ptosis on abduction—also occurs.

Ptosis associated with mouth opening (the inverse Marcus Gunn phenomenon) is a rare condition in which the ipsilateral eyelid closes when the external pterygoid muscle moves the jaw to the opposite side (Fig. 22.8). Patients with this condition have a mild degree of ptosis of the affected eyelid when the eyes are in primary position and the mouth is closed. EMG studies confirm that the associated ptosis is consequent to levator inhibition without contraction of the orbicularis oculi. This syndrome is an inverse of the Marcus Gunn jaw-winking phenomenon (see below) and represents a synkinesis between the oculomotor and trigeminal nerves.

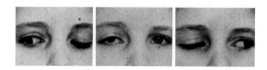

Figure 22.7. Congenital right ptosis with levator inhibition in left gaze and levator excitation in right gaze. Alternating lateral movements of the eyes produced the unusual appearance of seesaw lid movements. (Courtesy of Dr. H. Rose.)

Ptosis from Lesions of the Oculomotor Nucleus, Fascicle, or Nerve

Ptosis originating from a nuclear midbrain lesion is invariably bilateral and symmetric, usually complete, and commonly associated with other signs of mesencephalic dysfunction. In some cases, ptosis is the predominant manifestation, or it occurs as an isolated finding (Fig. 22.9). Rarely, mesencephalic ptosis is associated with a Cogan's lid twitch and fatigue, thus mimicking ocular myasthenia gravis. Midbrain ptosis also may be congenital, occurring as a consequence of dysplasia or aplasia of the oculomotor nucleus or nerve. Acquired causes include ischemia, inflammation, infiltration, compression, and metabolic and toxic processes.

Fascicular lesions of the oculomotor nerve present with partial or complete signs of oculomotor nerve dysfunction, often associated with a contralateral hemiplegia, cerebellar ataxia, or rubral tremor. In some cases, the associated signs of midbrain dysfunction are minimal and consist of nothing more than an oculomotor nerve palsy and an abnormal masseter reflex. Ptosis in patients with fascicular lesions is unilateral, of variable severity, and associated with weakness of one or more of the extraocular muscles innervated by the oculomotor nerve. Pupillary involvement is commonly but not invariably present.

The ptosis that accompanies a peripheral lesion of the oculomotor nerve is usually unilat-

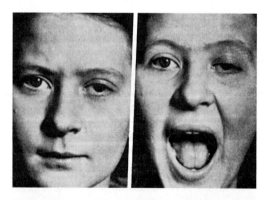

Figure 22.8. Inverse Marcus Gunn phenomenon. *Left:* There is mild left ptosis with the eyes directed straight ahead. *Right:* Inhibition of the left levator muscle occurs with opening of the mouth.

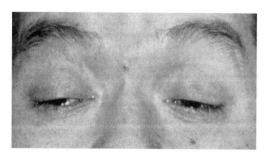

Figure 22.9. Isolated, bilateral ptosis in a patient with brainstem encephalitis and discrete inflammatory foci in the caudal mesencephalon. Ocular motility was normal. (Reprinted with permission from Conway VH, Rozdilsky B, Schneider RJ, et al. Isolated bilateral complete ptosis. Can J Ophthalmol 1983;18:37–40.)

eral and almost invariably accompanied by ophthalmoparesis or pupillary involvement. Rarely, however, ptosis precedes the other signs of oculomotor nerve dysfunction or occurs in isolation. ''Isolated'' ptosis caused by oculomotor nerve dysfunction can occur in patients with aneurysms, pituitary adenomas, meningiomas, and meningitis. Some of these cases are examples of truly isolated ptosis. In others, there are other symptoms, such as headache, or subtle signs of oculomotor dysfunction, such as a mildly dilated but reactive pupil, an incomitant phoria, or asymptomatic underaction of the superior rectus that is only evident on extreme upgaze.

Ptosis from Lesions of the Oculosympathetic Pathways

Lesions of the oculosympathetic pathway produce Horner's syndrome, a condition that is characterized in part by a partial, unilateral ptosis that usually can be differentiated from ptosis associated with oculomotor nerve dysfunction (see Chapter 15). The ptosis in Horner's syndrome is usually mild, variable, and associated with ipsilateral miosis. Involvement of smooth muscle located below the inferior tarsus results in ''upside-down'' ptosis of the lower eyelid. Other signs of Horner's syndrome include ipsilateral facial anhidrosis (in patients with first-order or second-order neuron lesions), ocular hypotony, heterochromia (in congenital and long-standing cases) and increased accommodative amplitude (Fig. 22.10). The ptosis occasionally observed after conjunctival instillation of timolol maleate, a β-adrenergic blocking agent, may be caused by Müller's muscle blockade. Similarly, both systemic and topical thymoxamine (an α-adrenergic blocking agent) may cause ptosis.

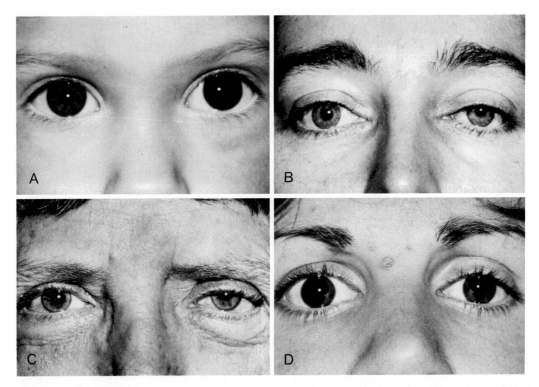

Figure 22.10.   Horner's syndrome in four patients. Note marked variability in ptosis. *A.* Congenital right Horner's syndrome. Note associated heterochromia iridis. *B.* Left Horner's syndrome after neck trauma. *C.* Left Horner's syndrome associated with apical lung (Pancoast) tumor. *D.* Left Horner's syndrome in a patient with Raeder's paratrigeminal neuralgia.

Ptosis from Defects of the Levator Aponeurosis

The most common cause of acquired ptosis in adults is a defect in the levator aponeurosis. The ptosis may be bilateral or unilateral and can vary in its severity. In the early stages, the ptosis may be barely evident in primary position, but because it typically worsens in downgaze, the eyelid may obstruct the visual axis when reading. The coincidental occurrence of anisocoria or strabismus, or the frequent worsening of symptoms at the end of the day, may lead to the erroneous diagnosis of oculomotor nerve palsy or myasthenia gravis. Nevertheless, the findings of normal levator excursion, an elevated or absent superior lid crease, a deep superior eyelid sulcus, worsening of ptosis in downgaze, and thinning of the skin above the tarsal plate should distinguish an aponeurotic ptosis from developmental, neurogenic, and myogenic causes (Fig. 22.11).

Levator aponeurotic defects commonly occur in the elderly from involutional or degenerative changes that result in dehiscence, disinsertion, or thinning of the aponeurosis. Among patients between ages 15 and 50, aponeurotic ptosis is most commonly associated with a long history of wearing rigid contact lenses. Repeated manipulation and traction of the upper eyelid while inserting or removing contact lenses may cause disinsertion of the levator aponeurosis.

A variety of mechanisms may lead to ptosis following eyelid trauma or eyelid surgery. Ptosis not infrequently occurs after cataract extraction, glaucoma surgery, radial keratotomy, orbital surgery, conjunctival procedures, enucleations, strabismus surgery, and blepharoplasty. In the case of orbital surgery or blepharoplasty in which there is deep orbital fat dissection or supratarsal fixation, it is likely that there is direct injury to the levator aponeurosis. The aponeurosis may be stretched or damaged from postoperative swelling, injection of an anesthetic into the upper eyelid, the use of a rigid lid speculum, ocular compression and massage, or attempts to open the eyelid against a tight patch. The myotoxic effects of anesthetic injections and trauma to the levator palpebrae superioris itself from bridle sutures or retrobulbar injections may also play a role.

Aponeurotic defects of the eyelid may be associated with blepharochalasis, thyroid orbitopathy, pregnancy, and chronic use of topical steroids. Aponeurotic defects may also occur after repeated eyelid trauma or after episodes of eyelid edema caused by allergic reactions. In rare cases, congenital ptosis is caused by defects of the levator aponeurosis.

Myopathic Ptosis

Ptosis that occurs from involvement of the levator palpebrae superioris muscle may be congenital (developmental) or acquired.

Congenital Myopathic Ptosis (Developmental Ptosis)

Although congenital ptosis is occasionally neurogenic (e.g., oculomotor nerve palsy, Mar-

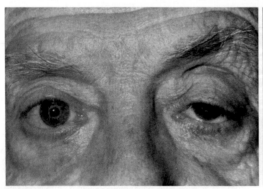 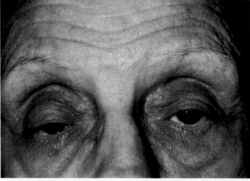

Figure 22.11. Ptosis from levator dehiscence. *Left:* Unilateral ptosis. Note the difference in location of the superior lid folds, with the left fold being much higher than the right. Also note the deepened superior sulcus on the left side.

Right: Bilateral ptosis from levator dehiscence. Both eyelids show high superior lid folds and deep superior sulci. (Courtesey of Dr. N.T. Iliff.)

cus Gunn jaw-winking phenomenon, Horner's syndrome) or traumatic (e.g., from a forceps delivery) in origin, the most common form is caused by a developmental myopathy of the levator palpebrae superioris muscle. A decrease

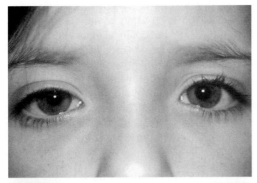

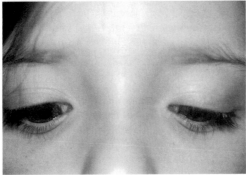

Figure 22.12.   Developmental ptosis showing mild lid lag in downgaze.

in striated muscle fibers, hyaline degeneration, fatty replacement, an increase in endomysial collagen, and loss of cross-striations characterize this disorder histopathologically. Because developmental ptosis may worsen with age, it may not be noticed until early infancy or even later in life. Childhood photographs are sometimes helpful in establishing onset. About 15% of the patients have a family history of congenital ptosis.

Developmental ptosis is characterized by a deficiency in levator excursion, an elevated or absent superior lid crease and, most importantly, lid-lag on downgaze (Fig. 22.12). The majority of cases are unilateral, but about 20% are bilateral. In severe cases, patients may exhibit a compensatory chin elevation or frontalis contraction.

Developmental ptosis may exist in isolation, or it may be associated with other ocular findings, including strabismic or occlusion (deprivation) amblyopia, astigmatism, and anisometropia. Because the levator derives embryologically from the same anlage as the superior rectus, it is not surprising that underaction of the superior rectus frequently accompanies developmental ptosis (Fig. 22.13).

Developmental ptosis may be associated with a variety of congenital ocular or systemic malformations. In some cases, the association is distinctive enough to constitute a well-defined syndrome, such as the blepharophimosis-epicanthus-ptosis syndrome, congenital fibrosis syndrome, or Goldenhar's syndrome. In other cases, developmental ptosis occurs in association with

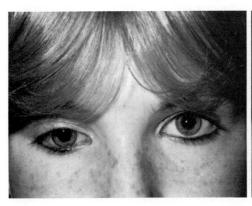

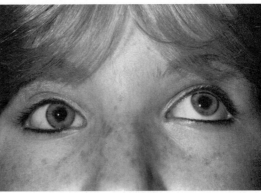

Figure 22.13.   Unilateral congenital ptosis with ipsilateral hypotropia and limitation of upward gaze. *Left:* In primary position, the patient has a moderate right ptosis and there is a slight right hypotropia. *Right:* On attempted upward gaze, the patient cannot elevate the right eye normally. (Courtesy of Dr. N.T. Iliff.)

less clearly defined entities, including anomalies of the brain, heart, urogenital, skeletal, or auditory systems.

Acquired Myopathic Ptosis

Ptosis occurs in a number of the mitochondrial cytopathies characterized by chronic progressive external ophthalmoplegia (CPEO) (see Chapter 20). In some patients, the ptosis is the presenting sign and may persist in isolation for months to years before the development of ophthalmoplegia. Ptosis of this type is usually bilateral, relatively symmetric, and very slowly progressive. Excessive wrinkling of the brow and backward head tilting are commonly employed to facilitate vision beneath the drooping lids. Orbicularis oculi function tested by forced lid closure is frequently weak. The superior palpebral lid fold may be completely absent. These patients are remarkably tolerant of their symptoms and thus generally present relatively late in the course. Bilateral partial ptosis contributes to the characteristic facies of patients with myotonic dystrophy (myotonia dystrophica) and may also occur in the various types of familial periodic paralysis.

The levator palpebrae superioris muscle may be damaged by a variety of inflammatory, ischemic, or infiltrative processes affecting the orbit. Occasionally, ptosis is the most prominent manifestation. Lymphoid infiltration, sarcoidosis, amyloidosis, and idiopathic inflammatory disease of the orbit can sometimes selectively affect the levator and spare the extraocular muscles. Patients with diabetes mellitus may develop unilateral or bilateral ptosis in association with other evidence of microangiopathic changes elsewhere in the body. Although most of these patients probably have a localized infarction in the midbrain that affects either the oculomotor nerve nucleus or fascicle, chronic hypoxia of the levator palpebrae superioris is responsible for this form of ptosis in some.

Neuromuscular Ptosis

Recognition of this type of ptosis depends in part on the absence of clinical signs of an oculomotor or sympathetic lesion and the presence of clinical signs of neuromuscular disease. Ptosis in myasthenia gravis may occur in isolation, but it is more often associated with diplopia, varying degrees of external ophthalmoplegia, and weakness of the orbicularis oculi (see Chapter 21).

Ultimately, ptosis occurs in the majority of patients with myasthenia gravis. Regardless of when it develops, the ptosis of myasthenia gravis may be unilateral or bilateral; when it is bilateral, it may be symmetric or asymmetric.

The hallmark of myasthenic ptosis is its fatigability and tendency to fluctuate in severity, although this feature is by no means pathognomonic. A similar tendency to fatigue (but not to the same degree) occurs in patients with aponeurotic defects and oculomotor nerve palsies. Patients with ptosis from myasthenia gravis, myasthenic syndromes, botulism, or drugs affecting neuromuscular transmission usually have sufficient signs and symptoms to allow the correct diagnosis to be made. Ptosis as a side effect of botulinum toxin type A therapy is discussed below.

Mechanical Ptosis

Any process that increases the weight of the eyelid or mechanically interferes with the normal excursion of the eyelid can result in ptosis. The most common causes are neoplastic infiltration or mass effect on the eyelid (e.g., neurofibroma, capillary hemangioma, metastatic lesions, basal cell carcinoma, lymphoid lesions) and edema (e.g., blepharochalasis, inflammatory disease of the lid and orbit, giant papillary conjunctivitis, after trauma). Isolated eyelid swelling can sometimes be the presenting feature of an orbital tumor or thyroid orbitopathy. Cicatricial changes from trauma and diseases such as trachoma, erythema multiforme, and pemphigoid may result in an adhesive or restrictive type of ptosis. Entrapment (e.g., from orbital roof fracture) or encroachment (e.g., from bony fragments, intraorbital foreign bodies, subperiosteal and intraorbital hematomas, mass lesions) of the levator palpebrae superioris can also mechanically interfere with the movement and position of the eyelid.

Pseudoptosis

Pseudoptosis is an apparent ptosis unrelated to defects in the neural, neuromuscular, or myopathic components of eyelid elevation. Pseudoptosis may be present on the side of an eye that is abnormal in size, shape, or position; e.g., in patients with anophthalmos, phthisis bulbi, microphthalmos, or enophthalmos. Conversely, patients who present with isolated unilateral lid retraction and proptosis from thyroid orbitopathy are sometimes mistakenly thought to have ptosis on the normal side. In some persons, excessively loose skin (dermatochalasis) or prolapsed orbital fat (blepharochalasis) causes the skin of the upper eyelid to overhang the lid margin, simulating ptosis (Fig. 22.14).

Pseudoptosis often occurs on the side opposite a fixating hypertropic eye. In patients with this

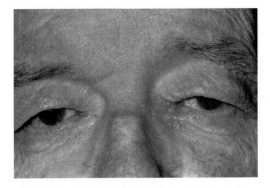

Figure 22.14. Pseudoptosis from dermachalasis in an elderly man. Note folds of skin from the superior eyelids that obscure the upper half of both corneas. (Courtesy of Dr. N.T. Iliff.)

disorder, the eyelids maintain the appropriate relationship with the eyes. When the hypertropic eye is covered, and the patient fixes with the previously hypotropic eye, the "ptosis" disappears (Fig. 22.15).

Pseudoptosis may occur in patients with downgaze paralysis. When such patients attempt to look downward, their eyes remain in the primary position, but their eyelids lower normally (Fig. 22.16).

Narrowing of the lid fissure from hemifacial contracture, hemifacial spasm, blepharospasm, or a previous facial nerve palsy may mimic ptosis (see below). In such patients, the presence of other evidence of abnormal facial movement usually permits the correct diagnosis.

Patients with nonorganic overactivity of the orbicularis oculi usually show mild or pronounced wrinkling of the eyelids proportional to the amount of narrowing of the fissure and depression of the brow (although occasionally the brow is elevated). Indicative of levator tone, the upper eyelid crease is present in primary gaze and may deepen in upgaze. In addition, one can often see—and always feel—fine tremors of the affected eyelid as the patient attempts to

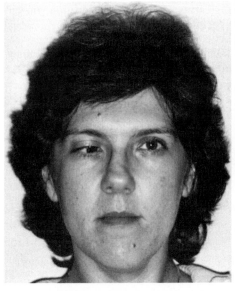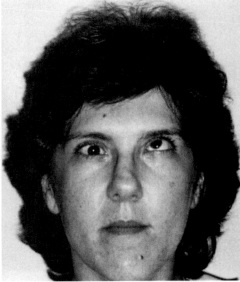

Figure 22.15. Unilateral pseudoptosis from vertical strabismus. *Left:* The patient has a marked right hypotropia and is fixating with the left eye. The right upper lid appears ptotic, but in fact the lid is in a position appropriate to the position of the eye. *Right:* When the patient fixates with her right eye, the "ptosis" disappears because the right eye is now in normal position. (Courtesy of J.E. Morris, C.O.)

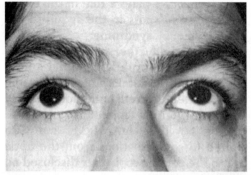

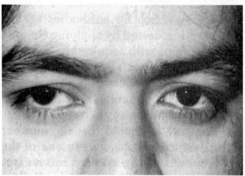

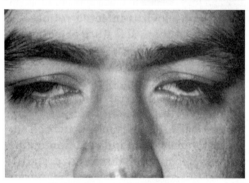

Figure 22.16. Bilateral pseudoptosis from bilateral down-gaze paralysis. On attempted downgaze, the patient's eyes remain looking straight ahead while the eyelids lower normally, resulting in pseudoptosis. *Top:* Upward gaze. *Middle:* Primary gaze. *Bottom:* Attempted downward gaze. (Reprinted with permission from LoBue TD, Feldon SE. Reverse Collier's sign: pseudoblepharoptosis associated with downgaze paralysis. Am J Ophthalmol 1983;95:120–121.)

maintain the ''ptotic'' lid position. Patients with organic ptosis do not show a delay in returning to their baseline lid position after manual elevation of the eyelid. In contrast, patients with nonorganic ptosis may sometimes exhibit a slight lag before the orbicularis oculi is factitiously

reactivated. Nonorganic ptosis may be unilateral or bilateral. It may occur in isolation or in association with other somatic complaints.

Treatment of Ptosis

Procedures used to treat ptosis include superior tarsectomy, repair or shortening of the levator aponeurosis and/or muscle, Müller's muscle resection, and slinging the eyelid to the frontalis muscle. The treatment for any individual patient depends on the etiology of the ptosis, the amount of levator function, and the preference of the surgeon.

INAPPROPRIATE ELEVATION OF THE UPPER EYELID: EYELID RETRACTION

Inappropriate and excessive elevation of the eyelids—**eyelid retraction**—makes a patient appear to be staring and also produces an illusion of exophthalmos. Mild degrees of lid retraction are frequently difficult to evaluate. The resting position of the upper lid is influenced by many factors, including age, alertness, and direction of gaze. Normal variations in resting lid position, or upper lid posture, are exemplified by the striking difference between infants and adults. The infant's eyelid, which barely touches the upper corneal limbus, may appear normal, whereas a similar lid position in an adult is abnormal and represents excessive lid elevation. In general, upper lid position is abnormal if it exposes sclera between the lid margin and the upper corneal limbus when the patient's head is straight and both of the patient's eyes are directed straight ahead.

Eyelid retraction may be unilateral or bilateral. It may result from inappropriate excitation or hyperactivity of levator neurons, the levator palpebrae superioris, or Müller's muscle, and also from disorders that produce shortening or contracture of the levator muscle or tendon. Thus, as with ptosis, causes of eyelid retraction may be classified as neuropathic, neuromuscular, myopathic, and mechanical.

Neuropathic Eyelid Retraction and Lid Lag

Eyelid Retraction from Supranuclear Lesions

Although true retraction of the eyelids does not usually occur from cerebral hemisphere damage, intermittent or prolonged inappropriate eyelid opening sometimes develops in patients with unilateral nondominant or bilateral cerebral hemisphere disease. Such patients may be unable to close their eyelids on command (i.e., compulsive eye opening), or they may close their eyes only briefly before opening them again (i.e., motor impersistence). These patients have a supranuclear disturbance of orbicularis control and have normal levator relaxation.

Supranuclear bilateral eyelid retraction or **Collier's sign** most commonly occurs with lesions of the dorsal mesencephalon. This type of lid retraction is almost invariably associated with other evidence of dorsal mesencephalic dysfunction, most often a deficiency of upward gaze but also convergence-retraction nystagmus and pupillary light-near dissociation. This condition, called Parinaud's syndrome, is discussed in Chapter 18 of this text. It suffices here to emphasize that the eyelid retraction that occurs with lesions of the dorsal mesencephalon is usually symmetric and sustained as long as the patient directs the eyes straight ahead or slightly upward (Fig. 22.17). On downward gaze, the lids follow the eyes in a normal fashion, which distinguishes this form of lid retraction from that seen in thyroid orbitopathy (see below), in which lid lag is invariably present in patients with lid retraction. In Parinaud's syndrome, the disparity between the position of the upper lids and the eyes increases as the patient looks up.

The nucleus of the posterior commissure (nPC) appears to be the premotor structure responsible for mesencephalic lid retraction (Fig. 22.18). Lesions that damage this structure generally produce bilateral lid retraction; however, they may also damage the oculomotor nerve fascicle on one side, producing a ptosis on the side of the fascicular damage. This results in a condition characterized by ptosis on one side and primary eyelid retraction (i.e., not secondary to the contralateral ptosis) on the other. This condition is called the "plus-minus syndrome" (Fig. 22.19). Imaging studies in patients with this syndrome show unilateral paramedian lesions, usually infarctions, dorsal and rostral to the red nucleus in the area of the nPC, extending ventrocaudally to the fascicle of the oculomotor nerve on the ptotic side. Thus, damage to the nPC apparently causes bilateral supranuclear lid retraction that may be masked on one side by an associated fascicular oculomotor nerve palsy.

Sustained eyelid retraction may be observed with any of the disorders known to produce a dorsal mesencephalic syndrome. In a series of 206 patients with this condition, 40% of whom had lid retraction, the most common causes were hydrocephalus (39%), stroke (26%), and tumor (22%). The remaining cases included infection (encephalitis, abscess), tentorial herniation, trauma, AVMs, congenital, Wernicke's syndrome, and Bassen-Kornzweig syndrome. Other causes of the dorsal mesencephalic syndrome are multiple sclerosis (MS) and shunt malfunction (Fig. 22.20).

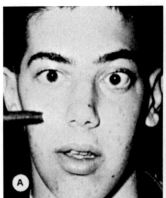 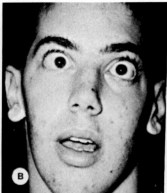 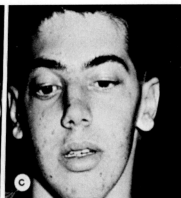

Figure 22.17.   Collier's sign: eyelid retraction with a lesion of the dorsal mesencephalon. *A.* The patient has mild bilateral eyelid retraction when looking straight ahead. *B.* On attempted upward gaze, the eyes do not elevate, but the eye lids elevate normally, producing marked eyelid retraction and stare. *C.* On attempted downward gaze, the eyelids move normally with the eyes, and the eyelid retraction and stare disappear.

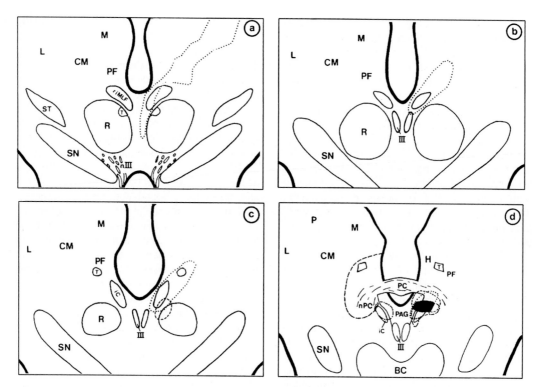

Figure 22.18. Lesion zones in four human cases with midbrain lid retraction and vertical gaze paralysis. *A–D:* Rostral to caudal, 2 mm cuts. The shaded area represents the area common to all four cases localizing to the nucleus of the posterior commissure (nPC). Key: ●●●● (Source: Pierrot-Deseilligny C, Chain F, Gray F, Serdaru M, Escourolle R, Lhermitte F. Parinaud's syndrome. Brain 1982;105: 667–696. Case 3.); - - - - (Source: Hatcher MA, Klintworth GK. The sylvian aqueduct syndrome: a clinicopathologic study. Arch Neurol 1966;15:215–222.); – – – – (Source: Collier J. Nuclear ophthalmoplegia, with especial reference to retraction of the lids and ptosis and to lesions of the posterior commissure. Brain 1927;50;488–498.); ● - ● - ● (Source: Andre-Thomas H, Schaeffer H, Bertrand I. Paralysie de l'abaissement du regard paralysie des inferogyres hypertonic des supergyres et des releveurs des paupières. Rev Neurol 1933;2:535–542.) *BC,* brachium conjunctivum; *CM,* nucleus centralis medialis thalami; *IC,* interstitial nucleus of Cajal; *H,* habenular nuclei; *IO,* inferior olive; *L,* lateral thalamic nuclei; *M,* nucleus medialis dorsalis thalami; *MB,* mammillary body; *MLF,* medial longitudinal fasciculus; *MT,* mammillothalamic tract; *nPC,* nuclei of the posterior commissure; *nIII,* oculomotor nerve; *nVI,* abducens nerve; *PAG,* periaqueductal grey; *PC,* posterior commissure; *PF,* nucleus parafascicularis thalami; *R,* nucleus ruber; *riMLF,* rostral interstitial nucleus of the medial longitudinal fasciculus; *SC,* superior colliculus; *SN,* substantia nigra; *ST,* nucleus subthalamicus; *T,* tractus retroflexus; *III,* oculomotor nucleus; *IV,* trochlear nucleus; *VI,* abducens nucleus. (Reprinted with permission from Schmidtke K, Buttner-Ennever JA. Nervous control of eyelid function. Brain 1992;115:227–247.)

Neurodegenerative conditions that cause supranuclear disturbances in upgaze may cause lid retraction. For example, lid retraction is common among patients with progressive supranuclear palsy, Parkinson's disease, and Machado-Joseph disease (spinocerebellar ataxia type 3). In addition, some patients with severe Landry-Guillain-Barré syndrome (GBS) demonstrate marked bilateral limitation of upper lid descent during the acute phase of their illness (Fig. 22.21). This phenomenon is not explained by associated facial weakness and may be caused by supranuclear levator dysfunction.

Lid retraction and slight downward gaze of both eyes in response to a sudden decrease in ambient light is a physiologic reflex seen in infants between 1 and 5 months of age. Sometimes called the "eye popping reflex" or "nonpathologic lid retraction," it is a useful way of assess-

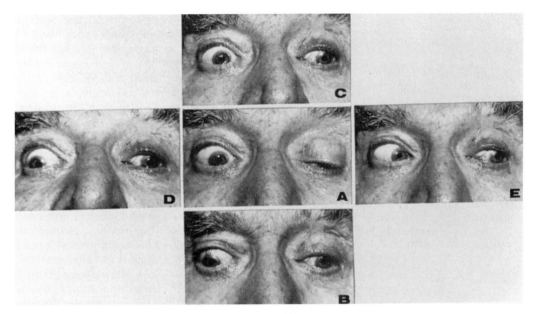

Figure 22.19. Plus-minus syndrome: left ptosis and right upper eyelid retraction. Note upward gaze paresis, left third nerve palsy and lid-lag on downgaze. CT scan showed a paramedian midbrain infarct located ventrally and laterally to the aqueduct, extending from the midline to the area of the red nucleus laterally. (Reprinted with permission from Gaymard B, Lafitte C, Gelot A, et al. Plus-minus syndrome. J Neurol Neurosurg Psychiatry 1992;55:846–848.)

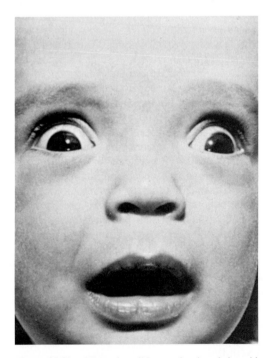

Figure 22.20. Bilateral eyelid retraction in a baby with communicating hydrocephalus. Upward following movements of the eyes were limited (the ''setting sun'' sign).

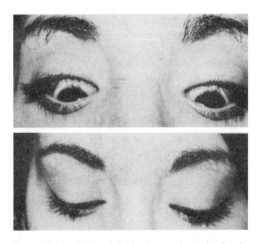

Figure 22.21. Bilateral lid-lag in a patient with Landry-Guillain-Barré syndrome. *Top:* Bilateral lid-lag on downward gaze. *Bottom:* Three months later, there is normal lid relaxation on downward gaze. (Reprinted with permission from Keane JR. Lid-lag in the Guillain-Barré syndrome. Arch Neurol 1975;32:478–479.)

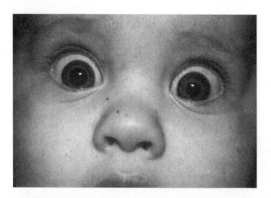

Figure 22.22. Eye popping reflex: lid retraction with a sudden decrease in ambient illumination. Anisocoria is physiologic. (Reprinted with permission from Bartley GB. The differential diagnosis and classification of eyelid retractions. Ophthalmology 1996;103:168–176.)

ing levator function in infants (Fig. 22.22). We have seen transient clonic bilateral lid retraction in several infants with spastic downward gaze deviation that resolved after several weeks. This may be a variant of the benign, transient, supranuclear disturbances of ocular motility that frequently occur in healthy neonates.

Coma and stupor are commonly associated with eyelid closure caused by an absence of levator tonus. Occasionally, however, levator tonus persists and produces the incongruous picture of intermittently open lids in an unresponsive patient (coma vigil). This sign usually indicates disease of the ventral mesencephalon and pons, but it may occur with diffuse hemisphere disease (persistent vegetative state). Comatose patients with Cheyne-Stokes respiration sometimes open their eyes during the rapid-breathing phase and close them during the slow-breathing phase. We have noted phasic lid opening that was synchronous with the inspiratory phase of respiration in comatose patients. Still another interesting reflexive opening of the eyelids may be demonstrated in some comatose patients by raising their head or turning it from side to side. Most commonly observed in infants and children, this phenomena seems analogous to the doll's head movements of the eyes. Rare comatose patients maintain constantly open, unblinking eyes caused by a failure of levator inhibition.

Some patients with extrapyramidal syndromes (postencephalitic parkinsonism, progressive supranuclear palsy, etc.) have defective inhibition

of their eyelids during downward gaze. Such patients have normal lid position when they look straight ahead; however, the lids lag behind briefly as the eyes follow an object downward. Patients with a unilateral midbrain lesion dorsal to the red nucleus may also exhibit lid lag without lid retraction. The lesion in these patients probably disrupts the pathways between the rostral interstitial nucleus of the MLF and the central caudal nucleus but spares the nPC.

Eyelid Nystagmus

Eyelid nystagmus is a rhythmic oscillation of the eyelids with a slow downward drift and a rapid upward phase that may be associated with convergence, gaze shifts, any form of vertical nystagmus, or oculopalatal myoclonus.

Convergence-evoked lid nystagmus occurs in patients with MS, cerebellar tumors invading the 4th ventricle, Miller Fisher syndrome, posttraumatic dorsal midbrain syndrome, and pontomedullary angiomas.

Gaze-evoked eyelid nystagmus is usually associated with damage to the brainstem, cerebellum, or both structures. For example, gaze-evoked eyelid and ocular nystagmus that is present only when looking at a distant, eccentrically placed object can occur in patients with the lateral medullary syndrome of Wallenberg (see Chapter 18). The nystagmus stops during a near eccentric fixation. Horizontal gaze-induced lid nystagmus can also develop in patients with intrinsic midbrain tumors, such as astrocytomas.

Upward jerking of the eyelids may occur synchronously with convergence-retraction nystagmus. This type of lid movement may be evoked when a patient with a pretectal or periaqueductal lesion (dorsal mesencephalic syndrome) attempts to make voluntary upward saccades, or as the patient watches downward-moving optokinetic stimuli. In such patients, upward gaze (particularly saccadic eye movements) is invariably defective. A similar phenomenon occurs in patients with a global paresis of gaze from Fisher's syndrome. The lid nystagmus in such cases may be precipitated by upward head rotations or downward optokinetic stimuli.

Eyelid Retraction from Paradoxic Levator Excitation

Eyelid retraction from paradoxic levator excitation may be congenital or acquired. It may

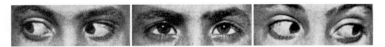

Figure 22.23. Physiologic synkinesis between normal eye movement and levator muscles. Subject with normal ocular motility shows elevation of both upper eyelids in extreme right and left horizontal gaze. (Reprinted with permission from Ticho U. Synkinesis of upper lid elevation occurring in horizontal eye movements. Acta Ophthalmol 1971;49: 232–238.)

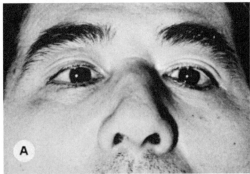

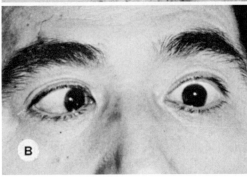

Figure 22.24. Eyelid retraction associated with left abduction paralysis. *A.* Primary position, the patient's upper eyelids are in normal and equal position. *B.* In attempted gaze left, there is elevation of the left upper lid and eyebrow.

occur from lesions of supranuclear, nuclear, or infranuclear pathways.

Elevation of the ipsilateral eyelid may be observed in normal subjects during abduction and, less commonly, on adduction (Fig. 22.23). The lid retraction on attempted abduction in patients with Duane's retraction syndrome and in patients with acquired abducens nerve palsies (Fig. 22.24) may represent an exaggerated expression of this physiologic synkinesis.

The **Marcus Gunn jaw-winking phenomenon** is an elevation of one eyelid that occurs during certain movements of the jaw. It is caused by a synkinesis between the pterygoid muscles and the levator palpebrae superioris. The associated movements of lid and jaw are termed a "trigemino-oculomotor" synkinesis and are subdivided into an external pterygoid-levator synkinesis and an internal pterygoid-levator synkinesis. Stimuli other than movement of the pterygoids can also produce the same kind of eyelid retraction.

Simultaneous contraction of the levator with the external pterygoid muscle is the most common trigemino-oculomotor synkinesis. The affected eyelid is usually ptotic, but it may appear normal or even retracted when the jaw muscles are active. Elevation of the upper lid can occur: (1) when the mandible is moved to the opposite side (contraction of the ipsilateral external pterygoid muscle); (2) when the mandible is projected forward or the tongue is protruded (bilateral contraction of the external pterygoid muscles); or (3) on wide opening of the mouth (i.e., strong depression of the mandible) (Fig. 22.25). The lid remains elevated as long as the jaw muscle contracts. The abnormal levator contraction is most evident when the patient is looking downward.

In most instances, the external pterygoid-levator synkinesis is congenital and is first recognized during the act of sucking soon after birth. The Marcus Gunn jaw-winking phenomenon improves with age in some patients but not in others.

Levator palpebrae synkinesias may involve cranial nerves other than the trigeminal nerve. For example, synkinetic overaction of the levator may be associated with teeth clenching, smiling, sternocleidomastoid contraction, tongue protrusion, inspiration, or voluntary nystagmus. Jaw movements may sometimes also induce movement of the extraocular muscles.

Patients with the Marcus Gunn phenomenon commonly have associated ocular abnormalities, including strabismus, amblyopia, anisometro-

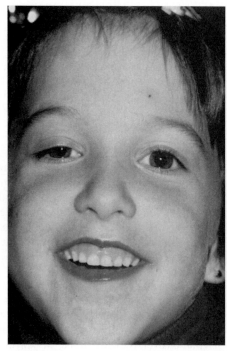 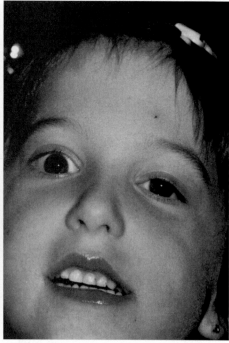

Figure 22.25. The Marcus Gunn jaw-winking phenomenon. *Left:* The patient has a congenital right ptosis. *Right:* When the patient moves her mouth to the left side, the right eyelid elevates and the ptosis disappears. (Courtesy of Dr. N.T. Iliff.)

pia, and congenital nystagmus. The most common ocular motor disturbances are double elevator palsy, unilateral superior rectus palsy, Duane's retraction syndrome, and adduction palsy with synergistic divergence. Rarely, trigemino-oculomotor synkinesis is associated with the triad of ipsilateral facial hemiatrophy, heterochromia, and poliosis.

The cause of the synkinesis between the pterygoid muscles and the levator muscle in the Marcus Gunn jaw-winking phenomenon is unknown. Although the possibility of a supranuclear synkinesis has been suggested, most investigators believe that a branch of the trigeminal nerve has been congenitally misdirected to the levator muscle. EMG studies are consistent with this concept, and histopathologic analysis of the levator palpebrae reveals evidence of neurogenic atrophy with aberrant reinnervation on the affected side and, to a lesser degree, the clinically unaffected side.

Treatment of patients with the Marcus Gunn jaw-winking phenomenon depends on their ophthalmologic and cosmetic status. Amblyopia should always be treated aggressively, and vertical strabismus should be corrected before attempting surgical repair of ptosis. Eyelid surgery should only be contemplated after the patient (when age permits), parents, and surgeon agree that the jaw winking, ptosis, or both are objectionable. Surgery usually consists of weakening the levator aponeurotic complex combined with a lid elevation procedure.

Other cases of **congenital oculopalpebral synkinesias** occur in which horizontal gaze induces reciprocal inhibition of one eyelid on abduction and excitation of the other on adduction, resulting in a gaze-induced seesaw-like movement of the eyelids. The inverse phenomenon, lid retraction on abduction, is most commonly seen in patients with Duane's retraction syndrome. EMG studies in such cases indicate that the ptosis on adduction is not caused by a mechanical retraction of the globe but rather by anomalous innervation. This seesaw-like synkinesis of the eyelid may, in rare cases, be induced by movements of the jaw from side to side. When the mouth is opened in such cases, both eyelids retract simultaneously (Fig. 22.26).

Eyelid retraction associated with misdirection of the oculomotor nerve usually occurs during attempted infraduction and adduction. During abduction of the affected eye, the eyelid becomes ptotic. This phenomenon is explained by reciprocal innervation. When the lateral rectus muscle contracts, both the ipsilateral medial rectus and the levator are inhibited.

One patient with bilateral traumatic oculomotor nerve palsies treated surgically subsequently (2 years later) developed bilateral alternating cyclic lid retraction that occurred every 1 to 2 minutes and lasted 5 seconds in each eye. Two other conditions that may cause periodic eyelid retraction are oculomotor palsy with cyclic spasms and ocular neuromyotonia (see Chapter 17). In both conditions, the eyelid retraction is usually unilateral and associated with pupillary dilation or spasms of one or more of the extraocular muscles innervated by the spastic nerve. Isolated lid retraction in these conditions has not been observed.

Patients with strabismus or amblyopia who fixate with the eye on the side of a unilateral ptosis may develop **pseudoretraction** of the eyelid on the opposite side. Depending on the technique used to detect this phenomenon, the frequency of pseudo-lid retraction varies from 2 to 66%. The methods include brief or prolonged occlusion of the eye on the side of the ptosis, manual elevation of the ptotic lid, or 2.5% phenylephrine applied to the eye on the side of the ptosis, while carefully observing the position of the contralateral retracted eyelid. Brief monocular occlusion is probably the least sensitive method, because the retracted eyelid may not reposition immediately. Pseudoretraction may be more easily detected if the ptotic eyelid is first manually closed, because release of the manually closed eyelid sometimes causes an appreciable upward flick of the contralateral eyelid as it resumes its retracted position.

The explanation for the phenomenon of eyelid retraction associated with contralateral ptosis is based on Hering's law. Intended to explain the conjugate movement of both eyes, Hering's law states that yoked extraocular muscles receive equal degrees of innervation. This law also applies to the levator muscles. Thus, in an attempt to maintain the normal position of a ptotic eyelid, the innervational drive on both lids increases, the ptotic lid assumes a more normal position, and the unaffected lid becomes retracted. Pseudoretraction of the eyelid is more likely to occur when ptosis is severe, acquired, and ipsilateral to the dominant eye (Fig. 22.27). The failure to recognize this phenomenon may lead to the erroneous diagnosis of thyroid orbitopathy.

The stimulus for Hering's law as it applies to the extraocular muscles is primarily sensory, that is, to maintain binocular fixation. Thus, the stimulus is probably a retinal error signal from one eye. Likewise, a decrease in retinal illumina-

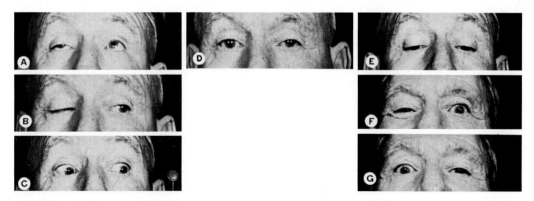

Figure 22.26. Synkinetic levator inhibition during conjugate gaze associated with paradoxic excitation with jaw opening resulting in bilateral jaw winking ("seesaw jaw winking"). *A.* Inhibition of the right levator in upgaze. *B.* Inhibition of the right levator in left gaze. *C.* Inhibition changes to bilateral levator excitation when mouth is open. *D.* Gaze straight ahead. *E.* Levator inhibition is normal in downward gaze. *F.* Elevation of left upper eyelid on jaw thrust to right. *G.* Elevation of right upper eyelid on jaw thrust to left.

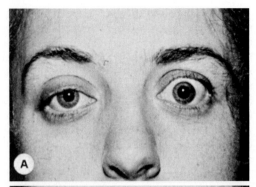

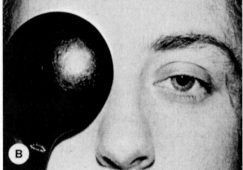

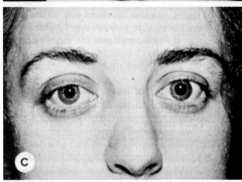

Figure 22.27. Paradoxic eyelid retraction with myasthenia gravis. *A.* The patient has moderate right ptosis and left upper eyelid retraction. *B.* When the right eye is covered, the left eyelid retraction disappears as levator tonus is reduced bilaterally. *C.* When intravenous edrophonium chloride (Tensilon) is administered to the patient, the right eyelid elevates and the left eyelid retraction disappears. Eyelid retraction occurs in this setting because Hering's law of equal innervation to agonist muscles applies to the levator muscles as well as to the extraocular muscles.

tion or contraction of the superior visual field may be the stimulus for increasing levator tone in patients with ptosis; however, levator tone is also influenced by the motor activity of the superior rectus. Thus, the levator palpebrae is unique in being subject to the influence of two yoke muscles: the contralateral levator palpebrae and the ipsilateral superior rectus. Any condition that limits the activity of the superior rectus and spares the levator can also result in lid retraction, as seen in patients with upgaze palsies, inferior rectus restriction, or underaction of the superior rectus.

Eyelid Retraction from Sympathetic Hyperfunction

Patients with neck trauma may develop a syndrome of recurrent throbbing headaches and oculosympathetic hyperactivity characterized by ipsilateral lid retraction, hyperhydrosis, and mydriasis (Claude-Bernard syndrome). During the headache-free interval, some of these patients have a Horner's syndrome. The syndrome is thought to be caused by sympathetic irritation or hyperactivity.

Sympathetic hyperactivity is also thought to be responsible for some cases of lid retraction observed in patients with thyroid orbitopathy (see below). Indeed, dilute solutions of both direct and indirect adrenergic stimulants (e.g., cocaine, hydroxyamphetamine, phenylephrine, apraclonidine, naphazoline) will widen the palpebral fissure in such patients.

Neuromuscular Eyelid Retraction and Lid Lag

Transient, spontaneous eyelid retraction occurs in patients with myasthenia gravis without evidence of thyroid dysfunction. This phenomenon, which usually occurs on return of the eyes from upward gaze to primary position, appears to be caused by post-tetanic facilitation of the levator palpebrae superioris (Fig. 22.28). Unlike the lid retraction of midbrain disease (Collier's sign), neuromuscular lid retraction is commonly asymmetric or completely unilateral. In addition, the levator muscle(s) usually fails to "relax" smoothly and completely, and the lid fold fails to smooth out as the eyes move downward. Momentary lid retraction also may be seen in patients with myasthenia after executing an upward saccade from downgaze

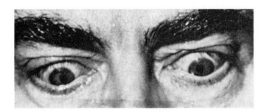

Figure 22.28. Transient, bilateral, asymmetric upper eyelid retraction in a patient with myasthenia gravis. This retraction occurred following prolonged upgaze. It persisted for several seconds and then disappeared. (Reprinted with permission from Puklin JE. Sacks JG, Boshes B. Transient eyelid retraction in myasthenia gravis. J Neurol Neurosurg Psychiatry 1976;39:44–47.)

to primary position (Cogan's lid twitch). Finally, patients with myasthenia may develop a pseudoretraction of the eyelid secondary to ptosis of the contralateral eyelid (see Fig. 22.27). Associated involvement of the extraocular muscles or the orbicularis oculi usually suggests the correct diagnosis, although in rare instances, the eyelid retraction is the initial sign of the neuromuscular disorder.

Lid retraction associated with the topical or systemic administration of drugs may be caused by effects at the neuromuscular junction. The anticholinesterase agents edrophonium chloride (Tensilon) and neostigmine methylsulfate (Prostigmin) produce eyelid retraction in some patients with myasthenia gravis. Subparalytic doses of succinylcholine can produce shortening of the levator muscle fibers associated with the depolarization effect of the drug, resulting in lid retraction.

Myopathic Eyelid Retraction and Lid Lag

Myopathic eyelid retraction occurs in both children and adults. Eyelid retraction that occurs in childhood may be caused by hyperthyroidism, misdirection of the oculomotor nerve, the dorsal midbrain syndrome, hydrocephalus, or the Marcus Gunn jaw-winking phenomenon. Thus, the diagnosis of congenital or developmental eyelid retraction should be made only after other causes have been excluded.

Congenital myopathic eyelid retraction can be unilateral or bilateral and may be associated with nonspecific strabismus, underaction of the superior rectus on the side of the retraction, or lower lid retraction. The condition may also be associated with other developmental anomalies, including optic disc hypoplasia, craniosynostosis, and Down syndrome. That levator excursion is normal and frequently shows lagophthalmos on downgaze indicates either failure in the levator to inhibit tonus appropriately or decreased elasticity of the levator or its suspensory ligaments. Routine histology of the levator muscle typically shows no specific abnormalities. In some cases, however, the medial and lateral horns of the levator aponeurosis appear thickened, and we are aware of one case in which the levator was fibrotic.

Thyroid orbitopathy with involvement of the levator muscle on one or both sides is the most common cause of acquired sustained lid retraction in adults (Figs. 22.29 and 22.30). The lid signs, which have a variety of names, are produced by pathologic shortening of the levator muscle, resulting in the inability of the muscle fibers to lengthen normally. Thus, patients with dysthyroid disease may show retraction of the upper eyelid associated with infrequent or incomplete blinking (Stellwag's sign), abnormal widening of the palpebral fissure (Dalrymple's sign), and lid lag (Graefe's sign) (see Figs. 22.29 and 22.30). On examination, the physician may have difficulty everting the patient's upper eyelid (Gifford's sign).

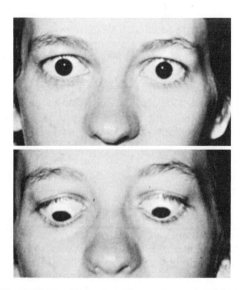

Figure 22.29. Bilateral eyelid retraction (*top*) and lid lag on downward gaze (*bottom*) in a patient with thyroid orbitopathy.

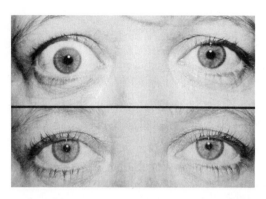

Figure 22.30. Patient with unilateral dysthyroid lid retraction. Patient was euthyroid at the time of the initial photo (*top*). After more than 4 years of lid retraction, the affected eyelid spontaneously returned to a normal position (*bottom*).

Patients with dysthyroid lid retraction may be chemically hyperthyroid, hypothyroid, or euthyroid. The retraction itself may be unilateral or bilateral and transient or persistent (see Fig. 22.30). It can occur in isolation, but it is more often associated with other signs of thyroid orbitopathy. If the lid retraction is mild and unassociated with other signs of thyroid orbitopathy, there may be difficulty in distinguishing lid retraction from pseudoptosis on the opposite side (see above). Levator excursion appears to be increased in patients with thyroid orbitopathy, and high-resolution sagittal computed tomographic (CT) scans show enlargement of the levator in most cases. In addition, EMG studies of the levator muscle demonstrate normal levator inhibition during downward gaze in patients with dysthyroid disease.

Multiple factors are involved in the genesis of dysthyroid lid retraction. Based on the inflammatory and fibrotic changes observed in the extraocular muscles, it would seem most likely that contracture or adhesive effects on the levator are the main reasons for persistent thyroid eyelid retraction; however, the levator muscle in some patients with dysthyroid lid retraction shows surprisingly little fibrosis or inflammation and is characterized instead by enlargement or hypertrophy of individual muscle fibers. Thus, the lid retraction that occurs in some patients with thyroid eye disease may result from some form of levator muscle "hyperactivity." Indeed, the spontaneous reversibility of lid retraction in some cases (see Fig. 22.30) and the development of ptosis after injections of botulinum toxin type

A in others would seem to argue against a restrictive fibrosis, in at least some cases.

Sympathetic stimulation induced by thyrotoxicosis or overmedication with thyroid replacement is probably responsible for lid retraction in some cases of thyroid orbitopathy. The lid retraction in such cases often resolves with improvement in thyroid status, and it responds transiently to topical sympatholytics, such as thymoxamine and guanethidine. Although sympathetic overstimulation infrequently plays a contributory role in lid retraction associated with thyroid orbitopathy, it does not explain the often asymmetric or unilateral cases, the absence of pupillary findings, and the fact that in some cases lid retraction persists as the patient becomes euthyroid.

Dysthyroid lid retraction results from restriction of the inferior rectus in some cases. Because the levator receives the same eye movement signal as the superior rectus, the increased drive on the superior rectus to overcome inferior rectus restriction causes excessive levator tonus. Recession of the inferior rectus in such cases results in a dramatic improvement in lid retraction.

In newborns with myopathic lid retraction, the retraction is usually the result of maternal hyperthyroidism. In such cases, the condition is transient and resolves in 2 to 3 weeks as the infant establishes its own endocrinologic equilibrium. There are also rare thyroid patients with ptosis (e.g., from myasthenia gravis, an aponeurotic defect from recurrent lid swelling, overcorrection from previous surgery for lid retraction) who develop pseudo-retraction of the contralateral eyelid.

The treatment of eyelid retraction in patients with thyroid orbitopathy is primarily surgical and consists of various levator-lengthening procedures, excision of Müller's muscle, and combined procedures on both muscles. Although topical sympatholytic agents (e.g., guanethidine, thymoxamine) may be used to overcome the retraction of the levator muscle by producing a sympathetic ptosis, these drugs are impractical for constant use. Guanethidine has a delayed effect and produces considerable corneal irritation. Topical thymoxamine, a selective α-adrenergic blocking agent, causes prompt ptosis, but it too causes considerable corneal irritation, and its long-term effects are unknown. Injection of botulinum toxin type A into the levator muscle may correct eyelid retraction for periods of 1 to 8 months.

Lid retraction occurs with increased frequency in patients with severe liver disease (Summerskill's sign). The appearance is similar to that seen in patients with thyroid orbitopathy.

Myotonic lid lag may be observed in patients with both hyperkalemic and hypokalemic familial periodic paralysis (Fig. 22.31). A similar myotonic lid lag may occur in patients with

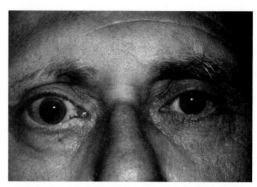

Figure 22.32. Upper and lower lid retraction due to right facial nerve palsy. (Reprinted with permission from Bartley GB. The differential diagnosis and classification of eyelid retractions. Ophthalmology 1996;103:168–176.)

myotonic dystrophy and in patients with congenital myotonia.

Mild lid retraction can occur in association with an ipsilateral facial nerve palsy because orbicularis oculi tonus contributes to the passive downward forces acting on the upper eyelid (Fig. 22.32). A similar mechanism may explain the lid retraction seen in some patients with ocular myasthenia gravis (see above and Chapter 21).

Mechanical Lid Retraction

The upper eyelid ordinarily maintains its position relative to the pupil even when an eye is proptosed by 10 mm or more. Thus, lid retraction associated with ipsilateral proptosis is almost invariably related to thyroid orbitopathy and not to an orbital mass. Nevertheless, various local processes can damage the eyelid and produce mechanical lid retraction.

Cutaneous cicatricial changes of the upper eyelid can produce eyelid retraction. The most common causes are burns and deep lacerations. Less commonly, cicatricial eyelid retraction occurs from damage to the eyelid from orbital cellulitis with necrosis (particularly from staphylococci and Group A streptococci), herpes zoster, scleroderma, or atopic dermatitis.

Lid retraction can occasionally be caused by contact lens wear. It resolves when the contact lens is removed. In some cases, a contact lens becomes displaced superiorly but is thought by the patient to have been lost. The retained lens

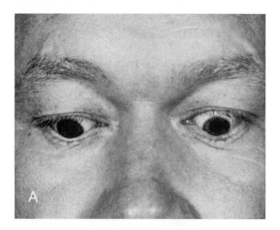

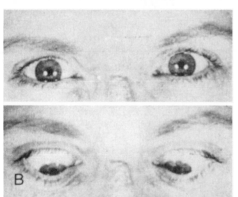

Figure 22.31. Myotonic lid-lag (levator myotonia) in patients with familial periodic paralysis. *A.* A patient with hypokalemic familial periodic paralysis. This photograph was taken following a period of upward gaze. The upper lids floated down about 20 seconds after the picture was taken. (Reprinted with permission from Resnick JS, Engel WK. Myotonic lid lag in hypokalemic periodic paralysis. J Neurol Neurosurg Psychiatry 1967;30:47–51.) *B.* A patient with hyperkalemic familial periodic paralysis. *Top:* Eyes in primary position. The eyelids are in relatively normal position. *Bottom:* On downward gaze, there is marked lag. (Reprinted with permission from Layzer RB, Lovelace RE, Rowland LP. Hyperkalemic periodic paralysis. Arch Neurol 1967;16: 455–471.)

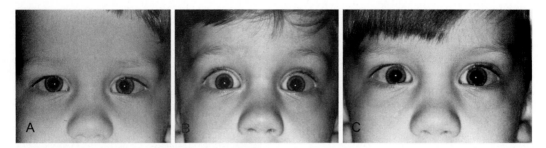

Figure 22.33. Bilateral upper eyelid retraction after surgery on the superior rectus muscles. *A.* Preoperative appearance. The patient has a V-pattern esotropia with bilateral overaction of the inferior oblique muscles. *B.* Postoperative appearance. After bilateral superior rectus recessions and inferior oblique weakening procedures, the patient has bilateral upper eyelid retraction. *C.* Six months following surgery, mild upper eyelid retraction remains. (Courtesy of Dr. D. Guyton.)

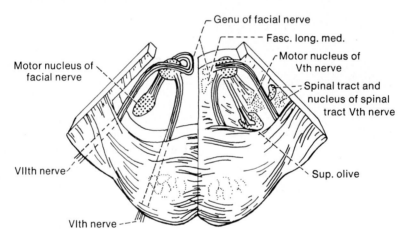

Figure 22.34. Anatomy of the facial nerve nuclei and fascicles. This diagram shows the intrapontine course of the facial nerve fascicles and their relationship to surrounding structures. *Fasc. Long. Med.,* medial longitudinal fasciculus. (Reprinted with permission from Brodal. Neurological Anatomy in Relation to Clinical Medicine. 3rd ed. New York, Oxford University Press, 1981:495.)

causes an inflammatory reaction in the superior fornix and eventually becomes embedded in an inflammatory cyst, the nature of which may not be appreciated until the cyst is opened surgically and the contact lens is found within it.

Postsurgical lid retraction is most often seen as an overcorrection after surgery for ptosis, although a variety of procedures, including vertical rectus muscle surgery (Fig. 22.33), trabeculectomy, cataract extraction, scleral buckling, blepharoplasty, myectomy for blepharospasm, orbital floor repair, and maxillectomy can also result in lid retraction. The mechanism is most often underaction of the superior rectus, restriction of the inferior rectus, cicatricial adhesion, or damage to the ligaments that create the passive downward eyelid forces. Levator motoneurons share the increased drive on superior rectus motoneurons that the nervous sytem employs to compensate for the decrease in superior rectus effectiveness.

Blowout fractures of the orbit may cause lid retraction by entrapment of the surrounding connective tissue. Lid retraction can also occur during an effort to elevate or fixate with a hypotropic or restricted eye.

ABNORMALITIES OF EYELID CLOSURE

As with eyelid opening, abnormalities of eyelid closure may occur from disorders involving any part of the pathway for contraction of the

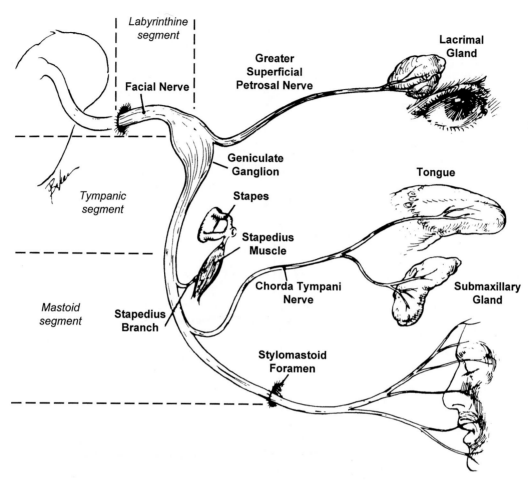

Figure 22.35.   Schematic drawing of the branches of the facial nerve showing the different functions of those branches. The branches and their functions include the greater superficial petrosal nerve (reflex tearing), the nerve to the stapedius muscle (stapedius reflex), the chorda tym-pani nerve (taste on the anterior two-thirds of the tongue and submaxillary gland secretion), and peripheral motor branches to the facial muscles. (Modified from Alford BR, Jerger JF, Coats AC, et al. Neurophysiology of facial nerve testing. Arch Otolaryngol 1973;97:214–219.)

orbicularis oculi, from the cerebral cortex to the muscle itself (Figs. 22.34 through 22.36). Such disorders may be congenital or acquired and may be caused by either hypofunction or hyperfunction.

INSUFFICIENCY OF EYELID CLOSURE

Insufficiency of Eyelid Closure Caused by Neuropathic Disease

Insufficiency of Eyelid Closure Caused by Supranuclear Disorders

Voluntary eyelid closure is mediated by the pyramidal system (see Fig. 22.36). Patients with cortical lesions of the precentral gyrus or more localized subcortical capsular lesions can usually close both eyes, although the force of closure is diminished, and the ability to wink may be lost on the contralateral paretic side (Revilliod's sign). In some cases, paresis is profound and yet spontaneous involuntary or emotional movements of the facial and orbicularis muscles remain undisturbed (automatic-voluntary dissociation) (Fig. 22.37).

Bilateral inability to voluntarily close the eyelids may result from a unilateral lesion, usually in the nondominant frontal lobe, but it more commonly develops with bilateral frontal lobe lesions. This phenomenon is called ''supranuclear paralysis of voluntary lid closure'' or **com-**

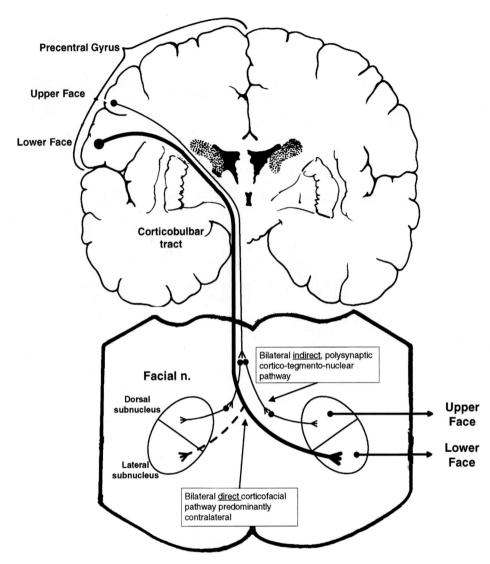

Figure 22.36. Diagram of the corticobulbar fibers serving the facial nuclei from their origin in the cerebral cortex, through the internal capsule into the brainstem at the level of the facial nucleus. Note that projections are bilateral along two pathways: (1) A direct, predominantly contralateral pro-jection to the lateral subnucleus responsible for lower facial muscles; and (2) an indirect pathway through the pontine reticular formation to the dorsal subnucleus that innervates the upper facial muscles.

pulsive eye opening. Patients with this syndrome are unable to initiate voluntary closure of either eyelid, even though they retain their ability to comprehend the task and have intact reflex eyelid closure (Fig. 22.38). Although some investigators consider this phenomenon to be an apraxia of eyelid closure, it is actually caused by true motor dysfunction. Supranuclear paraly-sis of eyelid closure can occur in patients with unilateral or bilateral infarcts or tumors in the frontal lobe, Creutzfeldt-Jakob disease, progressive supranuclear palsy, and motor neuron disease.

Motor impersistence of eyelid closure also occurs in patients with bilateral or unilateral hemispheric lesions. When such patients are re-

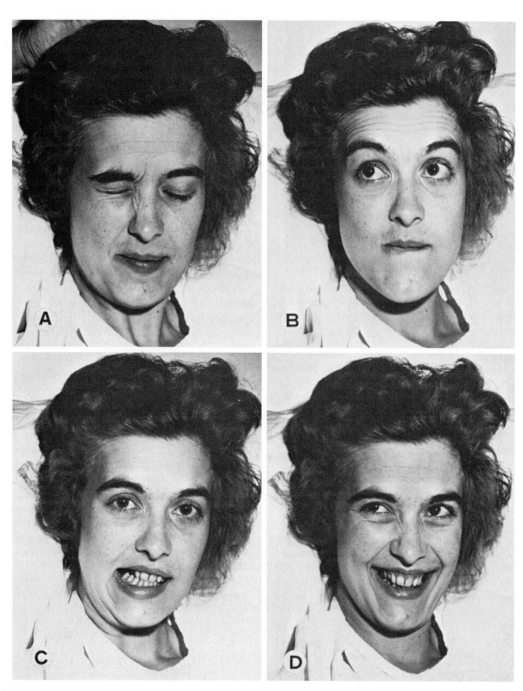

Figure 22.37. Central volitional paralysis of the orbicularis oculi after a subcortical hematoma. The patient also has a left hemiplegia. *A.* When the patient is told to close her eyes tightly, the left orbicularis oculi, left corrugator muscle, and the other muscles of the left lower side of the face fail to respond. *B.* Volitional control of the forehead is normal.

C. Left lower facial weakness is evident when the patient attempts to show her teeth. *D.* A spontaneous smile (emotional-extrapyramidal-facial innervation) evokes symmetric contraction of all facial muscles, including the orbicularis oculi.

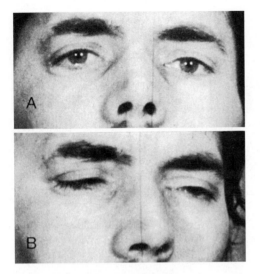

Figure 22.38. Supranuclear palsy (apraxia) of eyelid closure in a patient with Creutzfeldt-Jakob disease. *A.* Attempted voluntary eyelid closure to command. Note that the patient shows no clinical evidence of orbicularis activity at all. *B.* The patient shows some ability to blink to a visual threat. (Reprinted with permission from Ross Russell RW. Supranuclear palsy of eyelid closure. Brain 1980;103: 71–82.)

quested to close the eyelids and keep them closed, they are unable to obey. The eyelids close, often develop a fine tremor, and then almost immediately reopen. This phenomenon is most frequently seen in patients with a nondominant hemisphere stroke and is most evident during the first week after the stroke. Occasionally, the condition is unilateral.

It is likely that both supranuclear paralysis of eyelid closure (compulsive eye opening) and motor impersistence of eyelid closure have a common origin because they can coexist in the same patient and develop in similar clinical settings. EMG studies, however, have yielded conflicting results. In one patient with progressive supranuclear palsy, EMG showed both inadequate inhibition of the levator *and* insufficient orbicularis oculi activity. In another EMG study, patients with Parkinson's disease with motor impersistence showed a supranuclear disturbance of orbicularis control, rather than levator inhibition.

Cortical lesions may also affect involuntary lid closure. For example, the blink response to a threatening gesture is absent in patients with homonymous hemianopia when the gesture is presented in the blind field of vision. The blink to threat is also lost in patients with cortical blindness and may be absent in patients with profound visual inattention associated with large parieto-occipital or parietotemporal lesions. Loss of spontaneous blinking was described in a patient with Balint's syndrome caused by bilateral parieto-occipital lesions.

Insufficiency of Eyelid Closure from Facial Nerve Palsy: Topical Diagnosis

The insufficiency or weakness of eyelid closure associated with lesions of the facial nerve is usually combined with weakness of other facial muscles supplied by that nerve. A standardized clinical method of assessing the degree of facial palsy separates the severity into six grades (I to VI) based on the residual motion of the forehead, eyelid, and mouth, as well as the appearance of the face at rest. Grades I and II are generally considered mild or acceptable appearance and movement, whereas grade VI represents total paralysis. With respect to the eyelid, mild weakness (Grade II) of the orbicularis oculi from facial nerve paresis may be characterized by normal symmetry and tone, with only minimal effort being required to completely close the eyelid. The lower eyelid may be slightly retracted in patients with this grade of weakness. Patients with moderate paresis (Grade III) may close the eyes completely but only with extreme effort. Incomplete reflex and voluntary eyelid closure occurs with moderately severe (Grade IV) or severe (Grade V) dysfunction. In these severe cases, the lower eyelid sags, whereas the resting position of the upper eyelid remains unchanged or is slightly retracted (Figs. 22.32 and 22.39). Epiphora may occur in these patients from impaired lacrimal drainage and corneal exposure.

Topographic diagnosis of facial nerve paresis may be facilitated by the relationship of the facial nerve to surrounding structures and by the fact that during its course, the nerve gives off various branches that subserve specific functions. The facial nerve, in addition to innervating the facial musculature, is also responsible for reflex tearing (via the greater superficial petrosal nerve), hearing (via the nerve to the stapedius muscle), taste on the anterior two-thirds of the tongue (via the chorda tympani), and salivation (via nerve branches to the sublingual and sub-

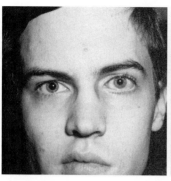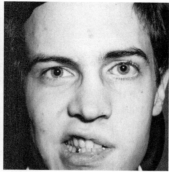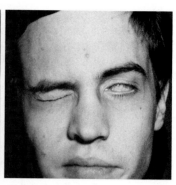

Figure 22.39. Peripheral facial nerve palsy in a 24-year-old man with an acoustic neuroma. *Left:* The patient has a complete left facial nerve palsy. Note the widened left lid fissure and sag of the left lower eyelid. *Center:* When the patient attempts to show his teeth, lower facial weakness is evident. This weakness did not improve when extrapyramidal facial innervation was stimulated. *Right:* On attempted eyelid closure, there is nearly complete paralysis of the left orbicularis oculi muscle. Note intact Bell's phenomenon.

mandibular glands) (see Fig. 22.35). In addition, various electrodiagnostic tests, including nerve excitability, electromyography, blink reflex, and electroneurography help determine the extent of dysfunction and prognosis for facial nerve recovery.

Unilateral weakness of eyelid closure and facial movement may result from unilateral damage to the facial nerve nucleus. In such instances, other evidence of brainstem disease is almost always present, including reduction in corneal sensation, ipsilateral abducens or horizontal gaze paralysis, and ipsilateral cerebellar ataxia.

Bilateral weakness of eyelid closure occurs as part of the facial diplegia that is caused by lesions of the pontine tegmentum. Such lesions may be congenital or acquired. Acquired processes include ischemia, inflammation, infiltration, and compression.

When insufficiency of eyelid closure results from damage to the facial nerve fascicle within the brainstem, there is usually complete facial paralysis associated with other signs of brainstem dysfunction, such as ipsilateral horizontal gaze palsy from damage to the ipsilateral abducens nucleus or paramedian pontine reticular formation, ipsilateral abduction weakness from damage to the ipsilateral abducens nerve fascicle, and contralateral hemiparesis from damage to the ipsilateral pyramidal tract (see Fig. 22.34). The combination of ipsilateral facial nerve palsy, ipsilateral abduction weakness, and contralateral hemiparesis is called the **Millard-Gubler syndrome** (see Chapter 17).

Lesions of the cerebellopontine angle (CPA) are characterized by signs and symptoms related to dysfunction of the vestibulocochlear, facial, and trigeminal nerves. Common manifestations include unilateral sensorineural hearing loss, tinnitus, vertigo, facial pain and numbness, corneal hypesthesia, and unsteadiness of gait. All of the components of the facial nerve may be affected. Less common manifestations include hemifacial spasm, nystagmus, evidence of cerebellar dysfunction (e.g., ataxia and tremor), and hydrocephalus. Although most patients with lesions in the CPA present with multiple neurologic findings, facial nerve paralysis may be the only manifestation, particularly in children. Tumors of the CPA include vestibular and trigeminal schwannomas, meningiomas, epidermoids, lipomas, arachnoid cysts, aneurysms, metastatic lesions, and glomus jugulare tumors.

A facial nerve lesion located between the internal auditory meatus and the geniculate ganglion produces many of the same signs as those encountered with disease in the CPA, except that brainstem signs are absent, and there is no evidence of dysfunction of the trigeminal nerve. Lesions between the geniculate ganglion and the branch to the stapedius muscle produce similar manifestations except that reflex lacrimation is preserved because the lesion is distal to the superficial petrosal nerve. Damage to the facial nerve between the branch to the stapedius muscle and the chorda tympani produces facial paralysis, loss of taste on the anterior two-thirds of the tongue, and diminution of salivary secretion.

Finally, a lesion of the facial nerve distal to the takeoff of the chorda tympani produces only facial motor paralysis. Facial neuropathies that localize to the intratemporal portion of the facial nerve may be caused by fractures of the temporal bone, herpes zoster (Ramsey Hunt syndrome), otitis media, and neoplasms. The condition called ''Bell's palsy'' belongs in this category (see below). Lesions distal to the stylomastoid foramen may affect one or more peripheral branches of the facial nerve and are usually caused by facial trauma, facial surgery, or disease of the parotid gland.

Distinguishing central and proximal peripheral lesions of the facial nerve from distal peripheral lesions is critically important. Unfortunately, although topographic analysis of facial nerve function often permits such differentiation, the findings in patients with lesions along the intratemporal segment of the facial nerve are often variable and inconsistent. This is particularly true in cases of Bell's palsy, in which magnetic resonance imaging (MRI) can show areas of demyelination anywhere from the brainstem to the periphery. The usefulness of precise localization along this segment of the facial nerve in diagnosis, management, and prognosis is limited.

The majority (about 50 to 70%) of isolated facial nerve palsies are idiopathic and are called **Bell's palsy.** The diagnosis of Bell's palsy is based on a constellation of findings and the exclusion of other known causes. The condition is usually unilateral, although bilateral cases occur in 0.1 to 1% of patients. About 60% of patients with a Bell's palsy have a history of a viral prodrome. The onset of facial motor weakness is acute and frequently accompanied by pain or numbness of the face, neck, or tongue. The pain is characteristically located in the retroauricular area. Hypesthesia or dysesthesia in the distribution of the trigeminal or glossopharyngeal nerve occurs in about 25 to 35% of patients. Sensory findings may precede the onset of facial paresis and usually do not persist beyond 7 to 10 days. Dysgeusia and dysacusis are fairly common accompaniments. Both subjective and objective signs of dry eye are present in 15 to 17% of patients. Epiphora from exposure or paralytic ectropion is common. The incidence of Bell's palsy is higher in adults than in children, and the condition occurs in both sexes with equal frequency. Familial cases are extremely unusual.

There is mounting evidence implicating a viral etiology in the pathogenesis of Bell's palsy:

1. Serologic studies that reveal evidence of a variety of infectious agents, particularly the herpes group of viruses, mumps virus, and rubella virus.
2. Polymerase chain reaction and in situ hybridization evidence of herpes simplex virus in the geniculate ganglion of adults with Bell's palsy.
3. Histopathologic evidence of inflammatory changes within the facial nerve.
4. Widespread subclinical disturbances in the peripheral nervous system and CNS indicative of a more widespread cranial polyneuropathy.
5. Epidemiologic studies.

Although it is likely that an immunologic response associated with infection is responsible in many cases, some authors maintain that the crucial factor is swelling of the facial nerve (from inflammation, ischemia, or both) within the facial canal.

In a study based on the untreated natural history of more than 1000 patients with Bell's palsy, it was found that among the 30% of patients with incomplete facial paresis, nearly all achieved complete recovery. Among the 70% with complete paralysis, the prognosis was still quite good if signs of recovery began within the first 3 weeks of onset.

Overall, 85% of patients with Bell's palsy eventually recover completely or are left with only slight residual deficits. The remaining 15% require 3 to 6 months before showing signs of improvement but have permanent deficits consisting of residual weakness, tonic contracture, synkinesis, spasms, or gustatory lacrimation (crocodile tears). Clinical factors that adversely affect recovery include advanced age (over 60), diabetes mellitus, complete paralysis, decreased tearing, hyperacusis, and delay in the onset of recovery. In 7 to 10% of cases, recurrences occur on the same side or alternate from side to side.

The efficacy of systemic corticosteroids in the treatment of Bell's palsy is somewhat controversial. Patients treated with prednisone have less denervation and greater improvement in functional grade at recovery than patients who are not treated. Although steroids may not entirely prevent partial denervation or contracture, their use may speed recovery and may also reduce the risk of gustatory lacrimation from autonomic synkinesis and of progression from incomplete to complete paralysis. Most physicians thus treat patients with Bell's palsy with prednisone in a dose of 1 mg/kg/day for 10 to 14 days followed by a rapid taper.

In addition, because herpes simplex virus is also implicated in the pathogenesis of Bell's palsy and because herpes zoster oticus can occur without a rash (zoster sine herpete), some clinicians recommend using acyclovir along with systemic corticosteroids in the treatment of patients with Bell's palsy. However, there is no difference in the outcome of patients treated with steroids alone compared with patients treated with both steroids and acyclovir.

There is strong pathologic, clinical, and neuroimaging evidence that the pathogenesis of facial nerve damage in patients with Bell's palsy is compression of the nerve at the meatal foramen and along its labyrinthine segment. Decompression procedures that expose more distal segments thus have been abandoned in favor of decompression of the meatal foramen and labyrinthine segment of the facial nerve via a middle fossa craniotomy. Nonetheless, the effectiveness of canal decompression in the treatment of Bell's palsy is unproven, and enthusiasm for the procedure is waning.

An isolated facial nerve palsy that may mimic Bell's palsy can occur in a large number of systemic disorders. These include infections and inflammations (herpes zoster oticus, acquired immune deficiency syndrome, otitis media, mastoiditis, Lyme disease, syphilis, sarcoidosis, tetanus), ischemia (diabetes mellitus, hypertension), and immune-mediated inflammatory diseases (periarteritis, GBS, postvaccination demyelination, MS). Neoplastic causes of isolated peripheral facial palsy include vestibular and facial nerve schwannomas, meningiomas, glomus jugulare tumors, lipomas, dermoids, epidermoids, parotid tumors, carcinomatous meningitis, cholesteatomas, metastatic tumors, and lymphoid lesions. Miscellaneous causes include toxic agents (thalidomide, ethylene glycol, organophosphate poisoning), trauma (temporal bone fractures, facial injuries, barotrauma from scuba diving), iatrogenic injuries (from local anesthetic blocks and facial surgery), amyloidosis, Paget's disease, and benign intracranial hypertension.

Because so many conditions can cause an acute, initially isolated, facial nerve paresis, progression of a facial palsy for greater than 3 weeks, lack of recovery after 3 to 6 months, development of hemifacial spasm, prolonged otalgia or facial pain, or recurrence of paralysis after recovery should prompt closer investigation of a "Bell's palsy" to rule out an underlying systemic inflammatory or infectious etiology or a neoplasm.

In patients with congenital or developmental facial nerve paresis, there may be other evidence of incomplete development (hypoplasia) or agenesis of the facial nerve. Such patients may have Möbius syndrome, congenital unilateral lower lip paralysis (CULLP), hemifacial microsomia, or other associated developmental defects, such as aural atresia and microtia. Acquired prenatal causes include birth trauma and exposure to thalidomide or rubella virus.

Less than 1% of all facial nerve palsies are bilateral and simultaneous. Such cases are usually idiopathic (i.e., Bell's palsy) or caused by Lyme disease, sarcoidosis, GBS, Fisher's syndrome, brainstem encephalitis, or neoplasia (e.g. carcinomatous meningitis, glioma). Less common causes include meningitis (e.g., from syphilis, tuberculosis, cryptococcus), diabetes mellitus, head trauma, pontine hemorrhage, systemic lupus erythematosus, ethylene glycol ingestion, benign intracranial hypertension, and Wernicke-Korsakoff syndrome.

The rehabilitation and supportive management of patients with a facial nerve palsy depends on the stage and severity of facial weakness. During the acute phase, treatment should be directed at preventing the complications of corneal exposure by using topical lubricants and, in some cases, cellophane wrap occlusive dressings or self-adhesive occlusive bubbles. If supportive therapy fails, a temporary or permanent tarsorrhaphy should be performed. When the facial nerve has been severed or severely damaged, and recovery is not likely to occur, procedures that juxtapose the upper and lower eyelids and improve eyelid (and other facial muscle) function should be considered, including permanent tarsorrhaphy, lateral canthoplasty to treat the effects of paralytic ectropion, and insertion of a gold weight or palpebral spring (cerclage) to reanimate the upper eyelid. Facial reanimation can sometimes be accomplished using a variety of techniques, including direct facial nerve

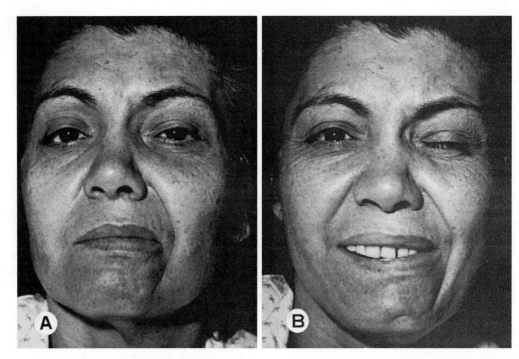

Figure 22.40. Facial contracture with misdirected regeneration of the left facial nerve following Bell's palsy. *A.* The patient has narrowed lid fissure and a deepened nasolabial groove on the left. *B.* Any movement, spontaneous or voluntary, produces co-movements in all muscles of the left side of the face. Movement of the corner of the left side of the mouth is associated with eyelid closure.

repair, autogenous nerve grafts, cross facial nerve grafting, and nerve crossovers using the hypoglossal nerve. In addition, temporalis muscle transfers, free-muscle grafts, and facial suspension with fascia lata, tendon, or alloplastic materials can be used.

Facial Nerve Misdirection (Aberrant Regeneration of the Facial Nerve)

Aberrant regeneration or misdirection of the facial nerve may occur after damage to the facial nerve, particularly after compression or trauma. It develops in about 10 to 20% of patients with Bell's palsy. The previously paralyzed side of the face is invariably weak and may appear contracted (Fig. 22.40). With each closure of the eye, a simultaneous twitch at the corner of the mouth occurs, accompanied by dimpling of the chin and contraction of the platysma. During forced lid closure, there is an exaggerated contraction of all facial muscles on the side of the previously paretic facial nerve. Both voluntary and involuntary movements of the lips or the corner of the mouth precipitate co-contraction of the orbicularis oculi on the affected side that may superficially resemble an inverse Marcus Gunn jaw-winking phenomenon (see above). However, unlike the inverse Marcus Gunn phenomenon, in which the eyelid closure is caused by levator inhibition, narrowing of the lid fissure in aberrant regeneration of the facial nerve is caused by inappropriate contraction of the orbicularis oculi muscle.

Insufficiency of Eyelid Closure Caused by Neuromuscular Disease

The orbicularis oculi is often weakened in diseases that affect the neuromuscular junction. Myasthenia gravis characteristically produces weakness of eyelid closure, usually combined with ptosis. This weakness of orbicularis function is responsible for the "peek phenomenon" in which a patient with myasthenia gravis is initially able to close the eyelids but as closure is maintained, the orbicularis fatigues and the eyelids separate, exposing the globe. Weakness of the orbicularis oculi in patients with neuromuscular disease may also be characterized by retraction of the lower eyelid. The diagnosis of neuromuscular disease, particularly myasthenia gravis, should be considered in any patient with weakness of eyelid closure associated with ptosis, ophthalmoparesis, or both. The weakness in such patients often improves transiently when the patients are given an intravenous injection of Tensilon or an intramuscular injection of Prostigmin.

Neuromuscular hypoexcitability of the muscles of eyelid closure is pronounced in neuromuscular disease other than myasthenia gravis, including botulism and toxic reactions to certain spider and snake bites.

Insufficiency of Eyelid Closure Caused by Myopathic Disease

The orbicularis oculi muscle is almost always weakened by any disease that weakens the facial musculature. Weakness of the orbicularis muscle may be characterized not only by weakness of spontaneous or forced eyelid closure but also by lack of upper facial expression, wasting of eyelid tissue, and fatigue of the eyelids during attempted sustained closure. In addition, there may be isolated retraction of the lower eyelid or paralytic ectropion (Fig. 22.41). Myogenic weakness of the orbicularis oculi is usually bilateral. Weakness in the pretarsal segment impairs blinking but must be significant before blinking is overtly impaired. Because lacrimal drainage depends in part on normal muscle action in the lower eyelid, weakness of contraction may result in epiphora. Patients with certain forms of congenital muscular dystrophy, myotonic dystro-

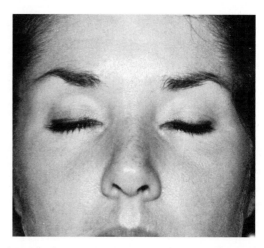

Figure 22.42.   Orbicularis oculi weakness in a patient with Kearns-Sayre syndrome. The patient is attempting to close her eyelids as tightly as possible.

phy, and the mitochondrial cytopathies associated with CPEO often have weakness of eyelid closure (Fig. 22.42).

EXCESSIVE OR ANOMALOUS EYELID CLOSURE: HYPERACTIVITY OF THE ORBICULARIS OCULI MUSCLE

Excessive Eyelid Closure of Cortical and Subcortical Origin

Essential Blepharospasm and the Blepharospasm-Oromandibular Dystonia Syndrome (Meige Syndrome; Brueghel Syndrome)

Blepharospasm is an involuntary closure of the eyelids evoked by contraction of the orbicularis oculi. When blepharospasm occurs in isolation without other evidence of neurologic or ocular disease, the condition is called **essential blepharospasm** (Fig. 22.43). When these focal dystonic eyelid movements spread to other cranial muscles, the syndrome is called blepharospasm-oromandibular dystonia or **Meige syndrome.** The disorder occurs most frequently in women over 50 years of age. Initially, there is an increased frequency of blinking, particularly in response to sunlight, wind, noise, movement, or stress. This blinking progresses to involuntary spasms, initially on one side, but inevitably on both. Certain maneuvers like touching the eyelid, coughing, vocalizing, or chewing gum may alleviate the spasms.

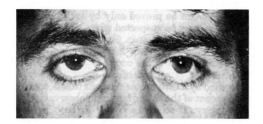

Figure 22.41.   Bilateral, symmetric lower eyelid retraction in a patient with myotonic dystrophy. (Reprinted with permission from Cohen MM, Lessell S. Retraction of the lower eyelid. Neurology 1979;29:386–389.)

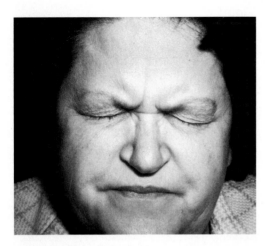

Figure 22.43. Essential blepharospasm. The patient first noted intermittent spasms of lid closure several years earlier. By the time she was examined, she was experiencing almost continuous, bilateral spasm of the orbicularis oculi muscles.

As the disorder progresses, the orbicularis oculi spasms increase in frequency and severity. Eventually, patients may experience involuntary chewing movements, lip pursing, trismus, wide opening of the mouth, spasmodic deviations of the jaw, abnormal tongue movements (protrusion, retraction, and writhing), spasmodic dysphonia, and even swallowing and respiratory difficulties.

In addition to orofacial spasms, patients with Meige syndrome may also have oculogyric crises, platysmal contractions, torticollis, retrocollis, or other forms of focal dystonia. Generalized dystonia is rare. Many patients stop reading, watching television, and driving; some become depressed, occupationally disabled and, in some cases, functionally blind. The disorder may plateau at any point along its progression. Remissions are rare but occur in about 11% of patients, almost always within 5 years of the onset of symptoms.

Most cases of Meige syndrome are sporadic, although there are familial occurrences. Thus, familial blepharospasm and craniocervical dystonia may be phenotypically heterogeneous and autosomal-dominantly inherited with incomplete penetrance. Patients with essential blepharospasm and Meige syndrome often have a family history of other movement disorders (e.g. essential tremor, Parkinson's disease, oromandibular dystonia, blepharospasm, habit tics) or

may give a past history of tics or excessive blinking, sometimes dating back to childhood.

Many patients with blepharospasm complain of dryness, grittiness, irritation, or photophobia. Such patients typically have evidence of dry eyes or ocular surface disease by slit lamp biomicroscopy or Schirmer testing. Indeed, disturbances of the ocular surface may be a precondition for blepharospasm in certain cases. Although there are scattered reports of an association between blepharospasm and certain autoimmune disorders (e.g., systemic lupus erythematosus, myasthenia gravis, rheumatoid arthritis, thyroid disease), there is no convincing evidence that autoimmunity is the underlying mechanism of idiopathic blepharospasm.

EMG studies of the orbicularis oculi show a variety of patterns in patients with blepharospasm. The most common finding is repetitive bursts that last 100 to 200 msec, with variable interburst intervals ranging from 200 to 800 msec. Some patients exhibit tonic spasms lasting 3 to 4 seconds or combinations of tonic and repetitive bursts. The characteristic lowering of the brow (Charcot's sign) may be absent among a subgroup of patients with blepharospasm in whom contractions are confined to the pretarsal portion of the orbicularis oculi.

The cause of blepharospasm and Meige syndrome is uncertain. Although psychologic factors are an important component of this disorder, there is abundant clinical and neurophysiologic evidence that essential blepharospasm and Meige syndrome are **focal dystonias** caused by dysfunction of the basal ganglia or brainstem. For example, blepharospasm can be a component of an assortment of extrapyramidal and brainstem disorders, and imaging studies show that focal lesions of the rostral brainstem, diencephalon, and basal ganglia may be associated with blepharospasm.

There is clear evidence of brainstem dysfunction in many patients with essential blepharospasm. About 30% of patients with essential blepharospasm exhibit abnormalities of the brainstem auditory-evoked response that localizes to the mid to upper brainstem. The reciprocal relationship between the orbicularis oculi and levator palpebrae may be altered, and there may be inappropriate episodes of levator inhibition or co-contraction. Although the latency of the blink and corneal reflex are normal in patients with essential blepharospasm, both amplitude and duration are abnormally increased. Patients with essential blepharospasm and patients with oromandibular dystonia have a more rapid R2 recovery cycle than normal control subjects, indicating that the brainstem interneurons that mediate the blink reflex are abnormally excitable. Similar findings can be documented in many patients with other cranial dystonias, even in the absence of blepharospasm. The basal ganglia, which plays a central role in the genesis of these movement disorders, is probably responsible for this facilitatory effect on brainstem interneurons.

Blepharospasm may be associated with a variety of eye movement disturbances that also occur in other extrapyramidal disorders. Using motion-picture or video analysis, one can observe impersistence of gaze, eyelid retraction, head tilt, head jerk, and tonic upward spasms of gaze in patients with essential blepharospasm. In addition, some patients experience episodes of prolonged involuntary conjugate spasmodic upward deviations lasting 1 to 10 seconds. These episodes are similar to those seen in patients with oculogyric crises. Abnormalities in saccadic eye movements also occur in patients with essential blepharospasm. They are nonspecific but consistent with extrapyramidal dysfunction.

The histopathologic findings in patients with essential blepharospasm are variable, although the basal ganglia are often abnormal. Some cases show microscopic abnormalities in the dorsal halves of the caudate and putamen that consist of neuronal cell loss and severe gliosis in a unique pattern that produces a "mosaic appearance." In others, there is mild to moderate cell loss in the pars compacta of the substantia nigra, the locus ceruleus, and several other areas in the brainstem. Some cases show no abnormalities or unrelated changes; however, the lack of morphologic changes does not necessarily imply normal function. For example, neurochemical analysis of the brain from a patient with Meige syndrome who had no significant neuropathologic findings at autopsy nevertheless demonstrated substantial increases in norepinephrine and dopamine in the red nucleus and substantia nigra.

Botulinum toxin type A is the primary form of therapy for patients with blepharospasm (see below). Other drugs can also be used to treat essential blepharospasm and Meige syndrome, but they are less efficacious. For example, in some patients with mild essential blepharo-

spasm, tranquilizers may be of short-term benefit. For patients with more severe disease, drugs that inhibit catecholamine synthesis (α-methyl-l-tyrosine), block dopamine receptors (phenothiazine, butyrophenones), deplete brain monoamines (Reserpine, tetrabenazine), or increase central cholinergic effects (physostigmine, Choline, lecithin) may suppress the abnormal movements. Tetrabenazine, clonazepam, trihexyphenidyl, lithium carbonate, and baclofen are of particular benefit in selected patients. In addition, selective inhibitors of serotonin re-uptake, such as fluoxetine (Prozac), may reduce facial and eyelid spasms in patients with severe blepharospasm, Meige syndrome, or both. L-dopa is occasionally useful in patients with blepharospasm related to parkinsonism, particularly that form induced by MPTP, but this drug is of little or no benefit in the treatment of essential blepharospasm.

Essential blepharospasm can be treated surgically, either by removing all or part of the orbicularis oculi muscle or by avulsing or otherwise destroying branches of the facial nerve. Complications, variable effectiveness, and frequent recurrence are major limitations of both procedures; however, comparisons of the two approaches indicate that myectomy may be preferable because it results in a more prolonged relief of symptoms, fewer recurrences requiring additional surgery, greater patient acceptance, and fewer complications than selective facial nerve avulsion. Nevertheless, complete healing may take 6 months or more after myectomy and may be associated with considerable facial swelling from lymphedema. With facial nerve avulsion, there is a fourfold increase in the need for secondary procedures in addition to the complications associated with facial paresis. We believe that surgery should be reserved for patients with disabling blepharospasm that does not respond to botulinum toxin, oral medications, or a combination of these treatments or for patients who cannot tolerate these treatments.

Patients with essential blepharospasm often have associated dermatochalasis, ptosis, or both. These can be treated with blepharoplasty and ptosis surgery, both of which often reduce the severity of the blepharospasm to some extent. However, these procedures are merely adjuncts to the treatment of blepharospasm and should not be considered as primary treatments for the condition.

Blepharospasm Associated with Lesions of the Brainstem and Basal Ganglia

Blepharospasm may be caused by a variety of lesions and disorders of the basal ganglia and mesodiencephalic region. These include strokes, demyelinating diseases, progressive supranuclear palsy, Parkinson's disease, MPTP-induced parkinsonism, Huntington's disease, Wilson's disease, Lytico-Bodig syndrome, Hallervorden-Spatz syndrome, olivopontocerebellar atrophy, communicating hydrocephalus, and encephalitis lethargica. Calcification of the basal ganglia associated with blepharospasm occurs in patients with Meige syndrome, pseudohypoparathyroidism, and ill-defined neurodegenerative disorders of unknown etiology.

The blepharospasm that follows a cerebrovascular accident frequently begins months to years after the stroke and is associated with other localizing signs, such as hemiplegia, midbrain ocular motor dysfunction, and extrapyramidal signs. The causative lesion may be unilateral or bilateral, but the blepharospasm is usually bilateral and symmetric. Delayed blepharospasm may also be associated with palatal myoclonus.

There are several possible explanations for the delay in onset of blepharospasm in patients with lesions of the brainstem and basal ganglia: (1) denervation supersensitivity of the facial nuclear complex, (2) disinhibition of facial nuclear and brainstem reflexes, and (3) delayed-onset dystonia caused by sprouting of surviving axons. If the basal ganglia plays a permissive role in the development of blepharospasm, this delay is not surprising because lid spasms would not develop until there was an adaptive increase in blink excitability from chronic trigeminal stimulation.

Blepharoclonus and Reflex Blepharospasm

Typical blepharospasm is characterized by repetitive episodes of tonic contractions of the orbicularis oculi, and EMG studies show that the orbicularis contractions in many such patients consist of rhythmic phasic bursts at a rate of 3 to 6 Hz. When such contractions of the orbicularis oculi result in visible repetitive upward jerks of the eyelids, the term **blepharoclonus** is used.

Blepharoclonus occurs in patients with brainstem syndromes caused by stroke or trauma, hydrocephalus from aqueductal stenosis in the setting of parkinsonism, and MS. In one case, blepharoclonus was precipitated by eccentric gaze and was not present when the patient looked straight ahead.

Reflex blepharospasm is a condition in which eyelid spasms are induced by voluntary lid closure or attempts to manually open the eyelids. It is a well-known finding in patients with recent, nondominant temporoparietal strokes, in which case it is associated with hemiplegia. The lid spasms are usually confined to the nonparalyzed side and are evoked when the examiner attempts to hold the eyelids apart. Some patients with spontaneous blepharospasm from extrapyramidal or brainstem lesions also have reflex blepharospasm during attempts by the examiner to open the eyelids. Likewise, gentle lid closure in some patients with Parkinson's disease will evoke a "lid tremor" that by EMG shows reciprocal contractions of the levator and orbicularis oculi muscles. Rarely, reflex blepharospasm is hereditary, with onset in early childhood.

Blepharoclonus and reflex blepharospasm are probably different manifestations of similar pathophysiologic processes. Although the origin of the primary stimulus may vary (e.g., extrapyramidal dysfunction, hemisphere or brainstem lesions, or stretching of the orbicularis), the final pathway is an increase in blink excitability. Suprasegmental disinhibition or adaptive responses to peripheral lesions enhance the neuronal activity of the blink pathways.

Although blepharoclonus and reflex blepharospasm usually occur in patients with cortical, extrapyramidal, brainstem, and trigeminal disturbances, some patients with these findings have no evidence of neurologic disease.

Ocular Blepharospasm

Blepharospasm is occasionally caused by irritative or painful ocular disease. Photophobia and lacrimation are also present in patients with this form of blepharospasm, often called **ocular blepharospasm.** The most common causes of ocular blepharospasm are disturbances of the eyelids (e.g., blepharitis, trichiasis, entropion), disturbances of the corneal epithelium, severe dry eyes, iritis, scleritis, and angle-closure glaucoma. Although less common, patients with ocular albinism, congenital achromatopsia, aniridia, or posterior subcapsular cataracts may experience blepharospasm and photophobia in response to bright light. Chemotherapeutic agents such as cyclophosphamide, doxorubicin, fluorouracil, tegafur (furanyl-5-fluorouracil), and mitomycin c may produce ocular irritation and severe blepharospasm, as may a variety of topical medications.

Rarely, patients with strabismus develop what appears to be a unilateral tonic blepharospasm to avoid diplopia. This is particularly common in patients with acquired paralytic strabismus and in patients with intermittent exotropia. It is most obvious in bright light.

In our experience, although patients with essential blepharospasm often have ocular surface abnormalities that may contribute to the spasms, true ocular blepharospasm is rare. Nevertheless, ocular causes of blepharospasm should always be excluded before a search is begun for a neurologic cause of blepharospasm or a diagnosis of essential blepharospasm is made.

Blepharospasm Associated with Drug-Induced Tardive Dyskinesia

Patients with **tardive dyskinesia** have blepharospasm and facial tics similar to those seen in patients with Meige syndrome (see above); however, patients with tardive dyskinesia have choreic movements of the extremities as opposed to the more sustained, dystonic movements observed in patients with Meige syndrome. The most important distinguishing feature of tardive dyskinesia, however, is that it is always drug-induced, usually developing about 1 to 2 years after starting the drug. In most instances, the responsible agents are antipsychotic or neuroleptic drugs, such as the dopamine-blocking or dopamine-stimulating drugs. Drug-induced dyskinesia can also occur after the use of antiemetics, anorectics, or nasal decongestants that contain sympathomimetic agents and antihistamines. Orofacial dyskinesia developed in one patient following an overdose of carbamazepine.

From 15 to 30% of patients on continuous neuroleptic therapy eventually develop tardive dyskinesia. The risk of acquiring this complication increases with higher drug doses, prolonged drug use, and increasing age. Women are more commonly affected than men.

The blepharospasm and facial tics of tardive dyskinesia may improve if the causative drug is identified and discontinued. If they do not do so, or if the drug cannot be stopped for medical reasons, botulinum toxin A can be used to control the spasms (see below).

In contrast to tardive dyskinesia, which occurs 1 to 2 years after beginning drug therapy, some patients develop an acute dystonic reaction after 2 to 5 days on neuroleptics. The reaction usually consists of abnormal postures and intermittent or sustained muscle spasms, but some patients develop blepharospasm or oculogyric crises. This reaction is more likely to occur among young patients on high doses of medication.

Facial Tics and Tourette Syndrome

In contrast to the sustained, dystonic movements typical of blepharospasm, facial tics are usually brief, clonic, and jerk-like. They tend to be stereotyped and repetitive. They can vary in frequency, increasing when the patient is bored, tired, or anxious. Eye-winking tics are most commonly observed in childhood, tend to be unilateral, and affect boys more often than girls. They resolve spontaneously after months or years.

When facial tics begin between 2 and 15 years of age, last more than 1 year, fluctuate in severity, and are associated with other motor multifocal tics, vocalizations (e.g., grunting, sniffing, barking, throat-clearing, utterance of obscenities), obscene gestures, and other aberrancies of behavior, **Tourette syndrome** (also called Gilles de la Tourette syndrome) should be considered. Ocular manifestations are common in this condition and include blinking, blepharospasm, forced staring, and involuntary gaze deviation.

Patients with Tourette syndrome have enhanced recovery cycles. In addition, tics and blepharospasm may coexist in the same patient and among other family members. These findings suggest that many of these disorders share common underlying mechanisms.

Nonorganic Blepharospasm

Nonorganic blepharospasm generally has a sudden onset and is usually preceded by an emotionally traumatic event. Although quite rare, it is more common among children and young adults with serious psychologic problems. The blepharospasm is frequently bilateral and may last for hours, weeks, or even months, at which point it may spontaneously resolve. The eyelids are sometimes gently, sometimes forcibly, closed. In some patients, psychotherapy, behavior therapy, hypnosis, or biofeedback are of benefit. In others, a single injection of botulinum toxin is sufficient to eliminate the spasms permanently.

Focal Seizures

Several eyelid phenomena are associated with seizures. An adversive (jacksonian) seizure from an irritative focus in the frontal eye fields can evoke contralateral spasmodic eyelid closure, twitching of the face, and "spastic" lateral gaze. Blinking or fluttering of the eyelids may also be observed in psychomotor or absence seizures. Blinking is usually bilateral and symmetric, although unilateral blinking ipsilateral to the seizure focus may occur.

A form of photomyoclonic epilepsy consists of the combination of eyelid "myoclonia" and absence spells. Upon eyelid closure, there is a marked blinking of the eyelids, upward deviation of the eyes, and a brief absence period during which electroencephalography shows bilateral 3 to 5 Hz spike-and-wave discharges. These seizures are triggered by the elimination of central fixation (fixation-off sensitive). The marked jerking of the lids and gaze deviation of eyelid myoclonia is usually easily distinguished from the slight flutter of the eyelids unassociated with any ocular deviation that is more typically seen in patients with pure absence seizures.

Seizures induced by eyelid closure or blinking represent a rare form of stimulus-sensitive epilepsy (usually absences or myoclonic attacks). The stimulus responsible for inducing the seizure in some cases is presumed to be the result of proprioceptive inputs. In other cases, a decrease in retinal illumination or a loss of central fixation brought on by eyelid closure precipitates the seizure (scotosensitive seizures). In some cases both the act of eyelid closure *and* a loss of central fixation are required.

Lid-Triggered Synkinesias

Eyelid closure occasionally triggers movements of muscles that are not innervated by the facial nerve, presumably from a central or supranuclear disturbance. In one patient with a progressive neurodegenerative condition, eyelid closure was associated with mouth opening and fanning of the fingers. In another case, eyelid closure was associated with closing of the hand.

Firm external stimulation of the cornea elicits a brisk anterolateral jaw movement to the side opposite the stimulus associated with eyelid closure: the **corneomandibular reflex.** An acquired palpebromandibular synkinesia occurs in which jaw movements, similar to the corneomandibular reflex, regularly accompany spontaneous eye blinks without an external corneal stimulus. This **palpebromandibular reflex** is associated with bihemispheric or upper brainstem pathology.

Facial Myokymia (with and without Spastic Paretic Facial Contracture)

The term **facial myokymia** refers to involuntary, fine, continuous, undulating contractions that spread across facial muscles. The contractions are usually unilateral. Electrophysiologically, affected muscles show brief tetanic bursts of motor unit potentials that recur in a rhythmic or semirhythmic fashion several times a second as singlets, doublets, or groups. These bursts recur at a rate of 3 to 8 Hz.

The most common type of facial myokymia occurs in otherwise normal persons and affects only the orbicularis oculi of the lower (or, occasionally, the upper) eyelid on one side. This eyelid myokymia often begins at times of excessive fatigue or stress. It usually lasts for several days, but it may persist for a few weeks and even for several months. During this time, it is usually intermittent, lasting for several hours at a time. Patients with this condition may become alarmed, particularly because they can feel the eyelid fasciculations. They often believe that their eye is "jumping," and some patients actually experience oscillopsia from the effects of the myokymic eyelid against the globe. Eyelid myokymia that persists continuously for several months is usually benign, but it may be a sign of dysfunction near the facial nerve nucleus in the dorsal pons.

Many disorders characterized by involuntary movements of the facial muscles can begin with eyelid myokymia, including essential blepharospasm, Meige syndrome, hemifacial spasm, and spastic-paretic facial contracture. This last disorder is characterized by myokymia that first begins in the orbicularis oculi muscle and gradually spreads to most of the muscles on one side of the face. At the same time, associated tonic contracture of the affected muscles becomes evident. Over a period of weeks or months, the nasolabial groove slowly deepens, the corner of the mouth is drawn laterally, the palpebral fissure narrows, and all the facial muscles become weak. As the contracture becomes more pronounced, voluntary facial movements on the affected side diminish (Fig. 22.44). Spastic-paretic facial contracture, like eyelid myokymia, is a sign of pontine dysfunction in the region of the facial nerve nucleus.

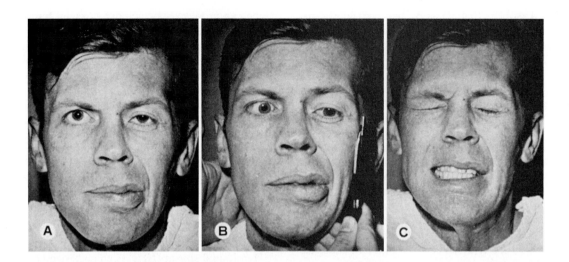

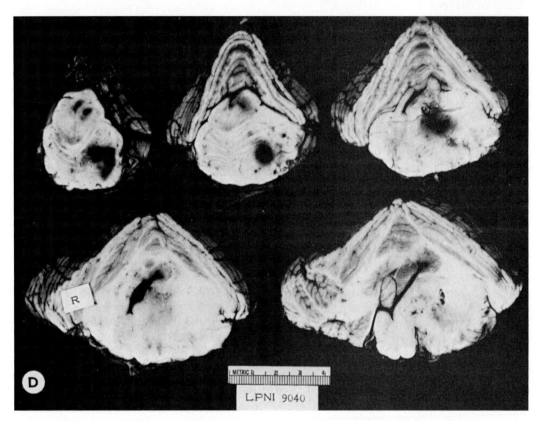

Figure 22.44. Spastic paretic facial contracture associated with a pontine astrocytoma. *A.* The patient's face is at rest. Note deepened nasolabial groove and narrowed palpebral fissure on the left. *B.* On attempted left gaze, the patient shows a horizontal gaze palsy. *C.* Voluntary forced eyelid closure exposes the paresis of the left orbicularis oculi and the left side of the face. *D.* The brainstem in this patient shows a left-sided astrocytoma. (Reprinted with permission from Sogg RL, Hoyt WF, Boldrey E. Spastic paretic facial contracture: a rare sign of brain stem tumor. Neurology 1963; 13:607–612.)

Disorders that are associated with spastic-paretic facial contracture and, to a much lesser extent, persistent eyelid myokymia, include MS, intrinsic brainstem neoplasms (particularly gliomas but also metastatic tumors), extra-axial neoplasms compressing the brainstem (e.g., chordomas), syringobulbia, brainstem vascular lesions, GBS, obstructive hydrocephalus, subarachnoid hemorrhage, basilar invagination, Machado-Joseph disease, brainstem tuberculoma, cysticercosis, and autosomal-dominant striatonigral degeneration. In most instances, the phenomenon and the pathology that causes it are unilateral, but bilateral facial myokymia from bilateral pontine disease may occur in patients with GBS, following cardiopulmonary arrest, during the course of a lymphocytic meningoradiculitis, and following exposure to a variety of toxins.

The pathophysiology of transient facial myokymia is unknown. MRI in patients with MS who have continuous facial myokymia often shows changes consistent with demyelination in the postgenu portion of the fascicle of the facial nerve in the dorsolateral pontine tegmentum. In all autopsy cases in which a brainstem tumor is responsible for the condition, the tumor infiltrates the pontine tegmentum, basis pontis, or both, sparing the facial nerve nucleus and its neurons. It has therefore been suggested that the lack of direct damage to the ipsilateral facial nerve nucleus in the presence of more rostrally placed lesions produces a functional deafferentation, possibly of local circuit neurons. This, in turn, results in hyperexcitability of facial nerve neurons, thus causing eyelid myokymia and spastic-paretic facial contracture. When the facial nerve nucleus itself is damaged by the pathologic process, the facial spasm resolves, leaving only facial paralysis and contracture. This hypothesis explains the phenomenon of facial myokymia and spastic-paretic facial contracture in patients with brainstem lesions but not in patients with peripheral neuropathies (see below).

Excessive Eyelid Closure of Peripheral Facial Nerve Origin

Facial Myokymia with Peripheral Neuropathy

The development of facial myokymia in patients with GBS, poliomyelitis, parotid gland tumor, and some peripheral nerve disorders indicates that damage to the peripheral facial nerve alone can produce hyperactivity of facial muscles. Other evidence that peripheral nerve injury can produce facial hyperactivity includes EMG studies that reveal that myokymia is common in patients with Bell's palsy, and the observation that timber rattlesnake envenomation causes facial myokymia from damage to the peripheral nerve. Thus, the occurrence of facial myokymia in a patient with apparent peripheral facial nerve dysfunction does not necessarily indicate an underlying central process. Myokymic discharges of peripheral nerve origin are usually attributed to spontaneous ectopic excitation arising in demyelinated fibers.

Hemifacial Spasm

Hemifacial spasm (HFS) is characterized by involuntary paroxysmal bursts of painless, unilateral, tonic or clonic contractions of muscles innervated by the facial nerve (Fig. 22.45). It occurs most commonly in middle-aged adults, but it may develop at any age, including infancy and childhood. The condition is almost always sporadic, but there are familial cases. Bilateral cases occur but are exceptionally rare.

HFS usually begins in the orbicularis oculi and then spreads slowly over months to years to the lower facial muscles. The spasms may be triggered by voluntary facial movements or positional changes, and they may worsen with fatigue, stress, or anxiety. Longstanding HFS is almost always associated with ipsilateral lower facial weakness, although this may be hard to detect, either because it is usually fairly mild or because of the constant spasms. In any event, facial movements between spasms usually appear normal. Most patients with HFS have clinical evidence, EMG evidence, or both, of synkinesis between the orbicularis oculi and orbicularis oris muscles.

There is considerable evidence, based primarily on direct observations at surgery, that most cases of HFS are caused by pulsatile compression of the proximal region of the facial nerve at the root entry zone (the transitional zone between central and peripheral myelin) by normal vessels in an aberrant location or dolichoectatic vessels. The blood vessels most commonly responsible for the compression are the anterior inferior cerebellar artery, the posterior inferior cerebellar artery, and the vertebral artery. Less commonly, one or more veins accompanying

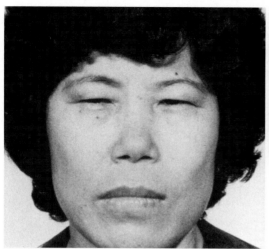
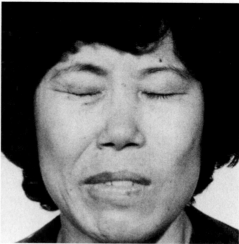

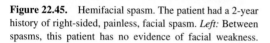

Figure 22.45.   Hemifacial spasm. The patient had a 2-year history of right-sided, painless, facial spasm. *Left:* Between spasms, this patient has no evidence of facial weakness.

Right: During a spasm, the right eyelid closes, and the right side of the face is drawn up.

these vessels seem to be responsible. A variety of imaging techniques, including CT scanning, MRI, MR angiography, and CT angiography may show ipsilateral displacement, tortuosity, or enlargement of the basilar or vertebral arteries in patients with HFS.

Although HFS appears to be caused by vascular compression from otherwise normal arteries or veins in over 99% of cases, vascular structures other than normal vessels can also compress the facial nerve at the root entry zone, producing HFS. These lesions include aneurysms, AVMs, intratemporal hemangiomas, and arterial dissections. Extra-axial tumors located in the CPA can produce HFS, including epidermoids, vestibular schwannomas (acoustic neuromas), meningiomas, cholesteatomas, and lipomas. Occasionally, HSF is produced by intraparenchymal brainstem lesions, including tumors and granulomas. Other rare causes include arachnoid cysts, MS, pontine infarction, hemosiderosis, arachnoiditis, and bony compression. HFS may occur as a false localizing sign in patients with tumors located in the contralateral CPA and in patients with pseudotumor cerebri. It may also occur after injury to the peripheral facial nerve. In some cases, HFS is associated with evidence of hyperfunction of other cranial nerves. The most common association is with trigeminal neuralgia.

Although there is general agreement regarding the importance of facial nerve decompression in the treatment of HFS (see below), the underlying neurophysiologic mechanism that produces the condition remains controversial. One theory is that HFS is the result of ephaptic transmission or crosstalk between branches of the facial nerve at the root entry zone where there is a focus of demyelination. Another theory, however, is that the facial motor nucleus changes in response to peripheral nerve injury. Central anatomic changes in response to peripheral nerve injury is a well-established phenomenon that could theoretically unmask synkinetic facial movements. It has also been suggested that chronic pulsatile arterial antidromic stimulation of the facial nerve increases the excitability of facial motor neurons through "kindling."

There still remains a subgroup of patients with HFS who have no obvious vascular compression yet improve after surgery. The improvement in such patients may be consequent to mild operative trauma and manipulation of the nerve rather than to the decompression itself. In addition, the severity of vascular compression observed in patients with HFS is extremely variable, ranging from obvious displacement and grooving of the facial nerve, to displacement without grooving, to touching without either displacement or grooving. That veins and, in some cases, venules, can cause HFS by apparent compression of the facial nerve is also problematic.

The only way to cure HFS is posterior fossa microvascular decompression. Although this procedure has a defined morbidity, the results are generally excellent. When performed by an experienced surgeon, the overall cure rate is 85 to 90%. Most patients whose condition is cured experience disappearance of HFS within 3 to 10 days after surgery, although a smaller group can take weeks to months to resolve. Among patients whose HFS persists after apparently successful surgery (i.e., the vessel compressing the nerve is identified and moved), 5 to 10% will be cured after a second operation.

Like the success rate, the complication rate of posterior fossa microvascular decompression for HFS varies according to the experience of the surgeon performing the operation. In some series, the complication rate is reported to be as high as 25%; in others, it is only 1 to 2%. The most common persistent complications are ipsilateral hearing loss (1 to 13%) and facial paralysis (1 to 6%). The mortality of this procedure is exceptionally low; however, death or disabling stroke from brainstem or cerebellar infarction can occur.

The results of medical therapy for HFS are generally disappointing. The most commonly used drugs are carbamazepine (Tegretol), diphenylhydantoin (Dilantin), and dimethylaminoethanol (Deanol).

Surgical procedures other than microvascular decompression produce similarly disappointing results. These procedures include intracanalicular facial nerve neurotomy and partial avulsion, section, longitudinal splitting, or radiofrequency destruction of the extracranial portion of the facial nerve. In some instances, section of the facial nerve is followed by a hypoglossal-facial anastomosis to relieve the resultant facial paralysis. None of these procedures is without complication, and the recurrence rate is considerable.

Intramuscular injections of botulinum toxin can be used to control, but not cure, HFS. In our opinion, this mode of therapy is the only effective alternative for those patients unwilling or unable to undergo posterior fossa microvascular decompression of the facial nerve (see below), although other injectable drugs, particularly doxorubicin (adriamycin) are under investigation.

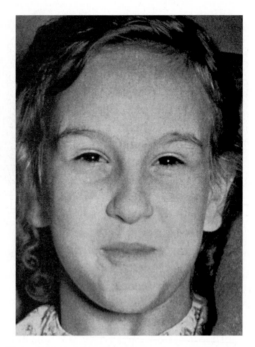

Figure 22.46. Mild risus sardonicus in a child with tetanus. Increased tone of all facial muscles is evident. Note that the child appears to be smiling. Her apparent bilateral ptosis is caused by myotonia of the orbicularis oculi muscles. (Reprinted with permission from Ford FR. Diseases of the Nervous System in Infancy, Childhood and Adolescence. 5th ed. Springfield, IL: CC Thomas, 1966:621.)

Excessive Eyelid Closure of Neuromuscular Origin

Neuromuscular hyperexcitability of the orbicularis oculi is usually part of a generalized disorder. The excitability may be latent, spasmodic, or constant. In hypoparathyroidism or during hyperventilation, a tap over the lateral orbital margin produces contraction of the ipsilateral orbicularis muscles and the surrounding facial muscles (latent hyperexcitability). Strychnine poisoning causes spasmodic hyperexcitability, and tetanus causes a constant or sustained neuromuscular hyperexcitability manifested in the facial muscles as risus sardonicus (Fig. 22.46).

Excessive Eyelid Closure of Myopathic Origin

Myotonia of the orbicularis oculi may occur in association with a number of disorders. For example, patients can develop eyelid myotonia in association with primary hypothyroidism. The

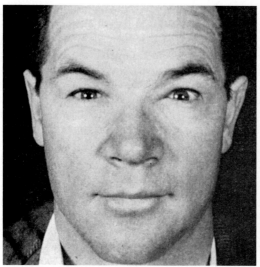
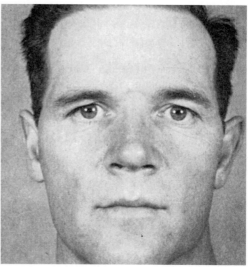
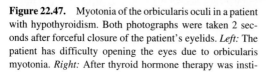

Figure 22.47. Myotonia of the orbicularis oculi in a patient with hypothyroidism. Both photographs were taken 2 seconds after forceful closure of the patient's eyelids. *Left:* The patient has difficulty opening the eyes due to orbicularis myotonia. *Right:* After thyroid hormone therapy was insti- tuted, the patient's myotonia disappeared. (Reprinted with permission from Sisson JC, Beierwaltes WH, Koepke GH, et al. "Myotonia" of the orbicularis oculi with myxedema. Arch Intern Med 1962;110:323–327.)

myotonia typically disappears after such patients are treated with replacement thyroid medication (Fig. 22.47).

Patients with both the congenital and adult forms of myotonic dystrophy may show myotonia of the orbicularis oculi. In one infant with congenital myotonic dystrophy, startle with a loud noise or a bright light caused tight eye closure followed by slow opening over many seconds. EMG studies demonstrate evidence of prolonged contraction in the orbicularis oculi following a blink in adults with myotonic dystrophy (see Chapter 20).

Myotonia of the orbicularis oculi may occur in patients with hyperkalemic familial periodic paralysis. Slowness of eyelid opening or temporary narrowing of the palpebral fissure may occur following sustained eyelid closure, application of ice to the lids, or administration of potassium salts. Eyelid myotonia can also occur in patients with chondrodystrophic myotonia (Schwartz-Jampel syndrome) (see Chapter 20).

Botulinum Toxin for Eyelid and Facial Spasms

Botulinum toxin is a neurotoxin produced by the anaerobic bacterium *Clostridium botulinum.* It exists in seven immunologically distinct serotypes (A, B, C1, C2, D, E, F, G). Type A is the most widely used for treatment. It is manufactured in the United States as Botox and in Europe as Dysport. Both Botox and Dysport are packaged as a freeze-dried powder in sterile, vacuum-sealed vials that contain 100 units of Botox (1 unit = 0.4 ng) or 500 units of Dysport. It has been estimated that 1 unit of Botox is equivalent to 3 units of Dysport in potency. Botulinum toxin type F is a potential alternative to botulinum toxin type A, but it is not available except on an experimental basis.

Locally injected toxin rapidly binds to peripheral cholinergic synapses at the neuromuscular junction, preventing the presynaptic release of acetylcholine. The histopathologic effects of botulinum toxin are consistent with denervation of muscle fibers; however, they are transient, and recovery is associated with sprouting of new nerve terminals and restoration of normal muscle morphology. Repeated injections over many years do not appear to cause irreversible changes in orbicularis oculi or other muscle fibers.

Botulinum toxin is an effective therapy for many conditions that cause abnormal localized muscle contractions or spasms. The toxin is injected intramuscularly or subcutaneously to treat a variety of disorders characterized by involuntary movements of the face, including blepharospasm, oromandibular dystonia, tardive dyskinesia, Tourette syndrome, HFS, postparalytic aberrant regeneration of the facial nerve, eyelid myokymia, apraxia of eyelid opening, and spastic entropion. Botulinum toxin can also be used to produce a temporary tarsorrhaphy in patients with facial nerve paresis and to transiently reduce or eliminate lid retraction in patients with thyroid orbitopathy. Botulinum toxin can be used to treat a variety of focal dystonias, including torticollis and spasmodic dysphonia. It can also be used to treat strabismus from a variety of causes, including ocular motor nerve palsies, gaze palsies, internuclear ophthalmoplegia, myasthenia gravis, and thyroid orbitopathy. Both congenital and acquired forms of nystagmus may be reduced by retrobulbar injection of botulinum toxin; however, a variety of side effects limit the usefulness of the drug in this setting (see Chapter 19).

The results of botulinum toxin treatment of eyelid spasms are remarkably consistent. Administered by injection in the vicinity of affected muscles, botulinum toxin type A produces weakening of the muscles within 1 to 5 days and achieves a maximum therapeutic effect within 1 to 2 weeks (Fig. 22.48). About 90 to 100% of patients experience a transient reduction in spasms that lasts 2 to 6 months. The duration is somewhat dose-dependent, but there is a maximum dose for any given patient beyond which a further increase does not result in either an increased reduction in spasms or an increased duration of effect. In addition, the development of side effects at higher doses limits the amount that can be effectively administered. Patients with HFS usually experience longer periods of relief, often 4 months or longer, than patients with essential blepharospasm.

Although nearly all patients experience some degree of weakening of muscles after injection of botulinum toxin, functional failures have been observed to occur in up to 23% of patients. In many instances, such failures are sporadic, and subsequent injections of the same dose or higher doses administered within 10 days to 4 weeks of the initial treatment will achieve the desired effect. Nevertheless, there remains a small group of patients with unusually refractory blepharospasm, who, even after receiving maximum dosages of botulinum toxin, ultimately require surgery.

Follow-up studies show that botulinum toxin type A maintains its efficacy for 10 years or more and that most patients do not develop intolerance or become refractory to the drug, although some patients do seem to become resistant to treatment. Patients injected chronically and frequently with large amounts of botulinum toxin for spasmodic torticollis may develop antibodies to the drug, and the disorder in some of these patients then may become refractory to this therapy. Immunoresistance has not been demonstrated in patients undergoing treatment for eyelid or facial spasms, probably because lower doses are used in the treatment of these conditions. Nevertheless, despite the lack of clear evidence of immunoresistance to botulinum toxin type A in patients treated for eyelid and facial spasms, it would seem prudent to administer the smallest possible dose and to minimize the number of short-term reinjections (within 1 month) at higher doses.

Despite minor side effects from injections of botulinum toxin, most patients with significant eyelid and facial spasms continue to undergo repeated injections of the drug to control their spasms. Side effects are usually mild, well-tolerated, and short-lived. The most common side effect is swelling of the upper or lower eyelid, sometimes accompanied by ecchymosis at the site of the injection. The ecchymoses typically resolve in several days to about 1 week. Weakening of the orbicularis oculi may produce subjective symptoms of dryness, more often in patients with HFS than in patients with blepharospasm. Lagophthalmos and ectropion can result in a mild exposure keratopathy characterized by irritation, redness of the eye, epiphora, and blurred vision. This effect generally resolves in 1 to 2 weeks and can be treated in the meantime with topical ocular lubricants.

Injections of botulinum toxin into the upper eyelid can spread to the levator muscle, producing a transient ptosis, whereas injections into either the upper or lower eyelid can spread to one of the extraocular muscles, producing diplopia. Both complications generally resolve in 1 to 3 weeks. Injecting facial muscles other than the orbicularis oculi can result in facial weakness that can be quite troublesome for the patient, particularly the patient with HFS who already has some degree of facial weakness (see above).

Complications, such as a flu-like illness, GBS, or aplastic anemia, have been described in rare

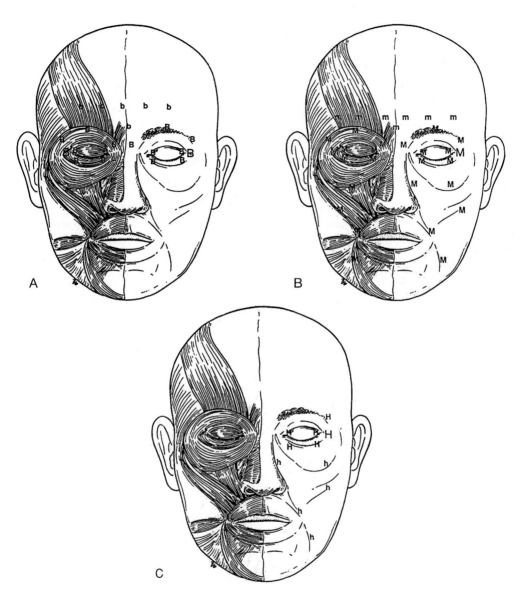

Figure 22.48. Sites of injections of botulinum toxin type A for blepharospasm, Meige syndrome and hemifacial spasm. *A.* Sites of injection for essential blepharospasm. Each site indicated by a small, uppercase *B* is injected with 2.5 to 5.0 units of Botox. The lateral canthal region is injected with 7.5 to 15 units of Botox (large, uppercase B). In selected patients, various sites in the forehead and in the region of the corrugator and procerus muscles may be injected with 2.5 to 5.0 units of Botox per site (lowercase b). *B.* Sites of injection for Meige syndrome with blepharospasm who require middle and lower facial injections. Each site indicated by a small, uppercase *M* is injected with 2.5 to 5.0 units of Botox. The lateral canthal region is injected with 7.5 to 15 units of Botox (large, uppercase *M*). In specific patients, various sites in the forehead and in the region of the corrugator and procerus muscles may be injected with 2.5 to 5.0 units of Botox per site (lowercase *m*). *C.* Sites of injection for left hemifacial spasm. Each site indicated by a small, uppercase *H* is injected with 2.5 units of Botox. The lateral canthal region is injected with 7.5 units of Botox (large, uppercase *H*). In selected patients, regions in the middle and lower face may be injected with 1.25 to 2.5 units of Botox (lowercase, *h*). (Reprinted with permission from Miller NR. Essential blepharospasm, Meige syndrome, atypical blepharospasm, and hemifacial spasm. In: Johnson RT, Griffin JW, eds. Current Therapy in Neurologic Disease. 5th ed. St Louis: CV Mosby, 1996:296–302.)

patients after botulinum toxin injections, but no causal relationship has been confirmed in such cases. Evidence of autonomic dysfunction can be detected in some patients after botulinum toxin injection, as can EMG abnormalities in muscles distant from the site of injection, but these effects are clinically asymptomatic.

Contraindications to the use of botulinum toxin include allergy to the drug, infection or inflammation at the site of injection, uncooperative patients, and coagulopathies. Large amounts of botulinum toxin should not be injected in patients with myasthenia gravis or the Lambert-Eaton syndrome, but small amounts, such as those used to treat strabismus, are perfectly safe. The safety of botulinum toxin during lactation or pregnancy is not established, but pregnant and postpartum women have been injected without adverse consequences to the fetus or neonate.

The optimum total dosage, the number and location of injection sites, and the volume per injection site vary within a limited set of parameters. There is no single combination of injection sites and dosage shown to be superior to any other; therefore, most physicians tailor therapy to the severity and distribution of facial spasms in the individual patient.

FOR MORE INFORMATION:
See Walsh & Hoyt's *Clinical Neuro-Ophthalmology,* 5th edition, Volume 1, Chapter 32, pp. 1509–1592.

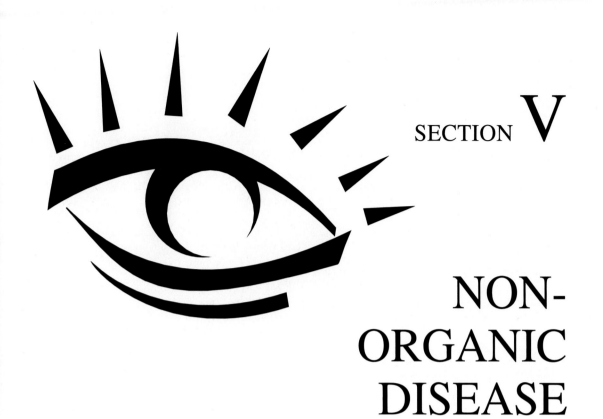

SECTION V

NON-ORGANIC DISEASE

CHAPTER 23

Neuro-Ophthalmologic Manifestations of Nonorganic Disease

Patients who have physical signs and symptoms for which no adequate organic cause can be found may receive any one of a large range of diagnostic labels, including functional illness, functional overlay, hysteria, hysterical overlay, conversion reaction, psychophysiological reaction, somatization reaction, hypochondriasis, invalid reaction, neurasthenia, psychogenic reaction, psychosomatic illness, malingering, and Münchausen's syndrome. This plethora of labels highlights the confusion that occurs when one tries to fit patients with nonorganic disease into a formal classification. For instance, it has been stated that ''la belle indifférence'' is one of the hallmarks of a conversion reaction; however, many ''hysterical'' patients do not show an indifferent attitude to their illness, and depression rather than indifference is present in about one-third of such patients. Certainly, it is difficult to classify various types of nonorganic disease.

Several issues need to be addressed in order to better define nonorganic disease. These issues include the nature of the symptom or symptoms, the somatic or physical aspect of the disorder, the ideation and affect of the patient, the patient's at-

titude toward those trying to diagnose and treat the condition, and the patient's motivation.

The **nature of the symptom** and the manner of its communication are crucial in the understanding of a nonorganic disorder. The patient may be stoic and restrained, or histrionic and dramatizing. The symptom may take the form of a physical dysfunction (e.g., strabismus) that is displayed with a minimum of verbal description, or the symptom may be described verbally during the examination. Therefore, one must determine the **nature of the physical dysfunction** and the degree of disability. It is important to determine why the symptoms have focused in a particular area (e.g., the visual system).

Another consideration is the amount of time a patient spends thinking about his or her symptoms and the precise nature of the thoughts in phenomenologic terms. This concept is called **ideation.** For example, is the patient phobic or deluded?

A patient's **affect** may tell the physician much about the patient's complaints. Some patients clearly are depressed, whereas others are truly indifferent, and still others are anxious. Of particular interest is a patient's **attitude toward those involved in the diagnosis and treatment of his or her condition.** These are persons with whom one would expect the patient to cooperate in an attempt to get well. Is the patient hostile, suspicious, fearful, flirtatious, pleading, aloof, or excessively cooperative and agreeable?

Understanding a patient's **motivation** or incentive for achieving the "sick role" and the degree to which he or she is conscious of it may be the most difficult part of the diagnostic process but may be the most crucial. The nature of motivation may range from an unconscious seeking of the dependency-gratifying and guilt-allaying aspects of the "sick role" to the overtly conscious attempt to obtain attention, sympathy, material gain, or a combination of these.

Considering these complicated issues, it is difficult to classify nonorganic illness clearly and concisely. For this reason, some authors consider all such disorders to be examples of **abnormal illness behavior.**

TERMINOLOGY

Most nonorganic disturbances are categorized by three types: malingering, Münchausen syndrome, and psychogenic.

MALINGERING

Patients whose symptoms are consciously and voluntarily produced are said to be **malingering.** A symptom reported by a malingerer, such as diplopia, is not psychogenic because the patient is not, in fact, experiencing the symptom. Malingering can be divided into several different categories, including (1) simulation of nonexistent disease, (2) elaboration of preexisting disease, and (3) attribution of a disability to a different cause, usually in the setting of potential compensation.

MÜNCHAUSEN SYNDROME

Malingering must be differentiated from **factitious disorder with physical symptoms,** also called the **Münchausen syndrome.** Patients with this condition intentionally produce physical symptoms and signs, some of which may be ocular. Symptoms might include swelling and redness of the conjunctiva simulating an orbital cellulitis, scarring of the eyelids and conjunctiva, and even chorioretinal scarring, all of which are then presented to members of the medical profession. Although the motivation for malin-

gering might be monetary compensation or avoidance of military service, patients with Münchausen syndrome are thought to harbor a psychologic internal need to adopt the role of the sick person.

PSYCHOGENIC DISTURBANCE

Patients whose symptoms seem truly independent of volition are said to have a somatoform disorder or **psychogenic disturbance.** Examples of psychogenic disturbances include: (1) body dysmorphic disorder, (2) conversion disorder (hysteria, conversion reaction), (3) hypochondriasis, and (4) somatization disorder.

A **body dysmorphic disorder** is characterized by a patient's perception of a single physical defect, most often in the facial region, including the eye. The patient is preoccupied with this sign even though it is minimal (e.g., a mild ptosis or anisocoria) or not present at all.

A **conversion disorder** is diagnosed if alterations or a loss of physical functioning are present that seem to express a psychologic conflict or need rather than indicating organic illness. This disorder comprises the clinical syndromes that were previously classified as "hysteria" or "conversion neurosis." Patients in whom such disorders occur may subconsciously obtain both primary gain (e.g., protection from trauma or reduction of stress) and secondary gain (e.g., increased attention).

Hypochondriasis is the fear of, or strong belief in, specific serious physical conditions accompanied by excessive self-observation and the reporting of numerous physical signs and symptoms. It differs from body dysmorphic disorder in that it includes both symptoms and signs from multiple organ systems throughout the body.

A **somatization disorder** features recurrent and multiple somatic complaints. As in hypochondriasis, multiple organ systems may be mentioned, but the patient's descriptions are vague, and anxiety or depression is usually present.

Unfortunately, there remains a large group of patients in whom a clear distinction among malingering, Münchausen syndrome, and psychogenic or somatoform disturbances simply cannot be made. In such cases, the physician must recognize that there is no organic basis for the patient's symptoms and signs and manage the patient accordingly.

SPECIFIC NONORGANIC NEURO-OPHTHALMOLOGIC DISORDERS

From a neuro-ophthalmologic standpoint, there are five areas that may be affected by nonorganic disease:

1. Vision, including visual acuity and visual field.
2. Ocular motility and alignment.
3. Pupillary size and reactivity.
4. Eyelid position and function.
5. Corneal and facial sensation.

The physician faced with a patient complaining of decreased vision or some other disturbance related to the afferent or efferent visual systems for which there is no apparent biologic explanation has two responsibilities. First, the physician must ascertain that an organic disorder is not present. Second, the physician should clinically challenge the patient to see or do something that would not be possible if the condition were organic in nature. To best achieve these goals, the physician must adopt an **empathetic** attitude toward the patient regardless of the patient's history, attitude of the patient toward the physician or the disease, or the clinical findings. If the physician has or is perceived to have a cynical, disbelieving, or confrontational attitude, the patient may not cooperate fully during the examination, and the results will be unsatisfactory.

NONORGANIC DISEASE AFFECTING THE AFFERENT VISUAL PATHWAY

Nonorganic disease that affects the afferent visual system may occur as monocular or binocular decreased visual acuity, abnormal visual fields, or both. Color vision often is abnormal in such patients (depending on the manner in which it is tested), but abnormal color vision is rarely a primary complaint.

Decreased Visual Acuity

Decreased visual acuity is probably the most common nonorganic disturbance in ophthalmology. It occurs most often in children and young adults, but it may be observed in older patients. It may be psychogenic or caused by malingering. Nonorganic visual loss that is psychogenic seems to be more common in children, with females being affected far more often than males.

Malingerers are most often adult males, perhaps because men are more often involved in motor vehicle and work-related accidents than are women.

Patients with nonorganic loss of visual acuity complain of a variable loss of vision in one or both eyes that is not accompanied by a refractive error, a disturbance of the ocular media, or objective evidence of retinal or optic nerve dysfunction. Abnormal color perception, an abnormal visual field, or both may accompany the visual loss.

In many cases, the physician may suspect that the patient's visual loss is nonorganic during the medical history interview, which is perhaps the most crucial aspect of the evaluation. In addition, the way the patient acts during the history taking may be helpful. Patients who are truly blind in both eyes tend to look directly at the person with whom they are speaking, whereas patients with nonorganic blindness, particularly patients who are malingering, often look in some other direction. Similarly, we have noted that patients claiming complete or nearly complete blindness often wear sunglasses, even though they do not have photophobia, and the external appearance of the eyes is perfectly normal.

Evaluation

The physician who suspects a nonorganic visual process may be able to orient the examination in a way to bring out the nonorganic nature of the visual disturbance. For example, if a patient claims no perception of light, light perception only, or perception of hand motions in one or both eyes, one can use a rotating optokinetic drum or horizontally moving tape to produce a horizontal jerk nystagmus that indicates intact vision of at least 20/400 (Fig. 23.1). It is important in this regard that the images on the tape or drum be sufficiently large that the patient is not able to look around them.

When testing a patient who claims complete loss of vision in one eye only, we begin the test by rotating the drum or moving the tape in front of the patient while he or she has *both* eyes open. Once we elicit good optokinetic nystagmus, we suddenly cover the unaffected eye with the palm of our hand or a hand-held occluder (see Fig. 23.1). The patient with nonorganic loss of vision in one eye will continue to show a jerk nystagmus. We are not comfortable estimating visual acuity in this setting by using an optokinetic

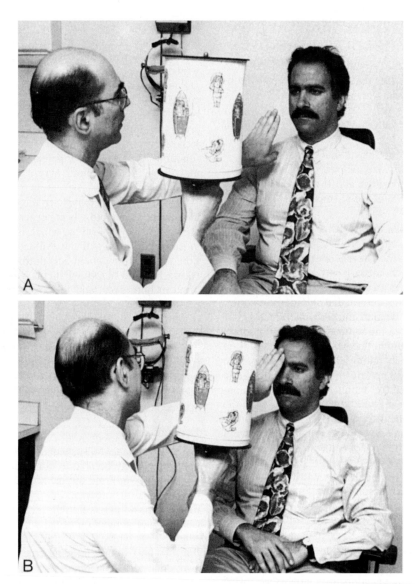

Figure 23.1. Use of optokinetic drum to detect nonorganic blindness. *A.* In a patient claiming bilateral blindness, the patient is asked to look straight ahead with both eyes open while the drum is rotated first in one direction, then in the other. *B.* In a patient claiming unilateral blindness, the drum is first rotated while the patient is instructed to look straight ahead with both eyes open. Once nystagmus is elicited, the examiner continues to rotate the drum and suddenly covers the ''normal'' eye with the palm of the hand and observes the ''blind'' eye for continued nystagmus.

drum with different-sized objects or placing neutral density filters in front of the patient's viewing eye until nystagmus disappears.

A second test that is helpful in detecting visual function in an eye or eyes that are said to have either no perception of light or light perception only is the ''mirror test.'' A large mirror is held in front of the patient's face, and the patient is asked to look directly ahead (Fig. 23.2). The mirror is then rotated and twisted back and forth, causing the images in the mirror to move. Patients with vision better than light perception will show a nystagmoid movement of the eyes, because they cannot avoid following the moving reflection in the mirror.

Some authors recommend placing an 8-prism diopter loose prism with the base directed inward in front of the affected eye of a patient with presumed monocular blindness and asking the patient to view a distant light or target. A report of diplopia indicates that the affected eye is not blind.

An interesting but somewhat extreme course of action taken in the past by some physicians in the Armed Forces when dealing with persons who claimed to have lost all vision in both eyes but in whom there was no organic evidence of disease was to place them at "retinal rest." The patients were told that the "retina was fatigued" and that the condition would only respond to rest. The patient would then be hospitalized with light-tight patches over both eyes placed in such a way that it would be immediately obvious if an attempt were made to remove or adjust them. The patient would not be allowed any sensory stimulation such as a radio, television, or compact disc player. No visitors were allowed, and visits by hospital personnel were kept to a mini-

mum. The patient's vision was checked once a day. This procedure invariably resulted in complete return of vision within a very short period of time.

Another way to detect nonorganic visual loss in a patient who claims to be unable to see shapes or objects in one or both eyes is to ask the patient to touch the tips of the first fingers of both hands together. If the patient claims loss of vision in one eye only, the opposite eye is patched before the test is performed. As every physician knows, the ability to touch the tips of the fingers of two hands together is based not on vision but on proprioception. Thus, patients with organic blindness can easily bring the tips of the first fingers of both hands together, whereas patients with nonorganic blindness, particularly those who are malingering, will not do so (Fig. 23.3). Similarly, a patient with organic blindness can easily sign his or her name without difficulty, whereas patients with blindness caused by malingering may produce an extremely bizarre signature.

Some physicians have tested patients who claim complete or severe loss of vision in one or both eyes by showing them photographs or cards with certain words or phrases that some

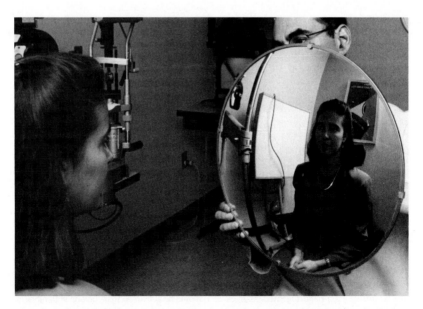

Figure 23.2. Use of a mirror to detect nonorganic blindness. The affected eye is occluded if the patient claims blindness in only one eye; otherwise, both eyes are left open. The patient is instructed to look straight ahead into the mirror, and the mirror is then rotated and turned from side to side. The development of nystagmus or a nystagmoid movement of the eyes indicates that the patient can see moving images in the mirror and thus is not blind.

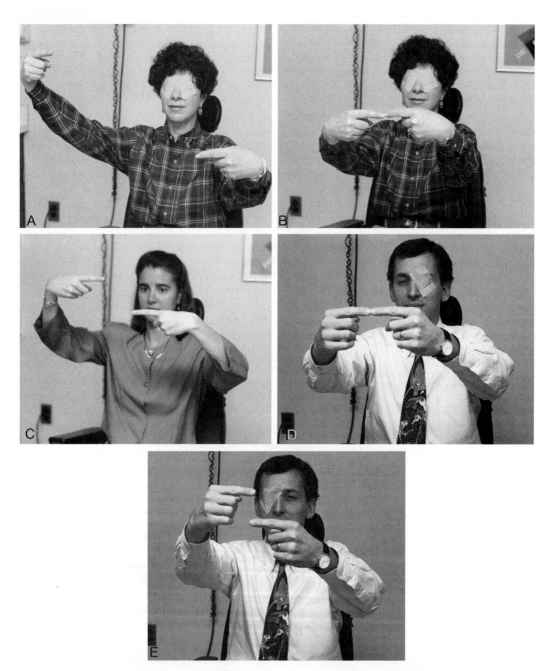

Figure 23.3. Testing nonorganic visual loss by asking a patient who claims monocular or binocular blindness to touch the tips of the first fingers of each hand together. *A–B*. A person who is truly blind can easily touch the tips of the fingers together, using proprioception, as the person in these photographs is doing despite having both eyes occluded. *C.* A woman with nonorganic loss of vision in both eyes is unable to touch the tips of the fingers together, even though she should be able to do so. A person with monocular nonorganic visual loss may touch the tips of the fingers together when viewing with the "normal" eye (*D*), but may claim to be unable to do so when viewing with the "blind" eye (*E*).

persons might consider "objectionable." The patient views this series of photographs or cards only with the "blind" eye or eyes, and the examiner observes the patient for a response to the content of the material being viewed. Gasps, smiles, or other responses suggest that the patient actually has vision in the affected eye. We consider this test too confrontational to recommend it.

A variety of tests may be performed in patients who claim vision in the range of 20/40 to hand motions in one or both eyes. None of these tests is invariably reliable, but one or more is usually sufficient to provide convincing evidence that visual acuity loss either is nonexistent or not as severe as the patient claims.

Visual acuity may be tested not by starting from the largest letters or numbers and moving progressively to smaller ones, but by beginning with the **smallest** line. Assuming that the patient cannot see this first line after being allowed to concentrate for several minutes, the physician tells the patient that the size of the print is now going to be "doubled," and the patient is shown the next larger line and given several minutes to read it. This process is continued until the patient is able to read the line. This method of testing often produces visual acuity better than that initially claimed by the patient. In addition, some projector slides have several 20/20 lines, and these lines may be shown to the patient in succession as the examiner tells the patient the size of the letters is increasing.

Testing of near vision is also important in patients claiming decreased acuity. A discrepancy in the distance and near visual acuity that is not attributable to a refractive error or a disturbance of the media, such as an oil-drop cataract, usually is evidence of a nonorganic disturbance.

The Potential Acuity Meter (Mentor of Norwell, Massachusetts) can be used to diagnose nonorganic visual disease. First, a determination is made of the patient's best corrected visual acuity in each eye. The patient's pupils are then dilated, and the patient is told that a test of potential visual function is going to be performed that bypasses or otherwise circumvents the visual problem and that gives the examiner knowledge of what the patient's vision would be if he or she did not have the reported visual problem. A significant improvement in vision in the affected eye or eyes that is unassociated with any abnor-

mality in the ocular media or retina indicates nonorganic visual loss.

Patients claiming decreased vision in one eye only may undergo a "refraction" in which the normal eye is fogged with a high plus lens (e.g., a + 5.00 or higher sphere), and a lens with minimal power (e.g., a + or −0.50 sphere or cylinder) or the patient's appropriate refraction is placed before the worse eye (Fig. 23.4). The patient is then told to read the chart with "both eyes." A variation of this test is the use of paired cylinders. A plus cylinder and a minus cylinder of the same power (usually from 2 to 6 diopters) are placed at parallel axes in front of the "normal" eye in a trial frame. The patient's normal correction is placed in front of the affected eye. The patient is asked to read with both eyes open a line that previously has been read with the normal eye but not with the affected eye. As the patient begins to read, the axis of one of the cylinders is rotated about 10° to 15°. The axes of the two cylinders thus will no longer be parallel, blurring vision in the normal eye. If the patient continues to read the line or can read it again when asked to do so, he or she must be using the affected eye.

Red-green glasses used with a red and green duochrome slide superimposed on the normal vision chart can be used to induce a patient to read with an eye that supposedly cannot see (or cannot see well) by making the patient think that he or she is using both eyes (Fig. 23.5). In this

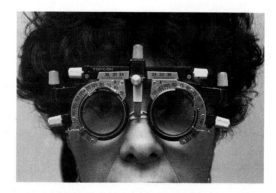

Figure 23.4. Use of a pseudorefraction to detect nonorganic uniocular decreased vision. A high plus lens (+ 7.00 sphere) has been placed in front of the unaffected left eye, and a lens with minimal power (−0.50 cylinder at axis 175°) has been placed in front of the eye with decreased vision. The patient is then told to read the chart with both eyes open.

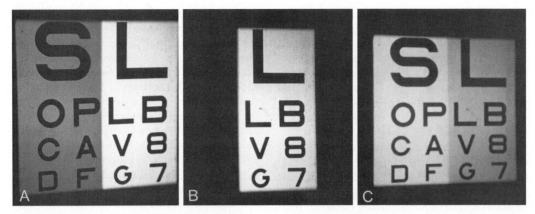

Figure 23.5. Use of red-green glasses with a red-green duochrome slide superimposed on a normal vision chart to detect uniocular nonorganic decreased vision. *A.* Appearance of the chart with superimposed red-green duochrome slide when viewed without red-green lenses. The left side of the chart is seen as red; the right side as green. *B.* The eye viewing through the green lens sees only the letters on the right (green) side of the chart. *C.* The eye viewing through the red lens sees both sets of letters. The lenses are arranged so that the red lens is over the eye with decreased vision, and the patient is asked to read the chart with both eyes open. If the patient reads the letters on both sides of the chart, he or she obviously is using the eye with decreased vision, because the unaffected eye that is viewing through the green lens should only be able to see the letters on one side of the chart.

test, the eye behind the red lens will see the letters on both sides of the chart, whereas the eye behind the green lens will see only those letters on the green side of the chart. The lenses are arranged so that the red lens is over the eye with decreased vision, and the patient is then asked to read the chart with both eyes open. If the patient reads the entire line, it is obvious that the abnormal eye must be functioning better than the patient claims.

A variant of the red-green glasses/duochrome chart test that employs the red-green glasses and Ishihara color plates can be performed in patients with presumed nonorganic monocular visual loss that is worse than 20/400. The patient should first be tested for "congenital" color vision as described below. Once it has been established that color vision is normal, the patient is asked to view the Ishihara color plates while wearing red-green glasses with the red lens over the affected eye. With the exception of plates 1 and 36, the numbers and lines on the Ishihara plates cannot be seen by the eye over which the green filter is placed. Even with visual acuity of 20/400, however, all of the color plates can be seen through a red filter. Thus, a patient who has normal color vision in at least the unaffected eye, who then views the plates through red-green

spectacles with the red lens in front of the affected eye, and who correctly identifies the figures on the plates, must have visual acuity of 20/400 or better in the affected eye.

Polarizing lenses can be used in several ways to detect nonorganic visual loss in a patient with decreased vision in one eye only (Fig. 23.6). In the American Optical Polarizing Test, the patient wears polarizing glasses, and the test object, a Project-O-Chart slide, projects letters alternately so that one letter is seen by both eyes, the next by the right eye, the next by the left eye, and so on. Another test uses a polarizing lens placed before a projector. The patient is asked to read the chart while wearing polarizing lenses, with one eye or the other being allowed to see the whole projected image at a time.

A prism that is 4 diopters in strength can be used to detect vision in an eye said to have reduced or no vision. The patient is asked to look with both eyes at the vision chart. A 4-prism diopter loose prism is then placed base out over the "affected eye." A patient with normal binocular vision will show a movement of both eyes toward the direction of the apex of the prism followed by a shift of the fellow eye back toward the center. A patient with true decreased or absent vision in the eye over which the prism is placed will show no conjugate movement at all, and when the prism is placed over the normal eye of a patient whose other eye truly is blind or has extremely reduced sight, only the first conjugate binocular shift will occur. There will be no compensatory movement of the blind eye back toward the center.

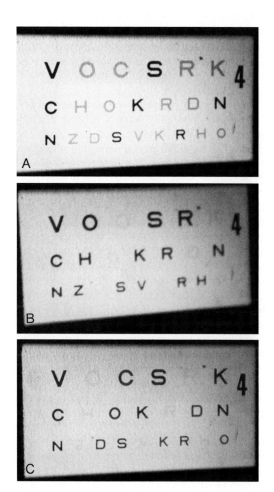

Figure 23.6.   Use of polarizing lenses and a Snellen chart with a superimposed polarizing filter to detect uniocular nonorganic decreased vision. The patient wears the polarizing glasses and is asked to view letters, some of which should be seen by both eyes, some only by the right eye, and some only by the left eye. *A.* Appearance of the entire chart when viewed without polarizing lenses. *B.* Appearance of same chart when viewed through one of the polarizing lenses. *C.* Appearance of chart when viewed through the other polarizing lens. Note that certain letters (e.g., V, S, C, K, N, S, and R) can be seen through both lenses, whereas others can be seen through one of the lenses but not the other.

Several **prism dissociation tests** can be used to detect mild degrees of nonorganic monocular visual loss. In these tests, the patient is first asked if he or she has experienced double vision in addition to loss of vision in the affected eye. If the answer is negative, the patient is told that the examiner will test the alignment of both eyes and that the test should produce vertical double vision. A 4-prism diopter loose prism is then placed base down in front of the unaffected eye at the same time that a 0.5-prism diopter loose prism is simultaneously placed with the base in any direction over the eye with decreased vision. In this way, the patient does not become suspicious that the examiner is paying specific attention to one eye or the other. A 20/20 or larger size Snellen letter is then projected in the distance, and the patient is asked if he or she has double vision. When the patient admits to diplopia, he or she is then asked whether the two letters are of equal quality or sharpness, and an assessment of visual acuity can then be made.

Patients in whom visual acuity is reduced and who have no evidence of a refractive error, disturbance of the ocular media, or a macular abnormality by ophthalmoscopic examination are often assumed to have an underlying optic neuropathy even if the optic disc appears normal. Patients with a true optic neuropathy, however, almost invariably have a disturbance of color vision that can be detected using various types of color plates, such as the Hardy-Rand-Rittler Pseudoisochromatic Plates or the Ishihara Color Plates. We have found it useful to "prepare" the patient suspected of having nonorganic visual loss for the test by asking if he or she was ever diagnosed as having "congenital color blindness." Assuming the patient gives a negative answer, he or she is told that the color vision test the physician is going to perform is a test of congenital color blindness and that the patient should therefore be able to see the figures or numbers.

Testing of stereopsis may be valuable in detecting nonorganic visual loss. There is a definite correlation between binocular visual acuity and stereopsis (Fig. 23.7 and Table 23.1). For instance, a patient with 20/20 vision in one eye and organic visual loss producing visual acuity of 20/200 in the fellow eye has stereoacuity of only about 180 seconds of arc, whereas a patient with 20/20 visual acuity in both eyes has ste-

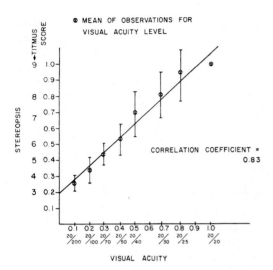

Figure 23.7. The relationship between visual acuity and level of stereopsis. Visual acuity is expressed as the fractional ratio of the Snellen acuity for near vision. Stereopsis is expressed as the fractional ratio of the smallest image disparity, 40 seconds, divided by the image disparity at the level at which a correct response was obtained. The Titmus test target associated with each response is indicated to the left of its fractional value. (Reprinted with permission from Levy NS, Glick EB. Stereoscopic perception and Snellen visual acuity. Am J Ophthalmol 1974;78:722–724.)

Table 23.1
Relationship of Visual Acuity and Stereopsis

VISUAL ACUITY	AVERAGE STEREOPSIS*
20/20	40
20/25	43
20/30	52
20/40	61
20/50	78
20/70	94
20/100	124
20/200	160

Modified from Levy NS, Glick EB. Stereoscopic perception and Snellen visual acuity. Am J Ophthalmol 1974;78:722–724.
* Measured in seconds of image disparity.

reoacuity of 40 seconds of arc. A variety of stereoacuity tests are available, all of which have advantages and disadvantages (Fig. 23.8).

Examination of pupillary responses can be helpful in diagnosing nonorganic visual loss. Patients who report complete blindness in both eyes should have pupils that do not react to light

stimulation unless the process affects the postgeniculate visual pathways. Thus, the pupils of a patient who cannot perceive light with either eye because of bilateral retinal, optic nerve, or optic tract lesions, or because of damage to the optic chiasm, do not react to light stimulation, whereas the pupils of a patient who is blind from bilateral lesions of the optic radiations or striate cortex will react relatively normally to light. Pupils that react to light stimulation in a patient who claims complete loss of vision in both eyes indicate either that the patient is cerebrally blind (usually from damage to the striate cortex; e.g., cortical blindness) or that the patient has nonorganic loss of vision.

Patients with unilateral or asymmetric optic neuropathy invariably have a relative afferent pupillary defect (RAPD) that can easily be detected by performing a swinging flashlight test (see Chapter 15). The absence of a RAPD in a patient with monocular visual loss indicates either that the patient does not have a unilateral optic neuropathy (and thus may support a diagnosis of nonorganic visual loss) or that the patient has a **bilateral** optic neuropathy that is asymmetric. It must be emphasized that patients with electrophysiologic evidence of bilateral optic neuropathy may nevertheless have very asymmetric visual acuity in the two eyes unassociated with a RAPD. Thus, if there is no indication of nonorganic disease in a patient with unexplained, unilateral visual loss without an obvious RAPD, the patient should undergo electrophysiologic testing, particularly full-field and macular electroretinography and pattern-reversal and flash-evoked visual-evoked potentials.

It must be remembered that although electroretinography is an objective test of overall retinal function, visual-evoked responses elicited by pattern reversal may be affected by a variety of factors other than organic disease of the central visual pathways. Some of these factors are related to the way the test is performed and include the size and color of the stimuli and the frequency with which they are presented, background illumination, and the state of dark adaptation. Other factors are related to the patient, including age, attention, concentration, pupil size, and fatigue. Indeed, both the amplitude *and* latency of the P100 peak can be consciously or unconsciously altered by a patient who is either not concentrating or not focusing continuously

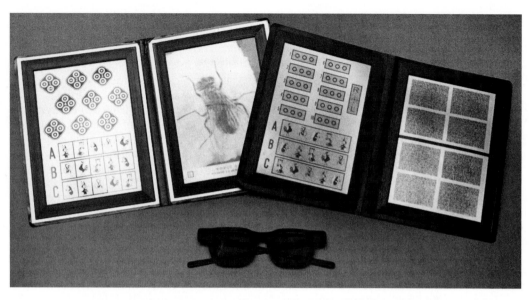

Figure 23.8.   Two tests of stereopsis useful in detecting nonorganic visual loss.

on the target. In addition, several investigators have reported cases in which normal responses were obtained from patients whose blindness was clearly organic in nature.

Management

The management of patients who have nonorganic loss of visual acuity is problematic and often depends on whether the patient is a child or an adult and whether the condition is thought to be psychogenic or caused by malingering.

In our experience, nonorganic visual loss in children occurs as a situational phenomenon caused by a wide range of academic, social, or familial difficulties. Once we are certain that the condition is nonorganic, we first attempt to ''cure'' the visual loss by informing the child that the only problem is a slight refractive error. A minimal correction is then placed into a trial frame or phoropter, and the patient is told that they ''should see normally'' with this set of glasses. If this is successful, the patient is told not to worry about the visual process and that the refractive error is sufficiently minimal that it probably is not necessary for glasses to be worn. If this maneuver is unsuccessful, we privately inform the parents of our findings so that they will not continue to be concerned about an organic process. We then inform the child that we are happy to report that there is **no irreversi-**

ble damage to the eyes and that vision should improve spontaneously with time. We do not specify a particular time frame during which we think this will occur, and we encourage the child to ''do as well as you can'' in school and at home until vision improves. In our experience, this approach seems to be sufficient to solve the problem in the vast majority of cases, and even works in some adults with psychogenic disease. Indeed, studies of children with nonorganic visual loss who are managed with only reassurance and follow-up indicate that 75 to 95% have resolution of symptoms and improvement in visual acuity. Parental support and encouragement are associated with more rapid resolution. Dealing with children whose visual loss is associated with complex interpersonal relationships within the family, such as sexual abuse or other social difficulties, is much more difficult and may require the services of a psychotherapist, child psychiatrist, or family counselor.

The treatment of adults with nonorganic loss of visual acuity is more complicated than the treatment of children, particularly when there is evidence of malingering, and the outcome usually is much less satisfactory. As long as there is a motivation for material secondary gain, it may be impossible to ''treat'' such a patient for his or her visual loss. In many cases, the physician must be content that the loss of vision is nonorganic and to record this fact in the patient's chart. We see no purpose in confronting the patient with our belief that the visual loss is nonorganic unless we can convince the patient that ultimately it is not in his or her best interest to continue the charade because we have proof that the visual loss is nonorganic and that such proof will eventually cost the patient time, money, or even freedom.

Visual Field Defects

Nonorganic visual field defects can be of several types. The most common nonorganic visual field defect is a nonspecifically constricted visual field. When the field is tested kinetically, using either a Goldmann perimeter or a tangent (Bjerrum) screen, the field may have a spiraling nature, becoming smaller and smaller as the test object is moved around the field (Fig. 23.9). Alternatively, the visual field may remain the same size or nearly the same size regardless of the size or brightness of the test stimulus (Fig. 23.10), or it may be inconsistent when tested repeatedly in one or more meridians. Other nonorganic visual field defects, however, include unilateral or bilateral central scotomas, unilateral hemianopias,

bitemporal hemianopias, binasal hemianopias, and even homonymous hemianopias.

Evaluation

A nonorganically constricted visual field may be diagnosed in a variety of ways. In some cases, the patient can be "cajoled" into enlarging the field. After completion of perimetry, the patient is told that he or she did fine but that it was clear to the examiner that the patient was responding only when he or she was "absolutely certain" that he or she saw the test object. The examiner then explains that the test is to be repeated and encourages the patient to respond at an earlier stage when he or she just barely detects the stimulus.

Nonorganic visual field constriction can also be detected by testing the field using a tangent screen with the patient at two different distances from the screen (usually 1 and 2 meters). The size of the test object is varied so that the ratio of the size of the test object and the distance of the patient from the screen remain constant; that is, a 9-mm diameter white test object is used when the patient is 1 meter from the screen, and an 18-mm diameter white test object is used

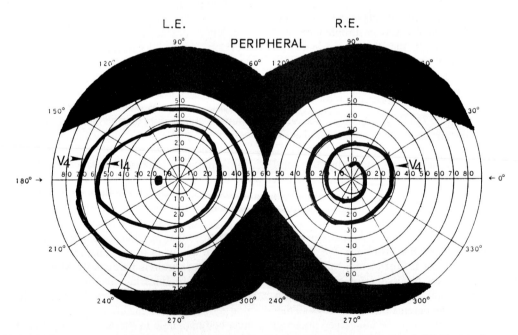

Figure 23.9. In a patient claiming visual difficulties in the right eye, there is a nonorganic spiral field when the eye is tested kinetically, using a Goldmann perimeter.

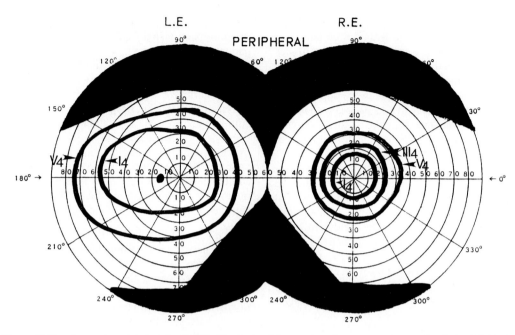

Figure 23.10.   In a patient claiming visual difficulties in the right eye, there is a nonorganic constricted visual field when the eye is tested kinetically, using a Goldmann perimeter.

when the patient is 2 meters from the screen. Patients with an organically constricted visual field (e.g., patients with retinitis pigmentosa) will show an increase in the absolute size of the visual field under these conditions when they are moved from 1 meter to 2 meters away from the screen, whereas patients with nonorganic visual field constriction will maintain the same absolute size of the field constriction.

Nonorganic monocular hemianopias and scotomas as well as both binasal and bitemporal hemianopic defects usually can be diagnosed by first performing visual field testing monocularly and then binocularly (Fig. 23.11). If the field defect is present in only one eye when the eyes are tested separately but is still present when binocular simultaneous field testing is performed, the defect can be assumed to be nonorganic. This method cannot distinguish between organic and nonorganic homonymous hemianopic defects or bilateral central scotomas.

One method for diagnosing nonorganic, monocular, paracentral visual field defects uses a red Amsler grid with red-green lenses. If the patient claims to have a paracentral scotoma when viewing with one eye but not with both eyes open, he or she is asked to map the scotoma while

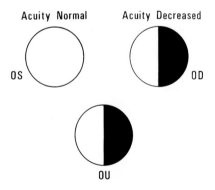

Figure 23.11.   Testing for nonorganic monocular hemianopia, using kinetic perimetry. *Left:* The visual field of the left eye is full. *Right:* The visual field of the right eye shows an apparent temporal hemianopsia. *Below:* The **binocular** visual field, which should be full, except for a missing right temporal crescent, shows an apparent temporal hemianopia. (Reprinted with permission from Keane JR. Neuro-ophthalmologic signs and symptoms of hysteria. Neurology 1982; 32:757–762.)

viewing a red Amsler grid. The patient then puts on the red-green glasses, with the red lens over the affected eye and is asked if he or she still sees the scotoma on the red Amsler grid. Because the eye behind the green lens will not see the grid, a patient with a real scotoma in the opposite eye should still see it; however, a patient with a nonorganic scotoma may think he or she is viewing with both eyes and will again state that the scotoma has disappeared.

A quick method of detecting nonorganic visual field loss of all types is to test saccadic eye movements into the supposedly absent portion of the field. The patient assumes that the eye movements and not the visual fields are being tested. This assumption is strengthened by first asking the patient if it hurts to move the eyes. Regardless of the patient's answer (which, interestingly, is often affirmative), the patient is told that the examiner is going to test the eye movements, and the patient is asked to pursue an object in various directions. The patient is then asked to look from the straight ahead position to an eccentric location where the examiner holds an object. The object is subsequently moved from one location to another with the patient being asked each time to look from the center to the object. If the patient complains that he or she "cannot see" that far in the periphery, the examiner explains that he or she understands and that is why the patient should look **directly** at the object rather than to try to see it in the peripheral vision.

It should be noted that patients can produce reproducible nonorganic visual field defects not only when tested with kinetic perimetry but also when tested using automated static perimetry (Fig. 23.12). Such patients do not necessarily show an increased number of fixation, false-positive, or false-negative errors.

Management

The management of patients with nonorganic visual field constriction is similar to that of patients with nonorganic visual loss. Children and adults who do not seem to be malingering are told that they will eventually improve, and this usually is the case, although we have been impressed that the percentage of patients who can be demonstrated to have normalization of, or significant improvement in, nonorganic visual field defects is substantially less than the percentage who have improvement in nonorganic

visual acuity loss. Studies report improvement in nonorganic visual field loss in 20 to 72% of patients.

It is our experience that most patients with nonorganic visual field loss deny that their visual field disturbance significantly limits their daily activities or state that despite their visual difficulties, they are able to maintain their normal life style. For this reason, we rarely recommend psychiatric or psychologic counseling for these patients. We generally do not advise confronting adults whose visual field defects are caused by malingering unless it seems likely that one can end the charade with a few well-chosen words.

Monocular Diplopia

Most patients who complain of double vision are suffering from misalignment of the visual axes. In such cases, the diplopia immediately resolves as soon as one eye is covered. Patients in whom diplopia remains despite occlusion of one eye are said to have **monocular diplopia.** This condition is caused most often by a refractive error, particularly uncorrected or improperly corrected astigmatism, by incorrectly fitted glasses, or by some disturbance of the cornea or lens. We have seen the condition particularly in patients with mild epithelial dystrophies and in patients with mild lenticular opacities or oil-drop cataracts. Most patients with this type of organic monocular diplopia will recognize a difference in the intensity of the two images that they see. One image will be fairly clear, but the second image will be perceived as "fuzzy" and may be described as a "ghost image" that overlaps the clear image. The "diplopia" in such cases usually resolves with a pinhole, a better refraction, or fitting of spectacles or a contact lens.

Rare examples of monocular diplopia and, more often, polyopia have been reported in patients with central nervous system disease such as migraine, stroke, and brain tumors. Patients with "cerebral polyopia" usually do not complain of overlapping images and generally see each image with equal clarity in both eyes; however, they complain bitterly of multiple images that may be of different sizes and shapes. Such patients usually have lesions in the parieto-occipital region, and most have obvious central nervous system disease (see Chapter 13).

True monocular diplopia (i.e., two separate and equal images of an object seen with one eye only) is almost never caused by organic disease. We and others have seen it most often in children

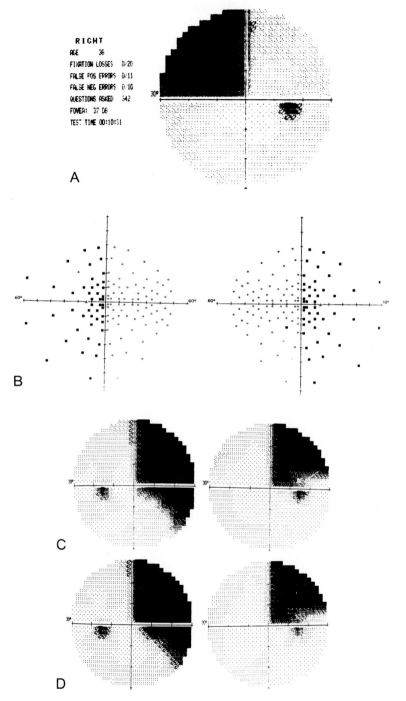

Figure 23.12. Fabricated visual field defects. *A.* Artificially produced quadrantanopia with the Humphrey field analyzer, using a 24–2 program. Note the excellent reliability. (Reprinted with permission from Glovinsky Y, Quigley HA, Bissett RA, et al. Artificially produced homonymous quadrantanopia in computed visual field testing. Am J Ophthalmol 1990;110:90–91.) *B.* Fabricated bitemporal hemianopia, using the Humphrey Full Field 120-point screening test (*left and right*). *C.* Fabricated incongruous right homony-

mous hemianopia, using Humphrey Central 30–2 threshold test (*left and right*). *D.* Fabricated visual fields recorded by the same subject 3 weeks later, attempting to reproduce an identical field defect (*left and right*). (*B–D:* Reprinted with permission from MacLeod JDA, Manners RM, Heaven CJ, et al. Visual field defects: how easily can they be fabricated using the automated perimeter? Neuro-ophthalmology 1994; 14:185–188.)

who have found themselves in stressful academic, social, or family situations. Once both the child and the parents are reassured as to the benign nature of the condition, it usually resolves within a short period of time.

NONORGANIC DISEASE AFFECTING FIXATION, OCULAR MOTILITY, AND ALIGNMENT

Disturbances of Fixation

Saccadic oscillations in most patients are involuntary eye movements caused by neurologic disease affecting the brainstem, cerebellum, or both (see Chapter 19). Nevertheless, some persons can produce saccadic oscillations that resemble nystagmus, ocular flutter, or opsoclonus.

Voluntary nystagmus is characterized by a rapid to-and-fro movement of the eyes that is willfully initiated. It can be sustained for only a few seconds. It can be produced by 5 to 8% of the population, and it may occur as a familial trait. It consists of rapidly alternating saccades with frequencies that range from 3 to 42 Hz and amplitudes that range from 0.5° to 35° (Fig. 23.13).

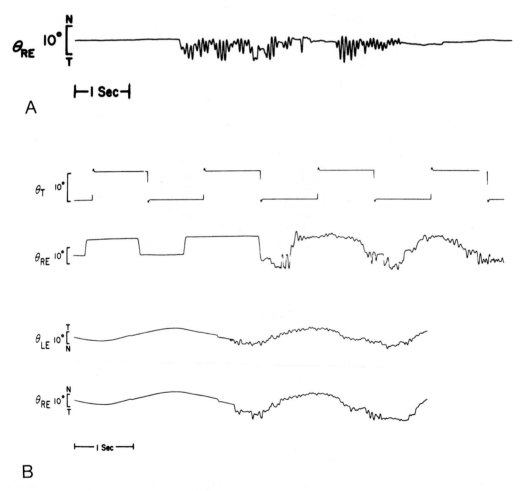

Figure 23.13. Voluntary nystagmus. Ocular motor recordings using a photoelectric method with infrared light. *A.* Voluntary nystagmus during binocular fixation. Note bursts of rapidly alternating saccades that vary in frequency and amplitude. θ_{RE}, eye position of right eye; *N,* nasal direction; *T,* temporal direction. *B.* Voluntary nystagmus during saccades (*top traces*) and pursuit (*bottom traces*). θ_{RE}, eye position of right eye; θ_{LE}, eye position of left eye; θ_{T}, position of target; *N,* nasal direction; *T,* temporal direction. (Reprinted with permission from Ciuffreda KJ. Voluntary nystagmus: new findings and clinical implications. Am J Optom Physiol Optics 1980;57:795–800.)

There is an inverse relationship between the frequency and the amplitude of the nystagmus.

Voluntary nystagmus usually is horizontal; however, it can be vertical or torsional. It can be produced in the light or dark and with the eyelids open or closed. It has even been reported as a monocular phenomenon, although we have not seen such a case.

Patients with voluntary nystagmus typically complain of oscillopsia and reduced vision. Such patients have fluttering of the eyelids and a strained facial expression during the episodes of nystagmus. In addition, the eyes tend to converge during the nystagmus, because the nystagmus seems to be produced in part by stimulation of normal convergence mechanisms. Patients who are able to produce voluntary nystagmus are also able to superimpose the nystagmus during normal tracking. Such persons often show transient nystagmoid movements associated with oscillopsia after an intense period of nystagmus.

Voluntary nystagmus has no pathologic significance. It may, however, be mistaken for certain pathologic conditions that affect fixation, including acquired nystagmus and saccadic intrusions.

Patients occasionally can produce large-amplitude to-and-fro **voluntary saccadic oscillations.** The movements are bursts of conjugate saccades in opposing directions, with no intersaccadic interval. Unlike the saccades of voluntary nystagmus, they are multidirectional (horizontal, vertical, or oblique), have amplitudes up to 40°, and sometimes have curvilinear trajectories. These characteristics are similar to those of ocular flutter and opsoclonus, involuntary movements that are caused by significant damage to the brainstem, cerebellum, or both; however, patients with true ocular flutter or opsoclonus generally have other neurologic manifestations. When saccadic oscillations that appear to be ocular flutter or opsoclonus are found in patients who do not have other neurologic signs or symptoms, a nonorganic basis should be considered.

Disorders of Ocular Motility and Alignment

Several nonorganic disorders of ocular motility and alignment may be observed in patients both with and without visual complaints. These disorders include insufficiency or paralysis of convergence, spasm of the near reflex, supranuclear horizontal and vertical gaze paresis, and forced downward deviation of the eyes.

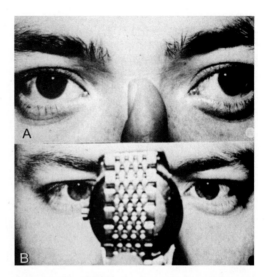

Figure 23.14.   Nonorganic convergence insufficiency. *A.* Inability to converge upon a near-target despite encouragement. *B.* Normal near-reflex elicited by asking patient to tell the time by looking at a wrist watch. (Reprinted with permission from Keane JR, Neuroophthalmologic signs and symptoms of hysteria. Neurology 1982;32:757–762.)

Insufficiency or Paralysis of Convergence

Convergence insufficiency or paralysis may be nonorganic in nature. We have seen several cases, usually in adolescents, but also in adults. Such patients often have associated insufficiency or paralysis of accommodation, although either disturbance may exist independently. Patients with apparent weakness of convergence may nevertheless show normal convergence when asked to read a paragraph at length during which the eyes are alternately covered. Asking the patient to perform other near tasks, such as telling time by looking at his or her wristwatch, may also be associated with normal convergence (Fig. 23.14). Convergence insufficiency may be misdiagnosed as myasthenia gravis.

Spasm of the Near Reflex

The most common nonorganic disturbance of ocular motility and alignment is **spasm of the near reflex** (Fig. 23.15). The syndrome is characterized by episodes of intermittent convergence, increased accommodation, and miosis. The degree of convergence is variable. Some patients exhibit marked convergence of both eyes, resulting in a marked esotropia. Other patients show a lesser degree of convergence such

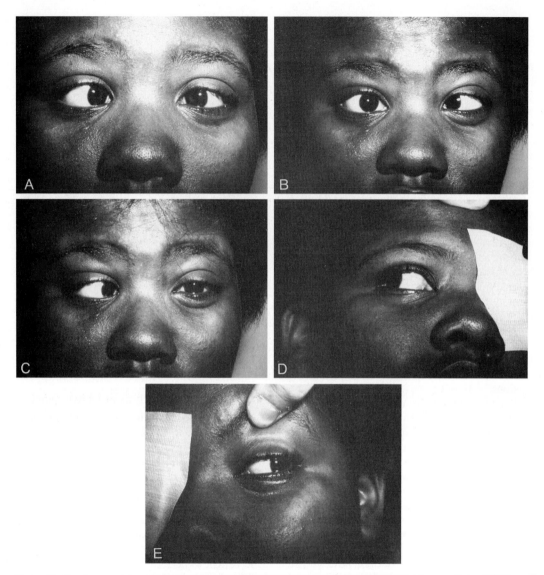

Figure 23.15. Spasm of the near reflex. The patient is a healthy 15-year-old girl. *A.* In primary position, the eyes are esotropic, and the pupils are constricted. *B.* On attempted right gaze, the right eye does not abduct, even to the midline, and the pupils become more constricted. *C.* On attempted left gaze, the left eye does not abduct beyond the midline, and the pupils become more constricted. *D.* When the left eye is patched and the patient is asked to pursue a target to the right or is asked to fixate a stationary target while the head is rotated to the left, the right eye abducts fully and the pupil becomes less constricted. *E.* When the right eye is patched and the patient is asked to pursue a target to the left or is asked to fixate a stationary target while the head is rotated to the right, the left eye abducts fully and the pupil becomes less constricted.

that one eye remains relatively straight while the other converges. In all cases, however, the patient seems to have unilateral or, more often, bilateral limitation of abduction during testing of versions although not necessarily during testing of ductions (see below). The degree of accommodation spasm also is variable. Some patients produce only a few diopters of myopia, whereas others produce 8 to 10 diopters of myopia. Miosis is invariably significant in patients who exhibit spasm of the near reflex regardless of the degree of accommodation and convergence spasm.

Spasm of the near reflex may be mistaken for unilateral or bilateral abducens nerve paresis, divergence insufficiency or paralysis, horizontal gaze paresis, or even myasthenia gravis. However, the lack of other neurologic deficits, the variability of the eye movements, and the constant occurrence of miosis associated with the adductive eye movements generally permit the correct diagnosis to be made. In addition, despite apparent unilateral or bilateral abduction weakness during testing of versions (with both eyes open), when ductions are tested directly with one eye occluded or indirectly using oculocephalic testing, both eyes invariably have full abduction, and the miosis seen when the eyes are in the esotropic position immediately resolves (see Fig. 23.15). Covering one eye during a typical spasm also may cause dramatic reversal of the miosis. Finally, refraction with and without cycloplegia during a period of spasm establishes the presence of pseudomyopia.

Several organic conditions, in addition to abducens nerve paresis and horizontal gaze paresis, may mimic spasm of the near reflex. Pretectal esotropia, also called pseudo-abducens paresis or pseudo-abducens nerve palsy, is a general disordered co-contraction of extraocular muscles and is not related to the near reflex. Convergence nystagmus jerks are not accompanied by miosis in this condition. Convergence substitution sometimes occurs when patients with supranuclear horizontal gaze paresis use convergence to move the adducting eye into the limited field of gaze. The resulting eye movement may suggest spasm of the near reflex. Finally, there are rare cases of true convergence spasm that have an organic basis. Most of these cases are unassociated with concomitant miosis, but exceptions exist. Typical spasm of the near reflex can occur in patients with intrinsic lesions of the mesencephalon or extrinsic lesions compressing the dorsal mesencephalon. Thus, the examiner who is unsure whether spasm of the near reflex is organic must be prepared to give the patient the benefit of the doubt.

MANAGEMENT

Management of persons with nonorganic spasm of the near reflex may consist only of reassurance. Psychiatric counseling may be appropriate in other cases. Some patients with spasm of the near reflex can be successfully treated with an Amytal (amobarbital) interview, during which it is suggested that the patient is orthophoric.

In other patients, symptomatic relief may be produced using a cycloplegic drug combined with bifocal spectacles or reading glasses. Glasses with an opaque inner third of the lens can also be used to treat patients with spasm of the near reflex. These spectacles occlude vision when the eyes are esotropic, thus presumably interrupting the spasm. Spasm of the near reflex should never be treated with strabismus surgery.

Horizontal and Vertical Gaze Paresis

We have seen several patients with nonorganic **paralysis of horizontal and vertical eye movements**. The patients would not make voluntary horizontal or vertical saccades or pursuit movements, and they would not fixate on a distant object to allow oculocephalic testing; however, when the patients were observed through a one-way mirror, they could be seen to make normal, purposeful pursuit and saccadic eye movements. In addition, measurements of eye movements during chair rotation in light and darkness indicated normal pursuit and saccadic systems.

Forced Downward Deviation of the Eyes

Forced downward deviation of the eyes can be used to help differentiate organic from nonorganic coma and seizures. The test is performed by moving the patient's head to one side and watching the movement of the patient's eyes. The head is then turned to the opposite side, again while watching the eye position.

The typical response of a patient with organic coma is either no movement of the eyes, such as occurs in patients with brainstem disease or drug-induced coma, or a smooth movement of the eyes in the direction **opposite** of the head turn (the normal "doll's eyes" response).

The eyes of a patient feigning a comatose state, however, will be deviated tonically toward the floor as if to avoid looking at the observer. On moving the head to the opposite side, the eyes will either saccade directly to the side facing the floor (i.e., in the **same** direction as the head turn), or they occasionally will dart from side to side before coming to rest.

Although a true seizure focus may certainly produce a deviation of the eyes to one side, turning the head from side to side in such a setting will not affect this deviation.

NONORGANIC DISORDERS OF PUPILLARY SIZE AND REACTIVITY

A variety of pupillary phenomena may be seen in patients with various types of psychiatric and psychogenic diseases. Investigators once hoped that certain disturbances of shape, size, and reactivity of one or both pupils could be used to diagnose specific psychiatric conditions. This has proved not to be the case. In general, patients who are anxious or having acute panic attacks may have bilaterally dilated pupils, often associated with generalized autonomic disturbances consistent with sympathetic hyperfunction, including profuse sweating, trembling, tachycardia, and tachypnea. The pupils of such patients appear normal between attacks.

Seesaw anisocoria can occur in "neurotic" patients. This phenomenon cannot be explained by the emotional or mental state of the patient, because psychosensory dilation is symmetric in such cases. In addition, seesaw anisocoria is transient and often reverses sides from one time to the next, so that it probably results from some type of temporary asymmetry in the central inhibitory neurons located in the mesencephalon.

Some patients can voluntarily dilate both pupils. We are aware of a patient who could dilate both pupils and accelerate his heart rate at will.

Perhaps the most common nonorganic pupillary disturbance seen in ophthalmologic practice is a unilateral (and occasionally bilateral) **fixed, dilated pupil** caused by topical administration of a mydriatic agent (Fig. 23.16). In some cases, the topical agent, usually atropine or scopolamine, has been administered by accident. For instance, patients who have been using a transdermal scopolamine patch to prevent seasickness or postoperative nausea may contaminate their fingertips during placement of the patch. The patients subsequently rub their eyes, and one or both pupils dilate. In addition, atropine and scopolamine are naturally occurring alkaloids produced in certain plants, such as deadly nightshade, henbane, jimson weed, and moonflower. Topical absorption after ocular contact with these agents in their natural form may occasionally occur, particularly in persons who work outdoors. Some patients, however, voluntarily place a topical parasympatholytic agent into one or both eyes and then present to a physician complaining of blurred vision.

Pharmacologically dilated pupils are extremely large and usually completely nonreactive to light or near stimulation (Figs. 23.16 and 23.17). They are unassociated with ptosis, diplopia, or strabismus unless there was a preexisting disturbance of eyelid function or ocular motility. The diagnosis of a pharmacologically dilated pupil is made by placing 1 to 2 drops of 1% pilocarpine in each lower cul-de-sac. A neurologically dilated pupil (i.e., oculomotor nerve paresis, tonic pupil) will constrict maximally within 30 minutes; however, a pharmacologically dilated pupil either is not affected and remains widely dilated (see Fig. 23.17) or constricts only minimally. Unresponsiveness or even partial responsiveness of a dilated, fixed pupil to a solution of pilocarpine that is of suffi-

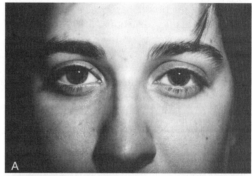

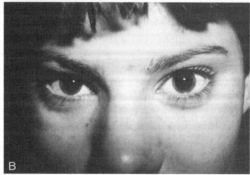

Figure 23.16. Pupillary dilation caused by voluntary use of a topical parasympathetic drug. *A.* Unilateral (left pupil). *B.* Bilateral. Note that in both cases, the affected pupils are extremely large. The size is much greater than that seen in patients with either oculomotor nerve paresis or tonic pupil syndromes.

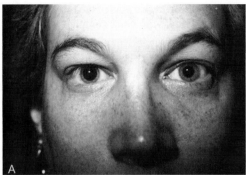

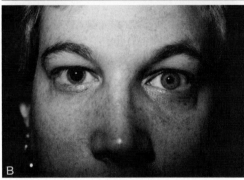

Figure 23.17. Testing for a pharmacologically dilated pupil, using a solution of 1% pilocarpine. *A.* Before testing. Note marked dilation of right pupil, compared with size of left pupil. *B.* At 45 minutes after placement of two drops of 1% pilocarpine into the lower cul-de-sac of *both* eyes, the left pupil is markedly constricted, but the right pupil is unchanged in size.

NONORGANIC DISTURBANCES OF EYELID FUNCTION

Nonorganic **ptosis** (pseudoptosis) is rare. When it occurs, one often can see and palpate spasm within the upper eyelid. There typically is relaxation of the elevators of the ipsilateral eyebrow, producing brow ptosis, a common finding in patients with psychogenic flaccid ptosis (Fig. 23.18).

Blepharospasm can occur as part of a more extensive neurologic disease, including Huntington's chorea, hepatolenticular degeneration, Hallervorden-Spatz disease, and postencephalitic parkinsonism. It may also develop after a brainstem stroke. Other causes of organic blepharospasm include drug toxicity with secondary tardive dyskinesia and ocular surface disease.

Some physicians believe that blepharospasm that is unassociated with overt neurologic or ocular disease is always a psychogenic disturbance. Although the condition called "essential blepharospasm" often worsens during periods of stress, it occurs most often in patients who do not have other psychogenic complaints. Nevertheless, we have seen several cases of blepharospasm that were clearly psychogenic in nature. Pressure over the supraorbital notch is often useful in inducing a person with nonorganic blepharospasm to raise the eyelids. Most cases of psychogenic blepharospasm occur in

cient strength to constrict the opposite, normally reacting pupil is absolute evidence of pharmacologic blockade, regardless of the patient's protestations to the contrary.

NONORGANIC DISTURBANCES OF ACCOMMODATION

The role of accommodation spasm in the condition called spasm of the near reflex is discussed above. In addition, however, nonorganic **weakness or paralysis of accommodation** may occur, primarily in children and young adults. Such patients are unable to read unless provided with an appropriate plus lens and even then may claim an inability to read clearly. Indeed, it is the failure of a patient with normal distance vision and an inability to read despite an appropriate reading aid that should alert the physician to the possibility that the condition is nonorganic.

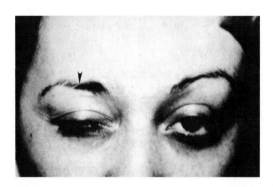

Figure 23.18. Nonorganic (voluntary) unilateral ptosis. Note that there is ptosis of both the eyelid and the **eyebrow** (*arrowhead*). The latter is virtually diagnostic of a nonorganic process unless there is true paralysis of the frontal branches of the facial nerve, in addition to damage to the levator palpebrae superioris muscle, Müller's muscle, or the nerves that innervate them. (Reprinted with permission from Keane JR. Neuro-ophthalmologic signs and symptoms of hysteria. Neurology 1982;32:757–762.)

children and young adults and seem to be triggered by a particular emotionally traumatic event.

We have seen no cases of nonorganic **eyelid retraction,** although patients who are anxious or upset often have variable bilateral eyelid retraction.

NONORGANIC DISTURBANCES OF OCULAR AND FACIAL SENSATION

Anesthesia of the skin of the eyelids and of one or both corneas may be nonorganic as may hypersensitivity, with the latter being associated with lacrimation, blepharospasm, photophobia, or a combination of these. Sensitive spots along the upper or lower margins of the orbits are common in patients with such complaints.

NONORGANIC DISTURBANCES OF LACRIMATION

Excessive secretion of tears may be nonorganic and may be associated with nonorganic blepharospasm. **Bloody tears** also may be associated with blepharospasm. Dr. Frank Walsh observed a patient who produced bloody tears by depositing blood from self-induced nosebleeds into the conjunctival sacs.

FOR MORE INFORMATION:
See Walsh & Hoyt's *Clinical Neuro-Ophthalmology,* 5th edition, Volume 1, Chapter 37, pp. 1765–1786.

Index

Page numbers in *italics* denote figures; those followed by a t denote tables.